ANTIBIOGRAM

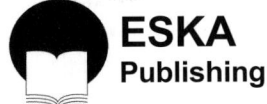

Cover photo:
"Antibiogram by agar diffusion of a *Klebsiella pneumoniae* strain producing extended-spectrum β-lactamase. AM, cefamandole; CAZ, ceftazidime; CB, carbenicillin; CTX, cefotaxime; FOX, cefoxitine; MZ, mezlocillin.

Published with the support of CNL - PARIS - FRANCE

All rights reserved.

No part of this publication may be reproduced, stored in a retrieval system, or transmitted in any means, electronic, mechanical, photocopying, recording, scanning, or otherwise, ewcept as expressly permitted by law, without either the prior written permission of the Publisher, or authorization through payment of the appropriat photocopy fee to thr Copyright Clearance Center. Requests for permission should be adressed to the Publisher, ESKA Publishing, Paul Lipscomb, 3808 SW Dosch Road, Portland, Oregon, 97239 - USA.
This publication is designed to provide accurate and authoritative information in regard to the subject matter covered. It is sold with the understanding that the publisher is not engaged in rendering professional services. If professionel advice or other expert assistance is required, the services of a competent professionel person should be sought.
Neither the authors nor the publisher are liable for any actions prompted or caused by the information presented in this book. Any views expressed herein are those of the authors and do not represent the views of the organizations they work for.

ESKA PUBLISHING, ASM PRESS © 2010
ISBN 978-2-7472-1545-9
PRINTED IN CANADA 2010

ESKA PUBLISHING
PAUL LIPSCOMB
3808 SW DOSCH ROAD
PORTLAND, OREGON
97239 - USA

We thank Ms Pascale SITBON and Sylvie BRÉMONT from the French National Reference Center for Antibiotic Resistance for preparation of manuscripts and iconography, respectively.

TABLE OF CONTENTS

Foreword, Yves-Achille CHABERT 11

First part:
PRINCIPLES AND METHODS OF ANTIBIOGRAM

1. Introduction. S. B. LEVY 15
2. Biochemistry of Resistance. P. PLESIAT 17
3. Genetics of Resistance. L. B. RICE 25
4. Bases for Clinical Categorization. D. BROWN, R. CANTON 37
5. Interpretive Reading. P. COURVALIN 47
6. Phenotypic Techniques. G. KAHLMETER, J. TURNIDGE 55
7. Genotypic Techniques. M.-C. PLOY 67
8. Antibiotic Assay. M.-D. KITZIS 75
9. Reporting of the Results. F.C. TENOVER, J. A. HINDLER 89

Second part:
ANTIBIOGRAM OF MAJOR BACTERIAL GROUPS

10. β-lactams and Staphylococci. V. CATTOIR, R. LECLERCQ 99
11. β-lactams and Streptococci (*pneumococcus*). M. R. JACOBS 109
12. β-lactams and Enterococci. J.-L. MAINARDI 127
13. β-lactams and Enterobacteria. R. BONNET, R. A. BONOMO 135
14. β-lactams and antibiotics and *Pseudomonas aeruginosa*. P. NORDMANN, T. NAAS 157
15. Antibiotic Resistance in other Nonfermentative Strict Aerobic Gram-negative Bacilli. A. PHILIPPON 175
16. Aminoglycosides and Gram-positive Bacteria. R. BISMUTH, P. COURVALIN 213
17. Aminoglycosides and Gram-negative Bacteria. T. LAMBERT 225
18. Quinolones and Gram-positive Bacteria. E. VARON 243
19. Quinolones and Gram-negative Bacteria. C.-J. SOUSSY 261
20. Glycopeptides and Staphylococci. R. LECLERCQ 275
21. Glycopeptides and Enterococci. P. COURVALIN 285
22. Lipopeptides, Lipoglycopeptides, and Glycolipodepsipeptides. H. S. FRAIMOW 295
23. Macrolides, Lincosamides, and Streptogramins. R. LECLERCQ 305
24. Tetracyclines. C. POYART 327
25. Oxazolidinones. R. LECLERCQ 339
26. Sulfonamides and Trimethoprim. F. GOLDSTEIN 347
27. Chloramphenicol, Fosfomycin, Fusidic Acid, and Polymyxins. V. CATTOIR 357
28. *Listeria monocytogenes*. O. F. JOIN-LAMBERT, S. KAYAL 373
29. Corynebacteria. Ph. RIEGEL 379
30. Bacillus. E. HERNÀNDEZ-GUINÀT 389
31. Lactic Acid Bacteria and *Erysipelothrix*. J. TANKOVIC 397
32. *Acinetobacter* and β-lactams. T. NAAS, P. NORDMANN 407

33.	*Acinetobacter* and other antibiotics. T. LAMBERT	421
34.	*Haemophilus influenzae*. O. GAILLOT	427
35.	*Neisseria meningitidis*. M.-K. TAHA, J.-D. CAVALLO	441
36.	*Neisseria gonorrhoeae*. J.-D. CAVALLO	451
37.	*Helicobacter pylori*. F. MEGRAUD	459
38.	*Campylobacter*. P. MC DERMOTT	479
39.	*Moraxella (Branhamella) Catarrhalis*. H. CHARDON	491
40.	*Pasteurella*. P.Y. DONNIO	501
41.	*Legionella*. S. JARRAUD, J. ETIENNE	503
42.	*Aeromonas*, *Vibrio*, and *Plesiomonas*. T. FOSSE	509
43.	*Mycoplasma*, *Ureaplasma*. C. BEBEAR	519
44.	*Chlamydia*. B. de BARBEYRAC	531
45.	Hacek and Dysgonic Fermenters. M. VERGNAUD	541
46.	Methods for Antimicrobial Susceptibility Testing of Anaerobic Bacteria. L. DUBREUIL	553
47.	Gram-positive Anaerobes. J.-L. PONS, F. BARBUT	567
48.	Gram-negative Anaerobes. L. DUBREUIL	577
49.	Mycobacteria. V. JARLIER	593
50.	*Bartonella, Borrelia, Brucella, Francisella, Ehrlichia, Rickettsia, Coxiella,* and *Treponema*. M. MAURIN	615
51.	*Nocardia*. P. BOIRON	643
52.	Antibiogram in Veterinary Practice. F. M. AARESTRUP	651

Third part:
PROTOCOLS FOR STUDY OF ANTIBIOTICS

1.	Antibiotics by Classes and Groups. P. COURVALIN, R. LECLERCQ	661
2.	Antibiotics by International Common Denomination. P. COURVALIN, R. LECLERCQ	665
3.	Preparation of Serial Dilutions of Antibiotics. P. COURVALIN, R. LECLERCQ	669
4.	Kinetics of Bactericidal Action. P. COURVALIN, R. LECLERCQ	671
5.	Antibiotic Combinations. P. COURVALIN, R. LECLERCQ	673
6.	Susceptibility Testing of Anaerobes. L. DUBREUIL	679

Fourth part:
APPENDICES

Definitions	685
Strain Storage	686
Abbreviations and Acronyms	687
Literature	690
Web Sites	691
Alphabetic Index	693

AUTHORS LIST

Franck AARESTRUP, Danish Veterinary Laboratory, Bulowsvej 27, DK-1790 Copenhagen V, Danemark. Tél. : +45 35 30 01 00 – Fax :+45 35 30 01 20 – E-mail :faa@food.dtu.dk

Bertille de BARBEYRAC, Université Victor Ségalen, Laboratoire de Bactériologie, EA 3671, Centre National de Référence des infections à Chlamydia, 146, rue léo Saignat, 33076 Bordeaux Cedex. France. Tél. : 05 57 57 16 33 – Fax : 05 56 79 56 11 – E-mail : bertille.de.barbeyrac@u-bordeaux2.fr

Frédéric BARBUT, Hôpital Saint-Antoine, Unité d'Hygiène et de Lutte contre les Infections Nosocomiales, 184, rue du faubourg Saint-Antoine, 75012 Paris. France. Tél. : 01 49 28 30 11 – Fax : 01 49 28 30 09 – E-mail : frederic.barbut@sat.ap-hop-paris.fr

Cécile BEBEAR, Université Victor Ségalen Bordeaux 2, Laboratoire de Bactériologie EA3671, 146, rue Léo Saignat, 33076 Bordeaux Cedex. France. Tél. : 05 57 57 16 25 – Fax : 05 56 93 29 40 – E-mail : cecile.bebear@u-bordeaux2.fr

Roland BISMUTH, Centre Hospitalo-Universitaire Pitié-Salpêtrière, Service de Bactériologie, 47, boulevard de l'Hôpital, 75634 Paris Cedex 13. France. Tél. : 01 42 16 20 87   Fax : 01 42 16 20 72 - E-mail : roland.bismuth@psl.ap-hop-paris.fr

Richard BONNET, Faculté de Médecine, Laboratoire de Bactériologie-Virologie, 28, place Henri Dunant, 63001 Clermont-Ferrand. France. Tél. : 04 73 17 81 50 – Fax : 04 73 27 74 94. E-mail : rbonnet@chu-clermontferrand.fr

Robert A. BONOMO, 2638 Edgerton Rd, University Heigh, OH, 44118-1643, USA. Tél. : 216 791 3800 – Fax : 216 844 6492 – E-mail : robert.bonomo@va.gov

Patrick BOIRON, Faculté de Pharmacie Rockefeller, Laboratoire de Mycologie, 8, avenue Rockefeller, 69373 Lyon Cedex 08. France. Tél. : 04 78 77 70 20 – Fax : 04 78 77 72 12 – E-mail : boiron@univ-lyon1.fr

Derek BROWN, 222 Broadway, Peterborough PE1 4DT, U.K. Tél. : +44 1733 349396 – E-mail : derek.brown222@btinternet.com

Rafael CANTÓN, Servicio de Microbiología, Hospital Universitario Ramón y Cajal, Carretera de Colmenar Km 9,1, 28034-Madrid, Spain. Phone : +34 913 368 330 – Fax : +34 913 368 809 – E-mail:rcanton.hrc@salud.madrid.org

Vincent CATTOIR, Centre Hospitalier Régional Universitaire de Caen, Laboratoire de Microbiologie, Avenue de la Côte de Nacre, 14033 Caen Cedex. France. Tél. : 02 31 06 45 72 – Fax : 02 31 06 45 73 – E-mail : cattoir-v@chu-caen.fr

Jean-Didier CAVALLO, Hôpital d'Instruction des Armées Bégin, Laboratoire de Biologie Médicale, 69, avenue de Paris, 94160 Saint-Mandé. France. Tél. : 01 43 98 47 34 – Fax : 01 43 98 53 36 – E-mail : hia-begin-biologie@worldonline.fr

Centre National de Référence Mycobactéries et Résistance des Mycobactéries aux Antituberculeux - Groupe Hospitalier La Pitié-Salpêtrière, Laboratoire de Bactériologie-Virologie, 47, boulevard de l'Hôpital, 75651 Paris Cedex 13. France. Tél. : 01 42 16 20 83 – Fax : 01 42 16 20 72 – E-mail : nicolas.veziris@upmc.fr

Yves A. CHABBERT, Villa Primavera, 15, avenue du Bassin, 33970 Lège Le Cap Ferret. France. Tél/Fax. : 05 56 60 41 95.

Hubert CHARDON, Centre Hospitalier Général, Laboratoire de Biologie, Avenue des Tamaris, 13616 Aix-en-Provence Cedex. France. Tél. : 04 42 33 50 87 – Fax : 04 42 33 51 84 – E-mail : hchardon@ch-aix.fr

Patrice COURVALIN, Centre National de Référence de la Résistance aux Antibiotiques, Unité des Agents Antibactériens, Institut Pasteur, 28, rue du Docteur Roux, 75724 Paris Cedex 15. France. Tél. : 01 45 68 83 20 – Fax : 01 45 68 83 19 – E-mail : patrice.courvalin@pasteur.fr

Pierre-Yves DONNIO, Hôpital Pontchaillou-CHRU, Laboratoire de Bactériologie-Virologie, Rue Henri Le Guillou, 35033 Rennes Cedex 09. France. Tél. : +33 2 99 28 42 76 – Fax : +33 2 99 28 41 29 – E-mail : pierre-yves.donnio@chu-rennes.fr

Luc DUBREUIL, Faculté de Pharmacie, Laboratoire de Microbiologie, 3, rue P. Laguesse, 59045 Lille. France. Tél. : 03 20 96 40 40 – Fax : 03 20 95 90 09 –E-mail : luc.dubreuil@univ-lille2.fr

Jérôme ETIENNE, Faculté RTH Laënnec, laboratoire Central de Microbiologie, 7, rue Guillaume Paradin, 69372 Lyon Cedex 08. France. Tél. : 04 72 11 05 94 – Fax : 04 72 11 07 61 – E-mail : jetienne@univ-lyon1.fr

Thierry FOSSE, Hôpital l'Archet, Laboratoire de Bactériologie, Route de Saint-Antoine de Ginestière, 06200 Nice. France. Tél. : 04 92 03 62 14 – Fax : 04 92 03 65 49 – E-mail : fosse@unice.fr

Henry FRAIMOW, Cooper Health University & Hospital, Department of Medicine Education and Research Building 401, Haddon Avenue Rm 274 , Camden, NJ 08103, USA. Phone : +1 856 757 7767 – Fax : +1 856 757 7803 – E-mail : fraimow-henry@cooperhealth.edu

Olivier GAILLOT, Centre Hospitalier de Lille, Laboratoire de Bactériologie, Hygiène Hospitalière, Centre de Biologie et Pathologie, 59034 Lille. France. Phone : +33 3 20 44 54 80 – Fax : +33 3 20 44 45 22 - E-mail : o-gaillot@chru-lille.fr.

Fred GOLDSTEIN, 81, allée du lac Inférieur, 78100 Le Vésinet. France. Tél. : 01 39 76 06 94 – Fax : 01 39 76 27 27 – E-mail : goldstein.fred@orange.fr

Eric HERNÀNDEZ-GUINÀT, Hôpital d'Instruction des Armées du Val de Grâce, Laboratoire de Biologie Médicale, 74, boulevard de Port Royal 75005 Paris. France. Tél. : 40 51 40 00 – Fax : 01 46 33 07 90 – E-mail : hnz.eric@free-surf.fr

Janet A. HINDLER, UCLA Medical Center, Los Angeles, CA 90095-1713, USA. Tél. : 310 794 2763 – Fax : 310 794 2765 – E-mail : jhindler@ucla.edu

Michael R. JACOBS, Case Western Reserve University, 11100 Euclid Ave, Cleveland, OH 44106-1712, USA. Tél. : 216 844 3484 - Fax : 216 844 5601 - E-mail : michael.jacobs@case.edu

Sophie JARRAUD, Hôpital Edouard Herriot, Laboratoire de Microbiologie, Bât. 10, Place d'Arsonval, 69437 Lyon Cedex 03. France. Tél. : 04 72 11 07 64 – Fax : 04 72 11 07 74 – E-mail : sophie.jarraud@chu-lyon.fr

Olivier JOIN-LAMBERT, Hôpital Necker-Enfants Malades, Laboratoire de Bactériologie, 149, rue de Sèvres, 75730 Paris Cedex 15. France. Tél. : 01 44 49 49 61 – Fax : 01 44 49 49 60 – E-mail : join@necker.fr

Gunnar KAHLMETER, Central Hospital, Clinical Microbiology, S-351 85 Växjö, Sweden. Tél. : 46 470587477 - Fax : 00 46 470587455 - E-mail : gunnar.kahlmeter@ltkronoberg.se

Samer KAYAL, Hôpital Necker-Enfants Malades, Laboratoire de Bactériologie, 149, rue de Sèvres, 75730 Paris Cedex 15. France. Tél. : 01 44 49 49 53 – Fax : 01 44 49 49 60 – E-mail : kayal@necker.fr

Marie-Dominique KITZIS, Hôpital Saint Joseph, Laboratoire de Microbiologie, 185, rue Raymond Losserand, 75674 Paris Cedex 14. France. Tél. : 01 44 12 36 38 – Fax : 01 44 12 32 38 – E-mail : mdkitzis@hopital-saint-joseph.org

Thierry LAMBERT, Hôpital Saint Michel, Laboratoire de Bactériologie, 33, rue Olivier de Serres, 75015 Paris. France. Tél. : 01 40 45 64 44 – Fax : 01 40 45 63 10 – E-mail : thierry.lambert@cep.u-psud.fr

Roland LECLERCQ, Centre Hospitalier Régional Universitaire de Caen, Laboratoire de Microbiologie, Avenue de la Côte de Nacre, 14033 Caen Cedex. France. Tél. : 02 31 06 48 95 – Fax : 02 31 06 45 73 – E-mail : leclercq-r@chu-caen.fr

Stuart B. LEVY, Tufts University School of Medicine, Department of Molecular Biology and Microbiology, 136 Harrison Avenue, Boston MA 02111-1800, USA. Phone :+1 617 636 6764 – Fax : +1 617 636 0458 – E-mail : stuart.levy@tufts.edu

Jean-Luc MAINARDI, Hôpital Européen Georges Pompidou, Laboratoire de Bactériologie, 20, rue Leblanc, 75908 Paris Cedex 15. France. Tél. : 01 56 09 39 52 – Fax : 01 56 09 24 46 – E-mail : jean-luc.mainardi@bhdc.jussieu.fr

Max MAURIN. Centre Hospitalo-Universitaire de Grenoble, Service de Bactériologie, BP 217, 38043 Grenoble Cedex 9. France. Tél. : 04 76 76 54 79 – Fax : 04 76 76 59 12 – E-mail : mmaurin@chu-grenoble.fr

Patrick McDERMOTT, Division of Animal & Food Microbiology, Office of Research, Center for Veterinary Medicine, U.S. Food & Drug Administration, 8401 Muirkirk Rd, Mod 2, Laurel, MD 20708, USA. Phone : +1 301 210 4213 – Fax : +1 301 210 4685 – E-mail: patrick.mcdermott@fda.hhs.gov

Francis MEGRAUD, Groupe Hospitalier Pellegrin, Laboratoire de Bactériologie, 1, place Amélie Raba Léon, 33076 Bordeaux Cedex. France. Tél. : 05 56 79 59 10 – Fax : 05 56 79 60 18 – E-mail : francis.megraud@chu-bordeaux.fr

Thierry NAAS, Hôpital de Bicêtre, Service de Microbiologie-Bactériologie, 78, avenue du Général Leclerc, 94275 Le Kremlin Bicêtre. France. Tél. : 01 45 21 20 19 – Fax : 01 45 21 63 40 – E-mail : thierry.naas@bct.aphp.fr

Patrice NORDMANN, Hôpital de Bicêtre, Service de Bactériologie-Virologie, 78, avenue du Général Leclerc, 94275 Le Kremlin Bicêtre. France. Tél. : 01 45 21 36 32 – Fax : 01 45 21 63 40 – E-mail : nordmann.patrice @bct.ap-hop-paris.fr

Alain PHILIPPON, Groupe Hospitalier Cochin-Port Royal, Service de Microbiologie, 27, rue du faubourg Saint-Jacques, 75674 Paris Cedex 14. France. Tél. : 01 58 41 15 60 – Fax : 01 58 41 15 48 – E-mail : alain.philippon@cch.ap-hop-paris.fr

Patrick PLESIAT, Hôpital Jean Minjoz, Laboratoire de Bactériologie, Boulevard Fleming, 25030 Besançon Cedex. France. Tél. : 03 81 66 85 81 – Fax : 03 81 66 89 14 – E-mail : patrick.plesiat@ufc-chu.univ-fcomte.fr

Marie-Cécile PLOY, Hôpital Universitaire Dupuytren, Laboratoire de Bactériologie-Virologie, 2, avenue Martin-Luther King, 87042 Limoges Cedex. France. Tél. : 05 55 05 67 27 – Fax : 05 55 05 67 22 – E-mail : marie-cecile.ploy@uni-lim.fr

Jean-Louis PONS, UER Médecine et Pharmacie de Rouen, Microbiologie-Pharmacie, 22, boulevard Gambetta, 76183 Rouen Cedex. France. Tél. : 02 35 14 84 52 – Fax : 02 32 88 80 24 – E-mail : Jean-Louis.Pons@univ-rouen.fr

Claire POYART, Groupe Hospitalier Cochin-Port Royal, Service de Microbiologie, 27, rue du faubourg Saint-Jacques, 75674 Paris Cedex 14. France. Tél. : 01 58 41 15 60 – Fax : 01 58 41 15 48 – E-mail : claire.poyart@cch.ap-hop-paris.fr

Louis B. RICE, V A Medical Center, Medical Service 111W, 10701 East Blvd, Cleveland, OH 44106, USA. Tél. :216-791-3800 x4806 ou 216-791-3800 x5818 Fax : 216 231 3289 – E-mail : Louis.Rice@med.va.gov ou vxl5@po.cwru.edu

Philippe RIEGEL, Institut de Bactériologie, 3, rue Koeberlé, 67000 Strasbourg. France. Tél. : 03 90 24 37 55 – Fax : 03 88 25 11 13 – E-mail : philippe.riegel@chru-strasbourg.fr

Claude-James SOUSSY, Hôpital Henri Mondor, Service de Bactériologie-Virologie, 51, avenue du Maréchal de Lattre de Tassigny, 94010 Créteil. France. Tél. : 01 49 81 28 31 – Fax : 01 49 81 28 39 – E-mail : claude-james.soussy@hmn.ap-hop-paris.fr

Muhamed-Kheir TAHA, Centre National de Référence des Méningocoques, Unité des *Neisseria*, Institut Pasteur, 25, rue du Docteur Roux, 75724 Paris Cedex 15. France. Tél. : 01 45 68 84 38 – Fax : 01 40 61 30 34 – E-mail : muhamed-kheir.taha@pasteur.fr

Jacques TANKOVIC, Hôpital Saint-Antoine, Service de Bactériologie-Virologie, 184, rue du faubourg Saint-Antoine, 75571 Paris Cedex 12. France. Tél. : 01 49 28 29 10 – Fax : 01 49 28 24 72 – E-mail : jacques.tankovic@sat.ap-hop-paris.fr

Fred C. TENOVER, Cepheid, 904 caribbean Drive, Sunnyvale, CA, 94089, USA. Tél. :408 400 4344 – Fax : 408 734 1260 – E-mail : fred.tenover@cepheid.com

John TURNIDGE, Women's & Children's Hospital, Microbiology and Infectious Diseases, 72 King William Road, North Adelaide SA 5006, Australia. Tél. : 61-8 8204 6873 – Fax : 61-8 8204 6051 – E-mail : john.turnidge@health.sa.gov.au

Emmanuelle VARON, Hôpital Européen Georges Pompidou, Laboratoire de Microbiologie, 20, rue Leblanc, 75908 Paris Cedex 15. France. Tél. : 01 56 09 39 52 – Fax : 01 56 09 24 47 – E-mail : Emmanuelle.Varon@hop.egp.ap-hop-paris.fr

Michel VERGNAUD, Centre Hospitalier Régional Universitaire de Caen, Laboratoire de Microbiologie, Avenue de la Côte de Nacre, 14033 Caen Cedex. France. Tél. : 02 31 06 48 96 – Fax : 02 31 06 45 73 – E-mail : vergnaud-m@chu-caen.fr

FOREWORD

Yves-Achille CHABBERT

« The important thing in Rugby is the basics »

Antibiotic susceptibility testing is sixty years old: the age of retirement or obsolescence? This book demonstrates the future of this technique, because antibiotic susceptibility testing is not a technique that can be superseded, but a concept that covers all of the methods used to study the activity of an antibiotic. Whether it is based on molecular studies of mechanisms of action or resistance « characters », or physiological effects observed « *in vitro* » at the sites of infection, or in cellular or non-cellular experimental models, the objective is to contribute to successful treatment. Resistance is not a cyclical or transient phenomenon, but an intrinsic property of the bacterial world. The variability of resistance is related to the capacity of mutation or accretion of foreign DNA. Penicillinase-producing staphylococci were found everywhere right from the start of antibiotic susceptibility testing. Transferable or nontransferable plasmid-mediated resistance was subsequently observed in wild animals in South Africa, desert dromedaries, and gate-post hens. The role of antibiotic pressure on selection of resistant bacteria is undeniable, but the universal presence of resistance ensures its persistence and justifies continuing research.

The future of antibiotics must be considered in the light of the past research. Around 1950 was the Golden Age of new antibiotics when the large drug companies collected soil samples from all over the world looking for the slightest « mycetes » activity. It was subsequently found to be very productive to submit β-lactams, quinolones, and other antibiotics to chemical processes. This resulted in broader activity spectra and several thousand-fold increased activity leading to a certain success, which even led some authors to imprudently claim that the problem of infectious diseases had been resolved. This approach appears to be running out of steam and new approaches need to be developed. Should we return to the empirical approach of the 1950s or develop « intelligent » antibiotics based on the hopes raised by a logical knowledge of bacterial metabolisms. As in other fields, we can always dream of a third alternative. The « basics » of antibiotic susceptibility testing are so well known that they will only be recalled briefly. « All antibiotics interfere directly with bacterial metabolism ». This direct link was obvious right from the discovery of the mechanism of action of sulphonamides despite certain authors who envisaged a link with immunity. The antibiotic consequently blocks bacterial growth. Very old technical and didactic habits distinguished bacteriostatic and bactericidal activities. A bacterial cell that does not divide dies. This process has been considered to constitute a birth-death process. The minimum inhibitory concentration (MIC), the pillar of antibiotic susceptibility testing, would represent the steady-state. This critical concentration measured *in vitro* by various techniques, which must nevertheless be correlated with each other, appears to have a value very close to that of the site of infection, which authorizes comparison of humoral and tissue pharmacological values. The continuing work of the « Breakpoint » Committees defines the breakpoints. That's for the basics. However, molecular and genetic studies over the last thirty years have demonstrated the very large number of resistance mechanisms. These mechanisms can be detected at the genes level and purely genetic antibiotic susceptibility testing has been proposed.

But are all of these resistance "characters" actually expressed? Although some are reflected in MIC, others are not, but would they have an effect on the antibiotic action under various environmental conditions? Certain bizarre effects are observed, either dependent on the inoculum or dependent on metabolic conditions. Some resistances are too short-lived to be explained genetically. Not all of these so-called physiological phenomena have been developed due to a lack of explanation at the molecular level; bridges must be made between all fields and, most importantly, research must focus on the varieties of responses of the bacterium according to its genome. In practice, the antibiotic therapy laboratory works in three fields. The first is classical and very clinical, and consists of using all possible ways (bacteriostatic action, bactericidal action, combinations, humoral and tissue levels, dynamics of the bacterial effect, etc.) to ensure the best possible treatment. In the early days, in view of the large numbers of new products and pharmacological uncertainties, a new specialty was created, « antibiotic therapy consultant » bridging the gap between the laboratory and clinical practice, as the « bacteriology results » tried to take precedence over other specialties. The choice of cases requiring such attention can only be based on confident cooperation with clinicians. In some diseases, for example lung infections, antibiotic therapy is not as effective as it should be due to the insufficient development of clinical bacteriology.

A second field has opened up over recent decades, that of new aetiologies and emergent bacteria, as extensively illustrated in this book. For a long time, too much interest was focused on staphylococci and enterobacteria; the bacterial realm has suddenly left the field of animal and human disease to acquire a global extension. Are we threatened by extremophiles? Do bacteria have an unsuspected aetiological role in certain diseases, as suggested by a recent example? All of these questions which must be addressed with the pioneer spirit of the 20th century and the basic principles of antibiotic therapy.However, the epidemiology of resistance has an essential practical role because it determines the list of antibiotics potentially active in a given infection and is or should be the guide to medical practice. It is also the justification for research on new products. Few patients receive tailored treatment based on antibiotic susceptibility testing. The vast majority of treatments are based on consensus guidelines founded on various bases: randomized clinical trials, the « authoritative experience » of clinicians, or meteorological situations of resistance, described by hospital working parties. This approach is certainly satisfactory, but possibly not sufficient, as some microbial groups are overrepresented due to their frequency, while others are orphans. This book is designed to fill in these gaps.Another important point concerns those specialties in which bacteriological studies are difficult and have never constituted a priority. Practitioners have very valid therapeutic practices, but sometimes routine is poorly adapted to bacterial evolution. The emphasis placed on the insufficient treatment of Gram-positive bacteria is an example.The pharmaceutical industry is following these epidemiological changes with interest and certainly wants to palliate their effects, particularly when the therapeutic field is sufficiently large. Over the last fifty years, there has been an ongoing war between antibiotics and resistance. For a long time, many battles were won, but the situation now appears to be at a standstill. Due to the difficulties of applying molecular genetics to medicine, many believe that biology is more complex than previously thought. This complexity also concerns the antibiotic action; bacterial death is the result of a cascade of metabolic events, a better understanding of which could lead to new approaches. I am nevertheless optimistic about the future of antibiotic therapy laboratory, as it plays an essential role in the fight against infectious diseases and the abundance and quality of participants in this book shows that there is no lack of soldiers in the field.

First Part:
PRINCIPLES AND METHODS OF ANTIBIOGRAM

INTRODUCTION

Stuart B. LEVY

With few new antibiotics in the pipeline, the appropriate use of our current ones is more important than ever before so as to both preserve their efficacy and control resistance to them. **Antibiogram**, a unique and widely-cited reference book now in its second French edition (2006) (the first was in 1985), has been an important resource for clinical microbiologists and others in the infectious diseases field. Here it appears in a totally new edition – this time in English. Many, including myself, have appreciated and benefited from the French editions and I am delighted that it is now available to English speaking clinicians, infectious disease experts, and microbiologists. It is a "state of the art" volume with many practical features, including in-depth presentations of each antibiotic, replete with details on appropriate choice in view of resistance. The authorship taps international resources, which provides a global feel and appeal as one peruses the volume chapters. Its content is comprehensive, having individual chapters devoted to each drug (and drug class) and to each organism (and its family members). The book combines common suggestions for drug use with how to interpret drug susceptibility tests. Expanding far beyond the meaning and clinical use of an "antibiogram", this is a resource that a wide audience of health-care providers will want in their offices and for their practices.

Readers of **Antibiogram** can easily find up-to-date information in both complementing drug and microbe areas in order to assess antibiotic susceptibility and to appreciate and understand the appropriate guidelines for antibiotic treatment. We encounter the antibiotic at different levels, from details on how to set up a drug test, to interpretation of test results, to deciding the best drug choice for treatment. The authors provide evaluations of the pros and cons of different tests and alternative treatment strategies. There is advice for treatment of all major microbial diseases and descriptions of a plethora of antimicrobial agents developed to cure infectious diseases. The major thrust of the book, as it has been in the past, is on human disease, but a chapter on drugs in veterinary practice is also included.

The book provides the reader with broad-ranged information on the drugs in terms of their names (generic and trade), which can vary from country to country, and their major mode of action. Relevant chapters delineate the spectrum of these drugs and whether they are bacteriostatic or bactericidal. Important features of the drug are emphasized, along with the salient details on drug dosing and expected disease response. Gram-positive and gram-negative bacterial pathogens are discussed separately. One chapter is devoted to some of the intra-cellular (atypical) organisms as well as *Treponema* and *Borrelia*. By pairing chapters on families of antibiotics with chapters describing families of bacteria, the reader and user of this book obtains a broad and deep understanding for the library of infectious organisms and of drugs to treat their infections.

Another feature that is addressed in this book, and that poses an increasing problem to health care providers, is the movement of commensals into the pathogen arena. As patients are becoming immunocompromised, *e.g.* through viruses such as AIDS or through chemotherapy for cancers, bacteria heretofore not on the clinical list of pathogens are now opportunistic causes of disease. Gram-negative commensals, such as *Pseudomonas*, *Acinetobacter* and *Burkholderia* continue to rise as new threats to our patients, carrying a "shadow" of drug resistance which can at times cover all drugs. We must become more familiar with infections caused by these organisms. This is an important point to convey since some of these bacteria have not been dealt with in the medical school training of numbers of practitioners throughout the world. While new antibiotics for gram-positive organisms have been introduced, none has appeared for treatment of gram-negative bacteria, in particular, the commensals as well as multidrug-resistant members of the *Enterobacteriaceae* such as *Klebsiella* and *E. coli*. There is mounting need, but lack of new drugs.

This book contains excellent presentations of tabular data, and instructive figures help the reader readily absorb and comprehend this very complex subject matter. In the present climate of internet access, **Antibiogram** will clearly compete in being an easy-to-read, user-friendly presentation of the subject, ranging from drug susceptibility to drug choice. Having this information compiled in a single volume to leaf through, especially with its thoughtful organization of the chapters, is a clear advantage. Reading through the index of the chapters, one appreciates the complexity of the microbial world in a text which combines microbiology with antibiotic treatment.

Bacteria respect no country boundaries. Likewise, this English edition of **Antibiogram** will go far in getting critically important information across to a wide audience. It caters to a demanding professional group, one that wants and needs up-to-date drug information and treatment options offered by top experts in the field. Readers will find how drugs work and how they are resisted – all packaged in a concise, available form. By advising how to approach a problem, from the microbiologic and infection viewpoints, this English edition will empower many new to the health-care area to make knowledgeable decisions about antibiotic choice and expected outcome.

Chapter 2. BIOCHEMISTRY OF RESISTANCE

Patrick PLESIAT

INTRODUCTION

Contrary to antiseptics, antibiotics act on bacteria by inhibiting specific physiological functions such as cell wall synthesis (β-lactams, glycopeptides, fosfomycin), DNA replication/transcription (4-quinolones, rifampin, sulfonamides, trimethoprim), protein synthesis (aminoglycosides, tetracyclines, macrolides group, chloramphenicol, oxazolidinones) or cellular respiration (polymyxins, daptomycin). To exert their action, antibiotics must bind to specific molecular targets, which are usually intracellular.

The intrinsic activity of an antibiotic against a given bacterial species depends on a complex combination of factors, notably the affinity of the antibiotic for its target, the number of target molecules to be inactivated and, lastly, the drug concentration in the vicinity of the target (C_{int}). The latter obviously depends on the drug concentration in the bacterial environment (C_{ext}), but is also influenced by the permeability of the bacterial membranes to the antibiotic (simple diffusion or active transport), the existence of activation or inactivation mechanisms, and the presence of bacterial efflux pumps which prevent the drug from accumulating inside the bacterial cell.

Bacteria also have the well-known ability to increase their resistance to antibiotics through a multitude of mechanisms, the nature and efficiency of which depend on the species and the particular antibiotic. The main strategies of bacterial resistance identified to date are described below and summarized in Table 1.

ENZYMATIC INACTIVATION OF THE ANTIBIOTIC

One of the most widespread and efficient mechanisms of resistance is the structural modification of the antibiotic by the bacteria, rendering the antibiotic unable to attach to, and consequently inhibit, its target. This mechanism relies on the production of enzymes which are either intrinsic to the bacteria (encoded by a chromosomal gene belonging to the species) or acquired (encoded by genes transferred by mobile genetic elements, plasmids, or transposons). The best known of these enzymes are the β-lactamases, which hydrolyze the β-lactam ring of β-lactam antibiotics, preventing these agents from covalently binding (acylation) to the active site of enzymes known as penicillin-binding proteins (PBPs), involved in cell wall synthesis. Since their discovery in the 1940s in penicillin G-resistant isolates of *Staphylococcus aureus*, several hundred β-lactamases have been identified in a wide variety of bacterial species, both pathogenic and nonpathogenic. These enzymes can be classified according to their spectrum of enzymatic activity (Richmond-Sykes or Bush classification scheme) or their amino acid sequence (Ambler classification). Their hydrolysis specificities determine in large part the β-lactam susceptibility of the bacteria which produce them. However, spontaneous mutations resulting in overexpression or introducing specific changes in the β-lactamase primary structure can increase the activity of these enzymes towards β-lactams that were otherwise relatively resistant to enzymatic hydrolysis. Thus, the 1990s saw the emergence of enzymes derived from restricted spectrum penicillinases (type SHV, TEM or OXA, for example) that were capable of inactivating third generation cephalosporins and therefore named extended-spectrum β-lactamases (ESBL) (26).

In the case of aminoglycosides, stereospecific bacterial enzymes modify the hydroxyl groups [phosphotransferases (APH); nucleotidyltransferases (ANT)] or amino groups [acetyltransferases (AAC)] present on aminoglycoside molecules, thereby blocking the interaction of these drugs with their ribosomal target. While it appears that many such enzymes were acquired by pathogenic bacteria through genetic exchange with environmental species (12), others appear to be intrinsic and have a physiological function other than resistance (36). The plethora of aminoglycoside-modifying enzymes observed in clinical isolates nonetheless argues for a defensive role of these enzymes against aminoglycosides (12). The example of acetyltransferase AAC(6')-Ib-cr illustrates how mutational events can extend the specificity of a modifying enzyme to several antibiotic classes, in

Table 1. Principal mechanisms of antibiotic resistance

Antibiotic	Mechanism	Main examples[a]	Frequency[b]
β-lactams	Enzymatic inactivation	β-lactamase production by many Gram + and -, with the exception of streptococci and rare in enterococci	+++
	Target modification	Mutations or recombination of PBP genes in *S. pneumoniae* and *H. influenzae*	+++
	Additional target	Acquisition of PBP2a by staphylococci	+++
	Active efflux	Overproduction of MexAB-OprM system in *P. aeruginosa*	++
	Membrane impermeability	Deficit of porin OprD in *P. aeruginosa* (carbapenems)	++
Aminoglycosides	Enzymatic inactivation	Acquisition of ANT, APH or AAC enzymes by many Gram + and -	+++
	Target alteration	Mutations in proteins S12 (streptomycin), S5 (spectinomycin)	+
	Target modification	Acquisition of 16S rRNA methylases	+/-
	Membrane impermeability	Defective active transport across cytoplasmic membrane	+/-
	Sequestration	Overproduction of inactivating enzymes vis-à-vis a non-substrate or production of periplasmic glycans	+/-
Macrolides group	Target modification	Acquisition of 23S rRNA methylases	+++
	Active efflux	Acquisition of exogenous systems (especially Gram +) or overproduction of intrinsic systems (especially Gram -)	++
	Target alteration	23S rRNA mutations in *H. pylori*, *Mycobacterium spp.* and *Mycoplasma*	+
	Enzymatic inactivation	Production of esterases or phosphotransferases	+/-
Oxazolidinones	Target alteration	23S rRNA mutations in enterococci and staphylococci	+/-
	Target modification	Acquisition of 23S rRNA methylase	+/-
Glycopeptides	Target modification	Acquisition of *van* determinants by enterococci and staphylococci	+/-
	Antibiotic sequestration	Overproduction of a rearranged peptidoglycan in *S. aureus*	+/-
Quinolones	Target alteration	Mutations in type II topoisomerases in Gram + and -	+++
	Active efflux	Overproduction of intrinsic systems in Gram + and -	++
	Target protection	Acquisition of *qnr* determinants by Gram -	+
	Enzymatic inactivation	Acquisition of acetyltransferase	+/-
Tetracyclines	Active efflux	Acquisition of exogenous systems (Tet proteins) or overproduction of intrinsic systems	+++
	Target protection	Acquisition of *tet*(O), *tet*(M) and *tet*(S) determinants by Gram +	+++
	Enzymatic inactivation	Acquisition of *tet*(X) determinants by anaerobes	+/-
Phenicols	Enzymatic inactivation	Production of acetyltransferases by many Gram + and -	++
	Active efflux	Acquisition of exogenous systems (CmlA, Flo proteins) or overproduction of intrinsic systems	++
	Target modification	Acquisition of 23S rRNA methylase	+/-
Rifampin	Target alteration	Mutations in RNA polymerase	++
	Enzymatic inactivation	Acquisition of ADP-ribosyl-transferase Arr-2 in Gram -	+/-
Fosfomycin	Membrane impermeability	Defect in glycerol-3-phosphate transport system	++
	Enzymatic inactivation	Acquisition of *fos* determinants	+/-
Isoniazid	Failure of enzymatic activation	Mutations in enzymes KatG, EthA, Ndh…	+
Ethionamide	Target alteration	Mutations in enzymes InhA, KasA	+
Pyrazinamide	Failure of enzymatic activation	Mutations in pyrazinamidase PazE	+
Metronidazole	Failure of activation	Deficit in redox systems in *H. pylori*	+/-
	Enzymatic inactivation	Acquisition of Nim determinants in *Bacteroides spp.*	+/-
Trimethoprim	Target alteration	Mutations in DHFR	++
	Additional target	Acquisition of low-affinity DHFR	+/-
	Target amplification	Overproduction of DHFR	+
Sulfonamides	Target alteration	Mutations in DHPS	++
	Additional target	Acquisition of low-affinity DHPS	+/-
Polymyxins	Membrane impermeability	Neutralization of LPS PO_4 groups in various Gram -	+/-

[a] AAC, aminoglycoside acetyltransferase; APH, aminoglycoside phosphotransferase; ANT, aminoglycoside nucleotidyltransferase; DHFR, dihydrofolate reductase; DHPS, dihydropteroate synthetase; LPS, lipopolysaccharide; PBP, penicillin binding protein; -, negative; +, positive.

[b] The frequency of the resistance mechanisms is given for information: rare (+/-), uncommon (+), common (++), very common (+++).

this case the aminoglycosides and the fluoroquinolones ciprofloxacin and norfloxacin (29).

Macrolides can be inactivated in pathogenic species such as *Escherichia coli* and *S. aureus* by esterases and phosphotransferases encoded by *ere* and *mph* genes transferred from phylogenetically distant microorganisms (21).

Another example of this type of strategy is the ADP-ribosyltransferase Arr-2. The gene encoding this enzyme, present on a type 1 integron, confers high-level rifampin resistance in various Gram-negative bacilli (33).

Fosfomycin is also a target of various enzymes including the metalloglutathione transferases FosA, FosB or FosX which catalyze the opening of the epoxide ring of the antibiotic to form an inactive glutathione-fosfomycin adduct (2). Here again, the genes encoding these enzymes are carried on plasmids or transposons (Tn*2921*, for example), although in some cases they are part of the genetic patrimony of the species, as for *Pseudomonas aeruginosa* (PA1129 locus).

Tetracycline is apparently the substrate of a single enzyme known as Tet(X), an NADPH-oxidoreductase identified in a strain of *Bacteroides* sp. harboring a transposon (7). However, the role of Tet(X) in tetracycline resistance in this strain appears marginal.

Finally, in the case of chloramphenicol and thiamphenicol, inactivating enzymes comprising a wide variety of type A or B acetyltransferases generally encoded by mobile genetic elements represent the main mechanism of resistance (31). Acetylation of the C-3 hydroxyl group prevents these drugs from interacting with the ribosomal peptidyltransferase domain and inhibiting protein synthesis. Florfenicol, which has a fluorine atom in place of the hydroxyl group, is unaffected by this modification and therefore remains active in acetyltransferase-producing strains.

FAILURE OF ANTIBIOTIC ACTIVATION

Some antibiotics are only active after being modified by bacterial enzymes. Examples include isoniazid (INH) and ethionamide (ETH), two major antituberculosis drugs which inhibit mycolic acid biosynthesis in the mycobacterial cell wall by blocking enoyl-ACP-reductase, InhA. In order to exert this action, these antibiotics must first be activated inside the cell by the catalase-peroxidase KatG and the monooxygenase EthA, respectively. Mutations which decrease the activity and/or expression of these two enzymes confer resistance to INH or ETH through a lack of prodrug activation (23). In an indirect and complementary manner, a decrease in the activity of Ndh, a type II NADH dehydrogenase responsible for NAD+ regeneration required for INH and ETH activation, can also increase resistance to these agents (34). A similar mechanism operates for pyrazinamide (PZA), whose antimycobacterial activity is abolished when the pyrazinamidase Pzase which converts it to active pyrazinoic acid is mutated (37).

Along similar lines, a failure to reduce the NO_2 group at position 5 of metronidazole by different redox systems (NADPH nitroreductase, RdxA; NAD(P)H:flavin oxidoreductase, FrxA) has been observed in resistant strains of the microaerophilic organism *Helicobacter pylori* (22). In *Bacteroides*, a plasmid-encoded reductase (NimA, B, C, D or E) converts the NO_2 group of metronidazole to an inactive NH_2 group, preventing formation of the NO- intermediate which is toxic to DNA.

TARGET MODIFICATION

Enzymatic

One common mechanism by which bacteria escape the action of antibiotics is to produce enzymes which modify cellular targets, leading to a loss of affinity for the antibiotic. In the case of macrolides, lincosamides, and streptogramin B (MLS_B group), enzymatic methylation of certain adenine residues (for example, A2058 in *E. coli*) of the 23S rRNA prevents these agents from correctly positioning in the peptidyltransferase domain and blocking progression of the nascent peptide in the ribosomal exit tunnel. The Erm methylases (*erythromycin ribosome methylases*) responsible for this cross-resistance (MLS_B phenotype) are encoded by genes often found on mobile elements and whose expression can be induced to different levels by MLS_B or rendered constitutive by mutations in their upstream sequence (3). This type of resistance does not affect linezolid, an oxazolidinone, because it does not interact with the same ribosomal sites as erythromycin. Resistance to linezolid may be conferred by another methylase encoded by the plasmid-borne *cfr* gene which adds a methyl group to adenine 2503 of the 23S RNA and affects the ribosomal binding of five different classes of antibiotics: phenicols, lincosamides, oxazolidinones, pleuromutilins, and streptogramins A (19).

More recently, another type of enzymatic alteration of ribosomal targets was described in aminoglycoside-resistant bacteria. Methylation of the

16S rRNA at position G1405 by the enzymes RmtA (35), RmtB, RmtC, RmtD, or ArmA (15) encoded by plasmid genes located on transposons is yet another example of target modification preventing interaction with the antibiotic and thus totally abolishing antibacterial activity. This modification conferring high-level resistance poses a potential threat to the future of aminoglycosides, since it affects virtually all members of this large class of therapeutic agents and is spreading to Gram-negative species (14).

The peptidoglycan is another target that can be altered in order to protect it from the action of antibiotics. For instance, in enterococci, the D-alanine-D-alanine sequence in the murein precursor UDP-N-acetylmuramic acid-pentapeptide can be converted to D-alanine-D-lactate or D-alananine-D-serine by the different Van enzymes, reducing, sometimes strongly, the affinity of the glycopeptides vancomycin and teicoplanin for this peptidoglycan precursor. The *vanA* and *vanB* genes, which are the main determinants of this resistance, spread within enterococcal populations by means of transposons which can be carried by plasmids.

Another example of target modification concerns polymyxin resistance (polymyxin B and colistin) in Gram-negative bacilli such as *E. coli*, *Salmonella* Typhimurium, and *P. aeruginosa*. To exert their depolarizing effect on the cytoplasmic membrane, polymyxins must first penetrate the outer membrane by displacing divalent cations (mainly Mg^{2+}) which link the phosphate groups of adjacent lipopolysaccharide (LPS) molecules. The main mechanism of resistance to these polycationic antibiotics is the overproduction of enzymes that can attach 4-amino-4-deoxy-L-arabinopyranose (L-Arap4N) or 2-aminoethanol residues to the phosphate groups of LPS, thereby preventing polymyxin penetration and binding (24). These enzymes, such as ArnA and ArnB, are encoded by chromosomal genes regulated by two-component systems that respond to environmental signals.

Mutational

Resistance to antibiotics can be caused by spontaneous mutations which introduce amino acid or nucleic acid substitutions in target molecules, leading to a loss of their affinity for the antibiotic. There are many examples of this type of mechanism in the literature concerning the different classes of antibiotics. However, this phenomenon can only occur easily if the target is encoded by a gene present in one or two copies on the chromosome. This means that single mutations in the 16S or 23S rRNA structural genes can only produce significant resistance to ribosomal inhibitors in species which have a low copy number of these genes, since the mutations are recessive to the wild-type alleles. This is why resistance due to rRNA mutations is observed mainly in *Propionibacterium acnes* (tetracycline), *H. pylori* (tetracycline, macrolides), the genus *Mycobacterium* (aminoglycosides, macrolides), *Mycoplasma hominis* (macrolides), and more rarely in *Streptococcus pneumoniae* (MLS_B, ketolides) (18). Oxazolidinone resistance associated with 23S rRNA mutations has been reported in some species including *Enterococcus faecium*, *S. aureus*, and *S. pneumoniae* (4). Ribosomal protein modifications have also been described in mutants of various species resistant to streptomycin (S12), spectinomycin (S5), MLS_B (L4, L22), or tetracycline (S10).

In a similar manner, β-lactam susceptibility can be reduced by mutations or rearrangements in PBP genes. This type of resistance is considered nonenzymatic because it does not depend on β-lactamase production. It has been widely documented in *S. pneumoniae* (modification of PBP1a, PBP2b, PBP2x) and *Haemophilus influenzae* (PBP3) but also in *Streptococcus pyogenes* (PBP2a', PBP5) (only in laboratory mutants), *E. faecium* (PBP5), *Neisseria gonorrhoeae* (PBP1, PBP2), *Neisseria meningitidis* (PBP2), *H. pylori* (PBP1), *Listeria monocytogenes* (PBP3), and *Proteus mirabilis* (PBP2) (17). The resistance conferred by these alterations varies according to the species, the type of modification (type of mutation, under- or overexpression of the corresponding proteins) and the specific affinities of β-lactams for the different PBPs.

The production of an extra PBP named PBP2a is the major mechanism of β-lactam resistance in methicillin-resistant staphylococci. This protein, encoded by the *mecA* gene located on an exogenous chromosomal sequence (SCC*mec*, for *Staphylococcal Cassette Chromosome mec*), is highly resistant to inhibition by β-lactams and is acylated approximately 1000 times more slowly than the PBPs intrinsically present in susceptible strains (6). Yet, other factors also contribute to methicillin resistance in staphylococci, including a plasmid-encoded β-lactamase as well as *fem* factors (*factors essential for methicillin resistance*) presumed to rearrange the structure of the peptidoglycan synthesized by PBP2a, the only PBP still functioning (6).

The main mechanism of resistance to 4-quinolones represents yet another example of target modification. In this case the targets are the type II topoisomerases: DNA gyrase and topoisomerase IV. These two tetrameric enzymes, respectively involved in DNA replication and chromosomal segregation during cell division, are each composed of two subunits: GyrA and GyrB for DNA gyrase, and ParC and ParE for topoisomerase IV (16). Different mutations in the genes encoding these subunits (*gyrA*, *gyrB*, *parC*, *parE*) have been identified in resistant strains. The impact of these mutations on the MICs of quinolones differs according to the type and number of amino acid substitutions, the type and number of subunits affected, and the bacterial species. Mutations in a precisely defined region of these subunits known as the QRDR (*Quinolone Resistance Determining Region*) prevents the quinolones from binding to and irreversibly blocking the DNA-enzyme complex. In general, DNA gyrase is the primary target of quinolones in Gram-negative organisms and topoisomerase IV in Gram-positive organisms (16).

Resistance to rifampin (modification of RNA polymerase β subunit, RpoB), trimethoprim (dihydrofolate reductase, DHFR), INH (NADH-enoyl-ACP reductase, InhA; β-keto-ACP synthase, KasA), mupirocin (isoleucyl-tRNA synthetase), and fusidic acid (elongation factor EF-G) are more examples of target modification identified in clinical mutants (17).

ANTIBIOTIC SEQUESTRATION AND TARGET PROTECTION

When there is no efficient way to inactivate the antibiotic or reduce the affinity of the target, bacteria may be forced to sequester the drug in order to neutralize its effects. This strategy has been evoked in an attempt to explain resistance to third generation cephalosporins (C3G) in "derepressed" mutants of Gram-negative bacilli overproducing the "chromosomal" cephalosporinase AmpC, due to the relative stability of these β-lactams to this enzyme (30). It is speculated that the antibiotic is neutralized by forming stable complexes with excess β-lactamase, resulting in an insufficient concentration to saturate PBPs.

Complex phenotypic alterations of the peptidoglycan have also been observed in *S. aureus* strains with reduced glycopeptide susceptibility (GISA, GRSA, VISA, hetero-VISA), including increased wall thickening, accumulation of cell wall precursors, inactivation of PBP4, reduction of murein crosslinking and muropeptide amidation (10). This resistance is accompanied by changes in the expression of roughly 200 genes, some of which are involved in peptidoglycan biosynthesis (9). Experimental overexpression of two of these genes – *graF* and *msrA2* – has been shown to raise the MICs of vancomycin and oxacillin and cause a characteristic increase in cell wall thickness (9). However, several mutations are needed for the bacterium to efficiently sequester glycopeptides by producing an amplified and remodeled target (11).

Another strategy involves bacterial production of a protein that can protect the target from interaction with the antibiotic. The Tet(O) and Tet(M) proteins, whose structure is similar to that of elongation factors EF-G and EF-U, can displace tetracycline from the ribosomal A site (aminoacyl-tRNA), thus allowing protein synthesis to continue normally (8). The *tet*(O) and *tet*(M) determinants underlying this mechanism are believed to have been recruited by mobile genetic elements from the natural producer of oxytetracycline, *Streptomyces rimosus* (8).

In 1994, a second protection mechanism came to light with the demonstration of transferable quinolone resistance in a *Klebsiella pneumoniae* isolate (20). Since then, several members of the pentapeptide repeat motif family (A[D/N]Lxx, where x represents any amino acid) have been implicated in low-level quinolone resistance. On the basis of studies on QnrA, it is hypothesized that these proteins (QnrA, QnrB, QnrC, QnrS) bind to the two GyrA and GyrB subunits (and probably also to ParC and ParE) upon formation of the DNA-enzyme complex and, by destabilizing this complex, block the inhibitory action of quinolones (32). The species *Shewanella algae* has been identified as the origin of the QnrA-like determinants (27).

LOSS OF MEMBRANE PERMEABILITY AND ACTIVE EFFLUX

With the exception of the polymyxins and perhaps the aminoglycosides, antibiotics active against Gram-negative bacteria penetrate the outer membrane by passive diffusion through channels known as porins. A quantitative decrease or modifications in the internal eyelet of these protein channels can slow drug entry into the cell and thereby cause low-level resistance to several antibiotic classes. These changes may provide considerable additional resistance to certain antimicrobials by potentiative the prevailing mechanisms (especially production of modifying enzymes).

Carbapenem resistance in *P. aeruginosa* represents the most typical and most frequent example of the type of resistance known as membrane impermeability. Indeed, carbapenems preferentially enter pyocyanic bacilli through a specific porin, OprD, whose natural function is to facilitate diffusion of basic amino acids and gluconate. A change or a defect in the synthesis of this porin due to mutations is, in the large majority of cases, the mechanism of resistance to imipenem in clinical isolates of *P. aeruginosa* (13, 25).

Impermeability may also affect the cytoplasmic membrane. For example, it has long been known that fosfomycin resistance is due mainly to a deficiency of the glycerol-3-phosphate active transport system which the antibiotic uses to enter the cytoplasm (1). More complex modifications affecting the respiratory chain or the quinone pool in the inner membrane have been described in aminoglycoside-resistant mutants with defective intracellular uptake of these agents. Nevertheless, many unknowns persist as to the type of defects and their role in the emergence of resistance (5).

A fairly widespread process by which living creatures maintain cellular homeostasis consists in actively expelling harmful agents outside the cell. These efflux systems, also known as pumps, were first described in tetracycline-resistant strains of *E. coli* by S. Levy in the 1980s. Since this first report, many other transporters have been found in virtually all bacterial species (28). Some are intrinsic while others have been acquired on mobile genetic elements. But their diversity does not stop there because, according to the case, they can be composed of one or three proteins, use the energy supplied by the cytoplasmic membrane electrochemical gradient or the hydrolysis of ATP, and expel a small number of similar antibiotics (tetracyclines, for example) or a wide variety of structurally unrelated agents. Hyperproduction of an active efflux system generally results in a moderate increase in MIC values (by a factor of 2 to 16) of the substrates for the efflux pump. The highest levels of resistance are seen in the species with the lowest permeability to antibiotics, such as *P. aeruginosa* (38).

CONCLUSION

Many bacterial resistance mechanisms have been described, some very recently such as aminoglycoside sequestration by periplasmic glycans, and others still latent or waiting to be discovered. Experience has shown that the strategies used by bacteria to escape the action of a new antiinfective agent involve processes that can be simple (spontaneous mutations, gene transfer) or complex (combinations of mechanisms), but in any case are usually unforeseeable. We must therefore come to terms with the idea that bacterial resistance is an inevitable phenomenon inherent to the adaptability of these microorganisms, but which we must try our best to control while waiting for novel therapeutic solutions.

REFERENCES

(1) **Arca, P., G. Reguera, and C. Hardisson.** 1997. Plasmid-encoded fosfomycin resistance in bacteria isolated from the urinary tract in a multicentre survey. J. Antimicrob. Chemother. **40**:393-399.

(2) **Arca, P., M. Rico, A.F. Brana, C.J. Villar, C. Hardisson, and J. Suarez.** 1988. Formation of an adduct between fosfomycin and glutathione: a new mechanism of antibiotic resistance in bacteria. Antimicrob. Agents Chemother. **32**:1552-1556.

(3) **Arthur, M., A. Brisson-Noël, and P. Courvalin.** 1987. Origin and evolution of genes specifying resistance to macrolide, lincosamide and streptogramin antibiotics: data and hypotheses. J. Antimicrob. Chemother. **20**:783-802.

(4) **Bozdogan, B., and P.C. Appelbaum.** 2004. Oxazolidinones: activity, mode of action, and mechanism of resistance. Int. J. Antimicrob. Agents. **23**:113-119.

(5) **Bryan, L.E.** 1989. Cytoplasmic membrane transport and antimicrobial resistance, pp. 35-57. *In* L. E. Bryan (ed.), Microbial resistance to drugs: handbook of experimental pharmacology. Springer Verlag, Berlin.

(6) **Chambers, H.F.** 1997. Methicillin resistance in staphylococci: molecular and biochemical basis and clinical implications. Clin. Microbiol. Rev. **10**:781-791.

(7) **Chopra, I., and M. Roberts.** 2001. Tetracycline antibiotics: mode of action, applications, molecular biology, and epidemiology of bacterial resistance. Microbiol. Mol. Biol. Rev. **65**:232-260.

(8) **Connell, S.R., D.M. Tracz, K.H. Nierhaus, and D.E. Taylor.** 2003. Ribosomal protection proteins and their mechanisms of tetracycline resistance. Antimicrob. Agents Chemother. **47**:3675-3681.

(9) **Cui, L., J.Q. Lian, H.M. Neoh, E. Reyes, and K. Hiramatsu.** 2005. DNA microarray-based identification of genes associated with glycopeptide resistance in *Staphylococcus aureus*. Antimicrob. Agents Chemother. **49**:3404-3413.

(10) **Cui, L., X. Ma, K. Sato, K. Okuma, F.C. Tenover, E.M. Mamizuka, C.G. Gemmel, M.N. Kim, M.C. Ploy, N. El'Sohl, V. Ferraz, and K. Hiramatsu.** 2003. Cell wall thickening is a common feature of vancomycin resistance in *Staphylococcus aureus*. J. Clin. Microbiol. **41**:5-14.

(11) **Cui, L., H.M. Neoh, M. Shoji, and K. Hiramatsu.** 2009. Contribution of *vraSR* and *graSR* point mutations to vancomycin resistance in vancomycin-inter-

mediate *Staphylococcus aureus*. Antimicrob. Agents Chemother. **53**:1231-1234.

(12) **Davies, J., and G.D. Wright.** 1997. Bacterial resistance to aminoglycoside antibiotics. Trends Microbiol. **5**:234-240.

(13) **Dib, C., J. Trias, and V. Jarlier.** 1995. Lack of additive effect between mechanisms of resistance to carbapenems and other beta-lactam agents in *Pseudomonas aeruginosa*. Eur. J. Clin. Microbiol. Infect. Dis. **14**:979-986.

(14) **Fritsche, T.R., M. Castanheira, G.H. Miller, R.N. Jones, and E.S. Armstrong.** 2008. Detection of methyltransferases conferring high-level resistance to aminoglycosides in enterobacteriaceae from Europe, North America and Latin America. Antimicrob. Agents Chemother. **52**:1843-1845.

(15) **Galimand, M., P. Courvalin, and T. Lambert.** 2003. Plasmid-encoded high-level resistance to aminoglycosides in *Enterobacteriaceae* due to 16S rRNA methylation. Antimicrob. Agents Chemother. **47**:2565-2571.

(16) **Hawkey, P.M.** 2003. Mechanisms of quinolone action and microbial response. J. Antimicrob. Chemother. **51** *(suppl. S1)*:29-35.

(17) **Lambert, P.A.** 2005. Bacterial resistance to antibiotics: modified target sites. Adv. Drug Deliv. Rev. **57**:1471-1485.

(18) **Leclercq, R., and P. Courvalin.** 2002. Resistance to macrolides and related antibiotics in *Streptococcus pneumoniae*. Antimicrob. Agents Chemother. **46**:2727-2734.

(19) **Long, K.S., J. Poehlsgaard, C. Kehrenberg, S. Schwarz, and B. Vester.** 2006. The Cfr rRNA methyltransferase confers resistance to phenicols, lincosamides, oxazolidinones, pleuromutilins, and streptogramin A antibiotics. Antimicrob. Agents Chemother. **50**:2500-2505.

(20) **Martinez-Martinez, L., A. Pascual, and G.A. Jacoby.** 1998. Quinolone resistance from a transferable plasmid. Lancet **351**:797-799.

(21) **Matsuoka, M., and T. Sasaki.** 2004. Inactivation of macrolides by producers and pathogens. Curr. Drug Targets Infect. Disord. **4**:217-240.

(22) **Mendz, G.L., and F. Mégraud.** 2002. Is the molecular basis of metronidazole resistance in microaerophilic organisms understood? Trends Microbiol. **10**:370-375.

(23) **Morlock, G.P., B. Metchock, D. Sikes, J.T. Crawford, and R.C. Cooksey.** 2003. *ethA, inhA,* and *katG* loci of ethionamide-resistant clinical *Mycobacterium tuberculosis* isolates. Antimicrob. Agents Chemother. **47**:3799-3805.

(24) **Nummila, K., I. Kilpelainen, U. Zahringer, M. Vaara, and I.M. Helander.** 1995. Lipopolysaccharides of polymyxin B-resistant mutants of *Escherichia coli* are extensively substituted by 2-aminoethyl pyrophosphate and contain aminoarabinose in lipid A. Mol. Microbiol. **16**:271-278.

(25) **Pai, H., J.-W. Kim, J. Kim, J.H. Lee, K.W. Choe, and N. Gotoh.** 2001. Carbapenem resistance mechanisms in *Pseudomonas aeruginosa* clinical isolates. Antimicrob. Agents Chemother. **45**:480-484.

(26) **Paterson, D.L., and R.A. Bonomo.** 2005. Extended-spectrum ß-lactamases: a clinical update. Clin. Microbiol. Rev. **18**:657-686.

(27) **Poirel, L., J.M. Rodriguez-Martinez, H. Mammeri, A. Liard, and P. Nordmann.** 2005. Origin of plasmid-mediated quinolone resistance determinant *qnrA*. Antimicrob. Agents Chemother. **49**:3523-3525.

(28) **Poole, K.** 2005. Efflux-mediated antimicrobial resistance. J. Antimicrob. Chemother. **56**:20-51.

(29) **Robicsek, A., J. Strahilevitz, and G.A. Jacoby.** 2006. Fluoroquinolone-modifying enzyme: a new adaptation of a common aminoglycoside acetyltransferase. Nat. Med. **12**:83-88.

(30) **Sanders, C.C., and W.E. Sanders Jr.** 1985. Microbial resistance to newer generation ß-lactam antibiotics: clinical and laboratory implications. J. Infect. Dis. **151**:399-406.

(31) **Schwartz, S., C. Kehrenberg, B. Doublet, and A. Cloeckaert.** 2004. Molecular basis of bacterial resistance to chloramphenicol and florfenicol. FEMS Microbiol. Rev. **28**:519-542.

(32) **Tran, J.H., G.A. Jacoby, and D.C. Hooper.** 2005. Interaction of the plasmid-encoded quinolone resistance protein Qnr with *Escherichia coli* DNA gyrase. Antimicrob. Agents Chemother. **49**:118-125.

(33) **Tribuddharat, C., and M. Fennewald.** 1999. Integron-mediated rifampin resistance in *Pseudomonas aeruginosa*. Antimicrob. Agents Chemother. **43**:960-962.

(34) **Vilcheze, C., T.R. Weisbrod, B. Chen, L. Kremer, M.H. Hazbon, F. Wang, D. Alland, J.C. Sacchettini, and W.R. Jacobs Jr.** 2005. Altered NADH/NAD+ ratio mediates coresistance to isoniazid and ethionamide in mycobacteria. Antimicrob. Agents Chemother. **49**:708-720.

(35) **Yokoyama, K., Y. Doi, K. Yamane, H. Kurokawa, N. Shibata, K. Shibayama, T. Yagi, H. Kato, and Y. Arakawa.** 2003. Acquisition of 16S rRNA methylase gene in *Pseudomonas aeruginosa*. Lancet **362**:1888-1893.

(36) **Zeng, L., and S. Jin.** 2003. *aph(3')-IIb*, a gene encoding an aminoglycoside-modifying enzyme, is under the positive control of surrogate regulator HpaA. Antimicrob. Agents Chemother. **47**:3867-3876.

(37) **Zhang, Y., and D. Mitchison.** 2003. The curious characteristics of pyrazinamide: a review. Int. J. Tuber. Lung Dis. **7**:6-21.

(38) **Ziha-Zarifi, I., C. Llanes, T. Köhler, J.-C. Pechère, and P. Plésiat.** 1999. *In vivo* emergence of multidrug-resistant mutants of *Pseudomonas aeruginosa* overexpressing the active efflux system MexA-MexB-OprM. Antimicrob. Agents Chemother. **43**:287-291.

Chapter 3. GENETICS OF RESISTANCE

Louis B. RICE

INTRODUCTION

The phenotype represented by the antibiogram is nothing more than the sum total of effects created by the genetic composition of the bacterial strain under study. Since susceptibility or resistance to antimicrobial agents is genetically defined, the emergence and spread of antimicrobial resistance in bacteria is no surprise, given their extraordinary genetic flexibility. In this chapter, I will discuss general concepts of bacterial genetics as they relate to antimicrobial resistance mechanisms, providing examples of how these mechanisms work individually and in concert to create phenotypic antimicrobial resistance.

All antibiotics act by interacting with bacterial target molecules (most often but not exclusively cellular enzymes) that are essential to cell growth, function, or both. This interaction results in inhibition of cell replication (bacteriostatic activity) or cell death (bactericidal activity). Critical to successful inhibition is the presence of inhibitory concentrations of antibiotic at the target. Antibiotics that have a very high affinity for their target molecule will require lower concentrations to inhibit growth, whereas those with lower affinity require higher concentrations. The ultimate goal of all resistance mechanisms is to insure that the concentration of antibiotic at the target site falls below the level required for effective inhibition. There are many mechanisms by which bacteria accomplish this goal, mechanisms which may be employed alone or in combination. The specific biochemical mechanisms of resistance are beyond the scope of this chapter, and will be discussed in detail in other chapters.

Antimicrobial resistance can be intrinsic or acquired. Intrinsic resistance is that which is recognized from the first development of an antibiotic, and is not a major clinical concern. Examples of intrinsic resistance include the resistance of all Gram-negative bacteria to glycopeptides due to inability of these large molecules to traverse the Gram-negative outer membrane, the resistance of anaerobic bacteria to the aminoglycosides because movement of aminoglycosides across the cytoplasmic membrane is an oxygen-dependent process, and the resistance of enterococci to trimethoprim-sulfamethoxazole due to their ability to absorb exogenous folate (thereby eliminating the need for the enzymes that are inhibited by these antimicrobial agents). These intrinsic resistances are simply accepted as part of the profile of a given antibiotic when it is introduced and are taken into account when designing empirical or specific therapies for infections.

Of interest to us in this chapter is resistance to antibiotics that is acquired by normally susceptible bacteria. Bacteria can acquire resistance through the mutation of cellular genes, the acquisition of foreign resistance genes, and through mutation of acquired genes. As we will show through the course of this chapter, highly resistant strains use a variety of these mechanisms to develop their resistance portfolio.

MUTATION TO RESISTANCE

Reduced target affinity

As antibiotic interactions with their targets are very specific, it stands to reason that alterations of critical sites in target molecules may impair effective interaction between the antibiotic and its target. The likelihood that target molecules will mutate in ways that lower affinity depends on the impact those changes have on the normal function of the molecule and the stability of the molecule in its new conformation. In practice, this limitation is only a relative one, as many molecules have been shown to change in ways that decrease the affinity for antibiotics but preserve sufficient function to allow survival of the cell. A prime example of this mutational resistance is resistance to rifampin. Rifampin is one of our most broadly active and bactericidal antibiotics. Its use in the clinical setting, however, is limited by the emergence of resistance at a high frequency. Resistance to rifampin in *Escherichia coli* emerges because point mutations in one of six highly conserved regions of the ß-subunit of the *rpoB* gene (22), encoding RNA polymerase, result in amino acid changes that reduce the rifampin activity without appreciably altering the cellular function of the enzyme. Similar mutations have been reported in a variety of species. It is important to recognize that rifampin does not cause these mutations to occur. Rather it selects for small sub-populations that have acquired the mutations by random chance. By rapidly killing off the susceptible population of microorganisms, rifampin creates an environment in which the resistant subpopulation can emerge dominant. In treating tuberculosis, this emergence of resistance can be avoided by using antimicrobial combinations designed to include agents (like INH) that will continue to have bactericidal activity against rifampin-resistant *Mycobacterium tuberculosis*. A similar strategy has not been effective at preventing the emergence of resistance to rifampin in other species of importance, such as *Staphylococcus aureus* (11). A recent comprehensive review suggested resistance to rifampin develops on average in 17% of cases when used to try to eliminate superficial colonization of *S. aureus*.

In reality, however, point mutations in target genes often only confer relatively modest levels of resistance to antimicrobial agents (18). In most cases, sequential mutations must be accumulated for a reduction in target affinity sufficient for expression of clinically significant levels of resistance (37). In order for these early, non-resistance conferring mutations to survive and accumulate, it is likely that bacteria must be subjected to subinhibitory concentrations of antibiotics for prolonged periods. In practice, such exposure is probably quite common. In some cases, antimicrobial agents are dosed below their optimal level. In others, exposure occurs in areas where the pharmacokinetic profile of the antibiotic is either unknown or suboptimal (such as the gastrointestinal tract or on the skin). In still others, antimicrobial exposure in non-human venues, such as in farm animals, promotes the accumulation of one or more resistance mutations. Over time, enough mutations may accumulate to allow the bacterium to survive in the presence of high concentrations of antibiotic, and clinically significant resistance ensues.

Cellular recombination mechanisms may also be used to amplify the expression of resistance caused by point mutations in target genes. Linezolid acts by inhibiting the initiation complex, the consortium of ribosome, mRNA and tRNA that synthesizes cellular proteins. A single point mutation (most commonly G2572A) in the 23S ribosomal RNA gene reduces linezolid binding affinity significantly. However, there are between 4 and 6 23S rRNA genes in enterococci and staphylococci, and the level of resistance expressed is directly related to the number of rRNA genes with this modification. Despite the need for mutations in multiple genes for expression of selectable resistance, resistance is readily observed in patients receiving linezolid. This emergence is due to recombination between the different rRNA genes in the cell, rapidly amplifying expression of resistance through a process known as gene conversion. As such, the first mutation becomes the rate-limiting step for the emergence of resistance. Consistent with this mechanism, cells with defective intracellular recombination mechanisms have a difficult time emerging resistant to clinically significant concentrations of linezolid.

Mutations in regulatory networks

Point mutations may also result in alterations of regulatory networks that control expression of resistance. *Enterobacter* spp. have chromosomal β-lactamase genes (*ampC*) that confer resistance to a range of β-lactam antibiotics when expressed at high levels. Under normal circumstances, expression of *ampC* is repressed by the regulatory protein AmpR, which is encoded immediately upstream from *ampC* in *E. cloacae*. AmpR can serve either as a repressor or an activator of *ampC* transcription, depending on whether it is bound with UDP-*N*-acetylmuramic acid (repressor) or 1,6-anhydro-*N*-acetylmuramic acid tri-, tetra-, and pentapeptides (activator). Under normal circumstances, 1,6-anhydro-*N*-acetylmuramic acid tri-, tetra-, and pentapeptides, which are recyclable products of cell wall turnover, are brought back into the cell through a permease designated AmpG. After entering the cell, the 1,6-anhydro-*N*-acetylmuramic acid tri-, tetra-, and pentapeptides are processed by a cellular amidase (AmpD), resulting in UDP-*N*-acetylmuramic acid, which interacts with AmpR in a manner that represses *ampC* transcription. In a small subpopulation of an *Enterobacter* culture there will be cells in which a point mutation results in an inactive AmpD. Under these circumstances, 1,6-anhydro-*N*-acetylmuramic acid tri-, tetra-, and pentapeptides cannot be converted to UDP-*N*-acetylmuramic acid, and AmpR thus acts as a persistent activator of *ampC* transcription (the "derepressed" mutants), resulting in very high levels of resistance to many β-lactam antibiotics. Treatment of *Enterobacter* infections with extended-spectrum cephalosporins has been shown to be associated with emergence of these derepressed mutants in the clinical setting.

It is worth noting that the above "stably derepressed" mutants of *Enterobacter* spp. emerge in the setting of an "inducible" resistance phenotype. Some β-lactam antibiotics (such as amoxicillin, cefoxitin, imipenem, and the inhibitor clavulanic acid) are potent inducers of AmpC expression. If these agents are highly susceptible to hydrolysis by AmpC (as is amoxicillin), very high MICs will be observed. Other β-lactams (notably the extended-spectrum cephalosporins) are poor inducers but are susceptible to hydrolysis by AmpC. When extended – spectrum cephalosporins were introduced into clinical practice, their failure to induce AmpC expression was considered a positive feature. It was soon recognized, however, that the failure to induce expression of these enzymes made them powerful selectors of derepressed mutants. As a consequence, extended spectrum cephalosporins are not recommended for the treatment of serious *Enterobacter* infections, despite apparent susceptibility on the antibiogram.

With the exception of *Salmonella* spp., all Gram-negative bacteria produce chromosomal β-lactamases. However, the genetics of regulation differ from species to species. *E. coli* lack an *ampR*, and so do not exhibit either the inducible or stably derepressed phenotype. *P. aeruginosa* have several copies of *ampD*, resulting in graded levels of derepression depending on how many of the *ampD* genes are inactivated. *Acinetobacter baumannii* also lack an *ampR*, but insertion of IS(Aba1) upstream from the chromosomal β-lactamase gene in many clinical isolates suggests that increased expression could result from a better promoter contributed by the IS element. Increased expression of a chromosomal β-lactamase in *Bacteroides fragilis* has also been attributed to upstream insertion of an IS element.

Mutations that reduce access

The Gram-negative bacterial membrane is a lipid-rich barrier that is penetrated by few antimicrobial agents. Consequently, most antibiotics enter into the bacterial periplasmic space (the space between the outer membrane and the cytoplasmic membrane) by passing through aqueous channels known as porins. Low levels of resistance in some Gram-negative species (*A. baumannii* and *P. aeruginosa* are two examples) has been attributed to their expression of "slow" porins. In other words, passage of solutes across these porins occurs at a lower rate than in more susceptible bacteria. Bacteria can also undergo mutations that reduce the quantity of these porins in the outer membrane, resulting in higher MICs than seen in strains with a full complement and quantity of porins. In general, such changes do not by themselves result in MIC increases sufficient to result in clinical resistance, but they can augment the resistance resulting from expression of other determinants. One well studied example of this phenomenon is the emergence of resistance to imipenem in *P. aeruginosa*. *P. aeruginosa* produces an inducible AmpC that has poor activity against imipenem, which traverses the *P. aeruginosa* outer membrane through a porin designated OmpD2. Imipenem, as noted above, is a good inducer of AmpC β-lactamase expression, but because it is a poor substrate resistance does not result. Exposure to imipenem, however, can select for reductions in expression of OmpD2. When combined with increased β-lactamase expression, these reductions in OmpD2 result in expression of clinically significant levels of imipenem resistance in *P. aeruginosa*. Such resistant mutants emerge in as many as half of *P. aeruginosa* pneumonias treated with imipenem.

Reduced access can also result from mutations that lead to increased expression of multi-drug efflux pumps. As with porin mutations, efflux pump expression frequently does not yield clinically selectable levels of resistance by itself, but can amplify resistance in the presence of other mechanisms.

ACQUIRED RESISTANCE

Most clinically important antimicrobial resistance results from the acquisition of exogenous resistance determinants by intrinsically susceptible organisms. This stands to reason, since antimicrobial agents for which mutational resistance emerges at high frequency are unlikely to make it to market. The ready availability of sophisticated genetic analysis has greatly increased our understanding of the mechanisms by which bacteria exchange DNA. For many years, we thought of genetic exchange as occurring in fixed units, such as discrete plasmids or transposons. These elements were most often found to carry antimicrobial resistance determinants, largely because these determinants were easiest to track in the laboratory. The advent of comparative genomic sequence analysis has shown us that discrete units of DNA and fixed transfer mechanisms represent a minority of genetic exchange, and that complex genetic exchange is the rule, rather than the exception, in the bacterial world. For years we have recognized that some strains of *E. coli* caused urinary tract infections, whereas others caused gastrointestinal illnesses. We now recognize that these differences are genetically determined through the differential acquisition of large pathogenicity islands that carry determinants that promote different pathologic processes. The first fully sequenced *Enterococcus faecalis* genome (V583) suggested that 25% of the chromosome was acquired or mobile DNA, indicating that enterococci are highly promiscuous. Surprisingly, the second completely sequenced *E. faecalis* genome (OG1X) revealed virtually no acquired DNA. Work by Rob Willems and colleagues has shown that a single clonal complex of *Enterococcus faecium* is responsible for most of the outbreaks and clinical infections worldwide, and that this clonal complex characteristically has many loci of common (presumably acquired) DNA that could significantly impact its ability to colonize and infect people (23). So while we will spend considerable space in this chapter discussing discrete mechanisms of gene movement and exchange, the majority of gene movement occurs by complex combinations of these mechanisms and, almost certainly, by mechanisms that have yet to be discovered.

Transformation

Transformation refers to the ability of some bacterial species to take up naked DNA and integrate that DNA into its genome across regions or relative or complete homology. This appears to be a relatively infrequent mechanism of gene exchange, primarily because few pathogenic bacteria are capable of natural transformation. Among the most important species with this capability are *Streptococcus pneumoniae* and *Neisseria* spp (49). Resistance to β-lactam antibiotics in *S. pneumoniae* is exclusively due to the expression of "mosaic" Pbps that have evolved through the acquisition of fragments of pbp genes from less susceptible viridans streptococcal species. Levels of β-lactam resistance expressed by such strains will vary depending on the number and nature of the *pbps* having the mosaic genotypes. Overall, resistance due to expression of mosaic genes in *S. pneumoniae* is relatively modest, given the modest MICs of the donor bacteria and the need for substantial homology with the native proteins. Resistance to penicillin in *Neisseria* spp. is also associated with mosaic genes, in this case derived from acquisition of DNA from other *Neisseria* spp. *Neisseria gonorrhoeae* may also express resistance to penicillins through the expression of a β-lactamase. Mosaic genes acquired through transformation are not restricted to pbps. Resistance to fluoroquinolones through mosaic topoisomerase genes has also been reported.

Plasmid exchange

Plasmids are autonomously replicating segments of DNA. They vary greatly in size, with the smallest being 1-2 kb and the largest being greater than 200 kb. Plasmids can move between cells by three known mechanisms. They may encode their own transfer functions, they may be mobilized by other mobile elements, or they may be transferred by bacteriophage (transduction). It is not known exactly how important transduction is to overall plasmid exchange, but the size limitations of phage heads (the typical phage genome is roughly 40 kb) likely limits the size and types of plasmids that can be incorporated. It is interesting that the typical β-lactamase-producing plasmid found in *S. aureus* is 40 kb in size or smaller. Since these plasmids generally do not encode their own transfer functions, it is tempting to speculate that the mechanism of rapid spread of β-lactamase production through *S. aureus* in the 1940s and '50s was due to generalized transduction mediated by the many bacteriophages known to be present in *S. aureus*. It is also unclear how often mobilization is a mechanism for exchange. The presence of small, mobilizable plasmids carrying resistance determinants in *S. aureus* has been recognized for years, and may be one mechanism for the spread of certain antimicrobial resistance genes in this genus.

In most recognized cases, plasmid exchange functions are encoded by the plasmids themselves. Recent work indicates that some of these mechanisms of transfer bear homology to Type IV secretion systems used by bacteria to transfer DNA and proteins into target cells. One of the earliest recognized exchangeable plasmids was the *E. coli* F (fertility) factor, which can exhibit 100% transfer to a suitable recipient within one hour *in vitro*. Factors encoded by the F plasmid that may be involved in genetic exchange include the F pilus, which draws donor and recipient cells together to facilitate the genetic exchange by other mechanisms. In *E. faecalis*, highly transferable plasmids respond to the elaboration of small peptide molecules known as pheromones by producing aggregation substance, which causes donor and recipient cells to clump together and thereby facilitate genetic transfer. Pheromone responsive plasmids, while interesting, are unlikely to play a major role in interspecies genetic exchange, since in most cases their host range appears to be restricted to *E. faecalis*. A second type of *E. faecalis* plasmid that

Chapter 3. GENETICS OF RESISTANCE

has been described is the "broad host-range" plasmid, exemplified by plasmids pAMß1 and pIP501. Broad host-range plasmids, as their name implies, can transfer between disparate species. Circumstantial evidence exists that the transfer of -lactamase production to *E. faecalis* and the transfer of vancomycin resistance to *S. aureus* both involved broad host-range plasmids .

Plasmids often carry determinants for resistance to antimicrobial agents, which greatly facilitates their study in the laboratory. There are several different models for exchange, but one of the most common is a "rolling circle" model (Fig.1) in which a nicking enzyme cleaves a single strand of the plasmid, one end of which then moves into the recipient cell, followed by replication of the complementary strand in both donor and recipient and repair of the strand break by cellular repair enzymes. In this manner, plasmid is received by the target cell without loss of plasmid from the donor cell. Whether the plasmid can survive in the recipient cell will depend upon whether its DNA structure is resistant to the recipient restriction enzymes and whether its replication machinery can function in the recipient. Whether or not the plasmid can replicate, some resistance determinants introduced by the plasmid can still survive if they are encoded on mobile DNA such as transposons.

The concept of plasmids as completely independent of the chromosome, and of each other, in bacterial cells is no longer viable. Plasmids can move in and out of the chromosome, and can cointegrate with other plasmids. When they remove themselves from the chromosome, they can take some chromosomal DNA with them, and leave pieces of themselves behind. They can accept transposons from the chromosome and deliver transposons to the chromosome. As such, it is best to consider bacterial genomes (chromosome and all plasmids) as fluid structures that comingle on a regular basis.

Transposons

Transposons are genetic segments that encode functions that allow them to move from one replicon to another within or between cells. Characteristic of most transposons are enzymes that mediate transposition (generally a transposase or a transposase plus a resolvase) and specific termini (often inverted or directly repeated DNA sequences) that are bound by the transposases during transposition. Transposons have no replication genes, and so they must integrate into a replicative structure (generally a plasmid or the chromosome) to survive. Transposition can be conservative, in which the transposon leaves one structure and enters another, or replicative, in which transposition occurs through a cointegrate intermediate (Fig. 2), with ultimate resolution of the cointegrate coming through the cellular homologous recombination machinery or through resolvase functions encoded by the transposons itself.

The smallest transposons encode only their transposition functions and are referred to as insertion sequences, or IS elements. IS elements are generally 1-2 kb in size and are found in many different bacteria. In most, but not all cases, IS elements transpose by a replicative mechanism, with resolution of the resulting cointegrates occurring by cellular recombination mechanisms. IS elements are major drivers of genetic evolution, facilitating rearrangements and cointegrations. They

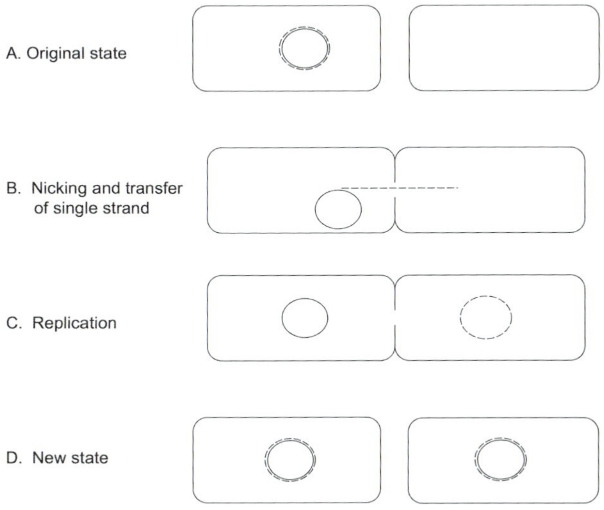

Fig. 1. Conjugation.

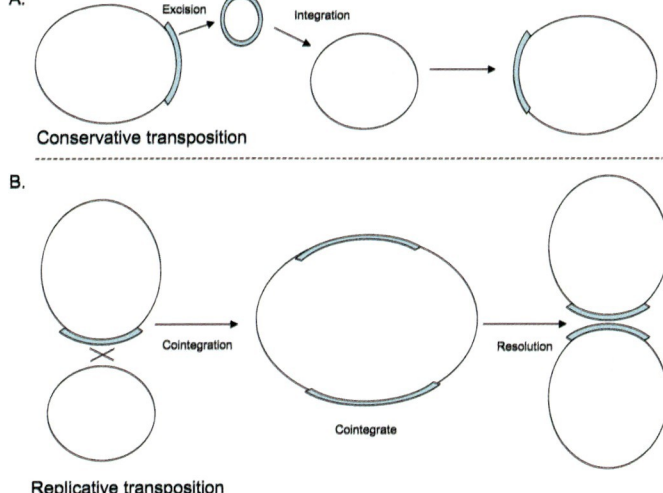

Fig. 2. Transposition.

can also impact the expression of cellular genes by supplying active promoters when they are integrated upstream from resistance genes that are, under normal circumstances, poorly expressed.

IS elements can also flank resistance or other genes, forming what is known as a "composite" transposon. Composite transposons owe their mobility to the activity of the tandem IS elements. Many composite transposons have been described. In staphylococci and enterococci, gentamicin resistance is most frequently encoded by the *aac-6'-aph-2"* aminoglycoside modifying enzyme gene, which in many strains is flanked by inverted copies of insertion sequence IS*256*. In staphylococci, this transposon is referred to as Tn*4001*, in enterococci as Tn*5281*. While some composite transposons like Tn*4001* appear repeatedly with a consistent structure, it is probably better to conceive of composite transposons as constantly evolving structures, since IS elements (in some cases not identical but just similar) located anywhere in the genome or on a plasmid can form composite transposons that (at least theoretically) can move from replicon to replicon.

Somewhat more complex than the simple composite transposons are the Tn*3*-family transposons. Tn*3*-family transposons employ a replicative transposition mechanism, encoding both a transposase and a resolvase. Tn*3* was one of the first transposons described, encoding ampicillin resistance in Gram-negative bacteria through expression of the bla_{TEM-1} β-lactamase gene. In Gram-positive bacteria, Tn*917* is a Tn*3*-family transposon that encodes resistance to macrolides, lincosamides and streptogramin B (MLS$_B$) through expression of the ErmB erythromycin ribosomal methylase. While all Tn*3*-family transposons conform to specific transposition structures, some can be quite complex in the resistance that they encode. Tn*1546* is a Tn*3*-family transposon that encodes resistance to vancomycin and teicoplanin through expression of the *vanA* resistance operon. The *vanA* operon is composed of seven open reading frames, two of which are regulatory genes, the rest of which encode proteins directly or tangentially involved in the vancomycin resistance mechanism. Extensive investigations indicate that all VanA-type resistance is encoded within Tn*1546*-like transposons, though many have their structures modified through the insertion of IS elements and associated deletions, etc. Movement of Tn*1546* from a broad host-range plasmid to staphylococcal plasmids is felt to be the mechanism underlying at least one example of transfer of vancomycin resistance from *E. faecalis* to *S. aureus*.

Tn*3* represents one branch of the so-called "class 2" transposons. Another branch is represented by Tn*21*, from which integrons were first described. Integrons are complex structures in which integrases "capture" circularized gene cassettes and functionalize them by lining them up downstream from a promoter. Several genes can be found in integron cassettes, with their expression often inversely related to their distance from the promoter. While integrons were first discovered encoding antimicrobial resistance within transposons, they are in reality very common elements in bacterial genomes and may play very important roles in bacterial genome evolution.

None of the transposons discussed to this point encode transfer functions. In order to move from cell to cell, they must be integrated into a replicon (generally a plasmid) that can transfer from cell to cell. There are, however, transposons that encode transfer functions. The first described of these were conjugative transposons Tn*916* (from *E. faecalis*) and Tn*1545* (from *S. pneumoniae*). Although Tn*916* and Tn*1545* are different in size (16 kb *vs.* 25.4, respectively) and in the resistance (they encode tetracycline/minocycline *vs* erythromycin, kanamycin and tetracycline/minocycline resistance, respectively), these transposons have identical ends and encode identical integrase and excisase. Tn*916*-family transposons move by a conservative mechanism in which the transposon is first excised from the donor molecule, forming a non-replicative circular intermediate. The "joint" region of the circular intermediate, where the two ends of the transposons are joined, is initially a heteroduplex consisting of single stranded DNA representing the previous junction sequences on each end of the integrated element. Although there is not universal agreement, compelling data exist for the resolution of the heteroduplex in enterococci, although not necessarily under experimental conditions in *E. coli*. The circular intermediate then either inserts in a separate area within the host strain, or transfers to a recipient strain as a single strand, followed by complementary strand synthesis and insertion in the recipient genome.

In most genera, Tn*916* target site selection is relatively non-specific, although there is a predilection for inserting into AT rich regions. This preference makes it a sub-optimal insertional mutagenesis tool, since it tends to insert in AT-rich promoter regions rather than within open reading frames. For years it was thought that all Tn*916*-like elements encoded Tet(M)-type tetracycline resistance. Analysis of genome sequences from a variety of Gram-positive bacteria indicates that Tn*916*-like transposons are more varied than previously suspected. Tn*5386*, for example, is a Tn*916*-family transposons that does not encode antimicrobial resistance, but rather what appears to a bacteriocin operon. Interestingly, Tn*5386* is able to function as one end of a composite transposon, with Tn*916* as the other end, facilitating excision from the chromosome and, in at least one instance, loss of 160 kb of DNA from *E. faecium*.

Conjugative transposons are now generally grouped within a larger class of transferable elements designated ICEs (Integrated Conjugative Elements). The prototypical ICEs from Gram-negative bacteria are the large chromosomal elements R391 (from *Proteus rettgeri*) and SXT (from *Vibrio cholerae*). SXT and R391 are 99.5 and 89 kb, respectively. The size difference largely reflects different modular components, with 65 kb of each element representing a "backbone" in which there is greater than 95% homology. Three modules of known function are common to the two elements – the integration module, the conjugation module, and the regulation module. SXT encodes several different antimicrobial resistances, including those to florfenicol, streptomycin, sulfamethoxazole, and trimethoprim whereas R391 encodes mercury and kanamycin resistance. There also appear to be three hotspots in which different insertions are found in the two elements.

Composites of different mobile elements

Large composite elements with varied constituents have been described in Gram-positive and Gram-negative species. One example from Gram-positives is Tn*5385*, an *E. faecalis* complex transposon that encodes resistance to ampicillin through expression of β-lactamase, erythromycin, gentamicin, mercury, streptomycin, and tetracycline (Fig. 3). The ends of this element are comprised of directly-repeated copies of insertion sequence IS*1216* and within it are several different independent transposons. Gentamicin resistance is encoded by a Tn*4001*-like element, which with a nearby IS*256* forms the ends of a larger erythromycin, gentamicin, and mercury resistance transposon designated Tn*5384*. Erythromycin resistance within Tn*5384*/Tn*5385* is encoded by a vestige of Tn*917* and resistance to mercuric chloride by a *merA* homologue flanked by directly-repeated copies of insertion sequence IS*257*. β-lactamase is encoded by a Tn*552*-like β-lactamase transposon, the regulatory gene *blaR1* of which is interrupted by the IS*256* forming the right end of Tn*5384*. At the left extreme of Tn*5385* lies a typical streptococcal streptomycin resistance determinant adjacent to Tn*5381*, a Tn*916*-family Tet(M)-encoding conjugative transposon. Finally, within the element lies an interrupted replication region characteristic of broad host-range plasmids. In summary, Tn*5385* is a composite of staphylococcal and enterococcal

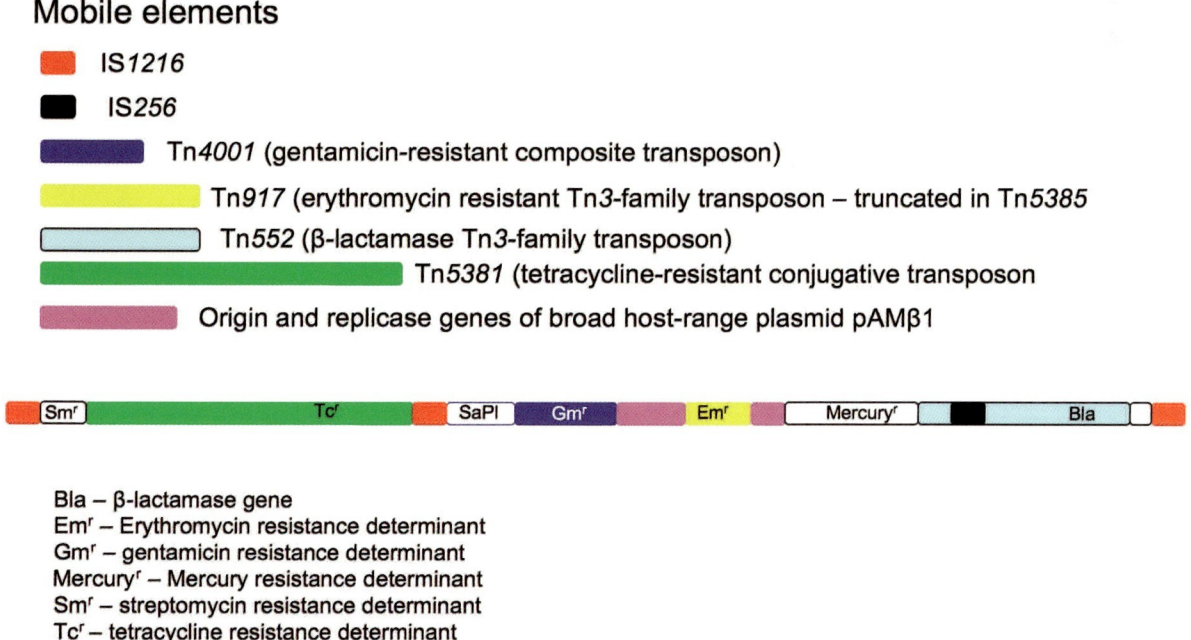

Fig. 3. Large composite element Tn*5385*.

plasmids and transposons linked together and mobilized by a variety of IS elements.

A similar example in Gram-negative bacteria is the recently described KQ element that confers resistance to a broad spectrum of β-lactam antibiotics, aminoglycosides and fluoroquinolones in *Klebsiella pneumoniae* (Fig. 4). The KQ element originated as Tn*3*, followed by insertion of three resistance genes [$aac(6')$-Ib, $aadA1$ and bla_{OXA-9}] within *tnpR*, creating Tn*1331*. Two subsequent insertions into Tn*1331*, Tn*4401* (encoding carbapenem resistance mediated by the ESBL KPC-3) into TnpA and Tn*5387* into bla_{OXA-9} yielded the KQ element, which when borne by a transferable plasmid insures transfer of multiple resistance determinants in a single transfer event. With the increase in whole genome sequences available, it is becoming clear that large composite resistance elements are extremely common. In one dramatic example, a multi-resistant *A. baumannii* strain was found to have an 86-kb genomic "resistance island" that encoded no fewer than 45 antimicrobial resistance genes. Interspersed among these resistance genes were a variety of transposases, integrases and IS elements.

Regulation of resistance expression

In general, expression of resistance comes at a cost to most bacteria, and this cost is commonly measured as a slower growth rate *in vitro* or an inability to successfully compete with susceptible bacteria *in vivo*. Among the putative costs of resistance expression include the cost of replication of the plasmid within which the resistance genes reside and the cost of expression of the resistance gene. These costs of resistance are often mitigated in bacteria by integration into the chromosome and by restricting the expression of resistance to circumstances where it will be useful. The VanA glycopeptide resistance determinant is tightly regulated in enterococci by two genes that are included in the operon encoding the resistance determinants. VanS is a sensor kinase that spans the bacterial cytoplasmic membrane a senses when vancomycin or teicoplanin is in the media. VanR is a cytoplasmic protein that acts as a repressor of VanA transcription when it is dephosphorylated, but as an activator of transcription when it is phosphorylated. Since the vancomycin resistance operon encodes and alternative ligase that contributes to formation of alternative peptidoglycan precursors that are resistant to vancomycin, the inducibility of VanA expression in the setting of lethal mutations in the normal cellular ligase can yield the curious phenomenon of "vancomycin dependence", in which cell wall precursors can only be synthesized in the presence of vancomycin.

The VanA resistance operon is activated by both vancomycin and teicoplanin. In contrast, the

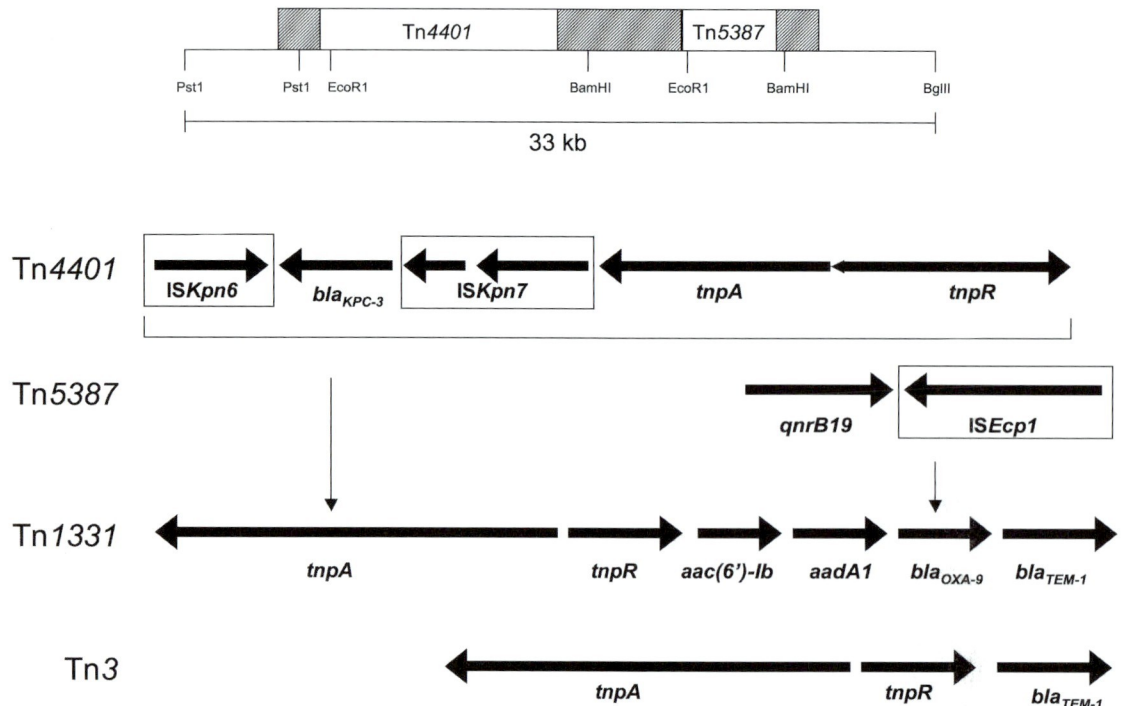

Fig. 4. The KQ element of *Klebsiella pneumoniae*.

enterococcal VanB operon is only activated by vancomycin, so strains expressing this operon appear susceptible to teicoplanin *in vitro*. Unfortunately, escape mutants that express resistance to teicoplanin as well are readily isolated *in vitro* and during therapy for infections. These resistant strains generally have mutations in the $vanS_B$ gene that either result in constitutive expression of the VanB operon, or that allow activation of $vanS_B$ by teicoplanin as well as vancomycin.

Another clinically important example of resistance regulation is the regulation of expression of the *erm* (A, B, and C) macrolide resistance determinants. Erm-expression confers resistance to macrolides, lincosamides (clindamycin) and streptogramins B. Expression of the *ermB* determinant in Tn917 and similar transposons is inducible by macrolides by a post translational attenuation mechanism. Clindamycin does not induce expression of this determinant, and so strains will appear susceptible to clindamycin on MIC testing. However, point mutations can occur that will result in constitutive expression of the *ermB* determinant, resulting in clindamycin resistance. In order to detect this type of resistance phenotypically, microbiologists have developed the "D" test, in which erythromycin and clindamycin disks are approximated on a plate. Erythromycin induces expression of the *ermB* determinant, blunting the normally circular zone surrounding the clindamycin disk (changing the shape of the zone from an "O" to a "D"). One recent study suggested a 14-fold increased rate of resistance emerging in *S. aureus* when inducible erythromycin resistance was caused by *ermC* in comparison to *ermA*. However, since information on the genetic basis for inducible resistance is not generally available at the time therapeutic decisions are made, clindamycin should be used with caution in D-test (+) strains of *S. aureus*.

Resistance augmenters

The above description of composite transposons indicates how bacteria can use combinations of genetic determinants to express resistance to multiple classes of antibiotics, and also how this multi-resistance can be transferred between strains. Perhaps not surprisingly, bacteria can use similar strategies to evolve resistance in settings where point mutations by themselves do not confer levels of resistance sufficient to result in selection in the clinical setting. The use of auxiliary mechanisms to amplify fluoroquinolone resistance associated with point mutations in the cellular topoisomerase genes is a case in point. Most clinically available fluoroquinolones target both the DNA gyrase and topoisomerase IV of Gram-negative bacteria. One of these enzymes will be the primary target, and mutations within the quinolone resistance determining regions of the primary target will have a greater impact on the MIC than will those in the secondary target. Still, single point mutations are often insufficient to confer levels of quinolone resistance in Gram-negative bacteria sufficient to prompt selection in the clinical setting. To augment the levels of resistance associated with these point mutations bacterial strains will often develop auxiliary mechanisms that, when combined with point mutations, result in selectable levels of resistance.

Perhaps the most common auxiliary mechanism used to augment fluoroquinolone resistance is the activation and increased expression of multidrug efflux pumps. Virtually all Gram-negative bacteria have one or more of these pumps, with the more resistance species having more than the susceptible strains. Scanning the *P. aeruginosa* genome suggests that there may be as many as twelve of the three-component Resistance-Nodulation-Cell Division pumps, several of which have already been shown to pump fluoroquinolones. Among the more interesting recent research findings is that these RND pumps have the capacity to vacuum substances from the peri-plasmic space as well as the cytoplasm, explaining the observed impact of their activation on β-lactam MICs. Expression of these pumps does not under normal circumstances confer selectable levels of resistance to fluoroquinolones, but their expression can augment the levels of resistance associated with single point mutations, potentially facilitating selection of single point mutants in the clinical setting.

Fluoroquinolone resistance can also be facilitated by a number of acquired genes. Most prominent among these are the *qnr* genes, which encode proteins that "protect" DNA from the action of the quinolones. Several *qnr* gene classes have now been described (*qnrA*, *B*, *C*, and *qnrS*) with variants within these classes. Fluoroquinolone resistance can also be augmented by acquisition of a modifying enzyme, aac(6')-Ib-cr, which is a point mutant of an aminoglycoside modifying enzyme gene. Resistance mediated by this enzyme is specific for ciprofloxacin and norfloxacin. Finally, an acquired efflux pump (QepA) can augment levels of quinolone resistance. Recent surveys looking for these resistance augmenters indicate the appearance of *qnrB* as early as 1991 and an increasing penetration of the *qnr* genes into important Gram-negative bacteria.

CONCLUSIONS

Bacteria access a variety of genetic tools to develop resistance to virtually any antibiotic with which they are confronted. If resistance cannot be acquired through mutation in intrinsic genes, the extensive social network that most bacteria operate within provides ample opportunity to acquire resistance from other species. The frequent use of antibiotics inside the hospital and in the community provides a virtually constant selective pressure for the evolution of resistance, with the emergence of clinically resistant strains frequently representing the final iteration of a continuous resistance acquisition process. Improving our ability to detect lower levels of resistance before they become clinically significant could help us in preventing clinical resistance, but no amount of information is likely to have an impact if we cannot develop more rational and parsimonious strategies for administering antimicrobial agents.

REFERENCES

(1) **Arthur, M., F. Depardieu, G. Gerbaud, M. Galimand, R. Leclercq, and P. Courvalin.** 1997. The VanS sensor negatively controls VanR-mediated transcriptional activation of glycopeptide resistance genes of Tn*1546* and related elements in the absence of induction. J. Bacteriol. **179:**97-106.

(2) **Arthur, M., C. Molinas, F. Depardieu, and P. Courvalin.** 1993. Characterization of Tn*1546*, a Tn*3*-related transposon conferring glycopeptide resistance by synthesis of depsipeptide peptidoglycan precursors in *Enterococcus faecium* BM4147. J. Bacteriol. **175:**117-27.

(3) **Arthur, M., and R. Quintiliani, Jr.** 2001. Regulation of VanA- and VanB-type glycopeptide resistance in enterococci. Antimicrob. Agents Chemother. **45:**375-81.

(4) **Beaber, J. W., V. Burrus, B. Hochhut, and M. K. Waldor.** 2002. Comparison of SXT and R391, two conjugative integrating elements: definition of a genetic backbone for the mobilization of resistance determinants. Cell. Mol. Life Sci. **59:**2065-2070.

(5) **Bourgogne, A., D. A. Garsin, X. Qin, K. V. Singh, J. Sillanpaa, S. Yerrapragada, Y. Ding, S. Dugan-Rocha, C. Buhay, H. Shen, G. Chen, G. Williams, D. Muzny, A. Maadani, K. A. Fox, J. Gioia, L. Chen, Y. Shang, C. A. Arias, S. R. Nallapareddy, M. Zhao, V. P. Prakash, S. Chowdhury, H. Jiang, R. A. Gibbs, B. E. Murray, S. K. Highlander, and G. M. Weinstock.** 2008. Large scale variation in *Enterococcus faecalis* illustrated by the genome analysis of strain OG1RF. Genome Biol. **9:**R110.

(6) **Caparon, M. G., and J. R. Scott.** 1989. Excision and insertion of the conjugative transposon Tn*916* involves a novel recombination mechanism. Cell **59:**1027-1034.

(7) **Chen, Y., X. Zhang, D. Manias, H. J. Yeo, G. M. Dunny, and P. J. Christie.** 2008. *Enterococcus faecalis* PcfC, a spatially localized substrate receptor for type IV secretion of the pCF10 transfer intermediate. J. Bacteriol. **190:**3632-3645.

(8) **Chow, J. W., M. J. Fine, D. M. Shlaes, and J. P. Quinn.** 1991. *Enterobacter* bacteremia: Clinical features and emergence of antibiotic resistance during therapy. Annals Internal Medicine **115:**585-590.

(9) **Daurel, C., C. Huet, A. Dhalluin, M. Bes, J. Etienne, and R. Leclercq.** 2008. Differences in potential for selection of clindamycin-resistant mutants between inducible erm(A) and erm(C) *Staphylococcus aureus* genes. J. Clin. Microbiol. **46:**546-50.

(10) **Evers, S., and R. Courvalin.** 1996. Regulation of VanB-type vancomycin resistance gene expression by the vanSB-VanRB two component regulatory system in *Enterococcus faecalis* V583. J. Bacteriol. **178:**1302-1309.

(11) **Falagas, M. E., I. A. Bliziotis, and K. N. Fragoulis.** 2007. Oral rifampin for eradication of *Staphylococcus aureus* carriage from healthy and sick populations: a systematic review of the evidence from comparative trials. Am. J. Infect. Control. **35:**106-114.

(12) **Fink, M. P., D. R. Snydman, M. S. Niederman, K. V. Leeper, Jr., R. H. Johnson, S. O. Heard, R. G. Wunderink, J. W. Caldwell, J. J. Schentag, G. A. Siami, et al.** 1994. Treatment of severe pneumonia in hospitalized patients: results of a multicenter, randomized, double-blind trial comparing intravenous ciprofloxacin with imipenem-cilastatin. The Severe Pneumonia Study Group. Antimicrob. Agents Chemother. **38:**547-557.

(13) **Fournier, P. E., D. Vallenet, V. Barbe, S. Audic, H. Ogata, L. Poirel, H. Richet, C. Robert, S. Mangenot, C. Abergel, P. Nordmann, J. Weissenbach, D. Raoult, and J. M. Claverie.** 2006. Comparative genomics of multidrug resistance in *Acinetobacter baumannii*. PLoS Genet. **2:**e7.

(14) **Gryczan, T. J., G. Grandi, J. Hahn, R. Grandi, and D. Dubnau.** 1980. Conformational alteration of mRNA structure and the posttranscriptional regulation of erythromycin-induced drug resistance. Nucleic Acids Res. **8:**6081-6097.

(15) **Hochhut, B., Y. Lotfi, D. Mazel, S. M. Faruque, R. Woodgate, and M. K. Waldor.** 2001. Molecular analysis of antibiotic resistance gene clusters in *Vibrio cholerae* O139 and O1 SXT constins. Antimicrob. Agents Chemother. **45:**2991-3000.

(16) **Hodel-Christian, S. L., and B. E. Murray.** 1991. Characterization of the gentamicin resistance transposon Tn*5281* from *Enterococcus faecalis* and comparison to staphylococcal transposons Tn*4001* and Tn*4031*. Antimicrobial. Agents Chemother. **35:**1147-1152.

(17) **Honore, N., M. H. Nicolas, and S. T. Cole.** 1986. Inducible cephalosporinase production in clinical isolates of *Enterobacter cloacae* is controlled by a regulatory gene that has been deleted from *Escherichia coli*. EMBO J. **5:**3709-3714.

(18) Hooper, D. C. 2001. Emerging mechanisms of fluoroquinolone resistance. Emerg. Infect. Dis. **7**:337-341.

(19) Jacobs, C., J.-M. Frere, and S. Normark. 1997. Cytosolic intermediates for cell wall biosynthesis and degradation control inducible β-lactam resistance in gram-negative bacteria. Cell **88**:823-832.

(20) Jacobs, C., B. Joris, M. Jamin, K. Klarsov, J. Van Beeumen, D. Mengin-Lecreux, J. van Heijenoort, J. T. Park, S. Normark, and J.-M. Frère. 1995. AmpD, essential for both β-lactamase regulation and cell wall recycling, is a novel cytosolic N-acetylmuramyl-L-alanine amidase. Mol. Microbiol. **15**:553-559.

(21) Jacoby, G. A. 2009. AmpC beta-lactamases. Clin. Microbiol. Rev. **22**:161-182.

(22) Jin, D. J., and C. A. Gross. 1988. Mapping and sequencing of mutations in the *Escherichia coli rpoB* gene that leads to rifampicin resistance. J. Mol. Biol. **202**:45-58.

(23) Leavis, H. L., R. J. Willems, W. J. van Wamel, F. H. Schuren, M. P. Caspers, and M. J. Bonten. 2007. Insertion sequence-driven diversification creates a globally dispersed emerging multiresistant subspecies of *E. faecium*. PLoS Pathog. **3**:e7.

(24) Lett, M. C. 1988. Tn3-like elements: molecular structure, evolution. Biochimie **70**:167-176.

(25) Livermore, D. M. 1992. Interplay of impermeability and chromosomal β-lactamase activity in imipenem-resistant *Pseudomonas aeruginosa*. Antimicrob. Agents Chemother. **36**:2046-2048.

(26) Lobritz, M., R. Hutton-Thomas, S. Marshall, and L. B. Rice. 2003. Recombination proficiency influences frequency and locus of mutational resistance to linezolid in *Enterococcus faecalis*. Antimicrob. Agents Chemother. **47**:3318-3320.

(27) Lomovskaya, O., H. I. Zgurskaya, M. Totrov, and W. J. Watkins. 2007. Waltzing transporters and 'the dance macabre' between humans and bacteria. Nat. Rev. Drug Discov. **6**:56-65.

(28) Lyon, B. R., J. W. May, and R. A. Skurray. 1984. Tn4001: a gentamicin and kanamycin resistance transposon in *Staphylococcus aureus*. Mol. Gen. Genetics **193**:554-556.

(29) Manganelli, R., S. Ricci, and G. Pozzi. 1997. The joint of Tn916 circular intermediates is a homoduplex in *Enterococcus faecalis*. Plasmid **38**:71-78.

(30) Marshall, S. H., C. J. Donskey, R. Hutton-Thomas, R. A. Salata, and L. B. Rice. 2002. Gene dosage and linezolid resistance in *Enterococcus faecium* and *Enterococcus faecalis*. Antimicrob. Agents Chemother. **46**:3334-3336.

(31) Mazel, D. 2006. Integrons: agents of bacterial evolution. Nat. Rev. Microbiol. **4**:608-620.

(32) Nikaido, H. 2003. Molecular basis of bacterial outer membrane permeability revisited. Microbiol. Mol. Biol. Rev. **67**:593-656.

(33) Paulsen, I. T., L. Banerjei, G. S. Myers, K. E. Nelson, R. Seshadri, T. D. Read, D. E. Fouts, J. A. Eisen, S. R. Gill, J. F. Heidelberg, H. Tettelin, R. J. Dodson, L. Umayam, L. Brinkac, M. Beanan, S. Daugherty, R. T. DeBoy, S. Durkin, J. Kolonay, R. Madupu, W. Nelson, J. Vamathevan, B. Tran, J. Upton, T. Hansen, J. Shetty, H. Khouri, T. Utterback, D. Radune, K. A. Ketchum, B. A. Dougherty, and C. M. Fraser. 2003. Role of mobile DNA in the evolution of vancomycin-resistant *Enterococcus faecalis*. Science **299**:2071-2074.

(34) Podglajen, I., J. Breuil, F. Bordon, L. Gutmann, and E. Collatz. 1992. A silent carbapenemase gene in strains of *Bacteroides fragilis* can be expressed after a one step mutation. FEMS Microbiol. Lett. **70**:21-29.

(35) Projan, S. J., and G. L. Archer. 1989. Mobilization of the relaxable *Staphylococcus aureus* plasmid pC221 by the conjugative plasmid pGO1 involves three pC221 loci. J. Bacteriol. **171**:1841-1845.

(36) Rice, L. B. 1998. Tn916-family conjugative transposons and dissemination of antimicrobial resistance determinants. Antimicrob. Agents Chemother. **42**:1871-1877.

(37) Rice, L. B., S. Bellais, L. L. Carias, R. Hutton-Thomas, R. A. Bonomo, P. Caspers, M. G. Page, and L. Gutmann. 2004. Impact of specific pbp5 mutations on expression of beta-lactam resistance in *Enterococcus faecium*. Antimicrob. Agents Chemother. **48**:3028-3032.

(38) Rice, L. B., and L. L. Carias. 1998. Transfer of Tn5385, a composite, multiresistance element from *Enterococcus faecalis*. J. Bacteriol. **180**:714-721.

(39) Rice, L. B., L. L. Carias, R. A. Hutton, S. D. Rudin, A. Endimiani, and R. A. Bonomo. 2008. The KQ element, a complex genetic region conferring transferable resistance to carbapenems, aminoglycosides, and fluoroquinolones in *Klebsiella pneumoniae*. Antimicrob. Agents Chemother. **52**:3427-3429.

(40) Rice, L. B., L. L. Carias, S. Marshall, S. D. Rudin, and R. Hutton-Thomas. 2005. Tn5386, a novel Tn916-like mobile element in *Enterococcus faecium* D344R that interacts with Tn916 to yield a large genomic deletion. J. Bacteriol. **187**:6668-77.

(41) Rowe-Magnus, D. A., A. M. Guerout, P. Ploncard, B. Dychinco, J. Davies, and D. Mazel. 2001. The evolutionary history of chromosomal super-integrons provides an ancestry for multiresistant integrons. Proc. Natl. Acad. Sci. USA **98**:652-657.

(42) Ruiz, M., S. Marti, F. Fernandez-Cuenca, A. Pascual, and J. Vila. 2007. Prevalence of IS(Aba1) in epidemiologically unrelated *Acinetobacter baumannii* clinical isolates. FEMS Microbiol. Lett. **274**:63-66.

(43) Schaefler, S. 1982. Bacteriophage-mediated acquisition of antibiotic resistance by *Staphylococcus aureus* type 88. Antimicrob Agents Chemother **21**:460-7.

(44) Schmidtke, A. J., and N. D. Hanson. 2006. Model system to evaluate the effect of ampD mutations on AmpC-mediated beta-lactam resistance. Antimicrob. Agents Chemother. **50**:2030-2037.

(45) Schmidtke, A. J., and N. D. Hanson. 2008. Role of ampD homologs in overproduction of AmpC in clinical isolates of *Pseudomonas aeruginosa*. Antimicrob. Agents Chemother. **52**:3922-3927.

(46) Shaw, J. H., and D. B. Clewell. 1985. Complete nucleotide sequence of macrolide-lincosamide-streptogramin B resistance transposon Tn917 in *Streptococcus faecalis*. J. Bacteriol. **164**:782-796.

(47) Shinabarger, D. L., K. R. Marotti, R. W. Murray, A. H. Lin, E. P. Melchior, S. M. Swaney, D. S. Dunyak, W. F. Demyan, and J. M. Buysse. 1997. Mechanism of action of oxazolidinones: effects of linezolid and eperezolid on translation reactions. Antimicrob. Agents Chemother. **41**:2132-2136.

(48) **Siguier, P., J. Filee, and M. Chandler.** 2006. Insertion sequences in prokaryotic genomes. Curr. Opin. Microbiol. **9:**526-531.

(49) **Spratt, B. G.** 1994. Resistance to antibiotics mediated by target alterations. Science **264:**388-393.

(50) **Stover, C. K., X. Q. Pham, A. L. Erwin, S. D. Mizoguchi, P. Warrener, M. J. Hickey, F. S. Brinkman, W. O. Hufnagle, D. J. Kowalik, M. Lagrou, R. L. Garber, L. Goltry, E. Tolentino, S. Westbrook-Wadman, Y. Yuan, L. L. Brody, S. N. Coulter, K. R. Folger, A. Kas, K. Larbig, R. Lim, K. Smith, D. Spencer, G. K. Wong, Z. Wu, I. T. Paulsen, J. Reizer, M. H. Saier, R. E. Hancock, S. Lory, and M. V. Olson.** 2000. Complete genome sequence of *Pseudomonas aeruginosa* PA01, an opportunistic pathogen. Nature **406:**959-964.

(51) **Swinfield, T.-J., L. Janniere, S. D. Ehrlich, and N. P. Minton.** 1991. Characterization of a region of *Enterococcus faecalis* plasmid pAMß1 which enhances the segregational stability of pAMß1-derived cloning vectors in *Bacillus subtilis*. Plasmid **26:**209-221.

(52) **Van Bambeke, F., M. Chauvel, P. E. Reynolds, H. S. Fraimow, and P. Courvalin.** 1999. Vancomycin-dependent *Enterococcus faecalis* clinical isolates and revertant mutants. Antimicrob. Agents Chemother. **43:**41-47.

(53) **Varon, E., and L. Gutmann.** 2000. Mechanisms and spread of fluoroquinolone resistance in *Streptococcus pneumoniae*. Res. Microbiol. **151:**471-473.

(54) **Weigel, L. M., D. B. Clewell, S. R. Gill, N. C. Clark, L. K. McDougal, S. E. Flannagan, J. F. Kolonay, J. Shetty, G. E. Killgore, and F. C. Tenover.** 2003. Genetic analysis of a high-level vancomycin-resistant isolate of *Staphylococcus aureus*. Science **302:**1569-1571.

(55) **Welch, R. A., V. Burland, G. Plunkett, 3rd, P. Redford, P. Roesch, D. Rasko, E. L. Buckles, S. R. Liou, A. Boutin, J. Hackett, D. Stroud, G. F. Mayhew, D. J. Rose, S. Zhou, D. C. Schwartz, N. T. Perna, H. L. Mobley, M. S. Donnenberg, and F. R. Blattner.** 2002. Extensive mosaic structure revealed by the complete genome sequence of uropathogenic *Escherichia coli*. Proc. Natl. Acad. Sci. USA **99:**17020-17024.

Chapter 4. BASES FOR CLINICAL CATEGORIZATION

Derek BROWN and Rafael CANTON

INTRODUCTION

Clinical categorization of antimicrobial susceptibility is normally required to guide clinical use of antimicrobial agents. This guidance is principally to predict the outcome of antimicrobial treatment of individual patients, but most antimicrobials are given empirically and accumulated susceptibility data are required to guide the selection of agents for empirical treatment (7, 26, 29). Although it is not the best way to perform resistance surveillance, clinical categorization is also used to monitor changes in antimicrobial susceptibility over time (12). Clinical categorization is not highly precise as there is variation in the *in vitro* tests used to determine susceptibility and the *in vitro* tests do not encompass the differences among micro-organisms, patients, and clinical conditions (19, 39, 42). Hence the clinical categorization of susceptibility provides guidance on likely outcome of therapy but should be used with information on the clinical condition of the patient.

DEFINITION OF CATEGORIES OF SUSCEPTIBILITY

The antimicrobial susceptibility of micro-organisms is traditionally categorized as susceptible (S), intermediate (I) or resistant (R). Various groups have used different definitions of the categories of susceptibility, which can lead to confusion, particularly with the intermediate category, and the International Organization for Standardization (ISO) (27) has defined susceptibility categories as follows:

Susceptible: A bacterial strain inhibited *in vitro* by a concentration of an antimicrobial agent that is associated with a high likelihood of therapeutic success

Intermediate: A bacterial strain inhibited *in vitro* by a concentration of an antimicrobial agent that is associated with uncertain therapeutic effect

Resistant: A bacterial strain inhibited *in vitro* by a concentration of an antimicrobial agent that is associated with a high likelihood of therapeutic failure

The definition of susceptible is based on use of the standard recommended dosage of the agent. The "uncertain therapeutic effect" in the intermediate category may be taken as a buffer zone where response is likely to be variable depending on the specific patient and micro-organism. The uncertainty has led some to describe the category as "indeterminate" rather than intermediate (24). The intermediate category is often taken to imply that an infection can be treated in body sites where the agent is physiologically concentrated, principally the lower urinary tract, or when a high dosage of drug can be used. In recognition of this, the category has sometimes been termed "moderately susceptible" or, particularly in antifungal susceptibility testing, "susceptible-dose dependent", but neither of these terms are widely accepted. An intermediate designation may also be taken as an indication that the micro-organism has acquired some degree of resistance (normally a low-level resistance mechanism) and that prediction of outcome is therefore difficult. In addition, the intermediate category has been used in calibration of antimicrobial susceptibility testing methods as a "buffer zone" to reduce the likelihood of technical variation causing major discrepancies in interpretation (4, 25, 34, 37, 38).

An additional categorization which can cause confusion is "non-susceptible". This term is used in some publications, particularly resistance surveillance studies, to indicate any organism that does not fall into the fully susceptible category, thereby combining the intermediate and resistant categories. It is also used by some antimicrobial susceptibility guidelines for new agents where no resistant micro-organisms have yet been described or when clinical correlation is still lacking for organisms displaying higher MICs than those obtained with susceptible ones. Any micro-organism with an MIC above the susceptible breakpoint is designated as "non-susceptible", which does not necessarily mean that there is a genotypic resistance mechanism in the micro-organism, but there is no clinical experience with such isolates in clinical trials. Other groups, *e.g.* EUCAST (22) do not accept the "non-susceptible" category because for practical purposes an organism that is not susceptible is effectively resistant until proven otherwise. EUCAST notes such situations with the comment that strains with MIC above the susceptible breakpoint are very rare or not yet reported and advises that the identification and susceptibility tests on any such isolate must be repeated. If the result is confirmed the isolate should be sent to a reference laboratory and, until there is evidence regarding clinical response, the prudent approach should be taken and the isolate reported resistant.

MIC BREAKPOINTS

The definitions of categories of susceptibility refer to concentrations of antimicrobial agents associated with therapeutic success or failure. The concentrations defining the borders of different categories are termed the breakpoint concentrations, presented by convention as MIC values based on a two-fold dilution series. The MIC breakpoints are the reference against which breakpoints in other clinical susceptibility testing methods, such as disk diffusion, are calibrated.

While conventional MICs may be limited by the fact that they use a two-fold dilution series, that the reproducibility is around ± one two-fold dilution for most micro-organism-antimicrobial agent combinations and that MICs are affected by the particular technique used, there is currently no better practical method of measuring antibacterial potency (42). The variation in MIC with test conditions has resulted in publication of several standard methods but it is only recently that an international standard was approved (27).

Several national and international groups currently publish MIC breakpoints for antimicrobial susceptibility testing. These include, among others, the British Society for Antimicrobial Chemotherapy (BSAC) (5), Comité de l'Antibiogramme de la Société Française de Microbiologie (CA-SFM) (10), Clinical and Laboratory Standards Institute (CLSI) (8), Commissie Richtlijnen Gevoeligheidsbepalingen) (CRG) (11), Deutsches Institut für Normung (DIN) (16), the European Committee on Antimicrobial Susceptibility Testing (EUCAST) (22), Norwegian Working Group on Antibiotics (NWGA) (6), and the Swedish Reference Group of Antibiotics (SRGA) (40). There may be considerable differences in breakpoints set by the different groups, even when dosing schedules are similar. These differences are largely related to different approaches to breakpoint setting and different weighting applied to the parameters used in setting breakpoints. Harmonization of breakpoints is clearly desirable and breakpoints will undoubtedly converge as modern approaches to setting breakpoints are applied by different groups. All the European groups mentioned above are now part of EUCAST and, through EUCAST, breakpoints for commonly used existing agents have been harmonized. Harmonized European breakpoints for new agents are set as part of the licensing process via the European Medicines Agency (EMEA) (22).

The format for presentation of the susceptible breakpoint by different groups is universally S ≤ x μg/ml. There is, however, variation in presentation of the resistant breakpoint, the European format being R > y μg/ml (22) and the CLSI format being R ≥ y μg/ml (8). Care must be taken when comparing resistance breakpoints as CLSI breakpoints may be mistakenly interpreted as one dilution higher than others.

Factors in breakpoint setting

Microbiological, pharmacological (pharmacokinetics/pharmacodynamics), and clinical data are important in setting breakpoints. The way the data are examined and the weighting applied to different factors is not an exact science (9, 22, 42), but more recently a better understanding of pharmacodynamic principles in particular has led to a more uniform approach to setting of breakpoints (1, 18).

Microbiological data

Microbiological data include data demonstrating the *in vitro* activity of the agent and information on resistance mechanisms. The *in vitro* activity of an agent is best represented by MIC distributions. The MICs should be determined by reference broth or agar dilution methods, or methods calibrated to reference methods. The test methods must be stated and data from different studies should not be combined unless quality control data are within range (if quality control limits have been established for a method) and wild type distributions are consistent. MIC distributions for individual species are desirable as species may differ in susceptibility and combining species may be misleading. Full MIC distributions are required, where possible with minimal truncation of ranges. This is particularly important at the lower end of the distribution so that the wild type population can be defined. At the upper end of the distribution the MIC range should at least extend above attainable concentrations at infection sites. Ideally, MIC ranges should be such that all tested micro-organisms are in range, but some truncation at the upper end of the range may be unavoidable and of little consequence as MICs for some species may be very high. MIC_{50} and MIC_{90} values are of no value in setting breakpoints as they hide important detail.

The characteristics of the source of organism populations should be defined, particularly for surveillance studies. If they are routine clinical isolates it should be stated whether they were consecutive isolates or selected in any way, which patient groups were sampled and from which geographical locations (12). If they are from culture collections the derivation of the collection should be given. When a new agent is a member of a group of related agents where resistance is established, the MICs of the new agent for organisms with known resistance mechanisms affecting the group should be investigated.

Examination of MIC distributions permits identification of the wild type population (organisms without acquired or mutational resistance). The wild type distribution is constant whatever the source of the organisms (different patient groups, different geographical locations, human or veterinary isolates) and does not change over time (31). The upper end of the wild type MIC distribution has been described as the "microbiological breakpoint", but this term is best avoided as it causes confusion with clinical breakpoints. EUCAST has defined this value as the "epidemiological cut-off" (ECOFF) (22) and it is also referred to as the wild type cut-off (42, 43). While the ECOFF can usually be defined simply by visual inspection of the MIC distribution, statistical analysis can also be applied, and may be particularly useful when low-level resistant strains overlap the wild type population (43). Clinical breakpoints should relate to clinical outcome whereas ECOFFs can be used for epidemiological surveillance and to provide a means of early detection and quantitative description of the emergence of resistance.

For some species and antimicrobial agents, e.g. Group A streptococci with penicillin G, MICs above the ECOFF are rare or not reported and the MIC distribution consists of only the wild type. This is also the current situation with daptomycin and Staphylococcus aureus (Fig. 1). With organism-antimicrobial agent combinations where MICs above the wild type distribution are seen the distribution may be essentially bimodal, e.g. Escherichia coli with tetracycline or ampicillin (Fig. 2), whereas with others the non-wild type isolates may merge into the wild type, e.g. E. coli with ciprofloxacin (Fig. 3), or be widely distributed, e.g. E. coli with piperacillin (Fig. 4).

When possible, clinical breakpoints should not split wild type populations as it is inappropriate to split a population that is essentially homogeneous in susceptibility. Also, from a practical point of view, it leads to irreproducible *in vitro* testing as replicate results will fall on either side of the breakpoint. Breakpoints that fall in the troughs of bimodal MIC distributions are likely to result in reproducible categorization of susceptibility (*e.g.* E. coli and ampicillin). Breakpoints in the middle of a distribution will result in poor reproducibility

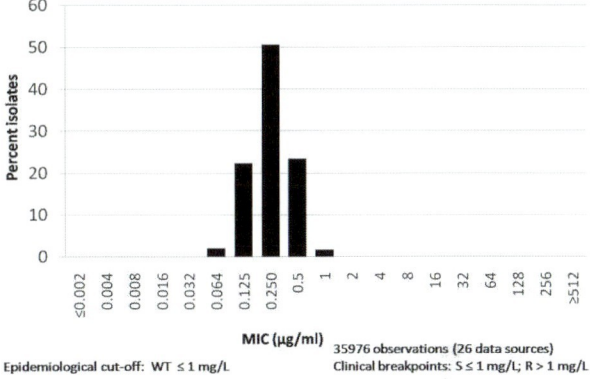

Fig.1. MIC distribution of daptomycin for *Staphylococcus aureus*, clinical breakpoints and epidemiological cut-off value (ECOFF). This is a unimodal distribution with the majority of MICs distributed ± 2 twofold dilutions around a mode MIC value of 0.25 μg/ml. Isolates with MICs above the ECOFF and the resistance breakpoint are rare (data from EUCAST website: http://www.eucast.org/mic_distributions_of_wild_type_microorganisms/). WT = wild type.

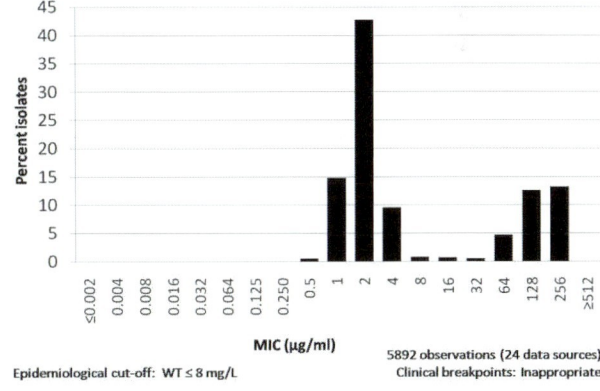

Fig. 2. MIC distribution of tetracycline for *Escherichia coli* and epidemiological cut-off value (ECOFF). This is a bimodal distribution with two different populations. The first belongs to the wild type whereas the second one has one or more resistance mechanisms (data from EUCAST website http://www.eucast.org/mic_distributions_of_wild_type_microorganisms/). No clinical breakpoints were defined by EUCAST as this species is a poor target for therapy with tetracycline. WT = wild type.

and it may be necessary to shift breakpoints slightly to reduce the impact of this problem (*e.g.* erythromycin and *Haemophillus influenzae*) (Fig. 5). Moreover, different species differ in their MIC distributions, and therefore it may be necessary to choose different breakpoints for different species (*e.g.* imipenem and *Enterobacteriaceae*) (Fig. 6).

Resistance mechanisms that are known to adversely affect clinical outcome most commonly result in MICs well above chosen breakpoints, but in some instances MICs may be low and it may be necessary to adjust breakpoints so that the organisms are reported intermediate or resistant, *e.g.* penicillin G breakpoints and penicillinase production in *Staphylococcus aureus*. Notably, and sometimes controversially, not all resistance mechanisms confer clinical resistance and there may be organisms with MICs above the ECOFF but which are still clinically susceptible with common dosage regimens, *e.g.* penicillin G and *Streptococcus pneumoniae* in treatment of pneumonia, where high doses are commonly used (28).

Pharmacokinetic/pharmacodynamic (PK/PD) data

Pharmacokinetics describes the concentration of an antimicrobial agent in the patient over time, whereas pharmacodynamics is the study of antimicrobial effects in terms of bacterial inhibition or killing over time (17). In the time-course of treatment of an infection, PK and PD are combined. PK/PD studies are a relatively recent development which is recognised as a major advance in the setting of clinical antimicrobial breakpoints, and values of PK/PD indices are used for the prediction of clinical outcome (9, 21, 34, 35, 42). The terminology used for PK/PD data can be confusing and inconsistent, and a standardized terminology has been proposed (36).

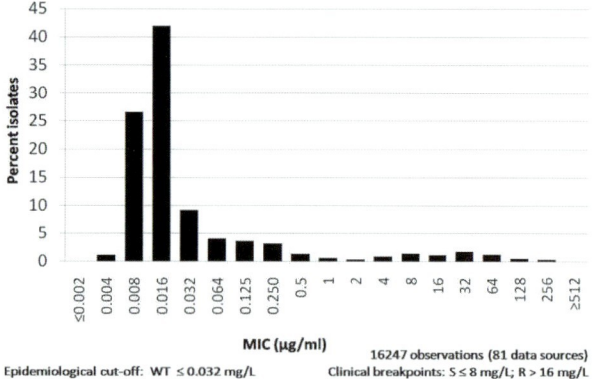

Fig. 3. MIC distribution of ciprofloxacin for *Escherichia coli*, clinical breakpoints and epidemiological cut-off value (ECOFF). This is a multimodal distribution with different populations. The first belongs to the wild type whereas the others have different resistance mechanisms variably expressed with isolates merged into the wild type population (from EUCAST website http://www.eucast.org/mic_distributions_of_wild_type _microorganisms/). WT = wild type.

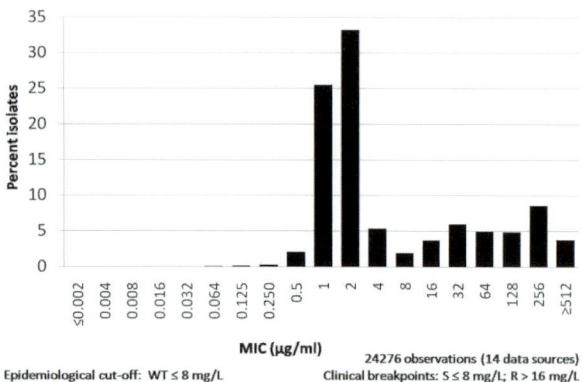

Fig. 4. MIC distribution of piperacillin for *Escherichia coli*, clinical breakpoints and epidemiological cut-off value (ECOFF). This is a multimodal distribution with different populations. The first belongs to the wild type whereas the others have different resistance mechanisms variably expressed and widely distributed beyond the ECOFF (data from EUCAST website http://www.eucast.org/mic_distributions_of_wild_type _microorganisms/). WT = wild type.

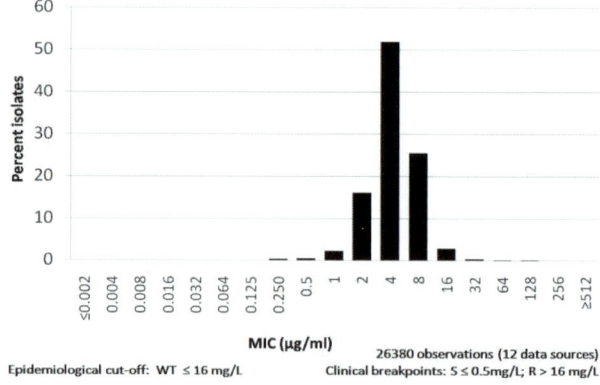

Fig. 5. MIC distribution of erythromycin for *Haemophilus influenzae*, clinical breakpoints and epidemiological cut-off value (ECOFF). This is a unimodal distribution. Isolates with MICs above the ECOFF are rare (data from EUCAST website http://www.eucast.org/mic_distributions_of_wild_type_microorganisms/). EUCAST susceptible and resistant breakpoints are below the ECOFF in order to categorise wild type *H. influenzae* isolates as intermediate due to the fact that the correlation between macrolide MICs and clinical outcome is weak for *H. influenzae*. WT = wild type.

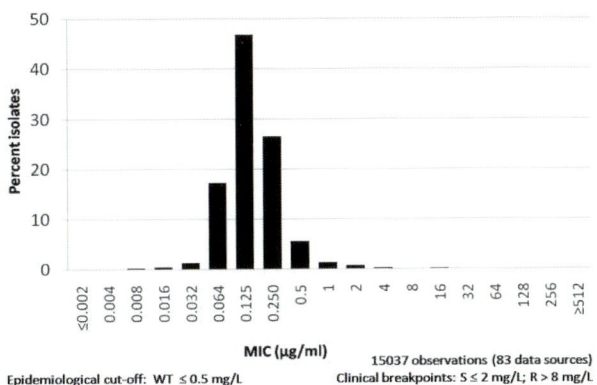

Fig. 6.a)

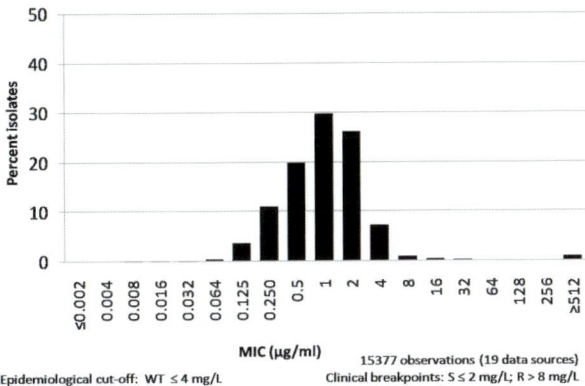

Fig. 6.b)

Fig. 6. MIC distributions of imipenem for *Escherichia coli* (6a) and *Proteus mirabilis* (6b), clinical breakpoints and epidemiological cut-off values (ECOFF). *P. mirabilis* shows a shift to higher MIC values and the corresponding ECOFF is higher than that for *E. coli* (data from EUCAST website : http://www.eucast.org/mic_distributions_of_wild_type_microorganisms/). Proteus species are considered poor targets for imipenem. WT = wild type.

Pharmacokinetic studies commonly examine the serum concentration as data for other sites, such as tissue concentrations and intracellular concentrations, are more difficult to collect. However, it is appropriate for data to be provided for particular sites if agents are targeted at infections in those sites, *e.g.* urinary tract, respiratory infection, cerebrospinal fluid. For a given dosage and route of administration the parameters usually specified include the maximum concentration (C_{max}, μg/ml), minimum concentration (C_{min}, μg/ml), total body clearance (L/h), the half life ($T_{1/2}$, h), the area under the time versus concentration curve over a 24 h period (AUC_{24}, mg.h/L), the degree of protein binding (%) and the volume of distribution (L).

Pharmacokinetics should, when possible, be based on data from relevant patient groups as, although it is not always the case, pharmacokinetics may be different in healthy volunteers. Numbers of individuals studied should be sufficient to provide reliable data as there may be considerable variation in pharmacokinetics between different individuals or with different underlying diseases (44). The characteristics of the groups used to study PK should be fully defined.

The PK/PD indices which have been shown to be predictive of clinical efficacy are (1, 13, 34):

- Time above MIC (T>MIC), expressed as the percentage of time during the dosing interval that the concentration of the agent is above the MIC of the micro-organism.
- The ratio of the area under the antimicrobial concentration-time curve over 24 h to the MIC (AUC_{24}/MIC).
- The ratio of the peak concentration to the MIC (C_{max}/MIC)

Relevant PK/PD indices for particular agents may be derived from *in vitro*, animal and clinical studies. *In vitro* "time-kill" and post-antibiotic effect (PAE) studies can be useful indicators of relevant PK/PD indices predicting *in vivo* efficacy (13, 15). Time-kill studies are used to examine the effects of fixed concentrations of agents on the inhibition and killing of clinically relevant micro-organisms over time (13). Agents tend to display either a concentration dependent effect, where the rate and degree of killing increases with the concentration of the agent above the MIC, or time dependent (sometimes referred to as concentration independent) effect, where the rate of kill increases little at concentrations above the MIC and the degree of killing depends on the time of exposure. Table 1 classifies current antimicrobial agents within these categories. The post-antibiotic effect (PAE) is the delay in re-growth following exposure to and then removal of the agent (15). The PAE may be very short or absent, or with some agents it is prolonged. Time-kill and PAE studies are affected by the test conditions, which should be clearly defined.

When *in vitro* studies show a time-dependent bactericidal activity with minimal PAE, T>MIC is usually the relevant PK/PD index. When *in vitro* studies show a time-dependent bactericidal or inhibitory activity with prolonged PAE, AUC/MIC is usually the relevant PK/PD index. When *in vitro* studies show a concentration-dependent bactericidal activity with prolonged PAE, AUC/MIC and/or C_{max}/MIC is usually the relevant PK/PD index. Examples are given in Table 1.

PK/PD studies in animal models are not only important in defining and/or confirming the PK/PD indices predictive of *in vivo* efficacy, but also give guidance on the magnitude of the index necessary for clinical effectiveness of the agent (3, 13, 45). The animal model should be relevant for the intended infection and target micro-organisms. The neutropenic mouse thigh and pneumonia models are widely used. Studies should be well controlled and include appropriate statistical analysis. As protein binding adversely affects the PK/PD index the free drug concentration should be used in analyses (14, 23).

Most clinical PK/PD studies are retrospective as it is difficult practically to include a sufficient range of dosages. Also it is unethical to plan clinical studies deliberately to include treatment failure, and failure as well as success is necessary for selection of the relevant PK/PD index. However, some clinical studies have examined PK/PD indices and these suggest similar indices to studies in animal models (42).

When the PK/PD index predictive of clinical outcome has been established it can be used to estimate a breakpoint by examining the probability of attaining the target value of the PK/PD index for relevant micro-organisms with different MICs. The probability of target attainment is commonly required to be above 90% so the PK/PD breakpoint (or cut-off) is the highest MIC for which the probability of target attainment is greater than 90%. A significant problem in making this estimate is the variability in PK values between different individuals, particularly populations of sick patients who may have underlying disease. Human PK studies are unlikely to include a sufficient range of patients to encompass the variation between individuals and this is overcome by application of Classification and Regression Tree Analysis (CART analysis) and Monte Carlo simulation (2, 32, 34). Both methods are statistical techniques which, based on PK data from a small number of patients, estimate the probability of achieving a specified PK/PD target for different MICs when a large population of patients is treated with a particular dosage regimen. CART analysis provides the value of the PK/PD index that distinguishes better from worse outcomes in a statistically significant fashion and the value can be selected based on what is regarded as an acceptable response rate. Fig. 7 illustrates CART analysis of tigecycline. The outcome of Monte Carlo simulation is dependent on the PK inputs and underlying assumptions, and these should be clearly stated. The simulation should also allow for variation in outcome between individuals, *e.g.* by including 95% confidence limits. Fig. 8 shows Monte Carlo simulation for ciprofloxacin treatment of infection due to *Enterobacteriaceae*.

Clinical data

The principal purpose of antimicrobial susceptibility testing is to predict outcome of treatment, yet data correlating outcome of treatment with MIC is often not available or is very limited. For new agents such data are required by regulatory authorities such as the EMEA and the United States Food and Drug Administration (FDA). Trials should be fully and clearly described prospective randomized studies with both clinical and bacteriological endpoints. It is, however, recognised that there are several constraints on the design of clinical outcome studies. Patients with resistant isolates are excluded from treatment or treatment is changed when resistance is recognised and therefore, as preliminary susceptibility breakpoints selected for use in trials tend to be conservative (*e.g* epidemiological cut-offs), data

Table 1. Pharmacokinetic/pharmacodynamic indices predicting clinical and microbiological efficacy of different antimicrobial agents

Antimicrobial agent	Bactericidal effect	Prolonged post-antibiotic effect	PK/PD Index
Aminogylycosides, fluoroquinolones	Concentration dependent	Yes	Cmax/MIC
β-Lactams, macrolides, clindamycin, linezolid	Time dependent	No	T/MIC
Tetracyclines, quinupristin/dalfopristin, glycopeptides, daptomycin, azithromycin, fluoroquinolones	Time dependent	Yes	AUC_{24}/MIC

Chapter 4. BASES FOR CLINICAL CATEGORIZATION

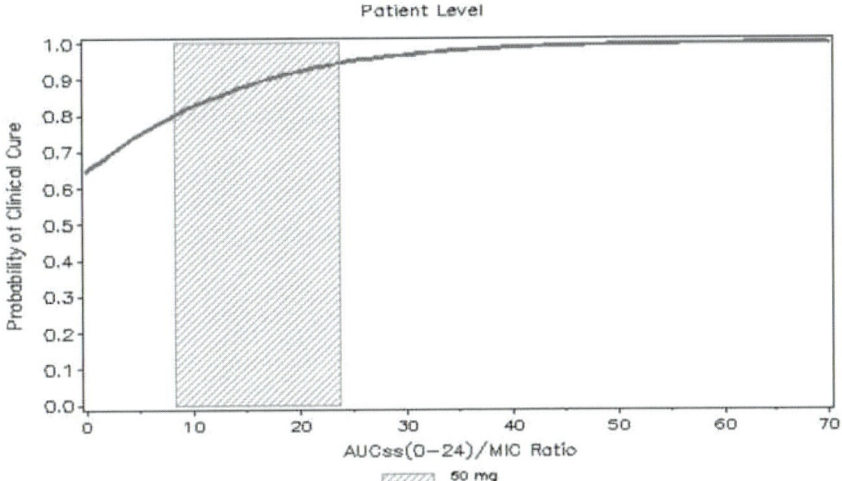

Fig. 7. Probability of response to tigecycline as a function of AUC/MIC ratio in patients with complicated intra-abdominal infection; Classification and Regression Tree (CART) analysis. The line represents the model-based predicted probability of clinical cure and the bar the 25th to 75th percentiles of the ratio distribution for the 50 mg dose group. This analysis shows that the AUC/MIC ratio that discriminates between populations with a good response from those with a poor response is 6.96 (data from the EUCAST Rationale Document for tigecycline, http://www.srga.org/eucastwt/MICTAB/RD/tigecyclinerationale1.0.pdf).

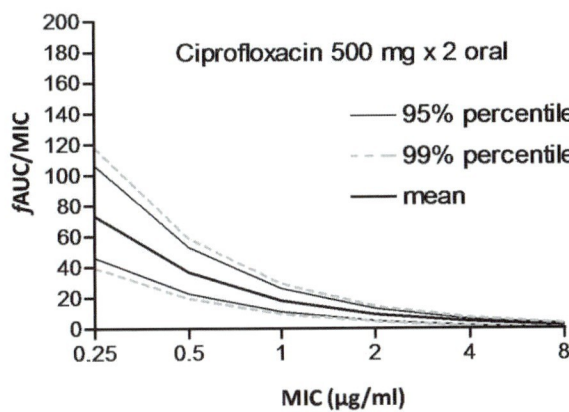

Fig. 8. Monte Carlo simulation of probabilities of target attainment (PTA) for ciprofloxacin with a 500 mg x 2 oral dose. A susceptibility breakpoint of 0.5µg/ml for Enterobacteriaceae gives close to 95% PTA for the AUC/MIC index of 30. This breakpoint allows low-level quinolone resistant Enterobacteriaceae to be categorized as susceptible to ciprofloxacin (see also Fig. 3). Data from EUCAST Rationale Document for ciprofloxacin.
(http://www.srga.org/eucastwt/MICTAB/RD/Ciprofloxacin%20rationale%201.9.pdf).

is scarce for response to treatment of infections caused by organisms with MICs in the critical range close to preliminary breakpoints. With a new agent the absence of resistant organisms may have the same effect. Also clinical studies do not usually take account of host defences (some patients with resistant organisms recover despite treatment) and not all relevant species may be well represented in clinical trials. Ideally, at least for a period after launch of an agent, data on clinical use, including failures and correlation with MICs, should be collected.

The process of 'setting' breakpoints for clinical categorization

Assessment and weighting of the microbiological, PK/PD, and clinical data that are the bases for clinical categorization is a subjective process which is dependent on the particular groups of individuals involved in setting the breakpoints. However, essentially the current approach involves examination of MIC distributions for relevant micro-organisms to establish ECOFFs and the MICs of organisms with resistance mechanisms; PK/PD studies *in vitro*, in animals, and in humans, with Monte Carlo simulation to estimate probability of target attainment in humans; checking PK/PD "breakpoints" against MIC distributions to ensure that wild type distributions are not split, and adjustment of breakpoints if necessary; and checking that clinical outcome studies are in line with PK/PD "breakpoints", and adjustment of breakpoints if necessary (9, 20, 21, 43). MIC breakpoints set by this process should be reviewed if there are new clinical (outcome studies) or microbiological (new resistance mechanisms) data indicat-

Table 2. Vancomycin breakpoints recommended over time by the Clinical and Laboratory Standards Institute (CLSI) and the European Committee for Antimicrobial Susceptibility Testing (EUCAST)

Year	CLSI		EUCAST	
	Susceptible (≤)	Resistant (≥)	Susceptible (≤)	Resistant (>)
Before 2006	≤ 4	≥ 32	-	-
2006	≤ 2	≥ 16	≤ 4	> 8
2009	≤ 2	≥ 16	≤ 2	> 2

ing that there may be a problem with existing breakpoints, if new dosage regimens are introduced, if clinical indications change, or if a new agent from an established group of agents is introduced. This has been the case with vancomycin and *S. aureus*, where breakpoints have been lowered (Table 2) due to the demonstration that patients with infections involving the so called VISA (Vancomycin Intermediate *S. aureus*) or GISA (Glycopeptide Intermediate *S. aureus*), or with higher MICs within the susceptible category, have a high probability of failure when treated with vancomycin (33, 41).

More recently, the process of clinical categorization has been more closely defined, particularly with the acceptance of the value of the PK/PD approach, and a consensus is developing (30, 42). Notably, the wide discrepancies seen in historical breakpoints are now not seen when breakpoints for new agents are set, and as the necessary process of revising breakpoints for older agents continues the desirable harmonization of breakpoints set by different groups will come closer to reality.

REFERENCES

(1) **Ambrose, P. G.** 2005. Antimicrobial susceptibility breakpoints: PK-PD and susceptibility breakpoints. Treat. Respir. Med. **4**(Suppl. 1):5–11.

(2) **Ambrose, P. G.** 2006. Monte Carlo simulation in the evaluation of susceptibility breakpoints: predicting the future: insights from the Society of Infectious Diseases Pharmacists. Pharmacotherapy **26**:129–134.

(3) **Ambrose, P. G., S. M. Bhavnani, C. M. Rubino, A. Louie, T. Gumbo, A. Forrest, and G. Drusano.** 2007. Pharmacokinetics-pharmacodynamics of antimicrobial therapy: it's not just for mice anymore. Clin. Infect. Dis. **44**:79–86.

(4) **Amsterdam, D.** 1991. Susceptibility testing of antimicrobial in liquid media, pp 53-105. *In* V. Lorian (ed.), Antibiotics in laboratory medicine. Third edition. Williams & Wilkins, Baltimore, MD.

(5) **Andrews, J.M. for the BSAC Working Party on Susceptibility Testing.** 2009. BSAC standardized disc susceptibility testing method (version 8). J. Antimicrob. Chemother. **64**: 454-489.

(6) **Arbeidsgruppen for Antibiotikaspørsmål.** 2006. AFAs brytningspunkter for bakteriers antibiotikafølsomhet, versjon 1.9. Arbeidsgruppen for Antibiotikaspørsmål, Tromso, Norway. .

(7) **Bergan, T., J.N. Bruun, A. Digranes, E. Lingaas, K.K. Melby, and J. Sander.** 1997. Susceptibility testing of bacteria and fungi. Report from "the Norwegian Working Group on Antibiotics". Scand. J. Infect. Dis. **103**(Suppl):1-36.

(8) **Clinical and Laboratory Standards Institute (CLSI).** 2009. Performance standards for antimicrobial susceptibility testing; 19th informational supplement. CLSI document M100-S19. CLSI, Wayne, PA.

(9) **Clinical Laboratory Standard Institute.** 2008. Development of in vitro susceptibility testing criteria and quality control parameters: approved guideline, 3rd edition, M23-A3. CLSI, Wayne, PA.

(10) **Comité de l'Antibiogramme de la Société Française de Microbiologie (CA-SFM).** 2009. Recommandations 2009. (edition de Janvier 2009) (Updates on http://. asso.fr)

(11) **Commissie Richtlijnen Gevoeligheidsbepalingen (CRG).** 2000. Interpretatie van gevoeligheidsonderzoek en gevoeligheidscriteria voor antibacteriële middelen in Nederland. Ned. Tijdschr. Med. Microbiol. **3**:79-81.

(12) **Cornaglia, G., W. Hryniewicz, V. Jarlier, G. Kahlmeter, H. Mittermayer, L. Stratchounski, F. Baquero and ESCMID Study Group for Antimicrobial Resistance Surveillance.** 2004. European recommendations for antimicrobial resistance surveillance. Clin. Microbiol. Infect. **10**:349-383.

(13) **Craig, W. A.** 1998. Pharmacokinetic/pharmacodynamic parameters: rationale for antibacterial dosing of mice and men. Clin. Infect. Dis. **26**:1–12.

(14) **Craig, W. A.** 2001. Does the dose matter? Clin. Infect. Dis. **33** (Suppl 3):S233-S237.

(15) **Craig. W. A., and S. Gudmundsson.** 1996. Postantibiotic effect, p. 296–329. *In* V. Lorian (ed.), Antibiotics in laboratory medicine, 4th ed. Williams and Wilkins, Baltimore, MD.

(16) **Deutches Institut für Normung (DIN).** 2004. Medical microbiology – susceptibility testing of pathogens to antimicrobial agents. 4. Evaluation classes of the minimum inhibitory concentration - MIC breakpoints of antibacterial agents. DIN document 58940 - supplement 1. Beuth Verlag GmbH, Berlin,

(17) **Drusano, G. L.** 2004. Antimicrobial pharmacodynamics: critical interactions of 'bug and drug'. Nat. Rev. Microbiol. **2**:289–300.

(18) **Dudley, M. N., and P. G. Ambrose.** 2000. Pharmacodynamics in the study of drug resistance and establishing in vitro susceptibility breakpoints: ready for prime time. Curr. Opin. Microbiol. **3**:515–521.

(19) **Ericsson, H.M., and Sherris J.C.** 1971. Antibiotic sensitivity testing. Report of an international collaborative study. Acta Pathol. Microbiol. Scand. B Microbiol. Imunol. **217** (Suppl.): 1–90.

(20) **European Committee for Antimicrobial Susceptibility Testing (EUCAST).** Information for pharmaceutical companies intending to bring new antimicrobial drugs to EUCAST for breakpoints (http://eucast.www137.server1.mensemedia.net/information_for_industry/)

(21) **European Committee for Antimicrobial Susceptibility Testing (EUCAST) of the European Society of Clinical Microbiology and Infectious Diseases (ESCMID).** 2000. Determination of antimicrobial susceptibility test breakpoints. Clin. Microbiol. Infect. **6**:570–572.

(22) **European Committee on Antimicrobial Susceptibility Testing (EUCAST)** (htttp://www.eucast.org)

(23) **Frei, C.R. and D.S. Burgess.** 2008. Pharmacokinetic/pharmacodynamic modeling to predict in vivo effectiveness of various dosing regimens of piperacillin/tazobactam and piperacillin monotherapy against gram-negative pulmonary isolates from patients managed in intensive care units in 2002. Clin. Ther. **30**:2335-2341.

(24) **Fuchs, P.C., A.L. Barry, C. Thornsberry, R.N. Jones, T.L. Gavan, E.H. Gerlach, and H.M. Sommers.** 1980. Cefotaxime: in vitro activity and tentative interpretive standards for disk susceptibility testing. Antimicrob. Agents Chemother. **18**:88-93.

(25) **Goldstein, F., C.J. Soussy, and A. Thabaut.** 1996. Definition of the Clinical Antibacterial Spectrum of Activity. Clin Microbiol Infect. **2** (Suppl 1):S40-S45.

(26) **Greenwood, D.** 1997. What's the use of susceptibility testing? J. Chemother. **9** (Suppl 1):7-12.

(27) **International Organization for Standardization (ISO).** 2006 Clinical laboratory testing and *in vitro* diagnostic diagnostic test systems – Susceptibility testing of infectious agents and evaluation of performance of antimicrobial susceptibility test devices – Part 1: Reference method for testing the *in vitro* activity of antimicrobial agents against rapidly growing aerobic bacteria involved in infectious diseases. International Standard 20776-1, ISO, Geneva.

(28) **Jacobs, M.R.** 2008. Antimicrobial-resistant *Streptococcus pneumoniae*: trends and management. Expert. Rev. Anti. Infect. Ther. **6**:619-635.

(29) **Jorgensen, J.H., and M.J. Ferraro.** 1998. Antimicrobial susceptibility testing: general principles and contemporary practices. Clin. Infect. Dis. **26**:973-980.

(30) **Kahlmeter, G., and D.F.J. Brown.** 2004. Harmonization of antimicrobial breakpoints in Europe – can it be achieved? Clin. Microbiol. Newsletter **26**:187-191.

(31) **Kahlmeter, G., D. F. J. Brown, F. W. Goldstein, A. P. MacGowan, J. W. Mouton, A. Österland, A. Rodloff, M. Steinbakk, P. Urbaskova, and A. Vatopoulos.** 2003. European harmonisation of MIC breakpoints for antimicrobial susceptibility testing of bacteria. J. Antimicrob. Chemother. **52**:145–148.

(32) **MacGowan, A., C. Rogers, and K. Bowker.** 2003. In vitro models, in vivo models, and pharmacokinetics: what can we learn from in vitro models? Clin. Infect. Dis. **33**(Suppl. 3):S214–S220.

(33) **Moise-Broder, P.A., G. Sakoulas, G.M. Eliopoulos, J.J. Schentag, A. Forrest, and R.C. Moellering Jr.** 2004. Accessory gene regulator group II polymorphism in methicillin-resistant *Staphylococcus aureus* is predictive of failure of vancomycin therapy. Clin. Infect. Dis. **38**:1700-1705.

(34) **Mouton, J. W.** 2002. Breakpoints: current practice and future perspectives. International J. Antimicrob. Agents. **55**:601-607.

(35) **Mouton, J. W.** 2003. Impact of pharmacodynamics on breakpoint selection for susceptibility testing. Infect. Dis. Clin. N. Am. **17**:579–598.

(36) **Mouton, J.W., M.N. Dudley, O. Cars, H. Derendorf, and G.L. Drusano.** 2005. Standardization of pharmacokinetic/pharmacodynamic (PK/PD) terminology for anti-infective drugs: an update. J. Antimicrob. Chemother. **55**:601-607.

(37) **Rex, J. H., M. A. Pfaller, J. N. Galgiani, M. S. Bartlett, A. Espinel-Ingroff, M. A. Ghannoum, M. Lancaster, F. C. Odds, M. G. Rinaldi, T. J. Walsh, and A. L. Barry.** 1997. Development of interpretive breakpoints for antifungal susceptibility testing: conceptual framework and analysis of in vitro-in vivo correlation data for fluconazole, itraconazole, and *Candida* infections. Clin. Infect. Dis. **24**:235–247.

(38) **Sirot, J., P. Courvalin, and C.J. Soussy.** 1996. Definition and determination of in vitro antibiotic susceptibility breakpoints for bacteria. Clin. Microbiol. Infect. **2** (Suppl 1):S5-S10.

(39) **Stratton, C.W.** 2006. In vitro susceptibility testing versus in vivo effectiveness. Med Clin North Am. **90**:1077-1088.

(40) **Swedish Reference Group of Antibiotics.** 1997. Antimicrobial susceptibility testing in Sweden. Scan& J. Infect. Dis. Suppl. **105**:5-31. (Updates on).

(41) **Tenover, F.C. and R.C. Moellering Jr.** 2007. The rationale for revising the Clinical and Laboratory Standards Institute vancomycin minimal inhibitory concentration interpretive criteria for *Staphylococcus aureus*. Clin Infect Dis. **44**:1208-1215.

(42) **Turnidge, J., and D.L. Paterson.** 2007. Setting and revising antibacterial susceptibility breakpoints. Clin Microbiol Revs. **20**:391-408.

(43) **Turnidge, J., G. Kahlmeter, and G. Kronvall.** 2006. Statistical characterisation of bacterial wild-type MIC value distributions and the determination of epidemiological cut-off values. Clin. Microbiol. Infect. **12**:418–425.

(44) **Verbeeck, R.K., and F.T. Musuamba FT.** 2009. Pharmacokinetics and dosage adjustment in patients with renal dysfunction. Eur. J. Clin. Pharmacol. **65**:757-773.

(45) **Vogelman, B., S. Gudmundsson, J. Leggett, J. Turnidge, S. Ebert, and W. A. Craig.** 1988. Correlation of antimicrobial pharmacokinetic parameters with therapeutic efficacy in an animal model. J. Infect. Dis. **158**:831–847.

Chapter 5. INTERPRETIVE READING

Patrice COURVALIN

Considerable progress has been made over the last twenty years in the understanding of bacterial resistance to antibiotics. The large number of antibiotics now available has allowed a precise description of resistance phenotypes and enzyme inhibitors have helped to elucidate certain resistance mechanisms. The study of the biochemical mechanisms of resistance of representative strains of various phenotypes has helped to elucidate cross-resistance and the study of large numbers of clinical isolates has provided information on antibiotic co-resistance. Detailed analysis of the bactericidal and bacteriostatic activity of single antibiotics and antibiotic combinations has revealed the limits of *in vitro* antibiotic susceptibility test techniques for the detection of resistance possibly responsible for treatment failure. The objective of combined molecular and therapeutic interpretation of *in vitro* antibiotic susceptibility testing of clinical isolates is to provide a logical basis for antibiotic therapy decision-making by taking into account progress in the understanding of bacterial antibiotic resistance.

PRINCIPLE

Molecular analysis and therapeutic interpretation, known as "interpretive reading", of in vitro antibiotic susceptibility testing consists of three steps: 1) characterization of the resistance phenotype with a carefully selected range of antibiotics belonging to the same family; 2) deduction of the observed phenotype from the corresponding biochemical resistance mechanism; and 3) inference of the predicted resistance phenotype from the inferred mechanism.

As shown in the examples provided in Table 1, this is the most useful approach for the detection and characterization of low-level resistance due to the production of a single enzyme. It also applies to combined phenotypes resulting from the co-existence, in the same host bacterium, of several different mechanisms conferring resistance to antibiotics belonging to the same family. However, the study of strains harboring two determinants conferring cross-resistance has generally showed that genes contribute in an additive fashion to the level of resistance, resulting in an easily detectable phenotype.

RATIONALE

Antibiotics are not isolated individuals but are members of tight families

The great majority of antibiotics used in human medicine can be assigned to a small number of families, such as β-lactams, aminoglycosides, quinolones, etc., which can be further subdivided into classes (for example, β-lactams comprise benzylpenicillin, the methicillin class, amino-carboxy-acylureido- and amidino-penicillins, carbapenems, cephalosporins and monobactams). As assignment to a group, family, or class is based on molecular structural criteria, antibiotics belonging to the same family or the same class are closely related structurally. This implies that they share similar mechanisms of action and activity spectra and that they are subject, although sometimes to varying degrees, to the same resistance mechanisms (cross-resistance). Some families, such as macrolides, lincosamides and streptogramins (MLS), although composed of chemically very different molecules, have the same intracellular target and can therefore be considered, for the purposes of interpretation of antibiotic susceptibility testing, as a single functional group.

This explains why antibiotic susceptibility test results must be analysed simultaneously for antibiotics belonging to the same family or class and not individually for each antibiotic considered separately. This concept has important implications for the selection of the antibiotics used in *in vitro* antibiotic susceptibility tests.

Limits of antibiotic susceptibility testing

Partly due to technical difficulties, particularly the limits of optical systems that do not allow quantification of bacterial populations less than 10^6-10^7 CFU/ml, routine antibiotic susceptibility tests only study the bacteriostatic activity of antibiotics. Under these conditions, the decreased activity of certain antibiotics on certain strains cannot be detected. This apparent absence of resistance is independent of the technique used because it is due to the resistance mechanism itself. This type of limitation is generally observed with antibiotics which are poor substrates for inactivating enzymes. For example, although the respective bacteriostatic activities of amikacin and netilmicin on Gram-positive cocci harboring an aminoglycoside 3'-phosphotransferase or a 6'-acetyltransferase-2''-phosphotransferase do not appear to be affected, the bactericidal activity of these two antibiotics is abolished and they are no longer synergistic with β-lactam antibiotics. They are inactive from a therapeutic point of view and these strains must therefore be reported as intermediate or resistant to each of these molecules (Table 1). Similarly, staphylococci with high-level resistance to lincomycin due to production of a lincomycin nucleotidyltransferase remain apparently susceptible to clindamycin. However, minimum bactericidal concentrations of clindamycin against these strains are increased and such isolates must therefore be considered to be resistant. Lowering the breakpoint concentrations that distinguish susceptible and resistant bacterial populations would not be of any use in these cases and would simply result in a distribution of the susceptible bacterial population into two clinical categories. These limitations or pitfalls of antibiotic susceptibility testing can be frequently avoided by complementary analyses (for example, use of a chromogenic cephalosporin for the detection of the β-lactamases) or, as indicated in Tables 1 and 2 and discussed below, by studying antibiotics not or no longer used in clinical practice or by interpreting the results obtained with other members of the same antibiotic family.

Co-resistance

Although they are due to different biochemical mechanisms, some types of resistance frequently coexist in the same strain. Apart from the context of epidemics of a particular strain, this phenomenon occurs in response to multiple selection pressures, disseminates as a result of favorable epidemiological conditions, and persists due to the coordinated expression of resistance genes that are frequently grouped along the genome. One can take advantage of this physical linkage between various determinants for the detection of resistance. For example, in some hospitals more than 90% of methicillin-resistant staphylococci are also resistant to fluoroquinolones. Due to phenotypic heterogeneity, the presence of methicillin resistance is difficult to confirm, while the presence of fluoroquinolone resistance, due to mutational alteration of the target, is easily detected. As the degree of correlation between the two characters is higher than the efficacy of the various phenotypic techniques for the detection of methicillin resistance, a fluoroquinolone is routinely used in these particular eco-systems for the detection of resistance to the β-lactams in strains of *Staphylococcus aureus*.

Clinical categorization is already interpretation

As indicated above, the limitations of antibiotic susceptibility testing are related to the fact that the increase of the MIC of an antibiotic due to a resistance mechanism is sometimes only minor and insufficient to induce a change of clinical category. This confirms the marked loss of information when the result obtained according to a system of multiple classes (MIC of antibiotics are usually determined by serial dilution according to a twofold geometric

Table 1. Examples of interpretive reading of antibiotic susceptibility tests

Host	Observed phenotype[a]	Inferred mechanism	Predicted phenotype[a]
Gram-positive cocci	Kan^{R}Tob^{S}Gen^{S}Ami^S	APH(3')-III	Kan^{R}Tob^{S}Gen^{S}Ami$^{I/R}$
	Kan^{R}Tob^{R}Gen^{S}Ami^S	ANT(4')	Kan^{R}Tob^{R}Gen^{S}Ami$^{I/R}$
	Gen^R	AAC(6')-APH(2'')	R to all aminoglycosides (except streptomycin)
Streptococcus	Em^{R}Lin^S without antagonism	Efflux	R to 14-/15-membered macrolides
	Em^{R}Lin^R	rRNA methylase	R to all 14-/15-/16-member macrolides
Enterobacteriaceae	Amino-carboxypénicillines^R	TEM1/2 or SHV1	Acylureidopenicillins$^{I/R}$ Mecillinam^R
	Amino-carboxypenicillins^R Synergy clavulanic acid + cefotaxime or ceftazidime	Extended-spectrum β-lactamase	R to all β-lactams except for cephamycins, carbapenems, moxalactam

[a] Abbreviations: Ami, amikacin; Em, erythromycin; Gen, gentamicin; Kan, kanamycin; Lin, lincomycin; Tob, tobramycin.

Table 2. Antibiotics and antibiotic combinations allowing optimal detection of certain resistance mechanisms

Antibiotic	Resistance to	Mechanism	Host
Oxacillin, cefoxitin, moxalactam	β-lactams	PLP2a	*Staphylococcus*
Oxacillin	Penicillins	PLP alteration	*S. pneumoniae*
Aminopenicillin Aminopenicillin + penicillinase inhibitor	Penicillins	Penicillinase	*Enterobacteriaceae*
Cefotaxime or ceftazidime or aztreonam + penicillinase inhibitor	β-lactams (except cephamycins, carbapenems)	Extended-spectrum β-lactamase	*Enterobacteriaceae* *P. aeruginosa* *Acinetobacter*
Kanamycin	Amikacin	APH(3') or ANT(4')	Gram-positive cocci
Gentamicin	Aminoglycosides (except streptomycin)	AAC(6')-APH(2")	
Erythromycin + lincomycin	MLS$_B$	rRNA methylase	Gram-positive cocci
Nalidixic acid	Quinolones	DNA gyrase	Gram-negatives
Tinidazole	Imidazoles	Reductase	Anaerobes

progression of the antibiotic) is expressed with three (susceptible, intermediate and resistant) or even only two (susceptible and resistant) classes. Concentrations of 0.006 and 1 mg/L of penicillin G are clearly distinct values, although the strains can be considered to be susceptible in both of these cases. One of the primary objectives of antibiotic susceptibility testing is to ensure more reliable detection of antibiotic resistance mechanisms by comparison of the phenotype of the clinical isolate with that of a susceptible strain of the same species. This approach must therefore be based on determination of MIC, or MIC equivalent for automated systems. Furthermore, as an international consensus has not been reached on interpretation breakpoints for antibiotic susceptibility testing, a system with a universal vocation cannot be based on local and subjective criteria, as resistance mechanisms and their bacterial hosts are the same all over the world. It should be remembered that in medical practice there are only two categories, success or failure, while the intermediate category is limited to antibiotics for which dosages can be significantly increased (for example β-lactams but not glycopeptides).

Facilitation of resistance

Therapists must be warned about situations in which the emergence of resistance can be expected. Mutations (for example in the *gyrA* gene) responsible for high-level resistance to nalidixic acid in enterobacteria also confer resistance to the other quinolones. However, the degree of cross-resistance depends on the intrinsic activity of the antibiotic and fluoroquinolones for which the MIC is only slightly increased remain clinically active.

Nevertheless, these strains possess a resistance mechanism to the quinolone family and therefore present an increased risk of becoming resistant to ciprofloxacin during monotherapy with this antibiotic following a second mutational event. For similar reasons, staphylococci with inducible MLSB resistance are good candidates for constitutive generalized cross-resistance to these antibiotics if they are treated with 16-member macrolides or lincosamides. On the other hand, it would be excessive to consider them as being resistant, as recommended by the CLSI and EUCAST.

IMPLICATIONS

Fixed menu or à la carte?

As all marketed antibiotics must not and cannot be studied, what are the best selection criteria for the antibiotics whose activity should be studied *in vitro*? The approach proposed here for the optimal detection and characterization of the resistance phenotype implies the study of a minimum of antibiotics belonging to the same family in the cases of various resistance mechanisms (for example aminoglycosides or MLS) or a representative of each class in the case of large families (for example β-lactams). As already mentioned, varying degrees of cross-resistance are often observed to antibiotics with closely related structures. The antibiotics most affected by a resistance mechanism and consequently the most suitable to detect resistance, are those with the lowest intrinsic activity compared to those of other members of the family. These molecules, as well as combinations of substrates and enzyme inhibitors must therefore be studied (Table 2). Antibiotics and combinations not or no longer used clinically must also be included (Table 2). Inversely, the activity of some antibiotics widely prescribed in human medicine must not be studied *in vitro* because they systematically provide erroneous results concerning their *in vitro* and *in vivo* efficacy (Table 3). Rational use of these antibiotics must be based on the study of other members of the same family (Table 1).

These various technical and biological constraints argue in favour of the use of fixed menus which can differ according to the Gram stain, species, and the site of isolation of the pathogen studied. As far as possible, they must include the most frequently prescribed antibiotics at the time of the examination. These molecules which exert a selection pressure are probably more suitable to rapidly detect the emergence of resistance. Provided they are established by experts, these menus will probably be more appropriate than those established by microbiologists who only occasionally perform antibiotic susceptibility tests. They should avoid redundancy and should contribute to standardization of *in vitro* testing, a prerequisite for comparison of results, epidemiological studies and effective quality control. The rigid selection of the antibiotics studied does not prevent adding other antibiotics as necessary according to the circumstances (patient, bacterium or environment factors), for the evaluation of new antibiotics, or for specific epidemiological studies.

The antibiotic family as a functional unit

The relationship between bacteria and antibiotics is more clearly defined at the species level due to the fact that the insusceptibility (intrinsic chromosomal resistance) resulting from a defect of penetration, active efflux, absence of the target for the antibiotic or the production of an inactivation enzyme tends to be species specific, rather than genus- or Gram stain-specific. Regarding acquisition of resistance by horizontal transfer of genetic information, this is due to the limited host spectrum of plasmids and barriers to the expression of heterologous genes, which mean that not all genes can be transferred or

Table 3. Antibiotics used in therapeutics, but which must not be studied *in vitro*

Antibiotic	Microorganism
Cloxacillin, dicloxacillin, flucloxacillin, nafcillin Cephalosporins Clindamycin	*Staphylococcus*
Amikacin Netilmicin	Gram-positive cocci

expressed in all hosts. On the other hand, as mentioned above, antibiotics belonging to the same group have the same activity spectrum and are subject to bacterial cross-resistance. For some combinations of bacterial species and antibiotic classes, it therefore appears justified (and even recommended) to report the results for the entire antibiotic family even when the in vitro activity was studied on only one member (Table 1).

Bacterial identification is required

Due to the multiple intrinsic or acquired resistances, which frequently co-exist, analysis of the biochemical mechanisms of resistance phenotypes is frequently impossible if the host bacterium has not been identified. Furthermore, the clinical significance of a particular resistance characteristic depends on the host. For example, acquisition of MLS resistance by members of the *Enterobacteriaceae* family is much less important than acquisition of MLS resistance by Gram-positive cocci. Finally, the level of phenotypic resistance due to the same determinant can vary considerably according to the host, as it may be easily detectable in one species and barely detectable in another. For example, aminoglycoside 6'-N-acetyltransferase induces extended-spectrum resistance in *Pseudomonas*, while it only confers resistance to a small number of antibiotics in *Escherichia coli*. Fortunately, effective techniques are available allowing the rapid identification of the bacterial species, which is essential for interpretive reading of antibiotic susceptibility tests. Inversely, speciation can lead to identification of intrinsic resistance mechanisms; for example, aminoglycoside 6'-N-acetyltransferase in *Enterococcus faecium* and *Serratia*, aminoglycoside 2'-acetyltransferase in *Providencia* and aminoglycoside 3'-phosphotransferase or efflux in *P. aeruginosa*.

Limitations

Not all medical microbiologists are experts in antibiotics. As interpretive reading requires a very extensive knowledge of antibiotics (chemical structure and mode of action, resistance mechanisms and corresponding phenotypes, intrinsic resistance, pharmacokinetics and pharmacodynamics, metabolism, MIC distribution of bacterial populations, correlation between **in vitro** results and therapeutic outcome, etc.), this approach remains confined to a few specialists. Given the large quantity of information required, interpretive reading is most effectively performed by computerized expert systems.

Several of these systems have been developed for routine use or for teaching purposes. The rapid diffusion of automats for determination of susceptibility and the use of computers in clinical laboratories has promoted the use of artificial intelligence applied to the evolution of antibiotic activities. In turn, this has led to improved quality and security of *in vitro* tests and has provided medical microbiologists with a better knowledge of antibiotic activities.

Not all resistance mechanisms have been identified

It is obvious that only those mechanisms that have already been described can be routinely analysed. Interpretive reading, by comparing bacterial identification and antibiotic susceptibility, is the most effective way to detect new resistance mechanisms, by drawing attention to discordant results that need to be verified. If they are confirmed, these discordant results can be due to a "new" mechanism which does not phenotypically mime an "old" mechanism. The detection of new resistance mechanisms leads to re-evaluation of clinical breakpoints (for example, reduction of the penicillin G breakpoint for pneumococci) and therefore contributes to improvement of *in vitro* methods. As indicated above, interpretation of resistance phenotypes is based on comparison of clinical isolates with "prototype" susceptible bacteria belonging to the same species and is therefore easier to perform with bacteria possessing a single resistance mechanism per class of antibiotic. However, the co-existence of various mechanisms conferring resistance to the same class of antibiotics is a common feature of human pathogens. As indicated above, this does not constitute a problem inasmuch as, in the majority of cases studied to date, these mechanisms are synergistic or additive and confer high-level resistance which is easily detected. A persistent limitation is the intrinsic resistance of new opportunistic pathogens, which has not been fully investigated.

Biochemical resistance and clinical resistance are not synonymous

Biochemical resistance is secondary to mutations or acquisition of exogenous DNA and refers to the parental strain considered to be susceptible. It is not always correlated with clinical resistance. For example, *Escherichia coli* produces a chromosomal cephalosporinase and, although aminocarboxypenicillins, acylureidopenicillins, and cephalosporins are less active on this species, these antibiotics remain effective in therapy. Conversely, penicillinase-producing *Staphylococcus*, *Haemophilus* and *Neisseria gonorrhoeae* must be considered to be clinically resistant to penicillins regardless of the MIC values.

Permeability mutants and active efflux

Resistance induced by production of an inactivating enzyme confers resistance to antibiotics of the same class. The MIC of antibiotics which are substrates for the enzyme are usually increased, while those of antibiotics which are not modified remain low, resulting in an easily recognizable "*in vivo* enzymatic substrate profile". Inversely, porin or lipopolysaccharide mutations which alter cellular permeability or active efflux of antibiotics can confer low-level cross-resistance to structurally unrelated antibiotics such as β-lactams, chloramphenicol, quinolones, tetracyclines, aminoglycosides, and trimethoprim. This resistance mechanism is therefore difficult to detect *in vitro* but also by molecular techniques which are not adapted to the detection of point mutations. In some cases, several frequently affected antibiotics can be helpful for the detection of this type of resistance (Table 2).

Inducible resistance

Glycopeptide resistance in *Enterococcus* represents a good example of the difficulty of detection of an inducible resistance mechanism. Various types of glycopeptide resistance have been identified and each one can be difficult to detect for different reasons. VanA type, which is a high-level resistance to vancomycin and teicoplanin, should be theoretically easy to detect phenotypically. However, this resistance is slowly inducible by glycopeptides, which explains why the VanA phenotype may not be detected by rapid automated systems. This phenomenon is even more pronounced and associated with genetic instability in *Staphylococcus* which explains why two of the nine strains of methicillin-resistant VanA type *S. aureus* isolated to date may appear to be susceptible to vancomycin. This is a particularly worrying problem, as use of a glycopeptide will induce resistance, which can be very high level. Finally, VanA type resistance is expressed to varying degrees after transfer to other bacterial genera. This observation at least partly explains the delayed detection of this resistance in other species.

CONSEQUENCES

Individualization of bacterial species

For the reasons indicated above, interpretation of antibiotic susceptibility tests cannot be dissociated from bacterial identification. For example, the modal MIC of ampicillin for susceptible pneumococci is 0.01 µg/ml and these bacteria are considered to be resistant when the MIC is ≥ 0.1 µg/ml, while the MIC of the same antibiotic for susceptible E. coli strains are 2 to 4 µg/ml. Inversely, some groups of bacteria must be identified to allow optimal in vitro studies. For each of these groups of microorganisms, various antibiotics must be studied and different breakpoints must be used. These requirements are at least partially recognized by the various national in vitro antibiotic susceptibility test committees. However, this subdivision introduces a supplementary degree of complexity in the analysis of the results which, once again, is best performed by expert systems

Aid to bacterial identification

If correct identification is required for analysis of antibiotic susceptibility tests, intrinsic resistance can be extremely useful to correct or confirm bacterial identification, which is why some antibiotics, which do not represent the best choice of treatment, must be studied *in vitro* in relation to certain bacterial genera or species (Table 4).

Improved and continuous quality control

By providing more logical results, one of the most important consequences of interpretive reading of antibiotic susceptibility tests is continuous quality control as a result of: 1) simultaneous analysis of bacterial identification and susceptibility profile of the clinical isolate, which ensures coherence between the two types of results obtained independently by means of different techniques and 2) critical interpretation of the observed resistance phenotype. This biological quality control is complementary to the technical quality control using control strains.

Impossible phenotypes

"Impossible phenotypes", although almost anything is possible in biology, actually correspond to resistance phenotypes that have not yet been observed in nature (Table 5). They are due to intrinsic resistance or susceptibility but also cross-resistance or co-resistance to antibiotics. The discovery of these phenotypes requires verification of bacterial identification and/or antibiotic susceptibility. When impossible phenotypes do not correspond to a new mechanism, they reflect an error of identification or determination of susceptibility, or mixed growth.

Abnormal and isolated susceptibility or resistance

In this situation, an isolated resistance or susceptibility determinant is discordant with the other results. This abnormality is usually associated with a technical error. For example, a microorganism susceptible to amoxicillin and resistant to the amoxicillin-clavulanic acid combination reflects instability of the antibiotic.

High incidence of rare phenotypes

Rare phenotypes (Table 6) represent resistance mechanisms that have been either recently detected (for example, vancomycin resistance in *S. aureus*) or that have not been epidemically successful (for example, lincosamide *O*-nucleotidyltransferase in *S. aureus*). Apart from clonal epidemics, for which they represent an excellent marker, a sudden change in the incidence of rare phenotypes is suspicious. For example, frequent isolation of a lincomycin-resistant *Staphylococcus* strain tends to suggest that the Gram-positive cocci examined may actually be an *Enterococcus*. Similarly, isolation of numerous strains of *Enterococcus faecium* with low-level resistance to vancomycin is suggestive of *Enterococcus gallinarum* or *E. casseliflavus-flavescens*. When a large number of trimethoprim-resistant isolates belonging to various species are detected, the thymidine content of the culture medium should be checked. The concept of rarity is obviously only relative and varies with the ecosystem considered. Penicillin-resistant *Enterococcus* due to penicillinase production are encountered with an increasing frequency in North America and South America, but have not been detected in Europe. Similarly, the same prevalence of resistance determinants is not expected in ICU patients and in inhabitants of rural communities.

Epidemiology of resistance determinants

A rational approach based on biochemistry replaces the study of the incidence of resistance mechanisms by the study of resistance to isolated antibiotics. This approach is much more subtle and informative and explains, for example, cross-selection of resistance due to cross-resistance and reveals how antibiotics only used in veterinary medicine can select resistance mechanisms subsequently

Table 4. Antibiotics useful for bacterial identification

Antibiotic	Microorganism
Amino-, carboxypenicillins	*Citrobacter diversus, Klebsiella*
Aminopenicillins,	*Citrobacter freundii, Enterobacter*
1st generation cephalosporins	*Morganella, Proteus vulgaris, Providencia, Serratia*
Cefoxitin	*C. freundii, Clostridium difficile, Enterobacter*
Cefalotin; cefotaxime	*Bacillus*
Clavulanic acid	*Campylobacter*
Sulbactam	*Acinetobacter, Burkholderia cepacia*
Carbapenems	*Stenotrophomonas maltophilia*
Aminoglycosides	*B. cepacia, S. maltophilia*, streptococci, anaerobes
Tetracycline	*Proteus mirabilis*
Lincomycin	*Eikenella corrodens, Enterococcus faecalis, Haemophilus, Staphylococcus xylosus, Listeria, Neisseria*, Gram-negative bacteria
Bacitracin	*Streptococcus pyogenes*
Colistin	Susceptibility: *P. aeruginosa*
	Resistance: *Proteus, Providencia, Serratia, B. cepacia*,
	Gram-negative bacteria
Trimethoprim	*Acinetobacter, Brucella* spp., *Campylobacter, Neisseria, Nocardia, Pseudomonas* spp.
Nitrofurans	*Proteus, Providencia, Acinetobacter*, micrococci
Novobiocin	*Staphylococcus saprophyticus, S. xylosus, S. cohnii*
Fosfomycin	*Acinetobacter, S. saprophyticus*
Vancomycin	*Erysipelothrix rhusopathiae, Lactobacillus, Leuconostoc, Nocardia, Pediococcus*, Gram-positive bacteria
Metronidazole	*Gardnerella vaginalis, Propionibacterium*, aerobes
Optochin[a]	Pneumococci
0/129[a]	Differentiation between *Micrococcus, Staphylococcus* Differentiation between enterobacteria, *Pasteurella, Vibrio*

[a] Not used in clinical therapy.

Table 5. Examples of impossible resistance phenotypes

Phenotype	Microorganism
Gentamicin[R] other aminoglycosides[S] Minocycline[R] tetracycline[S]	Gram-positive cocci
Methicillin[R] cephalosporins[S] carbapenems[S] Methicillin[R] penicillins[S]	*S. aureus*
Penicillins[R]	Group A, C, G streptococci
Teicoplanin[R], vancomycin[S]	Enterococci
Amino-carboxypenicillins[S]	*K. pneumoniae, C. diversus*
Cefamandole or cefuroxime[S]	*P. vulgaris, Serratia*
Cefoxitin[S]	*C. freundii, Enterobacter*
3rd generation cephalosporins[S], amino-carboxypenicillins[S] and/or 1st generation cephalosporins[S]	Enterobacteriaceae
Colistin[S]	*Proteus, Providencia, Serratia*
Kanamycin[S]	*P. aeruginosa*

Table 6. Examples of rare resistance phenotypes

Phenotype	Microorganism
Isolated lincosamide resistance	*Staphylococcus aureus*
Streptogramin resistance	
Vancomycin resistance	
Linezolid resistance	
Daptomycin resistance	
Cefotaxime-ceftriaxone resistance	*Streptococcus pneumoniae*
Penicillin resistance with penicillinase production	Enterococci
Isolated gentamicin resistance	
Isolated tobramycin resistance	
Carbapenem resistance	*Acinetobacter*, enterobacteria, *Bacteroides fragilis*
Amikacin resistance + tobramycin susceptibility	*Pseudomonas aeruginosa*, enterobacteria
Penicillin resistance with penicillinase production	*Neisseria meningitidis*
5-nitromidazole resistance	*Bacteroides fragilis*

revealed in clinical isolates in which they confer resistance to antibiotics used in human medicine (for example, gentamicin resistance due to production of an aminoglycoside 3-*N*-acetyltransferase selected by apramycin, Table 2).

CONCLUSION: THE END JUSTIFIES THE MEANS

The study of the biochemistry of antibiotic resistance has had two major applications: 1) design of new semisynthetic molecules which overcome certain resistance mechanisms and 2) a better understanding and therefore better detection of resistance.

Antibiotic susceptibility testing, like other laboratory tests, should provide objective quantitative results, *i.e.* diameters or MICs. For various historical reasons, it also provides subjective interpretation in the form of clinical categories. Interpretive reading of antibiotic susceptibility tests is an attempt to reconcile these two concepts with an interpretation based on the most recent knowledge in the field of antibiotics, particularly resistance mechanisms. Ideally, antibiotic susceptibility tests should allow the detection of resistance, particularly low-level resistance. This can be obtained by improved and more refined interpretation of the results and, in some cases, by genotypic techniques. The objective of this approach is to provide the clinician with the necessary results for the judicious choice of antibiotic therapy based on the available knowledge and to draw the clinician's attention to bacteria-antibiotic combinations presenting certain therapeutic risks. This approach should result not only in more adapted antibiotic therapy but also decreased selection of bacterial resistance and therefore a longer active half-life of antibiotics.

REFERENCES

(1) **Acar, J.F., and F.W. Goldstein.** 1991. Disk susceptibility test, pp.17-52. *In* V. Lorian. (ed.), Antibiotics in laboratory medicine. Williams & Wilkins. Philadelphia.
(2) **Courvalin, P.** 1992. Interpretive reading of antimicrobial susceptibility tests. ASM news **58** : 368-375.
(3) **Courvalin, P. F. Goldstein, A. Philippon, and J. Sirot.** 1985. L'antibiogramme. MPC-Videom, Paris.
(4) **Courvalin, P., J.P. Flandrois, F. Goldstein, A. Philippon, C. Quentin, and J. Sirot.** 1988. L'antibiogramme automatisé. MPC Vigot, Paris.
(5) **Livermore, D.M., T.G. Winstanley, and K.P. Shannon.** 2001. Interpretative reading: recognizing the unusual and inferring resistance mechanisms from resistance phenotypes. J. Antimicrob. Chemother. **48** (suppl. S1): 87-102.

Chapter 6. PHENOTYPIC TECHNIQUES

Gunnar KAHLMETER and John TURNIDGE

INTRODUCTION

Routine susceptibility testing can be conducted using a variety of established methods, including broth microdilution, agar dilution, disk diffusion, and semi-automated instrument-based methods. After many years of neglect, a reference method for determination of minimum inhibitory concentrations (MIC) in non-fastidious bacteria was finally developed in 2006 (14). All routine susceptibility testing methods in use should now conform to this reference method. However, the reference method does not address all phenotypic tests that might have roles in the routine laboratory, such as those designed to detect the presence of certain β-lactamases. Information on the current phenotypic techniques is provided in this chapter. This chapter does not deal with routine testing of mycobacteria, aerobic actinomycetes, mycoplasmas or obligate intracellular bacteria such as *Chlamydiaceae* or *Rickettsiae*.

METHODS

Recently, consensus was reached that broth microdilution employing Mueller-Hinton broth would be the international (ISO) reference standard for non-fastidious aerobic bacteria (14). This became the standard against which all other susceptibility tests on non-fastidious aerobic bacteria must now be compared (15). Fortunately, this is the method endorsed by the Clinical and Laboratory Standards Institute (CLSI) (1) and the European Committee on Antimicrobial Susceptibility Testing (EUCAST) (11). Both CLSI and EUCAST have produced a range of standards for antibacterial susceptibility testing, as shown in Table 1.

The authors of this chapter recommend following the methods found in the ISO, CLSI, and EUCAST documents. The rationale is that these are the most thoroughly evaluated methods and are the only methods that generate output to which all the modern interpretation of pharmacokinetic/pharmacodynamic parameters predicting efficacy have been developed.

Choices for routine

The choice of which method or methods to use is driven by considerations such as resources, workload, accessibility of reagents, skill, and training of staff and the degree of access to automation. The degree of sophistication increases with broth, and agar dilution methods and is most sophisticated with semi-automated methods available commercially. For cost and simplicity, disk diffusion techniques remain the most accessible and easiest to implement. If susceptibility testing for a large range of antimicrobial agents is required, agar dilution and semi-automated methods are often preferred, although disk testing in a large plate format is also possible.

Most laboratories choose to have access to at least two types of methodology, especially those with semi-automated equipment as the instruments are not capable of providing testing for all the bac-

Table 1. Currently recognized standards for antibacterial susceptibility testing

Target	Method	CLSI	Document	EUCAST	Document
Rapidly growing aerobic bacteria	Broth dilution	Standard	M7 (4)	Discussion document	E.Dis 5.1 (12)
	Agar dilution	Standard	M7 (1)	Definitive document	E.Def 3.1 (13)
	Disk diffusion	Standard	M2 (5)	Under development	
Infrequently isolated or fastidious bacteria	Broth dilution ± disk diffusion	Guideline	M45 (8)		
Anaerobic bacteria	Agar dilution and Broth microdilution	Standard	M11 (7)		

teria that the laboratory may wish to test. Having access to two methods also allows the laboratory to validate unusual results via an alternative method.

Applicability of methods

Non-fastidious rapidly-growing bacteria can generally be tested by any of the routine methods. Interpretive criteria are available for a wide range of bacteria of this type. For other bacterial types, some of the methods are unsuitable or have yet to be developed or standardized.

Broth microdilution

Standard method

Broth microdilution is generally conducted in conventional 96-well microtiter trays with rounded bottom wells (1). This format is quite flexible, permitting longer or shorter dilution ranges and can accommodate a moderately large number of drugs if short dilution ranges are used. Trays can be prepared in-house or purchased commercially. In-house manufacture is usually too demanding for small laboratories, requiring access to reagent grade antimicrobial agents (powders for injection for therapeutic use vary too much in their labeled content) and the quality control requirements are high. Commercially available trays can be purchased, and if there is sufficient demand, can be customized for the laboratory.

For in-house preparation, particular attention should be given to following the instructions for preparing stock solutions of the antimicrobial to be tested, especially those relating to the series of dilutions required for instillation into the individual microtiter tray wells. The recommendation dilution scheme is deliberately designed to reduce the compounding of error that would result for serial two-fold dilution.

The standard approach to broth microdilution is that described in the ISO document 20776-1 (14) to which the reader is referred for details. The basic features are: cation-adjusted Mueller-Hinton broth to a final volume of 100 μg/ml, an inoculum of approximately 5×10^4 bacteria, and incubation at 35°C for 18-24 h depending on the antimicrobial and species being tested. In general, the inoculum can be prepared by direct suspension of colonies from a plate or by a short period of incubation in a non-selective broth.

Quality control is an essential part of routine as well as reference testing. The recommendations should be followed to ensure that errors are detected. Considerable efforts have been applied over the years to ensure that the maximum benefit is gained for the minimum of effort.

Endpoints, or minimum inhibitory concentrations (MICs), are normally read as the first dilution which shows no visible growth. Some antimicrobial agents problems will be encountered with reading endpoints; these are discussed below.

Alternative media

For some species, the conditions of the test are varied to ensure that the organism grows sufficiently to be read. Test conditions for the different bacterial groups are listed in Table 3. With two exceptions, Mueller-Hinton is the basal medium for testing. Mueller-Hinton broth should always be used in its cation-adjusted form (CAMHB), meaning that the concentrations Ca^{++} and Mg^{++} are fixed at 20-25 and 10-12.5 μg/ml respectively. Cation-adjustment is required to ensure adequate concentrations of these two cations, both of which are known to affect the activity of aminoglyco-

Table 2. Appropriateness of routine susceptibility testing methods

Species where all routine methods are suitable	Species where all routine methods are suitable	Species where one or more of the routine methods is unsuitable	Species where no method described here is suitable
Staphylococcus spp.	*Streptococcus* spp.	*Helicobacter* spp.	*Bordetella* spp.
Enterococcus spp.	Anaerobes	*Aerococcus* spp.	*Bartonella* spp.
Bacillus spp.	*Campylobacter* spp.	*Lactobacillus* spp.	*Legionella* spp.
Coryneforms		*Listeria* spp.	
Enterobacteriaceae		*Neisseria* spp.	
Aeromonas spp.		*Haemophilus* spp.	
Vibrio spp.		*Moraxella* spp.	
Pseudomonas spp.		*Pasteurella* spp.	
Acinetobacter spp.			
Burkholderia spp.			
Stenotrophomonas spp.			

sides. CAMHB is readily available commercially. Haemophilus Test Medium (HTM) is CAMHB supplemented with β-NAD, bovine or porcine hematin, yeast extract, and (sometimes) thymidine phosphorylase. Lysed blood can replace hematin in this recipe. The ingredients for HTM are also readily available commercially. Brucella medium is required for testing *Brucella* spp. and anaerobes.

Supplements to the basal media, when used, are largely to ensure adequate growth within the recommended incubation period. Lysed horse blood is the commonest supplement for broth microdilution while sheep blood is preferred for agar dilution. Sodium chloride is added to CAMHB or MHA to enhance the expression of methicillin resistance when testing staphylococci against antistaphylococcal penicillins. Testing daptomycin requires special conditions. Ca^{++} concentrations require to be increased to 50 μg/ml to ensure accurate measurement of daptomycin activity. This is readily achieved with Mueller-Hinton broth but has so far not been achievable with Mueller-Hinton agar due to the variable concentrations of Ca^{++} introduced by agar itself. The nutritionally-defective Gram-positive species, *Abiotrophia* and *Granulicatella*, require supplementation with pyridoxal in order to grow.

Other susceptibility testing media that have been used in routine and investigative testing include Sensitest, Diagnostic Sensitivity Test, IsoSensitest and, for anaerobes, Wilkins-Chalgren media. Provided that results can be shown to be comparable to those obtained with the Mueller-Hinton based ISO standard using the ISO defined criteria (15), these can be used for routine testing, although they offer few or no advantages generally.

Issues

The commonest challenge in broth microdilution testing is endpoint reading. The most frequently observed problem is that of so-called trailing end points. Usually, the MIC is readily detected visually as the first well showing no visible growth. For some antimicrobial agents, particularly the folate antagonists and sometimes the tetracyclines, inhibition can be partial over a range of concentrations, resulting in a small number of wells manifesting reducing growth with increasing concentration, until a point of no visible growth is reached. By general agreement, the MIC is read as that concentration of antimicrobial that reduced growth by ≥ 80% compared to that of the growth control.

Another occasionally encountered phenomenon is that of skip wells. These are wells of no growth in between wells exhibiting growth. This could represent contamination, and the purity plate for this organism should be examined closely to rule out mixed cultures. If mixed growth can be ruled out, a single skip well in the series of wells exhibiting growth is ignored.

MBC determination

Occasionally, it is useful to determine whether an antimicrobial is bacteriostatic or bactericidal. The method for this is the determination of so-called minimum bactericidal concentration (MBC). In general, bactericidal agents have MBCs the same as or close to the MICs. Bacteriostatic agents have MBCs that are substantially higher than the MICs. Methods for MBC determination are well described (9). MBC determination is most useful in the initial phases of drug development to characterize the drug being investigated. However, it has almost no application currently in the clinical setting as to date there have been no clinical correlates shown between MBC and outcome.

Agar dilution

Standard method

Both CLSI and EUCAST provide a detailed description for susceptibility testing using the Mueller-Hinton agar dilution (1, 13). As with broth microdilution, conditions for testing need to be adjusted for certain organisms and antimicrobial agents; these are noted in Table 3.

Agar dilution retains many of the advantages of broth microdilution, including the capacity to generate MIC values and the ability to use shorter or longer ranges depending on the nature of the work. Since the development of the international reference method (14), rigorous comparison has not been undertaken to compare the results of agar dilution with the reference method. Nevertheless, there has been extensive experience over the years.

Agar dilution using a truncated series of concentrations relevant to interpretive breakpoints is an inexpensive option for routine use in large laboratories. As discussed below, not all antimicrobials can be tested in this manner.

Alternative media

As with broth microdilution, the conditions of the test are varied to ensure that the organism grows sufficiently to be read. Test conditions for

Table 3. Media and incubation conditions for antimicrobial susceptibility testing

Group	Broth[a]	Agar[b]	Supplement	Atmosphere	Incubation Temperature	Duration
Enterobacteriaceae	CAMHB	MHA	nil	Air	35 ± 2°C	16–20 h
P. aeruginosa	CAMHB	MHA	nil	Air	35 ± 2°C	16–20 h
Acinetobacter spp.	CAMHB	MHA	nil	Air	35 ± 2°C	20–24 h
B. cepacia complex	CAMHB	MHA	nil	Air	35 ± 2°C	20–24 h
S. maltophilia	CAMHB	MHA	nil	Air	35 ± 2°C	20–24 h
Other non-Enterobacteriaceae	CAMHB	MHA	nil	Air	35 ± 2°C	16–20 h
Staphylococcus spp.						
For oxacillin, methicillin and nafcillin	CAMHB	MHA	+2% NaCl for;	Air	35 ± 2°C	24 h
Staphylococcus spp. for daptomycin	CAMHB	nr	Added Ca^{++} up to 50 μg/ml	Air	35 ± 2°C	16–20 h
Staphylococcus spp. for vancomycin	CAMHB	MHA	nil	Air	35 ± 2°C	24 h
Staphylococcus spp. for all other agents	CAMHB	MHA	nil	Air	35 ± 2°C	16–20 h
Enterococcus spp. for daptomycin	CAMHB	nr	Added Ca^{++} up to 50 μg/ml	Air	35 ± 2°C	16–20 h
Enterococcus spp. for vancomycin	CAMHB	MHA	nil	Air	35 ± 2°C	24 h
Enterococcus spp. for all other agents	CAMHB	MHA	nil	Air	35 ± 2°C	16–20 h
H. influenzae and H. parainfluenzae	HTM	nr	nil	5% CO_2	35 ± 2°C	20–24 h
N. gonorrhoeae		GC	1% defined growth supplement	5% CO_2	36 ± 1°C	20–24 h
S. pneumoniae	CAMHB	nr	2.5–5% lysed horse blood	5% CO_2	35 ± 2°C	20–24 h
Streptococcus spp. for daptomycin	CAMHB		2.5–5% lysed horse blood and added Ca++ up to 50 μg/ml	5% CO_2	35 ± 2°C	20–24 h
Streptococcus spp. for other agents	CAMHB		2.5–5% lysed horse blood	5% CO_2	35 ± 2°C	20–24 h
Streptococcus spp. for agents other than daptomycin		MHA	5% sheep blood	CLSI: air or, if necessary, 5% CO_2, EUCAST: 5% CO_2	35 ± 2°C	20–24 h
Vibrio spp. including V. cholerae	CAMHB	nr	nil	Air	35 ± 2°C	16–20 h
N. meningitidis	CAMHB	nr	2.5–5% lysed horse blood			
N. meningitidis		MHA	5% sheep blood	5% CO_2	35 ± 2°C	20–24 h
Brucella spp.	Brucella	nr	pH adjusted to 7.1 ± 0.1	Air	35 ± 2°C	48 h
F. tularensis	CAMHB	nr	2% defined growth supplement	Air	35 ± 2°C	48 h
B. mallei	CAMHB	nr	nil	Air	35 ± 2°C	16–20 h
B. pseudomallei						
B. anthracis						
Y. pestis	CAMHB	nr	nil	Air	35 ± 2°C	24–48 h
H. pylori	nr	MHA	5% aged (≥ 2 weeks) sheep blood	Microaerobic ("campy")[c]	35 ± 2°C	3 days
Abiotrophia spp. Granulicatella spp.	CAMHB	nr	2.5–5% lysed horse blood; 1 μg/ml pyridoxal HCl	Air	35°C	20–24 h

Table 3. Media and incubation conditions for antimicrobial susceptibility testing (continued)

Group	Broth[a]	Agar[b]	Supplement	Atmosphere	Incubation Temperature	Duration
Aeromonas spp. *Plesiomonas* spp.	CAMHB	nr	nil	Air	35 ± 2°C	16–20 h
Bacillus spp. other than *B. anthracis*	CAMHB	nr	nil	Air	35 ± 2°C	16–20 h
C. jejuni and *C coli*	CAMHB		2.5–5% lysed horse blood	Microaerobic ("campy")[c]	36–37 °C or 42°C	48 h or 24 h
		MHA	5% sheep blood	Microaerobic ("campy")[c]	36–37 °C or 42°C	48 h or 24 h
Corynebacterium spp. for daptomycin	CAMHB	nr	2.5–5% lysed horse blood and added Ca++ up to 50 mg/L	Air	35°C	24–48 h
Corynebacterium spp. for agents other than daptomycin	CAMHB	nr	2.5–5% lysed horse blood	Air	35°C	24–48 h
E. rhusiopathiae	CAMHB	nr	2.5–5% lysed horse blood	Air	35°C	20–24 h
HACEK group[d]	CAMHB	nr	2.5–5% lysed horse blood	5% CO_2	35°C	24–48 h
Lactobacillus spp.	CAMHB	nr	2.5–5% lysed horse blood	Air	35°C	20–24 h
Leuconostoc spp.	CAMHB	nr	2.5–5% lysed horse blood	Air	35°C	20–24 h
L monocytogenes	CAMHB	nr	2.5–5% lysed horse blood	Air	35°C	20–24 h
M. catarrhalis	CAMHB	nr	nil	Air	35°C	20–24 h
Pasteurella spp.	CAMHB	nr	2.5–5% lysed horse blood	Air	35°C	18–24 h
		MHA	5% sheep blood	Air	35°C	18–24 h
Pediococcus spp.	CAMHB	nr	2.5–5% lysed horse blood	Air	35°C	20–24 h
Anaerobic bacteria		Brucella	5% laked sheep blood, 5 µg/ml hemin and 1 µg/ml vitamin K_1	Anaerobic (including 4-7% CO_2)	36 ± 1°C	42–48 h
Bacteroides fragilis group.	Brucella		5% lysed horse blood, 5 µg/ml hemin and 1 µg/ml vitamin K_1	Anaerobic (including 4-7% CO_2)	36 ± 1°C	46–48 h

[a] CA-MHB, cation-adjusted Mueller-Hinton broth.
[b] MHA, Mueller-Hinton agar; nr, not recommended.
[c] Microaerobic atmosphere, 10% CO_2, 5% O_2, 85% N_2.
[d] HACEK group, the *Aphrophilus* cluster of *Aggregatibacter* spp., *Actinobacillus actinomycetemcomitans*, *Cardiobacterium* spp., *Eikenella corrodens* and *Kingella* spp.

the different bacterial groups are listed in Table 3. Anaerobic bacteria can be tested on Brucella agar.

One widely used option for agar medium has been IsoSensitest agar (17). This medium is popular in Europe and forms the foundation of the methods from the British Society for Antimicrobial Chemotherapy (BSAC) and the Swedish Reference Group of Antibiotics (SRGA) (2, 18). It is possible to use other agar media and several have been tried around the world over the years, but with the listed exceptions, none using internationally accepted interpretive criteria.

Issues

Agar dilution has not been standardized for testing *Haemophilus influenzae*, *H. parainfluenzae* or *Burkholderia cepacia*, or a range of unusual or fastidious pathogens (8), as well as those listed as potential bioterrorism agents (*Brucella* spp., *Francisella tularensis*, *Burkholderia pseudomallei*, *Burkholderia mallei*, *Bacillus anthracis*, or *Yersinia pestis*) (1).

For some antimicrobial-organism combinations, MIC values generated using agar dilution can differ by one dilution from those seen with the reference method (1). This may relate to the slightly lower inoculum (~1 x 10^4) that results from the volumes deliver by the replicator pins. Laboratories that choose to use agar dilution as a routine technique should be aware of these differences and make suitable adjustments to interpretative criteria where necessary.

The trailing phenomenon noted above with broth microdilution can also sometimes be seen with agar dilution and with the same drug classes. Endpoint reading follows the same rules (>80%) reduction in visible growth. A concentration at which there is growth of a single colony should be ignored and the MIC read as the concentration immediately below.

An important difference between Mueller-Hinton broth and agar is the uncontrolled concentrations of Ca^{++} and Mg^{++} cations in MH agar. Therefore, testing of daptomycin is not possible on MH, as testing of this agent requires 50 μg/ml of Ca^{++} for optimum activity. Recently, similar issues have been demonstrated with manganese (Mn^{++}) ion concentrations and tigecycline (16).

Semi-automated methods

There are three major semi-automated commercial systems available for routine susceptibility testing: Siemens Microscan®, Biomerieux Vitek 2®, and BD Phoenix®. The underlying principle of these systems is the growth of the test organism in broth. Each system relies on frequent or continuous spectrophotometric or turbidometric reading to detect growth in wells containing antimicrobials at selected concentrations around breakpoint values, and comparing with growth in a control well. These systems are required by regulators to be comparable with the reference broth microdilution method (15). To ensure compliance with this standard, the developers engineer the software to facilitate correct interpretation of growth/no growth and MICs that would be obtained with the reference method.

Semi-automated instruments offer a range of advantages over broth and agar dilution methods. The reagents, in particular cards or plates, are provided by the manufacturer and if they have been transported and stored appropriately prior to use, they require only minimal quality control. The incubation/reading instruments come with associated software which undertakes interpretation of antibiograms in addition to interpreting growth endpoints. This can flag unusual results or the requirement for additional testing automatically, especially if the susceptibility testing is conducted simultaneously with instrument for organism identification. Semi-automated instruments also reduce the risk of variation in inoculum preparation and reader interpretation of endpoints. Most importantly, results are available more rapidly with instruments than with other methods of susceptibility testing. Typical times to generate results are in the range of 4-8 h. Laboratory working hours may need to be adjusted to get the benefit of these faster times because the susceptibility results must be communicated to the caring clinician who in turn needs to be available to receive them.

Issues

In general, the overall costs of running semi-automated instruments are higher on a per isolate basis than other phenotypic tests. Hence, it is not unusual to reserve their use to isolates where rapid results would be of greatest clinical benefit, *e. g.* blood culture isolates. Not all bacteria isolated in routine clinical laboratories will be able to be tested using semi-automated instruments. Hence, it is necessary to have other phenotypic testing methods available.

In published evaluations, semi-automated methods show a general good performance. One or the other is at times in disrepute from not picking up a specific resistance mechanism (low-medium level vancomycin resistance in staphylococci, carbapenemase production in a species, inducible clindamycin resistance in staphylococci). These issues are normally solved after a while but regulatory processes may result in delays.

The Phoenix® and the Microscan® methods perform a proper MIC-determination (growth or no growth in broth with 2-fold dilutions of the antibiotic in question) albeit in a limited series of concentrations one or two dilutions below and above the breakpoints. This is to save reagents and space on cards/trays. It results in a number of MIC values being listed as ≤ or ≥ the end-value of a truncated concentration series. The Vitek2® operates on "growth-curve algorithms", that is the growth dynamics in the presence of a few concentrations are calibrated to known MICs of strains used for calibration. Again series are truncated and many results are ≤ or ≥ the lowest and highest concentration. Other disadvantages to the semi-automated systems are a somewhat limited capacity, expert rules systems are dependent on the customer accepting the suggested antibiotics on cards or in trays, implementing changes in devices or cards/trays takes time, and once implemented technically and in the relevant software, it takes time to make the new package available to the customer. In some countries the processing of changes through regulatory authorities takes additional time. While waiting for revised breakpoints, breakpoints for new drugs, breakpoints to pick up new resistance mechanisms etc., laboratories often prefer to use a disk diffusion method. The latter can be rapidly adapted to new circumstances.

Disk diffusion methods

Standard methods

Disk diffusion remains the most widely used antimicrobial susceptibility testing method in routine clinical laboratories. It is suitable for testing the majority of bacterial pathogens, including the more common fastidious bacteria, such as streptococci, pneumococci, and *Haemophilus influenzae*. It is versatile in the range of antimicrobial agents that can be tested and requires no special equipment.

Disk diffusion is one of the oldest approaches to antimicrobial susceptibility testing and all currently used methods are based on the principles defined in the report of the International Collaborative Study of Antimicrobial Susceptibility Testing, 1972 (11) and the experience of expert groups worldwide.

Disk diffusion methods are based on an antibiotic concentration gradient being established in agar by the radial diffusion of the antibiotic from the diffusion centre, commonly a paper disk but in one method a tablet. The growth of the bacterium is inhibited by a certain concentration of the antibiotic and the distance from the edge of the disk at which this occurs is proportional to the MIC of the organism in a complex way (17). The concentration in the agar at the point of inhibition of growth is not known and interpretation therefore rests on the fact that the relationship between inhibition zones and MICs of representative organisms has been determined beforehand. This meets with three major problems :

- It is often not possible to guarantee the regression line in its full extent for each species and different species may well have different regression lines. The approximation obtained by using intrinsically resistant organisms in multi-species regression is inaccurate and in modern antimicrobial susceptibility testing (AST) both MICs and zone diameter breakpoints are species related to varying extent (17)
- Some antibiotics diffuse poorly (vancomycin, colistin) and for, these disk diffusion is often unsuitable.

Several breakpoint committees have developed and supported standardized disk diffusion methods; BSAC in the United Kingdom (18), CA-SFM in France (22), CLSI in the USA (5), and SRGA in Sweden (18). In each of these countries a vast majority of laboratories follow the national recommendations but with the exception of the CLSI disk diffusion method, few of the methods have followers outside the country of origin. The French and U.S. methods are both based on Mueller-Hinton agar but differ since the CA-SFM utilizes an inoculum which yields semiconfluent growth and CLSI an inoculum which yields confluent growth. The Swedish and UK methods are almost identical – both are based on Isosensitest medium and use inocula to yield semi-confluent growth. The two methods only differ on a few disk potencies.

The CLSI disk diffusion method is used widely outside the USA – in Europe, Canada, Asia, South-America and in many laboratories in Australia (5). It utilizes three types of agar; MH for non-fastidious rapidly growing micro-organisms, *Haemophilus* Test Medium (HTM) which is Mueller-Hinton agar or broth supplemented with X factor (hemin or hematin), V factor (nicotinamide adenine dinucleotide, NAD) and yeast extract, and for streptococci, including *Streptococcus pneumoniae*, MH with 5 % sheep blood. For various slow-growing microorganisms with special requirements for growth the reader is referred to the CLSI manuals. To determine the zone diameter correlates, CLSI follows the methods described in its M23 document (10).

The EUCAST is developing a disk diffusion test for routine antimicrobial susceptibility testing correlating inhibition zones to EUCAST clinical MIC breakpoints (23). The method is derived from the Kirby-Bauer method, variants of which are currently widely used in Europe. The method is based on two media, Mueller-Hinton agar without supplements (MH) for non-fastidious organisms, including enterococci, and MH with 5 % horse blood and 20 mg β-NAD/L (MH-F) for rapidly growing fastidious organisms, most importantly *Streptococcus* spp. including *Streptococcus pneumoniae* and *Haemophilus* spp. Apart from the fact that this method is calibrated to European breakpoints and that a different medium for fastidious organisms is used and that a few disk potencies are different, all other aspects of the European method are identical to the CLSI recommended disk diffusion method. This means that the two methods can be quality controlled to the same standards for non-fastidious organisms. It is assumed that laboratories in Europe will gradually embrace the European method during 2010 and 2011.

For more detailed descriptions of the respective methods we refer the reader to the manuals and web-pages of the respective methods.

Issues

Disk diffusion, like all other phenotypic susceptibility test methods, is relative and require the strictest standardization. In the laboratory it is essential not only to meticulously follow the description of how to set up the method but also to ensure that the end result meets the criteria of the standardized method. For this purpose there are published Tables of target values for all antibiotics and disk strengths encompassed by respective methods. MIC target values for non-fastidious organisms are part of the international standardization of microbroth dilution for MIC determination (14). Inhibition zone target values (and/or target ranges) are part of each of the standard methods for disk diffusion. The CLSI and EUCAST share targets for non-fastidious organisms for antibiotics where disk strengths are identical. For fastidious organisms they share MIC targets but not zone targets.

A complementary way of checking the standardization of methodology is to compare inhibition zone histograms generated in the local laboratory with those generated by the standards organization when calibrating disk diffusion to MIC-values. EUCAST makes these available on its website and they can be downloaded for comparison with locally generated histograms. That part of the distribution which represents wild type micro-organisms, *i. e.* organisms without resistance mechanisms, is readily identifiable in the graphs and its median and width serve as targets for routinely generated data (Fig. 1a and b).

Once the disk diffusion method has been validated in the routine laboratory, every day quality control to ensure the quality of media, disks, processing, etc. can be instituted.

For laboratories that wish to read zone diameter on a regular basis, there are commercially available zone readers with varying degree of automation. The most well known are Biomic®, Osiris®, and Aura®.

Gradient diffusion

In 1988 a new elegant way of measuring inhibitory concentrations was introduced (3). A plastic strip has antibiotic concentrations in variable size plastic disks attached to its backside. When placed on an agar surface preinoculated with the test bacterium, the diffusing antibiotic creates an "unlimited" series of concentration gradients in the agar. The further from the top of the strip the less antibiotic diffuses from the strip. The ensuing elipsoid inhibitory gradient results in a elipsoid inhibitory zone around the plastic strip, broad at the top and intersecting the strip at some point along the strip. The plastic strip is graded by subjecting each antibiotic strip to a number of strains with known MIC values. The original strip, produced by AB Biodisk, Sweden, was named E-test©. When the patent was void competitors developed similar strips but these have not yet been evaluated to the same extent as the E-test® which has become an integrated part of everyday microbiology.

Gradient diffusion tests are today available for many antibacterial and antifungal drugs. They have been evaluated not only for rapidly growing non-fastidious bacteria but also for more fastidious bacteria, such as anaerobes, some mycobacteria, and *Helicobacter*.

It is worth pointing out that although these tests appear easy to use and are instantly available to anyone with agar plates and a thermostat, they require knowhow on the part of the user, that the instructions of the manufacturer are followed, especially concerning media, inocula, and reading and they require that standard procedures for qua-

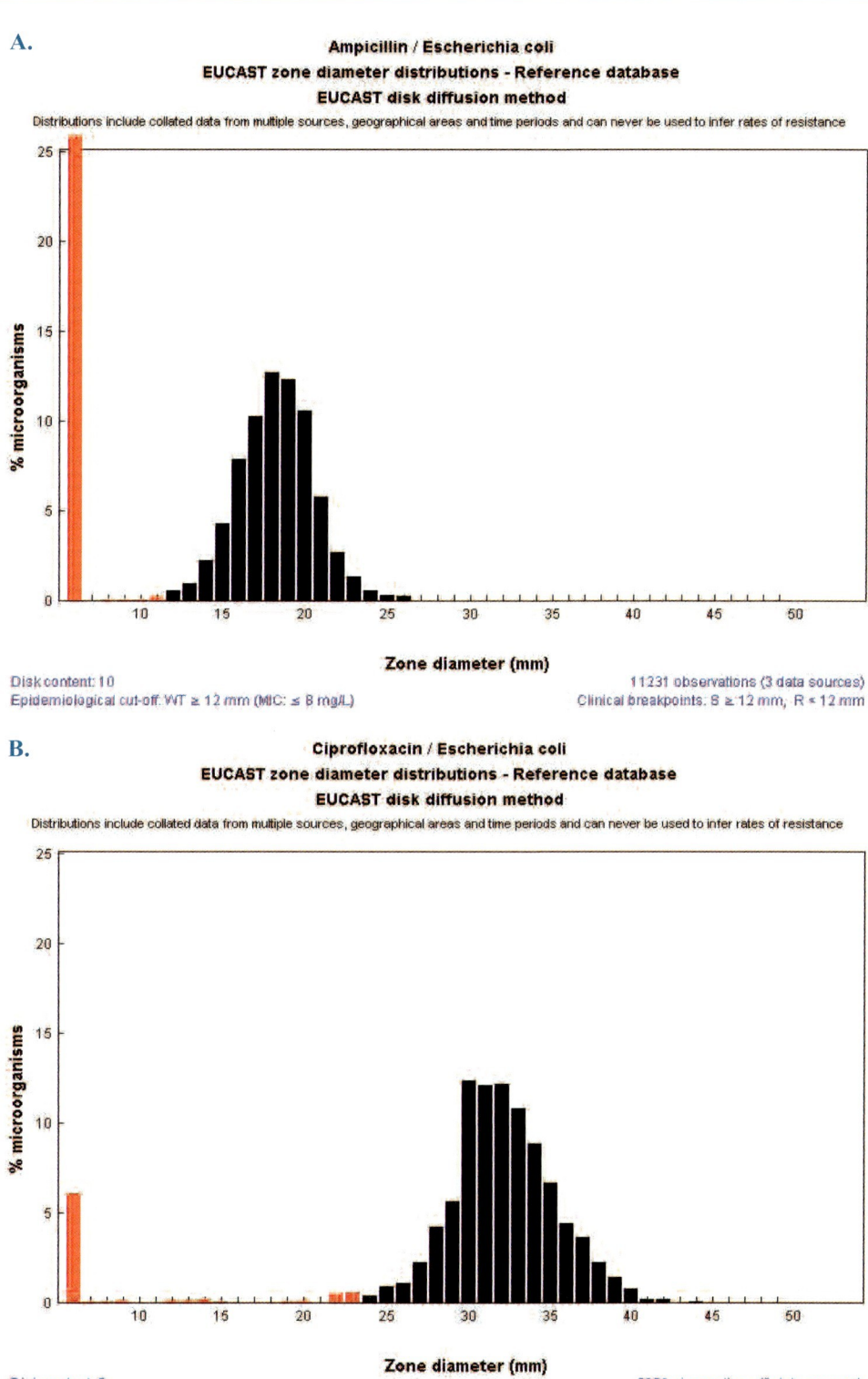

Fig. 1. *Escherichia coli* versus (A) ampicillin 10 μg and (B) ciprofloxacin 5 μg.
Inhibition zone diameter distributions on Mueller-Hinton agar using the standardized methodology of CLSI or EUCAST. Distributions are typically bell shaped and 10-14 mm wide (depending on antibiotic and disk content) with a clearly identifiable median, in the case of ampicillin 18 mm and ciprofloxacin 32 mm and epidemiological cut-offs of 12 mm for ampicillin and 26 mm for ciprofloxacin. If the method is well standardized, locally generated data should exactly match the width, the median, and the epidemiological cut-off of respective distributions.
From the EUCAST webpage (www.eucast.org).

lity control are followed. Aberrant results should always be checked. Systematically higher or lower values as compared to reference methods have been described (25).

Supplementary phenotypic tests

Not all resistance mechanisms of clinical importance can be detected satisfactorily using current dilution or diffusion methods. Alternative, so-called supplementary, tests are required or used for confirmation for these (19). Many phenotypic supplementary tests have been developed over the last few decades. The ones discussed in this section are those that have been shown to still have some practical value.

β-lactamase detection

Supplementary testing for the presence of β-lactamases in staphylococci, enterococci, *Haemophilus* spp., *Neisseria meningitidis*, *Moraxella catarrhalis,* and some Gram-negative anaerobic bacteria has been widely used in the past and still has occasional value, especially if a rapid result is required on positive cultures (19). Nitrocefin®, a chromogenic cephalosporin, has generally replaced older reagents/methods for detecting β-lactamases due to its simplicity of use. Laboratories may choose to use supplementary β-lactamase testing in selected circumstances, but in general, routine methods are designed to capture β-lactamase producing strains of the above species. The only exception to this are the very rare strains *Enterococcus faecalis* that produce β-lactamase, which routine methods fail to recognise.

Enterobacteriaceae – ESBL and carbapenemase confirmation

Standardized tests are available for the phenotypic confirmation of the presence of extended-spectrum β-lactamases (ESBLs) and carbapenemases. They are described in detail in the CLSI document M100 (6). Laboratories may choose to use these tests in addition to routine susceptibility. It is important to recognize that the ESBL tests as described do not identify the presence of plasmid-borne AmpC enzymes, which have positive screening test (are higher than the susceptible breakpoint) but a negative confirmation test. Furthermore, the CLSI carbapenemase confirmatory test (modified Hodge test) has only been thoroughly validated against KPC-producing strains, although it is known that many of the metallo-β-lactamases will be detected.

The need for confirmatory testing will largely be determined by the laboratories need to track these mechanisms of resistance for infection control purposes. With the current EUCAST breakpoints, and the new ones being published by CLSI, the great majority of strains of Enterobacteriaceae harboring these enzymes will be detected and categorized as non-susceptible by the breakpoint.

Enterococci – high-level aminoglycoside resistance

Strains of enterococci causing endocarditis should be tested for the presence of high-level aminoglycoside resistance by broth or agar screening (19). Semi-automated methods often include these tests in their panels. The combination of a cell wall active antimicrobial (β-lactam or glycopeptide) and an aminoglycoside (gentamicin or streptomycin) is synergistic for *Enterococcus* species and is considered essential to ensure the highest chance of curing endocarditis. Wild type strains of enterococci have MICs at or slightly above (e. g. gentamicin 4 – 32 µg/ml) the conventional breakpoints for aminoglycosides and cannot be treated with an aminoglycoside alone. However, synergy is preserved in these strains. Some strains harbor aminoglycoside-modifying enzymes and have very high MICs and synergy with cell wall active agents is lost. Testing endocarditis isolates of enterococci against a high gentamicin concentration (HLAR > 128 µg/ml for EUCAST and ≥ 500 µg/ml for CLSI) or streptomycin (HLAR ≥ 1000-2000 µg/ml) will detect high level resistance and predict lack of synergy. Both agents should be tested because it is usual for those strains that harbor high-level resistance to be resistant to only one of the two aminoglycosides.

Staphylococcus and Streptococcus - inducible lincosamide resistance

There is currently interest in screening staphylococci and streptococci for inducible resistance to lincosamides, lincomycin, and clindamycin (19). The rationale for this is twofold: strains of staphylococci and streptococci exist in some areas of the world which harbor the *msr*(A)-based resistance and *mef*(A)-based resistance which encode efflux pumps that generate resistance to macrolides but not lincosamides. This is in contrast to the more common *erm* gene resistance mechanism, which encodes ribosomal methylases which can either produce constitutive resistance to macrolides and lincosamides, or inducible resistance to macrolides and lincosamides inducible by macrolides. The combination of clindamycin with and without erythromycin, either in broth or as a disk approximation test, will detect whether which of the resistance patterns is expressed. It is commonly agreed that the detection of inducible lincosamide resistance should be accompanied by a warning against using lincosamides for treatment (6), especially for serious infections, due to the increased risk of treatment failure. Formal prospective studies to prove the validity of this warning are lacking.

Staphylococci – resistance and reduced susceptibility to glycopeptides

Strains of *Staphylococcus aureus* with vancomycin MICs of 4 of μg/ml (in broth or on agar, but not by gradient diffusion) are considered intermediate to vancomycin (by both CLSI and EUCAST). Teicoplanin MICs are often higher than this value for these strains. Unfortunately, there is no currently proven routine phenotypic method for the reliable detection of strains that are hetero-resistant to vancomycin, although the so-called macro E-test® looks the most promising as a screening method. Routine application of any screening test for the detection of hetero-resistance to vancomycin should only be considered if strains are considered to be prevalent in the institution(s) served by the laboratory.

REFERENCES

(1) **Amsterdam D.** 2005. Susceptibility testing in liquid media.. *In* V. Lorian (ed), Antibiotics in Laboratory Medicine. 5th ed. Lippincott Williams & Wilkins, Philadelphia PA.

(2) **Andrews, J. M.** 2001. Determination of minimum inhibitory concentrations. J. Antimicrob. Chemother. **48**:5-16.

(3) **Bolmström, A.** 1993. Susceptibility testing of anaerobes with E-test. Clin. Infect. Dis. **16** Suppl. 4:S367-370.

(4) **Clinical and Laboratory Standards Institute.** 2008. Methods for dilution antimicrobial susceptibility tests for bacteria that grow aerobically; Approved Standard–Eihth edition. CLSI document M07-A8. Clinical and Laboratory Standards Institute, Wayne, PA.

(5) **Clinical and Laboratory Standards Institute.** 2008. Performance Standards for Antimicrobial Disk Susceptibility Tests; Approved Standard–Tenth edition. CLSI document M02-A10. Clinical and Laboratory Standards Institute, Wayne, PA.

(6) **Clinical and Laboratory Standards Institute.** 2008. Performance Standards for Antimicrobial Susceptibility Testing; Approved Standard–Nineteenth edition. CLSI document M100-A19. Clinical and Laboratory Standards Institute, Wayne, PA.

(7) **Clinical and Laboratory Standards Institute.** 2007. Methods for Antimicrobial Susceptibility Testing of Anaerobic Bacteria; Approved Standard–Seventh edition. CLSI document M11-A7. Clinical and Laboratory Standards Institute, Wayne, PA.

(8) **Clinical and Laboratory Standards Institute.** 2006. Methods for Antimicrobial Dilution and Disk Susceptibility Testing of Infrequently Isolated or Fastidious Bacteria; Approved Guideline–First edition. CLSI document M45-A. Clinical and Laboratory Standards Institute, Wayne, PA.

(9) **Clinical and Laboratory Standards Institute.** 1999. Methods for Determining Bactericidal Activity of Antimicrobial Agents; Approved Guideline; Approved Guideline. CLSI document M26-A. Clinical and Laboratory Standards Institute, Wayne, PA.

(10) **Clinical and Laboratory Standards Institute.** 2008. Development of in vitro susceptibility testing criteria and quality control parameters; Approved Guideline–Third edition. CLSI document M23-A3. Clinical and Laboratory Standards Institute, Wayne, PA.

(11) **Ericsson, H. C., and J. C. Sherris**. 1971. Antibiotic sensitivity testing. Report of an international collaborative study. Acta Pathol. Microbiol. Scand. B Microbiol. Immunol. **217** Suppl B:1–90.

(12) **European Committee on Antimicrobial Susceptibility Testing (EUCAST).** 2003. Determination of minimum inhibitory concentrations (MICs) of antibacterial agents by broth dilution (EUCAST discussion document E.Dis 5.1). Clin. Microbiol. Infect. **9**:1-7.

(13) **European Committee on Antimicrobial Susceptibility Testing (EUCAST).** 2000. Determination of minimum inhibitory concentrations (MICs) of antibacterial agents by agar dilution (EUCAST discussion document E.Dis 3.1). Clin. Microbiol. Infect. **6**:509-515.

(14) **Fernández-Mazarrasa, C., O. Mazarrasa, J. Calvo, A. del Arco, and L. Martínez-Martínez** 2009. High concentrations of manganese in Mueller-Hinton agar increase MICs of tigecycline determined by E-test. J. Clin. Microbiol. **47**:827-829.

(15) **International Organization for Standardization (ISO).** 2006. Clinical laboratory testing and in vitro diagnostic test systems – Susceptibility testing of infectious agents and evaluation of performance of antimicrobial susceptibility test devices. Part 1: Reference method for testing the in vitro activity of antimicrobial agents against rapidly growing aerobic bacteria involved in infectious diseases. ISO 20776-1. Geneva: International organization for Standardization.

(16) **International Organization for Standardization (ISO)**. 2007. Clinical laboratory testing and in vitro diagnostic test systems — Susceptibility testing of infectious agents and evaluation of performance of antimicrobial susceptibility test devices. Part 2: Evaluation of performance of antimicrobial susceptibility test devices. ISO 20776-2. Geneva: International organization for Standardization.

(17) **Kronvall, G., and S. Ringertz.** 1991. Antibiotic disk diffusion testing revisited. Single strain regression analysis. Review article. APMIS **99**:295-306.

(18) **Kronvall G., G. Kahlmeter, E. Myhre, and M. F. Galas.** 2003. A new method for normalized interpretation of antimicrobial resistance from disk test results for comparative purposes. Clin. Microbiol. Infect. **9**:120–132.

(19) **MacGowan, A. P. and R. Wise.** 2001. Establishing MIC breakpoints and interpretation of *in vitro* susceptibility tests. J. Antimicrob. Chemother. **48** Suppl. S1:17-28. (updates on http://www.bsac.org.uk).

(20) **Prakash V, J. S.Lewis II, and J. H. Jorgensen.** 2008. Vancomycin MICs with methicillin-resistant *Staphylococcus aureus* (MRSA) isolates differ based upon the susceptibility test method used. Antimicrob. Agents Chemother. **52**:4528.

(21) **SFM Antibiogram Committee.** 2003 Comité de l'Antibiogramme de la Société Française de Microbiologie Report 2003. Int. J. Antimicrob. Agents. **21**:364-391. (updates on http//:www.sfm.asso.fr)

(22) **Swenson J. M., J. B. Patel, and J. H. Jorgensen.** 2007. Special phenotypic methods for detecting antibacterial resistance. *In* P. R. Murray, E. J. Barron, J. H. Jorgensen, M. L Landry, and M. A. Pfaller (ed.), Manual of clinical microbiology, 9th ed., ASM Press, Washington, DC.

(23) **The European disk diffusion test.** 2009. http://www.eucast.org

(24) **The Swedish Reference Group of Antibiotics.** 1997. Antimicrobial susceptibility testing in Sweden, Scand. J. Infect. Dis., Suppl. **105**:5-31. (updates on http://www.srga.org).

(25) **Turnidge J. D., and J. M. Bell.** 2005. Antimicrobial susceptibility on solid media. *In* V. Lorian (ed.), Antibiotics in Laboratory Medicine. 5th ed. Lippincott Williams & Wilkins, Philadelphia, PA.

Chapter 7. GENOTYPIC TECHNIQUES

Marie-Cécile PLOY

INTRODUCTION

Over the course of several decades, bacteria have acquired resistance to all the different classes of antibiotics, making it necessary for clinicians to rapidly identify the causal pathogen but also, and above all, to determine its susceptibility to antibiotics. This is especially true in the case of severe infections in frail patients, where a delay in antibiotic administration, or use of an inappropriate antibiotic, could be fatal (29, 48). Various biochemical and immunological methods, as well as automated systems, have considerably shortened the time required to detect resistance. However, all these techniques require isolation of the bacterial strain. New genotypic techniques for the detection of antibiotic resistance have been developed over the past ten years (10), but they have not yet forged a place as routine diagnostic methods in microbiology laboratories.

ADVANTAGES

Genotypic methods have advantages over phenotypic methods in the following circumstances:
- For slow-growing or fastidious bacteria such as anaerobes, *Helicobacter pylori, Chlamydia, Legionella, Mycobacterium, Rickettsia, Treponema, Brucella*. The use of genotypic methods shortens the response time and provides a more reliable result.
- These methods can be used directly on the pathological specimen.
- When a rapid response is needed, notably in the case of severe infections. For example, in staphylococcal infections, even automated systems cannot give a rapid response for methicillin susceptibility, whereas detection of the *mecA* gene by PCR takes only a few hours.
- In cases of low-level resistance. When resistance is weakly expressed *in vitro*, phenotypic techniques may not detect it even though a resistance gene is present. Yet this resistance may be more strongly expressed *in vivo*, resulting in treatment failure. This is more often the case when resistance is conferred by inactivating enzymes. For instance, with the aminoglycosides, the genes encoding certain inactivating enzymes such as *aac(6')-Ic* may be weakly expressed (40).
- Detection of a resistance gene has a universal value, as opposed to breakpoints which may not be the same in different countries, leading to different clinical categorizations of a same strain and a same antibiotic. In particular, genotypic methods can confirm the presence or absence of resistance in strains for which the MIC of an antibiotic is close to the upper critical concentration (22).
- Genotypic techniques are more informative than the antibiogram for the surveillance of epidemics caused by resistant bacteria. This is because one or more resistance genes carried on a plasmid or transposon may propagate among strains of different species. Genotypic methods not only detect the gene but also the genetic element that carries the gene, thereby identifying plasmid- or transposon-borne outbreaks.

DRAWBACKS

- Only known resistance genes can be detected. Genotypic methods cannot detect new resistance determinants, in contrast to the "conventional" antibiogram which examines the behavior of the strain with respect to the antibiotic, allowing detection of a novel phenotype. Furthermore, there are some resistances for which the genes have not been clearly identified or which are multifactorial. In such cases, genotypic methods will not be very informative. This is true for example in *Staphylococcus aureus* strains with reduced glycopeptide susceptibility (GISA), which are difficult to detect phenotypically but for which no genotypic test exists, since resistance appears to be mediated by multiple determinants.
- Phenotypic methods describe the behavior between the strain and the antibiotic and therefore reveal the level of expression. Unlike the

example of the aminoglycosides described earlier, in some situations it is more important to know the level of expression of resistance, *i.e.*, the MIC, than to detect the resistance genes themselves (22). For example, in pneumococcal infections, the probability of clinical success is directly related to the MIC of β-lactams for the strain and the site of infection. Different mosaic PBP genes with lower affinity have been described, but their presence does not predict the level of expression. Also, regulatory mutations causing overexpression of a chromosomal (housekeeping) gene and thereby conferring resistance are not detectable because they have not been identified.

- Genotypic methods only give information about resistance and not susceptibility. The absence of a resistance gene does not necessarily mean that the strain is susceptible to the antibiotic. Rolain et al. (38) used real-time PCR to study antibiotic susceptibility by quantifying the number of DNA copies in the presence or absence of antibiotics. Results were available in 2 h for Gram-negative bacilli and in 4 h for Gram-positive cocci.
- Genotypic methods have not been standardized, so sensitivity and specificity depend on the approach used.

METHODS

Antibiotic resistance can be due to the acquisition of a foreign gene or to mutations in structural or regulatory genes intrinsic to the bacteria. Accordingly, different strategies will be used. Many methods for the detection of resistance genes are based on amplification of the gene by PCR (46), sometimes confirmed solely by electrophoretic determination of the size of the amplification product, but usually by other methods including hybridization, restriction fragment length polymorphism (PCR-RFLP) or sequencing. Many publications describe oligonucleotide primer pairs specific for a resistance gene, while other groups have developed multiplex PCR methods allowing several resistance genes to be detected in a single reaction. Real-time PCR has also been used to detect antibiotic resistance. This technique has the advantage of a rapid response time and differs from conventional PCR because it quantifies DNA amplification in real time using a fluorescent reporter molecule (7). A number of resistance gene detection kits are now on the market; one example is the IDI-MRSA kit which detects methicillin-resistant *S. aureus* (MRSA) by PCR amplification of a product specific of the SCCmec cassette, which harbors the methicillin resistance gene. Recently, more highly automated systems have been developed, including Septifast® (Roche) and GeneXpert® (Cepheid). The latter integrates DNA extraction and amplification, delivering a result in under two hours directly from positive blood culture bottles, nasal or skin swabs (33, 39).

However, some antibiotic resistance genes may be variably expressed, depending on mutations in the promoter region or the presence of an upstream insertion sequence (11). The use of quantitative PCR techniques would therefore be useful to provide additional information on the amount of enzyme produced.

Other non-PCR amplification methods have been described, including the branched-DNA assay which uses several copies of a same probe amplifying the chemoluminescent signal and not the DNA (9, 14). Sequencing of PCR products, as well as restriction fragment length polymorphism, are also widely used to detect mutations. Some methods couple PCR with Single Strand Conformation Polymorphism (SSCP), based on denaturing electrophoresis that can distinguish a wild-type strain from a mutant strain by differences in electrophoretic mobility (9, 44), or Denaturing High Performance Liquid Chromatography (DHPLC), based on heteroduplex analysis (5). In all these cases, sequencing of amplification products is the reference method to characterize a PCR product. The availability of automatic sequencers will promote the use of this technique since costs have dropped considerably in the past few years. Other PCR-derived methods are used as well, including PCR-LiPA which consists in identifying the amplified fragment with a specific probe immobilized on a nitrocellulose strip; the biotinylated PCR product is then visualized with the aid of a chromogenic substrate (9).

Finally, the recent development of DNA chips containing thousands of probes has a definite advantage when it comes to detecting resistance genes or mutations, especially when resistance is due to different mechanisms or to an accumulation of mutations (4). PCR assays coupled to microchip technology have also been used to detect resistance genes and mutations (41, 50), although these tools have not yet been adapted for routine use in the microbiology laboratory.

β-LACTAMS

Staphylococci and methicillin resistance

The routine test most widely used by microbiology laboratories is detection of the staphylococcal methicillin resistance gene *mecA*. *mecA* resistance can be difficult to detect by phenotypic methods, especially when it is expressed in a heterogeneous manner, and moreover the strain may be falsely reported as resistant due to penicillinase hyperproduction. Several publications describe PCR assays to detect either *mecA* alone or multiplex PCR which detects the *mecA* gene and another gene specific to the genus *Staphylococcus* or the species *S. aureus* (*nuc, coa, femA, femB*, ARNr 16S,…) (9, 14). Real-time PCR has also been used for detection of the *mecA* gene; this method is rapid and thus very useful to the clinician, especially since it can be carried out directly on a specimen as in the case of Septifast® or GeneXpert® (16, 33, 36, 39, 40). Branched-DNA assays have also been used (19).

Pneumococci and β-lactam resistance

Six structural genes encoding penicillin binding proteins (PBPs) have been described in pneumococci. The mosaic genes *pbp*1a, 2b, and 2x encoding PBPs with lower affinity for β-lactams have been characterized. These genes are the result of DNA recombination between different pneumococcal strains or between pneumococci and other oropharyngeal commensal streptococci. PCR and PCR-RFLP techniques have been described to detect these mosaic genes (13, 14). However, in clinical practice it is more important to determine the level of resistance and therefore the MIC. Furthermore, a multitude of combinations are possible among these mosaic genes. For these reasons, molecular methods find their principal value in epidemiology for monitoring the dissemination of resistance genes between different strains over time.

Gram-negative bacteria and resistance due to β-lactamase production

Many β-lactamases have been identified and numerous PCR or hybridization methods have been described to detect the genes encoding these different enzymes (TEM, SHV, OXA, CARB, metalloenzymes, etc.) (for a review, see 14). In the case of the β-lactamases, two genotypic detection strategies exist side by side: detection of a resistance gene and detection of mutations. For example, in the case of the TEM or SHV penicillinases, the phenotype varies according to the mutations, particularly with respect to resistance to third generation cephalosporins. Hybridization methods using a panel of probes were first used to identify the different β-lactamase genes in 1990 (26). PCR coupled with restriction fragment length polymorphism or SSCP has also been used to differentiate these different mutations (14). More recently, real-time PCR methods have been proposed (35, 49). In the future, DNA chips which can contain a virtually unlimited number of probes will make β-lactamase detection even easier and faster, with response times under four hours (15).

AMINOGLYCOSIDES

Aminoglycoside resistance is attributable mainly to the acquisition of inactivating enzymes, of which there are three main classes: aminoglycoside phosphotransferases (APH), nucleotidyltransferases (ANT) and acetyltransferases (AAC). Several enzymes may coexist in the same bacterium, making their detection even more difficult by conventional phenotypic methods. Gram-positive organisms harbor few inactivating enzymes, so their detection by PCR is fairly simple. In Gram-negative bacteria, however, different resistance genes may be present in the same bacterium and, furthermore, some enzymes have many genetic determinants, as in the case of the AAC(6')-I genes where more than 25 structural genes encoding an acetyltransferase conferring the same resistance pattern have been identified. Several PCR and hybridization techniques have been described (9, 14). Multiplex PCR allowing identification of more than one gene, and degenerate primers allowing amplification of genes encoding related enzymes, are available (31, 34). Genotypic methods have an added advantage in the case of aminoglycosides because in some cases the level of resistance depends on regulatory genes. Thus, resistance may not be detected *in vitro* but be expressed *in vivo*. Direct detection of a resistance gene obviates this problem. Nonetheless, genotypic detection has its limitations. For instance, in the case of AAC(6')-I and AAC(6')-II, a point mutation causing a leucine/serine amino acid substitution changes the resistance phenotype (20). AAC(6')-I enzymes inactive netilmicin, tobramycin and amikacin but not gentamicin, while AAC(6')-II inactivate gentamicin but not amikacin. The PCR or hybridization methods employed for the genotypic detection of aminoglycoside resistance, described to date, do not test for this mutation. This illustrates how genotypic and phenotypic methods can complement each other, since in this case, it is the phenotype which suggests the genotype.

GLYCOPEPTIDES

Genotypic techniques have been widely used to study glycopeptide resistance, leading to the identification of the *van* alphabet in enterococci. The different *van* resistance determinants exist alongside their corresponding regulatory genes (11). The *vanA* operon can be readily detected by phenotypic methods because it confers high-level resistance to vancomycin and teicoplanin. However, other *van* determinants confer lower level resistance with MICs close to the breakpoint, making their detection more problematic. Specific primers allowing amplification of the different *van* genes have been described and multiplex PCR has been used (12). PCR can be followed by RFLP analysis (9). PCR detection of the *van* genes is a genotypic assay routinely carried out in several microbiology laboratories using "in-house" techniques. Real-time PCR kits for detection of the *vanA* and *vanB* genes have recently become available.

MACROLIDES - LINCOSAMIDES - STREPTOGRAMINS (MLS)

The distinct mechanisms of resistance to MLS antibiotics have been characterized. One of the first mechanisms to be described is target site modification by methylation of an adenine in the 23S rRNA, conferring an MLS_B phenotype. These methylases are encoded by *erm* genes (*e*rythromycin *r*ibosome *m*ethylation), more than 30 of which have been identified. Primers have been generated to amplify these genes by multiplex PCR or specific of each gene (14, 37), in some cases followed by hybridization or sequencing to confirm the results. Degenerate primers allowing amplification of several *erm* genes have also been described (2). DNA chips and real-time PCR (37) assays are still other techniques used to detect MSL resistance.

More recently, another resistance mechanism based on efflux has been identified. The resistance determinants identified in Gram-positive cocci are the genes *mef* [*mef(A)* described in *Streptococcus pyogenes* and *mef*(E) in *S. pneumoniae*], *msr* and *vga*. The *mef* genes confer resistance to macrolides but not to lincosamides or streptogramins, while the *msr* genes confer resistance to macrolides and type B streptogramins. Two genes, *msrA* and *msrB*, have been characterized in *S. aureus*. Two other putative efflux systems – the *vga* systems – have been described in *S. aureus* and confer resistance only to type A streptogramins. These various genes can be detected by PCR with the aid of specific primers (14, 24, 43, 55).

Macrolide resistance can also be due to inactivating enzymes (esterases, phosphorylases, transferases and hydrolyases) (37). The lyases that inactivate streptogramins B are encoded by the *vgb* genes and have been described in *Enterococcus* and *Staphylococcus*. The EreA and EreB esterases conferring erythromycin resistance have been found in Gram-negative organisms. The acetyltransferases which inactivate lincosamides and streptogramins A are encoded by different genes (*vat, sat*), while the phosphotransferases which inactivate macrolides are encoded by the *mph* genes and have been described in *S. aureus* as well as Gram-negative bacteria. The nucleotidyltransferases conferring lincomycin resistance are encoded by *lin* or *lnu* genes described in *Enterococcus* and *Staphylococcus*. Genotypic detection assays, mainly based on PCR, have been developed for some of these genes (14, 24, 42).

The final mechanism of MLS resistance is mutations that decrease the antibiotic's affinity for its target. Mutations in the 23S rRNA were initially described in *Mycobacterium avium* and *Helicobacter pylori*, then subsequently found in many other species (45). Mutations in riboproteins L22 and L4 have also been identified in different genera (37). To detect these mutations, the three genes coding for ribosomal proteins *rplD, rplV* and *rrl* must be characterized. Different groups have developed genotypic assays to detect these mutations; these tests are truly useful for routine diagnostics of *H. pylori*, a fastidious species for which the response time for phenotypic tests is long. Different strategies have been used, including PCR with confirmation by hybridization and visualization by ELISA, hybridization, PCR and sequencing, PCR-RFLP, or PCR-LiPA (14). In Gram-positive cocci, Canu et al. (5) described a PCR assay coupled with denaturing high performance liquid chromatography which allows automation of the method and delivers a rapid response (6 min per sample).

QUINOLONES

The targets of quinolones are the type II topoisomerases, DNA gyrase, and topoisomerase IV, each of which is composed of two subunits, A and B, encoded by the genes *gyrA* and *gyrB* (gyrase) and *parC* and *parE* (IV). The two main mechanisms underlying quinolone resistance are target modification due to mutations in the topoisomerase genes, and efflux.

PCR coupled with sequencing is the most widely used method for detection of topoisomerase mutations (14), although other resistance detection methods have been described, including PCR-SSCP (32) and PCR-RFLP. A PCR method using a primer specific for the Threonine86Isoleucine mutation, frequently found in *Campylobacter coli*, has been developed but has the drawback of only detecting this mutation (54). Another PCR method specific for mutations at defined positions has been described (14). Real-time PCR can be used to detect quinolone resistance (21, 52). Lastly, since the mutations map to well defined regions, the development of DNA chips should make them easier to detect (53). Recently, different plasmid-encoded quinolone resistance genes have been described: the *qnr* genes confer resistance through protection of DNA gyrase (6, 17, 27, 47); the *aac(6')-Ib-cr* gene [a derivative of *aac(6')-Ib*] codes for an inactivating enzyme resulting in resistance to aminoglycosides and quinolones, and *qepA* encodes an efflux protein. These different genes can be detected by PCR (25).

TETRACYCLINES

There are two main mechanisms of tetracycline resistance: efflux and ribosomal protection. The many *tet* genes which confer this resistance have been characterized (23) and different genotypic methods based on hybridization and especially PCR, alone or coupled with hybridization, have been proposed (1, 14). Multiplex PCR methods allowing the detection of 35 tetracycline resistance genes have been published (8). These methods are useful for slow-growing or fastidious bacteria, *Mycoplasma*, *Ureaplasma*, *Neisseria gonorrhoeae*. The only drawback is related to the multitude of *tet* genes, which requires the use of different primer pairs for their detection. DNA microarrays for simultaneous large-scale screening of many different probes have also been described (4).

TRIMETHOPRIM AND SULFONAMIDES

Trimethoprim resistance is due mainly to the acquisition of a dihydropteroate synthase *dfr* gene with no selectivity for trimethoprim. Many *dfr* genes have been described and many are carried by integrons. Genotypic detection methods based on hybridization or PCR have been developed (14) but an accurate identification of the *dfr* gene requires sequencing of the amplification product, since the different genes share a high level of homology.

Sulfonamide resistance is conferred by three genes: *sul1*, *sul2* and *sul3*. *sul1* is very common and is carried by integrons (28). Probes and primer pairs allowing the amplification of this gene have been described (14). Byrne-Bayley et al. (3) recently described a PCR method to detect the three *sul* genes.

SPECIAL CASE OF MYCOBACTERIA

Genotypic methods are particularly useful in the case of the mycobacteria. These organisms are difficult to cultivate and grow slowly, sometimes requiring several weeks before susceptibility test results become available. Genotypic tests for detection of resistance to rifampicin, isoniazid and pyrazinamide have been described (9, 30). Many techniques are available, including PCR-RFLP, PCR-SSCP, PCR and sequencing, real-time PCR, PCR-LiPA as well as other, more complex methods that are difficult to implement in a routine diagnostics laboratory (9, 51). PCR-SSCP has been coupled with *rpoB* gene sequencing for simultaneous identification of the species (18). It is very important to detect rifampin resistance because most resistant strains are also resistant to isoniazid. Several commercial kits are now available, for instance the INNOLIPA-Rif.TB® kit from InnoGenetics that uses the LiPA technique to detect rifampin resistance or the Xpert MTB/RIF® kit from Cepheid that concomitantly allows the identification of M. tuberculosis and the detection of the resistance to rifampin.

CONCLUSION

Genotypic methods have been widely used to detect resistance to antibiotics. Yet, few are in routine use today by microbiology laboratories, either because they are still too costly or because they are still too complex and laborious. In most cases, then, these methods complement the phenotypic approach and serve as an adjunct to the clinical reporting procedure. For some bacterial species, however, they provide the clinician with a rapid and reliable response. Today, the most widely used routine methods include *mecA* gene detection, testing for glycopeptide resistance in enterococci, and detection of rifampin resistance in *M. tuberculosis*.

If these methods are to become more widespread in the future, clinical studies will be needed to evaluate the outcomes of patients whose antibiotic therapy was guided in part by genotypic tests to detect resistance.

REFERENCES

(1) **Aminov, R.I., N. Garrigues-Jeanjean, and R.I. Mackie**. 2001. Molecular ecology of tetracycline resistance: Development and validation of primers for detection of tetracycline resistance genes encoding ribosomal protection proteins. Appl. Environ. Microbiol. **67**:22-32.

(2) **Arthur, M., C. Molinas, C. Mabilat, and P. Courvalin**. 1990. Detection of erythromycin resistance by the polymerase chain reaction using primers in conserved regions of *erm* rRNA methylases genes. Antimicrob. Agents Chemother. **34**:2024-2026.

(3) **Byrne-Bailey, K.G, W.H. Gaze, P. Kay, A.B. Boxall, P.M. Hawkey, and E.M. Wellington**. 2009. Prevalence of sulfonamide resistance genes in bacterial isolates from manured agricultural soils and pig slurry in the United Kingdom. Antimicrob. Agents Chemother. **53**:696-702.

(4) **Call, D.R., M.C. Bakko, M.J. Krug, and M.C. Roberts**. 2003. Identifying antimicrobial resistance genes with DNA microarrays. Antimicrob. Agents Chemother. **47**: 3290-3295.

(5) **Canu, A., A. Abbas, Malbruny, B. Malbruny, F. Sichel, and R. Leclercq**. 2004. Denaturing high-performance liquid chromatography detection of ribosomal mutations conferring macrolide resistance in Gram-positive cocci. Antimicrob. Agents Chemother. **48**: 297-304.

(6) **Cavaco, L.M., Hasman, H., Xia, S., and F.M. Aarestrup**. 2009. *qnrD*, a novel gene conferring transferable quinolone resistance in *Salmonella enterica* serovar Kentucky and Bovismorbificans strains of human origin. Antimicrob Agents Chemother **53**: 603-608.

(7) **Chomarat, M., et F. Breysse**. 2004. PCR en temps réel en bactériologie. Spectra Biol. **23**:59-61.

(8) **Chopra, I., and M. Roberts**. 2001. Tetracycline antibiotics: mode of action, applications, molecular biology, and epidemiology of bacterial resistance. Microbiol. Mol. Biol. Rev. **65**:232-260.

(9) **Cockerill, F.R.** 1999. Genetic methods for assessing antimicrobial resistance. Antimicrob. Agents Chemother. **43**:199-212.

(10) **Courvalin, P.** 1991. Genotypic approach to the study of bacterial resistance to antibiotics. Antimicrob. Agents Chemother. **35**:1019-1023.

(11) **Depardieu, F., M.G. Bonora, P.E. Reynolds, and P. Courvalin**. 2003. The *vanG* glycopeptide resistance operon from *Enterococcus faecalis* revisited. Mol. Microbiol. **50**:931-948.

(12) **Depardieu, F., B. Périchon, and P. Courvalin**. 2004. Detection of the *van* alphabet and identification of enterococci and staphylococci at the species level by multiplex PCR. J. Clin. Microbiol. **42**: 5857-5860.

(13) **Doit, C., C. Loukil, F. Fitoussi, P. Geslin, and E. Bingen**. 1999. Emergence in France of multiple clones of clinical *Streptococcus pneumoniae* isolates with high-level resistance to amoxicillin. Antimicrob. Agents Chemother. **43**:1480-1483.

(14) **Fluit, A.D.C., M.R. Visser, and F.J. Schmitz**. 2001. Molecular detection of antimicrobial resistance. Clin. Microb. Rev. **14**:836-871.

(15) **Grimm, V., S. Ezaki, M. Susa, C. Knabbe, R.D. Schmid, and T.T. Bachmann**. 2004. Use of DNA microarrays for rapid genotyping of TEM -lactamases that confer resistance. J. Clin. Microbiol. **42**:3766-3774.

(16) **Grisold, A.J., E. Leitner, G. Mühlbauer, E. Marth, and H.H. Kessler**. 2002. Detection of methicillin-resistant *Staphylococcus aureus* and simultaneous confirmation by automated nucleic acid extraction and real-time PCR. J. Clin. Microb. **40**:2392-2397.

(17) **Jacoby, G., V. Cattoir, D. Hooper, L. Martinez-Martinez, P. Nordmann, A. Pascual, L. Poirel, and M. Wang**. 2008. *qnr* gene nomenclature. Antimicrob. Agents Chemother. **52**: 2297-2299

(18) **Kim, B.J., K.H. Lee, Y.J. Yun, E.M. Park, Y.G. Park, G.H. Bai, C.Y. Cha, Y.H. Kook**. 2004. Simultaneous identification of rifampin-resistant *Mycobacterium tuberculosis* and nontuberculous mycobacteria by polymerase chain reaction-single strand conformation polymorphism and sequence analysis of the RNA polymerase gene (*rpoB*). J. Microbiol. Methods. **58**:111-118.

(19) **Kolbert, C.P., J. Arruda, P. Varda-Delmore, X. Zheng, M. Lewis, J. Kolberg, and D.H. Persing**. 1998. Branched-DNA assay for detection of the *mecA* gene in oxacillin-resistant and oxacillin-sensitive staphylococci. J Clin. Microbiol. **36**: 2640-2644.

(20) **Lambert, T., M.C. Ploy, and P. Courvalin**. 1994. A spontaneous point mutation in the *aac(6')-Ib'* gene results in altered substrate specificity of aminoglycoside 6'-*N*-acetyltransferase. FEMS Microbiol. Lett. **115**:297-304.

(21) **Lapierre, P., A. Huletsky, V. Fortin, F.J. Picard, P.H. Roy, M. Ouelette, and M.G. Bergeron**. 2003. Real-time PCR assay for detection of fluoroquinolone resistance associated with *grlA* mutations in *Staphylococcus aureus*. J. Clin. Microbiol. **41**:3246-3251.

(22) **Leclercq, R.** 2000. Détection moléculaire de la résistance aux antibiotiques, pp. 709-714. In J. Fréney, F. Renaud, W. Hansen, C. Bollet (eds). Précis de Bactériologie clinique. Eska, Paris.

(23) **Levy, S.B., L.M. McMurry, T.M. Barbosda, T.M.V. Burdett, P. Courvalin, W. Hillen, M.C. Roberts, J.I. Rood, and D.E. Taylor**. 1999. Nomenclature for new tetracycline resistance determinants. Antimicrob. Agents Chemother. **43**:1523-1524.

(24) **Lina, G., A. Quaglia, M.E. Reverdy, R. Leclercq, F. Vandenesch, and J. Etienne**. 1999. Distribution of genes encoding resistance to macrolides, lincosa-

mides, and streptogramins among staphylococci. Antimicrob. Agents. Chemother. **43**:1062-1066.

(25) **Ma, J., Z. Zeng, Z. Chen, X. Xu, X. Wang, Y. Deng, D. Lü, L. Huang, Y. Zhang, J. Liu, and M. Wang.** 2009. High prevalence of plasmid-mediated quinolone resistance determinants *qnr*, *aac(6')-Ib-cr*, and *qepA* among ceftiofur-resistant *Enterobacteriaceae* isolates from companion and food-producing animals. Antimicrob. Agents Chemother. **53**:519-524.

(26) **Mabilat, C., and P. Courvalin.** 1990. Development of "oligotyping" for characterization and molecular epidemiology of TEM -lactamases in *Enterobacteriaceae*. Antimicrob. Agents Chemother. **34**:2210-2216.

(27) **Martinez-Martinez, L., A. Pascual, and G.A. Jacoby.** 1998. Quinolone resistance from a transferable plasmid. Lancet **351**:797-799.

(28) **Mazel, D., B. Dychinco, V.A. Webb, and J. Davies.** 2000. Antibiotic resistance in the ECOR collection: integrons and identification of a novel *aad* gene. Antimicrob. Agents Chemother. **44**:1568-1574.

(29) **Meehan, T.P., M.J. Fine, H.M. Krumholz, J.D. Scinto, D.H. Galusha, J.T. Mockalis, G.F. Weber, M.K. Petrillo, P.M. Houck, and J.M. Fine.** 1997. Quality of care, process, and outcomes in elderly patients with pneumonia. JAMA. **278**:2080-2084.

(30) **Nachamkin, I., C. Kang, and M.P. Weinstein.** 1997. Detection of resistance to isoniazid, rifampin, and streptomycin in clinical isolates of *Mycobacterium tuberculosis* by molecular methods. Clin. Infect. Dis. **24**:894-900.

(31) **Noppe-Leclercq, I., F. Wallet, S. Haentjens, R. Courcol, and M. Simonet.** 1999. PCR detection of aminoglycoside resistance genes: a rapid molecular typing method for *Acinetobacter baumannii*. Res. Microbiol. **150**:317-322.

(32) **Ouabdesselam, S., D.C. Hooper, J. Tankovic, and C.J. Soussy.** 1995. Detection of *gyrA* and *gyrB* mutations in quinolone-resistant clinical isolates of *Escherichia coli* by single-strand conformational polymorphism analysis and determination of levels of resistance conferred by two different single *gyrA* mutations. Antimicrob. Agents Chemother. **39**:1667-1670.

(33) **Parta, M., M. Goebel, M. Matloobi, C. Stager, and D.M. Musher.** 2009. Identification of methicillin-resistant or methicillin-susceptible *Staphylococcus aureus* by GeneXpert in blood cultures and wound swabs. J. Clin. Microbiol. **47**:1609-1610.

(34) **Ploy, M.C., T. Lambert, H. Giamarellou, P. Bourlioux, and P. Courvalin.** Detection of *aac(6')-I* genes in amikacin resistant *Acinetobacter* spp. by the polymerase chain reaction. Antimicrob. Agents Chemother. **38**:2925-2928.

(35) **Randegger, C.C., and H. Hachler.** 2001. Real-time PCR and melting curve analysis for reliable and rapid detection of SHV extended-spectrum beta-lactamases. Antimicrob. Agents Chemother. **45**:1730-1736.

(36) **Reisch, U., H.J. Linde, M. Metz, B. Leppmeier, and N. Lehn.** 2000. Rapid identification of methicillin-resistant *Staphylococcus aureus* and simultaneous species confirmation using real-time fluorescence PCR. J. Clin. Microbiol. **38**:2429-2433.

(37) **Roberts, M.C.** 2004. Resistance to macrolide, lincosamide, streptogramin, ketolide, and oxazolidinone antibiotics. Mol. Biotechnol. **28**:47-62.

(38) **Rolain, J.M., Mallet M.N., Fournier P.E., and D. Raoult.** 2004. Real-time PCR for universal antibiotic susceptibility testing. J. Antimicrob. Chemother. **54**:538-541.

(39) **Rossney, A.S., C.M. Herra, G.I. Brennan, P.M. Morgan, and B. O'Connell.** 2009. Evaluation of the Xpert methicillin-resistant *Staphylococcus aureus* (MRSA) assay using the GeneXpert real-time PCR platform for rapid detection of MRSA from screening specimens. J. Clin. Microbiol. **46**:3285-3290.

(40) **Shaw, K.J., P.N. Rather, F.J. Sabatelli, P. Mann, H. Munayyer, R. Mierzwa, G.L. Petrikkos, R.S. Hare, G.H. Miller, P. Bennett, and P. Downey.** 1992. Characterization of the chromosomal *aac(6')-Ic* gene from *Serratia marcescens*. Antimicrob. Agents Chemother. **36**:1447-1455.

(41) **Strizhkov, B.N., A.L. Drobyshev, V.M. Mikhailovich, and A.D. Mirzabekov.** 2000. PCR amplification on a microarray of gel-immobilized oligonucleotides: detection of bacterial toxin-and drug-resistant genes and their mutations. Biotechniques. **29**:844-852.

(42) **Strommenger, B., C. Kettlitz. G. Werner, and W. Witte.** 2003. Multiplex PCR assay for simultaneous detection of nine clinically relevant antibiotic resistance genes in *Staphylococcus aureus*. J. Clin. Microb. **41**: 4089-4094.

(43) **Sutcliffe, J., T. Grebe, A. Tait-Kamradt, and L. Wondrak.** 1996. Detection of erythromycin-resistant determinants by PCR. Antimicrob. Agents Chemother. **40**:2562-2566.

(44) **Telenti, A., P. Imboden, F. Marchesi, T. Schmidheini, and T. Bodmer.** 1993. Direct automated detection of rifampin-resistant *Mycobacterium tuberculosis* by polymerase chain reaction and single-strand conformation polymorphism analysis. Antimicrob. Agents Chemother. **37**:2054-2058.

(45) **Vester, B., and S. Douthwaite.** 2001. Macrolide resistance conferred by base substitutions in 23S rRNA. Antimicrob. Agents Chemother. **44**:1-12.

(46) **Visser, M.R., and A.C. Fluit.** 1995. Amplification methods for the detection of bacterial resistance genes. J. Microbiol. Methods. **23**:105-116.

(47) **Wang, M., Guo, Q., Xu, X., Wang, X., Ye, X., Wu, S., and D.C. Hooper.** 2009. New plasmid-mediated quinolone resistance gene, *qnrC*, found in a clinical isolate of *Proteus mirabilis*. Antimicrob. Agents Chemother. **53**:1892-1897.

(48) **Weinstein, M.P., M.L. Towns, S.M. Quartey, S. Mirrett, L.G. Reimer, G. Parmigiani, and L.B. Reller.** 1997. The clinical significance of positive blood cultures in the 1990s: a prospective comprehensive evaluation of the microbiology, epidemiology, and outcome of bacteremia and fungemia in adults. Clin. Infect. Dis. **24**:584-602.

(49) **Weldhagen, G.F.** 2004. Rapid detection and sequence-specific differentiation of extended-spectrum -lactamase GES-2 from *Pseudomonas aeruginosa*. Antimicrob. Agents Chemother. **48**:4059-4062.

(50) **Westin, A., C. Miller, D. Vollmer, D. Canter, R. Radtkey, M. Nerenberg, and J.P. O'Connell.** 2001. Antimicrobial resistance and bacterial identification

utilizing a microelectronic chip array. J. Clin. Microbiol. **39**:1097-1104.

(51) **Williams, D.L., L. Spring, T.P. Gillis, M. Salfinger, and D.H. Persing.** 1998. Evaluation of a polymerase chain reaction-based universal heteroduplex generator assay for direct detection of rifampin susceptibility of *Mycobacterium tuberculosis* from sputum specimens. Clin. Infect. Dis. **26**:446-450.

(52) **Wilson, D.L., S.R. Abner, T.C. Newman, L.S. Mansfield, and J.E. Linz**. 2000. Identification of ciprofloxacin-resistant *Campylobacter jejuni* by use of a fluorogenic PCR assay. **38**:3971-3978.

(53) **Yu, X., M. Susa, C. Knabbe, R.D. Schmid, and T.T. Bachmann.** 2004. Development and validation of a diagnostic DNA microarray to detect quinolone-resistant *Escherichia coli* among clinical isolates. J. Clin. Microbiol. **42**:4083-4091.

(54) **Zirnstein, G., B. Li, B. Swaminathan, and F. Angulo**. 1999. Ciprofloxacin resistance in *Campylobacter jejuni* isolates: detection of *gyrA* resistance mutations by mismatch amplification mutation assay PCR and DNA sequence analysis. J. Clin. Microbiol. **37**:3276-3280.

(55) **Zolezzi, P.C., L.M. Laplana, C.R. Calvo, P.G. Cepero, M.C. Erazo, and R. Gomez-Lus.** 2004. Molecular basis of resistance to macrolides and other antibiotics in commensal viridans group streptococci and *Gemella* spp. and transfer of resistance genes to *Streptococcus pneumoniae*. Antimicrob. Agents Chemother. **48**:3462-3467.

Chapter 8. ANTIBIOTIC ASSAY

Marie-Dominique KITZIS

INTRODUCTION

The development of methods to quantitatively determine antibiotic concentrations in biological media went hand in hand with the discovery of antimicrobial agents due to the need to:
- determine the pharmacokinetic properties of these drugs,
- ensure that therapeutically effective and non-toxic concentrations are reached in patients (treatment monitoring).

As early as 1957, Y. Chabbert and A. Boulingre (2) recommended the use of antibiotic assays to monitor treatment in patients with serious infections: "There is no doubt as to the value of quantitatively determining antibiotic levels in patients with serious infectious diseases requiring complex antibiotic therapy, due to differences in metabolism from one patient to another, as well as differences in dosage and particular routes of administration". Unlike other drugs which act on an organ, antibiotics act on the bacteria which infect an organ. Antibiotic assays and treatment monitoring fall within the province of the microbiologist, who's job is to know the susceptibility of the causative bacteria and the dose-concentration-effect relationship of the different antibiotics.

Different antibiotic assay methods have been proposed, classically divided into two types:
- microbiological assay, based on the biological activity of antibiotics, which is the reference method.
- non-microbiological assays of which there are two types: immunological methods involving the ability of different haptens to compete for binding to an antibody, and chromatographic methods based on the physicochemical properties of antibiotics.

SAMPLING METHODS

Assays are carried out on serum or plasma. For aminoglycosides, heparinized sampling tubes are not recommended since these drugs are inactivated in the presence of high concentrations of heparin (32). Different studies have found either no interference from barrier gels or separators in the sampling tube, or on the contrary have described significant absorption (1). As these types of tubes have not been evaluated with all antibiotics, it is preferable to draw a blood sample into dry tubes when working with serum or EDTA tubes for plasma.

The sample should be promptly centrifuged and the serum or plasma separated and analyzed, or else stored at +4°C (several hours for aminoglycosides, glycopeptides, quinolones and macrolides), at –20°C (if the above are to be assayed more than 24 hours later), or at –80°C (for all β-lactams, including β-lactamase inhibitors). As imipenem is very unstable, the sample should be centrifuged, decanted and immediately frozen after sampling, or diluted in MES buffer in which it is stable.

ANTIBIOTIC ASSAY METHODS

Microbiological method

This reference method, which determines the overall microbiological activity of an antibiotic contained in a sample, was developed by Grove and Randall (11) and modified by Chabbert and Boulingre (2). Interestingly, antibiotic susceptibility testing by the diffusion method was derived from this technique.

Principle

Microbiological assay is based on comparing the inhibition zone diameters of a susceptible organism in agar medium obtained with a series of standard antibiotic concentrations, to the inhibition zone diameters obtained with the biological test sample. Virtually all antibiotics can be assayed by this method. The method is classically divided into three broad categories: one, two, and three-dimensional (16).
- One-dimensional assay: the agar inoculated with the indicator bacteria is placed in a test tube or capillary tube and is loaded with the sample onto the surface. Diffusion of the antibiotic into the agar defines a vertical inhibition zone.

- Two-dimensional assay: the indicator bacteria are swabbed on the agar surface and the antibiotic diffuses from a well or disk placed on the surface.
- Three-dimensional assay: the indicator bacteria are inoculated in the agar. The antibiotic which is placed in a cylinder or disk diffuses along the surface and through the thickness of the agar. This is the most widely used technique.

Methodology

The principle of microbiological assay is the same for all antibiotics, but the technical conditions (indicator bacteria, medium, incubation temperature) differ according to the characteristics of the antibiotic class or of each individual drug so as to achieve sufficient sensitivity (4, 16, 25).

Indicator bacteria

Selected for their susceptibility (ability to detect a low antibiotic concentration) and specificity (for only one antibiotic), the indicator bacteria must grow rapidly and correctly in the assay conditions so as to obtain clearly defined inhibition zones. One or two reference bacteria exist for each antibiotic or class of antibiotics (Table 1). However, in practice, other strains are also routinely used for the following reasons:
- patients frequently receive therapy with a combination of antibiotics,
- the antibiotics prescribed to a patient are often modified during the course of therapy according to the strains isolated and the patient's clinical course. This must be taken into account since some antibiotics, even after being discontinued, can cause interference. For example, a very long half-life (as in the case of ceftriaxone, quinolones, azithromycin, tetracyclines, fusidic acid, etc.) together with a clinical context of renal failure, dialysis or liver impairment, may result in slow or incomplete elimination of the antibiotic.

To circumvent these problems, multiresistant indicator bacteria are used. In most cases these are clinical strains harboring specific resistance phenotypes or else mutant strains specific for an antibiotic or a class of antibiotics. It is easy to mutate a bacterial strain for resistance to rifampin, fosfomycin, quinolones, fusidic acid, and macrolides, but more difficult for tetracyclines or teicoplanin. Likewise, reference strains can be mutated for resistance to certain antibiotics.

Clinical strains having more specific profiles are conserved, and can also be mutated in order to compensate for "unforeseeable" combinations of antibiotics. Examples include *Pseudomonas* for assaying ceftazidime in the presence of imipenem and quinolones; *Bacillus* mutants for assaying oxacillin or β-lactams in the presence of third generation cephalosporins and/or quinolones, macrolides, or fusidic acid; *Staphylococcus aureus* mutants for rifampin or fusidic acid in the presence of linezolid. These assays do not necessarily have the same sensitivity as with reference strains, but the mutant strains can serve as a rapid guide for making

Table 1. Medium, buffer and indicator bacteria according to the antibiotic to be assayed.

Antibiotic	Medium	Buffer (pH)	Indicator bacteria
β-lactams	Difco medium 2	Phosphate (6.6)	*B. subtilis* ATCC 6633
Aminoglycosides	Difco medium 5	Phosphate (8)	*B. subtilis* ATCC 6633
Fluoroquinolones	Difco medium 5	Phosphate (8)	*Klebsiella* B480m
Tetracyclines	Difco medium 8	Phosphate (4.5)	*S. aureus* 209P
			B. cereus ATTC 9634
Imipenem	Difco medium 1	MES (7)	*B. subtilis* ATCC 6633
Trimethoprim	Mueller-Hinton + hemolyzed blood (2.5 %)	Phosphate (7)	*B. pumilus* CN 607
			E. coli K12J5AzRif
Fusidic acid	Trypticase Soy	Phosphate (8)	*S. aureus* ATCC 25923
Macrolides	Difco medium 5	Phosphate (8)	*M. luteus* ATCC 9341
Rifampin	Difco medium 5	Phosphate (8)	*M. luteus* ATCC 9341
Clavulanic acid	Nutrient agar + 5g/l NaCl + penicillin 60 mg/l	Citrate (6.5)	*K. pneumoniae* NCTC 11228
Tazobactam	Nutrient agar + 5g/l NaCl + ampicillin 50 mg/l	Citrate (6.5)	*P. haemolytica* 59B010
Colistin	Difco medium 10	Phosphate (6) 10%	*B. bronchiseptica* ATCC4617

dosage adjustments so as to avoid underdosing or toxicity due to overdosing. Practically speaking, strains should be subcultured at least once a week, if not more often. When subculturing, it is important to check that resistance has been conserved (by using several antibiotic disks): suspensions should be prepared from colonies in contact with these disks.

A suspension is prepared using a recent culture of the strain, then standardized according to the microorganism and the antibiotic to be assayed in order to have a confluent culture (approximately 10^6 cells/ml of medium). Optical density is measured for each bacteria/antibiotic pair to maintain reproducibility over time.

For some indicator bacteria, exponentially growing cultures in broth medium are used (*K. pneumoniae* NCTC 11228 to assay clavulanic acid or *Pasteurella haemolytica* 59B010 to assay tazobactam, or *P. aeruginosa*). At the same time, several cultures of each strain should be stored at –80°C.

Media

Many different culture media are available. The composition and pH of the culture medium influence the growth of the indicator bacteria and the activity and diffusion of the antibiotic, thereby conferring different levels of sensitivity to the assay. Conventional media are listed in Table 1 (Difco media); they are derived from the media described by Grove and Randall (11). Agar, prepared according to the supplier's recommendations, is melted, cooled to 50°C (only sporulated indicator bacteria such as *Bacillus subtilis*, *Bacillus cereus*, and *Bacillus pumilus* tolerate higher temperatures) and inoculated, then poured into a horizontally held plate. Sterile 24.3 x 24.3 cm plastic trays are usually used (Nunc® distributed by VWR International or Dutscher). For optimum assay sensitivity, the agar is poured to about 1 mm thickness, which requires a level workbench (in optimum conditions) or an adjustable leveling tripod so as to keep the plate as horizontal as possible.

Series of standards

This is prepared from an antibiotic powder with defined potency (generally indicated by the manufacturer or available from Sigma). The powder is supplied with a certificate of analysis stating the potency, dissolution solvent, stability conditions and expiry date. A stock solution is prepared, usually at a concentration of 4000 or 5000 µg/mL, in the recommended solvent (water, methanol, water + HCl, water + NaOH, DMSO, etc.). The concentration range is then prepared by serial dilution in a matrix identical to the nature of the test sample: usually in human serum (particularly for drugs with concentration-dependent protein binding such as ceftriaxone), or serum + buffer (1:1 ratio using buffer specific for each antibiotic class), or buffer alone if the drug shows low protein binding (*e.g.*, fosfomycin) and for assays in CSF, urine, etc. The human serum used to prepare the standards or dilute the samples should first be tested on different microorganisms covering all antibiotic classes to check that it contains no antibiotics. The range of concentrations used for the standard curve is chosen for each antibiotic/test organism so as to give a linear regression line encompassing the concentrations likely to be found in the biological fluids under study.

Sample

The sample is diluted according to the clinical context (dosage, body weight, renal function, trough or peak, suspected overdose, etc.) so that inhibition zone diameters will fall on the standard curve. Sample dilutions should conserve the same matrix as the standard curve. The standards and samples are then treated as follows:
- the most widely used method is to apply 25 µl on sterile filter paper disks 6 mm in diameter (Schleicher & Schuell disks available from VWR International). Each standard concentration and each test sample disk is randomly placed on the same plate at least in triplicate (to account for variations in inoculum or agar thickness).
- 50-100 µl of sample are distributed into wells punched into the agar.
- 200-300 µl are loaded into metal cylinders placed on the agar surface.

Incubation

Plates are placed in an incubator for 18 hours, usually at a temperature of 35-37°C although some organisms such as *Micrococcus luteus* and certain staphylococcus strains have to be incubated at 30°C. A temperature of 30°C or 33°C allows some strains to grow more slowly and thereby provides greater sensitivity. Prediffusing the antibiotic by leaving the plates at room temperature or even at +4°C prior to incubation is another way to increase sensitivity.

Reading and interpretation

After incubation, the inhibition zone diameters are measured with the aid of a microfilm reader (Fischer Scientific) which projects the diameter onto

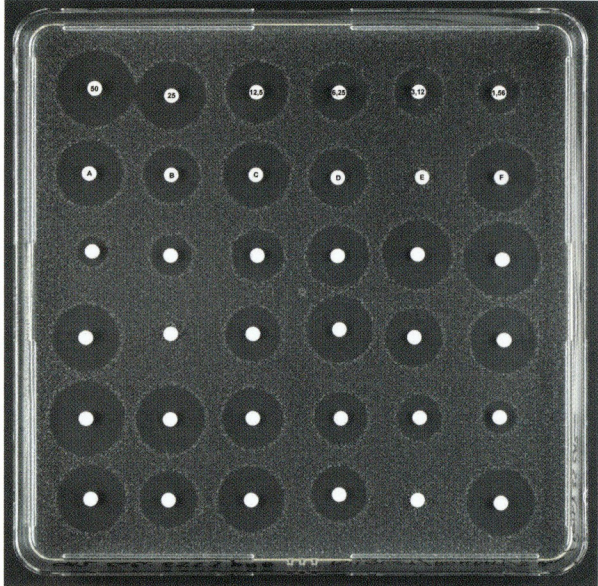

Fig. 1. Microbiological assay of ceftazidime. *E. coli* SJ6553; agar: medium 2. Lines A, C, E: standard curve from 50 to 1.56 µg/mL. Lines B, D, F: Patient 1, continuous concentrations: A, serum at 1/2; B, serum at 1/5. Patient 2, continuous concentrations: C, serum at 1/2; D, serum at 1/5. E, antibiotic-free control (serum used for standard curve); F, control point at 25 mg/l.

a graduated film after a minimum 6 to 8-fold magnification of the inhibition zone. Diameters read with a caliper or ruler are much less accurate (Fig. 1).

The mean of the measurements for each point is calculated and a regression line of log concentration versus diameter is plotted on semi-logarithmic paper or with the aid of a program that can be easily run using Excel®. The precision and accuracy of the regression line are given by the value of the correlation coefficient (ideally, equal to 1 but in any case always > 0.95), and by the coefficient of variation which estimates the standard deviation of the mean diameter for each assay. The diameters obtained with the test samples are plotted on the standard curve in order to calculate the concentration, which is then adjusted for the dilution used (Fig. 2).

Neutralization of antibiotics

This is often necessary to prevent interference with the antibiotic to be assayed.

The activity of some antibiotics can be sharply reduced by changing the pH or the composition of the agar.

Aminoglycosides

Aminoglycosides can be neutralized by adsorption on cellulose phosphate (Sigma): 100 mg cellulose phosphate are added to 0.5 ml pure or diluted serum (or any other biological matrix). The mixture is shaken and allowed to stand for 30 min, then centrifuged. The resulting supernatant is free of aminoglycosides (30).

Penicillins

Penicillins can be eliminated with penicillinase (Penase Difco™). 0.5 ml penicillinase is added to 0.5 ml serum. The mixture is shaken and allowed to stand for 30 min, after which the β-lactam is neutralized.

Cephalosporins

Cephalosporins are eliminated with cephalosporinase obtained from an exponentially growing culture of *Enterobacter cloacae* 99P or *Stenotrophomonas maltophilia*. The broth is centrifuged, the pellet washed several times and the bacteria lysed by ultrasonication.

Cephalosporinase, present in the supernatant, is then tested against different antibiotics (cefotaxime, ceftazidime, cefepime, imipenem, etc.) to determine the amount to be used to neutralize therapeutic concentrations of the antibiotic. A cephalosporinase is also available from Sigma.

Sulfonamides

Sulfonamides can be neutralized by adding 100 µg/mL para-aminobenzoic acid to the agar.

Trimethoprim

Trimethoprim is neutralized by adding 1 µg/mL thymidine to the agar.

Colistin and chloramphenicol

Colistin and chloramphenicol have little activity at therapeutic concentrations and generally do not interfere with the antibiotics to be assayed.

Pristinamycin

Pristinamycin binds to red blood cells and is inactive in serum.

In all cases, a point on the standard curve (usually the highest concentration) should be used to check that concomitant antibiotic(s) do not cause interference; no inhibition zone should be observed for this point.

Assay in fluids other than blood

Assays can be carried out in other biological fluids including CSF, pleural fluid, ascites, synovial fluid, urine, bronchial secretions, and lung, prostate, or bone biopsies.

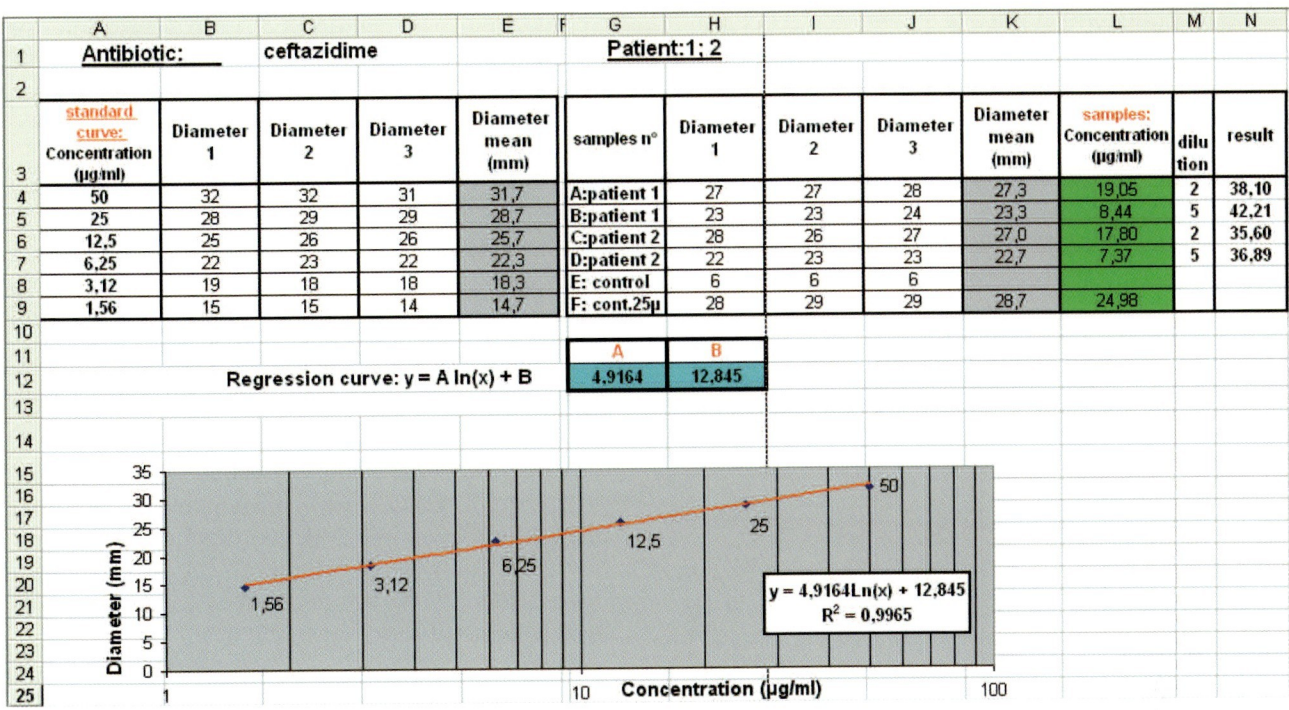

Fig. 2. Calibration curve and calculation of serum concentrations (with the aid of a program developed on Excel®).

Bronchial secretions are diluted in Sputazol®, shaken and incubated at 37°C for 30 min in a water bath before being assayed.

Bone biopsies are sponged off to remove as much contaminating blood as possible, then weighed, crushed, and placed in buffer for 24 h. The supernatant is assayed and the bone is again placed in fresh buffer, repeating this step until all antibiotic is released. The bone can also be cryoground in liquid nitrogen.

The standard concentrations should be prepared in a solvent having the same nature as the test sample, but this is rarely possible. Therefore, the standards are usually prepared in buffer. It is also useful to assay the infection site, particularly in cases of treatment failure. However, interpretation is not always straightforward because even if high antibiotic concentrations are found, the interpretation must take into account the fact that the organism will have a different susceptibility than that detected in the laboratory, due to local conditions at the infection site, particularly pH and anaerobiosis (leading to disagreement of *in vitro* and *in vivo* MICs).

Advantages and drawbacks

Microbiological assays offer the advantage of being inexpensive and easy to perform by trained technicians, in addition to a high throughput allowing many drugs to be tested each day. They also have the huge advantage of assaying both the antibiotic and its bacteriologically active metabolites without the need to separate them. The specificity of the method depends on an accurate knowledge of the antibiotics taken by the patient, to make sure that only one drug is assayed. The level of detection depends on the indicator bacteria. Microbiological assays have a precision of ± 10-15% depending on operator experience. The rapidity of results depends on culture times, usually 12-18 hours. This type of assay can be performed on a 24/7 emergency basis in case of severe infection or toxicity.

Non-microbiological assays

These fall into three categories:
- enzymatic assays
- immunoassays
- "physicochemical" assays (chromatography and the like)

Enzymatic and immunological methods

Radioenzymatic method (Radio-Enzyme Assay or REA)

This method has been used to assay aminoglycosides. The antibiotic is recognized by an inactivating enzyme (adenylyltransferase or acetyltransferase) present in resistant bacteria and specific for the antibiotic. The aminoglycoside contained in the sample is labeled with ^{14}C (acetyl-coenzyme A or ATP). After elimination of excess cofactor, the radioactivity in the sample is proportional to the amount of aminoglycoside it contains. REA is a specific, accurate and highly sensitive method, but the need to use radiolabeled reagents makes it fairly expensive and it is no longer routinely used.

Immunological methods

These methods are all based on the principle of specific recognition of the antibiotic by an antibody.

Radioimmunological method (Radio-Immuno Assay, RIA) (27).

The antibody is simultaneously contacted with the antibiotic contained in the sample (unlabeled antigen) and a known amount of radiolabeled antibiotic (labeled antigen). Labeled and unlabeled antibiotic compete for binding to the antibody. The antibody-antigen complexes are then precipitated in a second immunological reaction and radioactivity is measured in the supernatant. Due to competitive binding, the residual radioactivity is inversely proportional to the amount of antibiotic present in the sample. This method has high specificity and sensitivity but is costly and requires the handling of radioisotopes.

Immunoenzymatic assay (Enzyme Multiplied Immunoassay Technique, EMIT) (27, 28).

This method is based on competition between the antibiotic to be assayed, present in the sample, and a known amount of antibiotic conjugated to G-6-PD, an enzyme which catalyzes a color reaction. After antibiotic-antibody binding, the amount of G-6-PD in the supernatant is inversely proportional to the amount of antibiotic in the sample. G-6-PD is quantified by the intensity of the color reaction it catalyzes, measured by optical density (reduction of NAD to NADH). This method is used by Dade Behring on Cobas Mira and ACA analyzers to assay gentamicin, tobramycin, netilmicin, amikacin, and vancomycin.

CEDIA (Cloned Enzyme Immunodonor Assay)

This method, developed in the 1980s, makes use of two genetically engineered enzyme fragments: the enzyme acceptor fragment (EA) corresponding to 90% of the β-galactosidase sequence, and the enzyme donor fragment (ED) corresponding to the missing part of the sequence. Spontaneous association of EA + ED forms active β-galactosidase. The method is based on competition between the antibiotic present in the sample and ED-conjugated antibiotic for binding to antibody. When antibody blocks the antigen site, it prevents ED from associating with EA. Enzymatic activity of the β-galactosidase is directly proportional to the concentration of free antibiotic in the sample. CEDIA technology was developed by Roche for use on Hitachi analyzers to assay tobramycin and vancomycin.

Fluorescent Polarization Immuno Assay (FPIA)

This method, developed by Abbott in the 1970s, is based on competition between antibiotic present in the sample and fluorescein-labeled antibiotic for binding to an antibody directed against the antibiotic. The fluorescence polarization emitted by the antibiotic increases when it is bound to antibody (15, 28).

The method, which runs on Abbott's TDx and AxSym analyzers and on Roche's Cobas Integra, can be used to assay aminoglycosides and glycopeptides. Not all drugs can be assayed on all instruments; for example teicoplanin can only be assayed on the TDx.

Other assay techniques, based on heterogeneous phase competition, are also available:
- Fluorescent ImmunoAssay (FIA), developed by Dade Behring on the OPUS analyzer (vancomycin).
- Chemiluminescence, developed by Chiron on the ACS 180 analyzer and by DPC on the Immulite (gentamicin, tobramycin and vancomycin, depending on the instrument).
- Spectrophotometric analysis, developed by Bayer on the Immuno 1 (vancomycin).
- Turbidimetric analysis, developed by Dade Behring on the Dimension RLX and by Bayer on the Advia 1650 (gentamicin, tobramycin and vancomycin, depending on the instrument).

Uses, advantages and limitations

Immunological methods have several advantages: no pretreatment of the biological sample, low volume (100 µl), rapid response time (< 30 min), and good sensitivity and reproducibility thanks to automation (coefficient of variation < 5%).

One of the limitations is the need to produce antibodies which are specific for the test antibiotic and reproducible. The antibody does not allow differentiation between the antibiotic and its metabolites or the different antibiotic fractions (such as in the case of teicoplanin). These methods are routinely used to assay aminoglycosides, gentamicin, tobramycin, netilmicin and amikacin as well as the glycopeptides, vancomycin and teicoplanin. They give equivalent results for aminoglycosides. For vancomycin, FPIA gives higher values than EMIT or HPLC for renal insufficiency or dialysis patients in whom an inactive crystalline degradation product CDP-1 is assayed simultaneously. Results are 10-20% higher than with other methods (22, 31). Modification of the Abbot FPIA reagents on the TDx and AxSYM analyzers eliminates the problem of CPD-1 and gives similar results with the different methods (29).

These are fully automated methods which can rapidly assay several drugs for purposes of treatment monitoring or dosage adjustment. A limiting factor is the availability of commercial assay kits, the development of which is related to demand. At present, these methods and instruments cannot be used for all antibiotics. For example, teicoplanin can only be assayed by FPIA on Abbott's TDx.

Chromatographic methods

Chromatographic methods are based on the physicochemical properties of antibiotics. High performance liquid chromatography, or HPLC, was developed for antibiotic assay in the 1980s and can be used on all antibiotics and their potential metabolites present in biological samples. HPLC separates the compounds contained in a sample according to their different affinity for a solid stationary phase packed inside a column, and a liquid mobile phase running through the column. Once separated, the compounds can be quantified by UV or visible detection, fluorimetry (quinolones) or coulometry (macrolides).

HPLC assay of antibiotics comprises the following steps:
- Pretreatment of the biological sample: Very few biological media can be directly injected, due to the presence of high concentrations of endogenous compounds such as plasma proteins. The various types of sample pretreatment must not diminish the sensitivity of the assay through sample dilution or loss during extraction. Pretreatment can comprise a concentration step (evaporation of organic phase during liquid-liquid extraction). Proteins are precipitated in acidic medium (perchloric or trichloracetic acid) or by an organic solvent (acetonitrile, methanol), or else by ultrafiltration or liquid-liquid or solid-liquid extraction. Deproteinization allows both free and bound drug to be assayed. The pretreatment step must be as simple as possible, reproducible, and must not affect the stability of the antibiotic to be assayed. In light of this mode of sample preparation, the use of an internal standard is sometimes recommended to take into account variations related to the sample.
- Separation of the antibiotic, its metabolites and residual endogenous compounds by passage of the treated sample through a chromatography column. Several types of chromatography may be used:
  - Partition chromatography: "normal phase" if the stationary phase is polar with a low polarity mobile phase; "reverse phase" if the stationary phase is apolar with a polar mobile phase. The latter is more widely used.
  - Ion exchange chromatography.
  - Ion pair chromatography when the polarity of the test molecule is changed by adding an ion with the opposite charge (counter ion).
- Eluent detection at column exit: The detection system depends on the properties of the antibiotic being assayed:
  - UV spectrophotometry at fixed or variable wavelength detects many antibiotics.
  - Spectrofluorimetry: Many quinolones are naturally fluorescent and this detection method has good sensitivity.
  - Electrochemical detection is useful for compounds which do not absorb in the UV and which do not fluoresce but are easily oxidized or reduced. Macrolides can be assayed by this method.
- Antibiotic quantification: This is achieved by continuous measurement of the signal emitted by the detector. The baseline corresponds to the mobile phase while the peaks represent the compounds detected. Quantification is done by measuring peak height or peak area, which are proportional to concentration. To quantify an antibiotic, the signal must be compared to the signals at different points of a standard curve containing increasing amounts of antibiotic in the same biological medium as the test sample and assayed in the same manner.

HPLC systems comprise:
- A constant flow high pressure pump. Elution is usually isocratic, meaning that the composition of mobile phase does not change. However, during development or to separate several compounds, it may be necessary to elute with a polarity gradient, in which mobile phase com-

position changes over time. In this case a second pump is used and the entire system is programmed.
- An analytical chromatography column which separates the different compounds and which determines the resolution of the system. The efficacy of the column results from a very small (3-5 µm) and homogeneous particle size and the quality and stability of bonding. The most widely used columns are packed with silica covalently bonded with apolar side chains containing 8 or 18 carbon atoms (C8 or C18). In some cases the column may be heated (column oven).
- An injector, which is either manual (injection loop into which a syringe is inserted), or automatic.
- A detector, usually a UV detector, spectrophotometer (UV or UV-visible), fluorimeter, electrochemical or conductimetric detector. More sophisticated detectors include diode array for continuous multiwavelength measurements or mass spectrometer detection; these detection methods have higher specificity.
- An integrator, which measures peak height or peak area for the test antibiotic, both of which are proportional to concentration.

Uses, advantages, and limitations

HPLC can be used to assay the majority of antibiotics thanks to the variety of detection systems. It is used in research to evaluate new antibiotics and determine pharmacokinetic parameters, and is routinely used for treatment monitoring and dose adjustment. The method is specific, allowing to separately assay the antibiotic and its metabolites, as well as sensitive, reproducible and adaptable to different biological media. Precision is 5-10%. It requires trained operators and the instrumentation is costly. The many HPLC methods described for antibiotic assays differ solely in terms of the type of extraction, separation and detection. The optimum HPLC conditions for each antibiotic can be found in the many literature reviews and publications available on this subject (14, 19, 24, 25).

Capillary electrophoresis has been used to assay antibiotics for the past ten years or so. Advantages include a very small injection volume, very good separation and inexpensive consumables. This method appears to complement HPLC (6, 20).

Choosing an assay method

The choice depends on the antibiotic to be assayed and the context (Table 2). For aminoglycosides and glycopeptides, immunoassays are simple, rapid and can be used for treatment monitoring and dosage adjustment, important considerations for these drugs which have a narrow therapeutic margin.

For other classes of antibiotics, microbiological assay is simple when performed by qualified personnel. It has the advantage of being able to assay many different antibiotics but rapidity depends on bacterial growth, and the response time is 12-15 hours at best.

HPLC methods can be developed to assay a large number of antibiotics and separate the different metabolites. Results are available the same day but practically speaking this type of assay is not feasible on a 24/7 basis. Limitations include the instrumentation and operator training.

Recent advances in HPLC coupled with mass spectrometry, particularly the development of atmospheric pressure ionization sources and tandem quadripole analyzers (MS/MS), make it possible to envision the simultaneous assay of many molecules. Newly available workstation analytical tools which are reliable, robust, efficient, and easy to use have contributed to the development of this method.

Table 2. Comparison of assay methods

Criterion	Microbiological method	HPLC	Immunoenzymatic methods
Specificity	+ (metabolite)	++ (physicochemical)	++
Precision	+/- 10 %	5 - 10 %	5%
Robustness	++	+/-	++
Difficulty	Easy	+/-	Easy
Response time	12 to 18 h	2 h (ideally)	30 min
Cost	Inexpensive materials (technician time)	+++ (equipment)	++ to +++ (reagents)

UTILITY OF ANTIBIOTIC ASSAYS

Antibiotic assays are a routine part of new drug development which involves the study of pharmacokinetic properties, determination of antibiotic concentrations in different tissues and toxic levels, etc. In clinical practice, antibiotic assays should be performed in the following circumstances (10, 12):

- In patients with renal insufficiency or on dialysis or hemofiltration. All antibiotics can be assayed in order to optimize the dose: If the antibiotic is dialysable, to rule out underdosing; if it is only weakly or non-dialysable (oxacillin or cloxacillin), to avoid drug accumulation which can cause neurotoxicity (as in the case of β-lactams (8) or quinolones for example).
- For antibiotics with a narrow therapeutic margin, such as aminoglycosides: in these cases an increase in trough concentrations is a predictor of renal toxicity.
- To ensure that effective concentrations are reached when the causative organism has reduced susceptibility, in order to avoid failure of eradication or prevention of resistance. For instance, to eradicate *Pseudomonas* with a fluoroquinolone if the infection site concentration is just above the MIC, or to eradicate *S. aureus* (GISA) with vancomycin.
- In severe infections: endocarditis, meningitis, infectious osteoarthritis.
- In case of severe liver impairment, in order to adjust the dosage of antibiotics that are metabolized by the liver (clindamycin, metronidazole, tetracycline, cefotaxime, etc.).
- In heart failure, due to reduced hepatic and renal clearance resulting from lower cardiac output.
- Under special physiological conditions: neonates and premature infants as well as the elderly have different elimination rates than adults.
- For monitoring antibiotic efficacy in ICU patients, who often have an expanded volume of distribution and altered hepatic and renal function (longer half-life), making pharmacokinetic parameters difficult to predict.
- In cystic fibrosis patients, severe burn patients, or in the presence of severe ascites. Large variations in plasma volume with a decrease in the serum half-life and an increase in renal or extrarenal clearance require dosage adjustment in order to avoid underdosing.
- When there is no correlation between the administered dose and plasma levels (inter- and intra-individual variability), for example with the quinolones.
- In case of clinical failure, the infection site itself can be assayed: in CSF for example, where concentrations are hard to predict due to the existence of a diffusion barrier and excretion systems. Moreover, drug interactions are often discovered at this time. Examples include quinolones and iron salts (18) or quinolones and antacids, or during routine assays in severe bone and joint infections: interaction between benzodiazepines and fusidic acid (personal data, in press).
- To monitor treatment compliance.

Accidents related to antibiotic overdose

Aminoglycosides

Overdose from drug accumulation (elevated trough concentrations) is a predictor of renal toxicity which manifests as a reduction in renal clearance 24-72 hours after the increase in trough levels.

β-lactams

In renal insufficiency, ICU patients and the elderly, β-lactam accumulation in serum and high penetration into CSF, in the absence of inflammation, are often responsible for neurotoxicity and convulsions (8). This phenomenon has been described for all β-lactam antibiotics, particularly penicillins, cefepime and imipenem.

Fluoroquinolones

Neurotoxicity and convulsions have been reported with pefloxacin, ofloxacin, and ciprofloxacin, mainly in renal failure or elderly patients. In our personal experience, serum levels of pefloxacin, ofloxacin, levofloxacin, and ciprofloxacin greater than 20, 8, 8, and 4 µg/mL, respectively, have been found in patients presenting with neurological effects (status epilepticus, convulsions, myoclonia, confusion, aggressiveness, etc.). In most cases the patients were elderly and had impaired renal function (or were even on dialysis), and some had prolonged exposure to the antibiotic.

Problems related to antibiotic underdosing

Considering the risk of toxicity associated with certain antibiotics, it is not always possible to increase the dose. When serum levels (and especially infection site concentrations) are only slightly above the MIC, there is a risk of treatment failure and selection of resistant mutants. This is the case in *Pseudomonas aeruginosa* nosocomial pneumonia treated with ceftazidime which has an MIC of 16 or 32 µg/mL, where it is often illusory to achieve concentrations high enough to eradicate the microorganism without incurring a risk of toxicity.

Apart from the problem of multiresistant strains, resistant mutants can be selected during therapy in case of underdosing (quinolones, macrolides) (9).

A recent, unpublished retrospective study in ICU patients analyzed 196 β-lactam assays (only the first assay prescribed was analyzed). With respect to the susceptibility of the causative organism and the pathology to be treated, drug concentrations were satisfactory in 42.8% of samples, while drug concentrations indicated underdosing in 12.3% and overdosing in 44.9%.

INTERPRETATION OF RESULTS

Very specific data are needed to interpret the assay results. Required information includes age, weight, renal function: clearance, dialysis (when related to dosing time and sampling time, type of membrane), hemofiltration, peritoneal dialysis, liver function, dosage, dose schedule, route of administration, exact infusion time, sampling time, concomitant treatments particularly with other antibiotics, pathology, site of infection, susceptibility of the causative organism (MIC). The results can only be interpreted in close collaboration with the microbiology laboratory.

As a guide, recommended target concentrations are given below according to the type and susceptibility of the causative pathogen, the antibiotic used, and the site of infection.

TARGET SERUM CONCENTRATIONS FOR DIFFERENT ANTIBIOTICS

Glycopeptides

The bactericidal activity of glycopeptides is time-dependent (3). In a peritonitis model, Knudsen et al. (17) showed that predictors of glycopeptide efficacy include the period of time during which the drug levels are above the MIC (T > MIC). T > MIC and the ratio serum concentration/MIC (inhibitory quotient at the residual concentration) are important factors and the MIC is crucial.

In the treatment of severe infections, the administration of antibiotics should not be "one size fits all" but adapted to the patient's characteristics and to the susceptibility of the bacteria.

The goal is to obtain a trough serum level where the ratio serum concentration/MIC is not less than 8, as long as the level is below the toxicity range (13). In infections which are not bacteriologically documented, the lower critical concentration (c = 4 µg/mL) must be considered for calculation of target trough values which in this case are 30-35 µg/mL (8 times the MIC).

Vancomycin

In many countries vancomycin is usually given by 60-minute infusion of 1 g *bid* or 500 mg *qid*. In other contries, such as France a continuous infusion of 30-40 mg/kg (after a loading dose of 15 mg/kg in 60 min) is preferred so as to maintain serum levels as follows (9 b):
- Streptococci (including *S. pneumoniae*), enterococci: 10-20 µg/ml; for severe infections (endocarditis, bone-joint infections, meningitis, etc.) target concentrations are 20-30 µg/mL.
- Staphylococci: For a susceptible strain (MIC = 0.5-1 µg/mL), continuous concentrations of 15-20 µg/mL; for more severe infections (ICU patients, meningitis, bone-joint infections, endocarditis or *S. aureus* (GISA) with reduced vancomycin susceptibility (MIC ≥ 4 µg/mL), target levels are 30-35 or even 40 µg/mL (inhibitory quotient at the residual concentration ≥ 8).

These concentrations may seem high when compared with the American therapeutic range of 5-10 µg/mL, but are perfectly justified by the following considerations :
- the number of published (and unpublished) failures due to drug levels that are too low,
- the low toxicity of vancomycin,
- high protein binding,
- the fact that tissue concentrations do not exceed one-third of serum levels, and
- the inoculum effect, especially with *S. aureus* (GISA).

Teicoplanin

Due to high protein binding, steady state is achieved slowly and for this reason, trough levels after a unit dose and at steady state measured after several injections vary considerably (at 6 mg/kg/12h, trough levels are ≈ 4 µg/mL after the first dose and ≈ 15 µg/mL at steady state). Therefore, treatment should be initiated with a large loading dose in order to rapidly reach the therapeutic range. Then, since the half-life is very long (70-100 h), doses can be given at longer intervals while maintaining trough levels in the correct range. After the loading dose, trough concentrations of 15-20 µg/mL allow injections to be given at 24-h intervals (or longer in case of renal insufficiency).

In severe infections such as endocarditis, bone-joint infections, ICU patients or if the MIC of teicoplanin is increased from 4 to 16 µg/mL, a loading dose of 3-5 injections of 12 mg/kg/12h produces trough levels in the range of 30-40 µg/mL. However, when the MIC is 16 µg/mL, it is preferable to use another antibiotic.

Aminoglycosides

Bactericidal activity is directly correlated with the peak concentration (concentration-dependent) whereas toxicity [nephrotoxicity (usually reversible) and ototoxicity (often irreversible)] is related to accumulation and total duration of antibiotic exposure. Aminoglycosides exert a post-antibiotic effect on Gram-positive and Gram-negative bacteria which lasts for several hours. In an experimental model, it was shown that bacterial killing of *P. aeruginosa* and *Serratia marcescens* by netilmicin and amikacin was more rapid if the drug was given as a bolus (unit dose) as compared with three injections per day. A high aminoglycoside peak concentration (Cmax/MIC or inhibitory quotient at the residual concentration ≥ 10) was predictive of a rapid response to treatment and a shorter hospital stay (21). The desired profile for aminoglycosides is a high peak concentration (for efficacy) and a low trough concentration (to avoid accumulation). It is generally recommended to sample at the trough (predose) to detect any accumulation, and at the peak 30 min after stopping the 30-min infusion to evaluate efficacy. On the other hand, when treating streptococcal endocarditis, aminoglycosides must imperatively be administered twice daily to prolong the synergistic effect of β-lactams or vancomycin. Aminoglycoside target concentrations are shown in Table 3.

When administering unit doses of gentamicin and tobramycin, a nomogram (23) may be used to determine, on a sample taken 6-14h after injection, if the dose was sufficient and when the next dose should be given.

β-lactams

These antibiotics have a time-dependent effect and show little concentration-dependence (3). Many different studies have indicated that in severe infections (ICU patients with increased volume of distribution, nosocomial pneumonia, etc.), serum levels must be 4-5 times over the MIC of the causative organism and maintained 50% of the time between two injections (T > MIC). These levels are difficult to achieve with discontinuous dosing, especially when the causative organism has reduced susceptibility. Continuous infusion maintains constant concentrations which are always above the MIC. However, the advantages of continuous versus discontinuous dosing have only been demonstrated in animal models. Continuous infusion also has the advantage of avoiding subinhibitory concentrations which promote the emergence of resistance (5). To achieve continuous β-lactam concentrations when treating severe infections, one must therefore consider the MIC for the organism as well as the site of infection so as to obtain concentrations at least 4-5 times above the MIC. For instance, when treating nosocomial *Pseudomonas* pneumonia (MIC of ceftazdime = 2 µg/ml), concentrations in the range of 30-50 µg/ml by continuous infusion are necessary.

Fluoroquinolones

These drugs have concentration-dependent bactericidal activity and a post-antibiotic effect (3). In

Table 3. Target concentrations for aminoglycosides

Antibiotic	Twice dailydosage		Unit dose	
	Trough (µg/ml)	Peak (µg/ml)	Trough (µg/ml)	Peak (µg/ml)
Gentamicin, Tobramycin	< 0.5	5 - 6	< 0.5	15 - 25
Netilmicin	-	-	< 0.5	15 - 25
Amikacin	< 3	20 - 30	< 0.5	40 - 60
Tobramycin (cystic fibrosis: 8-10 mg/kg)	-	-	< 0.5	35 - 40

Table 4. Dosage, route of administration and target plasma concentrations in bone and joint infections

Antibiotic	Daily dosage	Frequency and route	Target concentrations (μg/ml)
Amoxicillin	100-150 mg/kg	4-6 slow i.v. injections	C_{max} 80 ; C_{min} < 20
Oxacillin-cloxacillin	100-150 mg/kg	or continuous infusion via electric syringe	50
Cefazolin	50-100 mg/kg		
Cefotaxime	100 mg/kg		
Ceftazidime	50-100 mg/kg		
Cefepime	150-200 mg/kg		Piperacillin 50-tazobactam 5-7 (i.v.s.e)
Piperacillin-tazobactam	100 mg/kg	4-6 slow i.v. injections	C_{max} 80 ; C_{min} < 20
Amoxicillin-clavulanic acid	30-35 mg/kg	1-2 slow i.v. injections	
Ceftriaxone	50-100 mg/kg	3-4 slow i.v. injections	C_{max} 20-30 ; C_{min} 1-3
Imipenem	40-60 mg/kg	continuous infusion via electric syringe	30-40
Vancomycin	12 mg/kg	1 slow i.v. injection	C_{min} 30-35
Teicoplanin	3 mg/kg	2 30 minute i.v. injections	C_{max} 4-6 ; C_{min} < 0,5
Gentamicin Tobramycin	15 mg/kg	2 30 minute i.v. injections	C_{max} 25-30 ; C_{min} < 3
Amikacin	800-1200 mg	2-3/day p.o. or i.v.	C_{max} 10 ; C_{min} 6-8
Pefloxacin	400-800 mg	2-3/day p.o. or i.v.	C_{max} 5 ; C_{min} 3
Ofloxacin	1500-2000 mg	2-3/day p.o. or i.v.	C_{max} 2-6 ; C_{min} 0,5-1,5
Ciprofloxacin	1800-2400 mg	3-4 slow i.v. injections 3 doses	C_{max} 15 ; C_{min} 5
Clindamycin	20 mg/kg	2-3 60 minute i.v. injections 2-3 doses	C_{max} 10-15 ; C_{min} 2-5
Rifampin	1500 mg	2-3 doses 2-3 slow i.v. injections	C_{max} 80 ; C_{min} 50
Fusidic acid	1500-200 mg/kg	continuous infusion via electric syringe	70-90
Fosfomycin		3-4 60-120 minute injections	
Linezolid	600 mg bid	p.o. or i.v.	

C_{max}: peak concentration, sample taken after injection (1 h after start of infusion for aminoglycosides, 15 min after the end of infusion for other antibiotics, 2 h after an oral dose).

C_{min}: trough concentration of antibiotic sampled immediately before next injection or dose. Rifampin should be assayed between days 8 and 10 of treatment, fluoroquinolones after approximately 5 days of treatment. The other assays can be done between 48 and 72 h, then at least once a week for glycopeptides and aminoglycosides. An assay after 1 week of treatment is desirable for β-lactams and fosfomycin administered by continuous infusion (risk of accumulation in renal failure or elderly).

For continuous infusion via electric syringe, treatment should always be initiated with a loading dose (1/4 the daily dose) administered over 30-60 minutes, followed by continuous infusion.

p.o., per os ; i.v. , intraveinous.

patients receiving ciprofloxacin, the AUC/MIC ratio must be > 125, or the Cmax/MIC ratio > 12, to obtain a satisfactory clinical and microbiological response (7). This can easily be attained with a ciprofloxacin dosage of 200 mg i.v. *bid* or *tid* or 500 mg per os *bid* for microbes such as *Haemophilus* spp. for which the MIC is < 0.01 mg/l, but a much higher dosage (400 mg i.v. *tid* or more often; or 750 mg per os *bid*) is required for *P. aeruginosa* and *S. aureus* (MIC of 0.25-0.5 µg/ml).

TARGET CONCENTRATIONS ACCORDING TO SITE OF INFECTION

Meningitis

Antibiotics often penetrate poorly into the cerebro-spinal fluid, even in case of inflammation. Considering that such infections can be fatal, it is essential that therapeutic concentrations be reached in CSF. Table 5 shows the extent of diffusion of the main antibiotics into the cerebro-spinal fluid. To ensure that CSF concentrations are high enough, the antibiotic should be assayed each time a lumbar puncture is done, and a serum assay should be performed at the same time for purposes of comparison.

Endocarditis

Endocarditis is difficult to treat because antibiotics penetrate poorly into the fibrinous vegetations and the bacteria therein have abnormal metabolism. The bacterial time-kill curves and the post-antibiotic effect of the antibiotic must be taken into account. For antibiotics with a slow bactericidal effect (β-lactams, quinolones), the dosing interval should be short. For those with rapid bactericidal activity (aminoglycosides) and a post-antibiotic effect, a longer dosing interval is acceptable. Antibiotic concentrations should be checked frequently, both at the start of parenteral therapy and when switching to the oral route. In *C. burnetii* endocarditis, a correlation has been found between the decline in antibody levels and the serum concentration/MIC ratio. A ratio > 1 predicts a positive outcome with serum levels > 3 µg/mL (26).

Bone and joint infections

Target serum concentrations for bone and joint infections are shown in Table 4 (33). Although some of these levels may seem high, it should be kept in mind that these are serum concentrations, and it is at the infection site that satisfactory concentrations must be reached, and infection site concentrations are often lower than those in serum.

REFERENCES

(1) **Alcantarilla, G., and D. Lozano.** 1996. Absorption of some aminoglycoside drugs by barrier gels in sampling tubes. Clin. Chem. **42**: 771.

(2) **Chabbert, Y., and H. Boulingre.** 1957. Modifications pratiques concernant le dosage des antibiotiques en clinique. Rev. Fr. Etud. Clin. Biol. **2**: 636-640.

(3) **Craig, W.A.** 1998. Pharmacokinetic/pharmacodynamic parameters: rationale for antibacterial dosing of mice and men. Clin. Infect. Dis. **26**: 29-35.

(4) **de Louvois, J.** 1982. Factors influencing the assay of antimicrobial drugs in clinical samples by the agar plate diffusion method. J. Antimicrob. Chemother. **9**: 253-265.

(5) **Fantin, B., R. Farinotti, A. Thabaut, and C. Carbon.** 1994. Conditions for the emergence of resistance to cefpirome and ceftazidime in experimental endocarditis due to *Pseudomonas aeruginosa*. J. Antimicrob. Chemother. **33**: 563-569.

(6) **Flurer, C.L.** 2003. Analysis of antibiotics by capillary electrophoresis. Electrophoresis. **24**: 4116-4127.

(7) **Forrest, A., D.E. Nix, C.H. Ballow, T.F. Goss, M.C. Birmingham, and J.J. Schentag.** 1993. Pharmacodynamics of intravenous ciprofloxacin in seriously ill patients. Antimicrob. Agents Chemother. **37**: 1073-1081.

(8) **Garrec, F., T. Bensousan, M.D. Kitzis, and B. Leclercq.** 1998. Evolution des concentrations de ceftazidime dans le LCR après surdosage au cours d'une insuffisance rénale aigue. Therapie **53**: 516-17.

(9) **Goldstein, F.W., B. Vidal, and M.D. Kitzis.** 2005. Telithromycin-resistant *Streptococcus pneumoniae*. Emerg. Infect. Dis. **11**:1489-1490.

(9b) **Kitzis, M.D., F.W. Goldstein.** 2006. Monitoring of vancomicyn serum levels for the treatment of staphylococcal infections. Clin. Microbiol. Infect. Jan. **12 (1)**:92-95

(10) **Gross, A.S.** 1998. Best practice in therapeutic drug monitoring. Br. J. Clin. Pharmacol. **46**: 95-99.

(11) **Grove, D.C., and W.A. Randall.** 1955. Assay methods of antibiotics: a laboratory manual: Medical Encyclopedia, New York.

(12) **Hammett-Stabler, C.A., and T. Johns.** 1998. Laboratory guidelines for monitoring of antimicrobial drugs. Clin. Chem. **44**: 1129-1140

(13) **Harding, I., A.P. McGovan, L.O. White, E.S. Darley, and V. Reed.** 2000. Teicoplanin therapy of *Staphylococcus aureus* septicemia: relationship between pre-dose serum concentrations and outcome. J. Antimicrob. Chemother. **45**: 835-841.

(14) **Jehl, F., C. Gallion, and H. Monteil.** 1990. High-performance chromatography of antibiotics. J. Chromatogr. **531**: 509-548.

(15) **Jolley, M.E., S.E. Stroupe, C.J. Swang, H.N. Panas, L. Keeganc, R.L. Schmidt, and K.S. Schwenzer.** 1981. Fluorescence polarization immunoassay I: monitoring aminoglycosides antibiotics in serum and plasma. Clin. Chem. **27**: 1190-1197.

(16) **Klassen, M., and S.C. Edberg.** 1996. Measurement of antibiotics in human body fluids : techniques and significance pp. 230-295. *In* V. Lorian (ed.) Antibiotics in Laboratory Medicine. 4th edition, Williams & Wilkins, Baltimore, Maryland, USA.

(17) **Knudsen, J.D., K. Fuursted, S. Raber, F. Espersen, and N. Frimodt-Moller.** 2000. Pharmacodynamics of glycopeptides in the mouse peritonitis model of *Streptococcus pneumoniae* or *Staphylococcus aureus* infection. Antimicrob. Agents Chemother. **44**: 1247-1254.

(18) **Le Pennec, M.P., M.D. Kitzis, M. Terdjman, S. Foubard, E. Garbarz, and G. Hanania.** 1990. Possible interaction of ciprofloxacin with ferrous sulphate. J. Antimicrob. Chemother. **25**: 183-185.

(19) **Levêque, D., C. Gallion-Renault, H. Monteil, and F. Jehl.** 1998. Analysis of recent antimicrobial agents in human biological fluids by high-performance liquid chromatography. J. Chromatogr. **A 815**: 163-172.

(20) **Levêque, D., C. Gallion-Renault, H. Monteil, and F. Jehl.** 1997. Capillary electrophoresis for pharmacokinetic studies. J. Chromatogr. **B 697**: 67-75.

(21) **Moore, R.D., P.S. Lietman, and C.R. Smith**. 1987. Clinical response to aminoglycoside therapy: importance of the ratio of peak concentration to minimal inhibitory concentration. J. Infect. Dis. **155**: 93-99.

(22) **Morse, G. D., D.K. Nain, J.S. Bertino, and J.J. Walshe.** 1987. Overestimation of vancomycin concentration utilizing fluoresence polarization immunoassay in patients on peritoneal dialysis. Ther. Drug Monit. **9**: 212-215.

(23) **Nicolau, D.P., C.D. Freeman, P.P. Belliveau, C.H. Nightingale, J.W. Ross, and R. Quintiliani.** 1995. Experience with a once-daily aminoglycoside program administered to 2184 adult patients. Antimicrob. Agents Chemother. **39**: 650-655.

(24) **Pehourcq, F., and C. Jarry.** 1998. Determination of third-generation cehalosporins by high-performance liquid chromatography in connection with pharmacokinetic studies. J. Chromatogr. A. **812**: 159-178.

(25) **Reeves, D.S., R. Wise, J.M. Andrews, and L.O. White.** 1999. Clinical Antimicrobial Assays. Oxford University Press. Oxford, UK.

(26) **Rolain, J.M., A. Boulos, M.N. Mallet, and D. Raoult.** 2005. Correlation between ratio of serum doxycycline concentration to MIC and rapid decline of antibody levels during treatment of Q fever endocarditis. Antimicrob. Agents Chemother. **49**: 2673-2676.

(27) **Rotschafer, J.C., C. Morlock, L. Strand, and K. Crossley.** 1982. Comparison of radioimmunoassay and enzyme immunoassay methods in determining gentamicin pharmacokinetic parameters and dosages. Antimicrob. Agents Chemother. **22**: 648-651.

(28) **Selepak, S.T., F.G. Witebsky. E.A. Robertson, and J.D. Mac Lowry.** 1981. Evaluation of five gentamicin assay procedures for clinical microbiology laboratories. J. Clin. Microbiol. **13**: 742-749.

(29) **Smith, P.F., W.P. Petros, M.P. Soucie, and K.R. Copeland.** 1998. New modified fluorescence polarization immunoassay does not falsely elevate vancomycin concentrations in patients with end-stage renal disease. Ther. Drug Monit. **20**: 231-235.

(30) **Stevens, P., and L.S. Young.** 1977. Simple method for elimination of aminoglycosides from serum to permit bioassay of other antimicrobial agents. Antimicrob. Agents Chemother. **12**: 286-287.

(31) **Trujillo, T.N., K.M. Sowinski, R.A. Venezia, M.K. Scott, and B.A. Mueller.** 1999. Vancomycin assay performance in patients with acute renal failure. Int. Care Med. **25**: 1291-1296.

(32) **Walterspiel, J.N., S. Feldman, R. Van, and W.R. Ravis.** 1991. Comparative inactivation of isepamicin, amikacin, and gentamicin by nine beta-lactam and two beta-lactamase inhibitors, cilastatin and heparin. Antimicrob. Agents Chemother. **35**: 1875-1878.

(33) **Zeller, V., L. Lhotellier, M.D. Kitzis, J.M. Ziza, P. Mamoudy, and N. Desplaces.** 2004. Traitement des infections osseuses sur matériel étranger. Lett. Infect. **19**: 204-216.

Chapter 9. REPORTING OF THE RESULTS

Fred C. TENOVER and Janet A. HINDLER

INTRODUCTION

Antimicrobial Susceptibility Testing (AST) is a critical task of microbiology laboratories. In an age where antimicrobial resistance among bacterial isolates is becoming more common and multiple drug resistance is emerging in many Gram-negative pathogens leaving few treatment options (12, 28), the importance of rapid and concise AST reports cannot be underestimated. In addition, AST results not only guide individual patient therapy but aggregate results can be used to guide the selection of empiric therapy (3, 7). All of these activities, however, presuppose that the AST results are reported accurately and effectively by the laboratory. Even when strict attention is paid to issues such as how organisms are selected for AST and how the susceptibility test is performed and interpreted, ineffective reporting can nullify the impact of any AST result (11). The way in which the laboratory communicates AST results to the physician is the subject of this chapter.

PRELUDE TO EFFECTIVE REPORTING - SELECTING ORGANISMS FOR AST

The first step to effective reporting involves developing protocols that specify which of the organisms isolated from clinical specimens will be subjected to AST and those organisms for which AST is not warranted. This will vary by specimen source and sometimes by patient age and gender. The decision to test should be based on the likelihood that the organism is causing an infection and does not have a predictable susceptibility profile. For example, when coagulase-negative staphylococci (CoNS) are present in large quantities in pure culture from multiple blood cultures in a patient with an indwelling central catheter, the CoNS should be tested for susceptibility to a variety of antimicrobial agents including vancomycin (24). However, when only a few colonies of CoNS are isolated from a superficial leg wound that also grows abundant amounts of *Staphylococcus aureus*, it is unlikely that the CoNS are contributing to the infection and AST should not be performed on these isolates. According to many physicians in informal surveys, AST results on a bacteriology report imply that the organism is causing an infection and that the physician should consider antimicrobial therapy for the patient. Reporting AST results on organisms that are unlikely to represent infection may result in unwarranted and inappropriate antimicrobial therapy that may put the patient at risk for an adverse drug reaction, or worse, a *Clostridium difficile* infection (14, 17). In addition, the physician may fail to search further to identify the true cause of the patient's infection. On the other hand, some bacterial species still have predictable antimicrobial susceptibility patterns to certain classes of antimicrobial agents and need not be tested. For example, *Streptococcus pyogenes* isolates remain susceptible to penicillin and, according to CLSI guidelines, need not be tested against this class of agents (6). However, the susceptibility of *S. pyogenes* isolates to erythromycin and clindamycin is not predictable and these agents should be tested, if the physician is considering using one of these classes of agents for therapy.

TIMELINESS OF AST REPORTS

A drawback to AST reporting is often the slow turnaround time of final results, which may require anywhere from 6 to 48 h beyond the time that the organism is available in pure culture. While most results are available in 18-24 h, the presence of extended-spectrum β-lactamases (ESBLs), possible resistance to vancomycin among *S. aureus* isolates, or the occurrence of an unusual antibiogram may delay release of results because confirmation of results is required. An exception to this involves molecular amplification tests that identify methicillin-resistant *S. aureus* (MRSA), *Mycobacterium tuberculosis*, or other bacterial pathogens directly in clinical specimens, such as blood cultures, wounds or respiratory samples, where results may be available within a few hours (13, 15, 21, 33). For other situations, the shortest time to AST results is with rapid automated AST systems where results may be available for some bacterial species 6-8 h after isolated colonies become available, or 24-32 h after a culture is obtained. From a practical standpoint, patients are often placed on broad-spectrum antimicrobial agents empirically until the AST report indicates that the isolate is susceptible to narrower-spectrum agents, indicating that therapy can be de-escalated.

Despite the slow turnaround, it is important to understand the potential impact of AST reports. For example, in cases of life-threatening disease, such as bacterial meningitis, endocarditis, or fulminate sepsis, rapid identification of the infecting agent and a rapid assessment of the bacterial susceptibility profile can dramatically influence the outcome of the disease (18, 27). This is particularly true if the pathogen is resistant to the antimicrobial agents commonly used for empiric therapy, such as in the case of ceftriaxone for bacterial meningitis. If a culture of cerebrospinal fluid reveals ceftriaxone-resistant *Streptococcus pneumoniae*, the laboratory should contact the physician immediately (19, 26). Similarly, if a wound culture from a patient in an intensive care unit grows a Gram-negative bacterium, such as *Klebsiella pneumoniae*, that is resistant to all agents commonly tested, including carbapenems, the patient's physician should be notified (12). In addition, because of the risk for spread of this multidrug resistant organism to other patients, infection control personnel should also be notified when a multidrug resistant organism is recovered from a patient (22, 34).

FORMATING THE AST REPORT

Measurements obtained from ASTs, which include either zone diameters from disk diffusion tests or MICs from dilution tests, are interpreted as susceptible, intermediate, or resistant using criteria published by standards-setting organizations, such as the Clinical and Laboratory Standards Institute (CLSI) (4, 5) or the European Union Committee on Antimicrobial Susceptibility Testing (EUCAST) [http://www.eucast.org/clinical_breakpoints/]. The final AST report may include qualitative interpretive results [susceptible (S), intermediate (I), or resistant (R)] only, or quantitative results (usually MIC values) together with S, I, or R interpretations. In addition, it is becoming increasingly common for AST reports to include one or more comments, qualifications, or further explanations.

Qualitative results

The qualitative or interpretive result (S, I, R) for each antimicrobial agent tested is the most critical piece of information on the AST report. Reports missing interpretations or with non-standardized interpretations (e.g., "conditionally susceptible" or "low-level resistance") are often confusing and either lead to telephone calls to the laboratory for an explanation, or the selection of another antimicrobial agent for therapy (such as one marked "S"). Making sure that the most current version of interpretive standards is used for interpretation of results (such as the M100 series, which is published annually by CLSI, or the EUCAST website) is critical, since both MIC and disk diffusion interpretive criteria (also known as breakpoints) may change from year to year. Two recent examples of breakpoint changes include the lowering of the vancomycin MIC breakpoints for *S. aureus* (6, 31) by one doubling dilution, and the addition of a new set of higher MIC breakpoints for parenteral penicillin for *S. pneumoniae* for non-meningitis indications (6).

Quantitative results

The MIC values on an AST report for a series of antimicrobial agents can be of considerable value to a physician, particularly when selecting therapy for a deep-seated infection, such as endocarditis or osteomyelitis (1, 16, 18, 20). In these cases, the limited penetration of some antimicrobial agents into heart tissue or bone can reduce the effectiveness of an agent, even when the AST result is in the susceptible range. Therefore, an antimicrobial agent that has an MIC at the lower end of the susceptible range would be preferred over an agent with a higher MIC. MIC results are particularly useful for physicians who use pharmacokinetic and pharmacodynamic principles to select anti-infective therapy.

Listing disk diffusion zone diameters on AST reports can be confusing for physicians, since some antimicrobial agents often give small zones of inhibition even for susceptible organisms. Although the laboratory should record zone diameters for each antimicrobial agent tested for internal use, they should not report zone diameter results without S, I, R interpretations to the physician, although this practice has been reported (30). Preferentially, the interpretation only (S, I, or R) is reported.

Cascade or selective reporting

Using antimicrobial agents wisely and judiciously goes beyond just prescribing the correct antimicrobial agent, at the correct dosage, for the correct period of time (23, 29). It often involves narrowing the spectrum of the antimicrobial agent given from broad coverage to more focused therapy (e.g., changing from imipenem to ampicillin for an ampicillin-susceptible *E. coli* isolate), while considering cost effectiveness and the selective pressure exerted by using that antimicrobial agent in that patient in that healthcare setting (23). While judicious antimicrobial use, also known an antimicrobial stewardship, is a strategic goal in many hospitals, and strongly supported by professional societies such as the Infectious Disease Society of America (10), many microbiology laboratories are reluctant to withhold any information from physicians regarding the antimicrobial susceptibility profiles of bacterial isolates. Deciding which susceptibility test results to report and which to suppress deserves careful consideration (11).

Ultimately, the purpose of cascade or selective reporting is to reserve the most potent, broadest spectrum antimicrobial agents as the agents of last resort. This is accomplished by directing physicians to use older, more narrow-spectrum agents that will be efficacious first. Other criteria that sometimes factor into selective reporting protocols include cost and potential toxicity of an agent (10). Keeping the selective pressure low for the emergence of vancomycin, linezolid, and daptomycin resistance in enterococci and staphylococci, and avoiding the development and spread of extended-spectrum beta-lactamase and carbapenemase-mediated resistance in enteric Gram-negative bacilli, *Acinetobacter* species, and *Pseudomonas* species is a critical goal of antimicrobial stewardship. Several key concepts of cascading are depicted in Table 1.

One caveat for cascade reporting involves reporting unexpected resistance. For example, a laboratory may suppress reporting of carbapenems among *Enterobacteriaceae* that are susceptible to cephalosporins. However, an isolate of *Serratia marcescens* that produces an SME carbapenemase may test susceptible to some cephalosporins but resistant to carbapenems. In this case, both cephalosporins and carbapenems should be reported, assuming that the carbapenem resistance phenotype is reproducible.

Suppressing agents inappropriate for the species isolated or specimen source

For cost-conscious and streamlined AST, many laboratories will only routinely test a limited number of antimicrobial agents, whether by MIC or disk diffusion testing. This is true also of laboratories using automated AST methods. It is commonplace to have separate MIC panels (or a set of disks for disk diffusion testing) for non-fastidious Gram-positive cocci (staphylococci and enterococci) and for non-fastidious Gram-negative rods (*Enterobacteriaceae* and glucose non-fermenters). Some laboratories may have an additional panel for streptococci, and another panel that contains agents that may require testing in selected situations (e.g., a *Pseudomonas aeruginosa* isolate that is resistant to all agents on the primary panel or from a cystic fibrosis patient). Depending on the species isolated and specimen source, not all of the antimicrobial agents on a panel may be appropriate for reporting. For example, a non-fastidious Gram-positive panel may include clindamycin, however, clindamycin should be suppressed for enterococcal isolates (since all enterococci are resistant to clindamycin). Similarly, trimethoprim-sulfamethoxazole would likely be included on most Gram-negative panels, but should not be reported for *P. aeruginosa*. Some agents, such as nitrofurantoin, should be suppressed for organisms

Table 1. Cascade reporting examples for *Enterobacteriaceae*[a]

Antimicrobial class	If organism is susceptible to:	Then do not report results for:
Aminoglycosides	Gentamicin	Tobramycin or amikacin
β-lactams	Ampicillin	Ampicillin-sulbactam
	Cephalothin or cefazolin	Ceftriaxone or cefepime
	Ceftriaxone and piperacillin-tazobactam	Imipenem

[a] Cascading rules are typically institution-specific and should be established only after consultation among the laboratory, the medical and infectious disease services, the pharmacy service, and infection control committee.

isolated from sources other than urine, and agents that do not penetrate the blood-brain barrier, such as narrow spectrum cephalosporins, should not be reported on isolates from cerebrospinal fluid. Thus, there are many caveats to consider in order to provide accurate reports and the optimal information to the physician.

Comments, qualifications, and further explanations

Although not all laboratory information systems have the ability to add free text or standardized comments to AST reports, such comments can be very useful to physicians. CLSI standards contain a series of comments that relate to specific results obtained from testing; other comments relate to therapeutic approaches (4-6). A comment on the report that "MRSA are resistant to all beta-lactams" would likely eliminate requests for testing cephalosporins or other beta-lactam agents for MRSA isolates. For enterococcal endocarditis, a comment suggesting combination therapy (e.g., a cell wall active agent and an aminoglycoside) may prevent clinicians from contemplating use of a cell wall active agent that tests susceptible as single agent therapy. For drugs where multiple dosing options are available, a comment regarding the recommendation of using high doses of a drug to treat meningitis may be useful. Reporting reduced susceptibility of *Salmonella* species to fluoroquinolones, as demonstrated by resistance to nalidixic acid (8, 9), can indicate that alternative therapy should be considered, particularly when the isolate is causing a systemic infection. All of these explanations could be communicated in supplemental comments on AST reports.

AST RESULTS REQUIRING FOLLOW UP

Results requiring additional tests or confirmation of initial results

Most antimicrobial susceptibility results generated by routine AST systems stand alone and can be reported to the physician once the technologist confirms that the results are accurate. However, there are some results that require additional attention.

Some types of resistance are difficult to detect with routine disk diffusion or MIC tests. Consequently, supplemental tests must be performed prior to reporting results (Table 2). For

Table 2. Examples of antimicrobial susceptibility test results that require supplemental testing prior to reporting. The routine method may be inadequate to detect resistance

Organism	Results requiring supplemental test	Test required	Rationale
Staphylococcus spp.	Penicillin MIC ≤0.12 µg/ml (interpreted as susceptible)	Induced β-lactamase test	Some staphylococci for which the penicillin MICs are ≤0.12 µg/ml produce beta-lactamase and would be considered penicillin-resistant
Coagulase-negative *Staphylococcus* spp.	Oxacillin MIC 0.5-2 µg/ml (interpreted as resistant)	Optional *mecA* assay or cefoxitin disk diffusion test	Oxacillin MIC lacks specificity for staphylococcal species other than *S. epidermidis*
Staphylococcus spp. *Streptococcus*, β group	Clindamycin for clindamycin susceptible and erythromycin resistant isolates	Inducible clindamycin resistance (disk diffusion or MIC)	Some isolates with *erm*-mediated clindamycin resistance test susceptible to clindamycin unless induced
Staphylococcus aureus	Vancomycin zone ≥7 mm by disk diffusion	Vancomycin MIC	Disk diffusion inadequate to distinguish vancomycin susceptible, intermediate, and resistant *S. aureus*
Streptococcus pneumoniae	Oxacillin zone ≤19 mm by disk diffusion (oxacillin disk diffusion screen for non-meningeal isolates only)	Penicillin MIC	*S. pneumoniae* producing zones of inhibition of ≤19 mm around an oxacillin disk may have penicillin MICs in the susceptible, intermediate, or resistant range
Enterobacteriaceae	Carbapenem zones of inhibition at the lower end (disk diffusion) or MICs at the upper end of the susceptible range	Carbapenem inactivation test	Current carbapenem CLSI interpretive criteria may not detect carbapenemase-producing Enterobacteriaceae

example, the addition of vancomycin macro E-test® results to an MRSA report, further clarifying the reduced susceptibility of the organism to vancomycin (i.e., the presence of the heteroresistance phenotype), can be of value when the patient is not responding to vancomycin therapy (31, 32).

In some cases of infection, suspicion of emerging resistance, where the bacterial isolate appears susceptible to an antimicrobial agent even though it contains subpopulations of cells with increased levels of resistance, the laboratory may be required to perform additional testing beyond the standard susceptibility testing panel to insure accurate reporting. Vancomycin heteroresistance in an isolate of *S. aureus* or hidden carbapenemase activity in *K. pneumoniae* isolates, are examples of "stealth" resistance phenotypes that challenge the microbiology laboratory. Such suspicions must be communicated to the physician early so that alternative treatment strategies can be considered if heteroresistance is confirmed.

Other AST results that are uncommon and that should be confirmed prior to reporting are listed in Table 3. For these, the method used to confirm the unusual findings could be a reference method (e.g., CLSI broth microdilution, agar dilution, or disk diffusion method) or a commercial method that has demonstrated accuracy for the results in question.

Reporting of critical AST values

Microbiologists should develop a "critical values" list for AST results that would include results that require immediate notification of the physician and, in some cases, infection control personnel. For example, suspicion that an *S. aureus* isolate may demonstrate high-level vancomycin resistance (i.e., vancomycin MIC ≥ 16 µg/ml) (2, 4, 6, 25) is a critical preliminary result for the

Table 3. Examples of antimicrobial susceptibility test results that should be confirmed prior to reporting; phenotype that are uncommon or not reported to date[a]

Organism	Results requiring confirmation
Enterococcus spp.	Daptomycin-non-susceptible
	Linezolid-resistant
Staphylococcus spp.	Daptomycin-non-susceptible
	Linezolid-non-susceptible
	Quinupristin-dalfopristin-intermediate or resistant
Staphylococcus aureus	Vancomycin-intermediate or resistant (MIC ≥ 4 µg/ml) or no zone around vancomycin disk[b]
Streptococcus pneumoniae	Linezolid-non-susceptible
	Carbapenem-intermediate or resistant[b]
	Quinupristin-dalfopristin-intermediate or resistant
	Vancomycin-non-susceptible[b]
Streptococcus, beta group	Ampicillin or penicillin-non-susceptible[b]
	Carbapenem-non-susceptible[b]
	Extended-spectrum cephalosporin-non-susceptible[b]
	Daptomycin-non-susceptible
	Linezolid-non-susceptible
	Quinupristin-dalfopristin-intermediate or resistant
	Vancomycin-non-susceptible[b]
Streptococcus, viridans group	Daptomycin-non-susceptible
	Linezolid-non-susceptible
	Quinupristin-dalfopristin-intermediate or resistant
	Vancomycin-non-susceptible[b]
Enterobacteriaceae	Carbapenem-intermediate or resistant[b]
Acinetobacter baumannii	Colistin/polymyxin-B resistant[b]
Pseudomonas aeruginosa	Colistin/polymyxin-B intermediate or resistant[b]
Stenotrophomonas maltophilia	Trimethoprim-sulfamethoxazole resistant
Neisseria meningitidis	Extended-spectrum cephalosporin non-susceptible[b]

[a] Does not imply all antimicrobial agent/organism combinations listed should be routinely tested.
[b] Critical results; immediate notification of physician and possibly infection control suggested. Information compiled in part from reference (6) and EUCAST website, Expert rules, Tables 5 and 6.

patient's physician and for the infection control service. A strain that shows no zone of inhibition around a vancomycin disk or yields a vancomycin resistant result using an automated testing system requires confirmation. Simply withholding the vancomycin result while confirming the phenotype may have devastating consequences both for the patient and the hospital should such a strain containing the *vanA* vancomycin resistance gene, emerge and spread. Preliminary reports, which inform the physician that additional testing is necessary or underway, are often underutilized by clinical microbiologists. A list of preliminary results that require confirmation, some of which are considered critical, is highlighted in Table 3.

TOOLS FOR GENERATING ACCURATE AND EFFECTIVE REPORTS - THE NEED FOR EXPERT SOFTWARE OR ARTIFICIAL INTELLIGENCE

AST reporting has become quite complex and there are many rules that must be considered, prior to reporting AST results. It is nearly impossible for the practicing clinical microbiologist to consistently apply all of these rules. Consequently, manufacturers of commercial AST systems have developed software that facilitates application of the rules. Additionally, a set of expert rules is available on the EUCAST website [http://www.eucast.org/expert_rules/]. Some laboratories may utilize their laboratory information system to maintain the rules. Typically, the software will automatically flag unusual results that require additional testing, immediate notification of the physician and/or reporting to infection control. In addition, the software can apply cascading or selective reporting rules, edit certain susceptible results to resistant, and add comments to the patient's report. In an era when there is a shortage of qualified and trained personnel to perform laboratory tests, it is critical that such software or expert rules are updated, readily available, and utilized to the maximum.

DECISIONS RELATED TO AST REPORTS

There are many decisions to be made with reporting AST results. These include selecting antimicrobial agents for the test panels, developing rules for reporting specific agents based on the species tested, body site and overall susceptibility profile, and adding comments to the report. In addition, decisions must be made for those results that should immediately be reported to the patient's physician, infection control, and possibly public health authorities. Laboratory personnel should review the various options with representatives of the infectious disease and pharmacy services to insure that their AST reporting protocols are consistent with pharmacy or infectious disease practice.

REFERENCES

(1) **Calhoun, J. H., and M. M. Manring.** 2005. Adult osteomyelitis. Infect. Dis. Clin. North. Am. **19:**765-786.
(2) **Chang, S., D. M. Sievert, J. C. Hageman, M. L. Boulton, F. C. Tenover, F. P. Downes, S. Shah, J. T. Rudrik, G. R. Pupp, W. J. Brown, D. Cardo, and S. K. Fridkin.** 2003. Infection with vancomycin-resistant *Staphylococcus aureus* containing the *vanA* resistance gene. N. Engl. J. Med. **348:**1342-1347.
(3) **Clinical and Laboratory Standards Institute.** 2009. Analysis and presentation of cumulative antimicrobial susceptibility test data; Approved Guideline - Third Edition M39-A3. Clinical and Laboratory Standards Institute, Wayne, PA.
(4) **Clinical and Laboratory Standards Institute.** 2009. Methods for dilution antimicrobial susceptibility tests for bacteria that grow aerobically; Approved standard- Eighth Edition M7-A8. Clinical and Laboratory Standards Institute, Wayne, PA.
(5) **Clinical and Laboratory Standards Institute.** 2009. Performance standards for antimicrobial disk susceptibility tests; Approved standard-Tenth Edition M2-A10. Clinical and Laboratory Standards Institute, Wayne, PA.
(6) **Clinical and Laboratory Standards Institute.** 2009. Performance standards for antimicrobial susceptibility testing; Nineteenth informational supplement; M100-S19. Clinical and Laboratory Standards Institute, Wayne, PA.
(7) **Critchley, I. A., and J. A. Karlowsky.** 2004. Optimal use of antibiotic resistance surveillance systems. Clin. Microbiol. Infect. **10:**502-511.
(8) **Crump, J. A., T. J. Barrett, J. T. Nelson, and F. J. Angulo.** 2003. Reevaluating fluoroquinolone breakpoints for *Salmonella enterica* serotype Typhi and for non-Typhi salmonellae. Clin. Infect. Dis. **37:**75-81.
(9) **Crump, J. A., K. Kretsinger, K. Gay, R. M. Hoekstra, D. J. Vugia, S. Hurd, S. D. Segler, M. Megginson, L. J. Luedeman, B. Shiferaw, S. S. Hanna, K. W. Joyce, E. D. Mintz, and F. J. Angulo.** 2008. Clinical response and outcome of infection with *Salmonella enterica* serotype Typhi with decreased susceptibility to fluoroquinolones: a United States foodnet multicenter retrospective cohort study. Antimicrob. Agents Chemother. **52:**1278-1284.
(10) **Dellit, T. H., R. C. Owens, J. E. McGowan, Jr., D. N. Gerding, R. A. Weinstein, J. P. Burke, W. C.**

Huskins, D. L. Paterson, N. O. Fishman, C. F. Carpenter, P. J. Brennan, M. Billeter, and T. M. Hooton. 2007. Infectious Diseases Society of America and the Society for Healthcare Epidemiology of America guidelines for developing an institutional program to enhance antimicrobial stewardship. Clin. Infect. Dis. **44:**159-177.

(11) **Diekema, D. J., K. Lee, P. Raney, L. A. Herwaldt, G. V. Doern, and F. C. Tenover.** 2004. Accuracy and appropriateness of antimicrobial susceptibility test reporting for bacteria isolated from blood cultures. J. Clin. Microbiol. **42:**2258-2260.

(12) **Endimiani, A., A. M. Hujer, F. Perez, C. R. Bethel, K. M. Hujer, J. Kroeger, M. Oethinger, D. L. Paterson, M. D. Adams, M. R. Jacobs, D. J. Diekema, G. S. Hall, S. G. Jenkins, L. B. Rice, F. C. Tenover, and R. A. Bonomo.** 2009. Characterization of *bla*KPC-containing *Klebsiella pneumoniae* isolates detected in different institutions in the Eastern USA. J. Antimicrob. Chemother. **63:**427-437.

(13) **Evans, J., M. C. Stead, M. P. Nicol, and H. Segal.** 2009. Rapid genotypic assays to identify drug-resistant *Mycobacterium tuberculosis* in South Africa. J. Antimicrob. Chemother. **63:**11-16.

(14) **Gerding, D. N., C. A. Muto, and R. C. Owens, Jr.** 2008. Measures to control and prevent *Clostridium difficile* infection. Clin. Infect. Dis. **46 Suppl 1:**S43-49.

(15) **Jones, M., D. Helb, E. Story, C. Boehme, E. Wallace, K. Ho, J. Kop, M. Owens, R. Rodgers, P. Banada, H. Safi, R. Blakemore, N. Lan, E. Jones-López, M. Levi, M. Burday, I. Ayakaka, R. Mugerwa, B. McMillan, E. Winn-Deen, L. Christel, P. Dailey, M. Perkins, D. Persing, and D. Alland.** 2009. Rapid detection of *Mycobacterium tuberculosis* and rifampin-resistance from sputum samples with an easy-to-use PCR test system with near-patient capability. Abstracts of the 19th European Congress of Clinical Microbiology and Infectious Diseases, Helsinki Finland:**0185.

(16) **Kaplan, S. L.** 2005. Osteomyelitis in children. Infect. Dis. Clin. North. Am. **19:**787-797.

(17) **Kelly, C. P., and J. T. LaMont.** 2008. *Clostridium difficile*--more difficult than ever. N. Engl. J. Med. **359:**1932-1940.

(18) **Kollef, M. H., G. Sherman, S. Ward, and V. J. Fraser.** 1999. Inadequate antimicrobial treatment of infections: a risk factor for hospital mortality among critically ill patients. Chest **115:**462-474.

(19) **Leggiadro, R. J., F. F. Barrett, P. J. Chesney, Y. Davis, and F. C. Tenover.** 1994. Invasive pneumococci with high level penicillin and cephalosporin resistance at a mid-south children's hospital. Pediatr. Infect. Dis. J. **13:**320-322.

(20) **Murdoch, D. R., G. R. Corey, B. Hoen, J. M. Miro, V. G. Fowler, Jr., A. S. Bayer, A. W. Karchmer, L. Olaison, P. A. Pappas, P. Moreillon, S. T. Chambers, V. H. Chu, V. Falco, D. J. Holland, P. Jones, J. L. Klein, N. J. Raymond, K. M. Read, M. F. Tripodi, R. Utili, A. Wang, C. W. Woods, and C. H. Cabell.** 2009. Clinical presentation, etiology, and outcome of infective endocarditis in the 21st century: the International Collaboration on Endocarditis-Prospective Cohort Study. Arch. Intern. Med. **169:**463-473.

(21) **Parta, M., M. Goebel, M. Matloobi, C. Stager, and D. M. Musher.** 2009. Identification of methicillin-resistant or methicillin-susceptible *Staphylococcus aureus* in blood cultures and wound swabs by GeneXpert. J. Clin. Microbiol. **47:**1609-1610.

(22) **Patel, G., S. Huprikar, S. H. Factor, S. G. Jenkins, and D. P. Calfee.** 2008. Outcomes of carbapenem-resistant *Klebsiella pneumoniae* infection and the impact of antimicrobial and adjunctive therapies. Infect. Control. Hosp. Epidemiol. **29:**1099-1106.

(23) **Rice, L. B.** 2008. The Maxwell Finland Lecture: for the duration-rational antibiotic administration in an era of antimicrobial resistance and *Clostridium difficile*. Clin. Infect. Dis. **46:**491-496.

(24) **Rogers, K. L., P. D. Fey, and M. E. Rupp.** 2009. Coagulase-negative staphylococcal infections. Infect. Dis. Clin. North. Am. **23:**73-98.

(25) **Sievert, D. M., J. T. Rudrik, J. B. Patel, L. C. McDonald, M. J. Wilkins, and J. C. Hageman.** 2008. Vancomycin-resistant *Staphylococcus aureus* in the United States, 2002-2006. Clin. Infect. Dis. **46:**668-674.

(26) **Sloas, M. M., F. F. Barrett, P. J. Chesney, B. K. English, B. C. Hill, F. C. Tenover, and R. J. Leggiadro.** 1992. Cephalosporin treatment failure in penicillin- and cephalosporin-resistant *Streptococcus pneumoniae* meningitis. Pediatr. Infect. Dis. J. **11:**662-666.

(27) **Somand, D., and W. Meurer.** 2009. Central nervous system infections. Emerg. Med. Clin. North. Am. **27:**89-100, ix.

(28) **Souli, M., I. Galani, and H. Giamarellou.** 2008. Emergence of extensively drug-resistant and pan-drug-resistant Gram-negative bacilli in Europe. Euro. Surveill. **13:**1-11.

(29) **Spellberg, B., R. Guidos, D. Gilbert, J. Bradley, H. W. Boucher, W. M. Scheld, J. G. Bartlett, and J. Edwards, Jr.** 2008. The epidemic of antibiotic-resistant infections: a call to action for the medical community from the Infectious Diseases Society of America. Clin. Infect. Dis. **46:**155-164.

(30) **Stevenson, K. B., M. Samore, J. Barbera, J. W. Moore, E. Hannah, P. Houck, F. C. Tenover, and J. L. Gerberding.** 2003. Detection of antimicrobial resistance by small rural hospital microbiology laboratories: comparison of survey responses with current NCCLS laboratory standards. Diagn. Microbiol. Infect. Dis. **47:**303-311.

(31) **Tenover, F. C., and R. C. Moellering, Jr.** 2007. The rationale for revising the Clinical and Laboratory Standards Institute vancomycin minimal inhibitory concentration interpretive criteria for *Staphylococcus aureus*. Clin. Infect. Dis. **44:**1208-1215.

(32) **Tenover, F. C., S. W. Sinner, R. E. Segal, V. Huang, S. S. Alexandre, J. E. McGowan, Jr., and M. P. Weinstein.** 2009. Characterisation of a *Staphylococcus aureus* strain with progressive loss of susceptibility to vancomycin and daptomycin during therapy. Int. J. Antimicrob. Agents **33:**564-568.

(33) **Wolk, D. M., M. J. Struelens, P. Pancholi, T. Davis, P. Della-Latta, D. Fuller, E. Picton, R. Dickenson, O. Denis, D. Johnson, and K. Chapin.** 2009. Rapid detection of *Staphylococcus aureus* and methicillin-resistant *S. aureus* (MRSA) in wound specimens and blood cultures: multicenter preclinical evaluation of the Cepheid Xpert MRSA/SA skin

and soft tissue and blood culture assays. J. Clin. Microbiol. **47:**823-826.

(34) **Yokoe, D. S., L. A. Mermel, D. J. Anderson, K. M. Arias, H. Burstin, D. P. Calfee, S. E. Coffin, E. R. Dubberke, V. Fraser, D. N. Gerding, F. A. Griffin, P. Gross, K. S. Kaye, M. Klompas, E. Lo, J. Marschall, L. Nicolle, D. A. Pegues, T. M. Perl, K. Podgorny, S. Saint, C. D. Salgado, R. A. Weinstein, R. Wise, and D. Classen.** 2008. A compendium of strategies to prevent healthcare-associated infections in acute care hospitals. Infect. Control. Hosp. Epidemiol. **29 Suppl 1:**S12-21.

Second Part:

ANTIBIOGRAM OF MAJOR BACTERIAL GROUPS

Chapter 10. β-LACTAMS AND STAPHYLOCOCCI

Vincent CATTOIR and Roland LECLERCQ

INTRODUCTION

Staphylococci are Gram-positive bacteria that are naturally susceptible to β-lactams (with the exception of monobactams). *Staphylococcus aureus* is responsible for numerous human infections of community and nosocomial origins. They have the incredible ability of adapting very rapidly to antibiotic pressure through acquired resistance. Following the introduction of penicillin G in clinical use in the early 40's, the first resistant strains emerged during subsequent years. Only two years after the 1959 clinical introduction of β-lactamase resistant penicillin-M, the first strains of *S. aureus* that were methicillin resistant (MRSA) were isolated. Among the coagulase-negative staphylococci (CNS), two species are above all multi-resistant to β-lactam antibiotics, *Staphylococcus epidermidis* and *Staphylococcus haemolyticus*.

MODE OF ACTION OF β-LACTAMS

β-lactams are time-dependent bactericidal antibiotics that act on the bacteria during the growth phase. Like glycopeptides, they interfere with the metabolism of peptidoglycan that is the principal component of the bacterial wall notably during the final stages of transpeptidation. They act by inhibiting the enzymes known as 'penicillin binding proteins' (PBP) which are implicated in the biosynthesis and modification of peptidoglycan (16). *S. aureus* has four natural PBPs: PBP1, PBP2, PBP3 and PBP4 (17). The PBPs of high molecular weight (PBP1, 2, and 3) are bi-functional enzymes with a C-terminal transpeptidase domain and a N-terminal transglycosylase domain (17). They are essential to the growth and the survival of the bacterial cell, and the β-lactams strongly bind to their transpeptidase domain (Table 1) (3, 6, 9). PBP4, the only PBP of low molecular weight, is non-essential to the survival of the bacteria and is not a privileged target for β-lactams (Table 1). In general, there is a direct correlation between the binding affinity of the β-lactam with the essential PBPs, and inhibition of bacterial growth. In *S. aureus*, anti-staphylococcal activity of a β-lactam correlates with the binding affinity to PBP1 that corresponds to the major transpeptidase, as well as to PBP3 that is implicated in septation. PBP2 is a transpeptidase that functions in stationary phase and PBP4 has carboxypeptidase activity (10).

In CNS, depending on the species, there are between two and five PBPs. Similarly to *S. aureus*, PBPs of high molecular weight with transpeptidase activity are primary targets of β-lactams.

Table 1. Binding of β-lactams to *S. aureus* PBPs (3, 6, 9).

Antibiotic	IC_{50} (μg/ml)[a]				
	PBP (85 kDa)	PBP2 (81 kDa)	PBP2a (78 kDa)	PBP3 (75 kDa)	PBP4 (45 kDa)
Penicillin G	0.1	0.03	17	0.01	13
Ampicillin	0.6	0.4	15	0.1	150
Oxacillin	1	0.2	300	0.1	4
Cefamandole	0.04	0.1	50	0.02	6
Cefoxitine	4	0.3	50	2	0.02
Cefotaxime	0.3	0.3	>1000	7	3
Ceftobiprole	0.1	0.5	0.9	0.05	1
Ceftaroline	0.25	0.14	0.9	0.5	86
Imipenem	0.07	0.07	60	0.05	0.02
Clavulanate	13	0.2	>1000	30	14

[a] IC_{50}, β-lactam concentration required to prevent 50 % binding to PBP.

The β-lactams display a strong structural analogy with peptidoglycan precursor motifs, D-Ala-D-Ala (Fig. 1). These antibiotics react like 'suicide' substrates for high molecular weight PBPs. After serine acetylation of the active site (S-X-X-K), a covalent complex is formed inactivating the enzyme; this, in turn, inhibits synthesis of peptidoglycan, stopping growth, morphological development and resulting in bacteriolysis by autolysin system induction (Fig. 2). In Gram-positive bacteria, the PBPs are located on the external side of the cytoplasmic membrane; thus β-lactams do not have to cross the membrane to reach their targets (17).

β-LACTAM ACTIVITY

Against wild-type strains not-producing penicillinase, the most active β-lactams are: penicillin G, ampicillin, and amoxicillin (Table 2). However, because of the high prevalence of penicillinase production, the M group penicillinases (oxacillin, cloxacillin, nafcillin) remain the most active. Among the cephalosporins, none has better *in vitro* activity than oxacillin considering that those of 3rd generation are generally less active than those of 1st and 2nd generations (Table 2) (1). Imipenem and other carbapenems display activity similar to that of oxacillin (Table 2) and are inactive against MRSA (19). Interest in new cephalosporins (ceftobiprole, ceftaroline) has been raised by the fact that they have strong affinity to PBP2a produced by MRSA. These cephalosporins are active on MRSAs with MIC_{90} similar to those of cefotaxime on MSSA (Table 2). All things considered, in absence of acquired resistance, oxacillin, cloxacillin, and nafcillin remain the reference β-lactams against *S. aureus*.

RESISTANCE MECHANISMS

There are two mechanisms of resistance to β-lactams in staphylococci: production of β-lactamase and modification of the target by either acquisition of an exogenous PBP, more frequently, or alteration of an endogenous PBP, more rarely.

Table 2. MIC (µg/ml) of β-lactams for *S. aureus* isolates suceptible (MSSA) or resistant (SARM) to metHicillin (1, 9, 18, 19).

β-lactam	MSSA		MRSA	
	MIC_{50}	MIC_{90}	MIC_{50}	MIC_{90}
Penicillins				
Penicillin	0.03[a]	0.06[a]	32	>32
Ampicillin	0.06[a]	0.12[a]	32	>32
Oxacillin	1	1	32	>32
Amoxicillin-clavulanate acid	1	2	>32	>32
Piperacillin-tazobactam				
Cephalosporins				
Cephalotin	0.25	0.5	32	>32
Cefamandole	0.5	1	8	8
Cefoxitine	2	4	32	>32
Cefotetan	8	8	>32	>32
Moxalactam	8	16	>32	>32
Cefotaxime	2	2	>32	>32
Ceftriaxone	4	4	>32	>32
Ceftazidime	16	16	>32	>32
Cefepime	2	4	>32	>32
Cefpirome	0.5	1	>32	>32
Ceftobiprole	0.25	0.5	1	2
Ceftaroline	0.25	0.25	1	2
Carbapenem				
Meropenem	0.01	0.03	32	32
Ertapenem	0.12	0.25	16	32
Doripenem	0.12	0.25	8	>32
	0.03	0.06	16	16

[a] Non producers of penicillinase

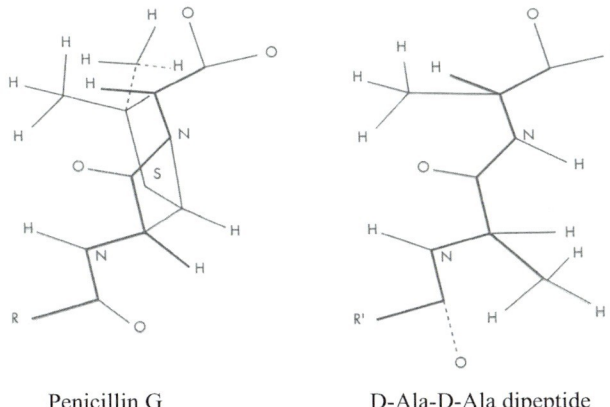

Fig. 1. Structures of D-Ala-D-Ala terminus of precursors and of penicillin G.

Penicillin Production

The β-lactamase enzymes catalyze penicillin inactivation through covalent binding to the β-lactam cycle. This reaction is similar to that occurring between the β-lactams and the active site of PBPs with the major difference that this reaction is irreversible (or extremely slow) with PBPs while it is reversible (and much more rapid) with β-lactamases (Fig 2) (17). According to Ambler's classification, there are four groups of β-lactamases, depending on their primary structure the nature of their active site, and the molecular weight; these are: serine-active enzymes (Class A, B, and D) and metallo-β-lactamases (Class B). It should be noted that the β-lactamase produced by staphylococci are all Class A enzymes (10). Serine-active enzymes are homologues of PBPs with conserved active sites (motif S-X-X-K). Furthermore, certain PBPs, such as PBP4 of S. aureus, have detectable β-lactamase activity whose clinical implication has not been demonstrated.

The capacity of a β-lactamase to hydrolyze its substrate can be evaluated by its catalytic efficiency: k_{cat} / K_m, in which k_{cat} is the number of substrate molecules degraded per second and per enzyme molecule; and K_m is the Michaelis-Menten constant which reflects the enzyme affinity for its substrate (Table 3) (21).

By immunological methods, four enzyme variants (A, B, C, and D) have been distinguished in *S. aureus*. The substrate profiles are similar with an hydrolysis of penicillin G, aminopenicillins (e.g., ampicillin, amoxicillin), carboxypenicillins (e.g. ticarcillin), and ureidopenicillins (e.g. piperacillin). Penicillin inhibitors (clavulanic acid > tazobactam > sulbactam) restore the activity of penicillins (21). Cefamandole, cefotaxime, oxacilline, and imipenem are relatively resistant to these penicillinases (21). Most strains produce both extra cellular isoforms and isoforms linked to the cytoplasmic membrane. After cleavage of its leader peptide sequence of 24 amino acids, the secreted penicillinase is an exoenzyme of 257 amino acids (MW 28 kDa) with a very basic pI (9.7-10.1) (10).

More often, the genetic basis of the structural gene for the penicillinase is a plasmid, even if in certain strains chromosomal location was identified. Certain plasmids contain as well, genes for resistance to heavy metals (e.g. cadmium), to antiseptics, and to other antibiotics (e.g. erythromycin, gentamicin) (10).

The synthesis of the enzyme is inducible in particular in the presence of oxacillin or cefotaxime, both among the most powerful inducers. This regulatory negative control involves a diffusible repressor (*blaI* gene product) which is linked to the *blaZ* structural gene. There is also an inactive antirepressor (*blaR1* gene product) synthesized in a

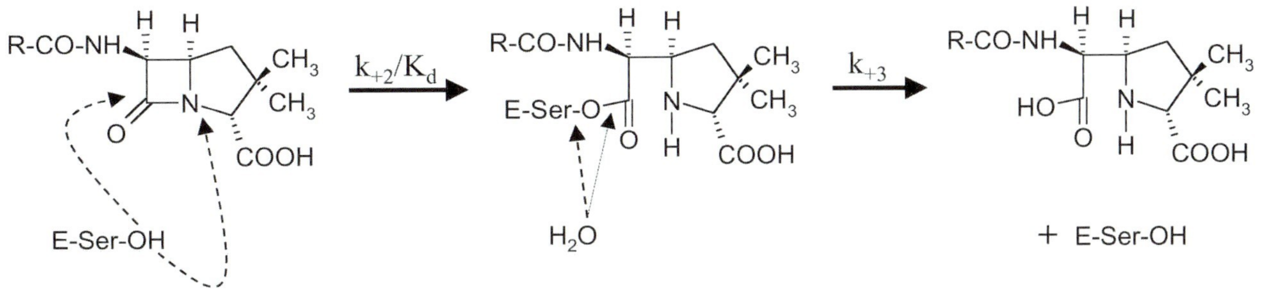

Fig. 2. Mode of action of penicillinases.

constitutive manner. In the presence of inducer, BlaR1 is able to inactivate the repressor by cleaving a 3 kDa fragment of BlaI, which results in an increase of penicillinase synthesis by 30 to 100 times (Fig. 3). It should be noted that in the chromosome, there is another gene (*blaR2*) that could code for a second anti-repressor (10).

Hyper-production of penicillinase has also been detected in strains that show decreased susceptibility to oxacillin (MIC = 2 µg/ml). Penicillinase inhibitors restore *in vitro* activity of penicillins against these so-called BORSA strains ('Borderline *S. aureus*'). In the presence of clavulanic acid, the MIC of penicillin G decreases from ≥ 128 to 2 µg/ml and the MIC of oxacillin, from ≥ 2 to 0.25 µg/ml. Mutations have been identified in regulatory regions (e.g. *blaI*, *blaR2*), which are responsible for large quantities of penicillinase production in a constitutive manner, even in the absence of inducer.

In coagulase-negative staphylococci, most clinical strains also produce a β-lactamase with a substrate profile similar to that of penicilinases produced by *S. aureus* strains.

Target modification

PBP2a acquisition

This resistance, also referred to as resistance to methicillin, is linked to an additional inducible PBP, known as PBP2a (or PBP2'), having very weak affinity to the penicillins M and other β-lactams (2, 20). It should be noted that there are affinity differences between the various β-lactams. In fact, penicillin G and ampicillin bind better than cefamandole and cefoxitin which themselves bind better that oxacillin and cefotaxime to PBPs (Table 1) (3). This additional PBP found in *S. aureus* and CNS, is encoded by a very conserved gene of 2.1 kb, *mecA*, which is part of a mobile genetic element called '*staphylococcal cassette chromosome*' (SCC*mec*); itself integrated within the *S. aureus* chromosome. This DNA fragment, present in all the strains of MRSA, varies in size from 20.9 to 66.9 kb and to date, eight types have been recognized (Table 4) (7, 20). While SSCmec types I, IV, V, VI and VI code only for resistance to β-lactams, SSCmec types II and III contain additional resistance genes originating from plasmids (e.g. pUB110, pI1258, and pT181) or transposons (e.g.

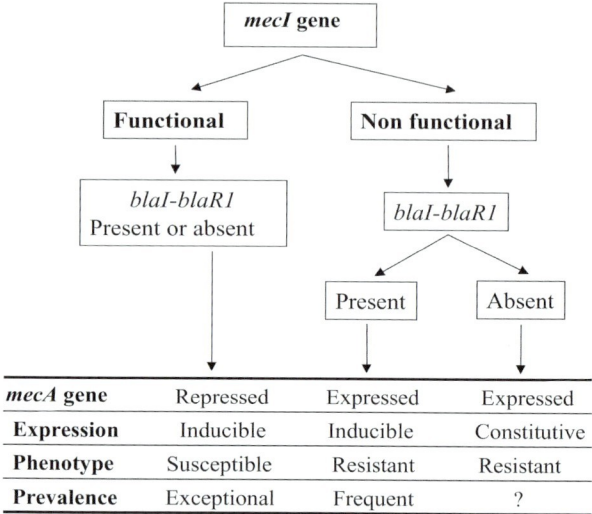

Fig. 3. Regulation of expression of resistance to methicillin.

Table 3. Kinetic parameters of type A β-lactamase from *S. aureus* (21)

Antibiotic	k_{cat}^a (s⁻¹)	K_m^b (µM)	k_{cat}/K_m^c (mM⁻¹ s⁻¹)	Stability^d
Penicillin G	171	51	3.4	1
Ampicillin	308	255	0.8	4.25
Methicillin	17	10000	0.0017	2000
Cephalothin	0.015	7	0.0021	1545
Cefamandole	0.057	5	0.011	309
Nitrocefin®	23	6	3.8	0.89

[a] K_{cat}, catalytic parameter which represents efficiency of the enzyme (number of catalytic cycles per second achieved by the enzyme)
[b] K_m, affinity parameter (Michaelis constant) which is characteristic of each enzyme for a given substrate. When weak, affinity of enzyme for the antibiotic is high.
[c] k_{cat}/K_m, parameter which represents the catalytic efficiency of an enzyme. It is weak for PBPs and high for β-lactamases, corresponding to rapid hydrolysis of the acyl-enzyme complex.
[d] Stability is expressed as a ratio of the stability of penicillin G, which was set at 1.

Tn554) (Table 4) (7). These SSCmec elements contain genes coding for recombinases (ccr for cassette chromosome recombinase) responsible for specific integration and excision at the chromosomal attBscc site near the origin of chromosome replication (at the 3' end of gene orfX). By PCR, it is possible to determine the type of SSCmec cassette in the MRSA strains for epidemiological purposes; many methods have already been described (7).

Since no homologue has been found in strains of S. aureus susceptible to methicillin, the most probable hypothesis is that the mecA gene has been acquired from a strain of coagulase-negative Staphylococcus. A mecA-like gene coding for an 88% similar protein was identified in the chromosome of a strain of Staphylococcus sciuri susceptible to methicillin (5).

Regulation of mecA gene expression is complex and depends on at least two systems of transcription regulation: the mecI and mecR1 genes located upstream from mecA and the blaI and blaR1 genes located upstream from the blaZ gene coding the penicillinase (2, 10). Indeed, the mecI and mecR1 encoded proteins present strong homology with the products of blaI and blaR1, respectively. A strain having a mecI-mecR1 functioning system can appear susceptible to oxacillin because the gene products more strongly repress transcription of mecA than BlaI-BlaR1 (Fig. 3). Actually, the majority of clinical isolates of MRSA have a non-functional mecI-mecR1 system (deletions, insertions or mutations in mecI). In strains containing mecA and producing penicillinase, the blaI-blaR1 system takes control of the expression of mecA and the transcription of the gene is inducible. Strains that do not produce penicillinase express the mecA gene in a constitutive manner (Fig. 3).

Some accessory genes such as fem (factor essential for resistance to methicillin resistance) and aux (auxiliary), which are normally present in the chromosome of S. aureus and play an important role in peptidoglycan synthesis, are also implicated in expression of methicillin resistance (2). Moreover, external factors can also influence resistance; such as temperature, NaCl concentration, pH, or the size of the bacterial inoculum (2).

PBP modifications

Resistance rarely results from the modification of endogenous PBPs. Such strains are called MODSA ('Modified PBP S.aureus'). This diminished affinity is mostly observed for PBP1 and PBP2. The strains express low-level oxacillin resistance (MIC from 1 to 4 μg/ml) (14). Finally, even if PBP4 is not essential to viability of S. aureus, hyper-expression may provoke a minor but reproducible augmentation of β-lactam resistance.

With regards to the new anti-MRSA cephalosporins, studies of resistance through successive passages in sub-inhibitory concentrations have shown that the selection frequency of in vitro mutants are very weak (18, 9). In fact, the development of high-level resistance to ceftobiprole in MRSA has been associated with the combination of at least seven mutations in the mecA gene.

Table 4. Various types of SSCmec cassettes (7, 20)

SSCmec type	mec complex	ccr genes	Size (kb)	Resistance(s) associated with methicillin-resistance[a]
I	B	A1/B1	34.3	-
II	A	A2/B2	53	Kan, Tob (ant(4') on pUB110) Ery (ermA on Tn554) Spc (aad(9) on Tn554)
III	A	A3/B3	66.9	Pen (blaZ on pI258) Ery (ermA on Tn554) Spc (aad(9) on Tn554) Tet (tet(K) on pT181)
IV	B	A2/B2	20.9-24.3	-
V	C	C	28	-
VI	B	A4/B4	20.9	-
VII	C2	C2. C8	35.9	-
VIII	A	A4/B4	32.2	Ery (ermA on Tn554) Spc (aad(9) on Tn554)

[a] -, None ; Ery, Erythromycin ; Kan, Kanamycin ; Pen, Penicillin ; G Spc, Spectinomycin ; Tet, Tetracycline ; Tob, tobramycin.

Finally, in the course of clinical development, no acquired resistance *in vivo* has been detected (18).

PENICILLINASE EXPRESSION AND DETECTION

The expression of plasmid penicillinase is inducible by β-lactams and results in a large MIC dispersion of penicillin G and amoxicillin. Antibiogram interpretation can be difficult for some borderline MICs. By disk diffusion, detection of this resistance is achieved, by using a penicillin disk containing 6 μg. The ampicillin test is not recommended.

- Strains susceptible to penicillin G have an inhibition zone diameter of ≥ 29 mm (and often larger) (CLSI recommendations) and the inhibition zone presents a remarkable outline formed by colonies growing smaller, becoming increasingly transparent leading to a "ghost zone" (Fig. 4A). In measuring the diameter only the clear growth end should be taken into account and not this "ghost zone". The MIC is ≤ 0.12 μg/ml.
- Strains resistant to penicillin G by penicillinase production have an inhibition zone diameter of ≤ 28 mm (often, 25 mm) (CLSI recommendations). The ghost zone is replaced by large-sized opaque colonies forming a clear border, though sometimes with "squatters" growing in the inhibition zone (Fig. 4B). This aspect is characteristic of production of a penicillinase. For certain penicillinase-producing strains, particularly coagulase-negative staphylococci, the inhibition diameter can remain just within the limits of susceptibility and thus can be categorized as penicillin G susceptible. The disappearance of the 'ghost zone' is equally observed in these difficult strains; this allows penicillinase production to be suspected.

For strains with MIC ≤ 0.12 μg/ml or having a ≥ 29 mm inhibition zone diameter, presence of a penicillinase should be verified by a β-lactamase test, a nitrocefin® test, for example. To avoid 'false-negatives' it is necessary to test the colonies induced for penicillinase production. To do so, tested colonies should be taken near a disk of penicillin G, or oxacillin, or cefoxitin. Automated system test critical concentrations of penicillin G and most include a penicillinase test. However, false-negatives exist particularly for coagulase-negative staphylococci, because the bacteria are tested without induction. It is necessary to check negative results by a nitrocefin test on induced colonies. Colonies from blood-agar plates made in parallel to check the purity of the inoculum can be used provided that a β-lactam disk has been placed (e.g. cefoxitin).

The European EUCAST committee (rule 8.2; http://www.escmid.org/sites/index_f.aspx?par=2.4)

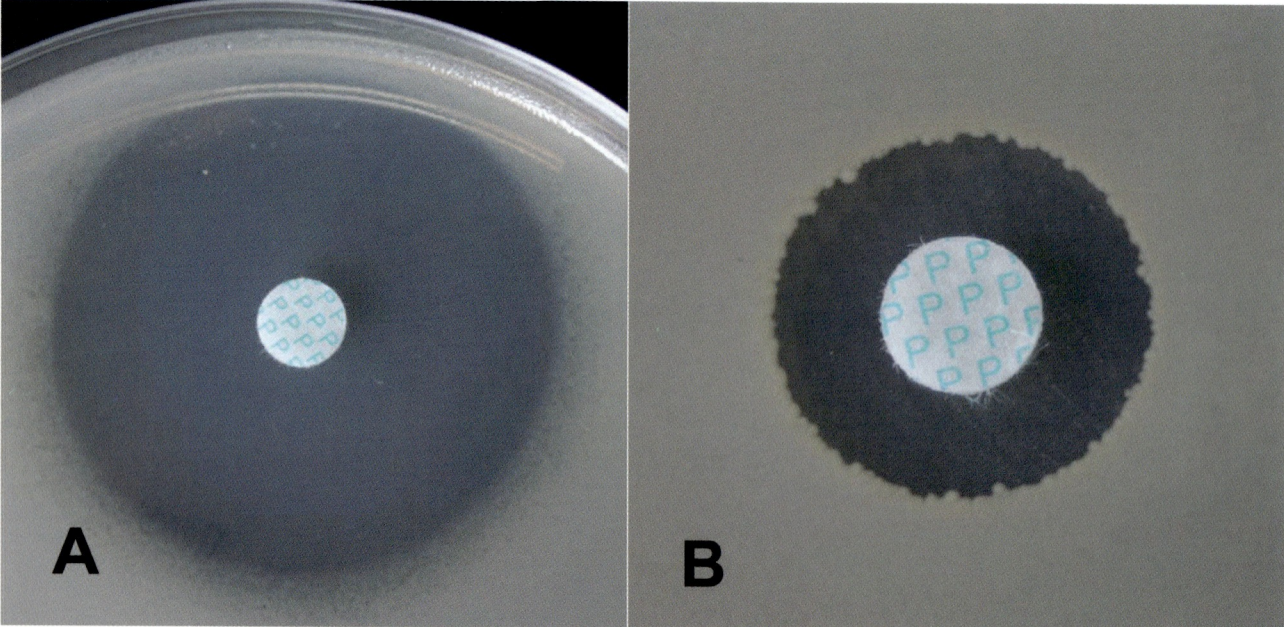

Fig. 4. Penicillin G tests: (A) *S. aureus* non–producing penicillinase; (B) *S. aureus* producing penicillinase

considers that in the countries with high prevalence of *S. aureus* penicillinase producers, it is possible to report all strains resistant to penicillin G, ampicillin, and amoxicillin because of the difficulty of detection and high risks of false-negatives.

Antibiogram interpretation

If resistance to penicillin G is detected, β-lactams susceptible to penicillinases are inactive: penicillin G, ampicillin, amoxicillin, carbenicillin, azlocillin, ticarcillin, and piperacillin. The combinations with penicillinase inhibitors (clavulanic acid, sulbactam, tazobactam) restore *in vitro* susceptibility to these antibiotics. The response for penicillin G predicts the response for all these antibiotics.

When methicillin (oxacillin) resistance is detected, the staphylococci should be reported as penicillin G resistant irrespective of the inhibition diameter or the MIC of penicillin G.

EXPRESSION AND DETECTION OF METHICILLIN RESISTANCE

The term 'methicillin resistance' was first used to describe resistance to penicillins stable to penicillinases. The term had been kept even though this antibiotic is no longer used and was replaced by oxacillin.

As previously mentioned, 'methicillin resistance' expression is modified by accessory genes and culture conditions. Resistance expression can be homogenous or heterogeneous. In the former, the entire population expresses resistance to a high level; in the latter, only a fraction of the population expresses a detectable resistance. Three classes of heterogeneity have been described by Tomasz *et al*. (15). Class I is characterized by the lowest level of oxacillin resistance, where the most resistant population is less that 10^{-6} of the total population and present an MIC that is not higher than 128 μg/ml. This resistance is the most difficult to detect. MIC determination by a standard technique classifies these strains as susceptible when in fact they have the *mecA* gene and should be reported as resistant.

Class II is also heterogeneous but with a larger resistant population (10^{-4} of the total population) and presents a higher MIC (1024 μg/ml).

Class III shows resistance that is only for a small part heterogeneous with a very high MIC; it is easily detectable.

Detection of methicillin resistance

Detection of methicillin heterogeneous resistance by disk diffusion has raised numerous difficulties since this resistance was described. Diverse techniques have been proposed seeking to obtain better *in vitro* expression. Oxacillin test rather than that of methicillin, a heavy inoculum, a lowering of incubation temperature to 30°C, use of a high salt medium, and the prolongation of incubation to 48 hours were all at different times recommended by various national committees.

Only recently the proposal of cefoxitin as a replacement marker for oxacillin allowed a detection in strains weakly expressing PBP2a *in vitro* (8). The cefoxitin test is the preferred routine test for detection of methicillin resistance by production of PBP2a. Resistance detection remains difficult for coagulase-negative staphylococci. Distinct recommendations were put forward for *S. aureus* and *Staphylococcus lugdunensis* on one hand and on the other, coagulase-negative staphylococci (other than *S. lugdunensis*), which are detailed below. For *S. aureus*, the presence of associated markers like fluoroquinolones resistance suggests methicillin resistance. Community-acquired methicillin-resistant *S. aureus* (CA-MRSA) were multi-susceptible to antibiotics, notably fluoroquinolones. However, this figure that was initially observed is rapidly changing for multiple resistance.

Molecular methods used to detect the presence of *mecA* or to find PBP2a are reference methods in case of doubt.

S. aureus and *S. lugdumensis*

MIC. The CLSI recommends determining the MIC of oxacillin (methicillin or nafcillin) by the microdilution technique in MH broth or by dilution in agar supplemented by 2 % NaCl with an 24 h incubation with temperature that does not exceed 35°C to allow better expression. The strains having a MIC ≥ 4 μg/ml (CLSI) or > 2 μg/ml (EUCAST) are resistant and very probably possess a *mecA* gene.

Disk diffusion. The oxacillin test remains recommended for *S. aureus* respecting the conditions and interpretive criteria indicated in the CLSI document (note: any growth in the inhibition zone indicates resistance) (4). It is possible to use Mueller-Hinton agar screening with 4% of NaCl and 6 μg/ml oxacillin (see CLSI document). The cefoxitin test (30 μg disk) is proposed as a screening method for *S. aureus* and *S. lugdunensis* because of a strong correlation with PBP2a expression. It has the advantage of being carried out in standard conditions (without exceeding an incubation temperature of 35°C for allowing better expression). Recent automated systems also include the test of cefoxitin. The strains having MIC of cefoxitin ≥ 8 µg/ml (CLSI) or > 4 µg/ml (EUCAST) are considered as possessing the *mecA* gene. Other anti-staphylococcal β-lactams which could give results of false susceptibility should not be tested.

In practice, the cefoxitin test is the preferable test, routinely recommended because of its sensitivity for the detection of heterogeneous strains, and should be preferred. Nonetheless, it should be emphasized that it does not detect oxacillin resistance strains by any other mechanism than PBP2a production (hyper-producing penicillinase strains or with PBP mutations). Therefore, it may also be useful to test oxacillin.

EUCAST is developing a diffusion method that will be available in 2010. The cefoxitin test will also be proposed.

Coagulase-negative staphylococci (other than *S. lugdunenis*). For both CLSI and EUCAST, strains having MIC ≤ 0.25 µg/ml are considered as susceptible and those having a MIC ≥ 0.5 as resistant. These low critical concentrations are at the origin of 'false resistance' in species other than *S. epidermidis*. In the case of severe infection due to coagulase-negative staphylococci (other than *S. epidermidis*), the CLSI recommends testing strains having a MIC between 0.5 and 2 µg/ml for the presence of the *mecA* gene or production of PBP2a according to the algorithm shown in Fig. 5.

Because of its weak sensitivity, oxacillin testing by disk diffusion is not recommended, especially for species other than *S. epidermidis* (Table 5). The cefoxitin test is recommended as a replacement of the oxacillin test (4). However, its sensitivity never reaches 100% (Table 5) (13).

Antibiogram interpretation and report

Susceptibility of oxacillin is reported according to the cefoxitin (or oxacillin) results. The strains

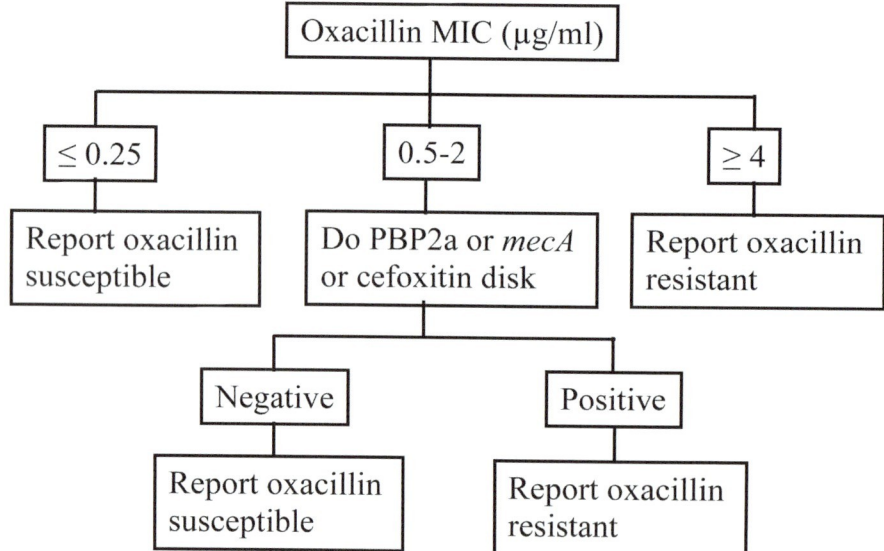

Fig. 5. Algorithm for determining susceptibility to oxacillin for coagulase-negative staphylococci (except *S. lugdunensis* et *S. epidermidis*) according to oxacillin MIC

Table 5. Detection of resistance to oxacillin with various methods in 196 clinical isolates of coagulase negative staphylococci (126 *mecA*-positive et 70 *mecA*-negative) (13).

Antibiotic (method)	Susceptibility (%)	Specificity (%)
Oxacillin (MIC)	98	91
Oxacillin (disk diffusion)	99	89
Cefoxitin (disk diffusion)	99	97

positive for the *mecA* gene or for PBP2a are reported as resistant to oxacillin.

In case of oxacillin resistance in *S. aureus* or coagulase-negative staphylococci, the other β-lactams (penicillins, penicillinase inhibitor associations, cephalosporins, carbapenems) should be reported as inactive. Ceftobiprole and ceftaroline, which have an affinity to PBP2a present an exception provided that they demonstrate clinical efficacy.

REFERENCES

(1) **Ayers, L. W., R. N. Jones, A. L. Barry, C. Thornsberry, P. C. Fuchs, T. L. Gavan, E. H. Gerlach, and H. M. Sommers.** 1982. Cefotetan, a new cephamycin: comparison of in vitro antimicrobial activity with other cephems, β-lactamase stability, and preliminary recommendations for disk diffusion testing. Antimicrob. Agents Chemother. **22:**859-877.

(2) **Chambers, H. F.** 1997. Methicillin resistance in staphylococci: molecular and biochemical basis and clinical implications. Clin. Microbiol. Rev. **10:**781-791.

(3) **Chambers, H. F., and M. Sachdeva.** 1990. Binding of β-lactam antibiotics to penicillin-binding proteins in methicillin-resistant *Staphylococcus aureus*. J. Infect. Dis. **161:**1170-1176.

(4) **Clinical and Laboratory Standards Institute.** 2009. Methods for Dilution Antimicrobial Susceptibility Tests for Bacteria That Grow Aerobically; Approved Standard-Eighth Edition & Performance Standards for Antimicrobial Susceptibiliy Testing; Nineteenth Informational Supplement, M07A8, M100S19.

(5) **Couto, I., H. de Lencastre, E. Severina, W. Kloos, J. A. Webster, R. J. Hubner, I. S. Sanches, and A. Tomasz.** 1996. Ubiquitous presence of a *mecA* homologue in natural isolates of *Staphylococcus sciuri*. Microb. Drug Resist. **2:**377-391.

(6) **Davies, T. A., M. G. Page, W. Shang, T. Andrew, M. Kania, and K. Bush.** 2007. Binding of ceftobiprole and comparators to the penicillin-binding proteins of *Escherichia coli*, *Pseudomonas aeruginosa*, *Staphylococcus aureus*, and *Streptococcus pneumoniae*. Antimicrob. Agents Chemother. **51:**2621-2624.

(7) **Deurenberg, R. H., and E. E. Stobberingh.** 2008. The evolution of *Staphylococcus aureus*. Infect. Genet. Evol. **8:**747-763.

(8) **Felten, A., B. Grandry, P. H. Lagrange, and I. Casin.** 2002. Evaluation of three techniques for detection of low-level methicillin-resistant *Staphylococcus aureus* (MRSA): a disk diffusion method with cefoxitin and moxalactam, the Vitek 2 system, and the MRSA-screen latex agglutination test. J. Clin. Microbiol. **40:**2766-2771.

(9) **Kanafani, Z. A., and G. R. Corey.** 2009. Ceftaroline: a cephalosporin with expanded Gram-positive activity. Future Microbiol. **4:**25-33.

(10) **Kernodle, D. S.** 2000. Mechanisms of resistance to β-lactam antibiotics, pp. 609-620. *In* V.A. Fischetti; R.P. Novick, J.J. Feretti, D.A. Portnoy, J.I. Rood (eds.), Gram-positive pathogens. American Society for Microbiology, Washington, D.C.

(11) **Lowy, F. D.** 2003. Antimicrobial resistance: the example of *Staphylococcus aureus*. J. Clin. Invest. **111:**1265-1273.

(12) **McDougal, L. K., and C. Thornsberry.** 1986. The role of beta-lactamase in staphylococcal resistance to penicillinase-resistant penicillins and cephalosporins. J. Clin. Microbiol. **23:**832-839.

(13) **Swenson, J. M., F. C. Tenover, and Cefoxitin Disk Study Group.** 2005. Results of disk diffusion testing with cefoxitin correlate with presence of *mecA* in *Staphylococcus* spp. J. Clin. Microbiol. **43:**3818-3823.

(14) **Tomasz, A., H. B. Drugeon, H. M. de Lencastre, D. Jabes, L. McDougall, and J. Bille.** 1989. New mechanism for methicillin resistance in *Staphylococcus aureus*: clinical isolates that lack the PBP2a gene and contain normal penicillin-binding proteins with modified penicillin-binding capacity. Antimicrob. Agents Chemother. **33:**1869-1874.

(15) **Tomasz, A., S. Nachman, and H. Leaf.** 1991. Stable classes of phenotypic expression in methicillin-resistant clinical isolates of staphylococci. Antimicrob. Agents Chemother. **35:**124-129.

(16) **Waxman, D. J., and J. L. Strominger.** 1983. Penicillin-binding proteins and the mechanism of action of β-lactam antibiotics. Annu. Rev. Biochem. **52:**825-869.

(17) **Zapun, A., C. Contreras-Martel, and T. Vernet.** 2008. Penicillin-binding proteins and β-lactam resistance. FEMS Microbiol. Rev. **32:**361-385.

(18) **Zhanel, G. G., A. Lam, F. Schweizer, K. Thomson, A. Walkty, E. Rubinstein, A. S. Gin, D. J. Hoban, A. M. Noreddin, and J. A. Karlowsky.** 2008. Ceftobiprole: a review of a broad-spectrum and anti-MRSA cephalosporin. Am. J. Clin. Dermatol. **9:**245-254.

(19) **Zhanel, G. G., R. Wiebe, L. Dilay, K. Thomson, E. Rubinstein, D. J. Hoban, A. M. Noreddin, and J. A. Karlowsky.** 2007. Comparative review of the carbapenems. Drugs **67:**1027-1052.

(20) **Zhang, K., J. A. McClure, S. Elsayed, and J. M. Conly.** 2009. Novel staphylococcal cassette chromosome mec type, tentatively designated type VIII, harboring class A *mec* and type 4 *ccr* gene complexes in a Canadian epidemic strain of methicillin-resistant *Staphylococcus aureus*. Antimicrob. Agents Chemother. **53:**531-540.

(21) **Zygmunt, D. J., C. W. Stratton, and D. S. Kernodle.** 1992. Characterization of four β-lactamases produced by *Staphylococcus aureus*. Antimicrob. Agents Chemother. **36:**440-445.

Chapter 11. β-LACTAMS AND STREPTOCOCCI

Michael R. JACOBS

INTRODUCTION

The streptococci addressed in this chapter, *Streptococcus pneumoniae*, β-hemolytic streptococci and viridans group streptococci, are the etiologic agents of a wide variety of infections. *S. pneumoniae* is an important cause of bacteremia and meningitis, and is one of the most common causes of acute, community-acquired bacterial respiratory infections, including bacterial rhinosinusitis, pneumonia, and otitis media (1-3,39,50). Pneumococci also cause septic arthritis, endocarditis, peritonitis and a variety of other infections. *S. pyogenes* (Lancefield group A) is a major bacterial cause of pharyngitis and superficial skin infections, and can also cause many other infections, including endocarditis and necrotizing fasciitis (1, 10, 49). *S. agalactiae* (Lancefield group B) is a major cause of neonatal bacteremia and meningitis, and also causes a variety of other infections, including urinary tract infections (50). Lancefield groups C, F and G β-hemolytic streptococci are occasional causes of a variety of infections, including endocarditis. Viridans group streptococci are common etiologic agents of native valve endocarditis, bacteremia in neutropenic patients and pyogenic infections (5). The most common species in this group are *S. sanguis*, *S. oralis (mitis)*, *S. salivarius*, *S. mutans*, the *S. anginosus* group and *Gemella morbillorum* (formerly *S. morbillorum*). Members of the *S. anginosus* group (*S. intermedius*, *S. anginosus*, and *S. constellatus*), also referred to as the *S. milleri* group, tend to cause pyogenic infections and can cause hematogenously disseminated infection, including abscesses, arthritis and osteomyelitis.

HISTORY

Sulfonamides were the first antibiotics put into wide use and the first to show efficacy in patients with lobar pneumonia, with the case fatality rate decreasing from 27% to 8% in patients treated with sulfapyridine in a study reported in 1938 (20). Unfortunately, within fewer than 5 years, sulfonamide-resistant strains of the pneumococcus emerged. Penicillin G, which had demonstrated extraordinary efficacy against streptococci reported in Alexander Fleming's 1929 paper introducing the antibiotic, was not initially developed because of production difficulties, in contrast to the relatively easily synthesized sulfonamides. With the increasing resistance to the sulfonamides, researchers turned to penicillin G, – and several studies published in the early 1940s showed excellent results using penicillin G to treat various streptococcal infections. The penicillins and other β-lactams are still the principal agents used to treat streptococcal infections.

Penicillins remained widely used, fully effective agents for treatment of streptococcal infections for over three decades before resistant strains began to be identified and reported in *S. pneumoniae*. Reports of resistance between 1950 and 1975 were infrequent, and little penicillin resistance of clinical significance was found. This situation changed drastically in 1977 with the isolation of penicillin resistant serotype 19A isolates from children with bacteremia and meningitis in South Africa (4, 31). These strains were highly resistant to penicillin G, ampicillin, and chloramphenicol, the agents of choice for empiric treatment of meningitis at that time. Many of the Johannesburg isolates were also multi-drug resistant (MDR), additionally resistant to macrolides, lincosamides, tetracycline, and trimethoprim-sulfamethoxazole. The penicillin G MICs of these "resistant" pneumococci (2-4 μg/ml) were up to 250-fold higher than MICs of wild-type strains (0.015 μg/ml). Nevertheless, over sixty years after its introduction, penicillin G and many other β-lactams remain effective agents for treatment of most infections caused by streptococcal species. However, multi-drug resistant replacement serotypes of *S. pneumoniae*, notably serotype 19A, the same serotype as the original MDR South African strains, have emerged following the introduction in the US of a conjugate pneumococcal vaccine in 2000 (6).

TREATMENT

The β-lactams recommended for treatment of the major diseases caused by these pathogens will be briefly reviewed.

Pneumonia

For inpatients recommended parenteral β-lactams are penicillin G, cefuroxime, cefotaxime, and ceftriaxone, while for outpatients recommended β-lactams are oral high-dose amoxicillin or amoxicillin clavulanate, cefpodoxime, or cefuroxime, or IM ceftriaxone (9, 39).

Meningitis

Ceftriaxone or cefotaxime are recommended, with meropenem and cefepime as alternatives for *S. pneumoniae* (50). Ampicillin or penicillin G, with ceftriaxone or cefotaxime as alternatives, are recommended for *S. agalactiae*.

Otitis media and sinusitis

High-dose amoxicillin-clavulanate, high-dose amoxicillin, cefpodoxime proxetil, cefuroxime axetil, or cefdinir are recommended (2, 3).

Pharyngitis

Penicillin G (10 days of oral therapy or one injection of intramuscular benzathine penicillin) is the treatment of choice for *S. pyogenes* pharyngitis because of low cost, narrow spectrum of activity, and effectiveness (10). Amoxicillin is equally effective and more palatable for children. First-generation cephalosporins such as cefadroxil and cephalexin are options in patients with some forms of penicillin allergy. Increased treatment failure with penicillin G has been reported, and some experts advocate the use of cephalosporins in all patients because of better eradication and effectiveness against chronic carriage.

Skin infections

Among the oral β-lactam drugs of choice for impetigo are dicloxacillin, cephalexin, and amoxicillin/clavulanic acid (49).

Endocarditis

Penicillin G, ampicillin or ceftriaxone is recommended for endocarditis caused by viridans group streptococci with penicillin MICs ≤ 0.12 μg/ml, with the addition of gentamicin if penicillin MICs are ≥ 0.25 μg/ml or if infection is due to *Abiotrophia defectiva*, *Granulicatella* species or *Gemella* species (5). The duration of antimicrobial treatment of endocarditis caused by members of the *S. anginosus* group may need to be longer than that for endocarditis caused by other viridans group streptococci. Patients with endocarditis caused by penicillin-susceptible *S. pneumoniae* should receive penicillin G, cefazolin, or ceftriaxone. High-dose penicillin or a third-generation cephalosporin can be used in patients with penicillin-resistant infection and without meningitis. In patients with endocarditis and meningitis, high doses of cefotaxime may be used. Penicillin G is the recommended treatment for endocarditis caused by *S. pyogenes* and other β-hemolytic groups, with cefazolin or ceftriaxone as alternatives.

MODE OF ACTION OF β-LACTAMS

β-lactams, including penicillins, cephalosporins, and carbapenems, prevent construction of the bacterial cell wall, leading to lysis and cell death (26). In the final step of the production of the cell wall peptidoglycan layer, cross linking of stem peptides from one polymer to the stem peptides of neighboring polymers provides integrity and structure to the bacterial cell wall. The peptide cross-linking is facilitated by enzymes called peptidases, which are located on the extracellular surface of the cell membrane. The active site of each peptidase enzyme catalyzes the formation of a covalent bond between amino acids and the natural substrates for these enzymes are the amino acids that comprise the stem peptides. Penicillin, the first β-lactam antibiotic, was shown to exert its antimicrobial effect by binding to these peptidases and interfering with their activity. Consequently, these peptidases have become known as penicillin binding proteins (PBPs). The chemical structure of β-lactams includes a β-lactam ring, a part of which is structurally similar to the D-Ala-D-Ala end of a stem peptide, allowing these antibiotics to mimic the natural substrates of the stem peptides competing for the same space at the active binding site and blocking cell wall peptidoglycan polymer cross-linkage (Fig.1). The various side chains found in the different β-lactams determine its spectrum of activity. There are six known PBPs in *S. pneumoniae*, each encoded by a *pbp* gene on the bacterial chromosome and often shared by (or acquired from) members of the viridans group of streptococci (23). These PBPs are differentiated by their molecular weight: the five high-molecular-weight PBPs [PBP 1a (79.7 kDa), PBP 1b (89.6 kDa), PBP 2x (82.3 kDa), PBP2a (80.8 kDa), and PBP 2b (82.3 kDa)], and one low molecular weight PBP [PBP3 (45.2 kDa)]. Four of the PBPs, PBP 1a, 2a, 2x, and 2b are transpeptidases that allow the formation of peptide bridges between the chains of peptidoglycan made of N-acetyl-muramic acid and N-acetyl-glucosamine. PBP 1a is a bifunctional enzyme that ensures both transglycosylation and transpeptidation. PBP 3, the smallest of the PBPs, is a carboxypeptidase with activity that influences the thickness of the peptidoglycan layer. The higher molecular weight PBPs, 1a, 2b, and 2x are the primary targets of β-lactams. These PBPs are made up of an N-terminal hydrophobic region, a central penicillin-binding domain, and a C-terminal domain. The active site of transpeptidase activity is formed by three conserved amino acid motifs, SXXK, SXN and KT(S)G. These motifs occur at amino acid positions 370-373, 428-430, and 557-559 in PBP1a, at positions 337-340, 395-397, and 547-549 in PBP2x, and at positions 385-388, 442-444, and 614-616 in PBP2b (Fig.2 and 3). Once the β-lactam binds to the PBP, peptido-glycan synthesis stops, leading to cellular lysis and death. Affinities of the various β-lactams differ for each of the PBPs and can also differ according to the concentration of the agent. Decreased affinity of PBP1a, 2x, and 2b for β-lactams plays an important part in resistance.

RESISTANCE MECHANISMS

S. pneumoniae

In contrast to many other organism groups, streptococcal resistance to β-lactams is mediated via alterations in the β-lactam-binding site of PBP1a, PBP2b and PBP2x. Changes in the motifs making up the active binding site, or in the positions flanking these motifs, are associated with low affinity variants of these PBPs. These changes are the result of point mutations, or of recombination of PBP genes with PBP genes of other pneumococci or viridans streptococci with point mutations in their PBP genes to form mosaic genes (22).

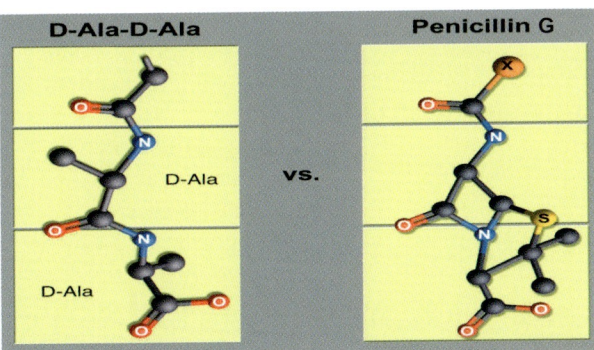

Fig. 1. Similarity between D-Ala-D-Ala of stem peptides and penicillin G. Copyright Michael R. Jacobs, used with permission.

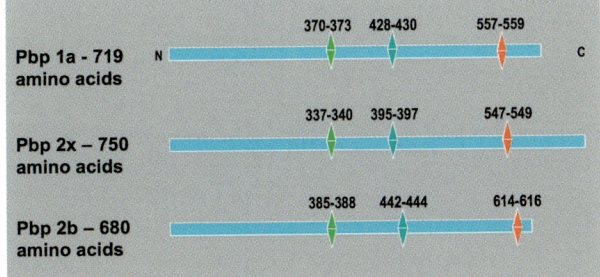

Fig. 2. Primary structures and positions of motifs making up the active transpeptidase sites of PBP1a, PBP2x and PBP2b of S pneumoniae. Copyright Michael R. Jacobs, used with permission.

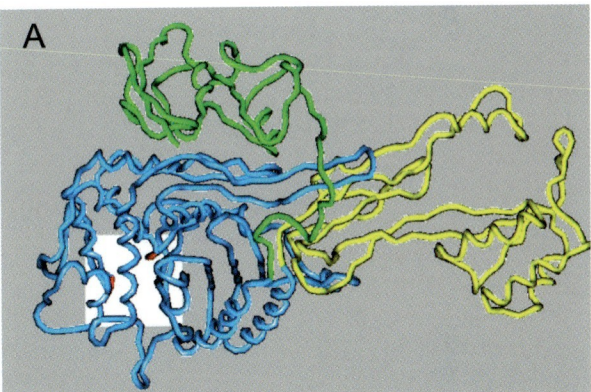

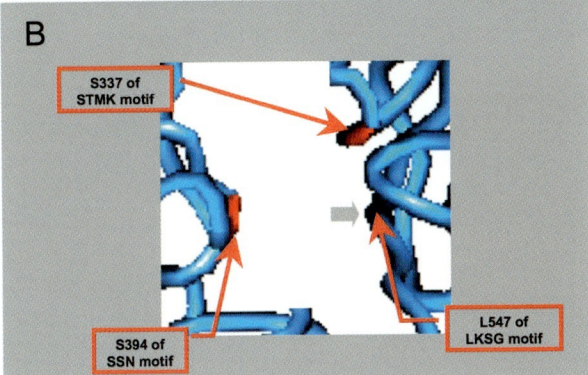

Fig. 3. A. Tertiary structure of Pbp2x of S pneumoniae, with the active binding site shown with a white background. B. Enlarged view of the active PBP binding site. Yellow, N-terminal domain; blue, penicillin-binding/transpeptidase domain; green, C-terminal domain and connecting loop. Copyright Blackwell Scientific Publications, used with permission (22).

Mutations in the genes encoding the PBPs disable proper folding of the proteins, inactivating the binding site and leading to antimicrobial resistance. These changes in the configuration of PBPs also reduce the affinity of PBPs for their natural linear stem peptide substrates, and the preferred substrates of altered PBPs are novel stem peptides. The *murMN* operon of *S. pneumoniae* is comprised of two genes (*murM* and *murN*) that encode enzymes involved in the assembly of stem peptides, and penicillin resistant strains have *murM* genes with a mosaic structure that code for enzymes involved in the production of novel stem muropeptides, such as D-Ala-D-Ser, as well as various branched variations (Fig.4). Thus, the ability to produce novel stem peptides is a necessary component for expression of penicillin resistance.

The effect of various changes in the key motifs making up the active binding sites of the key PBPs of *S. pneumoniae* on susceptibility to various β-lactams is shown in Table 1 (16). Wild type strains are susceptible to penicillin G, its derivatives, and the tested cephalosporins, with all β-lactam MICs being ≤ 0.03 µg/ml; these isolates do not have mutations in the penicillin-binding motifs of PBP1a, PBP2b, and PBP2x. Changes in the various motifs of the PBP genes lead to MICs increasing as much as 7 to 11 doubling dilution difference compared to wild type. Five genotypes of strains with altered PBPs have been described, with different spectra of resistance to various β-lactams. Genotype 1 strains are low-level penicillin intermediate (MICs 0.12 µg/ml) and susceptible to amoxicillin, cefuroxime, and third-generation cephalosporins and have a $T_{445}A$ substitution in the SSNT motif of PBP2b, which is also present in the other 4 genotypes. Genotype 2 isolates are high-level penicillin intermediate (MICs 1 µg/ml) and cefuroxime resistant, and have two additional substitutions, both in PBP2x – $L_{546}V$ in the LKSGT motif and $I_{371}T$ flanking the STMK motif. Genotype 3 strains are intermediate to third generation cephalosporins and have another substitution – $P_{432}T$ in the SRNVP motif PBP1a. Genotype 4 isolates are additionally resistant to amoxicillin, associated with a $A_{618}G$ substitution in the KTGTA motif of PBP2b. Genotype 5 strains are resistant to all of these agents, including third generation cephalosporins, that is associated with two substitutions in PBP2x – $M_{339}F$ in the STMK motif and $M_{400}T$ flanking this motif. Amoxicillin MICs against genotype 5 strains are usually higher than penicillin MICs, a feature only found in this genotype. Other substitutions frequently present in genotypes 3-5 include T → A or T → S in the STMK motifs of PBP1a and PBP2x, and $R_{384}G$ flanking the STMK motif of PBP2x.

Viridans group streptococci

Similar changes in PBPs and stem peptides to those described above are associated with resistance in this group, and indeed many of the resistance genes associated with pneumococcal resistance originate from viridans group streptococci (23).

β-hemolytic streptococci

Resistance has not been described in this group.

IN VIVO ACTIVITY OF β-LACTAMS

The activity of β-lactams *in vivo* has been shown to be dependent upon the time the serum concentration exceeds the MIC of the agent, with clinical success occurring when the unbound serum concentration of the agent exceeds the MIC of an infecting strain for more than 20 to 50% of the dosing interval (14). The proportion of the dosing interval needed varies by β-lactam class, with 20-25% needed for carbapenems, 30-40% for penicillins, and 40-50% for cephalosporins. Using standard dosing regimens and the blood pharmacokinetics of these agents, the unbound serum drug concentrations that are maintained for the appropriate proportion of the dosing interval can be determined and used as susceptibility breakpoints. The T > MIC value for β-lactams and extracellular pathogens like streptococci can be approximated using the free-drug concentration in serum, since it

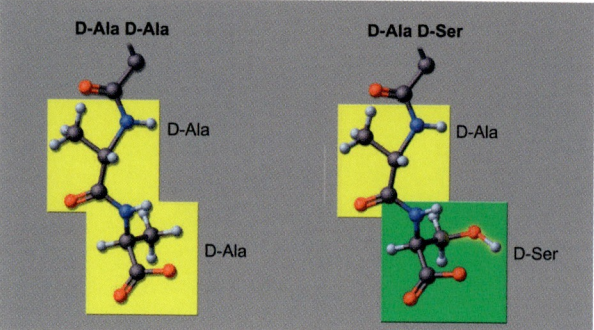

Fig. 4. *mur* genes in strains of *S. pneumoniae* with altered PBPs encode other stem peptide chains, such as D-Ala-D-Ser instead of D-Ala-D-Ala in penicillin-susceptible strains, that bind to PBPs and allow cross-linking of cell wall components in strains with altered PBPs. Copyright Michael R. Jacobs, used with permission.

Chapter 11. β-LACTAMS AND STREPTOCOCCI

Table 1. Genotypes based on PBP amino acid substitutions and β-lactam MICs of clinical isolates of *S. pneumoniae*. Dashes indicate no change from the wild type; boldface amino acids indicate differences from wild type. Adapted from Davies et al. (16)

Genotype	Phenotype[a]	MIC (μg/ml)[a]					PBP 1a[b]		PBP 2x[c]					PBP 2b[d]	
		PEN	AMC	CXM	CRO	CTX	370STMK	428SRNVP	337STMK	371I	384R	400M	546LKSGT	442SSNT	614KTGTA
Wild type	Susceptible	≤0.015	0.03	0.03	0.03	≤0.015	----	-----	----	-	-	-	-----	----	-----
1	PEN-I	0.12	0.06-0.12	0.25	0.06-0.12	0.06-0.12	----	-----	----	-	-	-	-----	---A	-----
		0.12	0.12	0.25	0.06	0.06	----	-----	----	-A-	-	G	-----	---A	-----
2	PEN-I, CXM-R	1	2	4	0.5	0.5	-S-	-----	-A-	T	G	-	V----	---A	-----
		1	1-2	4	0.5	0.5-1	----	-----	-A-	T	G	-	V----	---A	-----
3	PEN-R, CXM-R, TGC-I	2-4	2-4	2-16	0.5-2	0.5-2	-A-	---T	-A-	T	G	-	V----	---A	-----
4	PEN-R, AMC-R, CXM-R, TGC-I	8	8	8-16	1-2	2	-S-	---T	-A-	T	G	-	V----	---A	----G
5	PEN-R, AMC-R, CXM-R, TGC-R	8	16	32	4	8	-A-	---T	-AF-	T	G	T	V----	---A	----G
		8	8-16	32-64	4-8	8-16	-S-	---T	-AF-	T	G	T	V----	---A	----G
		8	16	64	16	16	-S-	---T	-AF-	T	G	T	V----	---A	----G

AMC, amoxicillin-clavulanic acid; CXM, cefuroxime; CRO, ceftriaxone; CTX, cefotaxime; I, intermediate; PEN, penicillin G; R, resistant; TGC, third generation cephalosporin.

[a] There were no substitutions in the 557KTG motif.
[b] There were no substitutions in the 393AHSSNV motif.
[c] There were no substitutions in the 385SVVK motif.

is generally proportional to that in the interstitial fluid surrounding the organism in non-meningeal infections. Consequently, the proportion of the dosing interval at which the free-drug concentration in serum is greater than the antibiotic MIC against the specific pathogen will reflect the concentration in most infection sites.

METHODS

Streptococci can be tested for antimicrobial susceptibility either using liquid or solid media (11, 12, 19). Broth microdilution is now generally recognized as the reference method and is performed using cation-adjusted Mueller-Hinton broth supplemented with 2.5-5% lysed horse blood according to standard methodologies (11, 19). Agar dilution is performed using Mueller-Hinton Agar (MHA) supplemented with 5% sheep blood, but is not included in the recommendations for *S. pneumoniae*. MHA with 5% sheep blood is also used for disk diffusion and E-test®. For broth microdilution, disk diffusion and E-test®, inoculation is with a direct colony suspension equivalent to a 0.5 McFarland standard, diluted appropriately if necessary, and incubation is at 35 ± 2 °C for 20-24 h. Agar dilution is performed with suspensions diluted to produce inocula of 10^4 CFU/spot. Broth-based tests are incubated in atmospheric air, while agar-based methods are incubated in atmospheric air supplemented if necessary for growth with 5% CO_2. *S. pneumoniae* is always incubated in atmospheric air supplemented with 5% CO_2 for agar-based methods. The recommended quality control strain for all streptococcal groups is *S. pneumoniae* ATCC 49619.

In the clinical laboratory, β-lactam susceptibility of *S. pneumoniae* can be screened using 1μg oxacillin disks (13). The oxacillin disk is placed on MHA with 5% sheep blood and inoculated with a direct colony suspension equivalent to a 0.5 McFarland standard and incubated as above. If a strain has an oxacillin zone of inhibition of ≥ 20 mm, it is considered penicillin susceptible based on the original breakpoint of 0.06 μg/ml and, consequently, susceptible to all appropriate β-lactams. A zone of < 20 mm indicates some degree of penicillin non-susceptibility and requires MIC testing of the agents of interest. In meningitis, MIC can be determined for penicillin G, cefotaxime, ceftriaxone, and meropenem. For non-meningeal infections, these agents can also be tested, while appropriate oral β-lactams can be tested when oral therapy is indicated (see treatment above).

RESISTANT PHENOTYPES

S. pneumoniae

Wild type pneumococci have unimodal MIC distributions for all β-lactams, with a modal value of 0.015 μg/ml for penicillin G (26). Isolates with higher MICs represent strains that have altered PBPs and bimodal or trimodal MIC distributions are frequently found. A few strains with decreased susceptibility to penicillin G with MICs of 0.1 – 0.5 μg/ml were reported in the 1960s from Australia and New Guinea and in the 1970s from patients with failure of penicillin in cases of meningitis in the USA. Strains isolated in 1977 in South Africa had penicillin G MICs as high as 2 μg/ml to 4 μg/ml (4, 31). Compared to fully susceptible isolates the most resistant of these strains were only inhibited by a more than 250-fold greater concentration of penicillin G and other β-lactams. Penicillin G MICs at this time were arbitrarily classified by MIC range as susceptible (MICs ≤ 0.06 μg/ml), intermediate (0.12-1 μg/ml), and resistant (MICs ≥ 2 μg/ml) as this had direct relevance to meningitis and to predicting susceptibility of penicillin susceptible isolates to other β-lactams (25, 31). However, this classification of penicillin MICs was confusing and led to inappropriate clinical applications, and "nonsusceptible" strains are best considered "β-lactam challenged," and this challenge can be overcome for many β-lactams based on clinically achieved levels. This situation has now largely been clarified by the development of clinically appropriate dosing regimens and susceptibility breakpoints for most β-lactams based on dosing regimen and site of infection, with breakpoints differing for meningeal and non-meningeal infections (13). The susceptible penicillin G breakpoint remains at ≤ 0.06 μg/ml for meningitis and for prediction of susceptibility to other β-lactams, while new susceptibility breakpoints for parenteral penicillin G in nonmeningeal infections have been established at ≤ 2 μg/ml, susceptible; 4 μg/ml, intermediate; and ≥ 8 μg/ml, resistant, based on 12 million units/day, with 18-24 million units/day recommended for treatment of patients with isolates in the intermediate category (13). Recent international surveillance studies have demonstrated that about 50% of *S. pneumoniae* still have penicillin G MICs in the "fully" susceptible range of ≤ 0.06 μg/ml, with 18-20% in the original intermediate range (0.12-1 μg/ml) and 12-33% in the original resistant range (≥ 2 μg/ml) (28, 32, 47). Application of the new, nonmeningitis penicillin G breakpoints to an extensive dataset results in 92.6% of isolates being susceptible (≤ 2 μg/ml), 7.1% intermediate (4 μg/ml) and 0.3% resistant (≥ 8 μg/ml), while only 68% are susceptible at the meningitis breakpoint (Fig. 5) (28). Although currently rare, highly penicillin G resistant strains with MICs ≥ 8 μg/ml are of concern should they proliferate (46). In general, the MIC distributions of all other β-lactams against *S. pneumoniae* also range over a greater than 200-fold concentration; however, there are significant differences among these agents with respect to the baseline activity and relationships to breakpoints, and each β-lactam is best considered as an independent agent with its own breakpoints based on its specific pharmacokinetics and dosing regimens (27). Susceptibility breakpoints and susceptibility to relevant β-lactams at these breakpoints for usual dosing regimens are shown in Tables 2 and 3.

MIC distributions of β-lactams against *S. pneumoniae*, with susceptibility breakpoints indicated, are shown in Fig. 6-9. These distributions are shown for strains classified according to the original penicillin breakpoints (susceptible, ≤ 0.06 μg/ml; intermediate, 0.12-1 μg/ml; and resistant, ≥ 2 μg/ml). Note that equal numbers of strains are shown in each of these three groups, so that the overall MIC distribution is not representative of sequentially collected clinical isolates. Penicillin G shows a trimodal MIC distribution, with peaks at 0.015, 0.12 and 4 μg/ml. Ampicillin shows a bimodal MIC distribution, with peaks at 0.06 and 4 μg/ml. Amoxicillin and amoxicillin-clavulanate have a more complex MIC distribution with peaks at 0.03 and 16 μg/ml. Piperacillin has the peaks at 0.06 and 4 μg/ml and ticarcillin at 1 and 64 μg/ml. MIC distributions of the cephalopsorins are generally complex, with considerable variations in potency in relation to penicillin G as well as to clinical breakpoints. The carbapenems imipenem and meropenem are highly potent against penicillin nonsusceptible isolates, while ertapenem is less potent.

Susceptibility of pneumococci to β-lactams and other drug classes varies widely by serotype, with several of the most drug resistant serotypes included or related to serotypes included in currently available pneumococcal vaccines. In a recent study the 9 most prevalent pneumococcal serotypes in children in the US were 19A, 6 A/C, 3, 19F, 35B, 23A, 15A, 33, and 22 (Table 4) (15). Serotype 19A has recently emerged as the predominant replacement serotype following the introduction of a 7-valent conjugate vaccine, and now accounts for about one third of strains isolated in most reports. It is often multi-drug resistant, though some strains are fully susceptible. In a recent report 50% or more of serotype 19A strains were resistant to penicillin G, cefdinir, and cefuroxime, and about one third were resistant to amoxicillin. Significantly, an additional 36% fell into the penicillin intermediate breakpoint range of 0.12-1 μg/ml. Serotype 6A and the newly identified serotype 6C accounted for about 10% of strains in this study with many (69%) penicillin intermediate strains and a few (8%) penicillin resistant. Serotype 3 was next in frequency, accounting for 7.4% of strains, but it was fully susceptible to all of the β-lactams tested. Pneumococcal protein conjugate vaccine serotype 19F was the next most frequently isolated serotype, two-thirds of which were resistant to penicillin G, cefdinir, and cefuroxime. The next five serotypes accounted for 2.5 to 3.8% of strains isolated. Among these, type 35B was susceptible to amoxicillin, but resistant to the other agents tested; type 23A was not resistant to any agent, but 43% were intermediate to penicillin G; type 15A were 93% intermediate to penicillin and 21% resistant to cefuroxime but susceptible to amoxicillin; serotypes 33 and 22 showed no resistance and only 8% of type 33 were intermediate to penicillin G.

β-hemolytic streptococci

Isolates of Group A and Group B β-hemolytic streptococci are consistently fully susceptible to penicillin G, cephalosporins, and penems. Susceptibility breakpoints and susceptibility to relevant β-lactams at these breakpoints are shown in Tables 5 and 6. MIC_{50}s of penicillin G are ≤ 0.03 μg/ml for Group A and Group B and ≤ 0.016 μg/ml for β-hemolytic streptococci including Groups A, B, C, F, G, and others. Occasional non-susceptible

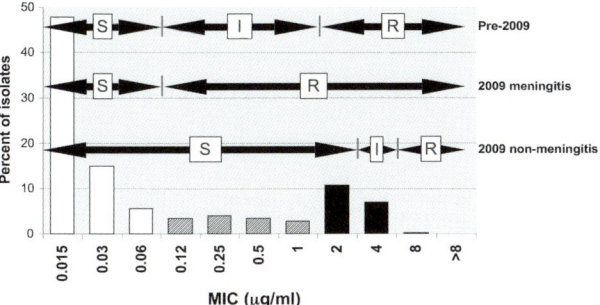

Fig. 5. Histogram of penicillin G MICs of 8,882 isolates of *S. pneumoniae* from 26 countries, 1998-2000, showing the effect of applying pre-2009 CLSI breakpoints and the 2009 CLSI breakpoints for meningitis and non-meningitis isolates. Data from Jacobs, et al. (28). Copyright Michael R. Jacobs, used with permission.

Table 2. Susceptibility breakpoints for *Streptococcus pneumoniae* to selected β-lactam antimicrobials based on CLSI, EUCAST and FDA guidelines (13, 18). Unless otherwise indicated CLSI breakpoints are shown.

Antimicrobial agent	MIC breakpoints (μg/ml)			Disk content (μg)	Disk diffusion breakpoints (mm)		
	Susceptible	Intermediate	Resistant		Susceptible	Intermediate	Resistant
Parenteral agents - meningitis							
Penicillin G	≤ 0.06	—	≥ 0.12	1[a]	≥ 20	—	—
Ceftriaxone	≤ 0.5	1	≥ 2	—	—	—	—
Cefotaxime	≤ 0.5	1	≥ 2	—	—	—	—
Cefepime	≤ 0.5	1	≥ 2	—	—	—	—
Meropenem	FDA ≤ 0.12	—	≥ 0.25	—	—	—	—
	EUCAST ≤ 0.25	0.5–1	≥ 2	—	—	—	—
Parenteral agents - nonmeningitis							
Penicillin G	CLSI ≤ 2	4	≥ 8	1[a]	≥ 20	—	—
	EUCAST ≤ 0.06	0.12–2	≥ 4	—	—	—	—
Ampicillin	EUCAST ≤ 0.5	1–2	≥ 4	—	—	—	—
Ceftriaxone	CLSI ≤ 1	1–2	≥ 4	—	—	—	—
	EUCAST ≤ 0.5	1–2	≥ 4	—	—	—	—
Cefotaxime	CLSI ≤ 1	1–2	≥ 4	—	—	—	—
	EUCAST ≤ 0.5	2	≥ 4	—	—	—	—
Cefepime	≤ 1	2	≥ 4	—	—	—	—
Cefuroxime	≤ 0.5	1	≥ 2	—	—	—	—
Meropenem	CLSI ≤ 0.25	0.5	≥ 1	—	—	—	—
	EUCAST ≤ 2	—	≥ 4	—	—	—	—
Ertapenem	CLSI ≤ 1	2	≥ 4	—	—	—	—
	EUCAST ≤ 1	—	≥ 2	—	—	—	—
Imipenem	CLSI ≤ 0.12	0.25–0.5	≥ 1	—	—	—	—
Doripenem	EUCAST ≤ 2	—	≥ 4	—	—	—	—
	EUCAST ≤ 1	—	≥ 2	—	—	—	—
Oral agents							
Penicillin V	CLSI ≤ 0.06	0.12–1	≥ 2	1[a]	≥ 20	—	—
	EUCAST ≤ 0.06	—	≥ 0.12	—	—	—	—
Amoxicillin	≤ 2	4	≥ 8	—	—	—	—
Amoxicillin/clavulanate	≤ 2	4	≥ 8	—	—	—	—
Cefaclor	≤ 1	2	≥ 4	—	—	—	—
Cefuroxime axetil	CLSI ≤ 1	2	≥ 4	—	—	—	—
	EUCAST ≤ 0.25	0.5	≥ 1	—	—	—	—
Cefpodoxime	CLSI ≤ 0.5	1	≥ 2	—	—	—	—
	EUCAST ≤ 0.25	0.5	≥ 1	—	—	—	—
Cefprozil	≤ 2	4	≥ 8	—	—	—	—
Cefdinir	≤ 0.5	1	≥ 2	—	—	—	—

[a] Using 1 μg oxacillin disks; for nonmeningitis *S. pneumoniae* isolates with oxacillin zones of ≥ 20 mm, indicate susceptibility to penicillin, ampicillin, ampicillin-sulbactam, cefaclor, cefdinir, cefditoren, cefpodoxime, cefprozil, ceftizoxime, cefuroxime, imipenem, loracarbef, and meropenem. Isolates with oxacillin zones of < 20 mm require determination of MICs against appropriate β-lactams.

Table 3. Adult and pediatric dosing regimens and susceptibility of antimicrobial agents used to treat pneumococcal infections (1-3, 24, 39)

Antimicrobial agent	Total daily dose (number of doses per day)[a]		Susceptible breakpoint (μg/ml)[b]	Percent susceptibility	Data source
	Adults	Infants and children			
Parenteral agents					
Meningitis					
Penicillin G	24 million units (6)	300,000-400,000 units/kg (4-6)	Penicillin ≤ 0.06	68.3	(28)
Ampicillin	12 g (6)	300 mg/kg (4)	Penicillin ≤ 0.06	68.3	(28)
Ceftriaxone	4 g (1-2)	100 mg/kg (1-2)	≤ 0.5	82.2-86.2	(28,34)
Cefotaxime	8-12 g (4-6)	225-300 mg/kg (4-6)	≤ 0.5	87.4	(34)
Cefepime	6 g (3)	150 mg/kg (3)	≤ 0.5	85.3	(34)
Meropenem	6 g (3)	120 mg/kg (3)	≤ 0.25	78.1-93.9	(43)
Parenteral agents					
Nonmeningeal infections					
Penicillin G (regular dose)	12 million units (6)	250,000-400,000 units/kg (4-6)	≤ 2[c]	92.6[d]	(28)
Penicillin G (high dose)	18-24 million units (6)	400,000 units/kg (4-6)	Penicillin ≤ 4	99.7[d]	(28)
Ampicillin	4-8 g (4)	50-100 mg/kg (4)		92.6	(28)
Ceftriaxone	1-2 g (1)	50-75 mg/kg (1-2)	≤ 1	95.2	(34)
Cefotaxime	3 g (3)	75-100 mg/kg (3-4)	≤ 1	95.1-96.5	(28,34)
Cefuroxime sodium	2.25 g (3)	50-100 mg/kg (3-4)	≤ 0.5	75.3	(34)
Cefepime	2 g (2)	100 mg/kg (2)	≤ 1	96.5	(34)
Meropenem	1.5-3 g (3)	60-120 mg/kg (3)	≤ 0.25	78.1-93.9	(43)
Imipenem	1-2 g (3-4)	60 mg/kg (4)	≤ 0.12	92.4-96.3	(43)
Ertapenem	1 g (1)	30 mg/kg (2)	≤ 1	93.2-93.3	(40,47)
Oral agents					
Penicillin V	1-2 g (3-4)	25-50 mg/kg (3-4)	≤ 0.06[c]	68.3	(28)
Amoxicillin (regular dose)	1.5 g (2-3)	45 mg/kg (2-3)	≤ 2	95.1	(28)
Amoxicillin/clavulanate (regular dose)	1.5 g/250 mg (2-3)	45/6.4 mg/kg (2-3)	≤ 2	95.5	(28)
Amoxicillin (high dose)	6 (3)	90 mg/kg (2-3)	≤ 4	97.9	(28)
Amoxicillin/clavulanate (high dose and extended release)	4 g/250 mg extended release (2)	90/6.4 mg/kg (2-3)	≤ 4	97.9	(28)
Cefaclor	750-1,500 mg (3)	20-40 mg/kg (3)	≤ 0.5	60.2	(28)
Cefuroxime axetil	500-1,000 mg (2)	20-30 mg/kg (2)	≤ 1	78.6	(28)
Cefixime	400 mg (1-2)	8 kg/kg (1-2)	≤ 1	68.3	(28)
Cefprozil	500-1,000 mg (2)	15-30 mg/kg (2)	≤ 1	79.7	(28)
Cefdinir	600 mg (1-2)	14 mg/kg (1-2)	≤ 0.5	76.5	(28)

[a] Dosing regimens are shown as total recommended daily dose and number of doses per day and should be used in conjunction with local prescribing information. Susceptibility data reflect overall findings from international studies and local susceptibility data should be taken into consideration as susceptibility patterns vary considerably.
[b] Susceptibility breakpoint for agent shown unless specified otherwise.
[c] Nonmeningeal isolates susceptible to penicillin G at this breakpoint can be considered susceptible to parenteral ampicillin, cefepime, cefotaxime and ceftriaxone. Nonmeningeal isolates susceptible to ≤ 0.06 μg/ml of penicillin G can be also considered susceptible to these parenteral agents, as well as to parenteral ertapenem, imipenem and meropenem and to oral ampicillin, amoxicillin, amoxicillin/clavulanate, cefaclor, cefdinir, cefditoren, cefprozil, cefuroxime and cefpodoxime.
[d] Includes penicillin G susceptible (92.6%) and intermediate (7.1%) isolates based on new, nonmeningeal, parenteral penicillin G susceptibility breakpoints (13).

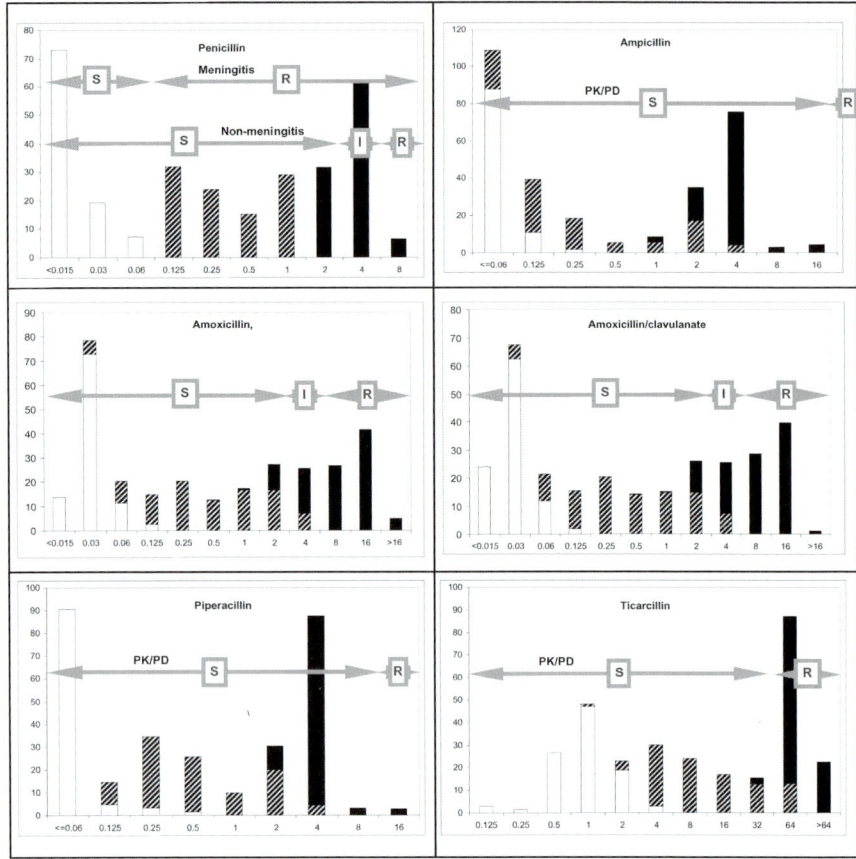

Fig. 6. Histograms of MIC distributions of penicillins for penicillin susceptible (□), intermediate (▨) and resistant (■) *S. pneumoniae* according to original penicillin G breakpoints. Equal numbers of isolates are shown in each category, and this does not represent the MIC distribution of any series of consecutive clinical isolates. Data from (29, 30, 42). Copyright Michael R. Jacobs, used with permission.

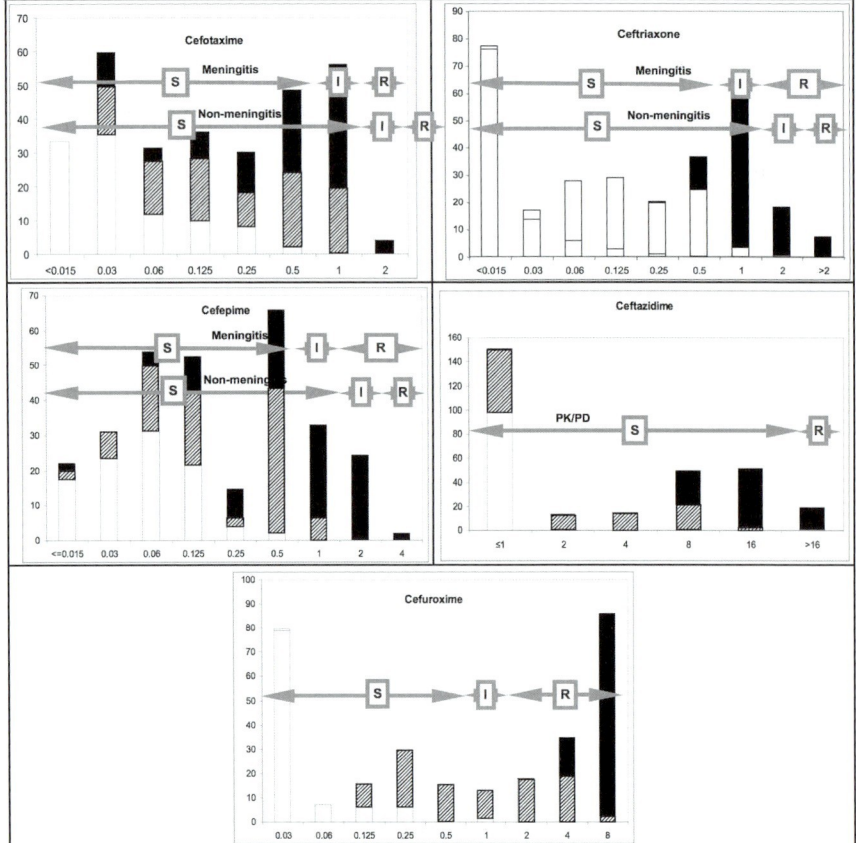

Fig. 7. Histograms of MIC distributions of parenteral cephalosporins for penicillin susceptible (□), intermediate (▨) and resistant (■) *S. pneumoniae* according to original penicillin breakpoints. Equal numbers of isolates are shown in each category, and this does not represent the MIC distribution of any series of consecutive clinical isolates. Data from refs. (29, 30, 33, 48). Copyright Michael R. Jacobs, used with permission.

Chapter 11. β-LACTAMS AND STREPTOCOCCI

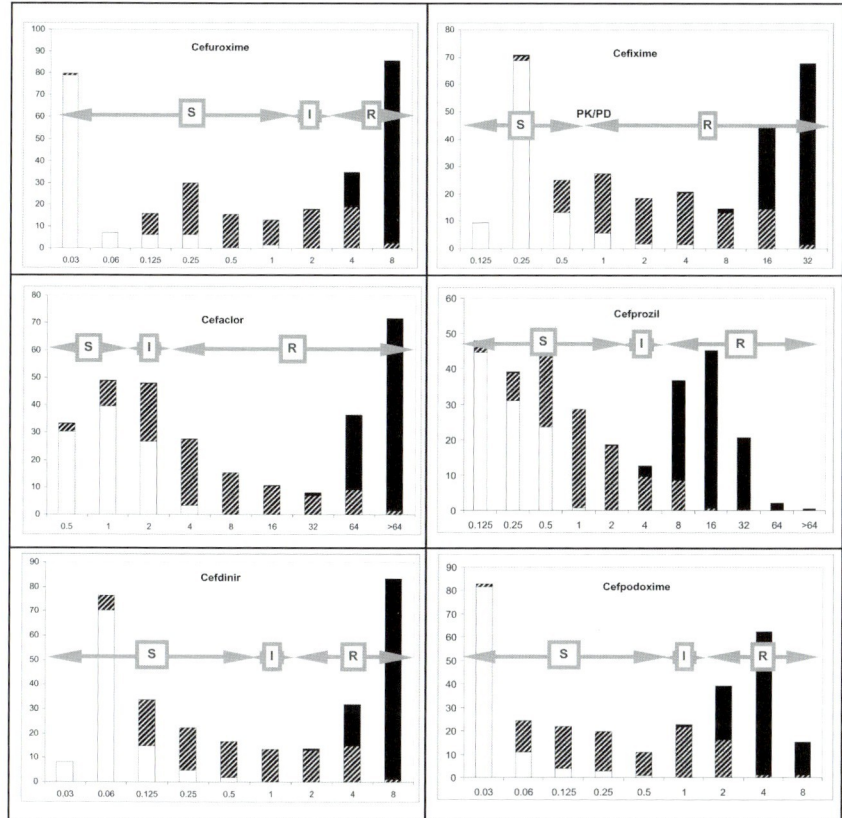

Fig. 8. Histograms of MIC distributions of oral cephalosporins for penicillin susceptible (□), intermediate (▨) and resistant (■) *S. pneumoniae* according to original penicillin G breakpoints. Equal numbers of isolates are shown in each category, and this does not represent the MIC distribution of any series of consecutive clinical isolates. Data from (28,29). Copyright Michael R. Jacobs, used with permission.

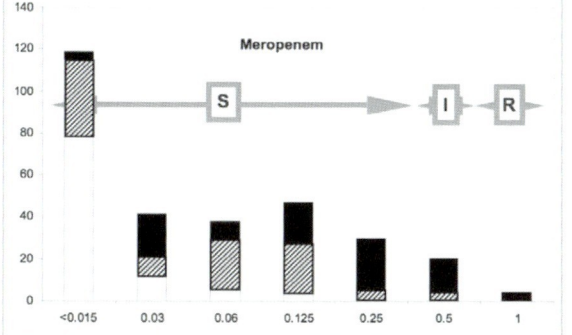
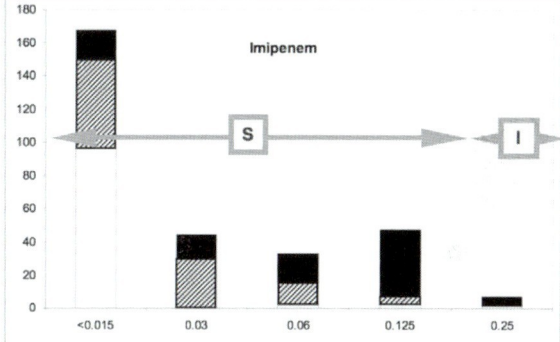

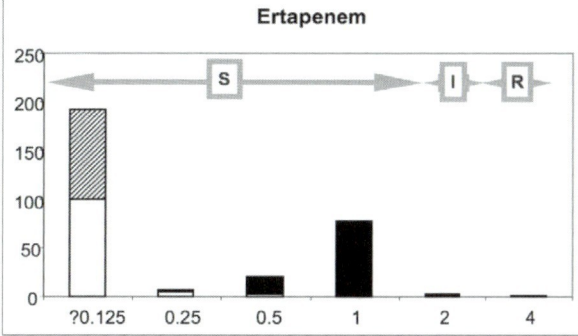

Fig. 9. Histograms of MIC distributions of carbapenems for penicillin susceptible (□), intermediate (▨) and resistant (■) *S. pneumoniae* according to original penicillin breakpoints. Equal numbers of isolates are shown in each category, and this does not represent the MIC distribution of any series of consecutive clinical isolates. Data from (33, 48) Copyright Michael R. Jacobs, used with permission.

Table 4. Antimicrobial susceptibilities for selected β-lactams of the nine most prevalent serotypes of *S. pneumoniae* collected from U.S. children in 2005-2006 (15).

Serotype	No. of isolates	Prevalence (%)	MIC_{90} in µg/ml (% of isolates susceptible/intermediate/resistant)[a] for:			
			Penicillin G	Amoxicillin/ clavulanate[b]	Cefdinir	Cefuroxime axetil
19A	120	30.5	4 (13/36/50)	8 (62/3/35)	> 8 (46/2/53)	16 (46/2/52)
6A/C	39	9.9	1 (23/69/8)	1 (97/0/3)	2 (59/26/15)	4 (64/23/15)
3	29	7.4	≤ 0.03 (100/0/0)	≤ 0.12 (100/0/0)	0.12 (100/0/0)	≤ 0.5 (100/0/0)
19F[c]	21	5.3	> 4 (33/0/67)	16 (47/5/48)	> 8 (33/0/67)	32 (33/0/67)
35B	15	3.8	2 (0/0/100)	2 (100/0/0)	4 (0/0/100)	4 (0/0/100)
23A	14	3.6	0.5 (57/43/0)	0.25 (100/0/0)	0.5 (93/7/0)	1 (93/7/0)
15A	14	3.6	0.5 (7/93/0)	0.25 (100/0/0)	1 (72/21/7)	4 (72/7/21)
33	12	3.1	≤ 0.03 (92/8/0)	≤ 0.12 (100/0/0)	0.12 (100/0/0)	≤ 0.5 (100/0/0)
22	10	2.5	≤ 0.03 (100/0/0)	≤ 0.12 (100/0/0)	0.12 (100/0/0)	≤ 0.5 (100/0/0)
All isolates	393	100	4 (49/26/25)	8 (84/2/14)	> 8 (68/4/28)	16 (68/4/28)

[a] Susceptible / intermediate / resistant breakpoints (µg/ml) used are: Penicillin, ≤ 0.06 / 0.12-1 / ≥ 2; amoxicillin/clavulanate, ≤ 2 / 4 / ≥ 8; cefdinir, ≤ 0.5 / 1 / ≥ 2; cefuroxime axetil, ≤ 1 / 2 / ≥ 4.
[b] Amoxicillin/clavulanate results are expressed as the amoxicillin component.
[c] Serotype included in 7-valent conjugate pneumococcal vaccine.

strains are seen among strains other than Groups A and B. Against amoxicillin, 99.1% of β-hemolytic strepotococci are susceptible, with all Groups A and B strains being susceptible, while 98.7% are susceptible to cefotaxime. Imipenem MIC_{50}s and MIC_{90}s for Group A isolates were both ≤ 0.06 µg/ml; for Group B, both values were ≤ 0.12 µg/ml. For meropenem, both values were 0.06 µg/ml for Group B isolates tested.

Viridans group streptococci

Strains of viridans group streptococci have decreased susceptibility to β-lactams compared with the β-hemolytic species (17, 35, 38, 41). Susceptibility breakpoints and susceptibility to relevant β-lactams at these breakpoints are shown in Tables 5 and 6. Reports of penicillin G MICs include $MIC_{50/90}$s of 0.06/2 µg/ml, respectively, with 66.7% of isolates susceptible. Amoxicillin MIC_{50} and MIC_{90} are reported at 0.12 and 4 µg/ml, respectively. Cefuroxime, ceftriaxone, and cefotaxime MIC_{50}s range from 0.12-0.25 µg/ml, with MIC_{90}s of 1-2 µg/ml and susceptibility of 90.7-93%. The meropenem MIC_{50} and MIC_{90} were 0.12 and 1 µg/ml, respectively, and 85% of isolates were susceptible. Histograms of MIC distributions of penicillin G and ceftriaxone for blood culture isolates of viridans group streptococci are shown in Fig.10 (17, 41).

SUGGESTED GROUPINGS OF AGENTS FOR ROUTINE TESTING OF STREPTOCOCCI

CLSI suggests groupings of antimicrobial agents with FDA clinical indications that should be considered for routine testing and reporting on streptococci by clinical microbiology laboratories in the USA (13). Agents listed also are required to have acceptable *in vitro* test performance. Agents are assigned to groups (A, B, and C) based on clinical efficacy, prevalence of resistance, minimization of emergence of resistance, cost, FDA clinical indications for usage, and current consensus recommendations for first-choice and alternative drugs. Agents are clustered together when inter-

Table 5. Susceptibility breakpoints for β-hemolytic and viridans group streptococci to selected β-lactam antimicrobials based on CLSI, EUCAST and FDA guidelines (13, 18). Unless otherwise indicated CLSI breakpoints are shown

Antimicrobial agent	MIC breakpoints (µg/ml)			Disk content (µg)	Disk diffusion breakpoints (mm)		
	Susceptible	Intermediate	Resistant		Susceptible	Intermediate	Resistant
β-hemolytic streptococci[a]							
Parenteral agents							
Penicillin G	CLSI ≤ 0.12	—	—				
	EUCAST ≤ 0.25	—	≥ 0.5				
Ampicillin	≤ 0.25	—	—	10	≥ 24	—	—
Cefepime, cefotaxime, ceftriaxone	≤ 0.5	—	—	30	≥ 24	—	—
Ertapenem	CLSI ≤ 1	—	—				
	EUCAST 0.5	—	≥ 1				
Meropenem	CLSI ≤ 0.5	—	—				
	EUCAST ≤ 2	—	≥ 4				
Imipenem	EUCAST ≤ 2	—	≥ 4				
Doripenem	EUCAST ≤ 1	—	≥ 2				
Oral agents							
Penicillin V	≤ 0.12	—	—	6	≥ 24	—	—
Viridans group streptococci[a]							
Parenteral agents							
Penicillin G	CLSI ≤ 0.12	—	—				
	EUCAST ≤ 0.25	—	≥ 4				
Ampicillin	CLSI ≤ 0.25	—	≥ 8				
	EUCAST ≤ 0.5	—	≥ 4				
Ceftriaxone	≤ 1	—	≥ 4	30	≥ 27	25-26	≤ 24
Cefotaxime	≤ 1	—	≥ 4	30	≥ 28	26-27	≤ 25
Cefepime	≤ 1	—	≥ 4	30	≥ 24	22-23	≤ 21
Ertapenem	CLSI 1	—	—				
	EUCAST ≤ 0.5	—	≥ 1				
Meropenem	CLSI ≤ 0.5	—	≥ 4				
	EUCAST ≤ 2	—	≥ 4				
Imipenem	EUCAST ≤ 2	—	≥ 4				
Doripenem	FDA[b] ≤ 0.12	—	—				
	EUCAST ≤ 1	—	≥ 2				

[a] The β-hemolytic group includes the large-colony-forming pyogenic strains of streptococci with Group A (*S. pyogenes*), B (*S. agalactiae*), C or G antigens. Small-colony-forming β-hemolytic strains with Group A, C, F or G antigens (*S. anginosus*, previously termed "*S. milleri*") are considered part of the viridans group, and interpretative criteria for the viridans group should be used
[b] FDA breakpoint, used only for *S. anginosus* group (*S. constellatus* and *S. intermedius*).

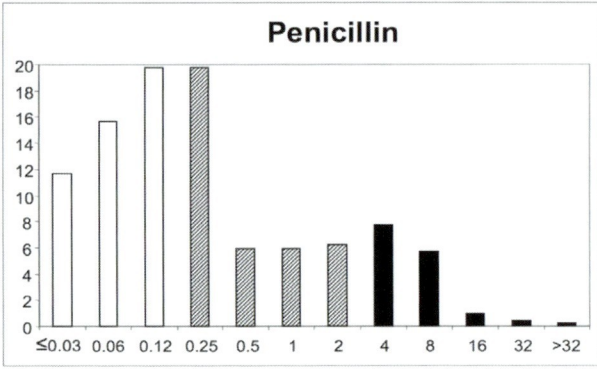

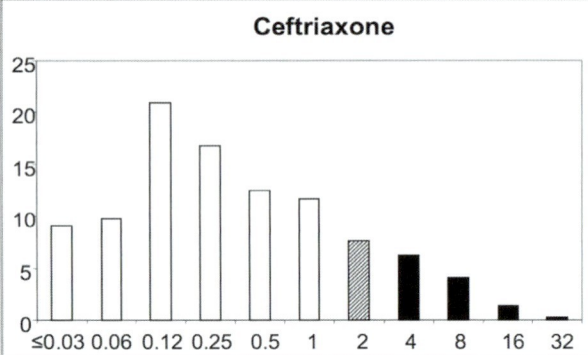

Fig. 10. Histograms of MIC distributions of penicillin and ceftriaxone for blood culture isolates of viridans group streptococci. Data from (17, 41).
Susceptible (□), intermediate (▨) and resistant (■)
Copyright Michael R. Jacobs, used with permission.

pretive results and clinical efficacy are similar. β-lactams suggested for streptococci are as follows (Table 7):

Group A. These agents are primary antimicrobial agents to be tested and reported. For *S. pneumoniae* penicillin G is the only agent listed and is tested by MIC determination or screened using the oxacillin disk method as discussed above. For viridans group and β-hemolytic streptococci, penicillin G or ampicillin are indicated, though susceptibility testing of penicillins and other β-lactams for treatment of *S. pyogenes* or *S. agalactiae* is not necessary for clinical purposes since resistant strains have not been identified. It is nonetheless valuable for pharmaceutical development, epidemiology, and monitoring of emerging resistance to do some susceptibility testing of these agents with these species. Any strains found to be intermediate or resistant should be referred to a reference laboratory for confirmation.

Group B. These are potential primary test agents, but reporting is done selectively, such as when the organism is resistant to agents of the same class in Group A. For *S. pneumoniae* cefepime, cefotaxime, and ceftriaxone are grouped together, and meropenem is also in this group. All of these agents are recommended for MIC testing,

Table 6. Antimicrobial susceptibilities of selected β-lactams for viridans group and β-hemolytic streptococci. Adapted from references (7, 8, 21, 35-38, 44, 45)

Agent	MIC$_{50/90}$ in µg/ml (% of isolates susceptible)			
	Viridans group	**Group A**	**Group B**	**All β-hemolytic groups**
Penicillin G	0.06/2 (66.7)	≤ 0.03/≤0.03 (100)	0.03/0.06 (100)	≤ 0.016/0.06 (100)
Amoxicillin	0.12/4 (79.4)	– [a]	–	0.12/0.25 (99.1)
Amoxicillin-clavulanate	–	≤ 0.03/≤ 0.03 (100)	0.06/0.06 (100)	–
Ampicillin	–	≤ 0.06/≤ 0.06 (100)	≤ 0.06/0.12 (100)	–
Cefuroxime	0.25/2 (NA)[b]	≤ 0.5/≤ 0.5 (100)	–	≤ 0.06/0.12 (NA)
Ceftriaxone	≤ 0.25/1 (90.7)	0.06/0.06 (100)	–	≤ 0.25/≤ 0.25 (100)
Cefotaxime	0.12/1 (93)	≤ 0.06/≤ 0.06 (100)	≤ 0.12/≤ 0.12 (100)	0.06/0.12 (98.7)
Cefepime	0.25/2 (NA)	0.03/0.06 (100)	–	0.12/0.25 (NA)
Ceftazidime	2/8 (NA)	–	–	–
Imipenem	–	≤ 0.06/≤ 0.06 (100)	≤ 0.12/≤ 0.12 (100)	–
Meropenem	0.12/1 (85)	–	0.06/0.06 (100)	–

[a] –, data not provided.
[b] NA, no CLSI interpretive criteria available.

as the disk diffusion test is unreliable for this organism. For β-hemolytic and viridans group streptococcal species, the agents in this group are cefepime, cefotaxime, and ceftriaxone. Any of the three is appropriate for the β-hemolytic streptococci, as these agents have nearly complete cross-resistance or cross-susceptibility. Disk diffusion is an acceptable method of testing these agents for β-hemolytic streptococci.

Group C. These are supplemental agents to be tested and reported selectively in institutions that harbor endemic or epidemic strains resistant to one or more of the primary drugs, particularly those in the same class. For *S. pneumoniae*, this group includes amoxicillin, amoxicillin/clavulanic acid, cefuroxime, ertapenem, and imipenem. There are no β-lactam agents in Group C for the other streptococcal species.

PHENOTYPIC DETECTION OF RESISTANCE

Resistance is detected in the clinical laboratory using disk diffusion, broth microdilution, or E-test® as described above. MIC breakpoints recommended by CLSI and EUCAST are summarized in Tables 2 and 5 (13, 18). Nonmeningeal isolates susceptible to ≤ 2 μg/ml of penicillin G can be considered susceptible to parenteral ampicillin, cefepime, cefotaxime and ceftriaxone. Nonmeningeal isolates susceptible to ≤ 0.06 μg/ml of penicillin G can be also considered susceptible to these parenteral agents, as well as to parenteral ertapenem, imipenem and meropenem and to oral ampicillin, amoxicillin, amoxicillin/clavulanate, cefaclor, cefdinir, cefditoren, cefprozil, cefuroxime and cefpodoxime. β-hemolytic and viridans group streptococci susceptible to penicillin G can, without further testing, be considered susceptible to ampicillin, amoxicillin, amoxicillin-clavulanic acid, ampicillin-sulbactam, cefaclor, cefazolin, cefdinir, cefepime, cefprozil, cefotaxime, ceftibuten (Group A streptococci only), ceftriaxone, cefuroxime, cefpodoxime, ceftizoxime, cephradine, cephalothin, cephapirin, ertapenem, imipenem, loracarbef, and meropenem.

GENOTYPIC DETECTION OF RESISTANCE

Genotypic testing for resistance is accomplished by sequencing PCR products of PBP genes

Table 7. Groupings of β-lactams with FDA clinical indications that should be considered for routine testing and reporting on streptococci (13).

| β-lactam group | *Streptococcus pneumoniae* | | *Streptococcus* spp. | Viridans group |
	Nonmeningitis	Meningitis	β-hemolytic group	streptococci
Group A: Primary test and report	Penicillin[a]	Penicillin[a]	Penicillin[b] or Ampicillin[b]	Ampicillin Penicillin
Group B: Primary test, report selectively	Cefepime Ceftriaxone[a] Ceftriaxone[a] Meropenem[a]	Cefotaxime[a] Ceftriaxone[a] Meropenem[a]	Cefepime or Cefotaxime or Ceftriaxone	Cefepime Cefotaxime Ceftriaxone
Group C: Supplemental, report selectively	Amoxicillin Amoxicillin-clavulanate Cefuroxime Ertapenem imipenem			

[a] Penicillin G and cefotaxime or ceftriaxone or meropenem should be tested by a reliable MIC method and reported routinely with CSF isolates of S. pneumoniae. With isolates from other sites, the oxacillin disk screening test may be used, and if the oxacillin zone size is ≤ 19 mm, penicillin and cefotaxime or ceftriaxone or meropenem MICs should be determined.

[b] Susceptibility testing of penicillins and other β-lactams approved by FDA for treatment of *Streptococcus pyogenes* or *S. agalactiae* is not necessary for clinical purposes and need not be done routinely, since resistant strains have not been recognized. Interpretive criteria are provided for pharmaceutical development, epidemiology, or monitoring for emerging resistance. Any strain found to be intermediate or resistant should be referred to a reference laboratory for confirmation.

to detect mutations in these genes and is not used in the clinical setting.

CONCLUSION

Considerable decreases in β-lactam susceptibility have occurred in pneumococci and viridans group streptococci. The clinical significance of these changes is evident in treatment recommendations for meningitis, endocarditis, pneumonia, sinusitis, and otitis media. To date β-lactam resistance has not developed in β-hemolytic streptococci, but if this occurs it will present significant challenges.

REFERENCES

(1) **American Academy of Pediatrics.** 2006. Section 3. Summaries of Infectious Diseases. Pneumococcal Infections. Red Book Online http://aapredbook.aap-publications.org/cgi/content/full/2006/1/3.100#T3.4.

(2) **American Academy of Pediatrics and American Academy of Family Physicians.** 2004. Subcommittee on Management of Acute Otitis Media. Diagnosis and management of acute otitis media. Pediatrics **113**:1451-65.

(3) **Anon, J. B., M. R. Jacobs, M. D. Poole, P. G. Ambrose, M. S. Benninger, J. A. Hadley, and W. A. Craig.** 2004. Antimicrobial treatment guidelines for acute bacterial rhinosinusitis. Otolaryngol Head Neck Surg **130**:1-45.

(4) **Appelbaum, P. C., A. Bhamjee, J. N. Scragg, A. F. Hallett, A. J. Bowen, and R. C. Cooper.** 1977. Streptococcus pneumoniae resistant to penicillin and chloramphenicol. Lancet **2**:995-7.

(5) **Baddour, L. M., W. R. Wilson, A. S. Bayer, V. G. Fowler, Jr., A. F. Bolger, M. E. Levison, P. Ferrieri, M. A. Gerber, L. Y. Tani, M. H. Gewitz, D. C. Tong, J. M. Steckelberg, R. S. Baltimore, S. T. Shulman, J. C. Burns, D. A. Falace, J. W. Newburger, T. J. Pallasch, M. Takahashi, and K. A. Taubert.** 2005. Infective endocarditis: diagnosis, antimicrobial therapy, and management of complications: a statement for healthcare professionals from the Committee on Rheumatic Fever, Endocarditis, and Kawasaki Disease, Council on Cardiovascular Disease in the Young, and the Councils on Clinical Cardiology, Stroke, and Cardiovascular Surgery and Anesthesia, American Heart Association: endorsed by the Infectious Diseases Society of America. Circulation **111**:e394-434.

(6) **Beall, B., M. C. McEllistrem, R. E. Gertz, Jr., S. Wedel, D. J. Boxrud, A. L. Gonzalez, M. J. Medina, R. Pai, T. A. Thompson, L. H. Harrison, L. McGee, and C. G. Whitney.** 2006. Pre- and post-vaccination clonal compositions of invasive pneumococcal serotypes for isolates collected in the United States in 1999, 2001, and 2002. J Clin Microbiol **44**:999-1017.

(7) **Betriu, C., M. C. Casado, M. Gomez, A. Sanchez, M. L. Palau, and J. J. Picazo.** 1999. Incidence of erythromycin resistance in Streptococcus pyogenes: a 10-year study. Diagn Microbiol Infect Dis **33**:255-60.

(8) **Betriu, C., M. Gomez, A. Sanchez, A. Cruceyra, J. Romero, and J. J. Picazo.** 1994. Antibiotic resistance and penicillin tolerance in clinical isolates of group B streptococci. Antimicrob Agents Chemother **38**:2183-6.

(9) **Bradley, J. S.** 2002. Management of community-acquired pediatric pneumonia in an era of increasing antibiotic resistance and conjugate vaccines. Pediatr Infect Dis J **21**:592-8; discussion 613-4.

(10) **Choby, B. A.** 2009. Diagnosis and treatment of streptococcal pharyngitis. Am Fam Physician **79**:383-90.

(11) **CLSI.** 2009. Methods for dilution antimicrobial susceptibility tests for bacteria that grow aerobically, 8th ed. Approved standard M7-A8. National Committee for Clinical Laboratory Standards, Wayne, PA.

(12) **CLSI.** 2009. Performance Standards for Antimicrobial Disk Susceptibility Tests; Approved Standard M02-A10 - Tenth Edition.

(13) **CLSI.** 2009. Performance Standards for Antimicrobial Susceptibility Testing; Nineteenth Informational Supplement. CLSI document M100-S19. Clinical and Laboratory Standards Institute, Wayne, PA.

(14) **Craig, W. A.** 1998. Pharmacokinetic/pharmacodynamic parameters: rationale for antibacterial dosing of mice and men. Clin Infect Dis **26**:1-10; quiz 11-2.

(15) **Critchley, I. A., M. R. Jacobs, S. D. Brown, M. M. Traczewski, G. S. Tillotson, and N. Janjic.** 2008. Prevalence of serotype 19A Streptococcus pneumoniae among isolates from U.S. children in 2005-2006 and activity of faropenem. Antimicrob Agents Chemother **52**:2639-43.

(16) **Davies, T. A., W. Shang, and K. Bush.** 2006. Activities of ceftobiprole and other beta-lactams against Streptococcus pneumoniae clinical isolates from the United States with defined substitutions in penicillin-binding proteins PBP 1a, PBP 2b, and PBP 2x. Antimicrob Agents Chemother **50**:2530-2.

(17) **Doern, G. V., M. J. Ferraro, A. B. Brueggemann, and K. L. Ruoff.** 1996. Emergence of high rates of antimicrobial resistance among viridans group streptococci in the United States. Antimicrob Agents Chemother **40**:891-4.

(18) **European Committee on Antimicrobial Susceptibility Testing (EUCAST).** 2009. Clinical breakpoints. http://eucast.www137.server1.mensemedia.net/index.php?id=59 accessed 25 June 2009.

(19) **European Committee on Antimicrobial Susceptibility Testing (EUCAST).** 2003. Determination of minimum inhibitory concentrations (MICs) of antibacterial agents by broth microdilution. http://eucast.www137.server1.mensemedia.net/fileadmin/src/media/PDFs/2News_Discussions/3Discussion_Documents/E_Def_5_1_03_2003.pdf accessed 25 June 2009.

(20) **Evans, G. M., and W. F. Gaisford.** 1938. Treatment of pneumonia with 2-(p-aminobenzene-sulphonamido)pyridine. Lancet **2**:14-19.

(21) **Fernandez, M., M. E. Hickman, and C. J. Baker.** 1998. Antimicrobial susceptibilities of group B streptococci isolated between 1992 and 1996 from patients with bacteremia or meningitis. Antimicrob Agents Chemother **42**:1517-9.

(22) **Hakenbeck, R., T. Grebe, D. Zahner, and J. B. Stock.** 1999. beta-lactam resistance in Streptococcus pneumoniae: penicillin-binding proteins and non-penicillin-binding proteins. Mol Microbiol **33:**673-8.

(23) **Hakenbeck, R., A. Konig, I. Kern, M. van der Linden, W. Keck, D. Billot-Klein, R. Legrand, B. Schoot, and L. Gutmann.** 1998. Acquisition of five high-Mr penicillin-binding protein variants during transfer of high-level beta-lactam resistance from Streptococcus mitis to Streptococcus pneumoniae. J Bacteriol **180:**1831-40.

(24) **Jacobs, M.** 2001. Optimisation of antimicrobial therapy using pharmacokinetic and pharmacodynamic parameters. Clinical Microbiology and Infection **7:**589-596.

(25) **Jacobs, M. R.** 2004. Anti-infective pharmacodynamics - maximizing efficacy, minimizing toxicity. Drug Discovery Today **1:**505-512.

(26) **Jacobs, M. R., J. Anon, and P. C. Appelbaum.** 2004. Mechanisms of resistance among respiratory tract pathogens. Clin Lab Med **24:**419-53.

(27) **Jacobs, M. R., S. Bajaksouzian, A. Zilles, G. Lin, G. A. Pankuch, and P. C. Appelbaum.** 1999. Susceptibilities of Streptococcus pneumoniae and Haemophilus influenzae to 10 oral antimicrobial agents based on pharmacodynamic parameters: 1997 U.S. Surveillance study. Antimicrob Agents Chemother **43:**1901-8.

(28) **Jacobs, M. R., D. Felmingham, P. C. Appelbaum, and R. N. Gruneberg.** 2003. The Alexander Project 1998-2000: susceptibility of pathogens isolated from community-acquired respiratory tract infection to commonly used antimicrobial agents. J Antimicrob Chemother **52:**229-46.

(29) **Jacobs, M. R., C. E. Good, S. Bajaksouzian, and A. R. Windau.** 2008. Emergence of Streptococcus pneumoniae serotypes 19A, 6C, and 22F and serogroup 15 in Cleveland, Ohio, in relation to introduction of the protein-conjugated pneumococcal vaccine. Clin Infect Dis **47:**1388-95.

(30) **Jacobs, M. R., C. E. Good, B. Beall, S. Bajaksouzian, A. R. Windau, and C. G. Whitney.** 2008. Changes in Serotypes and Antimicrobial Susceptibility of Invasive Streptococcus pneumoniae in Cleveland: a quarter-century experience. J Clin Microbiol.

(31) **Jacobs, M. R., H. J. Koornhof, R. M. Robins-Browne, C. M. Stevenson, Z. A. Vermaak, I. Freiman, G. B. Miller, M. A. Witcomb, M. Isaacson, J. I. Ward, and R. Austrian.** 1978. Emergence of multiply resistant pneumococci. N Engl J Med **299:**735-40.

(32) **Johnson, D. M., M. G. Stilwell, T. R. Fritsche, and R. N. Jones.** 2006. Emergence of multidrug-resistant Streptococcus pneumoniae: report from the SENTRY Antimicrobial Surveillance Program (1999-2003). Diagn Microbiol Infect Dis **56:**69-74.

(33) **Jones, R. N.** 2009. SENTRY Antimicrobial Surveillance Program platform (2004-2008; USA). JMI Laboratories, North Liberty, Iowa, USA.

(34) **Jones, R. N., A. H. Mutnick, and D. J. Varnam.** 2002. Impact of modified nonmeningeal Streptococcus pneumoniae interpretive criteria (NCCLS M100-S12) on the susceptibility patterns of five parenteral cephalosporins: report from the SENTRY antimicrobial surveillance program (1997 to 2001). J Clin Microbiol **40:**4332-3.

(35) **Kennedy, H. F., C. G. Gemmell, J. Bagg, B. E. Gibson, and J. R. Michie.** 2001. Antimicrobial susceptibility of blood culture isolates of viridans streptococci: relationship to a change in empirical antibiotic therapy in febrile neutropenia. J Antimicrob Chemother **47:**693-6.

(36) **Lindgren, M., J. Jalava, K. Rantakokko-Jalava, and O. Meurman.** 2007. In vitro susceptibility of viridans group streptococci isolated from blood in southwest Finland in 1993-2004. Scand J Infect Dis **39:**508-13.

(37) **Livermore, D. M., M. W. Carter, S. Bagel, B. Wiedemann, F. Baquero, E. Loza, H. P. Endtz, N. van Den Braak, C. J. Fernandes, L. Fernandes, N. Frimodt-Moller, L. S. Rasmussen, H. Giamarellou, E. Giamarellos-Bourboulis, V. Jarlier, J. Nguyen, C. E. Nord, M. J. Struelens, C. Nonhoff, J. Turnidge, J. Bell, R. Zbinden, S. Pfister, L. Mixson, and D. L. Shungu.** 2001. In vitro activities of ertapenem (MK-0826) against recent clinical bacteria collected in Europe and Australia. Antimicrob Agents Chemother **45:**1860-7.

(38) **Lyytikainen, O., M. Rautio, P. Carlson, V. J. Anttila, R. Vuento, H. Sarkkinen, A. Kostiala, M. L. Vaisanen, A. Kanervo, and P. Ruutu.** 2004. Nosocomial bloodstream infections due to viridans streptococci in haematological and non-haematological patients: species distribution and antimicrobial resistance. J Antimicrob Chemother **53:**631-4.

(39) **Mandell, L. A., R. G. Wunderink, A. Anzueto, J. G. Bartlett, G. D. Campbell, N. C. Dean, S. F. Dowell, T. M. File, Jr., D. M. Musher, M. S. Niederman, A. Torres, and C. G. Whitney.** 2007. Infectious Diseases Society of America/American Thoracic Society consensus guidelines on the management of community-acquired pneumonia in adults. Clin Infect Dis 44 Suppl **2:**S27-72.

(40) **Marchese, A., L. Gualco, A. M. Schito, E. A. Debbia, and G. C. Schito.** 2004. In vitro activity of ertapenem against selected respiratory pathogens. J Antimicrob Chemother **54:**944-51.

(41) **Marron, A., J. Carratala, F. Alcaide, A. Fernandez-Sevilla, and F. Gudiol.** 2001. High rates of resistance to cephalosporins among viridans-group streptococci causing bacteraemia in neutropenic cancer patients. J Antimicrob Chemother **47:**87-91.

(42) **Pankuch, G. A., M. R. Jacobs, and P. C. Appelbaum.** 1994. Susceptibilities of 200 penicillin-susceptible and -resistant pneumococci to piperacillin, piperacillin-tazobactam, ticarcillin, ticarcillin-clavulanate, ampicillin, ampicillin-sulbactam, ceftazidime, and ceftriaxone. Antimicrob Agents Chemother **38:**2905-7.

(43) **Pfaller, M. A., and R. N. Jones.** 1997. A review of the in vitro activity of meropenem and comparative antimicrobial agents tested against 30,254 aerobic and anaerobic pathogens isolated world wide. Diagn Microbiol Infect Dis **28:**157-63.

(44) **Pfaller, M. A., R. N. Jones, G. V. Doern, H. S. Sader, K. C. Kugler, and M. L. Beach.** 1999. Survey of blood stream infections attributable to gram-positive cocci: frequency of occurrence and antimicrobial susceptibility of isolates collected in 1997 in the United States, Canada, and Latin America

from the SENTRY Antimicrobial Surveillance Program. SENTRY Participants Group. Diagn Microbiol Infect Dis **33**:283-97.

(45) **Sader, H. S., R. N. Jones, M. G. Stilwell, M. J. Dowzicky, and T. R. Fritsche.** 2005. Tigecycline activity tested against 26,474 bloodstream infection isolates: a collection from 6 continents. Diagn Microbiol Infect Dis **52**:181-6.

(46) **Schrag, S. J., L. McGee, C. G. Whitney, B. Beall, A. S. Craig, M. E. Choate, J. H. Jorgensen, R. R. Facklam, and K. P. Klugman.** 2004. Emergence of Streptococcus pneumoniae with very-high-level resistance to penicillin. Antimicrob Agents Chemother **48**:3016-23.

(47) **Song, J. H., K. S. Ko, M. Y. Lee, S. Park, J. Y. Baek, J. Y. Lee, S. T. Heo, K. T. Kwon, S. Y. Ryu, W. S. Oh, K. R. Peck, and N. Y. Lee.** 2006. In vitro activities of ertapenem against drug-resistant Streptococcus pneumoniae and other respiratory pathogens from 12 Asian countries. Diagn Microbiol Infect Dis **56**:445-50.

(48) **Spangler, S. K., M. R. Jacobs, and P. C. Appelbaum.** 1994. Susceptibilities of 177 penicillin-susceptible and -resistant pneumococci to FK 037, cefpirome, cefepime, ceftriaxone, cefotaxime, ceftazidime, imipenem, biapenem, meropenem, and vancomycin. Antimicrob Agents Chemother **38**:898-900.

(49) **Stevens, D. L., A. L. Bisno, H. F. Chambers, E. D. Everett, P. Dellinger, E. J. Goldstein, S. L. Gorbach, J. V. Hirschmann, E. L. Kaplan, J. G. Montoya, and J. C. Wade.** 2005. Practice guidelines for the diagnosis and management of skin and soft-tissue infections. Clin Infect Dis **41**:1373-406.

(50) **Tunkel, A. R., B. J. Hartman, S. L. Kaplan, B. A. Kaufman, K. L. Roos, W. M. Scheld, and R. J. Whitley.** 2004. Practice guidelines for the management of bacterial meningitis. Clin Infect Dis **39**:1267-84.

Chapter 12. β-LACTAMS AND ENTEROCOCCI

Jean-Luc MAINARDI

INTRODUCTION

Enterococci are a leading cause of serious community-acquired and nosocomial infections. Of the twenty or so species, E. faecalis and E. faecium account for over 95% of clinical isolates and among these, E. faecalis is clearly predominant, representing more than 80% of isolated strains. However, in ICU in the USA, E. faecium can predominate.

The emergence of enterococci, particularly as nosocomial pathogens, is readily attributed to the existence in these bacteria of intrinsic multidrug resistance to antibiotics including aminoglycosides (low-level), cephalosporins (high-level), lincosamides and clindamycin (for E. faecalis). In addition to this intrinsic resistance, the emergence of acquired resistance to the three major antibiotic classes used to treat enterococcal infections - namely, penicillins, glycopeptides and aminoglycosides (used in combination with the former two) - poses serious problems in therapy and has driven the search for alternative treatments.

This chapter will review the behavior of enterococci, mainly the species E. faecalis and E. faecium, with respect to β-lactam antibiotics, the reference treatment for enterococcal infections.

β-LACTAM TARGETS: D,D-TRANSPEPTIDASES (PENICILLIN BINDING PROTEINS)

The β-lactams act by inhibiting D,D-transpeptidases, enzymes which catalyze the formation of crosslinks between two peptides attached to the polysaccharide backbone of the peptidoglycan. Because they also display affinity for β-lactams, the D,D-transpeptidases are known as penicillin binding proteins (PBP). PBPs are divided into multimodular and monomodular types (8). The D,D-transpeptidases are multimodular PBPs which fall into two classes (8). Class A PBPs have an N-terminal glycosyltransferase module and a C-terminal transpeptidase module. Class B PBPs have a non-catalytic N-terminal module whose function is unclear, and a C-terminal transpeptidase module. The profile and number of PBPs in enterococci is characteristic of each species. Analysis of the E. faecalis genome has revealed the presence of three class A PBP genes (pbpF, ponA and pbpZ) and three class B PBP genes (pbp5, pbpA and pbpB) (1, 8). Genes homologous to these PBPs have been identified in the E. faecium genome (1). β-lactam susceptibility in enterococci results from the ability of PBPs to bind to these antibiotics.

INTRINSIC β-LACTAM RESISTANCE

E. faecalis

E. faecalis harbors a PBP5 with intrinsically low affinity for penicillin G (1, 28), leading to a 10-100 fold increase in the MICs of penicillins, aminopenicillins, ureidopenicillins, carboxypenicillins and imipenem as compared to the MICs of these antibiotics for streptococci (Table 1). PBP5 is a class B PBP (B1) conferring high-level resistance to cephalosporins and oxacillin. In vitro deletion of the pbp5 structural gene restores susceptibility to penicillins and cephalosporins, with MICs of ampicillin decreasing from 2 to 0.5 µg/ml and ceftriaxone from > 1000 to 0.25 µg/ml (1).

E. faecium

Like E. faecalis, E. faecium harbors a PBP5 with low affinity for penicillins (29). Affinity is even lower than that of E. faecalis PBP5, leading to even higher MICs of penicillin (Table 1). As in the case of E. faecalis, deletion of the structural gene restores penicillin susceptibility with the MIC of ampicillin decreasing from 24 to 0.06 µg/ml and ceftriaxone from > 1000 to 2 µg/ml (13).

Other enterococcal species

The MICs for most other enterococcal species are the same or lower than for E. faecalis (Table 1).

On the other hand, *E. raffinosus* has higher penicillin G resistance (9, 10).

ACQUIRED RESISTANCE

E. faecalis

Production of penicillinase

The production of penicillinase sometimes encoded on transferable plasmids has been described in the United States, Argentina and Lebanon (19, 20, 21) but not in Europe. The responsible gene is identical to *blaZ*, the type A β-lactamase gene from *S. aureus* (31). In contrast to *S. aureus*, penicillinase expression in *E. faecalis* is constitutive. The MIC of penicillin G is 4-8 µg/ml and that of ampicillin is 2-4 µg/ml (21). This penicillinase is susceptible to the action of β-lactamase inhibitors (clavulanic acid, sulbactam, tazobactam) and the MICs of amoxicillin + clavulanic acid combinations are 1-2 µg/ml. This resistance is often associated with high level resistance to aminoglycosides.

Modification of PBP5

This mechanism is rare in clinical isolates of *E. faecalis* (3). In the few strains described, the MICs of ampicillin are 32 and 64 µg/ml. The mechanism is thought to involve an overproduction of PBP5, based on binding data of radiolabeled penicillin to PBP5.

E. faecium

Production of penicillinase

This resistance mechanism is very rare in *E. faecium* and only a few clinical isolates have been reported (4).

Modification of PBP5

Early studies suggested that the high-level ampicillin resistance in *E. hirae* (similar to that in *E. faecium*) was achieved *in vitro* by increasing levels of PBP5 expression. In *E. faecium* clinical isolates, intermediate β-lactam resistance (MIC ≤ 16 µg/ml) is usually related to a quantitative increase in PBP5 levels (7, 24). Conversely, high-level resistance (Table 1) is rarely associated with PBP5 overexpression but is more commonly due to mutations in the *pbp5* structural gene (24, 30). These mutations in close proximity to the catalytic site are presumed to decrease the affinity of PBP5 for β-lactam antibiotics, leading to higher MICs as a result. Studies with isogenic strains have revealed that a single amino acid substitution close to the conserved motifs, particularly of the active site serine, conferred a modest increase in MICs and, conversely, resistance levels were higher when some mutations were present in combination (22). In particular, the Met_{485} Ala substitution close to the active site serine, combined with the insertion of a serine at position 466 (situated in the loop forming the outer edge of the active site), was associated with high-level resistance to all β-lactams. Affinity for penicillin G generally correlated with the MICs for the utants, although this relationship was not strictly proportional (22). Using a strain containing a *pbp5* deletion, Rice et al. showed that *pbp5* is a transferable determinant, even in the absence of a vancomycin resistance mobile element (23).

Other enterococcal species

Data on other enterococcal species are scarce. Penicillin G-resistant strains of *E. hirae* have been obtained *in vitro*, presumably through a mechanism of increased PBP5 production. An *E. hirae*

Table 1. MIC (µg/ml) of the main penicillins and imipenem for enterococci[a]

Species	Penicillin G	Ampicillin	Amoxicillin	Piperacillin	Imipenem
E. faecalis	2 - 8	0.25 - 2	0.25 - 1	0.5 - 4	0.5 - 4
E. faecium	2 - 512	0.5 - 256	0.25 - 256	4 - 512	1 - 512
E. durans	0.25 - 8	0.12 - 4	ND[b]	ND	ND
E. gallinarum	1 - 4	1 - 2	ND	16 - > 16	1 - 2
E. avium	1 - 2	0.5 - 1	ND	16 - > 16	0.5 - 1
E. casseliflavus	0.5 - 4	0.5 - 2	ND	8 - > 16	0.5 - 4
E. hirae	2 - 8	2 - 4	ND	> 16	2
E. raffinosus	32	16	ND	> 16	8

[a] From 9, 11, 18, 24, 25, and 27.
[b] ND, not determined.

clinical isolate for which the MIC of penicillin G was 8 µg/ml associated with PBP5 overproduction has been described (18). Penicillin G resistance has been reported rarely in strains of *E. durans*, *E. raffinosus* and *E. gallinarum* (9, 10) and the mechanism is unknown.

TOLERANCE

The enterococci are considered to be tolerant to β-lactam antibiotics. Tolerance, defined as a MBC/MIC ratio ≥ 32, is present in 75% of *E. faecalis* strains. Detection of tolerance *in vitro* largely depends on the experimental conditions and its clinical significance has not been clearly established. Such strains also show a paradoxical phenomenon known as the Eagle effect, which is expressed after exposure to high antibiotic concentrations (20-30 times the MIC) and results in a 10-100 fold decrease in bactericidal activity relative to that seen in the presence of 2-5 times the MIC. In *E. faecalis*, the absence of an autolytic enzyme is thought to be responsible for the paradoxical effect (6).

NOVEL RESISTANCE MECHANISM

A novel mechanism of resistance to β-lactams was recently described in *E. faecium* (13, 17). HPLC and MS analysis of the peptidoglycan from an *E. faecium* mutant selected on ampicillin (MIC > 2000 µg/ml) from a parental strain devoid of PBP5 (MIC: 0.06 µg/ml) revealed a highly modified global structure with new, unidentified structures comprising a novel cross-link. This cross-link was the result of a new type of ampicillin-insensitive transpeptidation (L,D-transpeptidation), which replaced the classic D,D-transpeptidation normally inhibited by β-lactams (13). In addition to the L,D-transpeptidase which was identified and characterized (2, 15, 17), the formation of this new peptide cross-link was found to require the action of another enzyme, D,D-carboxypeptidase, also ampicillin-insensitive, for the L,D-transpeptidase to act and form the new cross-link (5, 14). This novel mechanism of β-lactam resistance in *E. faecium* might also be responsible for the emergence of high-level cross-resistance to glycopeptides (5), by replacing the terminal D-Ala$_4$-D-Ala$_5$ pentapeptide target of glycopeptides with the tetrapeptide generated by D,D-carboxypeptidase. Unexpectedly, the L,D-transpeptidase is inhibited by carbapenems (16).

BREAKPOINTS AND PREVALENCE OF RESISTANCE

EUCAST breakpoints for susceptibility and resistance to ampicillin or amoxicillin are MIC ≤ 4 µg/ml and MIC > 8 µg/ml, respectively (http://www.escmid.org/escmid_library/reports/eucast_reports/). The same breakpoints are proposed for imipenem. *E. faecalis* strains susceptible to ampicillin or amoxicillin are categorized as susceptible to piperacillin (with or without tazobactam) and imipenem. Penicillin-resistant *E. faecium* strains should be categorized as resistant to other β-lactams including imipenem. Ertapenem, another member of the carbapenem family, is ineffective against enterococci. Enterococci are intrinsically resistant to ticarcillin with or without clavulanic acid.

According to the CLSI (http://www.csli.org), for penicillin G and ampicillin an MIC ≤ 8 mg/ml (inhibition zone diameter ≥ 15 mm for a 10 µg disk) categorizes an enterococcal strain as susceptible while MIC ≥ 16 mg/ml (inhibition zone diameter ≤ 14 mm) is the breakpoint for resistance. However, enterococci for which the MIC of penicillin is ≤ 64 mg/ml or the MIC of ampicillin is ≤ 32 mg/ml may be susceptible to the synergistic effect of these penicillins in combination with gentamicin or streptomycin (if there is no high-level resistance to these aminoglycosides), if high penicillin doses are used. This synergy may not be efficient for higher MICs (MIC ≥ 128 mg/ml for penicillin G or ≥ 64 mg/ml for ampicillin).

Even when different breakpoints are used, clinical studies have shown that all *E. faecalis* strains are susceptible to amoxicillin (11, 25, 26, 27). On the other hand, in *E. faecium*, and depending on the study, only 58% of isolates are reported as susceptible (26). Lower rates of ampicillin susceptibility have been observed, particularly in the United States, highlighting the geographical differences in β-lactam susceptibility in this species (9, 11, 25, 27). In *E. faecium*, glycopeptide resistance and high-level gentamicin resistance are often associated with high-level resistance to ampicillin.

ANTIBIOTICS TO BE STUDIED

Antibiotic susceptibility testing by the diffusion or broth method efficiently detects penicillin-resistant enterococci in which resistance is due to modification of PBPs, but does not readily detect β-lactamase-producing strains, especially in the absence of a high inoculum. If the strain is suspected to be a β-lactamase producer, the CSLI recommends a nitrocefin® test (20) on isolates cultured from blood or meninges. A positive result predicts resistance to penicillin G, aminopenicillins, carboxypenicillins, and ureidopenicillins.

Ampicillin and amoxicillin are active against wild-type strains of enterococci and one of these two antibiotics should be included in the susceptibility test. However, penicillin G, ampicillin (or amoxicillin), the combination amoxicillin-clavulanic acid (or ampicillin-sulbactam), a first-generation cephalosporin and a third generation cephalosporin are often routinely tested against streptococci (especially blood isolates) before identification to the species and genus level (Fig. 1-5). If penicillin G is tested, enterococci susceptible to it are susceptible to ampicillin, amoxicillin, amoxicillin-clavulanic acid, piperacillin and piperacillin-tazobactam for non-β-lactamase-producing strains. However, ampicillin-susceptible enterococci cannot be interpreted as being susceptible to penicillin G. If penicillin G susceptibility

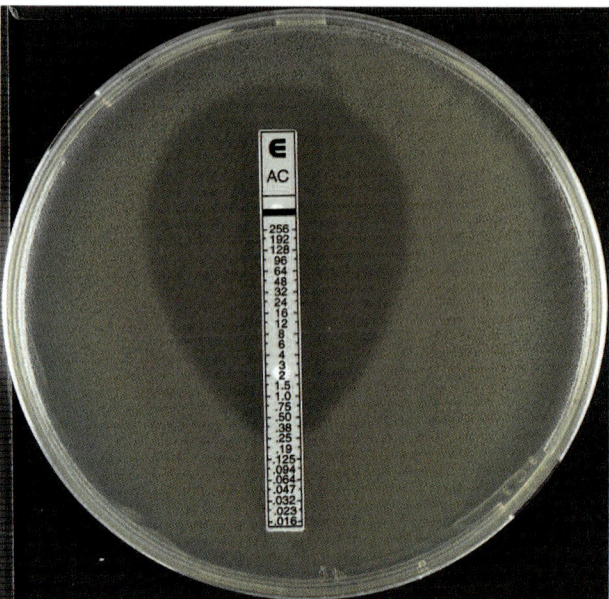

Fig. 1. Ampicillin-susceptible *E. faecalis* (MIC of amoxicillin = 0.5 µg/ml). Note the intrinsic cephalosporin resistance. P: penicillin G, AM: ampicillin, CTX: cefotaxime, CF: cephalothin, AMC: amoxicillin-clavulanic acid.

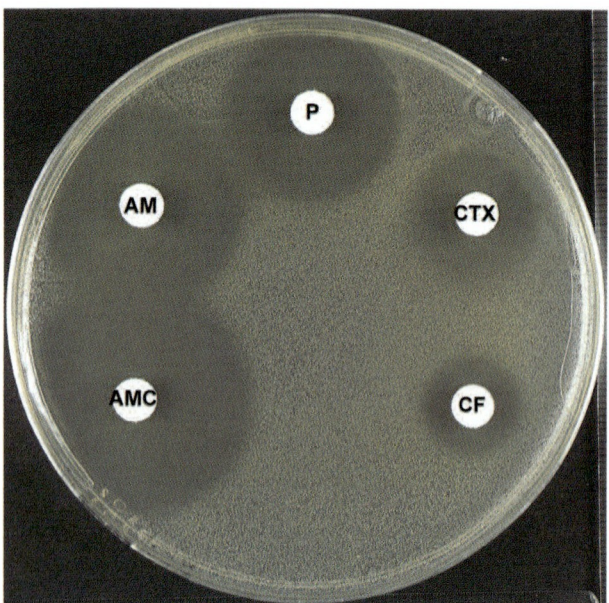
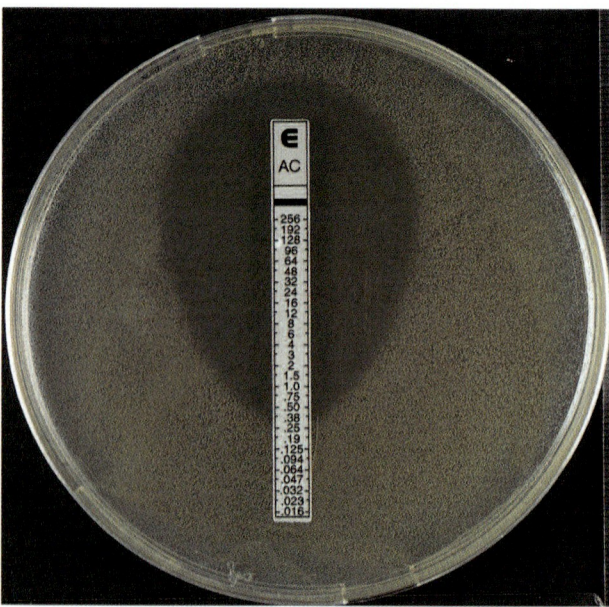

Fig. 2. Ampicillin-susceptible *E. faecium* (MIC of amoxicillin = 0.5 µg/ml). Like *E. faecalis*, *E. faecium* is intrinsically resistant to cephalosporins. P: penicillin G, AM: ampicillin, CTX: cefotaxime, CF: cephalothin, AMC: amoxicillin-clavulanic acid.

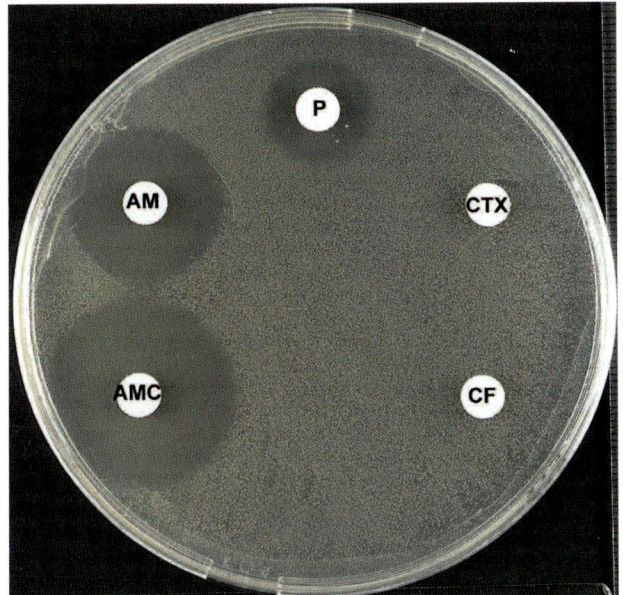
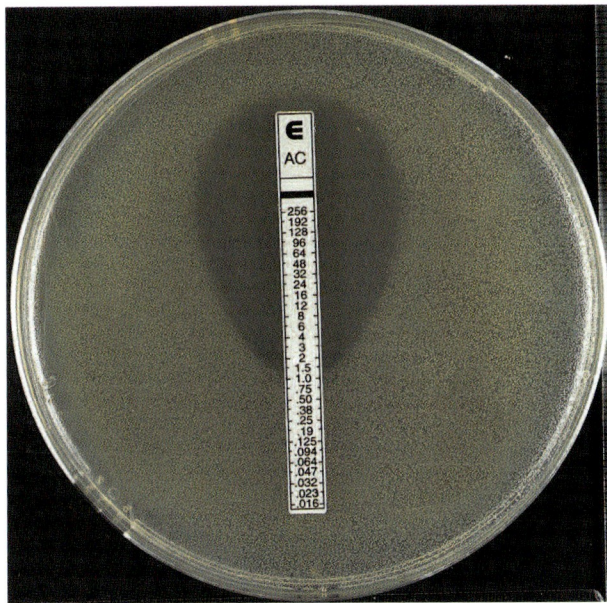

Fig. 3. Ampicillin-susceptible *E. faecium* (MIC of amoxicillin = 1.5 µg/ml) due to overproduction of low penicillin affinity PBP5 (24). P: penicillin G, AM: ampicillin, CTX: cephotaxime, CF: cefalothin, AMC: amoxicillin-clavulanic acid.

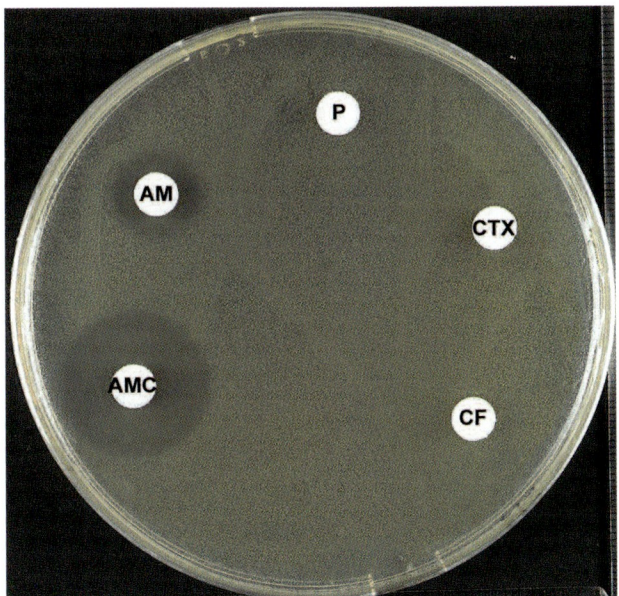
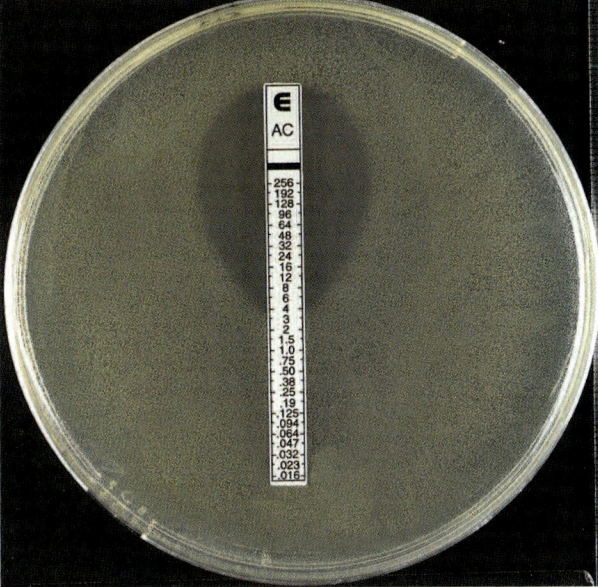

Fig. 4. *E. faecium* with MIC of amoxicillin = 12 µg/ml due to overproduction of low penicillin affinity PBP5 in combination with a $Met_{485}Thr$ substitution in close proximity to the conserved SDN motif of the protein (24). P: penicillin G, AM: ampicillin, CTX: cephotaxime, CF: cefalothin, AMC: amoxicillin-clavulanic acid.

must be known, it is recommended to test this antibiotic. There is no need to test for piperacillin or imipenem susceptibility, as the response to these two antibiotics is similar to that of ampicillin or amoxicillin only in *E. faecalis* and not in other species, particularly *E. faecium*, where the two drugs are less active.

In serious infections caused by *E. faecalis* (endocarditis, meningitis) and for *E. faecium*, in which susceptibility to ampicillin and amoxicillin is unpredictable, and especially in severe infections, the E-test® is justified for determining the MICs of ampicillin and amoxicillin (Fig. 1-5).

Cefotaxime and amoxicillin have shown synergy *in vitro* against *E. faecalis*, resulting from a complementary action of the two drugs on different PBPs (12). If testing is performed on blood agar, some strains of *E. faecalis* may test falsely susceptible to cefotaxime and should be reported as resistant to this antibiotic. If the laboratory does

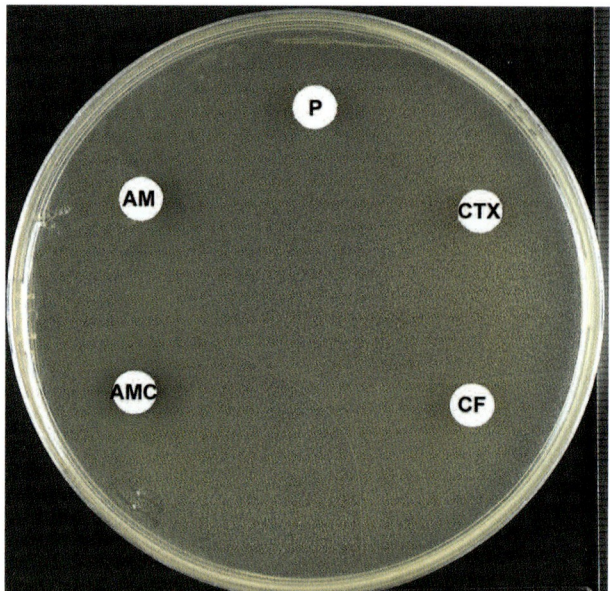
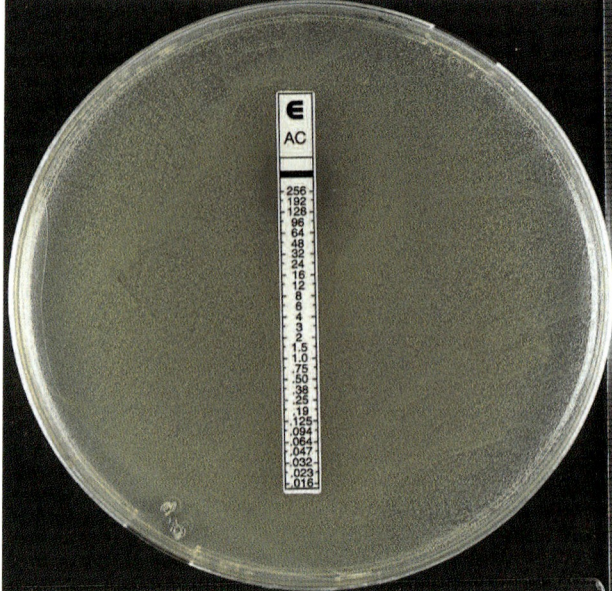

Fig. 5. Highly ampicillin-resistant *E. faecium* (MIC of amoxicillin = 96 µg/ml) harboring a very low penicillin G affinity PBP5 in combination with a Met$_{485}$ Ala substitution in close proximity to the conserved SDN motif of the protein (24). P: penicillin G, AM: ampicillin, CTX: cephotaxime, CF: cefalothin, AMC: amoxicillin-clavulanic acid.

not test cefotaxime, it may be useful to report resistance to the clinician so as to avoid the use of this antibiotic.

CONCLUSION

The majority of *E. faecalis* clinical isolates are susceptible to amoxicillin or ampicilin, the reference drugs for the treatment of enterococcal infections. β-lactamase-producing resistant strains are very rare. On the other hand, *E. faecium* clinical isolates show varied susceptibility to ampicillin and amoxicillin and in serious infections the MICs of these two drugs should be determined. The level of resistance to ampicillin or amoxicillin is an important factor in the potential use of these drugs and it may be necessary to use glycopeptides as an alternative if high-level ampicillin resistance is found.

REFERENCES

(1) **Arbeloa, A., H. Segal, J.E. Hugonnet, N. Josseaume, L. Dubost, J.P. Brouard, L. Gutmann, D. Mengin-Lecreulx, and M. Arthur.** 2004. Role of class A penicillin-binding proteins in PBP5-mediated beta-lactam resistance in *Enterococcus faecalis*. J. Bacteriol. **186** : 1221-1228.

(2) **Biarrotte-Sorin, S., J.E. Hugonnet, V. Delfosse, J.L. Mainardi, L. Gutmann, M. Arthur, and C. Mayer**. 2006. Crystal structure of a novel beta-lactam-insensitive peptidoglycan transpeptidase. J. Mol. Biol. **359**: 533-538.

(3) **Cercenado, E., M.F. Vicente, M.D. Diaz, C. Sanchez-Carrillo, and M. Sanchez-Rubiales**. 1996. Characterization of clinical isolates of beta-lactamase-negative, highly ampicillin-resistant *Enterococcus faecalis*. Antimicrob. Agents Chemother. **40** : 2420-2422.

(4) **Coudron, P.E., S.M. Markowitz, and E.S Wong**. 1992. Isolation of a beta-lactamase-producing, aminoglycoside-resistant strain of *Enterococcus faecium*. Antimicrob. Agents Chemother. **36** : 1125-1126.

(5) **Cremniter, J., J.L. Mainardi, N. Josseaume, J.C. Quincampoix, L. Dubost, J.E. Hugonnet, A. Marie, L. Gutmann, L.B. Rice, and M. Arthur**. 2006. Novel mechanism of resistance to glycopeptide antibiotics in *Enterococcus faecium*. J. Biol. Chem. **281**: 32254-32262.

(6) **Fontana, R., M. Boaretti, A. Grossato, E.A. Tonin, M.M. Lleo, and G. Satta**. 1990. Paradoxical response of *Enterococcus faecalis* to the bactericidal activity of penicillin is associated with reduced activity of one autolysin. Antimicrob. Agents Chemother. **34** : 314-320.

(7) **Fontana, R., M. Aldegheri, M. Ligozzi, H. Lopez, A. Sucari, and G. Satta**. 1994. Overproduction of a low-affinity penicillin-binding protein and high-level ampicillin resistance in *Enterococcus faecium*. Antimicrob. Agents Chemother. **38** : 1980-1983

(8) **Goffin, C., and J.M. Ghuysen**. 1998. Multimodular penicillin-binding proteins: An enigmatic family of orthologs and paralogs. Microbiol. Mol. Biol. Rev. **62** : 1079-1093.

(9) **Gordon, S., J.M. Swenson, B.C. Hill, N.E. Pigott, R.R. Facklam, R.C. Cooksey, C. Thornsberry, W.R. Jarvis, and F.C. Tenover**. 1992. Antimicrobial susceptibility patterns of common and unusual species of enterococci causing infections in the United States. Enterococcal Study Group. J. Clin. Microbiol. **30** : 2373-2378.

(10) Grayson, M.L., G.M. Eliopoulos, C.B. Wennersten, K.L. Ruoff, K. Klimm, F.L. Sapico, A.S. Bayer, and R.C. Moellering Jr. 1991. Comparison of *Enterococcus raffinosus* with *Enterococcus avium* on the basis of penicillin susceptibility, penicillin-binding protein analysis, and high-level aminoglycoside resistance. Antimicrob. Agents Chemother. **35** : 1408-1412.

(11) **Hallgren, A., H. Abednazari, C. Ekdahl, H. Hanberger, M. Nilsson, A. Samuelsson, E. Svensson, L.E. Nilsson, and Swedish ICU Study Group**. 2001. Antimicrobial susceptibility patterns of enterococci in intensive care units in Sweden evaluated by different MIC breakpoint systems. J. Antimicrob. Chemother. **48** : 53-62.

(12) **Mainardi, J.L., L. Gutmann, J.F. Acar, and F.W. Goldstein**. 1995. Synergistic effect of amoxicillin and cefotaxime against *Enterococcus faecalis*. Antimicrob. Agents Chemother. **39** :1984-1987.

(13) **Mainardi, J.L., R. Legrand, M. Arthur, B. Schoot, J. van Heijenoort, and L. Gutmann** 2000. Novel mechanism of beta-lactam resistance due to bypass of DD-transpeptidation in *Enterococcus faecium*. J. Biol. Chem. **275**: 16490-16496.

(14) **Mainardi, J.L., V. Morel, M. Fourgeaud, J. Cremniter, D. Blanot, R. Legrand, C. Frehel, M. Arthur, J. van Heijenoort, and L. Gutmann**. 2002. Balance between two transpeptidation mechanisms determines the expression of beta-lactam resistance in *Enterococcus faecium*. J. Biol. Chem. **277** : 35801-35807.

(15) **Mainardi, J.L., M. Fourgeaud, J.E. Hugonnet, L. Dubost, J.P. Brouard, J. Ouazzani, L.B. Rice, L. Gutmann, and M. Arthur**. 2005. Novel peptidoglycan cross-linking enzyme for a beta-lactam-resistant transpeptidation pathway. J Biol.Chem. **280**: 38146-38152.

(16) **Mainardi, J.L., J.E. Hugonnet, F. Rusconi, M. Fourgeaud M, L. Dubost, A. Nguekam Moumi, V. Delfosse, C. Mayer, L. Gutmann, L.B. Rice, and M. Arthur**. 2007. Unexpected inhibition of peptidoglycan L,D-transpeptidase from *Enterococcus faecium* by the beta-lactam imipenem. J. Biol. Chem. **282**: 30414-30422.

(17) **Mainardi, J.L., R. Villet, T.D. Bugg, C. Mayer, and M. Arthur**. 2008. Evolution of peptidoglycan biosynthesis under the selective pressure of antibiotics in Gram-positive bacteria. FEMS Microbiol. Rev. **32**: 386-408.

(18) **Massa, R., C. Bantar, M. Mollerach, F. Nicola, B.E. Murray, J. Smayevsky, and G. Gutkind**. 1998. Emergence *in vivo* of resistance to ampicillin in a clinical isolate of *Enterococcus hirae*. J. Antimicrob. Chemother. **4** : 559-561.

(19) **Murray, B.E**. 1990. The life and times of the *Enterococcus*. Clin. Microbiol. Rev. **3** :46-65.

(20) **Murray, B.E**. 1992. Beta-lactamase-producing enterococci. Antimicrob. Agents Chemother. **36** : 2355-2359.

(21) **Patterson, J.E., B.L. Masecar, and M.J. Zervos**. 1988. Characterization and comparison of two penicillinase-producing strains of *Streptococcus* (*Enterococcus*) *faecalis*. Antimicrob. Agents Chemother. **32** : 122-124.

(22) **Rice, L.B., S. Bellais, L.L. Carias, R. Hutton-Thomas, R.A. Bonomo, P. Caspers, M.G. Page, and L. Gutmann**. 2004. Impact of specific pbp5 mutations on expression of beta-lactam resistance in *Enterococcus faecium*. Antimicrob. Agents Chemother. **48** : 3028-3032.

(23) **Rice, L.B., L.L Carias, S. Rudin, V. Lakticová, A. Wood, and R. Hutton-Thomas**. 2005. *Enterococcus feacium* low-affinity pbp5 is a transferable determinant. Antimicrob. Agents Chemother. **49**: 5007-5012.

(24) **Rybkine, T., J.L. Mainardi, W. Sougakoff, E. Collatz, and L. Gutmann**. 1998. Penicillin-binding protein 5 sequence alterations in clinical isolates of *Enterococcus faecium* with different levels of ß-lactam resistance. J. Infect. Dis. **178** : 159-163

(25) **Schouten, M.A., A. Voss, and J.A. Hoogkamp-Korstanje**. 1999. Antimicrobial susceptibility patterns of enterococci causing infections in Europe. The European VRE Study Group. Antimicrob. Agents Chemother. **43** : 2542-2546.

(26) **Vachée, A., E. Varon, E. Jouy, D. Meunier, pour le conseil scientifique de l'Onerba**. 2008. Antibiotics susceptibility of *Streptococcus* and *Enterococcus*: Data of Onerba network. Pathol. Biol. In press.

(27) **Weinstein, M.P**. 2001. Comparative evaluation of penicillin, ampicillin, and imipenem MICs and susceptibility breakpoints for vancomycin-susceptible and vancomycin-resistant *Enterococcus faecalis* and *Enterococcus faecium*. J. Clin. Microbiol. **39** : 2729-2731.

(28) **Williamson, R., S.B. Calderwood, R.C. Moellering Jr, and A. Tomasz**. 1983. Studies on the mechanism of intrinsic resistance to beta-lactam antibiotics in group D streptococci. J. Gen. Microbiol. **129** : 813-822.

(29) **Williamson, R., C. LeBouguenec, L. Gutmann, and T. Horaud**. 1985. One or two low affinity penicillin-binding proteins may be responsible for the range of susceptibility of *Enterococcus faecium* to penicillin. J. Gen. Microbiol. **131** : 1933-1940.

(30) **Zorzi, W., X.Y. Zhou, O. Dardenne, J. Lamotte, D. Raze, J. Pierre, L. Gutmann, and J. Coyette**. 1996. Structure of the low-affinity penicillin-binding protein 5 PBP5fm in wild-type and highly penicillin-resistant strains of *Enterococcus faecium*. J. Bacteriol. **178** : 4948-4957.

(31) **Zscheck, K.K., and B.E. Murray**. 1991. Nucleotide sequence of the beta-lactamase gene from *Enterococcus faecalis* HH22 and its similarity to staphylococcal β-lactamase genes. Antimicrob. Agents Chemother. **35** : 1736-1740.

Chapter 13. β-LACTAMS AND *ENTEROBACTERIACEAE*

Richard BONNET and Robert A. BONOMO

INTRODUCTION

By virtue of their diversity, low toxicity, bactericidal action and broad spectrum of activity, β-lactams antibiotics are among the most widely used therapeutic agents in the treatment of infections caused by Gram-negative bacilli, especially the *Enterobacteriaceae*. The efficacy of β-lactams depends on three factors: the amount of antibiotic in contact with the target, the affinity of the antibiotic for the target (*i.e.*, penicillin binding proteins), and the production of antibiotic-inactivating β-lactamases.

Together, these factors can lead to resistance which is either intrinsic, and therefore present in all strains of a species, or acquired by certain strains as a consequence of mutations or the acquisition of genetic material such as plasmids, transposons or integrons. For each species, one can therefore distinguish *i*) a "wild-type" β-lactam resistance or susceptible phenotype, and *ii*) acquired resistance phenotypes or "resistant phenotypes". Resistance may be expressed at a low level *in vitro* but, nonetheless, be responsible for treatment failures.

Knowledge of resistance phenotypes makes it possible to:

a- establish the list of β-lactams to be tested for clinical investigations;

b- check the agreement between identification and resistance phenotype;

c- attenuate the flaws of *in vitro* susceptibility tests by applying interpretive criteria;

d- direct the choice of appropriate treatment.

Because of permeability considerations, enterobacteriaceae are intrinsically resistant to group G, V and M penicillins (*e.g.* penicillin G). Resistance phenotypes are therefore defined by β-lactams belonging to other groups, alone or combined with β-lactamase inhibitors: aminopenicillins (amoxicillin or ampicillin); carboxypenicillins (ticarcillin); ureidopenicillins (piperacillin); first generation cephalosporins (C1G) (cephalothin); second generation (C2G) (cefuroxime and, for the cephamycins, cefoxitin); third generation (C3G) (cefotaxime and ceftazidime); fourth generation (C4G) (cefepime and cefpirome); monobactams (aztreonam); and carbapenems (imipenem and meropenem).

MODE OF ACTION OF β-LACTAMS

The bacterial envelope of enterobacteria comprises the outer membrane, the peptidoglycan layer (murein sacculus), and the cytoplasmic membrane. The targets of β-lactams are located in the inner or the cytoplasmic membrane. The outer membrane is the major permeability barrier against penetration of β-lactams. For the most part, the β-lactams used against enterobacteria are hydrophilic and cannot diffuse to any significant extent across the enterobacterial outer membrane, which is rich in saturated fatty acids. Therefore, β-lactams cross the outer membrane mainly through aqueous channels formed by 35-40 kDa proteins known as porins (also known as outer membrane porins, Omps) (28). These porin channels allow passive diffusion of hydrophilic molecules smaller than 600 Da. The size, charge and hydrophibicity of β-lactams determines their ability to diffuse through porin channels.

The targets of β-lactams are membrane proteins known as penicillin binding proteins, or PBPs (42). Essentially, these are transpeptidases or transglycosidases that are the major proteins responsible for the construction of the cell wall. PBPs vary in number in different bacterial species. Ten PBPs have been detected in *Escherichia coli*: the high molecular weight PBPs 1A, 1B, 1C, 2, and 3, and the low molecular weight PBPs 4, 5, 6, 6b, and 7. The essential PBPs catalyze transglycosylation and/or transpeptidation reactions (bifunctional transglycosylase-transpeptidase PBPs 1A, 1B, and 1C; transpeptidase PBPs 2 and 3) to form polysaccharide chains and peptide cross-linkages in the peptidoglycan. The other PBPs are involved in the reorganization of these residues (PBP D,D-carboxypeptidases or D,D-endopeptidases 4, 5, 6, 6b and 7).

β-lactams are structural or «transition state» analogues of the D-Ala-D-Ala dipeptide, the natural substrate of PBPs, and behave as «suicide substrates» of these enzymes. β-lactams bind to the

PBP active site to form a pre-covalent complex (the Michaelis complex). The β-lactam ring undergoes nucleophilic attack and opens to form an irreversible covalent bond with the active serine in the PBP catalytic pocket (an acylated PBP). The potency of the β-lactam depends on its affinity (defined operationally as K_m) for the different PBPs. Ampicillin binds mainly to PBP 2 and 3, amoxicillin to PBP 1 and PBP 2, and the majority of cephalosporins to PBP 1A and PBP 3. On the other hand, β-lactams display low affinity for the low molecular weight PBPs. Inhibition of PBPs leads to an arrest of peptidoglycan biosynthesis and bacterial growth. The bactericidal effect of β-lactams results from poorly understood secondary phenomena triggered by the inhibition of PBPs. Cell wall lysis is initiated by an alteration in the peptidoglycan which is thought to deregulate the activation of autolytic cell wall hydrolases (murein hydrolase and endopeptidase), culminating in bacterial cell lysis.

METHODS

In current practice, the determination of β-lactam susceptibility in enterobacteria is based on the antibiogram. Data from the antibiogram are analyzed to identify the resistance mechanisms present in the strain under study. These data are then corrected according to the interpretive criteria established on the basis on available microbiological, genetic, biochemical and clinical data concerning the different resistance mechanisms by expert groups such as the Clinical and Laboratory Standards Institute (CLSI) (9), the British Society of Antimicrobial Chemotherapy (BSAC) (5), Comité de l'Antibiogramme de la Société Française de Microbiologie (CA-SFM) (10) and European Committee on Antimicrobial Susceptibility Testing - EUCAST (15).

Diffusion

Agar disk diffusion is used by many diagnostic laboratories. The reliability of the results is influenced by different parameters which must be rigorously controlled. The same techniques must be used to establish the correlation curves. Standardization is governed by the recommendations issued by working groups such as the CLSI in the United States (9), the BSAC in UK (5) , CA-SFM in France (10) and EUCAST (15).

Automated methods

Automated antimicrobial susceptibility testing systems have been developed to improve standardization and shorten run times for the diffusion method. These systems can read and interpret the results. In the best case scenario, results are available within four hours. Automated systems determine bacterial growth in liquid medium in the presence of one or more concentrations of antibiotics which discriminate susceptible from resistant bacteria. Bacterial growth is measured at a fixed time point by turbidity, or else over time by fluorimetry or colorimetry. For enterobacteria, the results obtained by diffusion and by automated systems show satisfactory concordance. However, this does not exclude the need to critically analyze the results and to use additional tests for specific detection of extended-spectrum β-lactamases or carbapenemases which may be expressed at low levels.

RESISTANCE MECHANISMS

Impermeability

The outer membrane of enterobacteria is composed of lipopolysaccharide (LPS), whose structure is hydrophilic due to its surface electrical charges, and whose core is very compact secondary to the presence of unsaturated fatty acids. This organization explains the intrinsic resistance to hydrophobic and/or high molecular weight antibiotics (penicillins G, V and M, macrolides, rifampin, fusidic acid and glycopeptides) (29).

Porins allow the exchange of nutrients and other substances between the periplasm and the external environment by passive diffusion. Hydrophilic β-lactams can also cross the outer membrane through porin channels (porins OmpF and OmpC in *E. coli* and their equivalents OmpK36, OmpD and Omp36 in *Klebsiella pneumoniae*, *Enterobacter aerogenes*, *Salmonella* Typhimurium). However, acquired resistance due to decreased cell wall permeability has been described in *E. coli*, *Proteus*, *Salmonella*, *Shigella*, *Klebsiella*, *Enterobacter*, *Citrobacter*, and *Serratia* as a result of a qualitative or quantitative alteration of porins. This mechanism generally confers low-level resistance, can affect many different antibiotic classes, and is often associated with other resistance mechanisms such as efflux systems and/or β-lactamase production. Porin alterations can also augment low level resistance mediated by modifying enzymes, *i.e.* β-lactamases.

Extrusion by efflux systems

Efflux systems in enterobacteria are generally composed of three proteins acting as a unit (29):

a- one embedded in the cytoplasmic membrane, the pump:

b- a second embedded in the outer membrane to ensure extrusion into the external medium:

c- a third, periplasmic protein which forms a bridge between the pump and the porin channel.

Indeed, efflux systems are «true pumps» which actively expel metabolic or toxic products, such as antibiotics, using proton-motive force PMF). When over-expressed, these systems, such as that encoded by the *mar*RAB genes in *E. coli*, cause generally low-level cross-resistance to different antibiotics including β-lactams, quinolones, chloramphenicol and tetracyclines (24). Resistance conferred by efflux systems is often accompanied by decreased outer membrane permeability resulting from reduced expression of porins [*e.g.*, through destabilization of a porin mRNA by *micF* antisense RNA from the *mar* operon (11)]. The combination of these two mechanisms can lead to high-level cross-resistance to structurally unrelated antibiotics, thereby conferring true multidrug resistance. There are five major superfamilies of efflux systems in prokaryotes: MFS (major facilitator superfamily); ABC (ATP binding casette); RND (resistance-nodulation-cell division superfamily); MATE (multi antimicrobial extrusion superfamily); and SMR (small multidrug resistance superfamily). Only the ABC superfamily are primary transporters (*i.e.* do not use PMF) (20).

Alterations in PBPs

Several factors can contribute to this type of resistance: loss of PBP affinity for β-lactams through amino acid substitutions, acquisition of genes or gene fragments encoding reduced affinity PBPs, or overproduction of normal PBPs. Isolates of *Proteus mirabilis* resistant to imipenem and mecillinam were found to harbor a PBP 2 with decreased affinity and had lower levels of PBP 1A (27). This type of resistance mechanism is uncommon in enterobacteria.

β-lactamase production

The production of inactivating enzymes is the most prominent mechanism of β-lactam resistance in enterobacteria. The most common enzymes act through a serine-based mechanism while the metallo-enzymes use a zinc-based mechanism (one or two Zn ions). In both cases β-lactam inactivation is due to hydrolytic opening of the β-lactam ring at the amide bond following activation of a water molecule.

The wide diversity of β-lactamases has prompted many different attempts to classify them. Two classifications are currently employed (Table 1): the structural classification of R. P. Ambler (1) based on the primary amino acid sequence of conserved elements in the active site, and the functional classification of K. Bush and G. A. Jacoby (6) based on the hydrolytic activity and susceptibility of β-lactamases to inhibitors such as clavulanate and EDTA, a divalent cationic chelator (www.lahey.org/studies/webt.htm).

The Ambler classification defines four enzyme classes, A to D. Class A, C and D enzymes have a serine active site while class B are zinc metallo-enzymes. The Bush and Jacoby classification takes into account the functional variations of the β-lactamases within these four structural classes, particularly in class A which is subdivided into six functional groups (Table 1):

Functional group 2a represents narrow spectrum penicillinases which hydrolyze benzylpenicillins only and are inhibited by clavulanic acid and tazobactam (IC_{50}s < 1 µM);

Functional group 2b represents broad spectrum penicillinases such as TEM-1, TEM-2 and SHV-1. They are inhibited by clavulanate and are capable of inactivating all the penicillins and, to a much lesser extent, second generation cephalosporins (C2G), excluding the cephamycins;

Functional group 2be corresponds to extended-spectrum β-lactamases (ESBLs) of molecular class A. They are inhibited by clavulanate and are able of inactivating all the penicillins and cephalosporins (including cefepime), with the exception of cephamycins. These enzymes (TEM an SHV) confer resistance to cefotaxime, ceftazidime, and aztreonam at a rate > 10% of benzylpenicillin. CTX-M ESBLs demonstrate substrate specificity for cefotaxime more than ceftazidime

Functional group 2br represents β-lactamases resistant to inhibitors (especially clavulanate, with

Table 1. Classification of β-lactamases (From R. P. Ambler and K. Bush[a])

Classification			Preferential inactivation of							Inhibited by	
Structural (Ambler)	Functional (Bush)	Enzyme	Penicillin	Carboxypenicillin	Oxacillin	C1G[b]	C3G	Aztreonam	Imipenem	Clavulanate	EDTA
Enzymes with active serine											
A	2a	Narrow spectrum penicillinases	+++[c]		-	+/-	-	-	-	+++	-
	2b	Broad spectrum penicillinases	+++	++	+	++	-	-	-	+++	-
	2be	Extended-spectrum β-lactamases	+++	++	+	++	++	++	-	+++	-
	2br	Inhibitor-resistant TEM	+++	++	+	+/-	-	-	-	-	-
	2c	Carbenicillinases	++	+++	+	+	-	-	-	+	-
	2e	Cefuroximases	++	++	-	++	+	-	-	+++	-
	2f	Carbapenemases	++	+	?	+++	+	+	++	+	-
C	1	Cephalosporinases	++	+	-	V[d]	V	-	-	-	-
D	2d	Oxacillinases	++	+	+++	++	V	-	-	V	-
Zinc metalloenzymes											
B	3	Carbapenemases	++	++	++	++	++	-	++	-	++

[a] From references 1, 6, 14.
[b] C1G, first generation cephalosporin; C2G, second generation cephalosporin.
[c] The enzymatic efficiency of β-lactamases and the activity of inhibitors are indicated semi-quantitatively by + et − signs.
[d] V, variable.

$IC_{50}s > 1$ μM), most group 2br β-lactamases are derived by point mutations in TEM-1 and TEM-2 penicillinases. These enzymes, known as Inhibitor Resistant TEMs (IRTs), have lower hydrolytic activity towards cephalosporins than TEM-1 or TEM-2 enzymes. There is also an increasing number of inhibitor resistant SHV β-lactamases being reported (five reported e.g., SHV-10, SHV-49, SHV-52, SHV-56 (35), SHV-92; the kinetic characterization of SHV-52 and SHV-92 awaits further study) (13, 14).

Functional group 2c represents carbenicillinases or CARB (or ESP) enzymes. They are characterized by a high activity against carboxypenicillins (ticarcillin).

Group 2e represents enzymes often referred to as cefuroximases. They are inhibited by clavulanate and have a high hydrolytic activity against aminopenicillins, first and second generation cephalosporins, with the exception of cephamycins (these are inducible chromosomal enzymes).

Group 2f includes carbapenemases from molecular class A. They are inhibited at low level by clavulanate. They inactivate penicillins, cephalosporins, aztreonam and carbapenems.

Class B enzymes or functional group 3 comprises carbapenemases resistant to inhibition by clavulanate but inhibited by EDTA. They have a broad substrate profile including penicillins, cephalosporins, carbapenems, but not aztreonam. There are three B subgroups (B1, B2, and B3). Some class B β-lactamases are plasmid encoded (bla_{IMP} and bla_{VIM}) that are sometimes found in enterobacteria and non-fermentors (P. aeruginosa and Acinetobacter baumannii).

Class C enzymes are AmpC cephalosporinases which form a heterogeneous group corresponding to Bush functional group 1. These enzymes are resistant to β-lactamase inhibitors. They hydrolyze aminopenicillins, C1G and, depending on the enzyme, C2G including cephamycins. AmpC enzymes also hydrolyze carboxypenicillins, ureidopenicillins and C3G to a lesser extent. Hyperproduction of these β-lactamases can efficiently inactivate these substrates. Generally, they do not confer resistance to carbapenems or C4G (cefepime and cefpirome), although rare mutant AmpC enzymes can inactivate C3G and C4G.

Class D enzymes comprise oxacillinases (OXA) corresponding to Bush functional group 2d. They inactive oxazolylpenicillins such as oxacillin more than benzylpenicillin. Most of these enzymes belong to group 2br due to their resistance to clavulanate and their spectrum of activity. However, oxacillinases can confer a reduction, albeit slight, in susceptibility to C4G, thus distinguishing them from IRT. The spectrum of some oxacillinases extends to C2G, C3G and C4G (ESBL from molecular class D), but such enzymes have not yet been described in enterobacteria. Others, like OXA-23 or OXA-48 have low carbapenemase activity.

RESISTANCE PHENOTYPES IN ENTEROBACTERIA

Intrinsic or "wild-type" resistance phenotype

Enterobacteria intrinsically produce various β-lactamases, allowing their classification into seven resistance phenotype groups (Table 2).

Group 0: "Susceptible" phenotype of species lacking β-lactamase genes

Salmonella spp. and *P. mirabilis* lack β-lactamase (*bla*) genes in their "wild-type" state and are intrinsically susceptible to aminopenicillins, carboxypenicillins, ureidopenicillins, aztreonam, cephalosporins and carbapenems. Inhibition zone diameters of imipenem are often smaller for the species *P. mirabilis*, as for other species from the phylum *Proteae*. This decrease is thought to be due to the low affinity of imipenem for the PBP 2 of these species. However, this reduced imipenem susceptibility is usually not clinically significant.

Group 1: "Susceptible" phenotype of species intrinsically producing a class C cephalosporinase

Like the previous species, *E. coli* and *Shigella* spp. are intrinsically susceptible to aminopenicillins, carboxypenicillins, ureidopenicillins, aztreonam, cephalosporins and carbapenems. However, they produce very low levels of a non-inducible chromosomal AmpC-type cephalosporinase (Bush-Jacoby group 1) which, in some strains, may lead to reduced susceptibility to aminopenicillins, aminopenicillin/clavulanate and/or C1G.

Group 2: "Low-level penicillinase" phenotype

Klebsiella pneumoniae, *Klebsiella oxytoca*, *Citrobacter koseri*, *Citrobacter amalonaticus* and *Escherichia hermannii* are intrinsic, constitutive (not induced by β-lactams, except in *C. amalonaticus*) producers of chromosomal class A enzymes susceptible to inhibitors:
- SHV-1 (functional group 2b) or LEN-1 (group 2a) for *K. pneumoniae*,
- OXY enzymes (group 2be) for *K. oxytoca*,
- CKO enzymes for *C. koseri*,
- CdiA enzyme (group 2b) for *C. amalonaticus*,
- HER-1 enzyme (group 2b) for *E. hermannii*.

These enzymes confer resistance to aminopenicillins and carboxypenicillins but often imperceptible resistance to ureidopenicillins. This so-called "low-level penicillinase" resistance phenotype is characterized by the persistence of an inhibition zone around aminopenicillin disks (contrary to the

Table 2. "Wild-type" β-lactam resistance phenotypes of enterobacteria

Antibiotic[a]	Phenotype group						
	0	1	2	3	4	5	6
Aminopenicillins	S	S/I	R	R	R	R	R/I [a]→I
Aminopenicillins/CLA[b]	S	S/I	S	R	R	S	S/I
Carboxypenicillins	S	S	R	S	R	S	R/I →I
Carboxypenicillins/CLA	S	S	S	S	S	S	S
Ureidopenicillins	S	S	S→I	S	S→I	S	I/S→I
Ureidopenicillins/TAZ[b]	S	S	S	S	S	S	S
Cephalosporin 1st generation	S	S/I	S	R	R	R	R/I
Cephalosporin 2nd generation	S	S	S	R/I/S[c]	S[d]	R	R/I/I→I
Cefoxitin	S	S	S	R/I/S[c]	S	S	S
Cephalosporin 3rd generation	S	S	S	S	S	S	S→I[e]/I
Cephalosporin 4th generation	S	S	S	S	S	S	S→I[e]/I
Carbapenems	S	S	S	S	S	S	S

[a] →, proposed interpretation.
[b] CLA, clavulanate; TAZ, tazobactam.
[c] Result depends on species and isolate.
[d] S→I or I for *S. fonticola*.
[e] If synergy test is positive for at least one third or fourth generation cephalosporin or aztreonam.

"high-level penicillinase or acquired penicillinase" phenotype characterized by an absence of inhibition zone around the disk). Penicillin/β-lactamase inhibitor combinations are active.

Interpretive criteria. Resistance to penicillins, and especially to ureidopenicillins, can be low-level. All "susceptible" results for these drugs should be reported as "intermediate" in species belonging to group 2 (5, 9, 10) according to CLSI and EUCAST.

Group 3: "Low-level cephalosporinase" phenotype

Enterobacteria in this group include producers of chromosomal class C cephalosporinase (AmpC, functional group 1) inducible by β-lactams (strong inducers include cefoxitin, imipenem, clavulanate). These cephalosporinases are quite widespread in clinical isolates of enterobacteria: *Enterobacter cloacae, Enterobacter aerogenes, Serratia marcescens* (and other species in this genus), *Citrobacter freundii, Morganella morganii, Hafnia alvei, Providencia stuartii, Providencia rettgeri,* and *Pantoea agglomerans.*

The "wild-type" phenotype of these species, often called "low-level cephalosporinase", comprises resistance to aminopenicillins, aminopenicillin/β-lactamase inhibitor combinations, and C1G. Their behavior towards C2G and cephamycins differentiates them into three subgroups: (i) species usually susceptible to cefuroxime (C2G) and cefoxitin (a cephamycin): *H. alvei, P. rettgeri, P. stuartii* and *P. agglomerans*; (ii) species more resistant to cefoxitin than to cefuroxime: *E. cloacae, E. aerogenes* and *C. freundii*; and (iii) species more resistant to cefuroxime than to cefoxitin: *S. marcescens* and *M. morganii*. The prevalence of the "wild-type" phenotype varies according to the species and the epidemiological situation at the particular place and time. Nonetheless the wild-type phenotype is more frequent in *H. alvei, P. rettgerii, Providencia* spp., and *M. morganii* than in *C. freundii, E. cloacae,* and *E. aerogenes*. The species *Proteus vulgaris* and *Proteus penneri* originally belonged to this group, but on the basis of phenotypic and molecular data it is now more suitable to include them in a new group 5, corresponding to the "cefuroximase" phenotype.

Group 4: Yersinia enterocolitica and Serratia fonticola

Y. enterocolitica and *S. fonticola* are intrinsic producers of an inducible class C cephalosporinase (functional group 1) and a class A enzyme. In *Y. enterocolitica,* the enzyme is a constitutive class A penicillinase produced at a low level (functional group 2b). In *S. fonticola,* the class A enzyme is an inducible β-lactamase from class 2be (SFO-1 and derivatives).

Y. enterocolitica is resistant to aminopenicillins, aminopenicillin/clavulanate, carboxypenicillins, and C1G. Ureidopenicillin resistance is usually not observed *in vitro.* *S. fonticola* has a similar resistance phenotype. However, cefuroxime is inactive and resistance to aminopenicillin/β-lactamase inhibitor, which should normally be induced by AmpC, is expressed very little or not at all *in vitro.*

Group 5: "Cefuroximase" phenotype

P. vulgaris and *P. penneri* intrinsically produce a class A cephalosporinase inducible by β-lactams and usually referred to as cefuroximase (functional group 2e). This phenotype is characterized by resistance to aminopenicillins, C1G and C2G (cefuroxime, cefamandole) with the exception of cephamycins (cefoxitin), and susceptibility to penicillin/β-lactamase inhibitor.

Group 6: "Extended-spectrum chromosomal β-lactamase" phenotype

The enterobacteria *Kluyvera ascorbata, Kluyvera cryocrescens, Kluyvera georgiana, Rahnella aquatilis, Citrobacter sedlakii* and *Erwinia persicina* intrinsically produce extended-spectrum β-lactamases from class A (group 2be). Often expressed at a low level, these ESBLs confer reduced susceptibility or resistance to aminopenicillins, carboxypenicillins, C1G and C2G except cephamycins. Resistance to ureidopenicillins or C3G is often not apparent. Interpretive criteria have not yet been proposed for these species. The activity of the enzymes suggests that "susceptible" results can be interpreted as "intermediate" for penicillins and also for C3G if the synergy test is positive (see below: "Extended-spectrum β-lactamase" phenotype).

Acquired resistance or "resistant" phenotypes

In addition to intrinsic β-lactam resistance, bacteria may express one or more mechanisms of acquired resistance. Acquired resistance due to β-lactamase production is the predominant mechanism in enterobacteria, although it is possible that the frequency of other types of resistance, often expressed at a low level, is underestimated.

"High-level penicillinase" or "Acquired penicillinase" phenotype

Phenotype (Table 3)

The "high-level penicillinase" phenotype is variably expressed according to the nature of the gene promoter, the gene copy number, number of bacterial β-lactamases present, and the bacterial species. Expression is usually low in *P. mirabilis*, *P. vulgaris*, *M. morganii*, and *Providencia*. The resistance phenotype therefore takes different forms which range between two extremes:

A low penicillinase activity responsible for minimal resistance to aminopenicillins (inhibition zone generally absent, as opposed to what is observed in the case of intrinsic resistance in group 2 species) and to carboxypenicillins. There is little or no effect on susceptibility to ureidopenicillins and C1G.

A high penicillinase activity conferring resistance to aminopenicillins, aminopenicillin/inhibitor combinations, carboxypenicillins, ureidopenicillins, and C1G (Fig. 1a). Reduced susceptibility is frequently observed for ticarcillin/clavulanate, and piperacillin/tazobactam. Resistance may extend to C2G, primarily in *Klebsiella* spp., *Enterobacter* spp., and *C. freundii*.

Interpretive criteria

Considering the enzymes underlying this phenotype, it is recommended that "susceptible" results are reported as "intermediate" for all penicillins if penicillinase production is suspected (5, 9, 10). The causative β-lactamases are plasmid-mediated class A broad spectrum penicillinases (functional group 2b): primarily TEM-1, and more rarely TEM-2 or SHV-1.

"Inhibitor-resistant penicillinase" phenotype

Phenotype (Table 4)

The "inhibitor-resistant penicillinase" phenotype was first described in 1991 in *E. coli*. Like the high-level penicillinase phenotype, this phenotype is characterized by resistance to aminopenicillins, carboxypenicillins and, to a lesser extent, ureidopenicillins. However "inhibitor-resistant penicillinases differ by its resistance to aminopenicillin or carboxypenicillin/β-lactamase inhibitor combinations, while C1G usually remain active (Fig. 1).

Interpretive criteria

When expression is low as in the case of some *P. mirabilis* strains, the ureidopenicillins may appear effective. In light of the activity of the enzymes underlying this phenotype, doubt persists

Table 3. "Acquired penicillinase" resistance phenotype of enterobacteria

Antibiotic	"Acquired penicillinase" phenotype from group:		
	0 and 1	2	3 and 5
Aminopenicillins	R	R	R
Aminopenicillins + clavulanate	S/I/R	S/I/R	R[a]
Carboxypenicillins	R (S → R/I)[b]	R	R
Carboxypenicillins + clavulanate	S/I (R)	S/I (R)	S/I (R)
Ureidopenicillins	S → I/I/R	I/R	I/R
Ureidopenicillins + tazobactam	S/I	S/I	S/I
Cephaloporin 1st generation	S/I/R	S/I/R	R
Cephaloporin 2nd generation	S	S (I)	S/I/R[c]
Cefoxitin	S	S	S/I/R[c]
Cephaloporin 3rd generation	S	S	S
Cephaloporin 4th generation	S	S	S
Carbapenems	S	S	S

[a] S/I/R for the species *P. vulgaris* and *P. penneri*.
[b] →, proposed interpretation; ( ), rarely observed data.
[c] Result depends on species and isolate.

Table 4. "Inhibitor resistant penicillinase" resistance phenotype of enterobacteria

Antibiotic	"Inhibitor resistant penicillinase" phenotype from group		
	0 and 1	2	3 and 5
Aminopenicillins	R	R	R
Aminopenicillins + clavulanate	R	R	R
Carboxypenicillins	R	R	R
Carboxypenicillins + clavulanate	R	R	R
Ureidopenicillins	S → I/I/R[a]	I/R	I/R
Ureidopenicillins + tazobactam	S → I/I (R)	S → I/I (R)	S → I/I (R)
Cephaloporin 1st generation	S	S	R
Cephaloporin 2nd generation	S	S	S/I/R[b]
Cefoxitin	S	S	S/I/R[b]
Cephaloporin 3rd generation	S	S	S
Cephaloporin 4th generation	S	S	S
Carbapenems	S	S	S

[a] →, proposed interpretation; ( ), rarely observed data.
[b] Result depends on species and isolate.

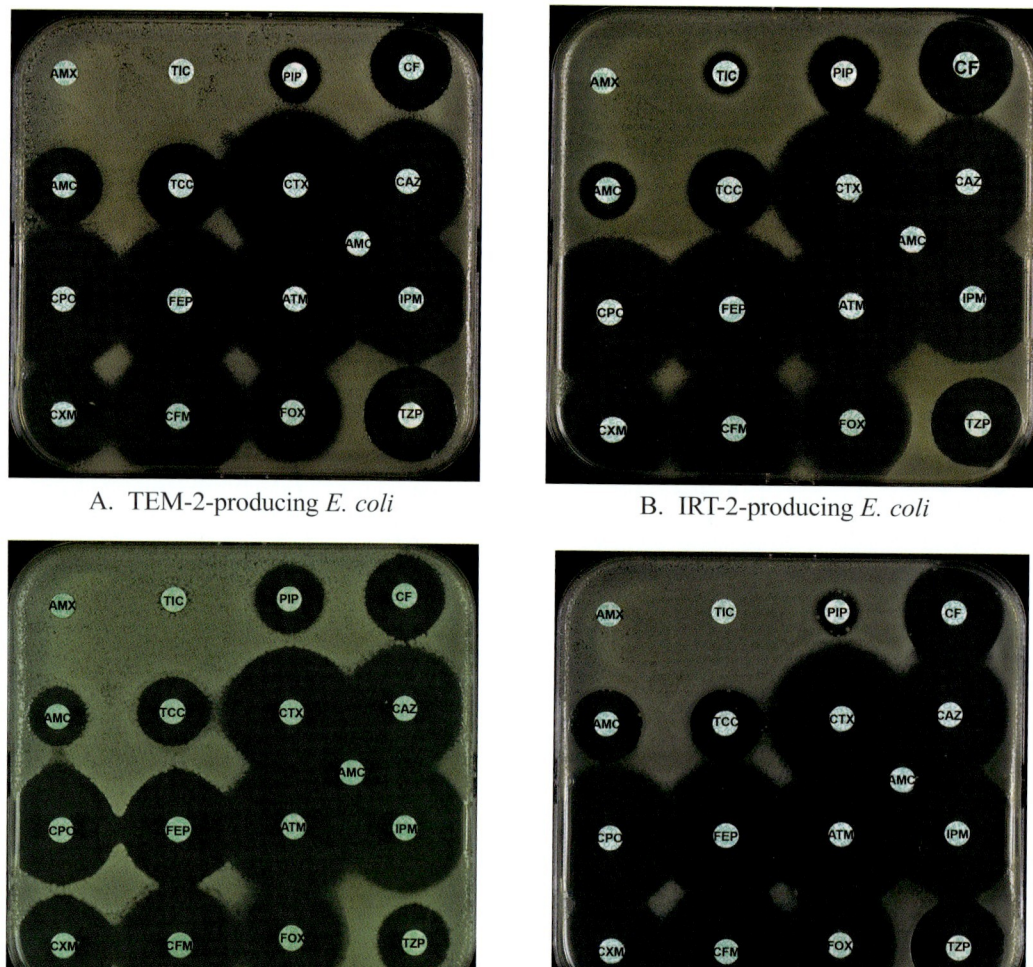

A. TEM-2-producing *E. coli* B. IRT-2-producing *E. coli*

C. OXA-1-producing *E. coli* D. CARB-2-producing *E. coli*

Fig. 1. Antibiograms of penicillinase-producing *E. coli*. AMC, amoxicillin clavulanate; AMX, amoxicillin; CAZ, ceftazidime, CF, cephalothin; CFM, cefixime; CPO, cefpirome; CTX, cefotaxime; CXM, cefuroxime; FEP, cefepime; FOX, cefoxitin; IPM, imipenem; PIP, piperacillin; TCC, ticarcillin clavulanate; TIC, ticarcillin; TZP, piperacillin tazobactam.

as to the true efficacy of these agents. Furthermore, time-kill experiments using penicillin/β-lactamase inhibitors sometimes show bacteriostasis (i.e are bacteriostatic) or a slight decrease in the bacterial population, followed by bacterial growth after 6-24 h of incubation. Therefore a prudent practice is to report "susceptible" results as "intermediate" for penicillins and penicillin/β-lactamase inhibitors.

The causative enzymes are usually (about 90% of the time) IRT (Inhibitor Resistant TEM), functional group 2br (Fig. 1b). The *bla* genes for these enzymes are harbored on non-conjugative plasmids. Strains which produce these enzymes are generally unrelated, suggesting the spontaneous emergence of mutant enzymes under selective pressure from penicillin/β-lactamase inhibitors. Mutations observed in IRT enzymes have been found in SHV-type enzyme and the *K. oxytoca* chromosomal enzyme IRKO, with the same effects on enzymatic activity and resistance phenotype (see above).

The oxacillinases (OXA, functional group 2d) and CARB enzymes (functional group 2c) confer a resistance phenotype similar to that associated with the IRT enzymes. Oxacillinases are the second largest group of inhibitor-resistant enzymes in enterobacteria (9%), after the IRTs (90%). They are distinguishable from the latter by their moderate activity on C4G (Fig. 1c) in some cases leading to an "intermediate" phenotype. CARB-2 is common in amoxicillin-resistant strains of *S.* Typhimurium (Fig. 1d). This resistance has spread considerably in recent years, to the point that 52% of strains in France in 1998 were not susceptible to amoxicillin/clavulanate (31). This increase is thought to be due to the clonal propagation of *S.* Typhimurium lysotype DT104.

"Extended"-spectrum β-lactamase" phenotype

Phenotype (Table 5)

The "extended-spectrum β-lactamase" phenotype is characterized by resistance to penicillins and cephalosporins with the exception of cephamycins (Fig. 2 and 3). Resistance to C3G, C4G and aztreonam is variable according to the enzyme and the strain (MICs range from < 1 to 128 µg/ml). As a rule, this resistance is evident for at least one of these agents, except when expression is very low as sometimes seen in *P. mirabilis* (Fig. 4). Most ESBLs are more susceptible to β-lactamase inhibitors than the broad spectrum penicillinases TEM-1 and SHV-1. Some ESBLs, including CMT enzymes (Complex Mutant TEM), nonetheless show reduced susceptibilities to inhibitors

Table 5. "Extended-spectrum β-lactamase" resistance phenotype of enterobacteria

Antibiotic	"Extended-spectrum β-lactamase" phenotype from group		
	0 and 1	2	3 and 5
Aminopenicillins	R	R	R
Aminopenicillins + clavulanate	S/I/R	S/I/R	R[a]
Carboxypenicillins	R	R	R
Carboxypenicillins + clavulanate	S/I/R	S/I/R	S/I/R
Ureidopenicillins	R	R	R
Ureidopenicillins + tazobactam	S/I (R)	S/I (R)	S/I (R)
Cephaloporin 1st generation	R	R	R
Cephaloporin 2nd generation	R	R	R
Cefoxitin	S	S	S/I/R[b]
Cephaloporin 3rd generation	R[c]/I/S → I[d]	Rc/I/S → I	Rc/I/S → I
Cephaloporin 4th generation	R/I/S → I	R/I/S → I	R/I/S → I
Carbapenems	S	S	S

[a] S/I/R for the species *P. vulgaris* and *P. penneri*.
[b] Result depends on species and isolate.
[c] At least one third generation cephalosporin is not susceptible except some species from the phylum *Proteae*, particularly *P. mirabilis*.
[d] →, proposed interpretation; ( ), rarely observed data.

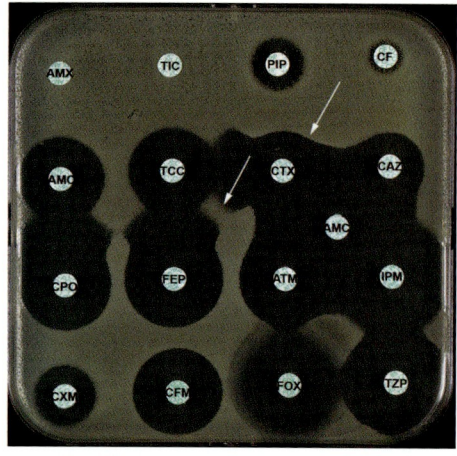
A. TEM-3-producing *E. coli*

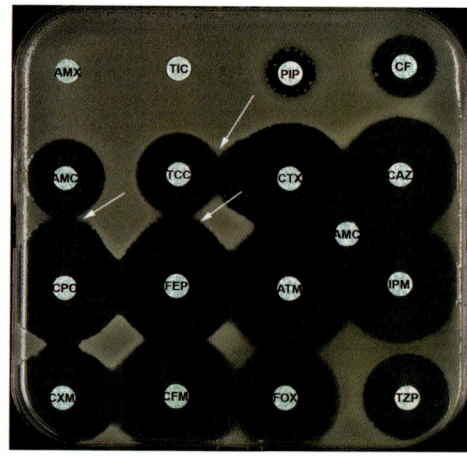
B. SHV-2-producing *E. coli*

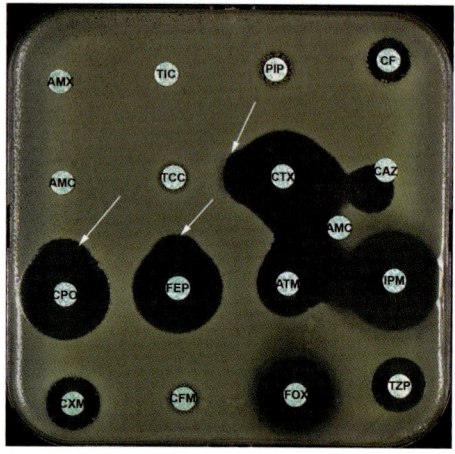
C. TEM-24-producing *E. coli*

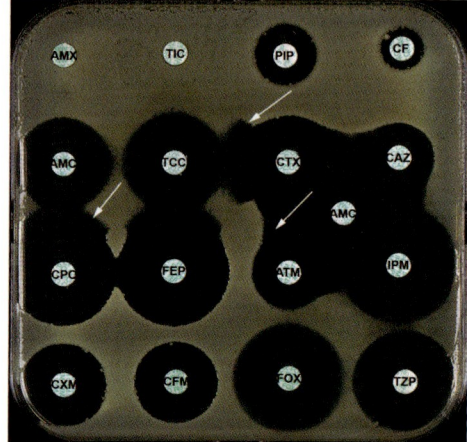
D. SHV-12-producing *E. coli*

Fig. 2. Antibiograms of ESBL-producing *E. coli*. The arrows indicate synergy pictures between clavulanate-containing disks and C3G or C4G-containing diks. AMC, amoxicillin clavulanate; AMX, amoxicillin; CAZ, ceftazidime, CF, cephalothin; CFM, cefixime; CPO, cefpirome; CTX, cefotaxime; CXM, cefuroxime; FEP, cefepime; FOX, cefoxitin; IPM, imipenem; PIP, piperacillin; TCC, ticarcillin clavulanate; TIC, ticarcillin; TZP, piperacillin tazobactam.

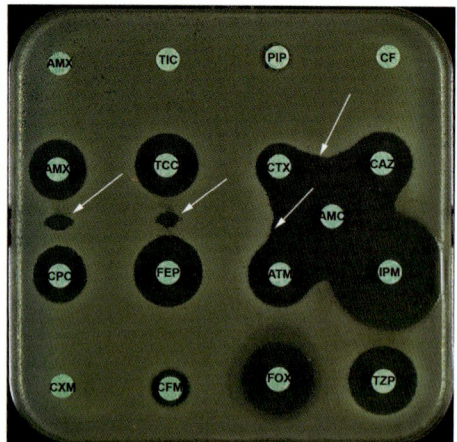
A. CTX-M-9-producing *E. coli*

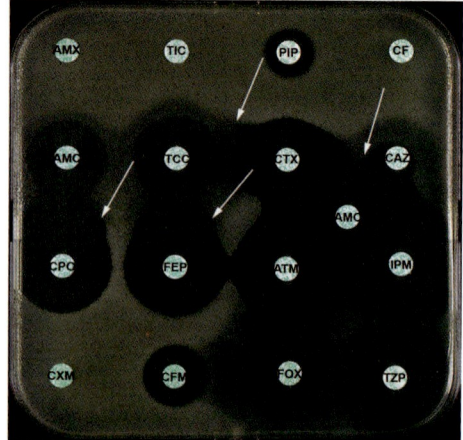
B. CTX-M-19-producing *E. coli*

Fig. 3. Antibiograms of *E. coli* producing the usual ESBL CTX-M-9 (A) or the point mutant Pro167Ser CTX-M-19 (B). The arrows indicate synergy pictures between clavulanate-containing disks and C3G or C4G-containing diks. AMC, amoxicillin clavulanate; AMX, amoxicillin; CAZ, ceftazidime, CF, cephalothin; CFM, cefixime; CPO, cefpirome; CTX, cefotaxime; CXM, cefuroxime; FEP, cefepime; FOX, cefoxitin; IPM, imipenem; PIP, piperacillin; TCC, ticarcillin clavulanate; TIC, ticarcillin; TZP, piperacillin tazobactam.

(Fig. 5). Penicillin/β-lactamase inhibitors are therefore not always effective, because efficacy depends on the type and level of production of the enzyme. However, susceptibility to β-lactamase inhibitors is generally sufficient to form the basis for the detection of this phenotype, which is characterized by a synergy between the β-lactamase inhibitor and the C3G and/or C4G and/or aztreonam.

Carbapenems and cephamycins are usually not substrates of ESBLs. However, reduced susceptibility to these agents was recently reported in *E. coli* and *K. pneumoniae* isolates in Europe and Japan. These strains produced enzymes with low carbapenemase activity derived from GES-type ESBL by single amino acid susbtitutions (see class A carbapenemase).

Interpretive criteria

In spite of some low MICs for C3G, ESBLs are the cause of numerous treatment failures. With the exception of combinations with β-lactamase inhibitors, cephamycins and carbapenems, β-lactams should be reported as "intermediate" rather than "susceptible" if the synergy test (see below) is positive (5, 9, 10).

Enterobacteria such as *S. fonticola*, *K. ascorbata*, *K. cryocrescens*, *E. persicina*, *R. aquatilis*, *C. sedlakii*, group 2 *Citrobacter*, *P. vulgaris*, and *P. penneri* intrinsically produce ESBLs. These ESBLs, often expressed at a low level, can either go undetected, or else give a positive synergy test.

In this case, it is desirable to apply the interpretive criteria previously indicated for acquired ESBL.

Epidemiology

ESBLs (functional group 2be) were initially described in western European hospitals in the mid-1980s (33). These enzymes had considerable success in intensive care wards where C3G were widely used. ESBLs are now observed worldwide, in hospitals and the community, although there are notable differences in temporal and geographical prevalence. The prevalence of ESBL is identical in France (1-3%) and Germany (1-5%) but higher in Italy (9-15%), Great Britain (7-22%) and Eastern Europe (Russia, Poland and Turkey: 39-47%) (17).

During the 1990s, ESBLs were described mainly as members of the TEM- and SHV-beta-lactamase families in *Klebsiella pneumoniae* causing nosocomial outbreaks. These first ESBLs derived from the penicillinases TEM-1, TEM-2 and SHV-1 by point mutations (4). These β-lactamases are generally encoded by conjugative plasmids, which facilitate their dissemination. The type of substitution determines the spectrum of activity of the β-lactamase and allows their separation into two main groups (Fig. 2): ceftazidimases which confer higher-level resistance to ceftazidime than to cefotaxime (eg., TEM-5, TEM-24, SHV-4, SHV-5), and cefotaximases which confer an equivalent level of resistance to both drugs (*e.g.*, TEM-3, SHV-2).

More recently, new ESBLs not derived from the TEM or SHV lineage have been described,

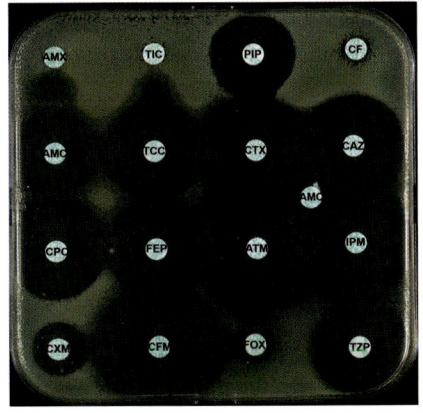
A.

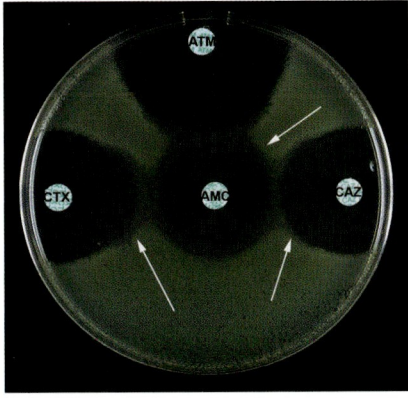
B.

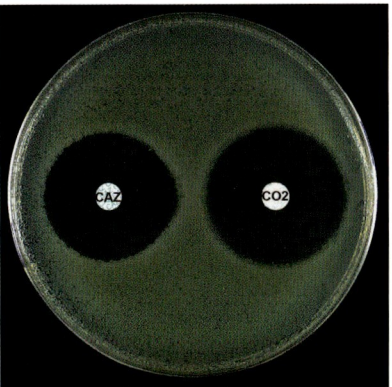
C.

Fig. 4. ESBL difficult to detect because of low expression : TEM-3-producing *P. mirabilis*.
A, Antibiogram with double disk synergy test using inter-disk distance of 2 and 3cm. B, Double disk synergy test using inter-disk distance of 4 cm. C, Synergy test using the combined disk method. The arrows indicate synergy pictures between clavulanate-containing disks and C3G or C4G-containing diks. AMC, amoxicillin clavulanate; AMX, amoxicillin; CAZ, ceftazidime, CF, cephalothin; CFM, cefixime; CO2, ceftazidime clavulanate; CPO, cefpirome; CTX, cefotaxime; CXM, cefuroxime; FEP, cefepime; FOX, cefoxitin; IPM, imipenem; PIP, piperacillin; TCC, ticarcillin clavulanate; TIC, piperacillin; TZP, ticarcillin tazobactam.

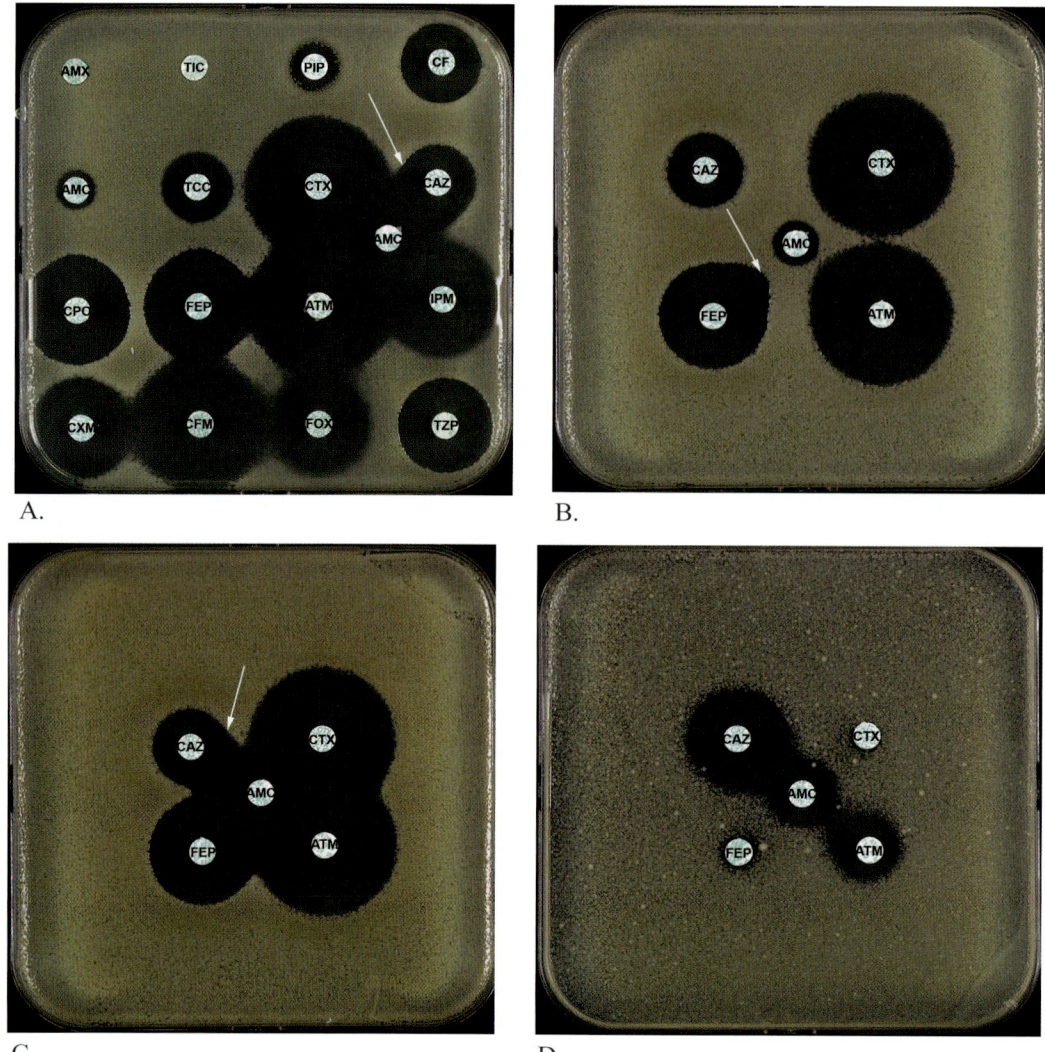

Fig. 5. ESBL difficult to detect. CMT-producing *E. coli* : A, Synergy test with the double-disk synergy test using an inter-disk distance of 2 and 3 cm; B and C, Synergy test with the double-disk synergy test using an inter-disk distance of 3 cm. D, CTX-M-producing *E. coli*, which overproduce AmpC-type enzyme : negative synergy test using the double-disk method with an inter-disk distance of 3 cm. The arrows indicate synergy pictures between clavulanate-containing disks and C3G or C4G-containing diks. AMC, amoxicillin clavulanate; AMX, amoxicillin; CAZ, ceftazidime, CF, cephalothin; CFM, cefixime; CO2, ceftazidime clavulanate; CPO, cefpirome; CTX, cefotaxime; CXM, cefuroxime; FEP, cefepime; FOX, cefoxitin; IPM, imipenem; PIP, piperacillin; TCC, ticarcillin clavulanate; TIC, ticarcillin; TZP, piperacillin tazobactam.

including CTX-M-type cefotaximases and PER, GES (or IBC), BES, and VEB-type ceftazidimases, to mention only the most common (4). PER-type enzymes have been observed mainly in Turkey (PER-1) and South America (PER-2), VEB-1 in Asia and GES-type enzymes in Europe and South America (BES-1 is found in Brazil). Nowadays, the ESBLs are mostly found in *E. coli* that cause community-acquired infections and with increasing frequency contain CTX-M enzymes (3, 7, 22). These are now considered the most prevalent ESBLs worldwide. They have been detected in all clinically relevant enterobacteria, including species such as *Salmonella* spp. and *Shigella spp.*. The origins of CTX-M genes have been elucidated. These are chromosomal genes naturally present in the species *K. ascorbata*, *K. gorgiana* and *K. cryocrescens*, where they are expressed at a very low level (as evidenced by the reduced susceptibility to cefuroxime and very slight synergy between clavulanate and cefotaxime). These CTX-M-type ESBLs confer higher resistance to cefotaxime than to ceftazidime. However, they are evolving through amino acid substitutions towards a greater activity against ceftazidime (Fig. 3).

"HyperOXY" phenotype

Phenotype

K. oxytoca are highly resistant to all penicillins, C1G and C2G with the exception of cephamycins, and show high or low level resistance to aztreonam. The synergy test with clavulanate is positive with aztreonam, variable with cefotaxime, and infrequently positive with C4G and ceftazidime. The level of resistance, which is always higher for aztreonam than for C3G and C4G, distinguishes the "hyperoxy" phenotype from the "ESBL" phenotype.

Epidemiology

This phenotype results from the intrinsic hyperproduction of chromosomal β-lactamase (OXY ESBL group 2be) by *K. oxytoxa* as a consequence of mutations in the promoter region of the gene encoding the enzyme. This phenotype is found in approximately 10% of hospital isolates.

Interpretive criteria

According to the CA-SFM (10), interpretation of the antibiogram should take into account the synergy test for each C3G and C4G. For C3G and C4G which appear active, the strain should be flagged as "intermediate" if the synergy test is positive for that agent.

"High-level cephalosporinase" phenotype

Phenotype (Table 6)

The "high-level cephalosporinase" phenotype is characterized by more or less marked resistance to penicillins, C1G, C2G, and at least one C3G or aztreonam. The synergy test is negative between C3G, C4G or aztreonam and β-lactamase inhibitors (Fig. 6). Cephamycins are inactive except in the species *H. alvei*, and C4G are usually active. C3G resistance can be partially or totally restored in the presence of cloxacillin 100 μg/ml.

Epidemiology

The prevalence of the "high-level cephalosporinase" phenotype has been gradually increasing since 1980. In Europe, the "high-level cephalosporinase" phenotype accounts for 5-40% of enterobacteria isolated in hospital (17). This phenotype is most common in the species *E. cloacae*, *E. aerogenes*, *S. marcescens*, *C. freundii* and *E. coli*.

In group 3 species which produce an inducible chromosomal AmpC (*Enterobacter* spp., *S. marcescens*, *C. freundii*, *Providencia* spp.), this phenotype is generally determined by constitutive hyperproduction of AmpC (functional group 1) due to mutations in the genes that regulate the synthesis of this enzyme. A very small number of *E.*

Table 6. "Hyperproduced cephalosporinase" resistance phenotype of enterobacteria

Antibiotic	"Extended-spectrum β-lactamase" phenotype from group		
	0 and 1	2	3 and 5
Aminopenicillins	R	R	R
Aminopenicillins + clavulanate	R	R	R
Carboxypenicillins	R (I)	R (I)	R (I)
Carboxypenicillins + clavulanate	R (I)	R (I)	R (I)
Ureidopenicillins	R (I)	R (I)	R (I)
Ureidopenicillins + tazobactam	R/I (S → I)[a]	R/I (S → I)	R/I (S → I)
Cephaloporin 1st generation	R	R	R
Cephaloporin 2nd generation	R/I (S → I)	R/I (S → I)	R/I (S → I)
Cefoxitin	R/I (S[b])	R/I (Sb)	R/I (S[b])
Cephaloporin 3rd generation	R[c]/I/S → I	Rc/I/S → I	Rc/I/S → I
Cephaloporin 4th generation	S (I/R)	S	S (I/R[d])
Carbapenems	S	S	S[e]

a →, proposed interpretation; ( ), rarely observed data.
b Intrinsic or acquired cephalosporinase hyperproduction in *H. alvei*.
c At least one third generation cephalosporin is not "susceptible".
d Mutant cephalosporinase capable of hydrolyzing fourth generation cephalosporins.
e I or R if there is also resistance due to impermeability.

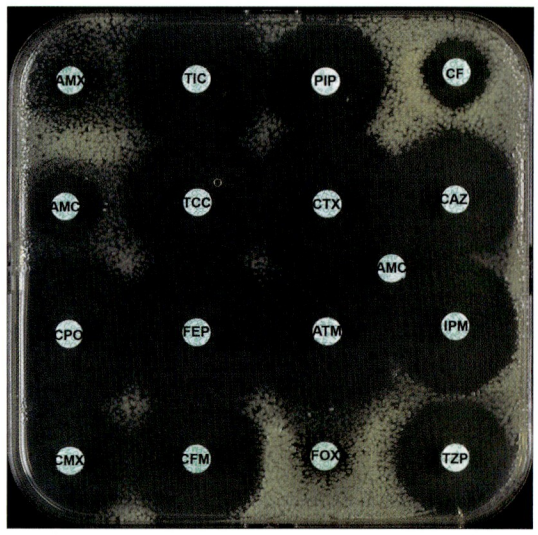
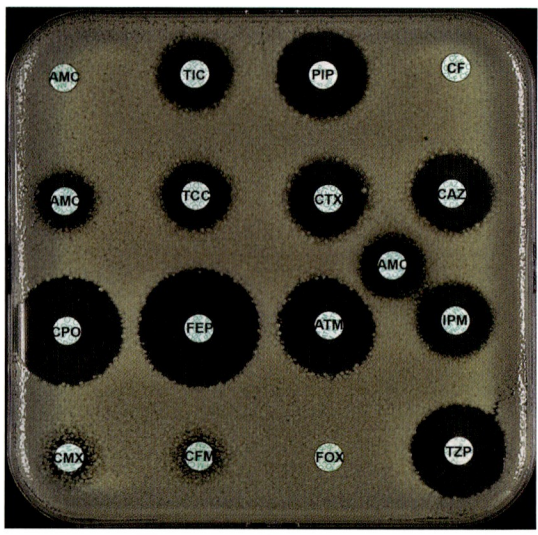

A. B.

Fig. 6. Antibiograms of wild-type *E. aerogenes* (A) and imipenem-resistant *E. aerogenes* (B) because of AmpC overproduction and impermability. AMC, amoxicillin clavulanate; AMX, amoxicillin; CAZ, ceftazidime, CF, cephalothin; CFM, cefixime; CPO, cefpirome; CTX, cefotaxime; CXM, cefuroxime; FEP, cefepime; FOX, cefoxitin; IPM, imipenem; PIP, piperacillin; TCC, ticarcillin clavulanate; TIC, ticarcillin; TZP, piperacillin tazobactam.

cloacae, *C. freundii* and *S. marcescens* strains produce AmpC mutants with increased activity towards C3G and C4G (37).

In *E. coli*, the "cephalosporinase" resistance phenotype is manifested in different ways ranging from the "low-level cephalosporinase" to the "high-level cephalosporinase" phenotype. β-lactamase production is not inducible; mutations in the promoter or attenuator region and/or gene duplications. AmpC mutants can have an increased activity towards C3G and C4G.

Lastly, the "high-level cephalosporinase" phenotype can result from acquisition of a plasmid-encoded bla_{ampC} gene (eg., CMY, FOX, MOX, ACT, DHA, etc.) (34). Mobilized by transposition, the *ampC* genes migrated from the chromosome of intrinsic AmpC-producing species on plasmids, usually conjugative, which then spread among the enterobacteria including *E. coli*, *K. pneumoniae*, *K. oxytoca*, *P. mirabilis* and *Salmonella* spp. These plasmid-borne enzymes are distributed throughout the world. In the United States, about 7% of C3G-resistant *E. coli*, *K. pneumoniae* and *K. oxytoca* strains isolated between 1992 and 2000 produced this type of plasmid-encoded β-lactamase (45% produced ESBLs).

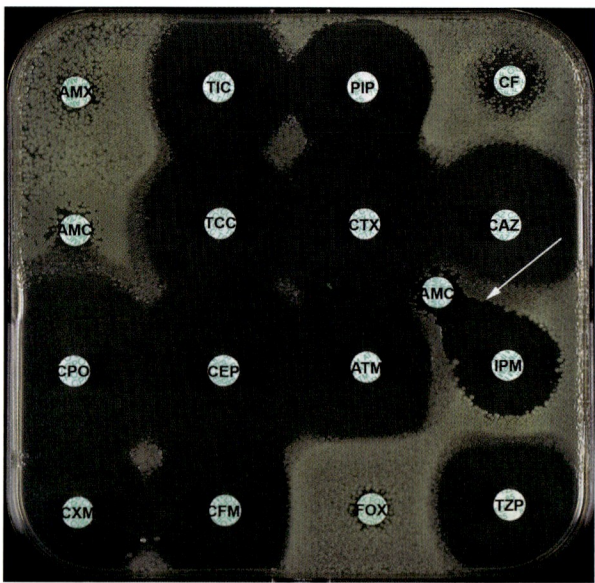

Fig. 7. NMC-A-producing *E. aerogenes*. The arrow indicate a synergy picture between clavulanate-containing disks and imipenem-containing diks. AMC, amoxicillin clavulanate; AMX, amoxicillin; CAZ, ceftazidime, CF, cephalothin; CFM, cefixime; CPO, cefpirome; CTX, cefotaxime; CXM, cefuroxime; FEP, cefepime; FOX, cefoxitin; IPM, imipenem; PIP, piperacillin; TCC, ticarcillin clavulanate; TIC, ticarcillin; TZP, piperacillin tazobactam.

Interpretive criteria

If an enterobacterial strain is resistant to at least one C3G and the synergy test is negative, β-lactams should not be reported as "susceptible", except C4G such as cefepime (5, 9, 10).

Carbapenem resistance

Overall, worldwide susceptibility to carbapenems is 98% among the *Enterobacteriaceae* (18, 48, 49). Rare strains of *E. cloacae*, *S. marcescens* and *S. fonticola* produce chromosomal class A carbapenemases inducible by β-lactams (the enzymes NMC-A, SME, IMI and SFC-1 in functional group 2f; Fig. 7) (30). These strains have reduced susceptibility or are resistant to penicillins, C1G, C2G, aztreonam and imipenem (MIC: 1 to ≥ 32 μg/ml). They are susceptible to C3G and C4G (Table 7).

Class A carbapenemases of the KPC ("*Klebsiella pneumoniae c*arbapenemase") and GES ("*Guyana Extended-Spectrum*") type (functional group 2f) are most worrisome because they are carried on plasmids which have allowed them to spread to numerous species. The discovery of KPC-2 in North Carolina in 1996 was quickly followed by several reports of this β-lactamase along the east coast of the United States (26, 41, 54). After this rapid expansion in the United States, KPC enzymes have been reported worldwide from Europe, South America, Middle East and Asia (36). They can confer resistance to all β-lactams, including cephamycins, C3G, C4G and carbapenems (Table 7) and the susceptibility to inhibitors is weak. The disks for the synergy test between clavulanate and imipenem disks should be placed close together (2 cm) or a combined disk method should be used.

GES-type ESBL harboring the substitution G170S have a weak carbapenemase activity (51). These enzymes have low susceptibility to inhibitors and imipenem resistance was expressed at a borderline detection level (MIC of imipenem, 8 μg/ml).

Plasmidic class B carbapenemases (VIM and IMP-type enzymes of the functional group 3) have been initially characterized in enterobacteria isolated in Japan and then worldwide. These enzymes hydrolyze all β-lactams with the exception of aztreonam (Table 7). The MICs of imipenem may be low (1 to > 16 μg/ml). Resistance is more constant for ceftazidime. These enzymes are resistant to β-lactamase inhibitors but can be inhibited by EDTA, thus producing a synergy image between imipenem or ceftazidime and EDTA disks.

As stated above, hyperproduction of cephalosporinase associated with membrane impermeability (altered porins) is a frequent cause of carbapenem resistance in enterobacteria. This combined resistance phenotype has been mainly observed in chromosomal cephalosporinase-producing strains of *E. aerogenes*, *E. cloacae* and *C. freundii* (Fig. 6b). Membrane impermeability in combination with the production of plasmid-mediated enzymes such as AmpC, OXA-type carbapenemase, and CTX-M- and SHV-type ESBLs can also confer resistance to carbapenems in *E. coli* and *K. pneumoniae* (25). Ertapenem can be

Table 7. Imipenem resistance phenotypes of enterobacteria due to carbapenemase production

Antibiotic	Carbapenemase		
	Class A		Class B
	Chromosome *S. marcescens*	Plasmid *E. coli*	Plasmid *E. coli*
Aminopenicillins	R	R	R
Aminopenicillins/clavunate	R	S/I/R	R
Carboxypenicillins	I/R (S → I)[a]	R (I)	R
Carboxypenicillins/clavunate	I/R (S → I)	S/I/R	R
Ureidopenicillins	I/S → I	R (I)	R/I (S → I)
Ureidopenicillins/tazobactam	S	S/I/R	R/I (S → I)
Cephalosporin 1st generation	R	R	R
Cephalosporin 2nd generation	R	R/I	R/I
Cefoxitin	I/R	R/I	R/I
Cephalosporin 3rd generation	S	R/I	R/I
Aztreonam	S	R/I	S
Cephalosporin 4th generation	S	R/I	R/I
Carbapenems	I/R (S → I)	I/R (S → I)	I/R (S → I)

[a] →, proposed interpretation; ( ), rarely observed data.

affected, whereas the MIC values of the other carbapenems are in the susceptibility range.

Other resistance phenotypes

The reduced susceptibility to cephamycins, C1G, C2G and, to a lesser extent, C3G observed in some strains of *E. coli*, *C. koseri*, *K. pneumoniae* and *P. mirabilis* is related to a porin deficiency which also leads to reduced susceptibility or resistance to quinolones, chloramphenicol, tetracyclines and trimethoprim. In *E. aerogenes*, alterations of porins can also cause resistance to C3G and C4G and reduced susceptibility to imipenem (45).

β-lactams to be studied

The choice of agents to be tested depends on the epidemiological situation, therapeutic practices, and the type of specimen. The CLSI documents provide recommendations (9). The CA-SFM recommends two standard test panels to meet the needs of hospitals (H) and community practice.

Standard antibiogram: amoxicillin or ampicillin, amoxicillin/clavulanate or ampicillin/sulbactam, mecillinam, cephalothin, cefixime, cefotaxime (H) or ceftriaxone (H).

Expanded antibiogram: amoxicillin or ampicillin, amoxicillin/clavulanate or ampicillin/sulbactam, ticarcillin (H), ticarcillin/clavulanate (H), piperacillin (H) or mezlocillin (H), piperacillin/tazobactam (H), mecillinam, cephalothin, cefuroxime (H) and/or cefamandole, cefixime or cefpodoxime/proxetil, cefoxitin (H) and/or cefotetan, (latamoxef, not commercialized), ceftazidime (H), cefotaxime (H) or ceftriaxone or ceftizoxime (H), cefepime (H) or cefpirome (H), aztreonam (H), imipenem (H).

Phenotypic detection of resistance

Fig. 8 is an algorithm for inferring the mechanisms of β-lactam resistance in enterobacteria. It is based on an analysis of the resistance phenotype and tests for the detection of ESBLs and carbapenemases. Confirmation of the type of resistance mechanism requires molecular analyses which go beyond the scope of the antibiogram.

Detection of ESBLs

In most cases ESBLs and overproduction of cephalosporinases confer resistance to one or several oxyiminocephalosporins. However, several ESBL producers have MIC values for extended-spectrum cephalosporins and aztreonam below the standard breakpoints for resistance (*e.g.*, between 1 and 8 µg/ml). Moreover, ESBLs and cephalosporinases behave differently with respect to C4G. For these reasons, it is essential to use specific tests by which to detect and distinguish the different enzymes. At the present time this distinction is based essentially on the detection of ESBL. Numerous strategies have been developed to detect ESBLs.

CLSI and BSAC recommend a two step strategy based on screening and confirmatory tests (5, 9). *E. coli*, *K. pneumoniae* and *K. oxytoca* strains with MIC ≥ 8 µg/ml for cefpodoxime or MICs ≥ 2 µg/ml against ceftazidime, cefotaxime, ceftriaxone, or aztreonam should be investigated using specific phenotypic confirmatory tests for ESBL production. For *P. mirabilis* isolates, confirmatory tests should be performed if strains demonstrate MICs ≥ 2 µg/ml for ceftazidime, cefotaxime or cefpodoxime. For the disk diffusion method, *E. coli*, *K. pneumoniae*, *K. oxytoca* and *P. mirabilis* with a zone inhibition diameter lower than the following values (cefpodoxime: ≤ 17 mm, ceftazidime: ≤ 22 mm, cefotaxime and aztreonam: ≤ 27 mm and ceftriaxone ≤ 25 mm) should be investigated with confirmatory tests. In the case of cefpodoxime, the critical inhibition diameter is ≤ 22 mm for *P. mirabilis*. BSAC suggests that all *Enterobacteriaceae* resistant to ceftazidime (MIC ≥ 4 µg/ml or zone inhibition ≤ 21 mm for *E. coli* and *Klebiella* spp. and ≤ 27 mm for the remaining species), cefotaxime (MIC ≥ 2 µg/ml or zone inhibition ≤ 29 mm), or cefpodoxime (MIC ≥ 2 µg/ml or zone inhibition ≤ 19 mm) should be evaluated by the ESBL confirmatory tests.

ESBL confirmatory testing based upon phenotype requires the use of both ceftazidime and cefotaxime alone and in combination with clavulanate. Typically, these disks contain 30 µg /disk of ceftazidime, cefotaxime with or without clavulanate (10 µg/disk). These discs are reported to have sensitivity and specificity of greater than 95% (8, 53). Screening and confirmatory tests for other *Enterobacteriaceae*, including those producing inducible AmpC chromosomal enzymes (*e.g.*, *Enterobacter* spp., *M. morganii*, *Providencia* spp., *Citrobacter freundii*, and *Serratia marcescens*), have not yet been established by the CLSI. ESBLs are more difficult to detect in these organisms because AmpC enzymes may be induced by clavulanate (which inhibits them poorly) and may increase resistance to cephalosporins, overcoming the synergy arising from inhibition of the ESBL (33). The BSAC advises the use of

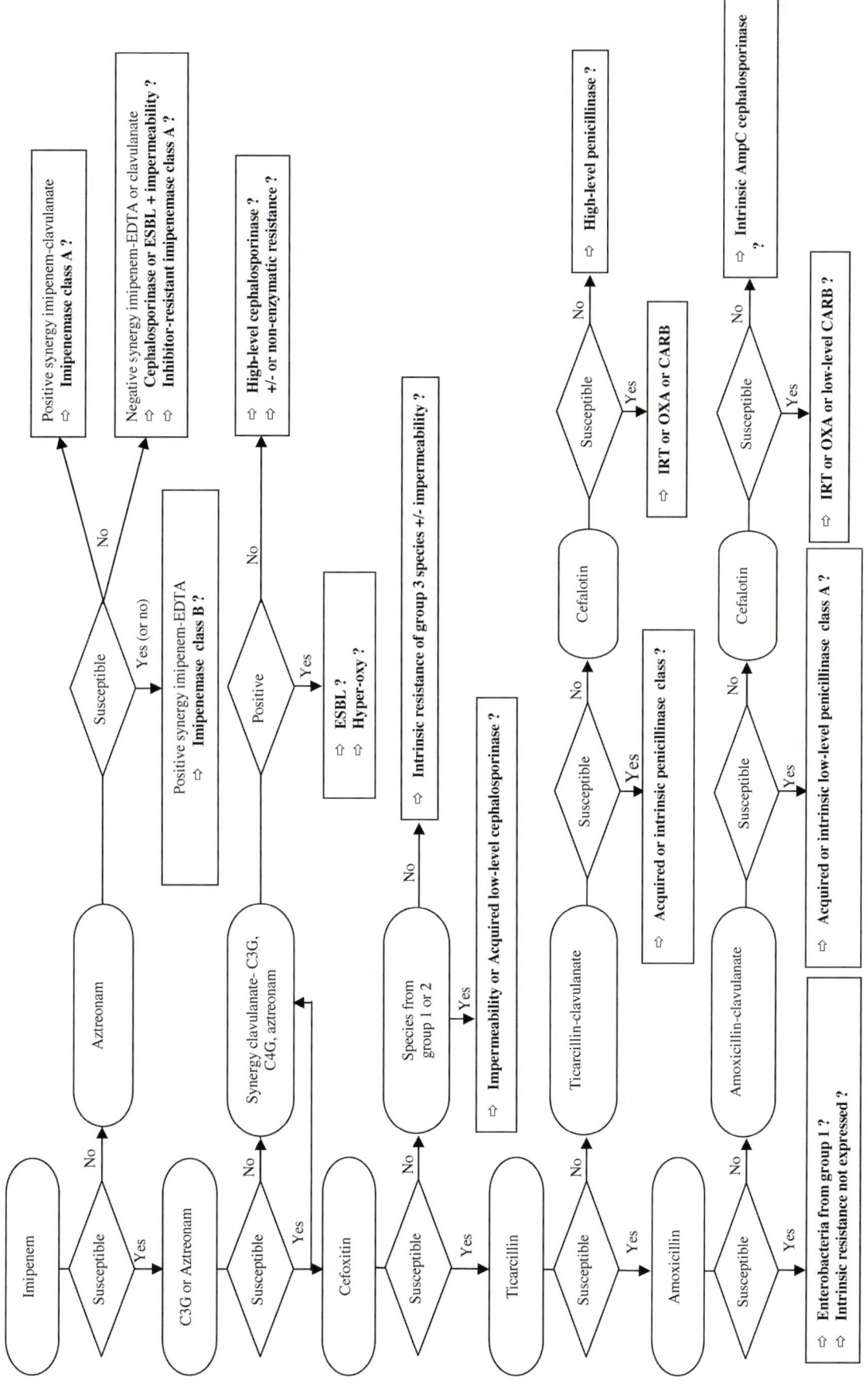

Fig. 8. Decision algorithm for inferring β-lactam resistance mechanisms in enterobacteria.

cefpirome/clavulanate combination disks (in addition to cefpodoxime/clavulanate) for *Enterobacter spp.* and *C. freundii* as a confirmatory test.

The E-test® method for ESBL detection determines MICs to extended-spectrum cephalosporins and their combinations to clavulanate (4 µg/ml). This method is suggested by the BSAC as a confirmatory test for ESBL production. ESBL production is inferred if the MIC ratio for cephalosporin alone/cephalosporin plus clavulanate MIC is ≥ 8. BASC recommends the cefepime/clavulanate E-test® for *Enterobacter spp.*. The cefepime/clavulanate strip is the only commercially available and highly reliable test that permits accurate detection of ESBLs within this group of organisms (44). The three available Etest strips and four disks combination (including ceftazidime, cefotaxime, cefpodoxime and cefpirome) showed sensitivity of 94% and 93%, and specificity of 85% and 81%, respectively (33).

The CA-SFM (10) proposes direct detection of ESBLs in all enterobacterial species. The method is based on the demonstration of synergy between cefotaxime, ceftazidime, cefepime or aztreonam disks and a clavulanate disk (Fig. 2 and 3). A center-to-center distance of 3 cm is usually recommended. If the enzyme has diminished sensitivity to inhibitors or if the ESBL is accompanied by hyperproduction of a class C cephalosporinase, the detection can be improved by separating the disk centers by 2 cm (50). In the case of a hyperproduced cephalosporinase, cefepime or cefpirome (which are poorly hydrolyzed by these enzymes) can also increase the sensitivity of detection and should therefore be used. If doubt persists, the synergy test and the complete antibiogram should be carried out in the presence of cloxacillin (50-300 *µ*g/ml) to inhibit the class C enzyme, particularly for group 3 enterobacteria. When ESBL production is low, as is often the case for the TEM-3 enzyme of *P. mirabilis* (Fig. 4), a center-to-center distance of 4 cm is more appropriate. As TEM-type ESBL are often associated with production of an AAC(6')-I enzyme, resistance to tobramycin, netilmicin and amikacin warrants a correspondingly modified synergy test, especially in species from the phylum Proteae. The double-disk test with ceftazidime, cefotaxime, cefpodoxime, and cefpirome showed the highest specificity and positive predictive value among all test methods (*i.e.*, 97% and 98%, respectively) (53). However, in routine practice the method is time-consuming and technically demanding.

Automated systems use different strategies to differentiate ESBL from hyperproduced cephalosporinases, based on comparing the resistance phenotype of the test strain with reference phenotypes and/or using specific tests based on the differences in sensitivity of cephalosporinases and ESBL to β-lactamase inhibitors. On the whole, automated systems give comparable performances and the percentage of correctly identified phenotypes averages ≥ 90% (23, 40), highlighting the usefulness of these technologies. However, this percentage varies according to the protocol and especially the strains used. It can be as high as 98-100% of strains for species like *E. coli* and *K. pneumoniae* (21, 23, 40) versus < 80-90% for cephalosporinase hyperproducers such as species from the genus *Enterobacter* (39, 43, 50).

Detection of carbapenemases

Carbapenemases do not always cause a sufficient increase in MICs to classify the strain as "resistant" or even "intermediate". Therefore, one should be watchful for any decrease in the susceptibility of enterobacteria to carbapenems (especially ertapenem). The ability of automated systems to detect these enzymes has been evaluated little or not at all. Consequently, expert systems can be imprecise (16).

Enterobacteria can produce two types of carbapenemases: class A carbapenemases susceptible to β-lactamase inhibitors, and class B carbapenemases inhibited by divalent cation chelators like EDTA, mercaptopropionic acid or percaptoacetic acid (2, 19). These properties can be exploited in synergy tests. Yet, few studies have been carried out to date, especially on the class A carbapenemases.

Production of a class A carbapenemase can be suspected if there is synergy image between a 10 µg clavulanate disk and a 10 µg imipenem disk (Fig. 7). Production of a class B carbapenemase can be suspected if a synergy image is observed between a 750 µg EDTA disk and a 10 µg imipenem or 30 µg ceftazidime disk. Addition of mercaptoacetic acid sodium to an EDTA disk improves sensitivity. In the absence of standardization, at least two inter-disk distances should be used: center-to-center distance between 1 and 2.5 cm. The combined disk method or MIC determination in the presence and absence of an inhibitor should help overcome the problem of distance. An E-test® is also available for specific detection of class B enzymes as imipenem/imipenem-EDTA and ceftazidime/ceftazidime-EDTA combinations. A positive test for a metallo-β-lactamase is interpreted as a threefold-or-greater MIC decrease in the presence of EDTA. This test strip produced a sensitivity of 94% and a specificity of 95% (52). However, false-negative results have been reported for the Etest when an isolate had an imipenem MIC of ≤ 4 µg/ml. It has also been observed that EDTA alone has inhibitory action against some bacteria due to permeabilization of the outer membrane and can lead to false positive results.

The true prevalence of KPC-producing *Enterobacteriaceae* may be under-appreciated due to difficulties with detection by the clinical laboratories. KPC β-lactamase production can be missed when laboratoires rely soley on automated methods as the MICs against the carbapenems may not be high enough to flag as resistant or intermediate. Some clinical laboratories use the modified Hodge test to detect KPC production. The modified Hodge test, a phenotypic test, has demonstrated high sensitivity detecting carbapenemase activity *in vitro*. In the Hodge test, a lawn of susceptibe *E. coli* (ATCC strain 25922) a carbapenem disks and a streak of the suspected KPC producer are placed upon an agar plate (Fig. 9).

In addition, limited data suggest that a novel chromogenic agar may help in early identification of KPC-producing strains with a sensitivity and specificity of 100% and 98.4% when compared with PCR. The CHROMagar KPC medium was compared to MacConkey agar with carbapenem disks and PCR for *bla*KPC gene for rapid detection of carbapenem Resistant *K. pneumoniae*. The sensitivity and specificity relative to PCR were 100 % and 98.4% for CHROMagar KPC and 92.7 % and 95.9% for MacConkey (38). In practical terms, the strains turn «red» with *E. coli* producing a carbapenemase is detected and «metallic blue» when *K. pneumoniae* produces a carbapenemase.

Boronic acid disks have also been used to detect KPC producers (12, 32, 46). In this assay, the boronic acid disks (*e.g.*, 3 aminophenylboronic acid) and has a senstitivity and specificity of 100%. As a clinically useful test boronic acid disks promise to accurately differentiate KPC-possessing *K. pneumoniae* isolates. In the assays reported by Tsakris *et al*. phenylboronic acid is used at a concentration of 20 µg/ml. From this solution, 20 µl (containing 400 µg of boronic acid) was dispensed onto commercially available antibiotic disks (47). A similar concentration is used by Doi *et al*. These assays can be performed more readily than others and can add to the current need to detect KPCs.

REFERENCES

(1) **Ambler, R. P.** 1980. The structure of beta-lactamases. Philos. Trans. R. Soc. Lond. B. Biol. Sci. **289**:321-331.

(2) **Arakawa, Y., N. Shibata, K. Shibayama, H. Kurokawa, T. Yagi, H. Fujiwara, and M. Goto.** 2000. Convenient test for screening metallo-beta-lactamase-producing gram-negative bacteria by using thiol compounds. J. Clin. Microbiol. **38**:40-43.

(3) **Bonnet, R.** 2004. Growing group of extended-spectrum beta-lactamases: the CTX-M enzymes. Antimicrob. Agents Chemother. **48**:1-14.

(4) **Bradford, P. A.** 2001. Extended-spectrum beta-lactamases in the 21st century: characterization, epidemiology, and detection of this important resistance threat. Clin. Microbiol. Rev. **14**:933-951.

(5) **Bristish Society of Antimicrobial Chemotherapy.** 1991. A guide to sensitivity testing. J. Antimicrob. Chemother. **27**(suppl.D):1-50.

(6) **Bush, K., G. A. Jacoby, and A. A. Medeiros.** 1995. A functional classification scheme for beta-lactamases and its correlation with molecular structure. Antimicrob. Agents Chemother. **39**:1211-1233.

(7) **Canton, R., and T. M. Coque.** 2006. The CTX-M beta-lactamase pandemic. Curr. Opin. Microbiol. **9**:466-475.

(8) **Carter, M. W., K. J. Oakton, M. Warner, and D. M. Livermore.** 2000. Detection of extended-spectrum beta-lactamases in Klebsiellae with the Oxoid combination disk method. J. Clin. Microbiol. **38**:4228-4232.

(9) **Clinical and Laboratory Standard Institute.** 2007. Performance standards for antimicrobial susceptibility testing: seventeenth informational supplement; M100-S17.

(10) **Comité de l'Antibiogramme de la Société Française de Microbiologie.** Communiqué 2009. http://www.sfm.asso.fr

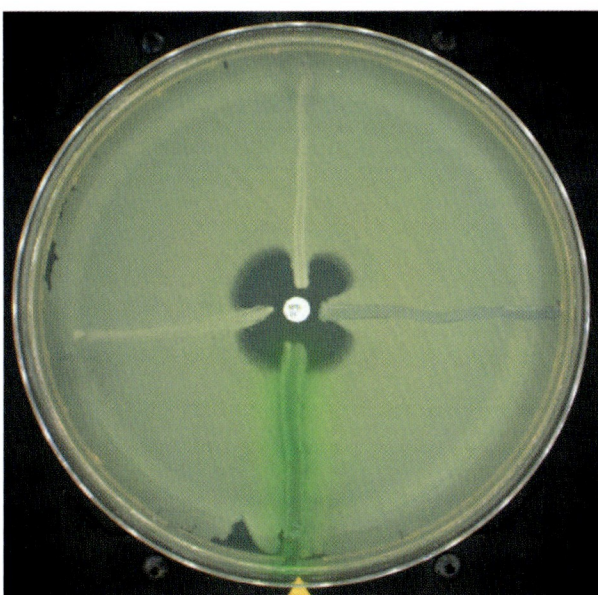

Fig. 9. Hodge test impregnated with to detect the presence of a carbapenemase in intact cells. The disk can be imipenem, ertapenem, or meropenem. Occasionally false positive tests can occur as a result of minor carbapenem hydrolysis by CTX-M or AmpC enzymes.

(11) **Delihas, N., and S. Forst.** 2001. *MicF*: an antisense RNA gene involved in response of *Escherichia coli* to global stress factors. J. Mol. Biol. **313**:1-12.

(12) **Doi, Y., B. A. Potoski, J. M. Adams-Haduch, H. E. Sidjabat, A. W. Pasculle, and D. L. Paterson.** 2008. Simple disk-based method for detection of *Klebsiella pneumoniae* carbapenemase-type beta-lactamase by use of a boronic acid compound. J. Clin. Microbiol. **46**:4083-4086.

(13) **Dubois, V., L. Poirel, C. Arpin, L. Coulange, C. Bebear, P. Nordmann, and C. Quentin.** 2004. SHV-49, a novel inhibitor-resistant beta-lactamase in a clinical isolate of *Klebsiella pneumoniae*. Antimicrob. Agents Chemother. **48**:4466-4469.

(14) **Dubois, V., L. Poirel, F. Demarthe, C. Arpin, L. Coulange, L. A. Minarini, M. C. Bezian, P. Nordmann, and C. Quentin.** 2008. Molecular and biochemical characterization of SHV-56, a novel inhibitor-resistant beta-lactamase from *Klebsiella pneumoniae*. Antimicrob. Agents Chemother. **52**:3792-3794.

(15) **European Committee on Antimicrobial Susceptibility Testing.** 2000. Determination of antimicrobial susceptibility test breakpoints. Clin. Microbiol. Infect. **6**:570-572.

(16) **Giakkoupi, P., L. S. Tzouvelekis, G. L. Daikos, V. Miriagou, G. Petrikkos, N. J. Legakis, and A. C. Vatopoulos.** 2005. Discrepancies and interpretation problems in susceptibility testing of VIM-1-producing *Klebsiella pneumoniae* isolates. J. Clin. Microbiol. **43**:494-496.

(17) **Goossens, H.** 2001. MYSTIC program: summary of European data from 1997 to 2000. Diagn. Microbiol. Infect. Dis. **41**:183-189.

(18) **Kiffer, C. R., C. Mendes, J. L. Kuti, and D. P. Nicolau.** 2004. Pharmacodynamic comparisons of antimicrobials against nosocomial isolates of *Escherichia coli*, *Klebsiella pneumoniae*, *Acinetobacter baumannii* and *Pseudomonas aeruginosa* from the MYSTIC surveillance program: the OPTAMA Program, South America 2002. Diagn. Microbiol. Infect. Dis. **49**:109-116.

(19) **Lee, K., Y. Chong, H. B. Shin, Y. A. Kim, D. Yong, and J. H. Yum.** 2001. Modified Hodge and EDTA-disk synergy tests to screen metallo-beta-lactamase-producing strains of *Pseudomonas* and *Acinetobacter* species. Clin. Microbiol. Infect. **7**:88-91.

(20) **Li, X. Z., and H. Nikaido.** 2009. Efflux-mediated drug resistance in bacteria: an update. Drugs **69**:1555-1623.

(21) **Linscott, A. J., and W. J. Brown.** 2005. Evaluation of four commercially available extended-spectrum beta-lactamase phenotypic confirmation tests. J. Clin. Microbiol. **43**:1081-1085.

(22) **Livermore, D. M., R. Canton, M. Gniadkowski, P. Nordmann, G. M. Rossolini, G. Arlet, J. Ayala, T. M. Coque, I. Kern-Zdanowicz, F. Luzzaro, L. Poirel, and N. Woodford.** 2007. CTX-M: changing the face of ESBLs in Europe. J. Antimicrob. Chemother. **59**:165-174.

(23) **Livermore, D. M., M. Struelens, J. Amorim, F. Baquero, J. Bille, R. Canton, S. Henning, S. Gatermann, A. Marchese, H. Mittermayer, C. Nonhoff, K. J. Oakton, F. Praplan, H. Ramos, G. C. Schito, J. Van Eldere, J. Verhaegen, J. Verhoef, and M. R. Visser.** 2002. Multicentre evaluation of the VITEK 2 Advanced Expert System for interpretive reading of antimicrobial resistance tests. J. Antimicrob. Chemother. **49**:289-300.

(24) **Maneewannakul, K., and S. B. Levy.** 1996. Identification for *mar* mutants among quinolone-resistant clinical isolates of *Escherichia coli*. Antimicrob. Agents Chemother. **40**:1695-8.

(25) **Martinez-Martinez, L.** 2008. Extended-spectrum beta-lactamases and the permeability barrier. Clin. Microbiol. Infect. **14**:82-89.

(26) **Miriagou, V., L. S. Tzouvelekis, S. Rossiter, E. Tzelepi, F. J. Angulo, and J. M. Whichard.** 2003. Imipenem resistance in a *Salmonella* clinical strain due to plasmid-mediated class A carbapenemase KPC-2. Antimicrob. Agents Chemother. **47**:1297-1300.

(27) **Neuwirth, C., E. Siebor, J. M. Duez, A. Pechinot, and A. Kazmierczak.** 1995. Imipenem resistance in clinical isolates of *Proteus mirabilis* associated with alterations in penicillin-binding proteins. J. Antimicrob. Chemother. **36**:335-342.

(28) **Nikaido, H.** 2000. Crossing the envelope: how cephalosporins reach their targets. Clin. Microbiol. Infect. **6 Suppl 3**:22-26.

(29) **Nikaido, H.** 1994. Prevention of drug access to bacterial targets: permeability barriers and active efflux. Science **264**:382-388.

(30) **Nordmann, P., and L. Poirel.** 2002. Emerging carbapenemases in Gram-negative aerobes. Clin. Microbiol. Infect. **8**:321-331.

(31) **ONERBA.** 2005. Base de donnees interactives des reseaux. http://www.onerba.org/bin/res/.

(32) **Pasteran, F. G., L. Otaegui, L. Guerriero, G. Radice, R. Maggiora, M. Rapoport, D. Faccone, A. Di Martino, and M. Galas.** 2008. *Klebsiella pneumoniae* Carbapenemase-2, Buenos Aires, Argentina. Emerg. Infect. Dis. **14**:1178-1180.

(33) **Perez, F., A. Endimiani, K. M. Hujer, and R. A. Bonomo.** 2007. The continuing challenge of ESBLs. Curr. Opin. Pharmacol. **7**:459-469.

(34) **Philippon, A., G. Arlet, and G. A. Jacoby.** 2002. Plasmid-determined AmpC-type beta-lactamases. Antimicrob. Agents Chemother. **46**:1-11.

(35) **Prinarakis, E. E., V. Miriagou, E. Tzelepi, M. Gazouli, and L. S. Tzouvelekis.** 1997. Emergence of an inhibitor-resistant beta-lactamase (SHV-10) derived from an SHV-5 variant. Antimicrob. Agents Chemother. **41**:838-840.

(36) **Queenan, A. M., and K. Bush.** 2007. Carbapenemases: the versatile beta-lactamases. Clin. Microbiol. Rev. **20**:440-458.

(37) **Raimondi, A., F. Sisto, and H. Nikaido.** 2001. Mutation in *Serratia marcescens* AmpC beta-lactamase producing high-level resistance to ceftazidime and cefpirome. Antimicrob. Agents Chemother. **45**:2331-2339.

(38) **Samra, Z., J. Bahar, L. Madar-Shapiro, N. Aziz, S. Israel, and J. Bishara.** 2008. Evaluation of CHROMagar KPC for rapid detection of carbapenem-resistant *Enterobacteriaceae*. J. Clin. Microbiol. **46**:3110-3111.

(39) **Sanders, C. C., M. Peyret, E. S. Moland, C. Shubert, K. S. Thomson, J. M. Boeufgras, and W. E. Sanders, Jr.** 2000. Ability of the VITEK 2 advanced expert system To identify beta-lactam phenotypes in isolates of

Enterobacteriaceae and *Pseudomonas aeruginosa*. J. Clin. Microbiol. **38**:570-574.

(40) **Sanguinetti, M., B. Posteraro, T. Spanu, D. Ciccaglione, L. Romano, B. Fiori, G. Nicoletti, S. Zanetti, and G. Fadda.** 2003. Characterization of clinical isolates of *Enterobacteriaceae* from Italy by the BD Phoenix extended-spectrum beta-lactamase detection method. J. Clin. Microbiol. **41**:1463-1468.

(41) **Smith Moland, E., N. D. Hanson, V. L. Herrera, J. A. Black, T. J. Lockhart, A. Hossain, J. A. Johnson, R. V. Goering, and K. S. Thomson.** 2003. Plasmid-mediated, carbapenem-hydrolysing beta-lactamase, KPC-2, in *Klebsiella pneumoniae* isolates. J. Antimicrob. Chemother. **51**:711-714.

(42) **Spratt, B. G.** 1975. Distinct penicillin binding proteins involved in the division, elongation, and shape of *Escherichia coli* K12. Proc. Natl. Acad. Sci. U.S.A. **72**:2999-3003.

(43) **Sturenburg, E., M. Lang, M. A. Horstkotte, R. Laufs, and D. Mack.** 2004. Evaluation of the MicroScan ESBL plus confirmation panel for detection of extended-spectrum beta-lactamases in clinical isolates of oxyimino-cephalosporin-resistant Gram-negative bacteria. J. Antimicrob. Chemother. **54**:870-875.

(44) **Sturenburg, E., I. Sobottka, D. Noor, R. Laufs, and D. Mack.** 2004. Evaluation of a new cefepime-clavulanate ESBL Etest to detect extended-spectrum beta-lactamases in an *Enterobacteriaceae* strain collection. J. Antimicrob. Chemother. **54**:134-138.

(45) **Thiolas, A., C. Bornet, A. Davin-Regli, J. M. Pages, and C. Bollet.** 2004. Resistance to imipenem, cefepime, and cefpirome associated with mutation in Omp36 osmoporin of *Enterobacter aerogenes*. Biochem. Biophys. Res. Commun. **317**:851-855.

(46) **Tsakris, A., I. Kristo, A. Poulou, F. Markou, A. Ikonomidis, and S. Pournaras.** 2008. First occurrence of KPC-2-possessing *Klebsiella pneumoniae* in a Greek hospital and recommendation for detection with boronic acid disc tests. J. Antimicrob. Chemother. **62**:1257-60.

(47) **Tsakris, A., I. Kristo, A. Poulou, K. Themeli-Digalaki, A. Ikonomidis, D. Petropoulou, S. Pournaras, and D. Sofianou.** 2009. Evaluation of boronic acid disk tests for differentiating KPC-possessing *Klebsiella pneumoniae* isolates in the clinical laboratory. J. Clin. Microbiol. **47**:362-367.

(48) **Turner, P. J.** 2004. Susceptibility of meropenem and comparators tested against 30,634 *Enterobacteriaceae* isolated in the MYSTIC Programme (1997-2003). Diagn. Microbiol. Infect. Dis. **50**:291-293.

(49) **Turner, P. J.** 2005. Trends in antimicrobial susceptibilities among bacterial pathogens isolated from patients hospitalized in European medical centers: 6-year report of the MYSTIC Surveillance Study (1997-2002). Diagn. Microbiol. Infect. Dis. **51**:281-289.

(50) **Tzelepi, E., P. Giakkoupi, D. Sofianou, V. Loukova, A. Kemeroglou, and A. Tsakris.** 2000. Detection of extended-spectrum beta-lactamases in clinical isolates of *Enterobacter cloacae* and *Enterobacter aerogenes*. J. Clin. Microbiol. **38**:542-546.

(51) **Wachino, J., Y. Doi, K. Yamane, N. Shibata, T. Yagi, T. Kubota, and Y. Arakawa.** 2004. Molecular characterization of a cephamycin-hydrolyzing and inhibitor-resistant class A β-lactamase, GES-4, possessing a single G170S substitution in the V-loop. Antimicrob Agents Chemother **48**:2905-10.

(52) **Walsh, T. R., A. Bolmstrom, A. Qwarnstrom, and A. Gales.** 2002. Evaluation of a new Etest for detecting metallo-β-lactamases in routine clinical testing. J Clin Microbiol **40**:2755-9.

(53) **Wiegand, I., H. K. Geiss, D. Mack, E. Sturenburg, and H. Seifert.** 2007. Detection of extended-spectrum beta-lactamases among Enterobacteriaceae by use of semiautomated microbiology systems and manual detection procedures. J Clin Microbiol **45**:1167-74.

(54) **Yigit, H., A. M. Queenan, J. K. Rasheed, J. W. Biddle, A. Domenech-Sanchez, S. Alberti, K. Bush, and F. C. Tenover.** 2003. Carbapenem-resistant strain of Klebsiella oxytoca harboring carbapenem-hydrolyzing beta-lactamase KPC-2. Antimicrob Agents Chemother **47**:3881-9.

Chapter 14. β-LACTAMS AND *PSEUDOMONAS AERUGINOSA*

Patrice NORDMANN and Thierry NAAS

INTRODUCTION

Pseudomonas aeruginosa, a Gram-negative bacillus, is a major pathogen mostly responsible for hospital-associated infections, generally difficult to treat, as pneumonia and bacteremia. It is also a community-acquired pulmonary pathogen in cystic fibrosis. *P. aeruginosa* produces endotoxins, exotoxins, and proteolytic enzymes that promote its pathogenicity, resulting in significant levels of morbidity and mortality. Distinctively characteristic is its high level of intrinsic resistance to antibiotics, in particular to β-lactams, as well as various acquired mechanisms of resistance to antibiotics, essentially enzymatic, which sometimes accumulate within the same strain.

METHODS

P. aeruginosa susceptibility to β-lactams may be measured basically by determining the MIC. The activity of β-lactams varies from one molecule to another within the same sub-family. In this way the MIC_{50} varies from 1 to 64 times for penicillins, from 1 to 16 times for cephalosporins and from 1 to 4 times for carbapenems (61). Anti-pseudomonal β-lactams are usually bactericidal having MBC values that are close to MIC values (61). The phenotype of colonies influence the *in vitro* susceptibility to β-lactams: in particular, the mucoid phenotype is usually associated with various susceptibilities. The inoculum effect remains the most important factor of variability when determining the MICs. This is shown for values greater then 10^7 cfu/ml and can be of clinical importance in the context of infection sites having a large quantity of infected cells. The β-lactams most susceptible to the inoculum effect are, in increasing order, imipenem, meropenem, ceftazidime, and ticarcillin. The latest critical MIC values recommended for β-lactams by EUCAST and CLSI are summarized in Table 1 (17 and http://www.escmid.org/escmid_library/reports/eucast_reports).

Table 1. MIC (µg/ml) breakpoints of β-lactams for *P. aeruginosa*

	CLSI			EUCAST		
	S	I	R	S	I	R
Piperacillin	≤ 64	-	≥ 128	≤ 16	-	> 16
Ticarcillin	≤ 64	-	≥ 128	≤ 16	-	> 16
Azlocillin	≤ 64	-	≥ 128			
Carbenicillin	≥ 128	256	≥ 512			
Piperacillin/tazobactam	≤ 64/4	-	≥ 128/4	≤16	-	> 16
Ticarcillin/clavulanic acid	≤ 64/2	-	≥ 128/2	≤ 16	-	> 16
Ceftazidime	≤ 8	16	≥ 32	≤ 8	-	> 8
Cefepime	≤ 8	16	≥ 32	≤ 8	-	> 8
Cefoperazone	≤ 16	32	≥ 64			
Monobactam	≤ 8	16-32	≥ 64			
Imipenem	≤ 4	8	≥ 16	≤ 4	-	> 8
Meropenem	≤ 4	8	≥ 16	≤ 2	-	> 8
Doripenem				≤ 1	-	> 4
Aztreonam				≤ 1	-	> 16

SUSCEPTIBLE PHENOTYPE

P. aeruginosa produces naturally relatively small amounts of cephalosporinase (AmpC) which contributes greatly to the intrinsic resistance of this species and naturally expresses at least four efflux systems, of which MexAB-OprM is the most important. It is resistant to many hydrophobic β-lactams (impermeability), such as benzylpenicillin and oxacillin, aminopenicillin; 1st and 2nd generation cephalosporins such as cephalothin, cefoxitin, cefuroxime ; several 3rd generation cephalosporins such as cefotaxime, and moxalactam and to a carbapenem, ertapenem, (http://www.escmid.org/escmid_library/reports/eucast_reports, expert rules in antimicrobial susceptibility testing). Wild-type *P. aeruginosa* is susceptible: to carboxypenicillins such as ticarcillin and carbenicillin; to ureidopenicillins, such as piperacillin; to several cephalosporins (cefsulodin, cefoperazone, and ceftazidime); to monobactams, such as aztreonam; and to carbapenems such as impenem, meropenem, and doripenem (Fig. 1A).

ACQUIRED RESISTANCE

Enzymatic resistance

A growing number of acquired β-lactamases have been described in *P. aeruginosa*. The first β-lactamases had a relatively narrow spectrum, whereas the more recent ones have a hydrolysis spectrum which extends to 3rd and 4th generation cephalosporins and/or to carbapenems. The different β-lactamases belong to classes A, B, C, D of Ambler's classification according to amino-acid sequence identities.

Overproduction of chromosomal cephalosporinase

P. aeruginosa has two natural β-lactamases (5, 32, 46). A narrow spectrum oxacillinase, OXA-50, has recently been described (32) but its contribution to the phenotype of intrinsic resistance is not significant. By contrast, natural cephalosporinase (AmpC) contributes to the phenotype of intrinsic resistance. The expression of AmpC is inducible, and the enzyme inactivates most inducer penicillins and cephalosporins.

Induction is mediated by a LysR (AmpR)-type system, as is the case with other species of Gram-negative bacilli that have inducible cephalosporinase *(Enterobacter cloacae, Morganella morganii, Serratia marcescens, Hafnia alvei,* etc.) (5, 46). Mutations in the regulatory system of this β-lactamase can occur at frequencies varying between 10^{-7} to 10^{-9} (46). They provoke a high-level stable production of AmpC which in turn affects the activity of the entire group of β-lactams with the exception of carbapenems (in the absence of associated impermeability) (Fig. 1B).

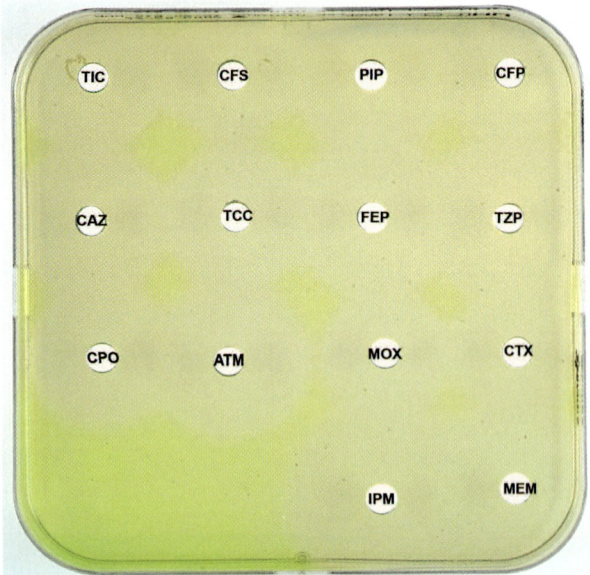

A. *P. aeruginosa* PAO38. Susceptible phenotype.

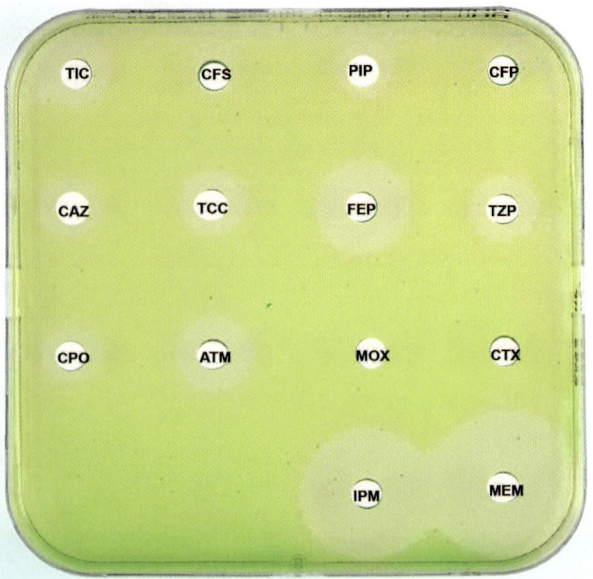

B. *P. aeruginosa* Momon. Phenotype for cephalosporinase over production.

Fig. 1. β-lactams and usual phenotypes of resistance to β-lactams. ATM, aztreonam; CAZ, ceftazidime; CFP, cefoperazone; CFS, cefsulodin; CPO, cefpirome; CTX, cefotaxime; FEP, cefepime; IPM, imipenem; MOX, moxalactam; MEM, meropenem; PIP, piperacillin; TCC, ticarcillin/clavulanic acid; TIC, ticarcillin; TZP, piperacillin/tazobactam.

Fourth generation cephalosporins (cefepime, cefpirome) are in theory more stable in regard to hydrolysis by cephalosporinases, but are in fact rarely effective on strains that overexpress AmpC because the association of a certain level of intrinsic resistance to cefepime-cefpirome with an overexpression of AmpC completely alters the effectiveness of these molecules (5, 46). Different levels of cephalosporinase expression have been observed, including also a moderate and a high constitutive level (5). The very precise mechanisms of overproduction of cephalosporinase have not yet been discovered - certain mechanisms being linked to mutations in the *ampD* gene (of an amidase) as in the case of the regulation of expression of cephalosporinases in enterobacteria (5). In all cases, the overproduction of cephalosporinase is linked to chromosomal mutations and no plasmid location for cephalosporinase gene in *P. aeruginosa* has yet been observed. The activity of this enzyme, as that of all cephalosporinases, is not inhibited by penicillinase inhibitors (clavulanic acid, tazobactam) (Table 2). Sequence variability of cephalosporinases is low in the *P. aeruginosa* species. However, certain "natural" cephalosporinases have a distinct structure that would explain why they are more likely to hydrolyze carbapenems (73). Overexpressing these enzymes permits a decreased susceptibility or a resistance to carbapenems resulting from a combination with other mechanisms of resistance to carbapenems.

Narrow spectrum β-lactamases

These β-lactamases are encoded by genes that are usually plasmid-borne although they are difficult to mobilize *in vitro* (non-conjugative plasmids, non-mobilizable plasmids…). These β-lactamases belong either to Ambler class A ("penicillinases") or to class D ("oxacillinases"). The class A β-lactamases with restricted spectrum are TEM-1/TEM-2, CARB-1 (PSE-4), CARB-2 (PSE-1), CARB-4 (6, 50). β-lactamases TEM-1 and TEM-2 differ by the substitution of only one amino acid. β-lactamases CARB-1/-2/-3 differ by one or two substitutions but differ from CARB-4 by more than 14% of residues (79, 80).

Class A β-lactamases activity is inhibited *in vitro* by penicillinase inhibitors, resulting in a more or less strong reduction of susceptibility to carbenicillins and cefsulodin (Table 2). A high level of production of carbenicillinase may also be associated with a resistance to penicillinase inhibitors and a fairly important decrease in susceptibility to cefepime or to cefpirome (Fig 1C). Restricted spectrum class D β-lactamases differ as well: OXA-1, -2, -4, -5, -9, 10, -13, -15, -18, -20, -31, -46, -47, LCR-1 (9, 20, 52, 79, 80) (Fig. 1D). The restricted spectrum of oxacillinases is, in fact, difficult to define for certain of these enzymes, which strongly hydrolyze cefepime without hydrolyzing ceftazidime. For example, this is true for OXA-31 (4) that is derived from OXA-1 (Table 2, Fig. 1E)

Table 2. Resistance phenotype to β-lactams and β-lactamases in *P. aeruginosa*

β-lactam	Overproduced Cephalo-sporinase	Penicillinase TEM/PSE (CARB)	Narrow spectrum Oxacillinase	Class A extended spectrum β-lactamase (PER, VEB)	Extended spectrum OXA type β-lactamase	Carbapenemase (IMP, VIM, SPM, GIM)
Ticarcillin	R[a]	R	R	R	R	R
Ticarcillin + clavulanic acid	R	I/S	I/R	S/I[b]	I/R	R
Piperacillin	I/R	I/R	I/R	I/R	I/R	I/S[b]
Piperacillin + tazobactam	I/R	I/S	I/R	S[b]/I	I/R	I/S[b]
Cefsulodin	I/R	I/R	I/R	R	I/R	R
Ceftazidime	I/R	S	S	R	I/R[b]	R
Cefpirome	I/R	S	I/R[c]	I/R	I/R	R
Cefepime	I/R	S	I/R	I/R	I/R	I/R
Aztreonam	I/R	S	S	R	S/I	S
Imipenem	S	S	S	S	S	R
Meropenem	S	S	S	S	S	R

[a] I, intermediate ; R, resistant ; S, susceptible.
[b] Phenotype observed *in vitro* and not interpreted.
[c] Certain oxacillinases of narrow spectrum cause resistance to 4th generation cephalosporins.

Extended-spectrum β-lactamases

This nomenclature includes class A and D β-lactamases with a spectrum more or less extended to 3rd and 4th generation cephalosporins and even carbapenems (Table 2).

Class A β-lactamases

The first extended-spectrum β-lactamase (ESBL) identified in *P. aeruginosa* was PER-1 (*P*seudomonas *E*xtended *R*esistance) from a Turkish patient hospitalized in France in 1991 (58) (Fig. 1F). This β-lactamase has subsequently been widely found in Turkey, in Southeast Asia and in many European countries (2, 25, 27, 53, 59). As in the case of enterobacteria, many other ESBLs have been identified: TEM-4, -21, -24, -42, SHV-2a, -5, -12 (26, 53, 54, 57, 93). Amongst other ESBLs, VEB-1 (*V*ietnamese *E*xtended-spectrum β-lacta-

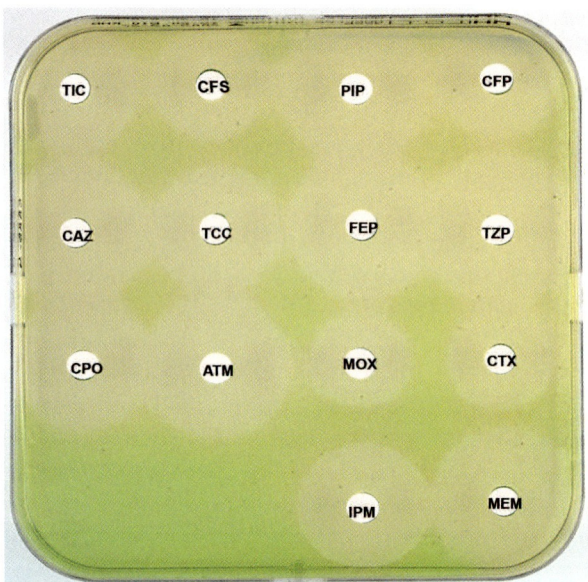

C. *P. aeruginosa* Carb. Carbenicillinase CARB-4.

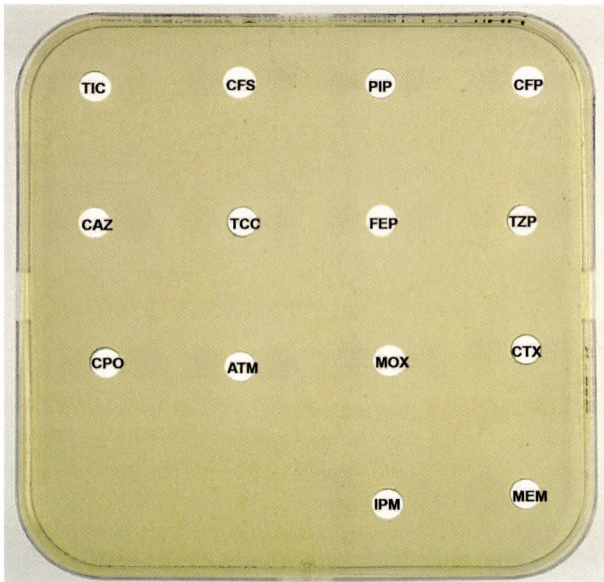

D. *P. aeruginosa* PAO38 (pMG90). Narrow spectrum type OXA-4 oxacillinase.

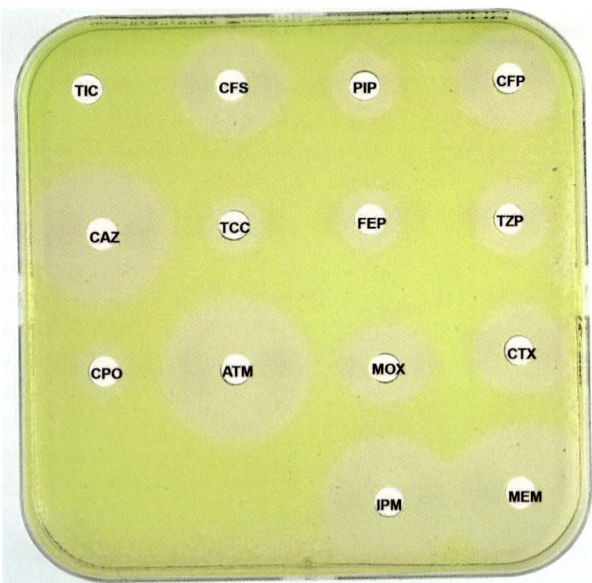

E. *P. aeruginosa* SOF-1. Narrow spectrum type OXA-31 oxacillinase.

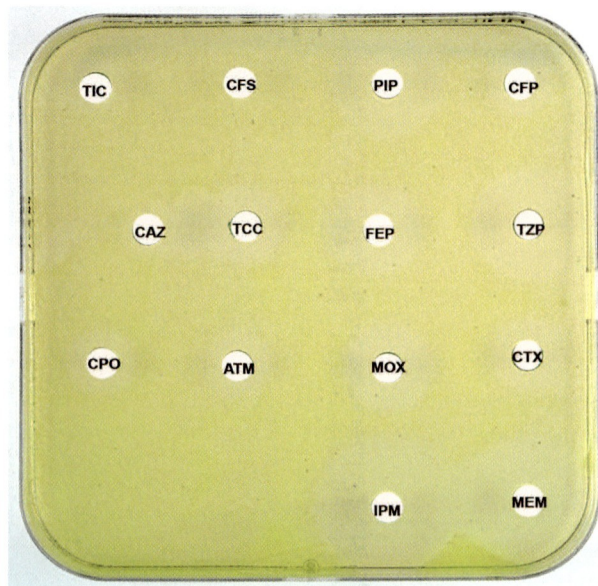

F. *P. aeruginosa* RNL-1. Extended-spectrum PER-1 β-lactamase.

Fig. 1. β-lactams and usual phenotypes of resistance to β-lactams. ATM, aztreonam; CAZ, ceftazidime; CFP, cefoperazone; CFS, cefsulodin; CPO, cefpirome; CTX, cefotaxime; FEP, cefepime; IPM, imipenem; MOX, moxalactam; MEM, meropenem; PIP, piperacillin; TCC, ticarcillin/clavulanic acid; TIC, ticarcillin; TZP, piperacillin/tazobactam.

mase) (31) has been identified in isolated areas of south Asia where it is particularly widespread, and has also been found in *P. aeruginosa* of Bulgaria (31,83, 94) (Fig. 1G). Only one other variant of VEB-1, VEB-2 has been identified in *P. aeruginosa*.

The ESBL GES-1, first identified in *Klebsiella pneumoniae* (66) was also found in *P. aeruginosa*. In contrast to the other class A ESBLs, GES-1/IBC-2 has a strong affinity, not only for 3rd and 4th generation cephalosporins but also for cefoxitin (93). GES type ESBLs have been very widely found in *P. aeruginosa* in many countries (13, 43, 92).

GES-2 was the first ESBL derived by a point mutation from another ESBL (GES-1) which gained extended activity on carbapenems. This β-lactamase has been identified in epidemic strains in South Africa (70, 71). One of the most recently identified ESBLs found in *P. aeruginosa* is BEL-1 (Belgium Extended β-lactamase), isolated in Belgium (64).

Furthermore, the emerging ESBLs widely recognized in enterobacteria are of the CTX-M type (10). They have also been seen, although more rarely, in strains of *P. aeruginosa* from strains isolated in South America and the Netherlands (3, 16, 63) (Fig. 1H). They belong to the CTX-M-1, CTX-M-2, and CTX-M-43 types.

All these ESBLs display, in fact, few similarity from a structural point of view (from 20 to 70% of identical amino acids). The reservoir of these genes may be environmental. The plasmid localization of the resistance genes, within integrons or transposons, promotes their diffusion contributing to the multiple resistance of *P. aeruginosa*.

Currently, KPC-type enzymes are the most powerful class A ESBLs since they hydrolyze almost all β-lactams and, most importantly, carbapenems (56). They are carbapenemases. These enzymes have been retrieved in *P. aeruginosa* isolates from South America and the Caribbean (Fig. 1I) (1, 89). Therefore, their diffusion is not just limited to enterobacteria.

Class D β-lactamases: extended-spectrum oxacillinases

OXA-18 and OXA-45 are the only oxacillinases activity of which is strongly inhibited by clavulanic acid and in which the resistance phenotype is, in all aspects, similar to that of class A ESBLs (62, 84, Fig. 1J). Most of the extended-spectrum oxacillinases in *P. aeruginosa* are derived by point mutations from OXA-2 (-15, -32) and OXA-10 β-lactamases (-11, -13, -14, -16, -17, -19, -28) (23, 46, 52, 65).

These variants hydrolyze 3rd generation cephalosporins (ceftazidime) or aztreonam to various degrees and their activity is not (or very little) inhibited by clavulanic acid (Fig. 1K). The hydrolysis of cefepime and of cefpirome is often pronounced. Plasmids or chromosomes are the underlying genetic support for these enzymes (at least for bla_{OXA-13}, bla_{OXA-17}, bla_{OXA-18}, bla_{OXA-20}) and most of these genes are part of class 1 integrons and are associated with genes of resistance to other families of antibiotics (essentially aminoglycosides) (68).

Although narrow-spectrum oxacillinases have been detected in many species of enterobacteria, the wide spectrum oxacillinases that strongly hydrolyze 3rd generation cephalosporins have only been identified, so far, in *P. aeruginosa*.

Class B carbapenemases

Although classes A, C, and D β-lactamases are very important effectors of resistance to β-lactams in *P. aeruginosa*, class B enzymes (carbapenemases) have the strongest catalytic activity and hydrolyze all the β-lactams except aztreonam (69, 90, 91) (Fig. 1L). The activity of these enzymes is not inhibited by clavulanic acid or by tazobactam. The strains that express these carbapenemases have several associated mechanisms of resistance to β-lactams, which explains why they are, in practice, most often resistant to all β-lactams, including aztreonam. The first enzyme of this type (IMP-1, IMiPenemase) was described in Japan in 1988 (90). Acquired carbapenemases currently form four groups: IMP, VIM (Verona IMipenamase), SPM (Sao Paulo Metallo-β-lactamase) and GIM (German IMipenamase) (14, 19, 34, 44, 65, 67).

Eighteen variants of the IMP group and twelve of the VIM group have been identified, most of them in *P. aeruginosa*, as well as a SPM-1 representative and a GIM-1. These four groups of enzymes are not really structurally related since they only have 20 to 30% of identical amino acids. They are also very different to natural metallo-β-lactamases found in species such as *Stenotrophomonas maltophilia* and *Chryseobacterium* spp (90, 91). The activity of these enzymes is linked to the presence of one or two zinc ions at the active site and is therefore inhibited by the addition of divalent ion chelating agents (EDTA). The structural genes of these enzymes are either plasmid- or chromosome-borne, located in transposons and most frequently associated with integrons.

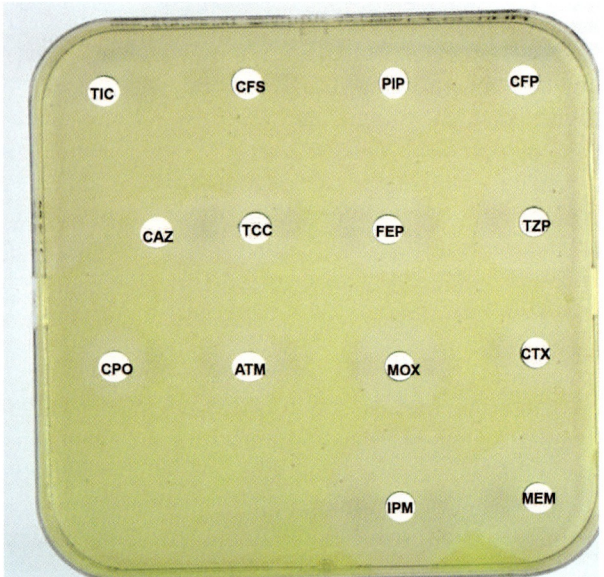

G. *P. aeruginosa* 15. Extended-spectrum VEB-1 β-lactamase.

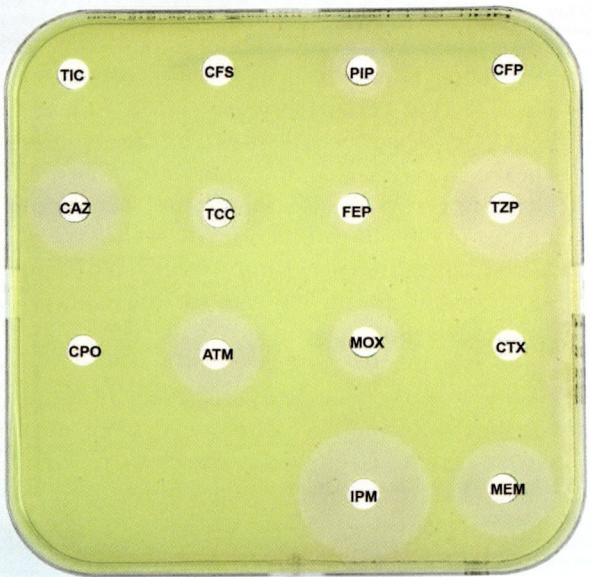

H. *P. aeruginosa* P6208. Extended-spectrum CTX-M-2 β-lactamase.

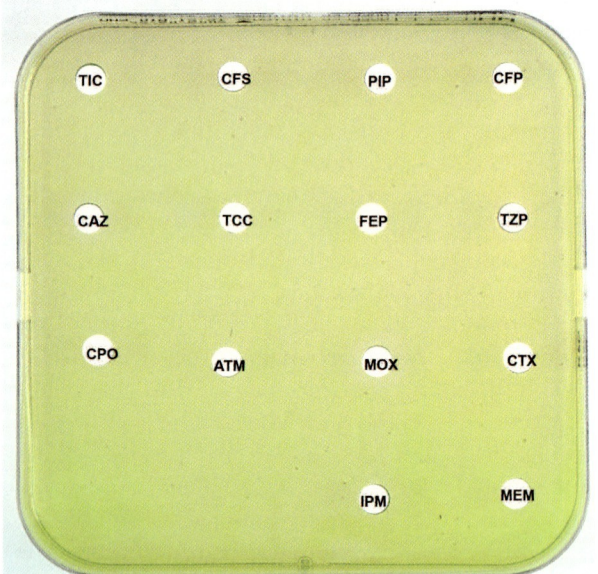

I. *P. aeruginosa* 2404. Carbapenemase KPC-2.

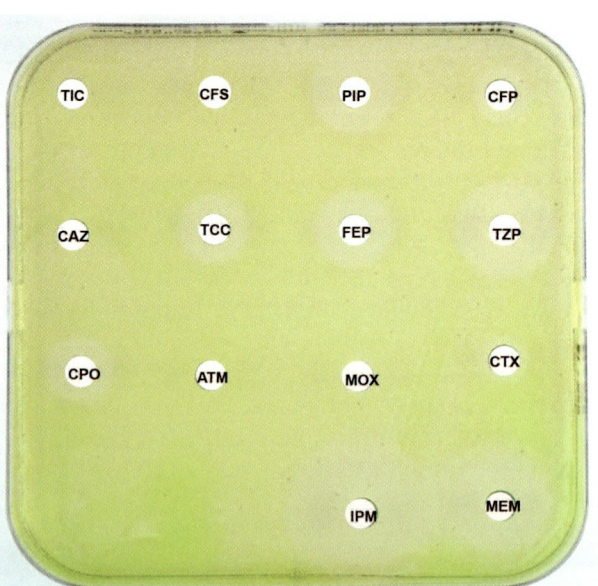

J. *P. aeruginosa* MUS. Extended-spectrum OXA-18 β-lactamase.

Fig. 1. β-lactams and usual phenotypes of resistance to β-lactams. ATM, aztreonam; CAZ, ceftazidime; CFP, cefoperazone; CFS, cefsulodin; CPO, cefpirome; CTX, cefotaxime; FEP, cefepime; IPM, imipenem; MOX, moxalactam; MEM, meropenem; PIP, piperacillin; TCC, ticarcillin/clavulanic acid; TIC, ticarcillin; TZP, piperacillin/tazobactam.

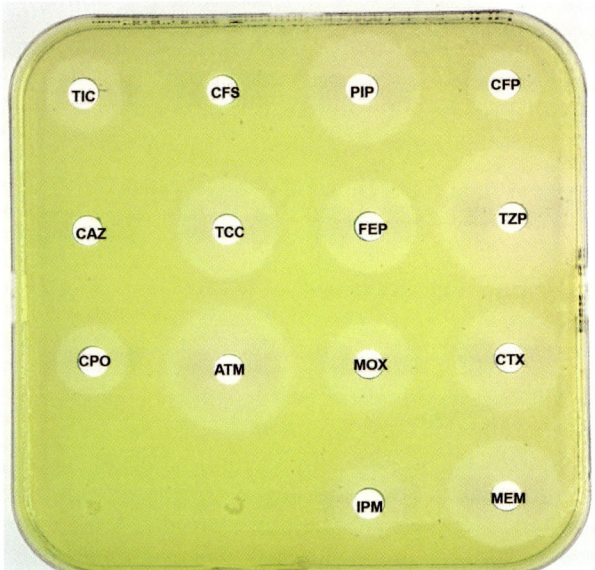
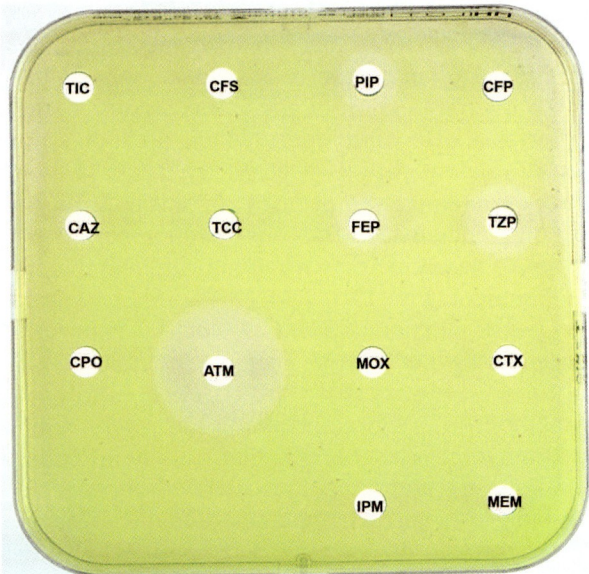

K. *P. aeruginosa* CY-1. Phenotype extended-spectrum OXA-32 oxacillinase.

L. *P. aeruginosa* COL-1. Phenotype type VIM-2 metallo-β-lactamase.

Fig. 1. β-lactams and usual phenotypes of resistance to β-lactams. ATM, aztreonam; CAZ, ceftazidime; CFP, cefoperazone; CFS, cefsulodin; CPO, cefpirome; CTX, cefotaxime; FEP, cefepime; IPM, imipenem; MOX, moxalactam; MEM, meropenem; PIP, piperacillin; TCC, ticarcillin/clavulanic acid; TIC, ticarcillin; TZP, piperacillin/tazobactam.

Non-enzymatic resistance

Imipenem resistance due to loss of porin OprD2

Porins play an important role in transmembrane penetration of β-lactams into Gram-negative enterobacteria. A qualitative modification or a production decrease in OprD2 porin brings about a selective resistance to imipenem (72) (Fig. 1M) (Table 2). OprD protein forms a specific channel that favors the entrance of basic amino acids, carbapenems, and to a very slight degree, meropenem but of no other β-lactams. Whereas the MICs for imipenem in strains deficient in OprD are 8 to 32 μg/ml, those for meropenem are 2-4 μg/ml. Resistance to imipenem is the result of a decrease in the penetration of the molecule through the external membrane associated with a partial hydrolysis by natural cephalosporinase whereas meropenem is much more stable to hydrolysis by cephalosporinase. The overexpression of the MexEF-OprN efflux system is associated with a decrease in the susceptibility to imipenem due to a decrease in the expression of the OprD2 porin (72).

Resistance to β-lactams due to target modification

The least frequent mechanism of resistance to β-lactams in *P. aeruginosa* is the modification of penicillin binding proteins (PBP). The modifications of PBP-2 and PBP-3 are responsible for acquired resistance to carbapenems, associated in certain cases, with protein modifications of outer membrane or the overexpression of efflux systems (33).

Overexpression of efflux systems

P. aeruginosa is usually less susceptible to most antibiotics than the enterobacteria. This difference in susceptibility, especially to β-lactams, is due to the natural expression of the efflux systems in association with a weak permeability.

Four efflux systems have been described in *P. aeruginosa*, Mex-A/ Mex-B/ OprM, MexC/ MexD/ OprJ, MexE/ MexF/ OprN, MexX/ MexY/OPrM that all belong to the RND (Resistance Nodulation Division) family of efflux systems (37, 39, 49, 72). They expel antibiotics into the external environment as would a pump, using the energy of the electrochemical gradient of the cytoplasmic membrane.

The first component of these 'pumps' is located within the cytoplasmic membrane (MexB, MexD, MexF, MexY). The second constituent is an external membrane protein (OprM, OprJ, OPrN and OprM). The third protein (MexA, MexC, MexE, MexX) is located in the peri-plasmic space and has the function of linking the other two proteins. MexA- MexB- OprM and MexY-OprM participate both in intrinsic resistance and acquired resistance while the other two pumps are only involved in acquired resistance. As indicated in Table 3, each of the efflux systems has substrate specificity.

The peculiar feature of resistance related to a stable overexpression of the efflux systems leads to resistance to antibiotics, which are not structurally related. In this way, MexAB-OprM overproduction leads to a decrease in susceptibility to certain β-lactams, to fluoroquinolones, to tetracyclines, to novobiocin, to trimethoprim, and to chloramphenicol (Fig. 1N).

Overproduction of MexCD-OprJ leads to resistance to zwitterionic β-lactams (cefepime, cefpirome) (Fig. 10), to fluoroquinolones, trimethoprim, chloramphenicol, tetracyclines and erythromycin. The MexEF-OprN system causes resistance to fluoroquinolones, trimethoprim, chloramphenicol, and tetracyclines; and the MexXY-OprM system to certain β-lactams (cefepime, cefpirome) (Fig. 1P), to aminoglycosides, to tetracyclines, and to erythromycin (37, 39, 40, 45, 46).

The levels of resistance to β-lactams that are the result of the overexpression of the efflux systems are moderate and weaker than those due to the presence of β-lactamase (Table 3). The overexpression of these efflux systems is often associated with other mechanisms of resistance.

Mutants that overproduce MexAB-OprM have decreased susceptibility to all β-lactams, except for imipenem, and particularly for ticarcillin, aztreonam and cefotaxime, whereas the activity of the other β-lactams is variable (Table 3). The activity of ceftazidime remains, in this case, greater than that of aztreonam; and chromosomal cephalosporinase remains inducible, which makes it possible to differentiate it from the phenotype of cephalosporinase overexpression. The stable derepression of system MexCD-OprJ or of system MexXY-OprJ leads to a decrease in susceptibility to zwitterionics, cephalosporins, cefepime and cefpirome (Table 3). The MexEF-OprN system does not, strictly speaking, pump out β-lactams, but resistance to imipenem, which is associated with it results in a negative co-regulation of the expression of the OprD porin (37, 39, 72) (Table 3).

FREQUENCY OF RESISTANCES

Enzymatic resistance

Overproduction of cephalosporinases

The overproduction of cephalosporinase continues to be the most frequent mechanism of resistance to 3rd generation cephalosporins in *P. aeruginosa*. Several studies have identified this resistance mechanism to broad spectrum cephalosporins in 50-80% of the cases of resistance to ceftazidime (24). The expression of extended-spectrum cephalosporinase, activity of which includes in part carbapenems, could in fact, be quite widespread (P. Nordmann unpublished).

Transferable β-lactamases
Narrow-spectrum β-lactamases

Studies that show evidence of the distribution of these β-lactamases in *P. aeruginosa*, are rare. (86). They have been identified in 12-13% of a collection of strains with a carbenicillinase (CARB), in the majority of cases and less frequently an oxacillinase (6). Another study identified OXA-32 (a OXA-2 derivative) as the main oxacillinase in strains resistant to ceftazidime, associated with other mechanisms of resistance (24). One study identified the presence of "transferable" β-lactamases in 7.1% of cases: with CARB 72%, TEM-2 10% and OXA 8% (15). However, this study did not identify the nature of the genes of these β-lactamases. Another study, focusing on strains resis-

Table 3. Consequences of the loss of porin OprD and overexpression of an efflux system on the susceptibility to β-lactams of *P. aeruginosa*

Mechanism	Ticarcillin	Piperacillin	Ceftazidime	Cefepime	Aztreonam	Imipenem	Meropenem
Susceptible	S[a]	S	S	S	S	S	S
Loss of porin OprD2	S	S	S	S	S	R	I/R
Overexpression of							
MexAB-OprM	I/R	S	S	S	I/R	S	S/I
MexCD-OprJ	S	S	S	I/R	S	S	S
MexEF-OprN	S	S	S	S	S	I	I
MexXY-oprM	S	S	S	I/R	S	S	S

[a] I, intermediate ; R, resistant ; S, sensitive.

tant to cefepime, underlined the strong prevalence of PSE-1 (38).

Extended-spectrum β-lactamases
Class A β-lactamases

First detected in France, the extended-spectrum β-lactamases (ESBLs) have been identified in *P. aeruginosa* in many countries and are often associated with strains with a strong epidemic power. The nature of these enzymes varies from one country to another, as does their prevalence. Thus, for example, the ESBL PER-1 - currently the most frequently isolated ESBL of *P. aeruginosa* in the world - has been identified in Turkey, Greece, France, Italy and Korea (27, 59, 74, 82, 93). SHV-type ESBLs are also frequently identified in the ESBL (+) strains of *P. aeruginosa* (Thailand,

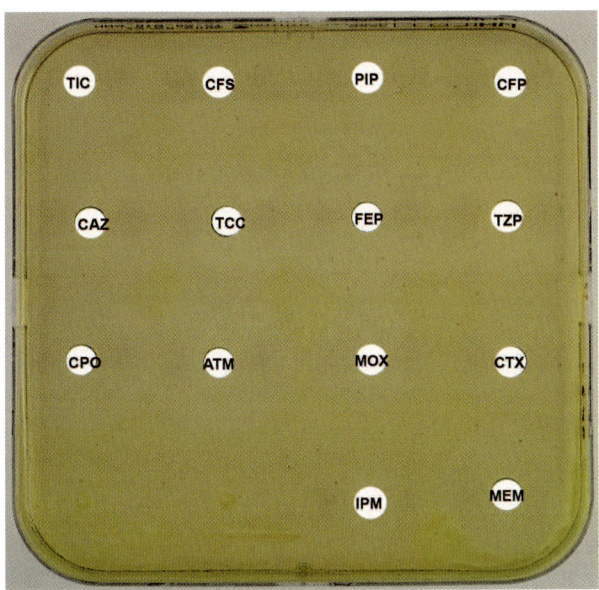

M. *P. aeruginosa* H729. Phenotype selective impermeability to imipenem; deficit in porin OprD2.

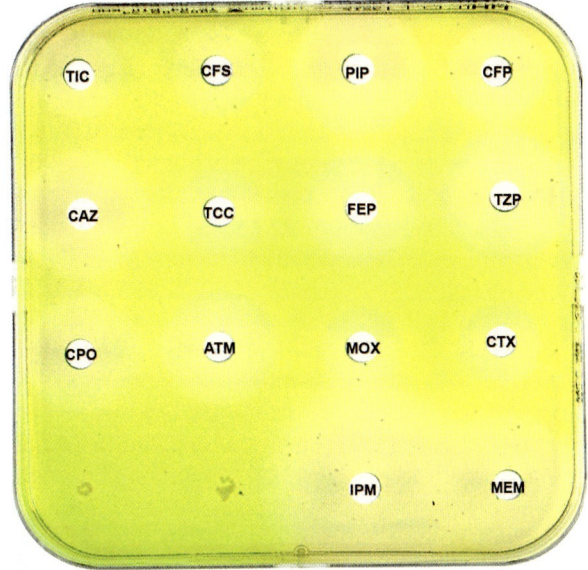

N. *P. aeruginosa* PAO4098E. Phenotype of over-expression of the MexAB-OprM efflux system.

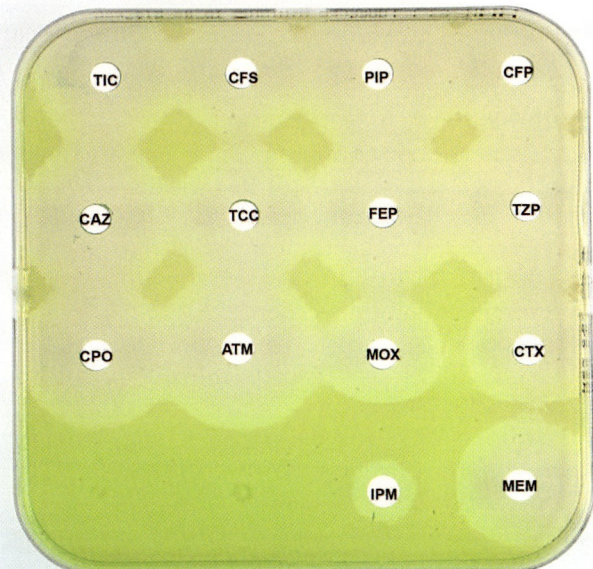

O. *P. aeruginosa* PAO-1 (ERYR). Phenotype over-expression of the MexCD-OprJ efflux system.

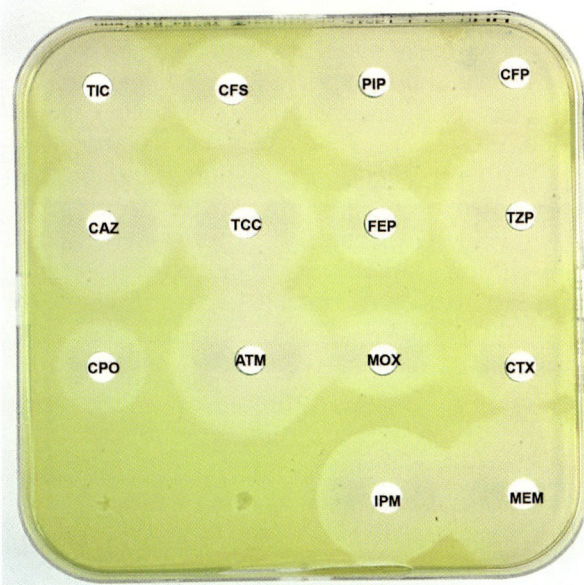

P. *P. aeruginosa* 12b (agrZ). Phenotype of over-expression of the MexXY-OprM efflux system.

Fig. 1. β-lactams and usual phenotypes of resistance to β-lactams. ATM, aztreonam; CAZ, ceftazidime; CFP, cefoperazone; CFS, cefsulodin; CPO, cefpirome; CTX, cefotaxime; FEP, cefepime; IPM, imipenem; MOX, moxalactam; MEM, meropenem; PIP, piperacillin; TCC, ticarcillin/clavulanic acid; TIC, ticarcillin; TZP, piperacillin/tazobactam.

France, Greece) as well as GES-type ESBLs (France, South America, Greece). The other types of ESBLs (TEM, BEL, VEB) may well have a more restricted dissemination (8, 93). In France, the limited group of studies on that subject indicates the presence of essentially, ESBL, PER-1.

Class D β-lactamases

The dissemination of these enzymes is also unknown. Most publications reporting the presence of these broad spectrum oxacillinases are based on the identification of only one strain and these reports essentially result from studies carried out by two teams (D. Livermore, London; P. Nordmann, Paris) and, notably, from a sole country, Turkey (23, 46, 52). So it is quite difficult to have a precise idea of the worldwide spread of these mechanisms of resistance. Recent studies report the identification of OXA-35 in a important number of strains resistant to cefepime (38) and OXA-18 (7).

Class B β-lactamases, metallo-β-lactamases

Of the four groups of metallo-β-lactamases, the most frequently isolated in *P. aeruginosa* are IMP and VIM (90, 91). The most widespread carbapenemase in *P. aeruginosa* is VIM-2. These carbapenemases have been detected on all continents though more prevalent in Asia and South America (29, 36, 48, 51, 75, 76, 77, 81, 85, 90, 91). In Europe, especially in France, the presence of these enzymes does not seem to modify the global rates of resistance to β-lactams in *P. aeruginosa*. However, many nosocomial outbreaks with this type of strain have been described, especially in Southern Europe (Italy, Greece, France, Portugal), in South America and in Asia (12, 18, 35, 48, 90, 91).

Long-term persistence in the same hospital environment of this type of strain has been demonstrated (90, 91). Recently, carbapenemase producing strains have been detected in patients suffering from cystic fibrosis.

Non-enzymatic resistance

Selective impermeability to imipenem

Modifications of porin D2 remain the main mechanism of resistance to imipenem in *P. aeruginosa* (35, 39). This mechanism could be present in 5-15% of strains of *P. aeruginosa*. This percentage varies considerably from country to country, particularly as it is most frequently associated with other mechanisms of resistance (efflux, overexpression of cephalosporinase, cephalosporinase with carbapenemase activity...).

Overexpression of efflux systems

The prevalence of overexpression of systems is very difficult to determine because it is very frequently associated with other mechanisms of resistance. Many studies describe the frequency of overexpression of the MexAB/OprM and MexY/OprM systems, particularly in association with other mechanisms in multi-resistant strains and in strains that are resistant to ticarcillin (35, 37, 30). Isolated resistance to cefepime has been associated with overexpression of the MexXY-OprM efflux system (37, 39).

Finally, one of the particularities of *P. aeruginosa* is that it is able to associate multiple mechanisms of resistance to antibiotics (β-lactamases, impermeability, efflux over-expression) with a much varied underlying genetic support mechanisms (plasmids, integrons, transposons). This explains the frequent isolation of strains with multiple resistance to families of antibiotics that are not structurally linked. Many studies have reported an increase in the frequency of isolation of this type of strain worldwide during the last five years (21, 22, 46, 75).

SUSCEPTIBILITY TO ANTIBIOTICS

The susceptibility of *P. aeruginosa* to β-lactams varies from one molecule to another and depends on many parameters. A study carried out on hospital strains showed a susceptibility of 80% to ceftazidime, cefepime imipenem, and meropenem with a slightly higher susceptibility to the combination of piperacillin/tazobactam (28). This susceptibility to β-lactams is less in most under-developed countries than in developed countries (Table 4) (60, 75, 95). In the USA, for example, a study of 600 strains in 1985 revealed a susceptibility to ceftazidime and to carbapenems in the order of 85% and to the piperacillin/tazobactam combination in the order of 90% (75).

In Europe, according to one of the latest studies (MYSTIC 2006), resistance to imipenem is in the order of 32% whereas it is in the order of 25% for ceftazidime, 22% for meropenem, and 15% for piperacillin/tazobactam (2006) (Table 5) (28). Other European data (EARSS,2007) reveals a large disparity between strains isolated in Northern Europe or in Switzerland in comparison with those isolated in Southern Europe. Thus, for example, the proportion of strains non-susceptible to imipenem varied from 5.4% in Switzerland to 32.5% in Italy and the rates of resistance varied in the same way for other antibiotics.

Table 4. Susceptibility to β-lactams (%) of *P. aeruginosa* according to the place of isolation by continent (after 75)

β-lactam	Europe	North America	Latin America	Asia-Pacific
Ticarcillin	74	78	58	76
Ticarcillin + clavulanic acid	78	78	59	75
Ceftazidime	80	80	66	79
Cefepime	80	83	67	83
Aztreonam	73	66	49	67
Imipenem	82	87	76	88
Meropenem	85	91	80	90

Table 5. Proportion of strains of *P. aeruginosa* not susceptible to certain β-lactams isolated in 23 European countries participating in a resistance to antibiotics surveillance system in Europe (EARSS, 2007)

Country	Proportion of strains not susceptible to:		
	Piperacillin[a]	Ceftazidime	Carbapenem[b]
Germany	48.5	24.4	31.5
Australia	7.1	9	13.7
Cyprus	28.8	15.4	21.1
Croatia	30.2	20.5	28.1
Denmark	4.8	4	3.9
Spain	8.1	15.2	18.4
Finland	7.3	7.7	9.4
France	20.5	18.6	18.4
Greece	38.4	44.8	50.5
Hungary	16.8	15.3	21.3
Ireland	11.8	10.3	11.2
Israel	15.2	13.3	14.9
Italy	27.2	41.4	32.1
Norway	3.1	6.7	14.5
Netherlands	5.2	5.6	5.4
Poland	35.8	22.7	22.4
Portugal	15.8	20.9	16.1
Czech Republic Tchèque	30	32.7	36
United Kingdom	5.4	14.1	17.2
Slovenia	12.5	13.6	20.4
Sweden	3.1	9.6	9
Switzerland	5	4.2	5.4
Turkey	32.4	31.3	31

[a] Tests performed with piperacillin or piperacillin/tazobactam.
[b] Tests performed with imipenem or meropenem.

The global rate of resistance increased from 1995 to 2005 (30, 41, 42, 55). However, in certain cases, some inversions of this trend have been noted, such as the increase of susceptibility to the piperacillin/tazobactam combination from 2002 to 2006 in Europe (80% versus 85%) and to ceftazidime from 70% to 75% (82).

The origin of the isolates conditions their level of resistance. Thus, the percentage of strains that are resistant to imipenem varies from 15% to 10% whether strains are isolated or not from intensive care units, respectively (41, 42). Similarly, the strains from bacteraemia are usually more resistant to β-lactams (87). A large number of studies have underlined the increase in the number of strains of *P. aeruginosa* multi-resistant to antibiotics, including β-lactams in the USA and Southern Europe. This evolution adversely affects the treatment of infections due to multi-resistant *P. aeruginosa* (22, 82).

PHENOTYPIC DETECTION OF RESISTANCE

A phenotypic approach to resistance to β-lactams could be proposed to detect the main mechanisms of resistance (88). G. Vedel proposed a simple detection method (Fig. 2). It used a limited number of molecules: ticarcillin, ticarcillin + clavulanic acid, cefotaxime, ceftazidime, cefsulodin, cefepime (or cefpirome), aztreonam, and imipenem.

Isolated resistance to imipenem is one of the most simple phenotypes to identify. Cefepime is a good marker of isolated MexCD-OprJ efflux system over-expression, but mutants of this type are very rarely found clinically. In fact, the low level of activity seen with cefepime in comparison to ceftazidime is very likely linked to the stable derepression of the MexXY-OprM system (37). Cefsulodin is a good marker to differentiate low from high levels of production of penicillinase. The inhibiting effect of clavulanic acid in the cases of certain narrow spectrum β-lactamases can be shown clearly by comparing the activity of ticarcillin and ticarcillin + clavulanic acid.

Detection of an extended-spectrum β-lactamase would benefit from an additional testing of disks impregnated with 3rd generation cephalosporins (ceftazidime, cefotaxime) or aztreonam and clavulanic acid at different distances (Fig. 3, panel A). It would also be useful to carry out an E-test® comparing ceftazidime/ceftazidime + clavulanic acid or cefepime/cefepime + clavulanic acid. Production of high levels of cephalosporinase may accompany a certain level of inducibility (ticarcillin + clavulanic acid zone diameter < ticarcillin zone diameter). In order to establish the difference between phenotypes of overproduction of cephalosporinase and of production of metallo-β-lactamase, it is possible to perform an imipenem/imipenem EDTA synergy test using an E-test® (Fig. 3, panel B).

The overexpression of the MexAB-OprM efflux system is sometimes difficult to differentiate from the production of certain extended-spectrum oxacillinases, often accompanied by significant cefepime hydrolysis.

Taking into account the multiplicity of mechanisms of resistance that can be observed in the same strain, it is possible in some cases to carry out disk diffusion tests on media containing oxacillin or cloxacillin (200 µg/ml). These antibiotics inhibit cephalosporinase activity allowing an extended-spectrum β-lactamase to be detected – when not easily suspected - in the presence of an overexpression of cephalosporinase; without these inhibitors, the detection would be less likely.

ANTIBIOTICS TO STUDY

A minimum antibiogram for an accurate phenotypic interpretation may include: ticarcillin, ticarcillin + clavulanic acid, piperacillin, piperacillin + tazobactam, ceftazidime, cefsulodin, cefotaxime, cefepime, aztreonam, and imipenem.

A more extended antibiogram would also include: cefoperazone, cefpirome, moxalactam, meropenem, and doripenem.

The ticarcillin/clavulanic acid disk should be placed near to the ceftazidime disk so as to show clearly any possible synergistic interaction. The detection of extended-spectrum β-lactamases can be made more easily, when using a disk diffusion technique, by placing the disks containing clavulanic acid near those containing ceftazidime, aztreonam, or cefepime (Fig. 3, panel A) or by performing an E-test® : ceftazidime and ceftazidime + clavulanic acid or cefepime and cefepime + clavulanic acid. The detection of metallo-β-lactamases can be done by using an E-test® with imipenem and imipenem + EDTA (Fig. 3, panel B).

GENOTYPE DETECTION

The acquired genes for extended-spectrum β-lactamases (class A, B and D) can be detected by PCR followed by sequence determination. Below we propose a technique for the extraction and amplification of DNA.

DNA Extraction

DNA is extracted from an 18 h trypticase soy broth culture. One ml of broth is centrifuged (10 min. at 7,000 rpm), the sediment is re-suspended in 500 µl of buffer SET [NaCl 75 mM, EDTA 25 mM, Tris 20 mM (pH 7.5)], 25 µl of SDS 20% and 1 µl of lysozyme (50 µg/ml) and incubated at 37°C for 1 h. 220 µl of NaCl (5M) and 700 µl of chloro-

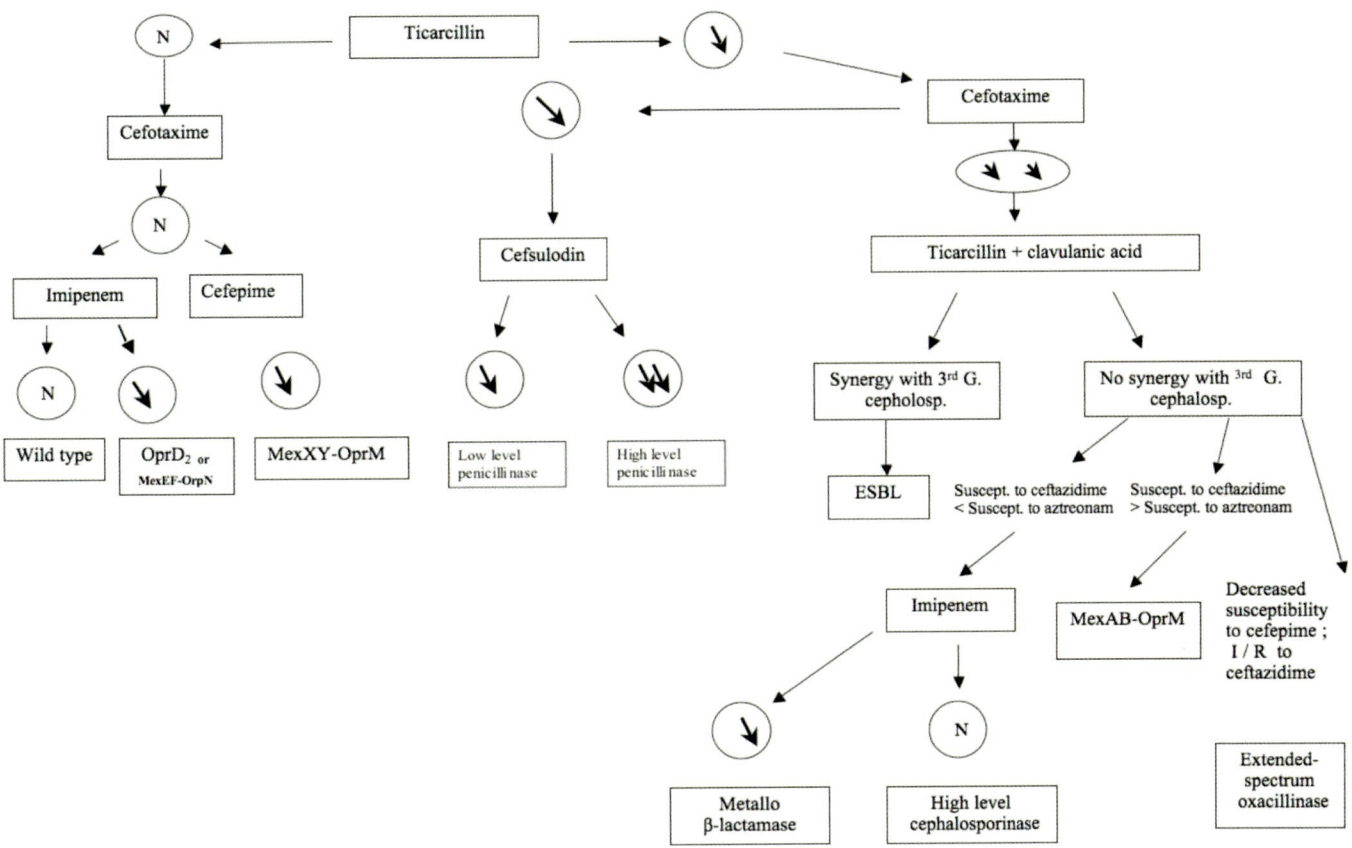

Fig. 2. Diagram to interpret the phenotypes of resistance to β-lactams in *P. aeruginosa*, adapted after G. Vedel (88). N, normal susceptibility; S, susceptiblity; I, intermediate; R, resistant.

form: isoamylalcohol are added and the mixture is vigorously shaken. After centrifugation for 10 min at 10,000 rpm, the DNA contained in the upper phase is collected and then precipitated by the addition of 700 µl of cold isopropanol for 1 h at 20°C. After centrifugation for 10 min at 10,000 rpm, the sediment is washed by the addition of cold 70% ethanol, centrifuged again and dried for 10 min at ambient temperature. The extracted DNA is re-suspended in 100 µl of distilled water.

Amplification Reaction by Polymerase Chain Reaction (PCR)

The reactions are performed as described by Sambrook *et al.* (78). The reactive mixture contains in addition to the DNA polymerase (Taq Gold polymerase, Roche Diagnostics): 0.2 mM of each dNTP, a reaction buffer (50 mM KCl, 10 mM Tris-HCl pH 8.5; 1.5 mM $MgCl_2$), 1 µM of each oligodeoxyribonucleotide and 0.1 to 1 µg of the DNA matrix. The list of primers for the detection of the genes of the β-lactamases' is indicated in Table 6. The reactions are carried out in an ABI 2700 thermal cycler (Applied Biosystems). A PCR reaction includes an initial stage of denaturation of the double stranded DNA for 12 min. at 94°C followed by 38 DNA amplification cycles (I min at 94°C (denaturation); 1 min. at 55°C (primer pairing); 1 min. at 72°C (elongation, variable time according to the size of the fragment to amplify) then a final stage of 10 min. at 72°C to finish the synthesis of the unfinished strands.

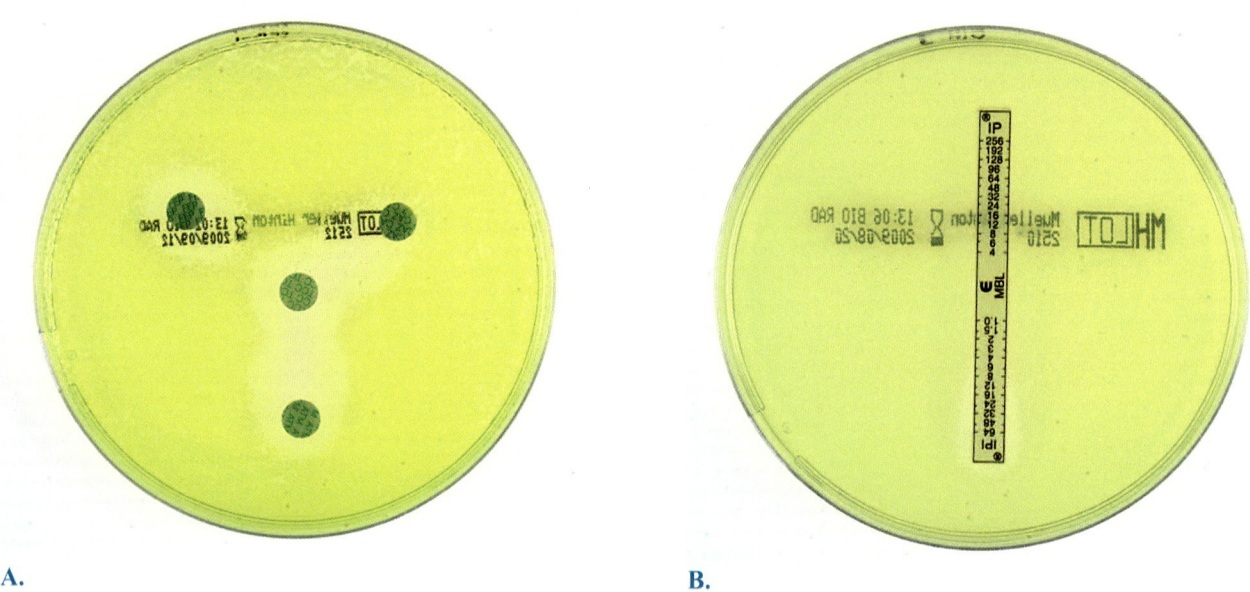

A. B.

Fig. 3. (A) Evidence of a β-lactamase of extended-spectrum type PER-1 due to synergy between the clavulanic acid in the ticarcillin + clavulanic acid disk and cefepime (FEP), ceftazidime (CAZ) or aztreonam (AZT); *P. aeruginosa* strain PER12 . (B) Display of a type VIM-2 metallo-enzyme using E-test®, imipenem (IP) synergy of imipenem + EDTA (IPI), *P. aeruginosa* strain COL-1.

Table 6. Deoxyribonucleotides for the amplification of the main genes of extended-spectrum β-lactamases

β-lactamases	Sequence from 5' to 3'	Gene
Extended-spectrum class A β-lactamase		
VEB-1A	CGACTTCCATTTCCCGATGC	bla_{VEB}
VEB-1B	GGACTCTGCAACAAATACGC	
PER-A	ATGAATGTCATTATAAAAGC	bla_{PER}
PER-B	AATTTGGGCTTAGGGCAGAA	
GES-1A	ATGCGCTTCATTCACGCAC	bla_{GES}
GES-1B	CTATTTGTCCGTGCTCAGG	
TEM-A	GAGTATTCAACATTTCCGTGTC	bla_{TEM}
TEM-B	TAATCAGTGAGGCACCTATCTC	
SWSHV-A	AAGATCCACTATCGCCAGCAG	bla_{SHV}
SWSHV-B	ATTCAGTTCCGTTTCCCAGCGG	
BEL-A1	CGACAATGCCGCAGCTAACC	bla_{BEL}
BEL-A2	CAGAAGCAATTAATAACGCCC	
Class B carbapenems		
IMP-2004	ACAYGGYTTGGTTGTTCTTG	bla_{IMP}
IMP-2004B	GGTTTAAYAAAACAACCACC	
VIM-2004A	GTTTGGTCGCATATCGCAAC	bla_{VIM}
VIM-2004B	AATGCGCAGCACCAGGATAG	
SPM-A	CTGCTTGGATTCATGGGCGC	bla_{SPM}
SPM-B	CCTTTTCCGCGACCTTGATC	
GIM-A	GGAGTATATCTTCATACCTCC	bla_{GIM}
GIM-B	TTCCAACTTTGCCATGCCCC	
Extended-spectrum class D β-lactamase		
OXA-2A	ATGGCAATCCGACTTCGC	bla_{OXA-2}
OXA-2B	TTATCGCGCTGCGTCCAGT	
OXA-10A	GTYCTTTCGAGTACGGCATTA	bla_{OXA-10}
OXA-10B	ATTTTCTTAGCGGCAACTTAC	
OXA-18A	ATTTCAACGGTTTGCCTTAG	bla_{OXA-18}
OXA-18B	TTGGCATCGGAAAGCGAACC	

ACKNOWLEDGEMENTS

We wish to thank collaborators and colleagues D. Aubert, C. De Champs, N. Fortineau, D. Girlich, D. Hocquet, A. Philippon, P. Plésiat, L. Poirel, J. M. Rodriguez-Martinez, and G. Vedel for having contributed in our Unit to the detection and characterization of new mechanisms of resistance to antibiotics in *P. aeruginosa*, for critical reading of this chapter, and for providing strains.

REFERENCES

(1) **Akpaka S. E., W. H. Swanston, H. N. Ihemere, A. Correa, J. A. Torres, J. D. Tafur, M. C. Montealegre, J. P. Quinn, and M. V. Villegas.** 2009. Emergence of KPC-producing *Pseudomonas aeruginosa* in Trinidad and Tobago. J. Clin. Microbiol. **47**:2070-2071.

(2) **Aktas Z., L. Poirel, M. Salcioglu, P.E. Ozcan, K. Midilli, C. Bal, O. Ang, and P. Nordmann.** 2005. PER-1- and OXA-10-like beta-lactamases in ceftazidime-resistant *Pseudomonas aeruginosa* isolates from intensive care unit patients in Istanbul Turkey. Clin. Microbiol. Infect. **11**:193-198.

(3) **Al Naiemi, N., B. Duim, and A. Bart.** 2006. A CTX-M extended-spectrum β-lactamase in *Pseudomonas aeruginosa* and *Stenotrophomonas maltophilia*. J. Med. Microbiol. **55**:1607-1608.

(4) **Aubert, D., L. Poirel, J. Chevalier, S. Léotard, J.M. Pagès, and P. Nordmann.** 2001. Oxacillinase-mediated resistance to cefepime susceptibility to ceftazidime in *Pseudomonas aeruginosa*. Antimicrob. Agents Chemother. **45**:1615-1620.

(5) **Bagge, N., O. Ciofu, M. Hentzer, J. I. Campbell, M. Givskov, and N. Holby.** 2002. Constitutive high expression of chromosomal β-lactamase in *Pseudomonas aeruginosa* caused by a new insertion sequence (IS*1669*) located in *ampD*. Antimicrob. Agents Chemother. **46**:3406-3411.

(6) **Bert, F., C. Branger, and N. Lambert-Zechovsky.** 2002 Identification of PSE and OXA β-lactamase genes in *Pseudomonas aeruginosa* using PCR-restriction fragment length polymorphism. J. Antimicrob. Chemother. **50**:11-18.

(7) **Blagui, S. K., A. Achour, M. S. Abbassi, M. Bejaoui, A. Abdeladhim, and A. B. Hassen.** 2007. Nosocomial outbreak of OXA-18-producing *Pseudomonas aeruginosa* in Tunisia. Clin. Microbiol. Infect. **13**:794-800.

(8) **Bogaerts, P., C. Bauraing, A. Deplano, and Y. Glupczynski.** 2007. Emergence and dissemination of BEL-1-producing *Pseudomonas aeruginosa* isolates in Belgium. Antimicrob. Agents Chemother. **51**:1584-1585.

(9) **Bojorquez, D., M. Belei, S. F. Delira, S. Sholly, J. Mead, and M. E. Tolmasky.** 1998. Characterization of OXA-9, a β-lactamase encoded by the multiresistance transposon Tn*1331*. Cell. Mol. Biol. **44**:483-491.

(10) **Cantón, R., and T. M. Coque.** 2006. The CTX-M beta-lactamase pandemic. Curr. Opin. Microbiol. **9**:466-447.

(11) **Cardoso, O., A. F. Alves, and R. Leitao.** 2008. Metallo beta-lactamase VIM-2 in *Pseudomonas aeruginosa* isolates from a cystic fibrosis patient. Int. J. Antimicrob Agents. **31**:375-379.

(12) **Carlos, J., A. Beceiro, O. Gutierrez, S. Alberti, M. Garau, J. L. Perez, G. Bou, and A. Oliver.** 2008. Characterization of the Nex Metalo-beta-lactamase VIM-3 and its integron-borne gene from a *Pseudomonas aeruginosa* clinical isolates in Spain. Antimicrob. Agents Chemother. **52**:3589-3596.

(13) **Castanheira, M., R. E. Mendes, T. R. Walsh, A. C. Gales, and R. N. Jones.** 2004. Emergence of the extended-spectrum-lactamase GES-1 in a *Pseudomonas aeruginosa* strain from Brazil: report from the SENTRY Antimicrobial Surveillance Program. Antimicrob. Agents Chemother. **48**:2344-2345.

(14) **Castanheira, M., M. A. Toleman, R. N. Jones, F. J. Schmidt, and T. R. Walsh.** 2004. Molecular characterization of a β-lactamase gene, *bla*GIM-1, encoding a new subclass of metallo- beta- lactamase. Antimicrob. Agents Chemother. **48**:4654-4661.

(15) **Cavallo, J. D., P. Plésiat, G. Couetdic, F. Leblanc, R. Fabre, and Groupe d'Etude de la Résistance de *Pseudomonas aeruginosa* aux β-lactamines (GERPB).** 2002. Mechanisms of β-lactam resistance in *Pseudomonas aeruginosa*: prevalence of OprM-overproducing strains in a French multicentre study (1997). J. Antimicrob. Chemother. **50**:1039-1043.

(16) **Celenza, G., C. Pellegrini, M. Caccamo, B. Segatore, G. Amicosante, and M. Perilli.** 2006. Spread of bla_{CTX-M}-type and bla_{PER-2} β-lactamase genes in clinical isolates from Bolivian hospitals. J. Antimicrob. Chemother. **57**:975-978

(17) **Clinical and Laboratory Standards Institute.** 2009. Performance standards for antimicrobial susceptibility testing; 19th informational supplement M100-S18. Clinical and Laboratory Standards Institute, Baltimore, MD, USA.

(18) **Cornaglia, G., M. Akova., G. Amicosante, R. Canton, R. Cauda., J.D. Docquier, M. Edelstein, J.M. Fuzi, M. Galleni., H. Giamarell, M. Gniadkowski, R. Koncon, B. Libisch, F. Luzzara, V. Miriagou, F. Navarro, P. Nordmann, L. Pagani, L. Peixe, L. Poirel, M. Souli, E. Taconelli, A. Vatoupoulos, and G.M. Rossolini. ESCMID Study Group for Antimicrobial Resistance Surveillance (ESGARS).** 2007. Metallo-β-lactamases as emerging resistance determinants in Gram-negative pathogens: open issues. Int. J. Antimicrob. Agents. **29**:380-388.

(19) **Cornaglia, G. , A. Mazzariol, A. Lauretti, G. M. Rossolini, and R. Fontana**. 2000. Hospital outbreak of carbapenem-resistant *Pseudomonas aeruginosa* producing VIM-1, a novel transferable metallo β-lactamase. Clin. Infect. Dis. **31**:1119-1125.

(20) **Couture, F., J. Lachapelle, and R. C. Levesque.** 1992. Phylogeny of LCR-1 OXA-5 with class A class D β-lactamases. Mol. Microbiol. **6**:1693-1705.

(21) **Cunha, B. A.** 2002. *Pseudomonas aeruginosa*: resistance and therapy. Semin. Respir. Infect. **17**:231-239.

(22) **D'Agata, E. M C.** 2004. Rapidly rising prevalence of nosocomial multidrug-resistant, Gram-negative bacilli: a 9-year surveillance study. Infect. Control. Hosp. Epidemiol. **25**:842-846.

(23) **Danel, F., L. M. C. Hall, D. Gür, and D. M. Livermore.** 1995. OXA-14, another extended-spec-

trum variant of OXA-10 (PSE-2) β-lactamase from *Pseudomonas aeruginosa*. Antimicrob. Agents Chemother. **39**:1881-1884.

(24) **De Champs, C., L. Poirel, R. Bonnet, D. Sirot, C. Chanal, J. Sirot, and P. Nordmann.** 2002. Prospective survey of beta-lactamases produced by ceftazidime-resistant *Pseudomonas aeruginosa* in a French Hospital in 2000. Antimicrob. Agents Chemother. **46**:3031-3034.

(25) **Docquier, J. D., F. Luzzaro, G. Amicosante, A. Toniolo, and G. M. Rossolini.** 2001. Multidrug-resistant *Pseudomonas aeruginosa* producing PER-1 extended-spectrum serine-beta-lactamase and VIM-2 metallo-beta-lactamase. Emerg. Infect. Dis. **7**:910-911.

(26) **Dubois, V., C. Arpin, P. Noury, C. Andre, L. Coulange, and C. Quentin.** 2005. Prolonged outbreak of infection due to TEM-21-producing strains of *Pseudomonas aeruginosa* and enterobacteria in a nursing home. J. Clin. Microbiol. **43**:4129-4138.

(27) **Empel, J., K. Filczak, A. Mrówka, W. Hryniewicz, D. M. Livermore, and M. Gniadkowski.** 2007. Outbreak of *Pseudomonas aeruginosa* infections with PER-1 extended-spectrum β-lactamase in Warsaw, Poland: further evidence for an international clonal complex. J. Clin. Microbiol. **45**:2829-2834.

(28) **Gales, A. C., R. N. Jones, and H. S. Sader.** 2006. Global assessment of the antimicrobial activity of polymyxin B against 54731 clinical isolates of Gram-negative bacilli: report from the SENTRY antimicrobial surveillance programme (2001-2004). Clin. Microbiol. Infect. **12**:315-321.

(29) **Gales, A. C., L. C. Menezes, S. Silbert, and H. S. Sader.** 2003. Dissemination in distinct Brazilian regions of an epidemic carbapenem-resistant *Pseudomonas aeruginosa* producing SPM metallo-β-lactamase. J. Antimicrob. Chemother. **52**:699-702.

(30) **Gaynes, R., J. R. Edwards, and the National Nosocomial Infections Surveillance System.** 2005. Overview of nosocomial infections caused by Gram-negative bacilli. Clin. Infect. Dis. **41**:848-854.

(31) **Girlich, D., T. Naas, A. Leelaporn, L. Poirel, M. Fennewald, and P. Nordmann.** 2002. Nosocomial spread of the integron-located *veb-1*-like cassette encoding an extended-spectrum beta-lactamase in *Pseudomonas aeruginosa* in Thailand. Clin. Infect. Dis. **34**: 603-611.

(32) **Girlich, D., T. Naas, and P. Nordmann.** 2004. Biochemical characterization of the naturally occurring oxacillinase OXA-50 of *Pseudomonas aeruginosa*. Antimicrob. Agents Chemother. **48**:2043-2048.

(33) **Giske, C.G., L. Buaro, A. Sundsfjord, and B. Wretlind.** 2008. Alterations of porin, pumps, and penicillin-binding proteins in carbapenem-resistant clinical isolates of *Pseudomonas aeruginosa*. Microb. Drug Resist. **14**:23-30.

(34) **Giuliani, F., J. D. Docquier, M. L. Riccio, L. Pagani, and G. M. Rossolini.** OXA-46, a new class D β-lactamase of narrow substrate specificity encoded by a bla_{VIM-1}-containing integron from a *Pseudomonas aeruginosa* clinical isolates. Antimicrob. Agents Chemother. **49**:1973-1980.

(35) **Gutierrez, O., C. Juan, E. Cernado, F. Navarro, E. Bouza, P. Coll, J. L. Pérez, and A. Oliver.** 2007. Molecular epidemiology and mechanisms of carbapenem resistance in *Pseudomonas aeruginosa* isolates from Spanish hospitals. **51**:4329-4335.

(36) **Hirakata, Y., K. Izumikawa, T. Yamaguchi, H. Takemura, H. Tanaka, R. Yoshida, J. Matsuda, M. Nakano, K. Tomono, S. Maesaki, M. Kaku, Y. Yamada, S. Kamihira, and S. Kohno.** 1998. Rapid detection and evaluation of clinical characteristics of emerging multiple-drug-resistant gram-negative rods carrying the metallo-β-lactamase gene bla_{IMP}. Antimicrob. Agents Chemother. **42**:2006-2011.

(37) **Hocquet, D., C. Llanes, I. Patry, F. El Garch, and P. Plésiat.** 2004. Two efflux systems expressed simultaneously in clinical *Pseudomonas aeruginosa*. Pathol. Biol. **52**:465-461.

(38) **Hocquet, D., P. Nordmann, F. El Garch, L. Cabanne, and P. Plésiat.** 2006. Involvement of the MexXY-OprM efflux system in emergence of cefepime resistance in clinical strains of *Pseudomonas aeruginosa*. Antimicrob. Agents Chemother. **50**:1347-1351.

(39) **Hocquet, D., M. Roussel-Delvallez, J. D. Cavallo, and P. Plésiat.** 2007. MexAB-OprM- and MexXY-overproducing mutants are very prealent among clinical strains of *Pseudomonas aeruginosa* with reduced susceptibility to ticarcillin. Antimicrob. Agents Chemother. **51**:1582-1583.

(40) **Jeannot, K., S. Elsen, T. Köhler, I. Attree, C. Van Delden, and P. Plésiat.** 2008. Resistance and virulence of *Pseudomonas aeruginosa* clinical strains overproducing the MexCD-OprJ efflux pump. Antimicrob. Agents Chemother. **52**:2455-2462.

(41) **Karlowsky, J. A., D. C. Draghi, M. E. Jones, C. Thornsberry, I. R. Friedland, and D. F. Sahm.** 2003. Surveillance for antimicrobial susceptibility among clinical isolates of *Pseudomonas aeruginosa* and *Acinetobacter baumannii* from hospitalized patients in the United States, 1998 to 2001. Antimicrob. Agents Chemother. **47**:1681-1688.

(42) **Karlowsky, J. A., M. E. Jones, C. Thornsberry, A. T. Evangelista, Y. C. Yee, and D. F. Sahm** 2005. Stable antimicrobial susceptibility rates for clinical isolates of *Pseudomonas aeruginosa* from the 2001-2003 tracking resistance in the United States today surveillance studies. Clin. Infect. Dis. **40**:S89-S98.

(43) **Labuschagne, C. J., G. F. Weldhagen, M. M. Ehlers, and M. G. Dove,** 2008. Emergence of class 1 integron-associated GES-5 and GES-5-like extended-spectrum beta-lactamases in clinical isolates of *Pseudomonas aeruginosa* in South Africa. Int. J. Antimicrob. Agents **31**:527-530.

(44) **Lauretti, L., M. L. Riccio, A. Mazzariol, G. Cornaglia, G. Amicosante, R. Fontana, and G. M. Rossolini.** 1999. Cloning and characterization of bla_{VIM}, a new integron-borne metallo-β-lactamase gene from a *Pseudomonas aeruginosa* clinical isolate. Antimicrob. Agents Chemother. **43**:1584-1590.

(45) **Livermore, D. M.** 2001. Of *Pseudomonas*, porins, pumps and carbapenems. J. Antimicrob. Chemother. **47**:247-250.

(46) **Livermore, D. M.** 2002. Multiple mechanisms of antimicrobial resistance in *Pseudomonas aeruginosa*: our worst nightmare? Antimicrob. Resist. **34**:634-640.

(47) **Maltezou, H. C.** 2009. Metallo-beta-lactamases in Gram-negative bacteria: introducing the era of pan-

resistance? Int. J. Antimicrob. Agents. **33**:405-e1-405e7.

(48) **Martin, A.F., A. P. Zavascki, P. B. Gaspareto, and A. L. Barth.** 2007. Dissemination of *Pseudomonas aeruginosa* producing SPM-1-like and IMP-1-like metallo-beta-lactamases in hospitals from Southern Brazil. Infection. **35**:457-460.

(49) **Masuda, N., E. Sakagawa, S. Ohya, N. Gotoh, H. Tsujimoto, and T. Nishino.** 2000. Substrate specificities of MexAB-OprM, MexCD-OprJ, and MexXY-oprM efflux pumps in *Pseudomonas aeruginosa*. Antimicrob. Agents Chemother. **44**:3322-3327.

(50) **Medeiros, A. A., M. Cohenford, and G. A. Jacoby.** 1985. Five novel plasmid-determined β-lactamases. Antimicrob. Agents Chemother. **27**:715-719.

(51) **Mesaros, N., P. Nordmann, P. Plésiat, M. Roussel-Delvallez, J. Van Eldere, Y. Glupczynski, Y. Van Laethem, F. Jacobs, P. Lebecque, A. Malfroot, P. M. Tulkens, and F. Van Bambecke.** 2007. *Pseudomonas aeruginosa*: resistance and therapeutic options at the turn of the new millennium. Clin. Microbiol. Infect. **13**:560-578.

(52) **Naas, T., and P. Nordmann.** 1999. OXA-type beta-lactamases. Curr. Pharm. Design **5**:865-879.

(53) **Naas, T., L. Poirel, and P. Nordmann.** 2008. Minor extended-spectrum beta-lactamases. Clin. Microbiol. Infect. **20**:42-52.

(54) **Neonakis, I. K., E. V. Scoulica, S. K. Dimitriou, A. I. Gikas, and Y. J. Tselentis.** 2003. Molecular epidemiology of extended-spectrum β-lactamases produced by clinical isolates in a university hospital in Greece; detection of SHV-5 in *Pseudomonas aeruginosa* and prevalence of SHV-12. Microb. Drug Resist. **9**:161-165.

(55) **Nicasio, A. M., J. L. Kuti, and D. P. Nicolau.** 2008. The current stage of multidrug-resistant Gram-negative bacilli in North America. Pharmacother. **28**:235-249.

(56) **Nordmann, P., G. Cuzon, and T. Naas**. 2009. The real threat of *Klebsiella pneumoniae* carbapenemase-producing bacteria. Lancet Infect. Dis. **9**:228-236.

(57) **Nordmann, P., and M. Guibert** 1998. Extended-spectrum β-lactamases in *Pseudomonas aeruginosa*. J. Antimicrob. Chemother. **42**:128-131.

(58) **Nordmann, P., and T. Naas.** 1994. Sequence analysis of PER-1 extended-spectrum beta-lactamase from *Pseudomonas aeruginosa* and comparison with class A beta-lactamases. Antimicrob. Agents Chemother. **38**:104-114.

(59) **Pagani, L., E. Mantengoli, R. Migliavacca, E. Nucleo, S. Pollini, M. Spalla, R. Daturi, E. Romero, and G. M. Rossolini.** 2004. Multifocal detection of multidrug-resistant *Pseudomonas aeruginosa* producing the PER-1 extended-spectrum beta-lactamase in Northern Italy. J. Clin. Microbiol. **42**:2523-2529.

(60) **Paterson, D. L.** 2006. The epidemiological profile of infections with multidrug-resistant *Pseudomonas aeruginosa* and *Acinetobacter* species. Clin. Infect. Dis. **43**:S43-S48.

(61) **Philippon, A., A. Thabaut, and P. Névot.** 1995. *Pseudomonas aeruginosa* et β-lactamines pp.103-110. *In* P. Courvalin, F. Goldstein, A. Philippon, J. Sirot (ed.), L'antibiogramme, MPC- videom, Paris, Bruxelles.

(62) **Philippon, L. N., T. Naas, A. T. Bouthors, V. Barakett, and P. Nordmann.** 1997. OXA-18, a class D clavulanic acid-inhibited extended-spectrum beta-lactamase from *Pseudomonas aeruginosa*. Antimicrob. Agents Chemother. **41**:2188-2195.

(63) **Picao, R., L. Poirel, A. C. Gales, and P. Nordmann.** 2009. Further identification of CTX-M-2 extended-spectrum β-lactamase in *Pseudomonas aeruginosa*. Antimicrob. Agents Chemother. **53**:2225-2226.

(64) **Poirel, L., L. Brinas L., Verlinde A., L. Ide, and P. Nordmann.** 2005. BEL-1, a novel clavulanic acid-inhibited extended-spectrum beta-lactamase, and the class 1 integron In120 in *Pseudomonas aeruginosa*. Antimicrob. Agents Chemother. **49**:3743-3748.

(65) **Poirel, L., P. Gerome, C. De Champs, J. Stephanazzi, T. Naas, and P. Nordmann.** 2002. Integron-located *oxa-32* gene cassette encoding an extended-spectrum variant of OXA-2 beta-lactamase from *Pseudomonas aeruginosa*. Antimicrob. Agents Chemother. **46**:566-569.

(66) **Poirel, L., I. Le Thomas, T. Naas, A. Karim, and P. Nordmann.** 2000. Biochemical sequence analyses of GES-1, a novel class A extended-spectrum beta-lactamase, and the class 1 integron In52 from *Klebsiella pneumoniae*. Antimicrob. Agents Chemother. **44**:622-632.

(67) **Poirel, L., T. Naas, D. Nicolas, L. Collet, S. Bellais, J. D. Cavallo, and P. Nordmann**. 2000. Characterization of VIM-2, a carbapenem-hydrolyzing metallo-β-lactamase and its plasmid- and integron-borne gene from a *Pseudomonas aeruginosa* clinical isolate in France. Antimicrob. Agents Chemother. **44**:891-897.

(68) **Poirel, L., T. Naas, and P. Nordmann.** 2008. Genetic support of extended-spectrum beta-lactamases. Clin. Microbiol. Infect. **14**:75-81.

(69) **Poirel, L., J. D. Pitout, and P. Nordmann.** 2007. Carbapenemases, molecular diversity clinical consequences. Future Microbiol. **2**:501-512.

(70) **Poirel, L., G. F. Weldhagen, C. De Champs, and P. Nordmann.** 2002. A nosocomial outbreak of *Pseudomonas aeruginosa* isolates expressing the extended-spectrum β-lactamase GES-2 in South Africa. J. Antimicrob. Chemother. **49**:561-565.

(71) **Poirel L., G. F. Weldhagen, T. Naas, C. De Champs, M. G. Dove, and P. Nordmann.** 2001. GES-2, a class A beta-lactamase from *Pseudomonas aeruginosa* with increased hydrolysis of imipenem. Antimicrob. Agents Chemother. **45**:2598-2603.

(72) **Poole, K.** 2004. Efflux-mediated multiresistance in Gram-negative bacteria. Clin. Microbiol. Infect. **10**:12-26.

(73) **Rodriguez-Martinez, J. M., L. Poirel, and P. Nordmann.** 2009. Extended-spectrum cephalosporinases in *Pseudomonas aeruginosa*. Antimicrob. Agents Chemother. **53**:1766-1771.

(74) **Rossolini, G. M., and E. Mantenggoli.** 2005. Treatment and control of severe infections caused by multiresistant *Pseudomonas aeruginosa*. Clin. Microbiol. Infect. **11**:856-857.

(75) **Rossolini, G. M., and E. Mantengoli.** 2008. Antimicrobial resistance in Europe and its potential impact on empirical therapy. Clin. Microbiol. Infect. **14**:2-8.

(76) **Rossolini, G.M., E. Mantengoli, J. D. Docquier, R. A. Musmanno, and G. Coratza.** 2007.

Epidemiology of infections caused by multiresistant Gram-negatives: ESBLs, MBLS, panresistant strains. New Microbiologica. **30**:332-339.

(77) **Sader, H. S., A. O. Reis, S. Silbert, and A. C. Gales.** 2005. IMPs, VIMs and SPMs: the diversity of metallo-β-lactamases produced by carbapenem-resistant *Pseudomonas aeruginosa* in a Brazilian hospital. Clin. Microbiol. Infect. **11**:73-76.

(78) **Sambrook, J., E. F. Fritsch, and T. Maniatis.** 2001. Molecular cloning: a laboratory manual, 2nd ed. Cold Spring Harbor Laboratory Press, Cold Spring Harbor. N.Y.

(79) **Sanschagrin, F., N. Bejaoui, and R. C. Lévesque.** 1998. Structure of CARB-4 and AER-1 carbenicillin-hydrolyzing beta-lactamases. Antimicrob. Agents Chemother. **42**:1966-1972.

(80) **Sanschagrin, F., F. Couture, and R. C. Lévesque.** 1995. Primary structure of OXA-3 phylogeny of oxacillin-hydrolyzing class D β-lactamases. Antimicrob. Agents Chemother. **39**:887-893.

(81) **Senda, K., Y. Arakawa, K. Nakashima, H. Ito, S. Ichiyama, K. Shimokata, N. Kato, and M. Ohta.** 1996. Multifocal outbreaks of metallo-β-lactamase producing *Pseudomonas aeruginosa* resistant to broad-spectrum-β-lactams, including carbapenems. Antimicrob. Agents Chemother. **40**:349-353.

(82) **Souli, M., I. Galani, and H. Giamarellou.** 2008. Emergence of extensively drug-resistant and pan-drug-resistant Gram-negative bacilli in Europe. Euro. Surveill. **13**:1-11

(83) **Strateva, T., V. Ouzounova-Raykova, B. Markova, A. Todorova, Y. Marteva-Proevska, and I. Mitov.** 2007. Widespread detection of VEB-1 type extended-spectrum β-lactamases among nosocomial ceftazidime-resistant *Pseudomonas aeruginosa* isolates in Sofia, Bulgaria. J. Chemother. **19**:140-145.

(84) **Toleman, M. A., K. Rolston, R. N. Jones, and T. R. Walsh.** 2003. Molecular biochemical characterization of OXA-45, an extended-spectrum class 2D β-lactamase in *Pseudomonas aeruginosa*. Antimicrob. Agents Chemother. **47**:2859-2863.

(85) **Toleman, M. A., K. Rolston, R. N. Jones, and T. R. Walsh.** 2004. bla_{VIM-7}, an evolutionarily distinct metallo-β-lactamase gene in a *Pseudomonas aeruginosa* isolate from the United States. Antimicrob. Agents Chemother. **48**:329-332.

(86) **Tirado, M., C. Roy, C. Segura, R. Reig, M. Hermida, and A. Foz.** 1986. Incidence of strains producing plasmid determined β-lactamases among carbenicillin resistant *Pseudomonas aeruginosa*. J. Antimicrob. Chemother. **18**:453-458.

(87) **Unal, S., R. Masterton, and H. Goossens.** 2004. Bacteraemia in Europe-antimicrobial susceptibility data from the MYSTIC surveillance programme. Int. J. Antimicrob. Agent. **23**-155-163.

(88) **Vedel, G.** 2005. Simple method to determine β-lactam resistance phenotypes in *Pseudomonas aeruginosa* using the disc agar diffusion test. J. Antimicrob. Chemother **56**:657-664.

(89) **Villegas, M. V., K. Lolans, A. Correa, J. N. Kattan, J. A. Lopez, and J. P. Quinn.** 2007. First identification of *Pseudomonas aeruginosa* isolates producing a KPC-type carbapenem-hydrolyzing β-lactamase. Antimicrob. Agents Chemother. **51**:1553-1555.

(90) **Walsh, T. R.** 2008. Clinically significant carbapenemases: an update. Curr. Opin. Infect. Dis. **21**:367-371.

(91) **Walsh, T. R., M. A. Toleman, L. Poirel, and P. Nordmann**. 2005. Metallo-beta-lactamases: the quiet before the storm? Clin. Microbiol. Rev. **18**:306-325.

(92) **Wang, C., P. Cai, D. Chang, and Z. Mi.** 2006. A *Pseudomonas aeruginosa* isolate producing the GES-5 extended-spectrum beta-lactamase. Antimicrob. Agents Chemother. **57**:1261-1262.

(93) **Weldhagen, G. F., L. Poirel, and P. Nordmann.** 2003. Ambler class A extended-spectrum beta-lactamases in *Pseudomonas aeruginosa*: novel developments and clinical impact. Antimicrob. Agents Chemother. **47**:2385-2389.

(94) **Woodford, N., J. Zhand, M. E. Kaufmann, S. Yarde, M. Del Mar Tomas, C. Faris, M. S. Vardhan, S. Dawson, S. L. Cotterill, and D. M. Livermore.** 2008. Detection of *Pseudomonas aeruginosa* isolates producing VEB-type extended-spectrum beta-lactamases in the United Kingdom. J. Antimicrob. Chemother. **62**:1265-1268.

(95) **Zhanel, G. G., M. DeCorby, N. Laing, B. Weshnoweski, R. Vashisht, F. Tailor, K. A. Nichol, A. Wierzbowski, P. J. Baudry, J. A. karlowsky, P. Lagacé-Wiens, A. Walkty, M. McCraken, M. R. Mulvey, J. Johnson, The Canadian Antimicrobial Resistance Alliance (CARA), and D. J. Hoban.** 2008. Antimicrobial-resistant pathogens in intensive care units in Canada: results to the Canadian National Intensive Care Unit (CAN-ICU) Study, 2005-2006. Antimicrob. Agents Chemother. **52**:1430-1437.

Chapter 15. β-LACTAM RESISTANCE IN OTHER NON-FERMENTATIVE STRICT AEROBIC GRAM-NEGATIVE BACILLI

Alain PHILIPPON

INTRODUCTION

The nonfermentative strictly aerobic Gram-negative bacilli are an extremely diverse group, as evidenced firstly by the multitude of names given to certain species and, secondly, by the number of genera and species currently identified within the order Burkholderiales in particular (class betaproteobacteria) (Table 1). Recent progress in taxonomy, mostly through molecular approaches, has resulted in the continual emergence of new designations. These taxonomic upheavals are confusing for clinicians and even microbiologists, who periodically have to go back and learn the correct terminology (http://www.ncbi.nlm.nih.gov/). For example, the genus *Achromobacter*, renamed *Alcaligenes*, was recently subdivided, reinstating the genus name *Achromobacter* to species such as *A. xylosoxydans spp xylosoxydans* and *A. piechaudii*, while the genus *Alcaligenes* was maintained for several species including *A. faecalis*.

Several factors may account for the emergence of certain species (Table 1), including their high nutritional versatility (processing up to 160 hydrocarbon substrates), which is consistent with the large number of ecological niches they inhabit and especially their intrinsic multi-antibiotic resistance (including β-lactams and aminoglycosides) and antiseptics.

These bacteria can be encountered in the hospital environment, where they are often responsible for endemic or epidemic infections through their presence in various fluids like saline or glucose, or other solutions such as parenteral nutrition, heparin, eosin, chlorhexidine, dialysis fluid, contact lens storage solution, etc. They affect inpatients, often those who have been in hospital for several days or weeks, with an underlying disease. Finally, many of these patients are catheterized or intubated, these devices providing a portal of entry for bacteria. Infection should be distinguished from colonization (of the skin for example) or from transient presence of bacteria (pseudobacteremia). From an epidemiological point of view, the existence of a common source of contamination will frequently result in the sudden simultaneous onset of a number of cases.

The treatment strategies are limited because of resistance to antibiotics including β-lactams, the

Table 1. Main bacterial genera and species studied

Group	Genus	Species
betaproteobacteria	*Achromobacter*	*A. denitrificans, A. xylosoxydans*
betaproteobacteria	*Alcaligenes*	*A. faecalis*
betaproteobacteria	*Bordetella*	*B. bronchiseptica*
betaproteobacteria	*Burkholderia*	*B. cepacia, B. pseudomallei, B. mallei*
CFB group	*Chryseobacterium*	*C. indologenes*
betaproteobacteria	*Delftia*	*D. acidovorans*
CFB group	*Elizabethkingia*	*E. meningoseptica*
CFB group	*Empedobacter*	*E. breve*
CFB group	*Flavobacterium*	*F. johnsoniae*
CFB group	*Myroides*	*M. odoratus, M. odoratimimus*
alphaproteobacteria	*Ochrobactrum*	*O. anthropi*
betaproteobacteria	*Ralstonia*	*R. pickettii*
gammaproteobacteria	*Shewanella*	*S. putrefaciens, S. oneidensis*
gammaproteobacteria	*Stenotrophomonas*	*S. maltophilia*

most resistant species being *Chryseobacterium meningosepticum*, *Chryseobacterium indologenes*, *Burkholderia cepacia*, and *Stenotrophomonas maltophilia*. Conversely, the most susceptible species, which are isolated more rarely, are *Alcaligenes faecalis* and *Delftia acidovorans* (Fig. 1).

From 1985, the existence of at least four natural β-lactam resistance phenotypes in enterobacteria which are important to be aware of in interpretative reading, led to research to characterize natural resistance phenotypes in this bacterial group. Furthermore, curious synergies were observed between a third generation cephalosporin or a monobactam (aztreonam) and a combination of amoxicillin or ticarcillin and clavulanic acid, suggesting the existence of a chromosomally encoded extended-spectrum β-lactamase (ESBL). Antibiotic susceptibility testing by disk diffusion, sometimes combined with multivariate analysis, has been used to characterize the resistance phenotypes of several species, thereby assisting in their identification (Fig. 2) (Susceptibility patterns of non fermentative Gram-negative bacilli, Intern. Congr. of Chemother., Stockholm, July 1993). Several natural resistance phenotypes were later validated by the Comité de l'Antibiogramme de la Société Française de Microbiologie (CA-SFM) from 1995 onwards, then in 2008 by the European Committee on Antimicrobial Susceptibility Testing (http://eucast.www137.server1.mensemedia.net/).

Methodological advances from 1997 onwards have improved our understanding of enzyme-mediated resistance, in particular that responsible for intrinsic β-lactam resistance, with the characterization of new species-specific chromosomal β-lactamases belonging to the four Ambler classes A, B, C, and D. The chromosomal β-lactamases that have been identified within this heterogeneous group include class A BPS, BOR-1, CGA-1, PenA, PENA-1 and L2, class B BlaB, CGB-1, GOB-1, IND-1, MUS-1 and TUS-1, class C OCH-1, and class D OXA-22, -54, -55, -57, -59, etc. (Fig. 3).

Finally, PCR and sequencing have enabled the identification of β-lactamases involved in acquired resistance, such as VEB-1, IMP-1, IMP-10, VIM-1, etc.

However, the other suspected mechanisms of resistance, particularly of intrinsic resistance, such as impermeability and efflux have not yet been adequately explored.

MAIN PHENOTYPES

The main β-lactam-susceptible phenotype observed *in vitro* before interpretation varies considerably between species (Table 2). β-lactam resistance may be associated with resistance to other antibiotics, such as aminoglycosides and polymyxins. This bacterial group is frequently

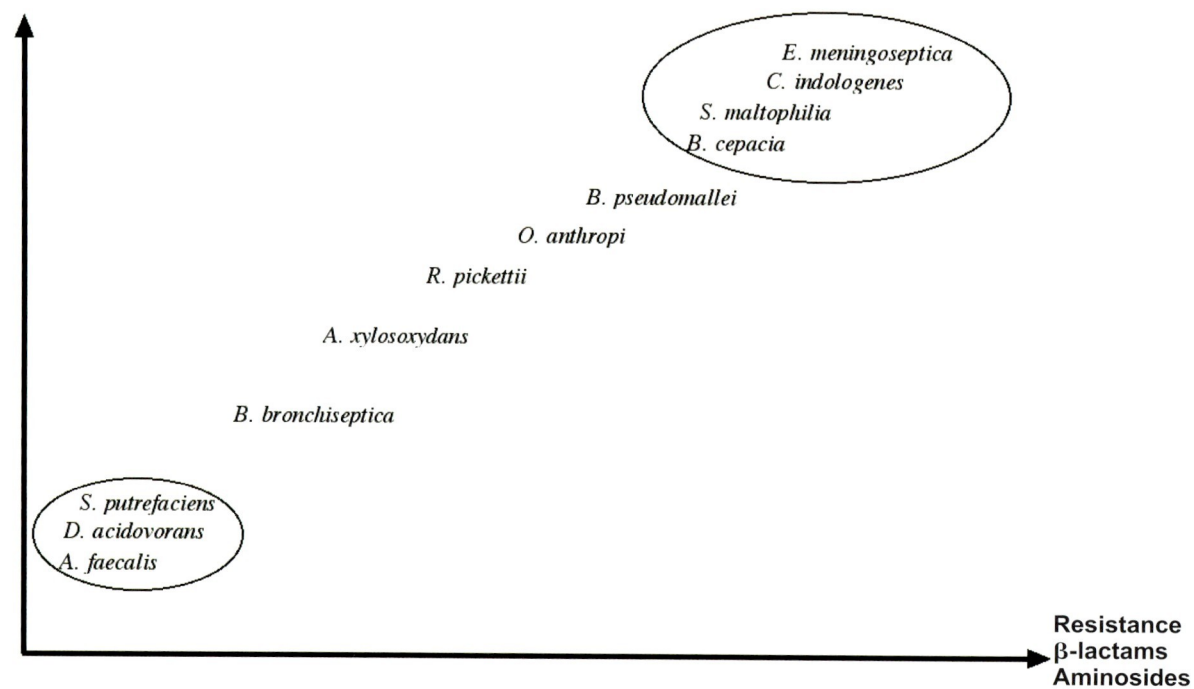

Fig. 1. Non fermentative Gram-negative bacilli: antibiotic susceptibility

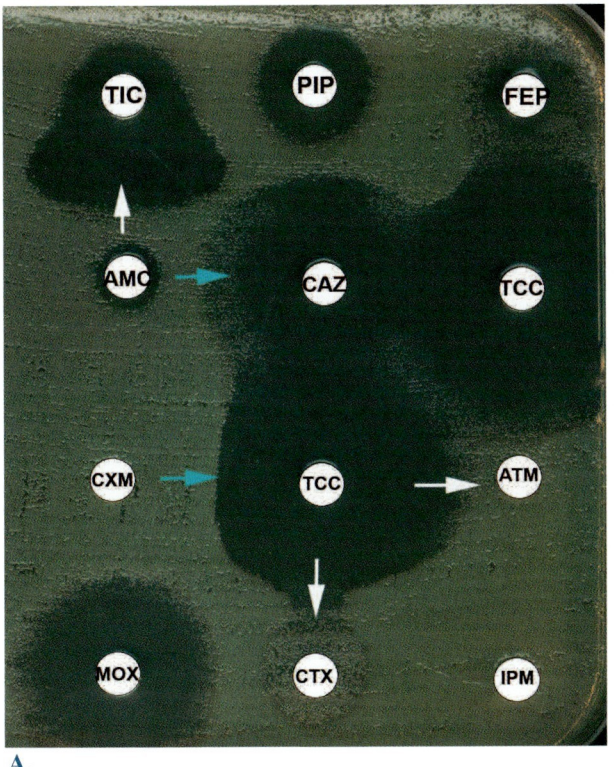 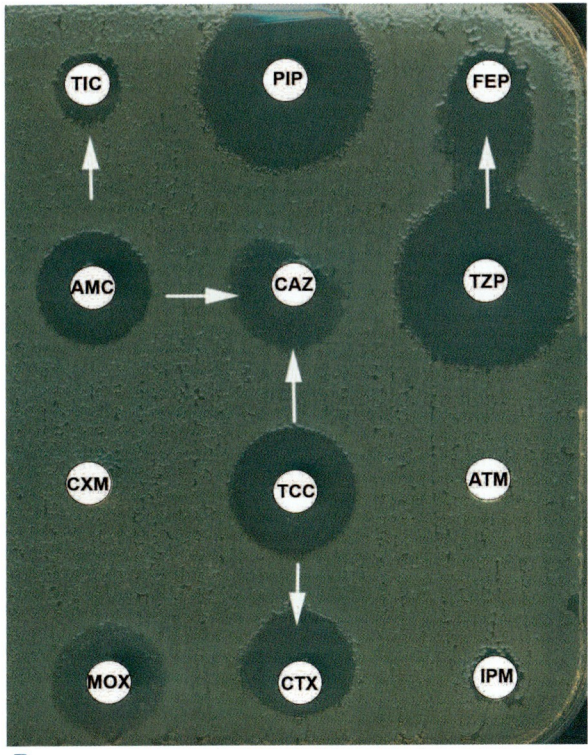

A. B.

Fig. 2. Antimicrobial susceptibility testing by disk diffusion: detection of synergy (blue arrow) and antagonism (white arrow)
A *Stenotrophomnas maltophilia*
AMC, amoxicillin + clavulanic acid; ATM, aztreonam; CAZ, ceftazidime; CTX, cefotaxime; CXM, cefuroxime; FEP, cefepime; FOX, cefoxitin; IPM, imipenem; MOX, latamoxef; PIP, piperacillin; TCC, ticarcillin + clavulanic acid; TIC, ticarcillin.
B. *Elizabethkingia (Chryseobacterium) meningoseptica*.
AMC, amoxicillin + clavulanic acid; ATM, aztreonam; CAZ, ceftazidime; CTX, cefotaxime; CXM, cefuroxime; FEP, cefepime; FOX, cefoxitin; IPM, imipenem; MOX, latamoxef; PIP, piperacillin; TCC, ticarcillin + clavulanic acid; TIC, ticarcillin; TZP, piperacillin + tazobactam.

characterized by reduced susceptibility to the following β-lactam antibiotics: first and second generation cephalosporins, mecillinam, aztreonam, and ertapenem, clearly distinguishing them from the natural susceptibility patterns of the other Gram-negative bacilli, the enterobacteria and *Pseudomonas aeruginosa*.

METHODS, ANTIBIOTICS TO BE STUDIED AND BREAKPOINTS

The following should be borne in mind: reported variation in susceptibility for the bacterial species being tested, the method of determination (slow, rapid), the growth medium used (Mueller-Hinton, Isosensitest), the concentration of certain ions in the medium, and finally the incubation temperature (22, 40, 46, 75, 93). Unfortunately, the expert committees (the CA-SFM, the BSAC (British Society for Antimicrobial Chemotherapy)

and the CLSI (Clinical and Laboratory Standards Institute) for example) do not always recommend the same media. In the absence of new arguments, Mueller-Hinton broth (cation-adjusted) would be the preferred choice, using the same methodology as for an enterobacterium (inoculum, temperature, incubation time). The only notable difference concerns the choice of method, for example disk diffusion or determination of the MIC. Disk diffusion is not recommended for all antibiotics but it can be of taxonomic value. The growth of many species in this group is suboptimal at 35-37°C. Therefore, determination of the MIC will be necessary for certain antibiotics that are useful for treatment. A dilution method should therefore be used, because disk diffusion leads to major interpretive errors, as illustrated in Fig. 4 (93). However, MIC determination (broth microdilution, agar dilution, or E-Test®) can show notable differences (Table 3) (40). Finally, the CLSI has only issued recommendations on which antibiotics to test (β-lactams in par-

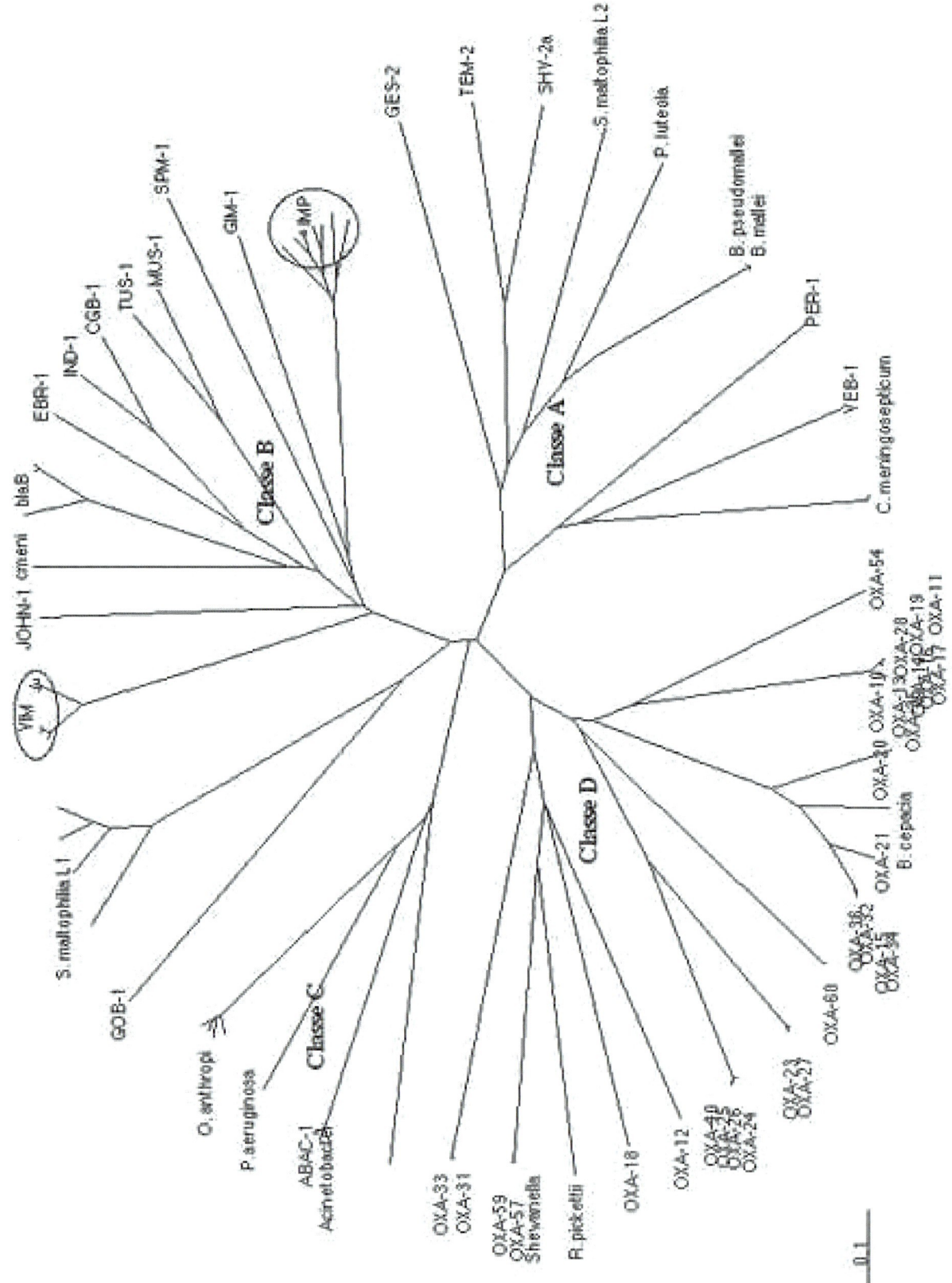

Fig. 3. Alignment of one hundred sequences of β-lactamases from nonfermentative strictly aerobic Gram-negative bacilli.

Table 2. Main resistance phenotypes of the nonfermentative strictly aerobic bacteria determined by diffusion

Species	Antibiotic											
	AMX[a]	AMC	FOX	TIC	TCC	PIP	CTX	CAZ	ATM	MOX	IMP	CS
A. faecalis	I/S[b]	S[c]	S	S	S[c]	S	S	S	I/S	S	S	S
A. xylosoxydans	I/S	S[c]	R	S	S	S	R	S/I	R	S/I	S	S
B. cepacia[d]	R	R	S	R	R	S	I/R	S	R	R	R	R
B. pseudomallei	R	S[c]	R	R	S[d]	S	I	S	I/R		S	R
B. bronchiseptica	I/R	I/R	R	S	S	S	R	S/I	R	S	S	S
E. meningosepticum	R	I/R	S/I	R	R	S	I/R	R	R	I/R	R	R
D. acidovorans	R	S[c]	S[e]	I/R	S[c]	S	S	S	S/I	S	S	R
O. anthropi	R	R	R	R	R	R	R	R	R	S	S	S
S. maltophilia	R	R	R	R	S[c]	R	R	S/I	I/R	S	R	R

[a] AMC, amoxicillin + clavulanic acid; AMX, amoxicillin; ATM, aztreonam; CAZ, ceftazidime; CS, colistin; CTX, cefotaxime; FOX, cefoxitin; IMP, imipenem; MOX, latamoxef; PIP, piperacillin; TCC, ticarcillin + clavulanic acid; TIC, ticarcillin.
[b] I, intermediate; R, resistant; S, susceptible.
[c] S, synergy
[d] Excellent susceptibility (diameter of inhibition zone > 35mm).
[e] Susceptibility to sulbactam.

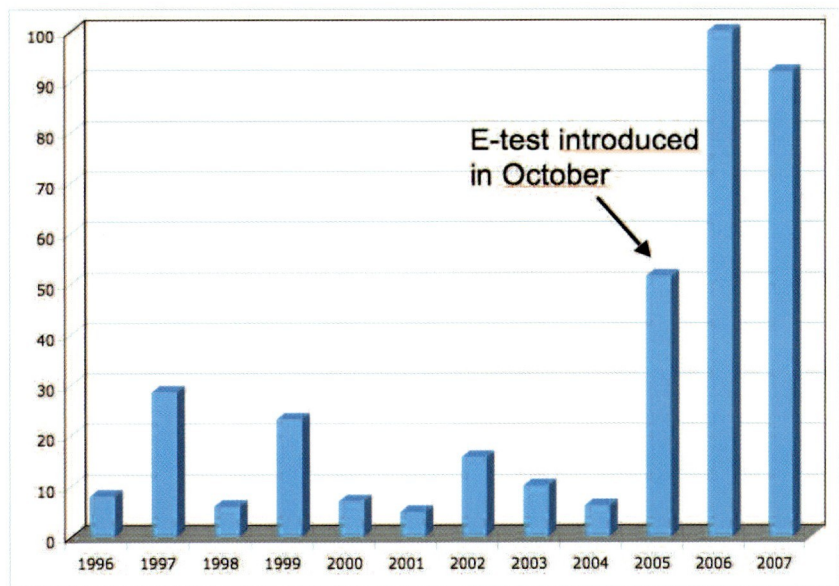

Fig. 4. *Burkholderia pseudomallei*: variation in susceptibility to co-trimoxazole depending on the method.

ticular) for a few species including *S. maltophilia*, *B. cepacia*, *B. mallei,* and *B. pseudomallei* (Table 4) (21). In the majority of cases, the MIC will need to be determined directly, because disk diffusion is not recommended. However, the EUCAST (European Committee on Antimicrobial Susceptibility testing) has been publishing interpretive rules since 2008 for five species (*A. xylosoxydans*, *B. cepacia* complex, *C. meningosepticum*, *O. anthropi*, and *S. maltophilia*) (Table 5) [http://www.srga.org/eucastwt/MICTAB/index.html]. For example, ceftazidime should be interpreted as being inactive in the latter species.

Table 3. MICs of antibiotics against *Burkholderia mallei*

Antibiotic	MIC (µg/ml) determined by			
	Broth dilution		E-test®	
	50%	90%	50%	90%
Ampicillin	64	64	4	6
Amoxicillin + clavulanic acid (2:1)	2	4	0.25	0.25
Piperacillin	4	8	0.25	0.38
Cefuroxime	64	64	3	6
Cefoxitin	32	32	8	16
Ceftriaxone	32	32	3	12
Ceftriaxone	32	32	3	12
Ceftazidime	2	4	0.25	0.5
Aztreonam	32	32	4	12
Imipenem	0.12	0.25	0.094	0.125
Gentamicin	0.5	0.5	0.064	0.094
Amikacin	1	2	0.5	0.5
Ofloxacin	1	8	0.5	1
Ciprofloxacin	0.5	1	0.12	0.25
Doxycycline	<0.3	0.12	0.23	0.32
Azithromycin	0.5	1	0.25	0.5
Co-trimoxazole	16	32	0.032	0.125
Chloramphenicol	16	32	3	8

Table 4. Antibiotics to test according to bacterial species (CLSI guidelines)

Antibiotic	Bacterial species				
	S. maltophila	B. cepacia	B. mallei	B. pseudomallei	Other[a]
Amoxicillin + CLA[b]			+[c]		+[c]
Ticarcillin + CLA	+[c]	+[c]			+[c]
Piperacillin					+[c]
Piperacillin + TAZ[b]					+[c]
Cefotaxime					+[c]
Ceftriaxone					+[c]
Ceftazidime	+[c]	+	+[c]	+[c]	+[c]
Aztreonam					+[c]
Imipenem			+[c]	+[c]	+[c]
Meropenem		+			+[c]
Gentamicin					+[c]
Tobramycin					+[c]
Tetracycline			+[c]	+[c]	+[c]
Doxycycline			+[c]	+[c]	
Minocycline	+	+			
Ciprofloxacin					+[c]
Ofloxacin					
or Lomefloxacin					+[c]
Norfloxacin					+[c]
Levofloxacin	+	+[c]			+[c]
Co-trimoxazole	+	+		+[c]	+[c]
Sulfafurazole					+[c]
Chloramphenicol	+[c]	+[c]			+[c]

[a] Other species of nonfermentative Gram-negative bacilli.
[b] CLA, clavulanic acid (2 µg/ml); TAZ, tazobactam (4 µg/ml).
[c] No critical diameters, determine the MIC.

Table 5. Interpretative rules according to bacterial species proposed by EUCAST

Antibiotic	A. xylosoxydans	B. cepacia	C. meningosepticum	O. anthropi	S. maltophilia
Ampicillin	R[a]	R	R	R	R
Amoxicillin + CLA[b]		R		R	R
Ticarcillin		R	R	R	R
Ticarcillin + CLA		R	R	R	
Piperacillin				R	R
Piperacillin + TAZ[b]				R	R
Cefazolin		R	R	R	R
tCefotaxime	R		R	R	R
Ceftriaxone	R		R	R	R
Ceftazidime	R		R	R	R
Ertapenem	R	R	R	R	R
Imipenem		R	R		R
Meropenem			R		R
Aminoglycosides		R			
Ciprofloxacin		R			
Chloramphenicol		R			
Trimethoprim		R			
Fosfomycin		R			
Tetracyclines/Tigecycline					
Polymyxin B/Colistin		R	R		

[a] R, resistant.
[b] CLA, clavulanic acid (2 µg/ml); TAZ, tazobactam (4 µg/ml).

Stenotrophomonas maltophilia

S. maltophilia (formerly *Pseudomonas* and later *Xanthomonas*) was characterized in 1981. It is a ubiquitous bacterium whose isolation in hospital practice has become much more frequent in recent years, particularly in nosocomial infections in immunosuppressed or vulnerable subjects (28). This opportunistic nosocomial (and more rarely community-acquired) bacterium (89) is weakly pathogenic and has an unusual aptitude to adhere (pili/fimbriae) and therefore to persist (23). Its "final" designation was attributed in 1996, and derives from the small number of substrates it uses («steno» and «troph»). It is the third most commonly isolated species of the strictly aerobic Gram-negative bacilli, after *P. aeruginosa* and *A. baumannii*.

Susceptible phenotype

One of the reasons for emergence is natural resistance to many antibiotics, such as aminoglycosides and β-lactams, including broad-spectrum penicillins such as ticarcillin, first and second generation cephalosporins, cefotaxime, and imipenem. This species is naturally more resistant to antibiotics than *P. aeruginosa* and *A. baumannii*.

Table 6 shows the activity of antibiotics against *S. maltophilia*. The *in vitro* susceptibility of the organism is increased by the combinations ticarcillin/clavulanic acid and especially trimethoprim/sulfamethoxazole, certain fluoroquinolones, and tetracyclines such as doxycycline. Multiple β-lactam resistance in disk diffusion rapidly guides the diagnosis towards this species (Fig. 5). In addition to resistance to various β-lactams including imipenem, the diamond-shaped image around the ticarcillin-clavulanic acid disk is characteristic firstly of synergy between ticarcillin and clavulanic acid, and secondly of antagonism between cefuroxime and ticarcillin/clavulanic acid (induction) suggesting the production of two β-lactamases.

Resistance phenotypes and mechanisms

The characterization of distinct β-lactam resistance phenotypes may be explained by variations in the expression of the two inducible chromosomal β-lactamases, L1 and L2, probably due to mutations, along with one or more permeability- or efflux-based mechanisms, which can be combined in several ways in different mutants (Table 7).

The L1 β-lactamase (BlaS or L1) is a chromosomal inducible zinc-enzyme with activity against a broad spectrum of β-lactams including peni-

Table 6. MICs (µg/ml) of antibiotics against *Stenotrophomonas maltophilia*

β-lactam	MIC	Other antibiotic	MIC
Ampicillin	> 16	Kanamycin	>64
Ampicillin + SUL[a]	16	Tobramycin	>64
Amoxicillin	> 16	Gentamicin	>64
Amoxicillin + CLA[a]	> 16	Netilmicin	>64
Ticarcillin	8-128	Amikacin	>64
Ticarcillin + CLA	4-16	Nalidixic acid	8-16
Piperacillin	16	Pefloxacin	4
Piperacillin + TAZ[a]	32-128	Norfloxacin	>8
Cefalotin	> 64	Ofloxacin	1-2
Ceftibuten	8-16	Ciprofloxacin	2
Cefamandole	> 64	Gatifloxacin	0.5
Cefuroxime	> 64	Levofloxacin	1
Cefoxitin	> 64	Clinafloxacin	0.25
Cefoperazone	2-8	Moxifloxacin	0.25
Cefotaxime	>16	Levofloxacin	1
Ceftazidime	2-8	Tetracycline	8-16
Cefepime	> 32	Doxycycline	2
Latamoxef	2	Minocycline	0.25-0.5
Aztreonam	>32	Tigecycline	0.5
Imipenem	>16	Sulfamethoxazole	2
Meropenem	>16	Trimethoprim	R[b]
Doripenem	>16	Co-trimoxazole	0.25-0.5
Ertapenem	> 8	Chloramphenicol	8-16
		Fosfomycin	64
		Polymyxin B	2
		Colistin	2
		Rifampicin	8

[a] CLA, clavulanic acid (2 µg/ml); SUL, sulbactam (8 µg/ml); TAZ, tazobactam (4 µg/ml).
[b] R, resistant.

cillins, third generation cephalosporins, and imipenem, belonging to class B (metallo-enzyme); it is therefore insensitive to clavulanic acid but is inhibited by both dipicolinic acid and EDTA (65).

The L2 β-lactamase is a chromosomal inducible class A (and therefore clavulanic acid-inhibited) enzyme which inactivates penicillins, third generation cephalosporins, and aztreonam (chromosomal ESBL). This explains the synergy usually observed with ticarcillin (Fig. 5). In addition, hyperproduction of this β-lactamase relative to L1 is responsible for the synergy obtained between ceftazidime, cefotaxime, or aztreonam and clavulanic acid.

The multiplicity of acquired β-lactam resistance phenotypes suggests that regulation of L1 and L2 production is not coordinated. *In vitro* isolation of mutants that constitutively express L1 or L2 has been reported (3). The possibility of the L1 and L2 genes being located on a plasmid has not been confirmed (4, 23).

Efflux mechanisms must also be involved in the expression of multiple resistance to β-lactams and to other antibiotics (104). As far as β-lactam resistance is concerned, the involvement of the two β-lactamases remains the norm.

The hypersusceptible phenotype has become rare and is associated with very low production of the L2 enzyme (Table 7). *In vitro*, these strains are susceptible to several β-lactams, including ticarcillin, cefotaxime, and ceftazidime and there is no synergy between ticarcillin and clavulanic acid. Constant resistance to imipenem is always related to induction of LI.

The main susceptible phenotype (over 50% of isolates) is characterized by high susceptibility to ticarcillin/clavulanic acid and to latamoxef. Two subtypes (CAZ^S and CAZ^R) are characterized on the basis of the quantity of L2 produced. Aztreonam resistance is found in the majority of cases (MIC$_{50}$ > 128 µg/ml) but susceptibility is quite frequently restored by clavulanic acid

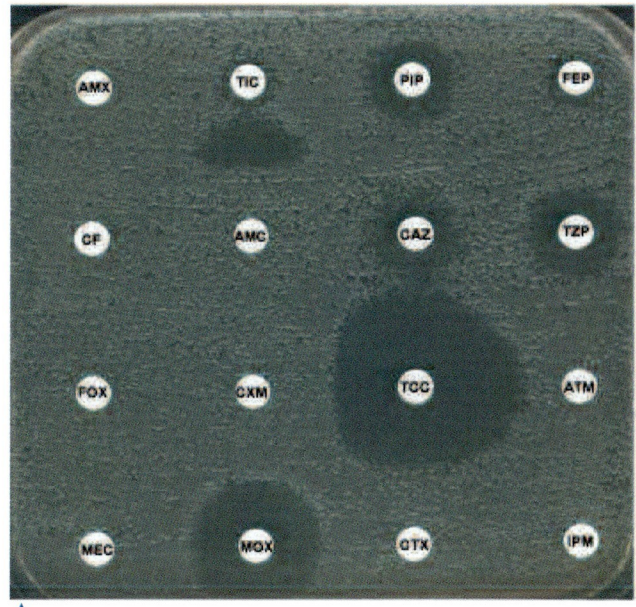
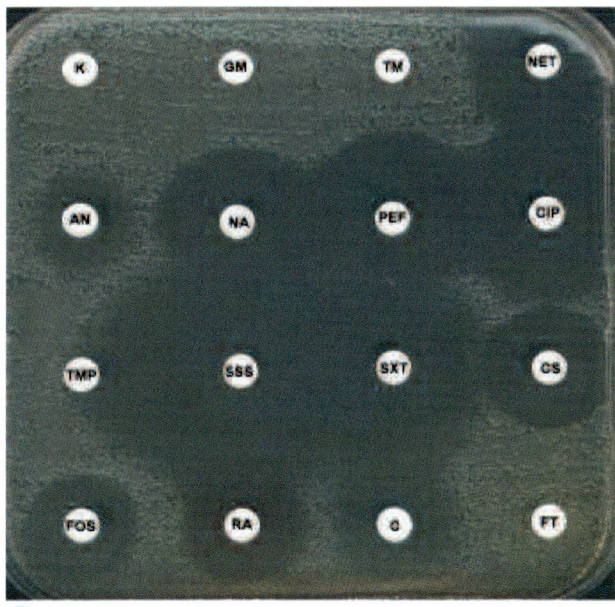

A. B.

Fig. 5. *Stenotrophomonas maltophilia* typical phenotype.
A, AMC, amoxicillin + clavulanic acid; AMX, amoxicillin; ATM, aztreonam; CAZ, ceftazidime; CF, cefalotin; CTX, cefotaxime; CXM, cefuroxime; FEP, cefepime; FOX, cefoxitin; IPM, imipenem; MEC, mecillinam; MOX, latamoxef; PIP, piperacillin; TCC, ticarcillin + clavulanic acid; TIC, ticarcillin; TZP, piperacillin + tazobactam. **B,** AN, amikacin; C, chloramphenicol; CIP, ciprofloxacin; CS, colistin; FOS, fosfomycin; FT, nitrofurans; GM, gentamicin; K, kanamycin; NA, nalidixic acid; NET, netilmicin; PEF, pefloxacin; RA, rifampicin; SSS, sulfonamides; SXT, trimethoprim+ sulfamethoxazole; TM, tobramycin; TMP, trimethoprim

Table 7. β-lactam resistance phenotypes of *Stenotrophomonas maltophilia*

Antibiotic	Phenotype				
	Hypersusceptible	Susceptible		Imipenem^S	Other
		Ceftazidime^S	Ceftazidime^R		
Amoxicillin	R	R	R	R	R
Amoxicillin + clavulanic acid	R	R	R	S	R
Ticarcillin	S	R	R	R	R
Ticarcillin + clavulanic acid	S	S	S	S	V
Ceftazidime	S	S	R	S	R
Latamoxef	S	S	S	S	I/R
Aztreonam	S	S	R	S	R
Imipenem	R	R	R	S	R
β-lactamase activity[b]					
L1 (clavulanic acid-resistant)	i	i	i	-	V
L2 (clavulanic acid-inhibited)	-	i	c	i	V

[a] I, intermediate; S, susceptible; R, resistant.
[b] Little or no detection; i, inducible; c, constitutive; V, activity highly variable.

(MIC_{50} of 2 µg/ml). L2 is inhibited by clavulanic acid but is relatively insensitive to other inhibitors (tazobactam, sulbactam). Finally, resistance to imipenem is constant (L1 induced).

The imipenem-susceptible phenotype remains very rare (and is probably associated with lack of significant L1 production). It is characterized by susceptibility to a combination of amoxicillin or ticarcillin and clavulanic acid (production of L2) and to latamoxef. The activity of ureidopenicillins, for example piperacillin, is always low.

Other resistance phenotypes have been observed, associated with altered permeability and/or one or more efflux systems, as well as with variable hyperproduction of LI and L2, with loss of activity of latamoxef and of ticarcillin/clavulanic acid combination. These multidrug resistant variants are isolated during β-lactam therapy.

Another type of acquired resistance is due to a TEM-2 β-lactamase (5). Recently, a search for ESBL genes by amplification in strains in which synergy was found between third generation cephalosporins and clavulanic acid, has demonstrated the presence of CTX-M-15 (60). Other strains produce TEM-1 or TEM-2. The presence of CTX-M had already been reported in the Netherlands (72).

Several multidrug resistance efflux pumps have been identified in this species. SmeDEF (2), when overexpressed, results in enhanced resistance to β-lactams, tetracyclines, chloramphenicol, erythromycin, norfloxacin, and ofloxacin. A mutation in the repressor gene *sme*T appears to be responsible for hyperproduction.

Later SmeABC and SmeDEF systems were identified, which can be responsible for resistance to meropenem and ciprofloxacin (2). The sequencing of the genome of a strain belonging to the dominant phylogenetic group A indicated the presence of at least nine RND-type (Resistance-Nodulation-Division) efflux system genes in addition to the smeABC and smeDEF operons (23). The deletion of RND efflux pump genes lowers resistance to certain aminoglycosides, tetracyclines, and fluoroquinolones, but none markedly.

Various mechanisms have been suggested for aminoglycoside resistance, such as enzyme-mediated inactivation, MDR systems, modification of porins or even PLP or LPS. An *N*-acetyltransferase (AAC(6')-I) and an *O*-phosphotransferase (APH(3')-II) have been characterized (see the chapter on aminoglycosides and Gram-negative bacteria).

Acquired resistance to fluoroquinolones is chromosomally encoded and usually related to changes in th outer membrane protein profile, to MDR systems, or to mutation in the of DNA gyrase. This type of mutant is observed *in vitro* but also appears clinically during therapy.

Finally, although resistance to sulfonamides or trimethoprim remains infrequent and varies between countries, it is emerging. Several mechanisms have been implicated, such as efflux. More recently, the presence of transposable *sul1* (class 1 integron) and *sul2* (ISR element) genes has been demonstrated (96).

Treatment

The treatment options are very limited (Tables 4 and 5). *S. maltophilia* infections are difficult to treat due to multidrug resistance and the clinical background on which they occur (31, 34, 75). First-line therapy remains trimethoprim-sulfamethoxazole, as more than 80% to 90% of isolated strains are susceptible to this combination. An alternative is the ticarcillin-clavulanic acid combination; it is recommended particularly in patients experiencing adverse effects with co-trimoxazole. However there is a greater risk of resistance.

The newer fluoroquinolones such as levofloxacin, gatifloxacin, and moxifloxacin, etc. are especially valuable because they have much higher *in vitro* bactericidal activity than the older members of the class and because the frequency of resistance remains below 2% to 15% (96). Considering the tetracyclines, minocycline has high activity, the frequency of susceptibility being greater than 80%. In spite of its high activity *in vitro*, tigecycline is still infrequently prescribed. Finally, the polymyxins should be mentioned, as polymyxin-resistance in *S. maltophilia* is low (< 20% of strains); however, there have been very few clinical studies involving large patient series.

Combining several antibiotics remains controversial, especially since the publications on the subject have been inadequate and the methods used and results presented differ. Various combinations have been studied using the checkerboard technique or time-kill curves, and the results vary depending on the technique and the author. Co-trimoxazole has been combined with ceftazidime, the ticarcillin/clavulanic acid combination, polymyxin B, colistin alone or combined with rifampin. The other combinations tested include gatifloxacin with a β-lactam, piperacillin or cefepime or levofloxacin with ceftazidime or cefoperazone. Finally, aztreonam appears to enhance the *in vitro* activity of the ticarcillin/clavulanate combination.

Burkholderia cepacia

The genus *Burkholderia*, which was validated in 1993, belongs to the betaproteobacteria class, and is phylogenetically distant from the genus *Pseudomonas* which has been placed in the gamma subdivision. *B. cepacia* was formerly called *Pseudomonas kingii* and *P. multivorans* on account of the large number of carbon sources it can assimilate, related to its soil habitat. This species was first described by Burkholder in 1950 as a phytopathogen causing a type of onion rot (hence the name *cepa* = onion). It was recently subdivided into nine species, which complicates routine identification. *B. cepacia* was, in fact, a collection of genomospecies («*cepacia* complex») and the species *B. cepacia sensu stricto* (genomospecies I), *B. multivorans* (genomospecies II), *B. cenocepacia* (genomospecies III) and *B. vietnamiensis* (genomospecies V) for example were created. These bacteria are mainly isolated from sputum and tracheal swabs in cases of bronchial colonization and infection, particularly in cystic fibrosis patients, from pus of various sources (major burns), from blood (septicemia and bacteremia after surgery) and from urine (particularly in patients with an indwelling catheter) (90). Outside from cystic fibrosis, with the spread of certain electrophoretic types (ET12, for example), *B. cepacia* is a cause of nosocomial infections and is regularly responsible for small epidemics in hospitals. The presence of a multiresistant genomovar III with enhanced virulence, the genome of which has just been sequenced, has been associated with a very poor prognosis in cystic fibrosis (cepacia syndrome) (44).

Susceptible phenotype

The recent division of *B. cepacia* into several species has not evidenced species-specific differences in susceptibility. Table 8 summarizes the usual behavior of this "species" before its subdivision: multiple resistance to most β-lactams including imipenem, aminoglycosides, and polymyxins was practically universal. Only a few β-lactams have *in vitro* activity against these bacteria: piperacillin, ceftazidime, cefotaxime and curiously sulbactam (a β-lactamase inhibitor which usually has no antibacterial activity). Low-level imipenem resistance is constant but there is no cross-resistance to meropenem. The effect of acid pH that follows incubation in the presence of 5% CO_2 is noticable for β-lactams (22).

The usual pattern of resistance to β-lactams and other antibiotic classes (Fig. 6) includes, as for *P. aeruginosa*, resistance to the aminopenicillins and first and second generation cephalosporins (cefuroxime, cefoxitin). However, the phenotype of *B. cepacia* differs in its natural resistance to ticarcillin (alone or in combination with clavulanic acid) and to imipenem (low-level resistance) whereas there is susceptibility to piperacillin. Finally, antagonism is observed between disks of imipenem and cefotaxime or ceftazidime, suggesting regulation of the expression of at least one β-lactamase. The fluoro-

Table 8. MIC (μg/ml) of antibiotics against *Burkholderia cepacia*

β-lactam	MIC	Other antibiotic	MIC
Ampicillin	> 64	Kanamycin	> 32
Amoxicillin	> 32	Gentamicin	> 32
Amoxicillin + CLA	> 32	Tobramycin	> 16
Ticarcillin	> 512	Amikacin	32
Ticarcillin + CLA	> 512	Tetracycline	4-8
Piperacillin	4	Norfloxacin	8
Piperacillin + TAZ	4	Ofloxacin	4-8
Azlocillin	16	Ciprofloxacin	1-2
Sulbactam	2-3	Sparfloxacin	1
Cefalotin	> 16	Levofloxacin	1-2
		Tigecycline	2-4
		Chloramphenicol	8-16
Cefuroxime	> 32	Trimethoprim	1-2
		Sulfamethoxazole	16-32
		Co-trimoxazole	2-4
Cefoxitin	> 32	Polymyxin E	> 32
Cefotaxime	16	Colistin	> 32
Cefoperazone	> 32	Rifampicin	8-16
Ceftazidime	2-4	Nalidixic acid	8-16
Cefepime	16	Azithromycin	32-64
Cefpirome	8		
Latamoxef	128	Doxycycline	4
Aztreonam	16		
Imipenem	4-8		
Meropenem	1-2		
Doripenem	0.5-1		

quinolones, including ciprofloxacin and sparfloxacin, exhibit activity *in vitro* as do trimethoprim alone or in combination with sulfamethoxazole, certain tetracyclines, and chloramphenicol, albeit to a lesser degree.

Resistance phenotypes and mechanisms

Intrinsic multiple resistance to β-lactams, including penicillins, but no synergy with clavulanic acid, tazobactam, or sulbactam suggests that several mechanisms are involved, such as impermeability, efflux, and enzyme-mediated inactivation. The first studies showed the existence of an inducible β-lactamase with an alkaline isoelectric point (pI > 7.9) that was present in many strains. A 23-kDa enzyme with a pI of 9.3 was characterized; it has a broad substrate profile including penicillins (ampicillin) and cephalosporins (cefuroxime, cefotaxime). A gene, called *penA*, has been identified which encodes a class A enzyme similar to that found in *B. mallei* and *B. pseudomallei* (97). PENA synthesis is regulated by an *ampR* gene, like *cumA* of *Proteus vulgaris* and *Yersinia enterocolitica*. An inducible narrow-spectrum penicillinase with an alkaline pI (PENA-1) was cloned very recently from *B. cenocepacia* (83). It appears to have a minor role in β-lactam resistance. Another inducible class C β-lactamase (cephalosporinase) had been postulated, but with no solid evidence.

A narrow-spectrum penicillinase was found in the *cepacia* group with a number of structural variations. The enzymes PENA and PENA-1 are found in the species *B. multivorans* while different enzymes (PEN-C, PEN-D, PEN-E, PEN-F, etc.) have been identified in other species of this group (44), enabling the use of genomic diagnosis in this bacterial group. Based on genome analysis, such as that of *B. cenocepacia* J2315, other β-lactamases (another class A, class C, class D) exist although their roles have yet to be elucidated (44). However, the existence of inducible metallo-β-lactamase PCM-I (*Pseudomonas cepacia* metallo-enzyme I) identified in several strains of "*P. cepacia*" does not appear to have been established with certainty.

Other mechanisms that play a major role in the natural resistance of this species include impermeability to hydrophilic antibiotics, LPS composition, and the mexAB-OprM or MexXP-OprM efflux systems. These mechanisms are mainly involved in resistance to other antibiotic classes: aminoglycosides, tetracyclines, fluoroquinolones, phenicols and trimethoprim (16, 73, 104). Genome sequences indicate that there could be many efflux systems of the MFS (Major Facilitator Superfamily), ABC (ATP Binding Cassette), RND, MATE (Multidrug and Toxic Compound Extrusion) and SMR (Small Multidrug Resistance) types (39, 44).

Finally, study of different strains from the *cepacia* complex isolated from cystic fibrosis patients has shown the existence of class 1 integrons containing the gene for an acetyltransferase, AAC(6')-1A, and other cassettes conferring resistance to β-lactams by production of an oxacillinase (class D) and to sulfonamides by production of a dihy-

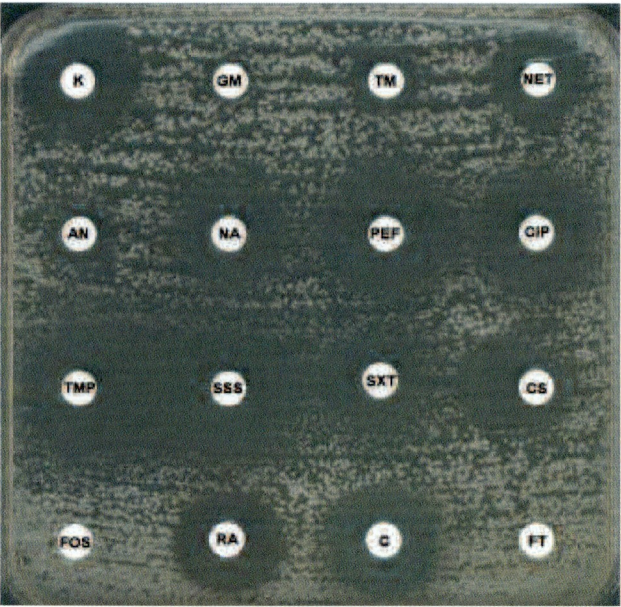

Fig. 6. *Burkholderia cepacia* phenotype.

Legend A and B: see Fig.5.

drofolate reductase (24). Two chromosomal genes for an aminoglycoside 3'-*O*-phosphotransferase and an aminoglycoside-3'-*O*-adenylyltransferase have been identified in *B. cenocepacia* (44).

Treatment

The intrinsic multidrug resistance of *B. cepacia* to several antibiotic classes (β-lactams, aminoglycosides, polymyxins) and its acquired resistance, particularly in cystic fibrosis patients, mean that the treatment options are limited to a few antibiotics such as piperacillin alone or in combination with tazobactam (low-level synergy), ceftazidime, meropenem, fluoroquinolones (ciprofloxacin) or trimethoprim-sulfamethoxazole (Tables 4 and 5). Antimicrobial susceptibility testing is required in order to choose the most appropriate treatment, followed by an investigation of combinations, especially since antagonism is possible (90). Due to lack of clinical trials means, the therapeutic efficacy has not been determined and the *in vitro* results have not been validated. Treatment of primary colonization with intravenous triple-antibiotic therapy (tobramycin, meropenem, and ceftazidime) followed by several months of local aerosols can eradicate *B. multivorans*. Some therapeutic prospects have yet to be explored, such as subinhibitory doses of bismuth-thiol adjuvants for example which lessen resistance to aminoglycosides.

Burkholderia pseudomallei

B. pseudomallei, or Whitmore's bacillus, is the agent responsible for melioidosis or pseudoglanders and was first described in Rangoon, Burma in 1912. This bacterium is isolated from muddy water and soil in wet tropical regions (paddy-fields), particularly in South-East Asia, and has also been isolated in the Middle East, Australia, and Africa as well as in temperate countries, albeit much more rarely (19). Humans and animals acquire the infection transcutaneously (abraded skin or mucous membranes) or through ingestion from stagnant water in tropical regions. The clinical manifestations are highly variable but are mainly pulmonary (where they can resemble tuberculosis) or septicemic (sometimes fulminant with numerous peripheral abscesses). The diagnostic value of antimicrobial susceptibility testing for this species is obvious, especially since it is infrequently isolated in temperate countries.

Susceptible phenotype

The typical susceptibility pattern of *B. pseudomallei* is indicated in Tables 9 and 10 (19, 52, 95). Its intrinsic resistance to polymyxins, aminoglycosides, β-lactams such as penicillins (amoxicillin, ticarcillin), first, second, and third generation cephalosporins with the exception of ceftazidime and carbapenems including imipenem should be noted. This species is relatively susceptible to combinations of amoxicillin or ticarcillin and clavulanic acid, piperacillin and tazobactam, thereby defining a «penicillinase» phenotype with resistance to cephalosporins, including cefuroxime, cefotaxime, and aztreonam. Few other antibiotics have activity against this organism: it is occasionally observed with chloramphenicol, certain tetracyclines (doxycycline, minocycline), and more rarely the trimethoprim-sulfamethoxazole combination. Finally, the *in vitro* antibacterial activity of fluoroquinolones including ciprofloxacin appears mediocre. The usual pattern of β-lactam resistance (Fig. 7) is very different from that seen in other strictly aerobic nonfermentative bacterial species.

Resistance phenotypes and mechanisms

β-lactams

The usual phenotype, which is easily detected, is low-level production of penicillinase with resistance to certain penicillins (amoxicillin, ticarcillin) and susceptibility to ureidopenicillins (piperacillin). High synergy is observed between clavulanic acid and amoxicillin or ticarcillin, but synergy between piperacillin and tazobactam is rarely detectable. Low-level synergy is occasionally observed between cefotaxime and inhibitors such as clavulanic acid and tazobactam, suggesting a very broad-spectrum, chromosomal β-lactamase (Table 10, Fig. 7).

Acquired resistance to ceftazidime and to the amoxicillin-clavulanic acid combination is observed. Although it was described a long time ago it remains rare, and three resistance phenotypes have been characterized (Table 11) (37, 98):

Following ceftazidime therapy, resistance to this antibiotic can appear, detected by synergy between ceftazidime and clavulanic acid. This synergy suggests the production of an ESBL.

Table 9. MIC (µg/ml) of antibiotics against *Burkholderia pseudomallei*

β-lactam	MIC	Other antibiotic	MIC
Amoxicillin	64	Kanamycin	16
Amoxicillin + CLA [a]	2	Tobramycin	8-16
Ampicillin	32	Gentamicin	8-16
Ampicillin + SUL [a]	4	Amikacin	8-16
Ticarcillin	128	Norfloxacin	8
Ticarcillin + CLA [a]	2	Ofloxacin	4
Piperacillin	1	Ciprofloxacin	4
Piperacillin + TAZ [a]	1	Temafloxacin	4
Azlocillin	12	Moxifloxacin	2
Cefalotin	> 256	Chloramphenicol	8
Cefoxitin	> 256	Rifampicin	8
Cefuroxime	16-32	Co-trimoxazole	0.5
Cefoperazone	16	Chloramphenicol	8
Cefotaxime	4	Tetracycline	4
Ceftriaxone	4	Azithromycin	32
Ceftazidime	2		
Cefixime	2		
Aztreonam	8-16		
Carumonam	2		
Imipenem	0.5-1		
Meropenem	1		
Ertapenem	8		

[a] CLA, clavulanic acid (2 µg/ml); TAZ, tazobactam (4 µg/ml); SUL, sulbactam (8 µg/ml).

Table 10. Comparison of the susceptibility of *Bhurkholderia pseudomallei* and *Bhurkholderia mallei*

β-lactam	B. pseudomallei	B. mallei	Other antibiotic	B. pseudomallei	B. mallei
Amoxicillin	64	64	Tobramycin	128	2
Amoxicillin + CLA [a]	8	0.12	Gentamicin	32	2
Ticarcillin	64	64	Netilmicin	128	0.12
Ticarcillin + CLA [a]	8	4	Amikacin	64	32
Piperacillin	4	4	Nalidixic acid	16	16
Piperacillin + TAZ [a]	0.25	0.25	Pefloxacin	8	2
Cefoxitin	>128	>128	Norfloxacin	32	8
Cefsulodin	>128	>128	Ofloxacin	4	2
Cefoperazone	16	8	Ciprofloxacin	2	2
Cefotaxime	16	8	Levofloxacin	2	1
Cefotaxime + CLA [a]	8	4	Gatifloxacin	2	0.5
Cefotaxime + TAZ	4	2	Chloramphenicol	8	2
Ceftazidime	4	2	Doxycycline	1	0.12
Aztreonam	2	32	Minocycline	1	0.12
Imipenem	1	0.25	Rifampicin	16	2
			Co-trimoxazole	8/152	2
			Fosfomycin	>128	>128
			Erythromycin	> 64	0.25
			Clindamycin	>128	>128

[a] CLA, clavulanic acid (2 µg/ml); TAZ, tazobactam (4 µg/ml).

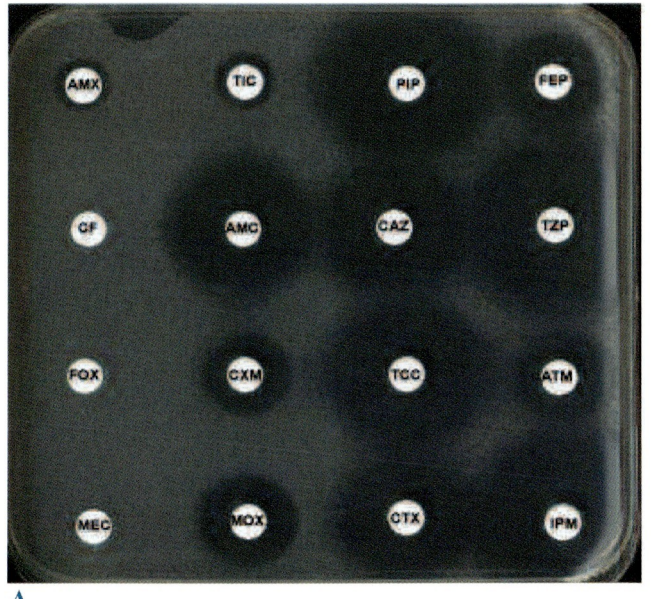
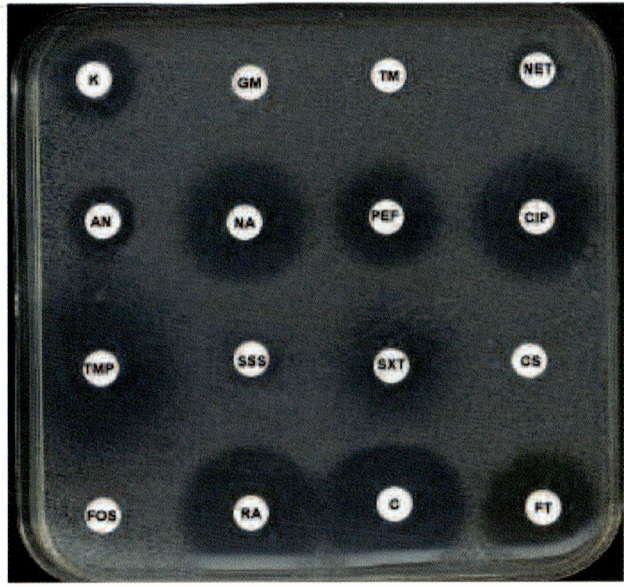

A.   B.

Fig. 7. *Burkholderia pseudomallei* typical phenotype.   Legend A and B: see Fig.5.

Nota Bene: RA is replaced by TE, tetracycline; This is the only difference compared to the other antimicrobial susceptibility tests.

Table 11. Resistance to β-lactams (MIC, µg/ml) of *Burkholderia pseudomallei*

β-lactam	Susceptible[a]	CAZ[R]	AUG[R]	ESBL
Amoxicillin	64	256	256	> 256
Amoxicillin + CLA [b]	2	2	256	> 256
Ticarcillin	128	256	256	> 256
Ticarcillin + CLA	2	4	256	> 256
Piperacillin	1	2	4	16
Azlocillin	16	2	4	32
Temocillin	8	8	4	8
Cefuroxime	16	16	4	256
Cefotaxime	4	8	16	64
Ceftriaxone	4	8	16	64
Ceftazidime	2	64	4	32
Cefixime	2	16	8	32
Cefetamet	2	4	4	16
Aztreonam	16	16	64	256
Imipenem	1	1	4	8

[a] AUG, amoxicillin - clavulanic acid; ESBL, synergism between 3rd generation cephalosporin and amoxicillin - clavulanic acid; CAZ, ceftazidime; R, resistant; S, susceptible; Susceptible, susceptible phenotype.
[b] CLA, clavulanic acid (2 µg/ml);

Following therapy with amoxicillin/clavulanic acid, resistance to this combination appears to be rather uncommon (fewer than 5%). There is cross-resistance with ticarcillin in combination with clavulanic acid as well as with certain cephalosporins (cefotaxime, ceftriaxone).

Finally, following therapy with β-lactams other than ceftazidime and amoxicillin/clavulanic acid, combined resistance to these antibiotics as well as to other β-lactams can occasionally develop.

Intrinsic resistance is related to the presence of a poorly inducible "chromosomal cefuroximase" that inactivates penicillins (amino-, carboxy-, and ureido-penicillins) and certain cephalosporins (cefalotin, cefaloridine, cefotaxime, and cefuroxime). Two class A clavulanic acid-inhibited enzymes, BPS-1 and PENA, have been characterized and are identical to those produced by *B. mallei* and similar to those of *B. cepacia* (Fig. 3) (20, 43). These enzymes can be hyperproduced or, alternatively, can evolve by mutation to confer resistance to either third generation cephalosporins (ceftazidime) or combinations involving clavulanic acid and a penicillin, thereby explaining the above phenotypes (20, 37, 98). Thus, a mutation in BPS-1 (Pro$_{167}$Ser) confers resistance to penicillins and to ceftazidime. It could therefore be described as a mutation-derived chromosomal ESBL.

Finally, the presence of an oxacillinase (OXA-42, -43, -57, -59, etc.) could explain resistance to ceftazidime and to imipenem (through hyperproduction) (53, 76). These enzymes are phylogenetically similar to the chromosomal enzyme of *R. pickettii* OXA-22. Two other β-lactamase genes belonging to class B (carbapenemase) and C (cephalosporinase) were discovered in the genome of this bacterium, although their respective roles have not been clearly established.

Although enzyme-mediated inactivation appears to have the most important role in explaining intrinsic and acquired resistance, other mechanisms must be involved, such as impermeability (for resistance to first generation cephalosporins) or efflux.

Other antibiotics

β-lactam resistance does not usually produce cross-resistance to other antibiotic classes. Intrinsic resistance to macrolides, aminoglycosides, and fluoroquinolones is due to RND-type efflux systems (AmrAB-OprA, BpeAB-OprB, or BpeEF-OprC) which can be overexpressed, in some cases associated with mutations of the DNA gyrase B gene (17, 57, 68, 99). Genome analysis suggests the existence of other efflux systems but their roles are yet to be elucidated.

Treatment

Treatment of melioidosis is based on β-lactams (Table 4). It is complex, prolonged (at least 20 weeks), and the effect is not particularly spectacular (the fever abates slowly over at least nine days on average). The advent of ceftazidime was a turning point in the treatment of melioidosis, and has since been based on double or even triple-antibiotic therapy, starting with intravenous acute-phase treatment with ceftazidime, imipenem, or meropenem, alone or combined with a second antibiotic, such as doxycycline or the trimethoprim-sulfamethoxazole combination in accordance with European guidelines (www.emea.europa.eu/pdfs/human/bioterror/10.GlandersMelioidosis.pdf, 19, 78). Next, the maintenance phase involves oral antibiotic therapy until the end of the 20-week period with a combination of doxycycline, trimethoprim-sulfamethoxazole, and chloramphenicol (only eight weeks). Alternative effective regimens using the amoxicillin-clavulanic acid combination exist. They are prescribed for pregnant women and children. There is currently no vaccine.

Burkholderia mallei

Among the other species of *Burkholderia*, *B. thailandensis* shows many similarities with *B. pseudomallei*, as evidenced by the presence of the same PEN β-lactamase (98). The only difference is that this soil-dwelling species is only weakly pathogenic in man.

However, *B. mallei* is responsible for glanders and is a possible bioterrorism threat. Glanders is a serious and sometimes fatal infectious disease that mainly affects equids. Other animals (cats, dogs, goats, etc.) can contract the infection accidentally through ingestion of contaminated food or water, as can humans. The clinical manifestations are variable but are dominated by fever and severe inflammation of the nasal fossae with discharge. Without treatment, death through septicemia results within days. Although it has been eradicated in North America, Australia, and most of Europe, this disease remains endemic in several continents (Africa, Asia, the Middle East, Central and South America). *B. mallei* is a zoonotic agent communicable by direct contact with infected animals through skin abrasions, through the surface of the oral and nasal mucosae, or by inhalation.

Susceptible phenotype

The susceptibility pattern is comparable to that of *B. pseudomallei*, particularly with respect to β-lactams (40, 54, 95). It has intrinsic resistance to polymyxins, certain β-lactams including penicillins (amoxicillin, ticarcillin) and first, second and even third generation cephalosporins, with the exception of ceftazidime (Table 10) (95). This species is susceptible to the combinations amoxicillin or ticarcillin with clavulanic acid, thereby defining a «low-level penicillinase» phenotype. The only important difference with *B. pseudomallei* is its high susceptibility to certain aminoglycosides (gentamicin, tobramycin). The difference in susceptibility is less marked for other antibiotics:

chloramphenicol, macrolides, quinolones, tetracyclines, or rifampin.

Resistance phenotypes and mechanisms

The usual penicillinase-type phenotype with resistance to cephalosporins, similar to that of *B. pseudomallei*, is due to comparable mechanisms (enzyme-mediated inactivation, efflux). The PENA β-lactamase is similar (98). The intrinsic resistance to other antibiotics has not yet been studied in details, but probably involves efflux (99). Finally, acquired resistance remains marginal.

Treatment

Glanders, like melioidosis, is an infectious disease caused by a bacterium closely related to *B. pseudomallei*. These diseases are endemic in some tropical regions and can cause a broad spectrum of shared clinical manifestations. It is a potential bioterrorism agent and these diseases must be diagnosed and treated rapidly. The antibiotics to test are limited (Table 4). The European guidelines on the treatment and prophylaxis of glanders (www.emea.europa.eu/pdfs/human/bioterror/10.GlandersMelioidosis.pdf) recommend amoxicillin/clavulanic acid, tetracyclines, or trimethoprim-sulfamethoxazole in the localized form treated for 60 to 150 days. In the pulmonary form, acute treatment is with imipenem or meropenem (intravenous route). It should be continued for 6 to 12 months. The septicemic form must be treated for 2 weeks intravenously, then with oral medication for a total of 6 months.

Prophylaxis is still controversial and is based on the trimethoprim-sulfamethoxazole combination after bacterial exposure in the event of biological warfare. There is no vaccine against glanders.

Ralstonia pickettii

This species was formerly classified in the genus *Burkholderia* and later reclassified to the new genus *Ralstonia*. It is naturally resistant to polymyxins. *R. pickettii* is isolated in hospitals quite frequently, for example in various patient care solutions and antiseptic solutions such as aqueous chlorhexidine (88). There is therefore a risk of contamination, colonization, and nosocomial infection such as septicemia, or pseudobacteremia in compromised patients. The recent characterization of new species (*R. insidiosa, R. mannitolytica*) raises the issue of identification in daily practice, the best being genomic approaches as well as differences in resistance profiles (25). This species is isolated more rarely than those previously discussed, sometimes as several clustered cases (nosocomial infections). It is more susceptible to antibiotics than the above-mentioned species belonging to the genus *Burkholderia*.

Susceptible phenotype

The β-lactam resistance phenotype is quite characteristic with, firstly, low-level resistance to penicillins (amoxicillin, ticarcillin) and, secondly, no synergy when they are combined with clavulanic acid (Fig. 8) (35, 36). Susceptibility to piperacillin, cefoxitin, cefuroxime, and other cephalosporins (third generation cephalosporins, for example) or imipenem is observed. There is high resistance to aztreonam (Table 12). As far as other antibiotic classes are concerned, there is natural resistance to polymyxins and aminoglycosides. Susceptibility to trimethoprim-sulfamethoxazole and to certain fluoroquinolones is common.

Resistance phenotypes and mechanisms

We have no accurate data on the frequency of acquired resistance, particularly to certain β-lactams such as the third generation cephalosporins and carbapenems.

Intrinsic low-level penicillin resistance and the absence of synergy between penicillins and clavulanic acid may be due to the production of chromosomal inducible oxacillinase β-lactamases OXA-22 and OXA-60 (Table 12) (35, 36, 77). Their role in resistance was assessed by obtaining variants deficient in one of either of these enzymes. The only notable difference could be the stability of imipenem to hydrolysis by OXA-60. Natural resistance to aztreonam is enzyme-mediated. The possibility of obtaining mutants that hyperproduce either one or both of these OXA enzymes could be due to a mutation in the -35 consensus sequence of their respective gene or to modification of an upstream ORF-RP3 regulatory region (36). The failure of ceftriaxone therapy in a case of septic arthritis may have been due to a hyperproducing variant (103).

Achromobacter (Alcaligenes)

The genus *Alcaligenes* has also been subdivided with the genus *Achromobacter* being reinstated and containing the main species *A. xylosoxydans (Alcaligenes denitrificans subsp.*

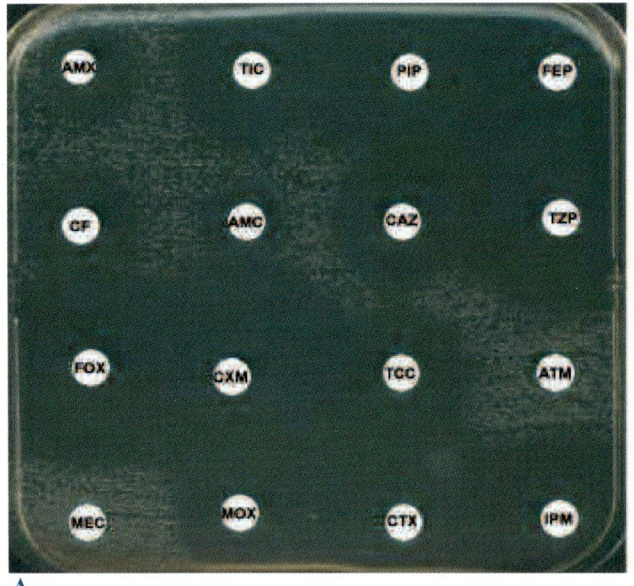
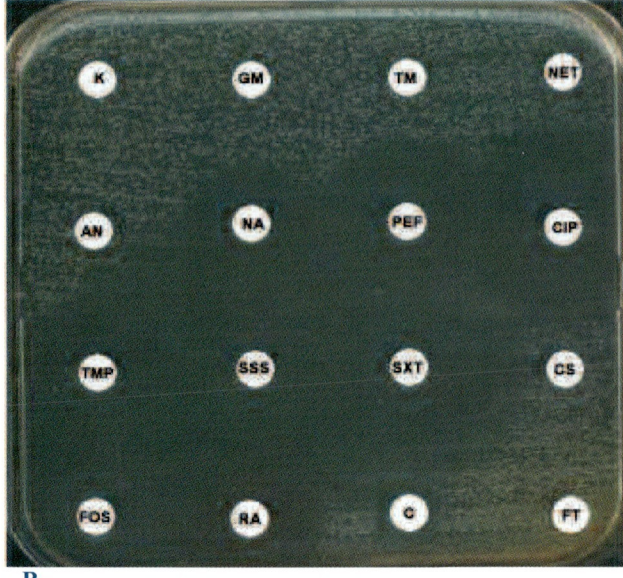

A. **B.**

Fig. 8. *Ralstonia pickettii* typical phenotype.   Legend A and B: see Fig.5.

Table 12. MICs of β-lactams (μg/ml) for *Ralstonia pickettii* isolates and *Escherichia coli* before and after transfer of genes coding for β-lactamases OXA-22 and OXA-60.

Antibiotic	*Ralstonia pickettii*		*Escherichia coli*		
	Isolates (5)	CIP103413	Recipient	pOXA-60[a]	pOXA-22[a]
Amoxicillin	8-64	128	4	256	64
Amoxicillin+CLA[b]	8-64	128	4	256	8
Ticarcillin	8-64	256	4	256	64
Ticarcillin+CLA	8-64	256	4	256	16
Piperacillin	2-4	32	1	2	64
Piperacillin+TAZ[b]	0.5-1	2	1	2	32
Cephalothin	4-8	64	2	2	16
Cefuroxime	8	2	0.5	4	16
Cefoxitin	1-4	8	1	4	4
Ceftazidime	4-16	4	0.5	0.5	0.5
Cefotaxime	0.5-2	2	0.12	< 0.06	0.12
Cefepime	0.5-1	8	0.03	< 0.06	0.25
Moxalactam	8-16	32	0.12	< 0.06	0.5
Aztreonam	128-256	128-256	0.25	0.12	1
Imipenem	0.5-1	1	0.12	0.5	0.25

[a] pOXA-60, plasmid encoding β-lactamase OXA-60; pOXA-22 plasmid encoding β-lactamase OXA-54.
[b] CLA, clavulanic acid (2 μg/ml); TAZ, tazobactam (4 μg/ml).

xylosoxidans) found in nosocomial or other infections in patients with particularly high exposure. It is characterized by its natural resistance to antibiotics and its presence in the external environment including the hospital aqueous environment (1, 38, 74). The species *A. denitrificans* and *A. piechaudii* are implicated less frequently. Only the species *A. faecalis* has been left in the genus *Alcaligenes*. As such bacteria are isolated infrequently, differential diagnosis remains a problem for bacteriologists with little experience of identifying *Achromobacter* species or related bacteria.

Susceptible phenotype

A. xylosoxydans and *A. denitrificans* are easily recognizable by their natural resistance to numerous antibiotics: β-lactams (cefalotin, cefoxitin, cefuroxime, cefotaxime, ceftriaxone, cefepime, aztreonam for example), aminoglycosides (gentamicin, tobramycin, amikacin), trimethoprim, fosfomycin, and quinolones (Table 13).

The characterization of the main susceptible phenotype shows high susceptibility to certain penicillins, such as ticarcillin, piperacillin, mezlocillin, and azlocillin, and low synergy between amoxicillin and clavulanic acid (Fig. 8) or cefoperazone and sulbactam. This species is susceptible to cefamandole, ceftazidime, imipenem, meropenem and fluoroquinolones (for example ciprofloxacin) and to trimethoprim-sulfamethoxazole.

Resistance phenotypes and mechanisms

Acquired resistance to broad-spectrum penicillins (ticarcillin, piperacillin for example) is due to the production of β-lactamases (12, 26, 27, 64, 81). The main acquired resistance phenotypes are summarized in Table 14.

High-level resistance to certain penicillins was initially reported in three Japanese strains. It is due to a species-specific penicillinase with a very alkaline pI (33).

In Europe, acquired resistance to amino-, carboxy-, and ureido-penicillins has been observed (64). The production of a PSE-1/CARB type β-lactamase has been detected (26). Marked synergy is obtained between these penicillins and clavulanic acid, and between cefoperazone and clavulanic acid (Table 14).

Other clinical isolates with resistance to penicillins have been reported (64). This resistance was not reversed by clavulanic acid (Table 14) and was due to an oxacillinase of a non specified type.

Very recently, the structural gene for oxacillinase OXA-114 was sequenced from a strain exhibiting a susceptible phenotype and for which synergy between amoxicillin and clavulanic acid was observed. The enzyme conferred resistance to amoxicillin but also to the inhibitory effect of clavulanic acid (29). This non-inducible chromosomal enzyme has been found in other strains of this species. It is uncertain whether it plays a major role in the natural resistance of this species to β-lactams, as has been reported in other strictly aerobic species such as *P. aeruginosa* (OXA51/69) and *A. baumannii* (OXA50-like).

Resistance to penicillins and third generation cephalosporins, particularly ceftazidime, was reported during treatment of a case of meningitis in the 1990s (27). Possible hyperproduction of chromosomal β-lactamase was proposed, unfortunately in the absence of genotypic identification.

Table 13. MIC (μg/ml) of antibiotics against *Achromobacter xylosoxydans*

β-lactam	MIC	Other antibiotic	MIC
Ampicillin + SUL [a]	6		
Amoxicillin	16	Tobramycin	> 32
Amoxicillin + CLA [a]	4	Amikacin	> 32
Ticarcillin	1-2	Gentamicin	> 32
Ticarcillin + CLA [a]	1-2	Netilmicin	> 32
Azlocillin	0.25	Nalidixic acid	> 16
Piperacillin	0.5	Pefloxacin	4-8
Imipenem	1-2	Ciprofloxacin	2-4
Cefalotin	128	Chloramphenicol	8
Cefamandole	8-16	Sulfonamides	0.5
Cefuroxime	> 64	Trimethoprim	> 8
Cefoxitin	32-64	Colistin	8
Cefotaxime	32-64	Fosfomycin	> 8
Ceftazidime	2-4	Co-trimoxazole	0.032
Cefoperazone			
Cefepime	> 16		
Latamoxef	2		
Aztreonam	> 32		
Imipenem	2		

[a] CLA, clavulanic acid (2 μg/ml); SUL, sulbactam (8 μg/ml).

Table 14. MIC (µg/ml) of β-lactams against *Achromobacter xylosoxydans*

β-lactam	MIC (µg/ml)				
	S[a]	HP	CARB	OXA	ESBL
Amoxicillin	2	>512	>512	256	1024
Ticarcillin	2	>512	>512	32	256
Ticarcillin + CLA[b]	2	32	32	4	8
Piperacillin	0.5	64	128	8	-
Piperacillin + CLA	0.5	1	1	0.5	-
Cefuroxime	> 1024	> 1024	> 1024	> 1024	-
Cefoxitin	512	128	256	256	-
Cefotaxime	64	128	128	128	> 512
Cefotaxime + CLA	64	32	128	128	256
Cefoperazone	2	64	32	16	-
Ceftazidime	8	8	4	32	512
Ceftazidime + CLA	8	4	4	8	16
Latamoxef	2	1	0.5	1	-
Imipenem	0.5	1	0.5	1	-

[a] ESBL, extended-spectrum β-lactamase VEB-1; CARB, PSE-1 type carbenicillinase; HP, cephalosporinase hyperproducer; OXA, oxacillinase. S, susceptible type
[b] CLA, clavulanic acid (2 µg/ml).

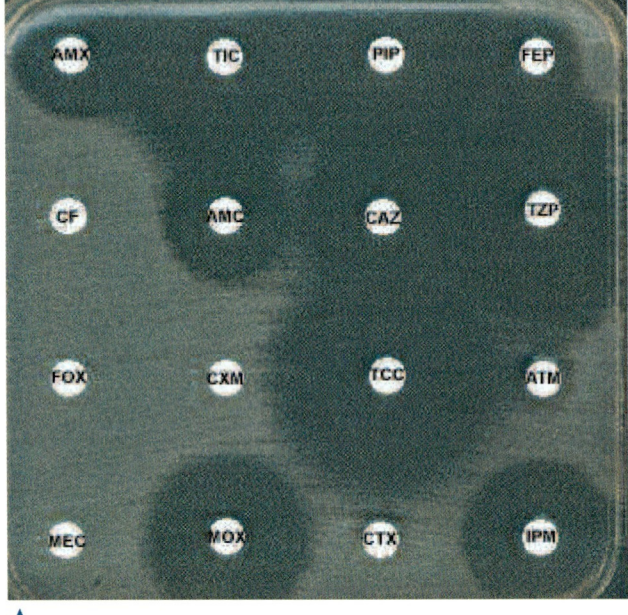

Fig. 9. *Achromobacter xylosoxydans* typical phenotype.

Legend A and B: see Fig. 5.

More recently, a novel example of acquired resistance to penicillins and third generation cephalosporins (particularly ceftazidime and cefepime) due to a transferable VEB-1 ESBL was reported in France in a cystic fibrosis patient (74).

Finally acquired resistance, in particular to third generation cephalosporins (ceftazidime) and carbapenems (imipenem), has been linked to other transferable β-lactamases that had already been identified in *P. aeruginosa*, in particular class B metallo-β-lactamases such as IMP-1, IMP-10 49 or VIM-1 (85). IMP-10 differs from IMP-1 by a single substitution ($G_{145}T$). The expression of imipenem resistance may be of low-level (MIC 8 µg/ml). Therefore, these β-lactamases could be detected by specific inhibition using 2-mercaptoacetic acid or EDTA, then by PCR (see chapters on enterobacteria, *P. aeruginosa*, and *Acinetobacter*).

Thus, acquired resistance to broad-spectrum penicillins, then to ceftazidime, and finally to carbapenems involves various β-lactamases that have previously been identified in enterobacteria and *P.*

aeruginosa. However, the mechanism underlying intrinsic resistance, in particular to cephalosporins including cefotaxime and ceftriaxone, remains unknown.

Treatment

There are no recommendations for antimicrobial susceptibility testing for these species, which have much higher susceptibility than the species discussed above (Tables 4 and 5). Empiric treatment is based mainly on penicillins, including piperacillin alone or in combination with tazobactam, carbapenems, and even ceftazidime. The treatment duration is one to two weeks. Antimicrobial susceptibility testing will enable to alter the choice of antibiotics, with co-trimoxazole as an alternative. Combinations such as piperacillin-gentamicin and ciprofloxacin-imipenem have been proposed. More recently, synergy has been reported *in vitro* between various combinations (azithromycin-trimethoprim-sulfamethoxazole, azithromycin-ceftazidime, azithromycin-doxycycline). They should be used in susceptibility testing when multidrug resistant strains are isolated, particularly in cystic fibrosis.

Alcaligenes faecalis

Susceptible phenotype

The species *A. faecalis*, which produces an aromatic odor, is sometimes isolated in a context of colonization or more rarely of skin, urinary, or ocular infection. This low frequency is probably due to its much greater susceptibility to antibiotics than *Achromobacter* species (formerly *Alcaligenes*), particularly to β-lactams, aminoglycosides, fluoroquinolones (ciprofloxacin, for example) or the trimethoprim-sulfamethoxazole combination (Table 15, Fig. 10) (12, 13).

Resistance phenotypes and mechanisms

Natural resistance to aminopenicillins is low-level and even more so to carboxypenicillins, and therefore difficult to detect. Synergy between amoxicillin or ticarcillin and clavulanic acid should be tested, the latter being more difficult to detect. Although susceptibility to first generation cephalosporins, cefamandole, and third cephalosporins generation is constant, there is however high-level resistance to cefuroxime (12, 13) (Fig. 10). This results in a clearly distinct natural resistance phenotype (taxonomic value). Unfortunately, a penicillinase described as inducible and probably of class A, and which curiously exhibits little clavulanic acid inhibition, has not yet been identified genomically.

Acquired resistance is still rare. It should be noted, however, that a PER-1 extended-spectrum β-lactamase has been identified in one strain with acquired resistance to third generation cephalosporins (79). This enzyme is mostly observed in Turkey in *P. aeruginosa* or *Acinetobacter*. More recently, a TEM-21 ESBL

Table 15. MIC (µg/ml) of antibiotics against *Alcaligenes faecalis*

Antibiotic	MIC range	MIC$_{50}$	MIC$_{90}$
Amoxicillin	2-1024	16	64
Amoxicillin + CLA [a]	0.5-128	2	4
Ticarcillin	1-512	16	64
Ticarcillin + CLA [a]	0.5-32	2	8
Piperacillin	1-256	4	16
Cefalotin	2-128	2-8	32
Cefoxitin	2-128	4	8
Cefotaxime	0.5-128	2	8
Aztreonam	32-128	32	32
Kanamycin	4-512	128	256
Gentamicin	32-512	32	64
Netilmicin	1-256	8	16
Nalidixic acid	128	128	128
Pipemidic acid	8-512	256	256
Ciprofloxacin	0.5-8	2	16

[a] CLA, clavulanic acid (2 µg/ml).

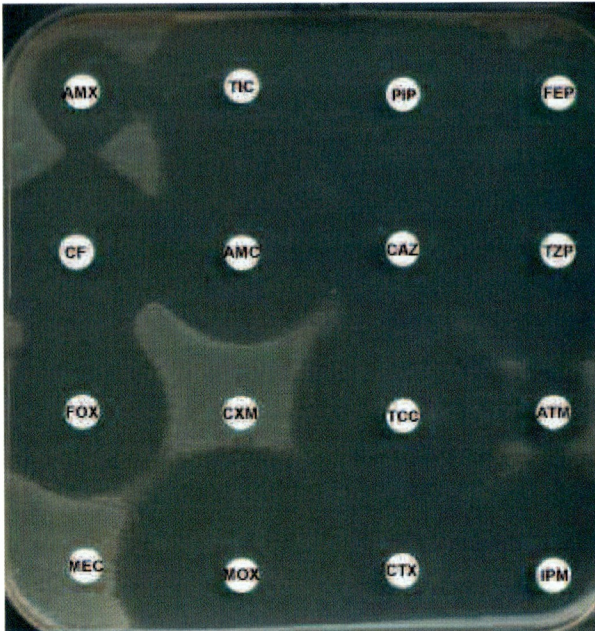

Fig. 10. *Alcaligenes faecalis* typical phenotype.
Legend A and B: see Fig. 5.

was identified in one strain, which was responsible for high-level resistance to broad-spectrum penicillins (amoxicillin, ticarcillin) and to cephalosporins including the third (cefotaxime, ceftazidime) and fourth generation cephalosporins (cefepime) with the exception of the cephamycins (30). Excellent synergy is observed in combination with clavulanic acid (2 µg/ml). This plasmid-encoded enzyme was detected during an endemic outbreak in the same unit in enterobacteria and *P. aeruginosa*. Genes corresponding to these two β-lactamases carried on different transposons could not be transferred by conjugation (30, 63).

Bordetella bronchiseptica

This species, which tends to be encountered in respiratory infections in animals such as pigs, is isolated more rarely in humans. Biochemically, it is a type of *Alcaligenes* with hydrolytic activity (urease positive). *B. bronchiseptica* was in fact initially classified in the genus *Alcaligenes*. This species is a rare cause of sporadic infection in patients with a serious underlying condition. Although it has colonizing potential, it is occasionally responsible for a variety of infections (septicemia, meningitis, pneumonia, otitis) particularly in immunocompromised patients (102). Finally, it is probably selected due to its multiple antibiotic resistance, and particularly to β-lactams including certain third generation cephalosporins such as cefotaxime. Generally no animal contact is established.

Susceptible phenotype

This bacterium is easily identified by its antimicrobial susceptibility pattern, which differs from that of *A. xylosoxydans* in its susceptibility to aminoglycosides; it is characterized by low-level resistance to aminopenicillins and weak susceptibility to carboxypenicillins, especially to ureidopenicillins such as piperacillin (50, 59, 69, 80, 105). Synergy is observed between aminopenicillins and clavulanic acid. Finally, imipenem susceptibility is a constant finding (Table 16, Fig. 11). The intrinsic resistance phenotype is similar to that of the *Achromobacter*, giving a rapid indication of its identity. Constant resistance to certain β-lactams (mecillinam, cefalotin, cefoxitin, cefuroxime, cefotaxime, cefepime, and aztreonam), trimethoprim, fosfomycin, and certain quinolones is an important feature. The only significant difference between *B. bronchiseptica* and *A. xyloxydans* and *A. denitrificans* is that it is typically susceptible to aminoglycosides such as gentamicin, tobramycin, and amikacin, with the exception of streptomycin and spectinomycin.

Resistance phenotypes and mechanisms

The basis for intrinsic resistance to certain cephalosporin-type β-lactams has not been fully elucidated, especially since a single clavulanic acid-inhibited penicillinase, BOR-1, has been identified as being responsible for resistance to broad-spectrum penicillins (59). The same enzyme has been found in *B. parapertussis*, which is usually much more susceptible, like *B. avium*. A recent study confirmed the existence of this penicillinase in eight out of 159 strains of *B. bronchiseptica* of porcine origin (99% identity) (51). Moreover, a class 1 integron containing a penicillinase cassette (bla_{OXA-2}) has been identified on a conjugative plasmid in several isolates. Its role in penicillin resistance (ampicillin) is minor. Although the BOR-1 β-lactamase partially explains resistance to broad-spectrum penicillins (ampicillin, MIC 32 µg/ml) other mechanisms are involved in natural resistance to cephalosporins, as suggested by the impermeability of this species to these antibiotics.

Ochrobactrum anthropi

O. anthropi, formerly classified as CDC group Vd, is a bacillus oxidase positive, motile, characterized by a strong urease activity. This species widely distributed in water and hospital environments has been isolated in some cases from water-

Table 16. MIC (µg/ml) of antibiotics against *Bordetella bronchiseptica*

β-lactam	MIC$_{50}$	MIC$_{90}$	Other antibiotic	MIC$_{50}$	MIC$_{90}$
Ampicillin	8	16	Gentamicin	2	2-4
Ampicillin + SUL[a]		8-16	Tobramycin		6
Amoxicillin + CLA[a] (2:1)	2	4	Neomycin	8	8
Ticarcillin		64	Amikacin		16
Mezlocillin		16	Streptomycin	64	256
Piperacillin		4	Chloramphenicol	4	8
Piperacillin + TAZ[a]		2	Florfenicol	2	4
Cefalotin	8	32	Tetracycline	0.25	0.5
Cefazolin		> 32	Doxycycline		< 1
Cefoxitin		64	Nalidixic acid	8	16
Cefuroxime		> 32	Enrofloxacin	0.25	0.5
Cefoperazone		8	Pefloxacin	4	
Cefotaxime		> 32	Sulfonamides	< 2	
Ceftriaxone		> 32	Trimethoprim	4	16
Ceftazidime		16	Trimethoprim+		
Cefepime	8-16		sulfamethoxazole	0.12	4
Cefpodoxime	16-32		Rifampicin		2
Ceftiofur	16	> 16			
Aztreonam		16-64			
Imipenem	0.25-0.5				
Meropenem	2				

[a] CLA, clavulanic acid ; SUL, sulbactam; TAZ, tazobactam.

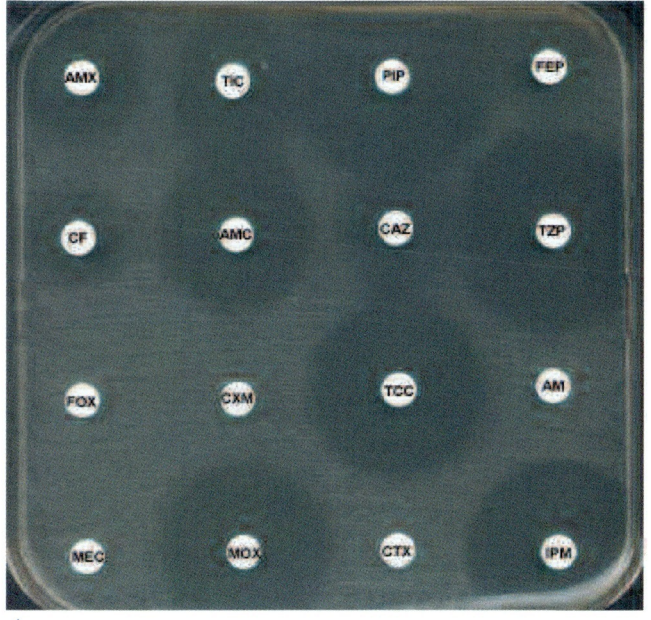

A.

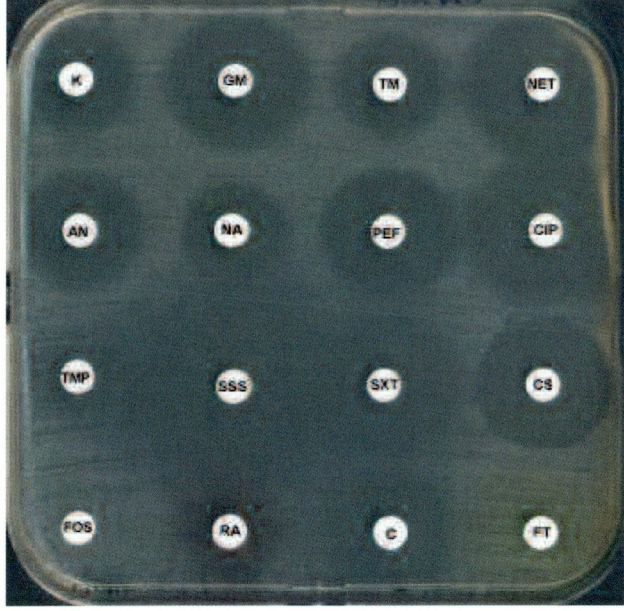

B.

Fig. 11. *Bordetella bronchiseptica* typical phenotype.　　　　　　　　　　　　　　　　Legend A and B: see Fig. 5.

based environments in hospitals (antiseptic solutions, dialysis fluids). It has often been found on human clinical material, adheres to catheters, but pacemakers, intraocular lenses, and silicon tubing may also become infected. Although only weakly virulent, *O. anthropi* causing hospital-acquired infections often in immunocompromised hosts plays a predominant role in this genus (94).

Susceptible phenotype

A typical susceptibility pattern is high level resistance to β-lactams and susceptibility to the other antibiotics tested against Gram-negative bacteria (Fig. 12). Thus, this species is usually resistant to most β-lactams (MICs from 64 to > 128 μg/ml), such as broad-spectrum penicillins (amoxicillin, ticarcillin, piperacillin), cephalosporins including oxyimino cephalosporins (42, 70). β-lactamase inhibitors are inactive (clavulanic acid) or have only weak activity (tazobactam) in restoring susceptibility to the penicillins. This species is generally susceptible to moxalactam, carbapenems, including meropenem (MICs imipenem 0.25-1 μg/ml, meropenem 0.19-0.25 μg/ml), aminoglycosides (tobramycin MICs 1-2 μg/ml), trimethoprim-sulfamethoxazole (MIC 0.1 μg/ml), quinolones including fluoroquinolones such as ciprofloxacin, tetracyclines (MIC 0.25 μg/ml) and rifampin (Fig. 12).

Resistance phenotypes and mechanisms

High level resistance to β-lactams is associated with an inducible class C β-lactamase (cephalosporinase) (42, 70). *E. coli* harboring the structural gene is resistant to all β-lactams (intermediate resistance to piperacillin and aztreonam) except cefepime (Table 17). Since cefepime is known not to be affected by class C β-lactamases, resistance to this drug is likely to be due to impermeability or efflux. The OCH-1 enzyme confers resistance to all β-lactams except cefepime and imipenem. The level of resistance to extended-spectrum cephalosporins is high and comparable to that in *Enterobacteriaceae* overproducing the chromosomal class C β-lactamase; it is therefore not possible to observe the inducible effect of cefoxitin or imipenem by diffusion. Comparison of deduced AmpC sequences from strains of *O. anthropi* showed β-lactamases with sequences 96 to 99% identical. Finally, immediately upstream from the *ampC* gene and in opposite orientation there is a gene 45 to 60% identical to *ampR* (70).

Among the other species characterized by 16S rDNA analysis, *Ochrobactrum intermedium* is also reported as opportunistic pathogen in humans. Surprisingly, 16S rDNA-based phylogeny, protein profiling, and AFLP analysis, place this species closer to *Brucella spp.* than to any other member of the genus *Ochrobactrum*. The recent study of Tessier *et al.* demonstrated that *O. intermedium* has identical β-lactam susceptibility pattern suggesting that a β-lactamase of the same class, or the same enzyme, could be present in this species (94).

Susceptibility to gentamicin, rifampin, fluoroquinolones, and trimethoprim-sulfamethoxazole is observed. But resistance, in all strains examined,

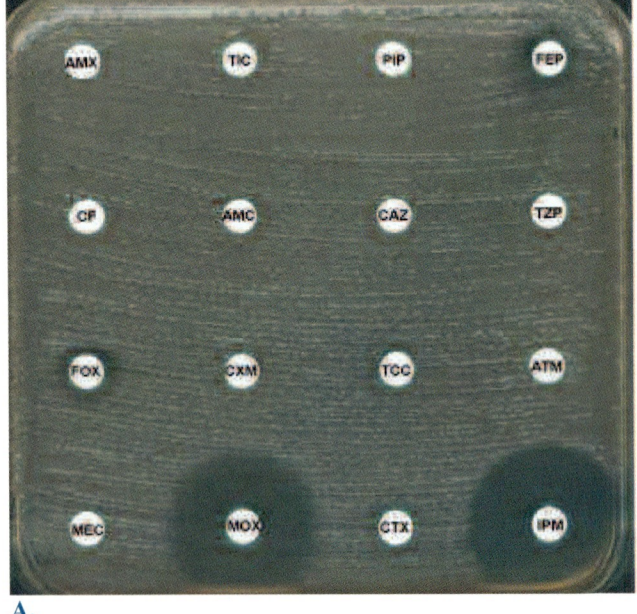

A.

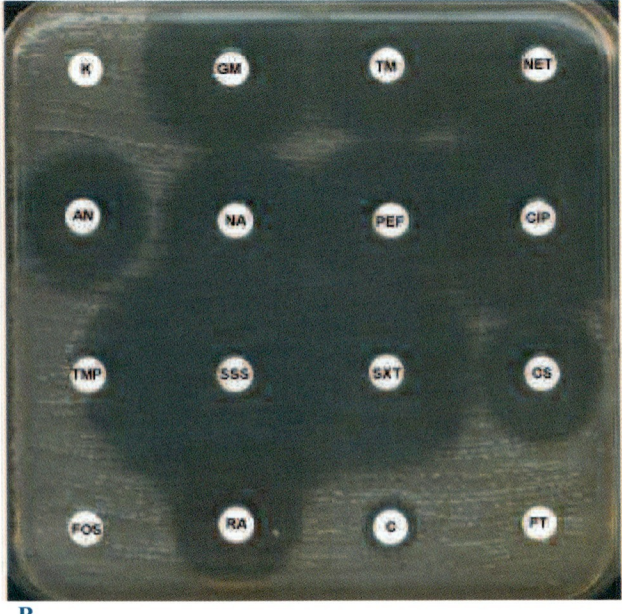

B.

Fig. 12. *Ochrobactrum anthropi* typical phenotype.

Legend A and B: see Fig. 5.

Table 17. MICs (μg/ml) of β-lactams for an *O. anthropi* isolate and an *E. coli* recipient before and after transfer of the gene for β-lactamase OCH-1

Antibiotic	Clinical isolate	Escherichia coli		
		Recipient	pOCH-1[a]	pOCH-1[b]
Amoxicillin	≥128	4	≥128	≥128
Amoxicillin + CLA[c]	≥128	1	128	≥128
Ticarcillin	≥128	0.5	≥128	≥128
Ticarcillin + CLA	≥128	0.12	≥128	≥128
Piperacillin	≥128	0.5	64	16
Piperacillin + TAZ[c]	≥128	0.25	16	8
Cephalothin	≥128	4	≥128	≥128
Cefamandole	≥128	0.5	≥128	≥128
Cefuroxime	≥128	0.5	≥128	≥128
Cefixime	≥128	0.25	64	≥128
Cefoxitin	128	2	≥128	128
Ceftazidime	≥128	0.12	128	≥128
Cefotaxime	≥128	0.06	64	32
Cefepime	≥128	0.06	0.5	0.5
Aztreonam	≥128	0.06	16	8
Imipenem	0.5	0.5	0.25	0.12

[a] Multicopy plasmid expressing β-lactamase OCH-1 (in the absence of a regulatory gene),
[b] Multicopy plasmid expressing β-lactamase OCH-1 (in the presence of a regulatory gene)
[c] CLA, clavulanic acid (2 μg/ml); TAZ, tazobactam (4 μg/ml).

has been reported for netilmicin, tobramycin, and colistin (94). So far, urease activity, mucoidy of the colonies, growth at 45°C, and susceptibility to tobramycin, netilmicin, and colistin, should be considered as characteristics for differentiation of *O. anthropi* and *O. intermedium*.

For both species, the most effective antimicrobial agents for treating human infections are imipenem, trimethoprim-sulfamethoxazole, and ciprofloxacin, sometimes in conjunction with catheter removal.

Shewanella putrefaciens

This species, which owes its names to the putrid odor of the cultured bacterium, had also been called *P. rubescens* on account of the salmon pink pigmentation of the colonies. This halotolerant bacterium is isolated very rarely from humans, and more frequently from warm- and cold-blooded animals such as saltwater and freshwater fish, foodstuffs (spoilage bacterium) or from fresh and sea water. More recently a new species, *Shewanella algae*, has been characterized by 16S rRNA sequencing. It can now be diagnosed phenotypically and it appears that the latter species is isolated more frequently from humans (45).

Susceptible phenotype

S. putrefaciens is considered susceptible to most antibiotics with activity against Gram-negative bacteria (β-lactams, aminoglycosides, quinolones, fluoroquinolones, tetracyclines, co-trimoxazole, or colistin/polymyxin B) with the exception of constant resistance to the first generation cephalosporins cefalotin and cefazolin, and fosfomycin (Fig. 13). This phenotype is constant with low-level production of a cephalosporinase. A few differences in the susceptibility profiles of these two bacterial species have been reported, *S. algae* appearing to be more resistant to penicillin G, tetracycline, and colistin (45).

Resistance mechanisms

Acquired resistance to β-lactams is uncommon, although a few such strains have been isolated during therapy, for example with imipenem (55). The only current resistance mechanism appears to be enzyme-mediated, rare β-lactamases having been characterized (Table 18). An AmpC type β-lactamase has been identified solely by genomic means in a strain of *S. algae* (Genbank AY069931). A «clavulanic acid-resistant penicillinase» phenotype with reduced susceptibility to imipenem but unal-

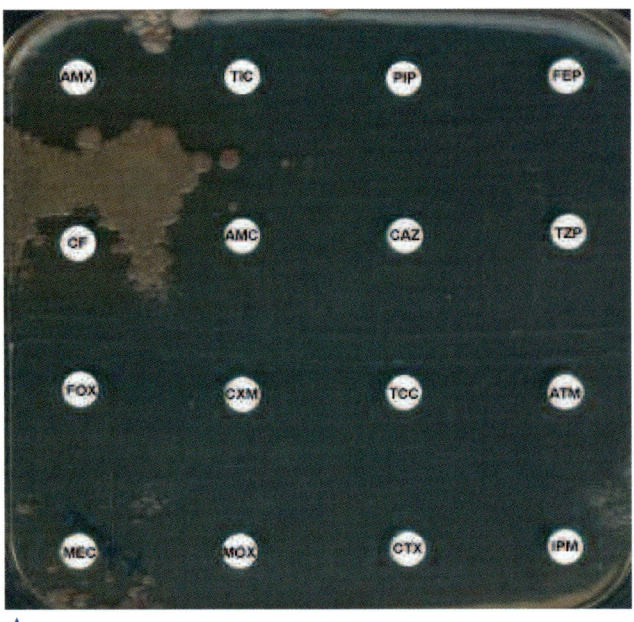
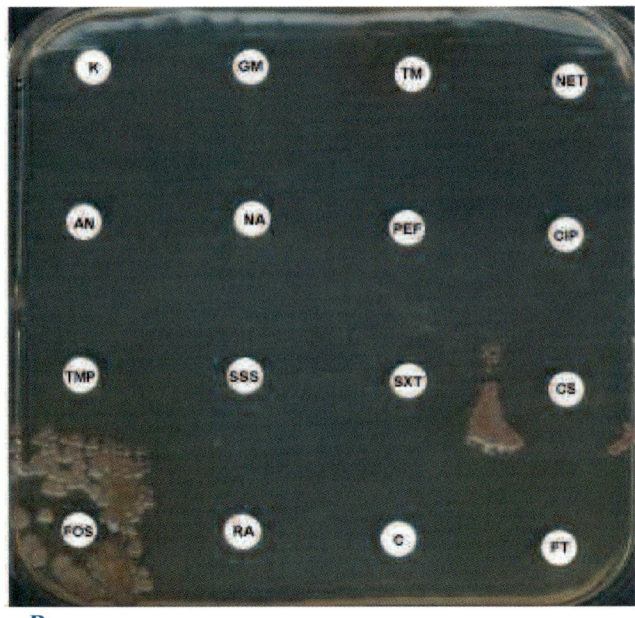

A.

B.

Fig. 13. *Shewanella putrefaciens* typical phenotype.

Legend A and B: see Fig. 5.

tered meropenem susceptibility was obtained *in vitro* in *S. algae* and *S. oneidensis* (Table 18) (41, 82). This marked resistance to penicillins (amoxicillin, ticarcillin) is associated with the presence of chromosomal oxacillinase enzymes that are relatively insensitive to clavulanic acid inhibition (OXA-54, OXA-55) (41, 82). The chromosomal oxacillinase OXA-54 identified in *S. oneidensis* could be the progenitor of the oxacillinases found in other bacterial genera such as *Acinetobacter* or *Klebsiella*, which mediate resistance to carbapenems (OXA-48). Thus, the OXA-54 gene and the gene encoding the plasmid enzyme OXA-48 share 92% identity.

Delftia (Comamonas) acidovorans

Very few articles have been published about this weakly pathogenic and recently named bacterium and they contain little information about its antibiotic susceptibility (58, 84, 92, 100). Its natural susceptibility phenotype categorizes it as a moderately susceptible species and differs from that of the other bacteria of this highly heterogeneous group, in particular in its response to β-lactams (Table 19, Fig. 14). Clinical isolates exhibit natural (occasionally low-level) resistance to certain β-lactams (ampicillin, amoxicillin, ticarcillin, and cefalotin) and are usually susceptible to the other antibiotics of this class and synergy is observed between clavulanic acid and amoxicillin or ticarcillin, in particular. High susceptibility to cefoxitin is a marker to consider. However, resistance to aminoglycosides (MIC > 64 µg/ml for gentamicin, tobramycin, netilmicin, and amikacin), trimethoprim and colistin appears to be constant. Finally, this bacterium is susceptible to tetracyclines, sulfonamides, nalidixic acid, and fluoroquinolones (MIC 0.25 µg/ml for ciprofloxacin and ofloxacin).

Acquired resistance, to β-lactams in particular, has been observed both *in vivo* and *in vitro* for broad-spectrum penicillins, cephalosporins including of third generation, and aztreonam (Table 20) (84). An inducible β-lactamase was found in a susceptible strain and the two resistant mutants that were selected *in vitro* exhibited different kinetic parameters; unfortunately genomic studies were not conducted.

Flavobacterium - Chryseobacterium - Elizabethkingia - Empedobacter - Myroides, etc.

The former «*Flavobacterium*» group, initially defined as strictly aerobic, Gram-negative, non-motile, oxidase-positive bacilli, and often yellow- or orange-pigmented, has undergone various overhauls and continues to do so with the constant creation of new taxonomic subdivisions. More than 80 genera have been proposed within the *Flavobacteriaceae* family since 1994: *Chryseobacterium*, *Elizabethkingia*, *Empedobacter*, *Myroides*, *Sphingobacterium*. (http://www.ncbi.nlm.nih.gov/). Their involvement in clinical bacteriology is still very rare and only a few species, including *Elizabethkingia*

Table 18. MICs (µg/ml) of β-lactams for *S. algae, S. putrefaciens,* and *E. coli* before and after transfer of genes for β-lactamases OXA-55 and OXA-54

Antibiotic	Shewanella		Escherichia coli		
	S. algae	*S. putrefaciens*	Recipient	OXA-55[a]	OXA-54[a]
Amoxicillin	16-32	32	4	128	512
Amoxicillin +CLA[b]	8-16	32	4	128	512
Ticarcillin	2-4	4	4	512	512
Ticarcillin+CLA	2-4	4	4	256	512
Piperacillin	1	1	2	4	32
Piperacillin +TZB[b]	1	1	2	4	32
Cephalothin	256-512	64	4	4	4
Cefuroxime	4	2	4	4	4
Cefoxitin	16	4	4	1	4
Ceftazidime	0.25	0.25	0.06	0.12	0.12
Cefotaxime	0.12	0.06	0.06	0.12	0.06
Cefepime	0.12	0.06	0.06	0.06	0.06
Cefpirome	0.06	0.06	0.06	0.25	0.06
Moxalactam	2	2	0.06	0.12	2
Aztreonam	0.25	0.25	0.06	0.06	0.12
Imipenem	4	1	0.06	0.25	1
Meropenem	0.25	0.06	0.06	0.06	0.12

[a] *E. coli* with recombinant plasmid expressing β-lactamase OXA-55 from *S. algae* or OXA-54 from *S. oneidensis*.
[b] CLA, clavulanic acid at a fixed concentration of 2 µg/ml; TZB, tazobactam at a fixed concentration of 4 µg/ml.

Table 19. Typical susceptibility patterns of *Delftia acidovorans*

β-lactam	Diameter[a]	Clinical categorization[b]	Other antibiotics	Diameter[a]	Clinical categorization
Amoxicillin	< 6	R	Gentamicin	9 ± 8	R
Amoxicillin + CLA[c]	25 ± 7	S	Tobramycin	9 ± 8	R
Ticarcillin	< 6	R	Netilmicin	9 ± 8	R
Ticarcillin + CLA	31 ± 7	S	Amikacin	9 ± 8	R
Piperacillin	26 ± 5	S	Nalidixic acid	29 ± 11	S
Piperacillin + TAZ[c]	31 ± 5	S	Norfloxacin	28 ± 10	S
Cefalotin	< 6	R	Pefloxacin	29 ± 10	S
Cefamandole	12 ± 9	R	Ciprofloxacin	34 ± 12	S
Cefuroxime	11 ± 9	R	Colistin	13 ± 4	R
Cefoxitin	39 ± 1	S	Trimethoprim	< 6	R
Cefotaxime	30 ± 6	S	Co-trimoxazole	31 ± 9	S
Ceftazidime	33 ± 5	S	Fosfomycin	< 6	R
Latamoxef	37 ± 2	S	Rifampicin	12 ± 4	I
Cefepime	20 ± 9	I/S	Tetracycline	20 ± 7	S
Cefpirome	16 ± 10	I/S	Chloramphenicol	15 ± 7	I/R
Aztreonam	20 ± 8	I/S			
Imipenem	33 ± 3	S			

[a] Diffusion as described in the recommendations of the CA-SFM (the French national breakpoint committee), results expressed as mean ± standard deviation
[b] I, intermediate; R, resistant; S, susceptible.
[c] CLA, clavulanic acid; TAZ, tazobactam

(Chryseobacterium) meningoseptica will therefore be considered, as more is known about their antibiotic susceptibility (Table 1).

These saprophytic bacteria live in soil, water, and the hospital environment. They account for fewer than 10% of the nonfermentative, non-pyocyanic bacteria isolated from human pathology samples. Only a few species are responsible for infectious diseases, including *E. meningoseptica* which is of particular importance in infants and premature babies. This species can cause septicemia and extremely serious epidemic meningitis in intensive care units. Death rates of about 50% have been reported, with major sequelae such as hydrocephalus and hearing impairment. Infections in adults are mainly iatrogenic and their prognosis is generally satisfactory in the absence of any adverse factors (14, 48, 61). The other species are isolated in the hospital environment. They can be exogenous contaminants of various pathology samples and more rarely can cause opportunistic infections.

Susceptible phenotypes

Antibiotic susceptibility within this highly heterogeneous group is mainly characterized by natural multiresistance to a variety of antibiotics including the β-lactams, aminoglycosides and polymyxins (Fig. 15-17). Various resistance phenotypes have been characterized, particularly with regards to the β-lactams, and synergy between clavulanic acid and amoxicillin or ticarcillin has been demonstrated very occasionally (66, 67). Most noteworthy however is their resistance to third generation cephalosporins and carbapenems (imipenem, meropenem), to aminoglycosides such as gentamicin, tobramycin, and amikacin and finally to the polymyxins. Yellow or orange pigmentation of colonies is suggestive of a bacterium from this group, with the exception of the main species *E. meningoseptica*.

The latter species is naturally resistant to many antibiotics that usually have activity against Gram-negative bacteria: β-lactams including imipenem and meropenem, aminoglycosides, tetracyclines, and polymyxins (Table 21). In routine practice, disk diffusion can be of taxonomic value (unique multiresistance phenotype) (Fig 17) (66, 67). Firstly, this species grows best at 30°C and does not acquire pigmentation within 24 h, and furthermore, in addition to the multiresistance mentioned above various synergies can be observed between

Table 20. MICs (μg/ml) of β-lactams against *Delftia acidovorans*

	Clinical isolate		*In vitro* mutant	
	PAC-1	PAC-9	PAC-9M	PAC-9M2
Ticarcillin	256	4	256	256
Piperacillin	32	1	128	64
Cefoperazone	256	8	256	256
Cefotaxime	16	0.25	8	16
Aztreonam	64	2	64	64
Imipenem	0.5	0.25	0.5	1

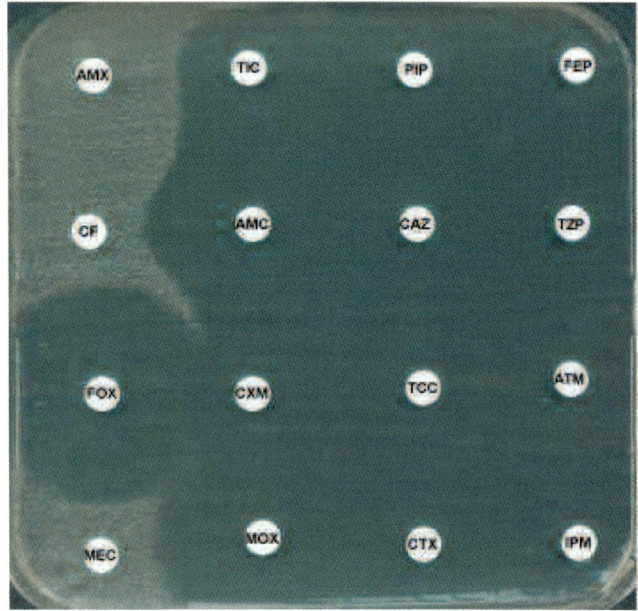

A.

B.

Fig. 14. *Delftia (Comamonas) acidovorans* typical phenotype.

Legend A and B: see Fig. 5.

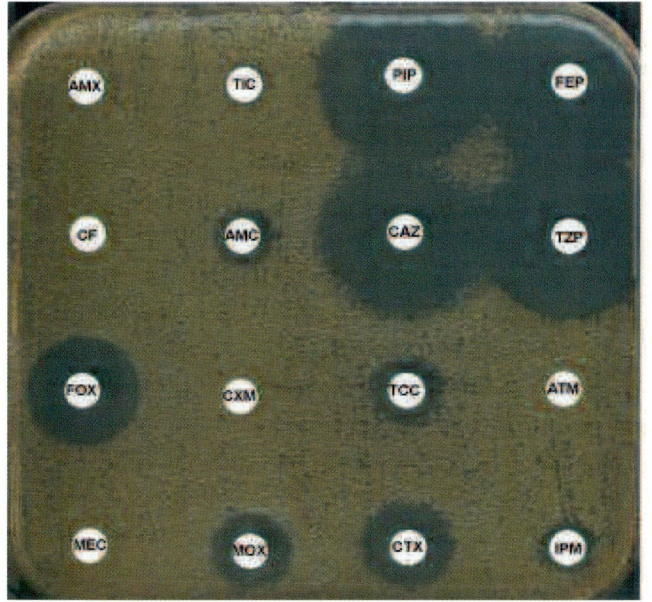
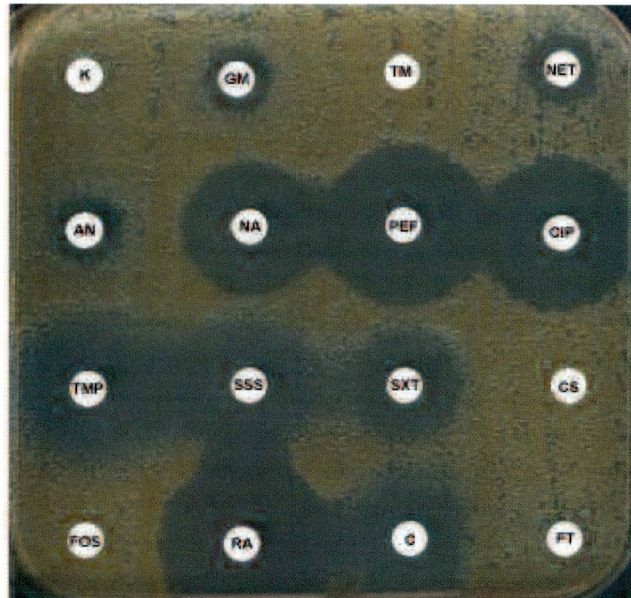

Fig. 15. *Chryseobacterium indologenes* typical phenotype. Legend A and B: see Fig. 5.

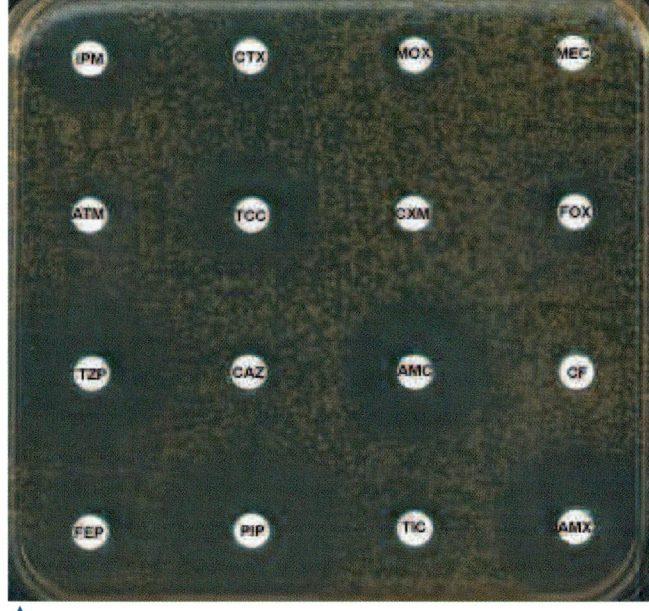
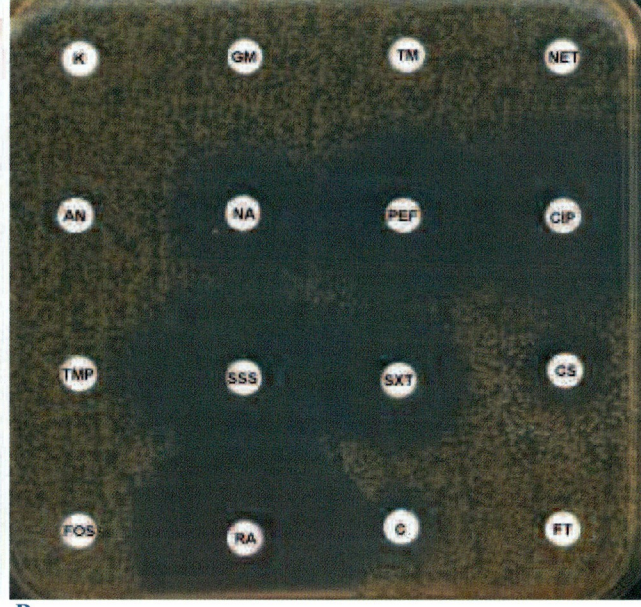

Fig. 16. *Myroides odoratus* typical phenotype. Legend A and B: see Fig. 5.

β-lactams, including third generation cephalosporins, and clavulanic acid, cefoxitin, or imipenem (Fig. 18). Table 22 shows the synergy between clavulanic acid and cephalosporins, and even third generation cephalosporins (67).

However, paradoxical susceptibility to antibiotics with activity against Gram-positive bacteria, such as vancomycin, novobiocin, erythromycin, and clindamycin has been reported. However, various studies have clarified the inconsistencies which were due to the technique used (diffusion or dilution). Thus, from as early as the 1980s, in a study on 52 strains of *C. meningosepticum*, Bruun *et al.* observed a marked difference for vancomycin and fusidic acid which appear to have activity against this species when diffusion is used but not by dilution (15). The idea of vancomycin susceptibility should therefore be abandoned (32).

A few differences are seen, related to greater susceptibility of other species in the group (*C. indologenes*, *C. gleum*, *M. odoratus*, *M. odoratissimus*). However, insufficient clinical isolates have

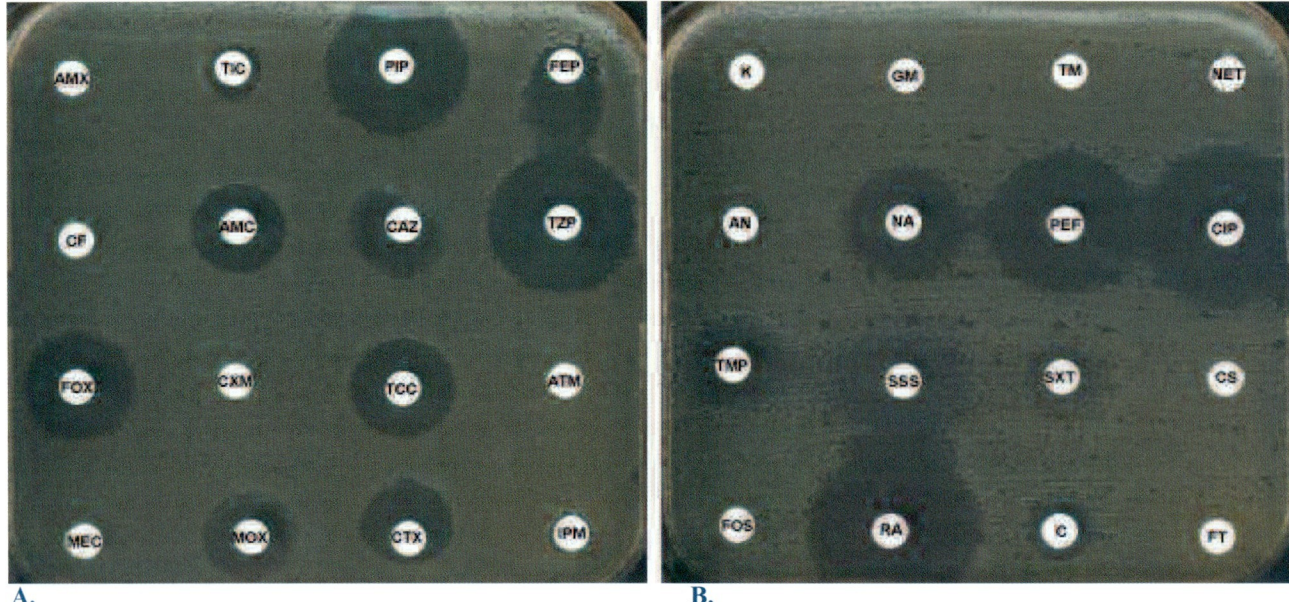

A. B.

Fig. 17. *Elizabethkingia (Chryseobacterium) meningoseptica* typical phenotype.
Legend A and B: see Fig. 5.

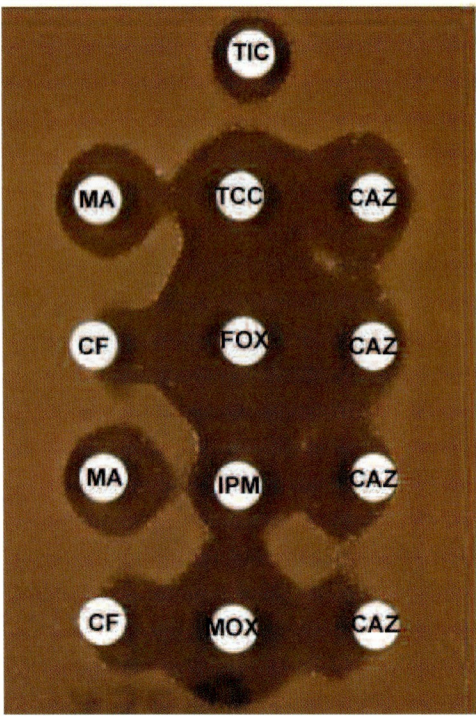

Fig. 18. *Elizabethkingia meningoseptica*. Synergy in disk diffusion testing (white arrow). CAZ, ceftazidime; CF, cefalotin; FOX, cefoxitin; IPM, imipenem; MA, cefamandole; TCC, ticarcillin + clavulanic acid; TIC, ticarcillin.

been collected for conclusions to be drawn about the true susceptibility patterns with regards to the β-lactams and other antibiotic classes (18, 32, 47, 48, 56, 66).

Resistance phenotypes and mechanisms

E. meningoseptica has a very unusual multiresistance pattern to β-lactams which is of very high predictive value in the identification of this species (see susceptibility phenotype) (66, 67). This phenotype is due to the production of species-specific chromosomal β-lactamases.

A noninducible ESBL that inactivates a broad spectrum of antibiotics (penicillins, cephalosporins including third generation cephalosporins, aztreonam) (Table 23) has been identified as being a class A enzyme (CME-1, CME-2) and therefore susceptible to various inhibitors (clavulanic acid, tazobactam, sulbactam, cefoxitin, latamoxef and imipenem) (11, 86).

Two EDTA-inhibited class B carbapenemases or metallo-enzymes have been characterized. The BlaB1 type inactivates a broad profile of antibiotics including the cephamycins and the carbapenems, even this is not obvious in the MICs (Table

Table 21. MIC (µg/ml) of antibiotics against *Elizabethiakingia meningospetica*

β-lactam	MIC	Other antibiotic	MIC
Ticarcillin	>128	Norfloxacin	>8
Ticarcillin + CLA[a]	>128	Ofloxacin	4
Piperacillin	8	Ciprofloxacin	1-2
Piperacillin-TAZ[a]	8	Gatifloxacin	0.5
Cefotaxime	> 8	Levofloxacin	1-2
Ceftriaxone	> 8	Sparfloxacin	0.25-0.5
Ceftazidime	>16	Clinafloxacin	0.5-1
Cefepime	>8	Moxifloxacin	0.25
Cefpirome	>32	Levofloxacin	0.5-1
Aztreonam	>32	Trovafloxacin	1
Imipenem	>8	Doxycycline	8
Meropenem	>8	Minocycline	0.25-1
Tobramycin	>16	Tigecycline	0.5
Gentamicin	>16	Co-trimoxazole	2-4
Netilmicin	>16	Chloramphenicol	8-32
Amikacin	>16	Rifampin	0.5-2
Polymyxin B	> 32		
Chloramphenicol	> 8		
Vancomycin	16-32		
Teicoplanin	16-32		
Erythromycin	4 ->32		
Azithromycin	>16		
Lincomycin	>32		
Clindamycin	8		
Quinupristin/dalfopristin	>8		
Linezolid	>16		

[a] CLA, clavulanic acid (2 µg/ml); TAZ, tazobactam (4 µg/ml).

23). BlaB1 and BlaB3 (87% homology) belong to the B1 subclass (87, 101).

Finally, another type of class B carbapenemase, GOB-1, has a narrower substrate profile and its sequence differs from that of BlaB (6). The existence of two chromosomal class B enzymes in a bacterial species is very unusual. Their inconstant presence in clinical isolates that are highly resistant to imipenem and even meropenem suggests the presence of another, as yet uncharacterized, resistance mechanism.

Within the genus *Chryseobacterium*, *C. gleum* (formerly *Flavobacterium* IIb) has a resistance phenotype different from that of *E. meningosepticum* and also naturally produces a chromosomal (class B) carbapenemase with a broad substrate spectrum (CGB-1) as well as a class A extended spectrum β-lactamase (CGA-1) (Table 23) (8, 9).

The intrinsic resistance of the other «*Flavobacterium*» species such as *C. indologenes*, *E. breve*, *F. johnsoniae*, *M. odoratum*, and *M. odoratimimus* to β-lactams including imipenem is now partly correlated with natural production of metallo-β-lactamases (class B) such as EBR-1 for *E. breve* (7), IND-1 for INDologenes (10), JOHN-1 for JOHNsoniae (71), TUS-1 for odoraTUS and MUS-1 for odoratimiMUS (previously *Flavobacterium odoratum*) (62) (Table 23). These enzymes share properties, for example do not hydrolyze aztreonam and are inhibited by EDTA, suggesting classification in the same functional group 3a (Bush classification).

Their intrinsic resistance to other antibiotic classes has not been studied.

Testing methods - choice of antibiotics - breakpoints

It is worth repeating that conflicting results can arise, depending on the technique used for antimicrobial susceptibility testing (broth microdilution, E-test®, disk diffusion) especially as some species in

Table 22. MIC (μg/ml) of 10 β-lactams against 21 isolates of *E. meningoseptica*

Antibiotic \ MIC	2	4	8	16	32	64	128	256	512	1024
Amoxicillin							13	7	1	
Ticarcillin							1	16	3	1
Ticarcillin +CLA[a]						3	14	4		
Piperacillin	12	8	1							
Cefalotin						4	12		4	1
Cefalotin +CLA				9	7	1	2			
Cefoxitin	2	14			2	3				
Cefamandole					1	12	5	2	1	
Cefamandole +CLA		1	17	3						
Cefotaxime				14	4	3				
Cefotaxime +CLA	12	7		2						
Ceftazidime							2	16	3	
Ceftazidime +CLA		4	9	8	2					
Latamoxef		1	11	9						
Imipenem		3	16	2						

[a] CLA, clavulanic acid at a fixed concentration of 2 μg/ml.

Table 23. MICs of β-lactams (μg/ml) for *E. coli* before (recipient) and after transfer of gene coding for some β-lactamases

β-lactamase	Recipient	Class A					Class B			
		CME-2	CGA-1	blaB-1	GOB-1	CGB-1	IND-1	THIN-1	EBR-1	JOHN-1
Amoxicillin/Ampicillin	<4	512	512	128	64	512	>512	16	>512	>512
Amoxicillin +CLA[a]	<4	4	16			256		32	>512	
Ticarcillin	<4	512	256	64	64	>512	>512		>512	>512
Ticarcillin +CLA[a]	<4	8	4			>512				
Piperacillin	<1	8	8	4	2	8	64	4	8	
Piperacillin +TAZ[a]	<1	4	2			8				8
Cefalothin	<2	256	64	16	32	32	128	64	32	256
Cefuroxime	<1		64			256		128	128	
Cefoxitin	<4	4	8	2	16	16	16	128	8	128
Ceftazidime	<0.25	32	16	0.5	16	0.5	8	32	0.5	16
Cefotaxime	<0.12	4	0.5	0.12	0.25	1	16	4	0.5	4
Cefepime	<0.06	0.5	0.5	0.03	0.06	0.06	0.06	0.12	0.12	0.25
Moxalactam	<0.12	0.25	1	0.12	1	0.12	0.12		1	32
Aztreonam	<0.25	16	16	0.25	0.25	0.06	0.25	0.25	0.12	0.06
Imipenem	<0.12	0.25	0.25	0.5	0.5	0.25	2	0.5	0.5	1
Meropenem	<0.06		0.06	0.12	0.12	0.25	0.5	0.5	0.25	0.25

[a] CLA, clavulanic acid at a fixed concentration of 2 μg/ml; TAZ, tazobactam at a fixed concentration of 4 μg/ml.

this group grow better at 30°C than at 35-37°C (32). However the CLSI and EUCAST guidelines remain limited (21, http://eucast.www137.server1.mensemedia.net/). It looks as if a dilution method ought to be proposed for determination of MIC values or E-test® if this is not possible. However, first-line antimicrobial susceptibility testing by disk diffusion is still of taxonomic value. Antibiotics of the β-lactam class are most probably not a treatment option; the choice will be between a fluoroquinolone, a macrolide, or trimethoprim-sulfamethoxazole.

CONCLUSIONS

Four species of nonfermentative strictly aerobic Gram-negative bacteria are predominantly isolated in clinical practice: *P. aeruginosa*, *A. baumannii*, *S. maltophilia*, and *B. cepacia*. This group is nevertheless extremely complex, which has led to its perpetual reclassification by taxonomists to the great displeasure of clinical bacteriologists. This taxonomic complexity was initially reflected by the characterization of a variety of intrinsic antibiotic resistance phenotypes, including to β-lactams. These environmental bacteria are isolated infrequently in clinical practice but reports regularly appear in the international literature where a case (or more usually several cases) of nosocomial infection has been caused by contamination of a fluid (an infusion solution, antiseptic, drug, dialysis fluid, contact lens cleaning solution, etc.) with these bacilli, particularly in compromised patients. The persistence of these bacteria is partly related to their intrinsic multi-antibiotic resistance (to β-lactams, aminoglycosides, and polymyxins) and some of these mechanisms, especially the enzyme-mediated ones (β-lactamases) have now been better characterized. Many of these bacteria have natural multi-drug resistance that probably involves other mechanisms such as efflux, impermeability, etc., which need to better characterized. The fact that they are generally soil-dwelling and the frequent absence of virulence factors have prevented their emergence in clinical bacteriology, until recently, especially since their optimum growing temperature is around 30°C rather than 37°C. This culture characteristic is useful for defining the methodology of susceptibility testing.

REFERENCES

(1) **Aisenberg, G, K. V. Rolston, and A. Safdar.** 2004. Bacteremia caused by *Achromobacter* and *Alcaligenes* species in 46 patients with cancer (1989-2003). Cancer **101**:2134-2140.

(2) **Alonso, A., G. Morales, R. Escalante, E. Campanario, L. Sastre, and J. L. Martinez.** 2004. Overexpression of the multidrug efflux pump SmeDEF impairs *Stenotrophomonas maltophilia* physiology. J. Antimicrob. Chemother. **53**:432-434.

(3) **Avison, M. B., C. S. Higgins, P. J. Ford, C. J. von Heldreich, T. R. Walsh, and P. M. Bennett.** 2002. Differential regulation of L1 and L2 β-lactamase expression in *Stenotrophomonas maltophilia*. J. Antimicrob. Chemother. **49**:387-389.

(4) **Avison, M. B., C. S. Higgins, C. J. von Heldreich, P. M. Bennett, and T. R. Walsh.** 2001. Plasmid location and molecular heterogeneity of the L1 and L2 beta-lactamase genes of *Stenotrophomonas maltophilia*. Antimicrob. Agents Chemother. **45**:413-419.

(5) **Avison, M. B., C. J. von Heldreich, C. S. Higgins, P. M. Bennett, and T. R. Walsh.** 2000. A TEM-2 β-lactamase encoded on an active Tn*1*-like transposon in the genome of a clinical isolate of *Stenotrophomonas maltophilia*. J. Antimicrob. Chemother. **46**:879-884.

(6) **Bellais, S., D. Aubert, T. Naas, and P. Nordmann.** 2000. Molecular and biochemical heterogeneity of class B carbapenem-hydrolyzing β-lactamases in *Chryseobacterium meningosepticum*. Antimicrob. Agents Chemother. **44**:1878-1886.

(7) **Bellais, S., D. Girlich, A. Karim, and P. Nordmann.** 2002. EBR-1, a novel Ambler subclass B1 β-lactamase from *Empedobacter brevis*. Antimicrob. Agents Chemother. **46**:3223-3227.

(8) **Bellais, S., T. Naas, and P. Nordmann.** 2002. Molecular and biochemical characterization of Ambler class A extended-spectrum β-lactamase CGA-1 from *Chryseobacterium gleum*. Antimicrob. Agents Chemother. **46**:966-970.

(9) **Bellais, S., T. Naas, and P. Nordmann.** 2002. Genetic and biochemical characterization of CGB-1, an Ambler class B carbapenem-hydrolyzing β-lactamase from *Chryseobacterium gleum*. Antimicrob. Agents Chemother. **46**:2791-2796.

(10) **Bellais, S., L. Poirel, S. Leotard, T. Naas, and P. Nordmann.** 2000. Genetic diversity of carbapenem-hydrolyzing metallo-β-lactamases from *Chryseobacterium (Flavobacterium) indologenes*. Antimicrob. Agents Chemother. **44**:3028-3034.

(11) **Bellais, S., L. Poirel, T. Naas, D. Girlich, and P. Nordmann.** 2000. Genetic-biochemical analysis and distribution of the Ambler class A β-lactamase CME-2, responsible for extended-spectrum cephalosporin resistance in *Chryseobacterium (Flavobacterium) meningosepticum*. Antimicrob. Agents Chemother. **44**:1-9.

(12) **Bizet, C., K. Mensah., and A. Philippon.** 1990. Sensibilité de *Alcaligenes faecalis* vis-à-vis de 31 antibiotiques - comparaison avec celle de *Alcaligenes denitrificans subsp. xylosoxydans*. Méd. Mal. Inf. **20**:148-152.

(13) **Bizet, C., F. Tekaia, and A. Philippon.** 1993. In-vitro susceptibility of *Alcaligenes faecalis* compared with those of other *Alcaligenes spp.* to antimicrobial agents including seven β-lactams. Antimicrob Chemother. **32**:907-910.

(14) **Bloch, K. C., R. Nadarajah, and R. Jacobs.** 1997. *Chryseobacterium meningosepticum*: an emerging pathogen among immunocompromised adults: report of 6 cases and literature review. Medicine **76**:30-41.

(15) **Bruun, B.** 1987. Antimicrobial susceptibility of *Flavobacterium meningosepticum* strains identified by DNA-DNA hybridization. Acta Pathol. Microbiol. Immunol. Scand. **95**:95-101.

(16) **Burns, J. L, C. D. Wadsworth, J. J. Barry, and C. P. Goodall.** 1996. Nucleotide sequence analysis of a gene from *Burkholderia (Pseudomonas) cepacia* encoding an outer membrane lipoprotein involved in multiple antibiotic resistance. Antimicrob. Agents Chemother. **40**:307-313.

(17) **Chan, Y. Y., and K. L. Chua.** 2005. The *Burkholderia pseudomallei* BpeAB-OprB efflux pump: expression and impact on quorum sensing and virulence. J. Bacteriol. **187**:4707-4719.

(18) **Chang, J. C., P. R. Hsueh, J. J. Wu, S. W. Ho, W. C. Hsieh, and K. T. Luh.** 1997. Antimicrobial susceptibility of *Flavobacteria* as determined by agar dilution and disk diffusion methods. Antimicrob. Agents Chemother. **41**:1301-1306.

(19) **Cheng A. C., and B. J. Currie**. 2005. Melioidosis: epidemiology, pathophysiology, and management. Clin. Microbiol. Rev. **18**:383-416.

(20) **Cheung, T. K., P. L. Ho, P. C. Woo, K. Y. Yuen, and P. Y. Chau**. 2002. Cloning and expression of class A β-lactamase gene *blaA*(BPS) in *Burkholderia pseudomallei*. Antimicrob. Agents Chemother. **46**:1132-1135.

(21) **Clinical and Laboratory Standards Institute.** 2009. Performance Standards for Antimicrobial Susceptibility Testing. 19th Informational supplement. M100-A4_S19. Clinical and Laboratory Standards Institute, Wayne, Pa.

(22) **Corkill, J. E., J. Deveney, J. Pratt, P. Shears, A. Smyth, D. Heaf, and C. A. Hart**. 1994. Effect of pH and CO_2 on in vitro susceptibility of *Pseudomonas cepacia* to β-lactams. Pediatr. Res. **35**:299-302.

(23) **Crossman, L. C., V. C. Gould, J .M. Dow, G. S. Vernikos, A. Okazaki, M. Sebaihia , D. Saunders, C. Arrowsmith, T. Carver, N. Peters, E. Adlem, A. Kerhornou, A. Lord, L. Murphy, K. Seeger, R. Squares, S. Rutter, M. A. Quail, M. A. Rajandream, D. Harris C. Churcher, S. D. Bentley, J. Parkhill, N. R. Thomson, and M. B. Avison**. 2008. The complete genome, comparative and functional analysis of *Stenotrophomonas maltophilia* reveals an organism heavily shielded by drug resistance determinants. Genome Biol. **9**:R74.

(24) **Crowley, D., M. Daly, B. Lucey., P. Shine, J. J. Collins, B. Cryan, G. Buckley, and S. Fanning**. 2002. Molecular epidemiology of cystic fibrosis-linked *Burkholderia cepacia* complex isolates from three national referral centres in Ireland. J. Appl. Microbiol. **92**:992-1004.

(25) **Daxboeck, F., M. Stadler, O. Assadian, E. Marko, A. M. Hirschl, and W. Koller**. 2005. Characterization of clinically isolated *Ralstonia mannitolilytica* strains using random amplification of polymorphic DNA (RAPD) typing and antimicrobial sensitivity, and comparison of the classification efficacy of phenotypic and genotypic assays. J. Med. Microbiol. **54**:55-61.

(26) **Décré, D., G. Arlet, E. Bergogne-Bérèzin, and A. Philippon**. 1995. Identification of a carbenicillin-hydrolyzing β-lactamase in *Alcaligenes denitrificans subsp. xylosoxydans*. Antimicrob. Agents Chemother. **39**:771-774.

(27) **Décré, D., G. Arlet, C. Danglot, J. C. Lucet, G. Fournier, E. Bergogne-Bérèzin, and A. Philippon**. 1992. A β-lactamase-overproducing strain of *Alcaligenes denitrificans subsp. xylosoxydans* isolated from a case of meningitis. J. Antimicrob. Chemother. **30**:769-779.

(28) **Denton, M, and K. G. Kerr**. 1998. Microbiological and clinical aspects of infection associated with *Stenotrophomonas maltophilia*. Clin. Microbiol. Rev. **11**:57-80.

(29) **Doi, Y., L. Poirel., D. L. Paterson, and P. Nordmann**. 2008. Characterization of a naturally occurring class D β-lactamase from *Achromobacter xylosoxidans*. Antimicrob. Agents Chemother. **52**:1952-1956.

(30) **Dubois, V, C. Arpin, L. Coulange, C. André, P. Noury, and Quentin C**. 2006. TEM-21 extended-spectrum β-lactamase in a clinical isolate of *Alcaligenes faecalis* from a nursing home. J. Antimicrob. Chemother. **57**:368-369.

(31) **Falagas, M. E., P. E. Valkimadi, Y. T. Huang, D. K. Matthaiou, and P. R. Hsueh**. 2008. Therapeutic options for *Stenotrophomonas maltophilia* infections beyond co-trimoxazole: a systematic review. J. Antimicrob. Chemother. **62**:889-894.

(32) **Fraser, S. L., and J. H. Jorgensen**. 1997. Reappraisal of antimicrobial susceptibilities of *Chryseobacterium* and *Flavobacterium* species and method for reliable susceptibility testing. Antimicrob. Agents Chemother. **41**:2738-2741.

(33) **Fujii, T, K. Sato, M. Inoue, and S. Mitsuhashi**. 1985. Purification and properties of a β-lactamase from *Alcaligenes denitrificans subsp. xylosoxydans*. J. Antimicrob. Chemother.**16**: 297-304.

(34) **Garrison, M. W., D. E. Anderson, D. M. Campbell, K. C. Carroll, C. L. Malone, J. D. Anderson, R. J. Hollis, and M. A. Pfaller**. 1996. *Stenotrophomonas maltophilia*: emergence of multidrug-resistant strains during therapy and in an in vitro pharmacodynamic chamber model. Antimicrob. Agents Chemother. **40**:2859-2864.

(35) **Girlich, D., T. Naas, and P. Nordmann**. 2004. OXA-60, a chromosomal, inducible, and imipenem-hydrolyzing class D β-lactamase from *Ralstonia pickettii*. Antimicrob. Agents Chemother. **48**:4217-4225.

(36) **Girlich, D., T. Naas, and P. Nordmann**. 2006. Regulation of class D β-lactamase gene expression in *Ralstonia pickettii*. Microbiology **152**:2661-2672.

(37) **Godfrey, A. J., S. Wong, D. A. Dance, W. Chaowagul, and L. E. Bryan**. 1991. *Pseudomonas pseudomallei* resistance to β-lactam antibiotics due to alterations in the chromosomally encoded β-lactamase. Antimicrob. Agents Chemother. **35**:1635-1640.

(38) **Gómez-Cerezo, J., I. Suárez, J.J. Ríos, P. Peña, M. J. García de Miguel, M. de José, O. Monteagudo, P. Linares, A. Barbado-Cano, and J. J. Vázquez**. 2003. *Achromobacter xylosoxidans* bacteremia: a 10-year analysis of 54 cases. Eur. J. Clin. Microbiol. Infect. Dis. **22**:360-363.

(39) **Guglierame, P., M. R. Pasca, E. De Rossi, S. Buroni, P. Arrigo, G. Manina, and G. Riccardi**. 2006. Efflux pump genes of the resistance-nodulation-division family in *Burkholderia cenocepacia* genome. BMC Microbiol. **6**:66.

(40) **Heine, H. S., M. J. England, D. M. Waag, and W.R. Byrne**. 2001. In vitro antibiotic susceptibilities of *Burkholderia mallei* (causative agent of glanders) determined by broth microdilution and E-test. Antimicrob. Agents Chemother. **45**:2119-2121.

(41) **Héritier, C., L. Poirel, and P. Nordmann**. 2004. Genetic and biochemical characterization of a chromosome-encoded carbapenem-hydrolyzing ambler class D β-lactamase from *Shewanella algae*. Antimicrob. Agents Chemother. **48**:1670-1675.

(42) **Higgins, C. S., M. B. Avison, L. Jamieson, A. M. Simm, P. M. Bennett, and T. R. Walsh**. 2001. Characterization, cloning and sequence analysis of the inducible *Ochrobactrum anthropi* AmpC β-lactamase. J. Antimicrob. Chemother. **47**:745-754.

(43) **Ho, P. L., T. K. Cheung, W. C. Yam, and K. Y. Yuen**. 2002. Characterization of a laboratory-generated variant of BPS β-lactamase from *Burkholderia*

pseudomallei that hydrolyses ceftazidime. J. Antimicrob. Chemother. **50**:723-726.

(44) **Holden, M. T., H. M. Seth-Smith, L. C. Crossman, M. Sebaihia, S. D. Bentley, A. M. Cerdeño-Tárraga, N. R. Thomson, N. Bason, M. A. Quail, S. Sharp, I. Cherevach, C. Churcher, I. Goodhead, H. Hauser, N. Holroyd, K. Mungall, P. Scott, D. Walker, B. White, H. Rose, P. Iversen, D. Mil-Homens, E. P. Rocha, A. M. Fialho, A. Baldwin, C. Dowson, B. G. Barrell, J. R. Govan, P. Vandamme, C. A. Hart, E. Mahenthiralingam, and J. Parkhill.** 2009. The genome of *Burkholderia cenocepacia* J2315, an epidemic pathogen of cystic fibrosis patients. J. Bacteriol. **191**:261-277.

(45) **Holt, H. M., B. Gahrn-Hansen, and B. Bruun B.** 2005. *Shewanella algae* and *Shewanella putrefaciens*: clinical and microbiological characteristics. Clin. Microbiol. Infect. **11**:347-352.

(46) **Hsueh, P. R., J. C. Chang, L. J. Teng, P. C. Yang, S. W. Ho, W. C. Hsieh, and K. T. Luh.** 1997. Comparison of E-test and agar dilution method for antimicrobial susceptibility testing of *Flavobacterium* isolates. J. Clin. Microbiol. **35**:1021-1023.

(47) **Hsueh, P. R., L. J. Teng, P. C. Yang, S. W. Ho, and K. T. Luh.** 1997. Susceptibilities of *Chryseobacterium indologenes* and *Chryseobacterium meningosepticum* to cefepime and cefpirome. J. Clin. Microbiol. **35**:3323-3324.

(48) **Hung, P. P., Y. H. Lin, C. F. Lin, M. F. Liu, and Z. Y. Shi.** 2008. *Chryseobacterium meningosepticum* infection: antibiotic susceptibility and risk factors for mortality. J. Microbiol. Immunol. Infect. **41**:137-144.

(49) **Iyobe, S., H. Kusadokoro, A. Takahashi, S. Yomoda, T. Okubo, A. Nakamura, and K. O'Hara.** 2002. Detection of a variant metallo-β-lactamase, IMP-10, from two unrelated strains of *Pseudomonas aeruginosa* and an *Alcaligenes xylosoxidans* strain. Antimicrob. Agents Chemother. **46**:2014-2016.

(50) **Kadlec, K., C. Kehrenberg, J. Wallmann, and S. Schwarz.** 2004. Antimicrobial susceptibility of *Bordetella bronchiseptica* isolates from porcine respiratory tract infections. Antimicrob. Agents Chemother. **48**:4903-4906.

(51) **Kadlec, K, I. Wiegand, C. Kehrenberg, and S. Schwarz.** 2007. Studies on the mechanisms of β-lactam resistance in *Bordetella bronchiseptica*. J. Antimicrob. Chemother. **59**:396-402.

(52) **Karunakaran, R, and S. D. Puthucheary.** 2007. *Burkholderia pseudomallei*: in vitro susceptibility to some new and old antimicrobials. Scand. J. Infect. Dis. **39**:858-861.

(53) **Keith, K. E., P. C. Oyston, B. Crossett, N. F. Fairweather, R. X. W. Titball, T. R. Walsh, and K. A. Brown.** 2005. Functional characterization of OXA-57, a class D β-lactamase from *Burkholderia pseudomallei*. Antimicrob. Agents Chemother. **49**:1639-1641.

(54) **Kenny, D.J., P. Russell, D. Rogers, S. M. Eley, and R. X. W. Titball.** 1999. In vitro susceptibilities of *Burkholderia mallei* in comparison to those of other pathogenic *Burkholderia spp*. Antimicrob. Agents Chemother. **43**:2773-2775.

(55) **Kim, D. M., C. I. Kang, C. S. Lee, H. B. Kim, E. C. Kim, N. J. Kim, M. D. Oh, and K. W. Choe.** 2006. Treatment failure due to emergence of resistance to carbapenem during therapy for *Shewanella algae* bacteremia. J. Clin. Microbiol. **44**:1172-1174.

(56) **Kirby, J. T., H. S. Sader, T. R. Walsh, and R. N. Jones.** 2004. Antimicrobial susceptibility and epidemiology of a worldwide collection of *Chryseobacterium* spp.: report from the SENTRY Antimicrobial Surveillance Program (1997-2001). J. Clin. Microbiol. **42**:445-448.

(57) **Kumar, A, M. Mayo, L. A. Trunck, A. C. Cheng, B. J. Currie, and H. P. Schweizer.** 2008. Expression of resistance-nodulation-cell-division efflux pumps in commonly used *Burkholderia pseudomallei* strains and clinical isolates from northern Australia. Trans R. So. Trop. Med. Hyg. **102** Suppl 1:S145-S151.

(58) **Lair, M. I., S. Bentolila, D. Grenet, P. Cahen, and P. Honderlick.** 1996. *Oerskovia turbata* and *Comamonas acidovorans* bacteremia in a patient with AIDS. Eur. J. Clin. Microbiol. Infect. Dis. **15**:424-426.

(59) **Lartigue, M. F., L. Poirel, N. Fortineau, and P. Nordmann.** 2005. Chromosome-borne class A BOR-1 β-lactamase of *Bordetella bronchiseptica* and *Bordetella parapertussis*. Antimicrob. Agents Chemother. **49**:2565-2567.

(60) **Lavigne, J.-P., J. B. Gaillard, G. Bourg, C. Tichit, E. Lecaillon, and A. Sotto.** 2008. Étude de souches de *Stenotrophomonas maltophilia* sécrétrices de BLSE : détection de CTX-M et étude de la virulence. Path. Biol. **56**:447-453.

(61) **Lin, P. Y., C. Chu, L. H. Su, C. T. Huang, W. Y. Chang, and C. H. Chiu.** 2004. Clinical and microbiological analysis of bloodstream infections caused by *Chryseobacterium meningosepticum* in nonneonatal patients. J. Clin. Microbiol. **42**:3353-3355.

(62) **Mammeri, H., S. Bellais, and P. Nordmann.** 2002. Chromosome-encoded β-lactamases TUS-1 and MUS-1 from *Myroides odoratus* and *Myroides odoratimimus* (formerly *Flavobacterium odoratum*), new members of the lineage of molecular subclass B1 metalloenzymes. Antimicrob. Agents Chemother. **46**:3561-3567.

(63) **Mantengoli, E., and G. M. Rossolini.** 2005. Tn*5393d*, a complex Tn*5393* derivative carrying the PER-1 extended-spectrum β-lactamase gene and other resistance determinants. Antimicrob. Agents Chemother. **49**:3289-3296.

(64) **Mensah, K, A. Philippon, C. Richard, and P. Névot.** 1990. Susceptibility of *Alcaligenes denitrificans subspecies xylosoxydans* to β-lactam antibiotics. Eur. J. Clin. Microbiol. Infect. Dis. **9**:405-409.

(65) **Mercuri, P. S., Y. Ishii, L. Ma, G. M. Rossolini, F. Luzzaro, G. Amicosante, N. Franceschini, J. M. Frere, and M. Galleni.** 2002. Clonal diversity and metallo-β-lactamase production in clinical isolates of *Stenotrophomonas maltophilia*. Microb. Drug Resist. **8**:193-200.

(66) **Moulin, V., J. Freney, W. Hansen, and A. Philippon.** 1992. Comportement phénotypique de 121 souches de *Flavobacterium* dont *F. meningosepticum* vis-à-vis de 39 antibiotiques. Méd. Mal. Inf. **22**:902-908.

(67) **Moulin, V., G. Arlet, J. Freney, W. Hansen, Ph. Lagrange and A. Philippon.** Susceptibility pattern of *Flavobacterium meningosepticum* to antimicrobial agents including 10 β-lactams. 1992, ICAAC, C1275.

(68) **Moore, R. A, D. DeShazer, S. Reckseidler, A. Weissman, and D. E. Woods.** 1999. Efflux-mediated aminoglycoside and macrolide resistance in *Burkholderia pseudomallei*. Antimicrob. Agents Chemother. **43**:2332.

(69) **Mortensen, J. E., A. Brumbach, and T. R. Shryock.** 1989. Antimicrobial susceptibility of *Bordetella avium* and *Bordetella bronchiseptica* isolates. Antimicrob. Agents Chemother. **33**:771-772.

(70) **Nadjar, D., R. Labia, C. Cerceau, C. Bizet, A. Philippon, and G. Arlet.** 2001. Molecular characterization of chromosomal class C β-lactamase and its regulatory gene in *Ochrobactrum anthropi*. Antimicrob. Agents Chemother. **45**:2324-2330.

(71) **Naas, T., S. Bellais, and P. Nordmann.** 2003. Molecular and biochemical characterization of a carbapenem-hydrolysing β-lactamase from *Flavobacterium johnsoniae*. J. Antimicrob. Chemother. **51**:267-273.

(72) **Naiemi, N., B. Duim, and A. Bart.** 2006. A CTX-M extended-spectrum β-lactamase in *Pseudomonas aeruginosa* and *Stenotrophomonas maltophilia*. J. Med. Microbiol. **55**:1607-1608.

(73) **Nair, B. M., K. J. Jr Cheung, A. Griffith, and J.L. Burns.** 2004. Salicylate induces an antibiotic efflux pump in *Burkholderia cepacia* complex genomovar III (*B. cenocepacia*). J. Clin. Invest. **113**:464-473.

(74) **Neuwirth, C., C. Freby, A. Ogier-Desserrey, S. Perez-Martin, A. Houzel, A. Péchinot, J.M. Duez, F. Huet, and E. Siebor.** 2006. VEB-1 in *Achromobacter xylosoxidans* from cystic fibrosis patient. Emerging Infect. Dis. **12**:1737-1739.

(75) **Nicodemo, A. C., and J. I. Paez.** 2007. Antimicrobial therapy for *Stenotrophomonas maltophilia* infections. Eur. J. Clin. Microbiol. Infect. Dis. **26**:229-237.

(76) **Niumsup, P., and V. Wuthiekanun.** 2002. Cloning of the class D β-lactamase gene from *Burkholderia pseudomallei* and studies on its expression in ceftazidime-susceptible and -resistant strains. J. Antimicrob. Chemother. **50**:445-455.

(77) **Nordmann, P., L. Poirel, M. Kubina, A. Casetta, and T. Naas.** 2000. Biochemical-genetic characterization and distribution of OXA-22, a chromosomal and inducible class D β-lactamase from *Ralstonia* (*Pseudomonas*) *pickettii*. Antimicrob. Agents Chemother. **44**:2201-2204.

(78) **Peacock, S. J., H. P. Schweizer, D. A. Dance, T. L. Smith, J. E. Gee, V. Wuthiekanun, D. DeShazer, I. Steinmetz, P. Tan, and B. J. Currie B.** 2008. Management of accidental laboratory exposure to *Burkholderia pseudomallei* and *B. mallei*. Emerg. Infect. Dis.**14(7)**:e2.

(79) **Pereira, M., M. Perilli, E. Mantengoli, F. Luzzaro, A. Toniolo, G. M. Rossolini, and G. Amicosante.** 2000. PER-1 extended-spectrum β-lactamase production in an *Alcaligenes faecalis* clinical isolate resistant to expanded-spectrum cephalosporins and monobactams from a hospital in Northern Italy. Microb. Drug Resist. **6**:85-90.

(80) **Philippon, A., G. Arlet, F. Chebbi, and N. Guiso.** 1991. Sensibilité aux antibiotiques de *Bordetella bronchiseptica*: différentiation phénotypique avec *Alcaligenes faecalis* et *Alcaligenes xylosoxydans*. Méd. Mal. Inf. **21**:627-632.

(81) **Philippon, A., K. Mensah, G. Fournier, and J. Freney.** 1990. Two resistance phenotypes to β-lactams of *Alcaligenes denitrificans subsp. xylosoxydans* in relation to β-lactamase types. J. Antimicrob. Chemother. **25**:698-700

(82) **Poirel, L., C. Heritier, and P. Nordmann.** 2004. Chromosome-encoded ambler class D β-lactamase of *Shewanella oneidensis* as a progenitor of carbapenem-hydrolyzing oxacillinase. Antimicrob. Agents Chemother. **48**:348-351.

(83) **Poirel, L., J. M. Rodriguez-Martinez, P. Plésiat, and P. Nordmann.** 2009. Naturally occurring Class A β-lactamases from the *Burkholderia cepacia* complex. Antimicrob. Agents Chemother. **53**:876-882.

(84) **Ravaoarinoro, M., and C. Therrien.** 1999. β-lactamases and outer membrane investigations in β-lactam-resistant *Comamonas acidovorans* strains. Int. J. Antimicrob. Agents. **12**:27-31.

(85) **Riccio, M. L., L. Pallecchi, R. Fontana, and G. M. Rossolini.** 2001. In70 of plasmid pAX22, a *bla*(VIM-1)-containing integron carrying a new aminoglycoside phosphotransferase gene cassette. Antimicrob. Agents Chemother. **45**:1249-1253.

(86) **Rossolini, G. M., N. Franceschini, L. Lauretti, B. Caravelli, M. L. Riccio, M. Galleni, J. M. Frère, and G. Amicosante.** 1999. Cloning of a *Chryseobacterium* (*Flavobacterium*) *meningosepticum* chromosomal gene *blaA*(CME) encoding an extended-spectrum class A β-lactamase related to the *Bacteroides* cephalosporinases and the VEB-1 and PER β-lactamases. Antimicrob. Agents Chemother. **43**:2193-2199.

(87) **Rossolini, G. M., N. Franceschini, M. L. Riccio, P. S. Mercuri, M. Perilli, M. Galleni, J. M. Frere, and G. Amicosante.** 1998. Characterization and sequence of the *Chryseobacterium* (*Flavobacterium*) *meningosepticum* carbapenemase: a new molecular class B β-lactamase showing a broad substrate profile. Biochem. J. **332**:145-152

(88) **Ryan, M. P., J. T. Pembroke, and C. C. Adley.** 2006. *Ralstonia pickettii*: a persistent gram-negative nosocomial infectious organism. J. Hosp. Infect. **62**:278-284.

(89) **Safdar, A., and K. V. Rolston.** 2007. *Stenotrophomonas maltophilia*: changing spectrum of a serious bacterial pathogen in patients with cancer. Clin. Infect. Dis. **45**:1602-1609.

(90) **Segonds, C., and G. Chabanon.** 2001. *Burkholderia cepacia*: dangers of a phytopathogen organism for patients with cystic fibrosis. Ann. Biol. Clin. (Paris). **59**:259-269.

(91) **Shibata, N., Y. Doy, K. Yamane, T. Yagi, H. Kurokawa, K. Shibayama, H. Kato, K. Kai, and Y. Arakawa.** 2003. PCR typing of genetic determinants for metallo-β-lactamases and integrases carried by gram-negative bacteria isolated in Japan, with focus on the class 3 integron. J. Clin. Microbiol. **41**:5407-5413.

(92) **Stonecipber, K. G., H. G. Jensen, P. R. Kastl, A. Faulkner, and J. J. Rowsey.** 1991. Ocular infections associated with *Comamonas acidovorans*. Am. J. Ophthalmol. **1**:46-49.

(93) **Tan, A. L., and M. L. Tan.** 2008. Melioidosis: antibiogram of cases in Singapore 1987-2007. Trans. R. Soc. Trop. Med. Hyg. **102** Suppl **1**:S101-S102.

(94) **Teyssier, C., H. Marchandin, H. Jean-Pierre, I. Diego, H. Darbas, J. L. Jeannot, A. Gouby, E. Jumas-Bilak.** 2005. Molecular and phenotypic features for identification of the opportunistic pathogens *Ochrobactrum spp*. J. Med. Microbiol. **54**:945-953.

(95) **Thibault, F. M., E. Hernandez, D. R. Vidal, M. Girardet, and J. D. Cavallo.** 2004. Antibiotic susceptibility of 65 isolates of *Burkholderia pseudomallei* and *Burkholderia mallei* to 35 antimicrobial agents. J. Antimicrob. Chemother. **54**:1134-1138.

(96) **Toleman, M. A., P. M. Bennett, D. M. Bennett, R. N. Jones, and T. R. Walsh.** 2007. Global emergence of trimethoprim/sulfamethoxazole resistance in *Stenotrophomonas maltophilia* mediated by acquisition of *sul* genes. Emerg. Infect. Dis. **13**:559-565.

(97) **Trépanier, S., A. Prince, and A. Huletsky.** 1997. Characterization of the *penA* and *penR* genes of *Burkholderia cepacia* 249 which encode the chromosomal class A penicillinase and its LysR-type transcriptional regulator. Antimicrob. Agents Chemother. **41**:2399-2405.

(98) **Tribuddharat, C., R. A. Moore, P. Baker, and D. E. Woods.** 2003. *Burkholderia pseudomallei* class a β-lactamase mutations that confer selective resistance against ceftazidime or clavulanic acid inhibition. Antimicrob. Agents Chemother. **47**:2082-2087.

(99) **Viktorov, D. V., I. B. Zakharova, M. V. Podshivalova, E. V. Kalinkina, O. A. Merinova, N. P. Ageeva, V. A. Antonov, L. K. Merinova, and V. V Alekseev.** 2008. High-level resistance to fluoroquinolones and cephalosporins in *Burkholderia pseudomallei* and closely related species. Trans. R. Soc. Trop. Med. Hyg. **102** Suppl 1:S103-S110.

(100) **Wen, A., M. Fegan, C. Hayward, S. Chakraborty, and L.I. Sly.** 1999. Phylogenetic relationships among members of the *Comamonadaceae*, and description of *Delftia acidovorans* (den Dooren de Jong 1926 and Tamaoka et al. 1987) gen. nov., comb. nov. Int. J. Syst. Bacteriol. **49**:567-576.

(101) **Woodford, N., M. F. Palepou, G. S. Babini, B. Holmes, and D. M Livermore.** 2000. Carbapenemases of *Chryseobacterium (Flavobacterium) meningosepticum*: distribution of *blaB* and characterization of a novel metallo-β-lactamase gene, *blaB3*, in the type strain NCTC 10016. Antimicrob. Agents Chemother. **44**:1448-1452.

(102) **Woolfrey, B. F., and J. A. Moody.** 1991. Human infections associated with *Bordetella bronchiseptica*. Clin. Microbiol. Rev. **4**:243-255.

(103) **Zellweger, C, T. Bodmer, M. G. Täuber, and K. Mühlemann.** 2004. Failure of ceftriaxone in an intravenous drug user with invasive infection due to *Ralstonia pickettii*. Infection. **32**:246-248.

(104) **Zhang L, X. Z. Li, and K. Poole.** 2001.Fluoroquinolone susceptibilities of efflux-mediated multidrug-resistant *Pseudomonas aeruginosa*, *Stenotrophomonas maltophilia* and *Burkholderia cepacia*. J. Antimicrob. Chemother. **48**:549-552.

Chapter 16. AMINOGLYCOSIDES AND GRAM-POSITIVE BACTERIA

Roland BISMUTH and Patrice COURVALIN

INTRODUCTION

Aminoglycosides are composed of several glycosidic rings linked to an aminocyclitol (ring with six carbon atoms). The aminocyclitol may be streptidine [streptomycin (Sm), spectinomycin (Sp)] (Fig. 1) but in most cases it is 2-deoxystreptamine (2-DOS). The 2-DOS ring may be substituted at positions 4 and 5 [neomycin (Nm), lividomycin and paromomycin] (Fig. 2) or at positions 4 and 6 [kanamycin (Km) group and derivatives: tobramycin (Tm), dibekacin, amikacin (Ak), arbekacin and isepamicin (Is) Fig. 3); and gentamicin (Gm) group and derivatives, sisomicin and netilmicin (Nt)] (Fig. 4).

Aminoglycosides are highly stable, cationic, hydrophilic antibiotics with a broad antimicrobial spectrum and rapid bactericidal action.

Entry of an aminoglycoside into a Gram-positive bacterium takes place in three steps (2, 3, 24): the first step across the peptidoglycan is passive, rapid and nonspecific; in the next two steps known as EDP-I and EDP-II (Energy Dependent Phase), the aminoglycoside crosses the cytoplasmic membrane by active transport requiring the protonmotive force generated by the respiratory chain and the electron translocator ATPase. The second step, EDP-I, allows translocation across the cytoplasmic membrane and slow accumulation in the cytoplasm; this step depends on the extracellular concentration of the antibiotic. As the aminoglycoside gradually attaches to ribosomal proteins, the third step (EDP-II) takes place, characterized by accelerated uptake and saturation of ribosomal binding sites. This step is essential for bactericidal activity and only occurs in susceptible strains (14). This active mechanism of aminoglycoside uptake explains why bacteria devoid of respiratory chain enzymes show little or no susceptibility to aminoglycosides; such bacteria include strict anaerobes (*Clostridium*) as well as oxygen-tolerant anaerobes (streptococci, including pneumococci, and enterococci).

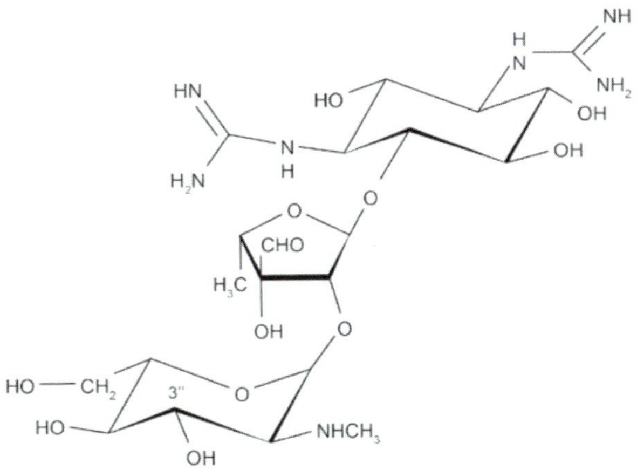

RESISTANCE MECHANISMS

Two mechanisms of unequal importance underlie acquired resistance in Gram-positive bacteria: alteration of the ribosomal target and structural modification of aminoglycosides by enzymes acquired by the bacteria.

Ribosomal alteration

This mechanism mainly concerns streptomycin which, because it binds to a single ribosomal protein, enables the selection of highly resistant mutants in a single step. Such mutants have been found in *S. pneumoniae* and *E. faecalis*. On the other hand, mutants resistant to other aminoglycosides (2-DOS derivatives) are rarely isolated in clinical practice because their selection implies that multiple mutations have taken place, since they have several, non-overlapping binding sites.

Enzymatic modification

This is the principal mechanism of acquired resistance. The synthesis of aminoglycoside-modifying enzymes encoded on plasmids or transposons is governed by endogenous housekeeping genes (23). There are three classes of enzymes catalyzing three types of reactions: aminoglycoside *N*-acetyltransferases (AAC) catalyze acetylation of an amino group; aminoglycoside *O*-phosphotransferases (APH) catalyze phosphorylation a

Fig. 1. Structure of streptomycin.

Deoxystreptamines substituted at 4.5

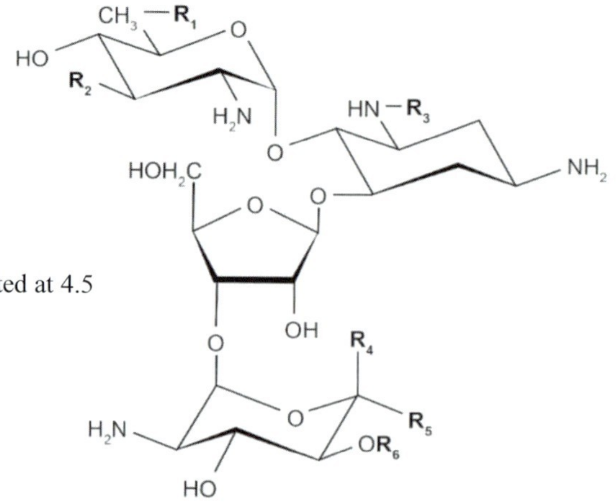

	R_1	R_2	R_3	R_4	R_5	R_6
Neomycin B	NH_2	OH	H	CH_2NH_2	H	H
Neomycin C	NH_2	OH	H	H	H	H
Lividomycin A	OH	H	H	CH_2NH_2	H	α-D-Mannose pyranosyl
Lividomycin B	OH	H	H	CH_2NH_2	H	H
Paromomycin I	OH	OH	H	CH_2NH_2	H	H
Paromomycin II	OH	OH	H	H	CH_2NH_2	CH_2NH_2

Fig. 2. Structures of neomycins, lividomycins, and paronomycins. Commercialized neomycin complex is *ca.* neomycin B 80-90%, C 20-10%.

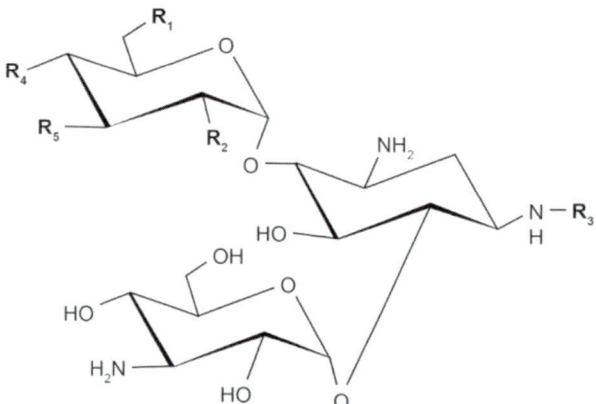

	R_1	R_2	R_3	R_4	R_5
Kanamycin A	NH_2	OH	H	OH	OH
Kanamycin B	NH_2	NH_2	H	OH	OH
Kanamycin C	OH	NH_2	H	OH	OH
Amikacin	NH_2	OH	$COCHOH(CH_2)_2NH_2$	OH	OH
Didekacin	NH_2	H	H	H	H
Habekacin	NH_2	NH_2	NH_2	H	H
Tobramycin	NH_2	NH_2	NH_2	OH	OH

Fig. 3. Structure of kanamycins and derivatives. Commercialized kanamycin complex is *ca.* kanamycin A 96-99%, B 4-1%.

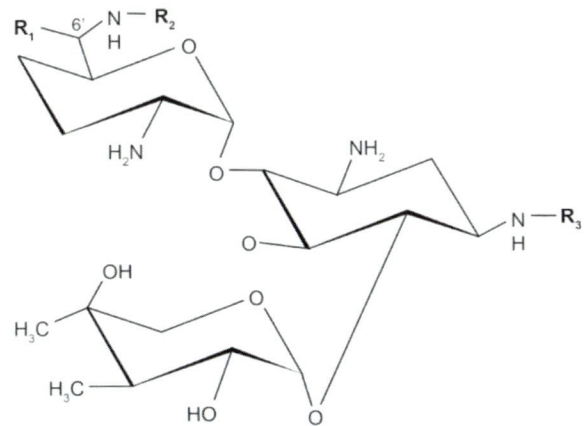

	R_1	R_2	R_3
Gentamicin C1	CH_3	CH_3	H
Gentamicin C1A	H	H	H
Gentamicin C2	CH_3	H	H
Sisomicin	NH_2	H	H
Netilmicin	NH_2	H	C_2H_5

Fig. 4. Structures of gentamicins and derivatives. Commercialized gentamicin complex is *ca.* gentamicin C1a 25%, C1 40%, and C2 33%.

hydroxyl group, and aminoglycoside nucleotidyltransferases (ANT) catalyze nucleotidylation of a hydroxyl group (Table 1).

Each of these classes can be divided into subclasses according to the position of the carbon atom bearing the amino or hydroxyl group which is modified (Arabic numerals). In some subclasses, certain enzymes have different substrate specificities and thus several distinct isoenzymes exist (Roman numerals). Each enzyme recognizes and modifies a given number of substrates, thereby conferring a unique resistance phenotype.

These enzymes are constitutive and intracellular: the aminoglycoside is only modified after entering the bacterial cell. This modification prevents it from binding to the ribosome which is necessary at the third step of cell entry (EDP-II). The resultant level of resistance differs according to the enzyme (APHs, unlike AACs and ANTs, confer high-level resistance) and the host cell, which means that the presence of an enzyme may not necessarily cause a sufficient increase in the MIC for the strain to be reported as resistant on the basis of critical values (breakpoints) that delineate the clinical categories. If the enzyme has low affinity for its substrate or if access to the catalytic site is hindered by the antibiotic's structure (e.g., amikacin), some of the drug molecules may remain unmodified and reach their ribosomal target, allowing the antibiotic to conserve much of its bacteriostatic activity while losing some of its bactericidal activity since the EDP-II step cannot take place.

Some enzymes have been found only in Gram-positive cocci [APH(2")], others only in Gram-negative bacilli [ANT(2"), AAC(3)] and still others, such as APH(3') and AAC(6'), in both types of organism. However, these latter enzymes are encoded by different genes and have different substrate specificities. For instance, APH(3')-I and –II which are present in Gram-negative bacilli modify kanamycin and neomycin but not amikacin, while APH(3')-III present in Gram-positive cocci modifies kanamycin, neomycin and also amikacin.

To date, five enzymatic activities have been described in Gram-positive microorganisms (23):

- **ANT(6)-I** confers resistance to streptomycin; **Sm phenotype**
- **ANT(9)-I** confers resistance to spectinomycin; this enzyme has only been detected in staphylococci.
- **APH(3')-III** confers high-level resistance to kanamycin and neomycin; **KmNm phenotype**. This enzyme also phosphorylates amikacin (13) and isepamicin (23) although strains harboring it are susceptible to these two drugs. This is because the enzyme has low affinity for these two substrates which are phosphorylated very slowly and which therefore conserve their bacteriostatic activity while losing their bactericidal activity (11, 14). This enzyme has been found in staphylococci (13), enterococci (28), streptococci, pneumococci (5) and *Bacillus* (6). Lividomycin has no hydroxyl group at position 3' and is modified on the 5" hydroxyl group; hence the enzyme is named APH(3')(5")-III (11).
- **ANT(4')-I** confers high-level resistance to kanamycin and especially to tobramycin; **KmTm phenotype**. It also modifies neomycin and dibekacin although they are poor substrates. Dibekacin does not have a 4' hydroxyl group and is modified on the 4" hydroxyl group, hence the name ANT(4')(4")-I (11). Amikacin and isepamicin are substrates for this enzyme if present at high concentrations, otherwise their structure hinders them from reaching the active site. Strains harboring this enzyme are therefore susceptible to these two aminoglycosides. The enzyme was originally detected in *S. aureus* (19) and *S. epidermidis*

Table 1. Substrate profiles of aminoglycoside modifying enzymes[a]

Aminoglycoside	Enzymes												
	Phosphotransferase (APH)					Nucleotidyltransferase (ANT)					Acetyltransferase (AAC)			
	(6)	(3')	(2")	(3")	(5")	(6)	(9)	(2")	(3")(9)	(4')	(1)	(3)	(2')	(6')-I
NeomycinB	-	+	-	-	(+)	-	-	-	-	+	(+)	(+)	(+)	+
Paromomycin	-	+	-	-	(+)	-	-	-	-	+	+	-	(+)	+
Lividomycin A	-	(+)	-	-	(+)	-	-	-	-	+	+	-	(+)	+
Ribostamycin	-	+	-	-	+	-	-	-	-	+	+	+	(+)	+
Butirosin	-	(+)	-	-	(+)	-	-	-	-	+	(+)	(+)	-	-
Kanamycin A	-	+	(+)	-	-	-	-	+	-	+	-	+	(+)	+
Kanamycin B	-	+	(+)	-	-	-	-	+	-	+	-	+	(+)	+
Kanamycin C	-	+	(+)	-	-	-	-	+	-	+	-	+	(+)	+
Tobramycin	-	-	(+)	-	-	-	-	+	-	+*	-	+	(+)	+
Dibekacin	-	-	(+)	-	-	-	-	+	-	(+)	-	+	(+)	+
Amikacin	-	(+)	(+)	-	-	-	-	-	-	+	-	-	-	+
Habekacin	-	-	(+)	-	-	-	-	-	-	-	-	-	-	-
Isepamicin	-	(+)	(+)	-	-	-	-	-	-	+	-	-	+	+
Gentamicin C1[a]	-	-	+	-	-	-	-	+	-	-	-	+	+	-
Gentamicin C1	-	-	+	-	-	-	-	+	-	-	-	+	+	+
Gentamicin C2	-	-	+	-	-	-	-	+	-	-	-	+	+	+
Sisomicin	-	-	+	-	-	-	-	+	-	-	-	(+)	+	+
5-episisomicin	-	-	-	-	-	-	-	-	-	-	-	(+)	+	+
Netilmicin	-	-	+	-	-	-	-	-	-	-	-	(+)	(+)	+
2-N-ethylnetilmicin	-	-	+	-	-	-	-	-	-	-	-	(+)	+	+
6'-N-ethylnetilmicin	-	-	+	-	-	-	-	-	-	-	-	(+)	+	-
Streptomycin	+	-	-	+	-	-	-	-	+	-	-	-	-	-
Spectinomycin	-	-	-	-	-	-	+	-	+	-	-	-	-	-
Apramycin	-	-	-	-	-	-	-	-	-	-	+	(+)	-	-
Fortimicin	-	-	-	-	-	-	-	-	-	-	-	(+)	-	-

[a] +, substrate; (+), substrate for certain isozymic forms of the enzyme; -, non substrate. The fact that an antibiotic is a substrate in vitro for an enzyme does not imply that strains producing that enzyme are necessarily resistant to this antibiotic.

but also in a few enterococcal strains (7) and *Bacillus* spp. (1).
- **AAC(6')-APH(2")** confers high-level resistance to kanamycin, gentamicin and tobramycin; **KmGmTm phenotype**. The two enzymatic activities are mediated by a bifunctional protein whose amino terminal has an AAC(6') domain and whose carboxy terminal has an APH(2") domain (17). APH(2") modifies kanamycin, gentamicin, tobramycin efficiently and netilmicin moderately, but it does not act upon amikacin or isepamicin (23). AAC(6') efficiently modifies kanamycin and tobramycin, but not gentamicin, and it modifies netilmicin, amikacin and isepamicin moderately (23). This explains why strains harboring this enzyme are susceptible to amikacin and neomycin. The enzyme was originally found in *S. aureus* (11), *E. faecalis* (17), *S. epidermidis*, *S. agalactiae* (group B streptococcus) (4) and *E. faecium*. The sequences of the genes isolated from these different species are highly conserved (22).

AAC(6') and APH(2") have been found alone in enterococci. *aac(6')* is a chromosomal gene which has been detected in all *E. faecium* strains (10). APH(2") has been found in a few enterococcal strains (15). The features of these aminoglycoside-modifying enzymes are summarized in Table 2.

Table 2. Aminoglycoside modifying enzymes in Gram-positive cocci

Enzyme	Gene	Resistance phenotype[a]
ANT(6)-I[b]	*ant*(6)Ia	Sm
ANT(9)-I	*ant*(9)Ia	Sp
APH(3')-III	*aph*(3')IIIa	KmNm(Ak,Is)[c]
ANT(4')-I	*ant*(4')Ia	KmTm(Nm,Ak,Is)
AAC(6')-APH(2")-I	*aac*(6')Ie	KmGmTm(Ak,Is,Nt)
	aph(2")Ia	
AAC(6')-Ii	*aac*(6')Ii	KmTm(Ak,Is,Nt)
APH(2")-Ib,d	*aph*(2")Ib,d	KmGmTmNt(Ak)
APH(2")-Ic	*aph*(2")Ic	KmGmTm

[a] Ak, amikacin; Gm, gentamicin; Is, isepamicin; Km, kanamycin; Nm, neomycin; Nt, netilmicin; Sm, streptomycin; Sp, spectinomycin; Tm, tobramycin.
[b] AAC, aminoglycoside acetyltransferase; ANT, aminoglycoside nucleotidyltransferase; APH, aminoglycoside phosphotransferase.
[c] ( ) poor substrates.

Resistance phenotypes in staphylococci

Five phenotypes can be distinguished:
- susceptible
- Sm ANT(6)
- KmNm APH(3')
- KmTm ANT(4')
- KmGmTm AAC(6')-APH(2")

Five combined phenotypes can be distinguished: Sm+KmNmANT(6)+APH(3'), Sm+KmGmTmANT(6)+AAC(6')-APH(2"), Sm+KmTm ANT(6)+ANT(4'), Sm+KmNm+KmGmTm and Sm+KmTm+KmGmTm. The first three result from combination of an Sm phenotype with a KmNm, KmGmTm or KmTm phenotype. On the other hand, there are three possible genotypes that can confer a KmGmTmNm (± Sm) phenotype: KmNm+KmGmTm: APH(3')+AAC(6')-APH(2"), KmTm(Nm)+KmGmTm: ANT(4')+AAC(6')-APH(2"), KmNm+KmTm+KmGmTm: APH(3')+ANT(4')+AAC(6')-APH(2").

Taking into account the behavior of each strain in the simultaneous presence of different aminoglycosides allows deduction of the resistance mechanism(s) underlying the phenotype, even when resistance is low-level.

Phenotypic analysis requires a minimum of three aminoglycosides: kanamycin, gentamicin and tobramycin and a maximum of seven: streptomycin, kanamycin, neomycin, gentamicin, tobramycin, amikacin and netilmicin.

Susceptible phenotype

S. aureus and coagulase-negative staphylococci are usually susceptible to aminoglycosides (Fig. 5A, 5B), the latter to a greater extent than the former. This explains why resistance phenotypes are more difficult to detect in coagulase-negative staphylococci. MIC values are given in Tables 3 and 4.

Sm phenotype [ANT(6)]

This high-level streptomycin resistance phenotype alone (Fig. 5C) is due to the presence of either an ANT(6) or a ribosomal mutation. By including spectinomycin in the susceptibility test it is possible to detect the presence of ANT(9) alone or combined with ANT(6).

KmNm phenotype [APH(3')]

This phenotype confers high-level resistance to kanamycin and neomycin. It is due to the presence of an APH(3')-III which modifies these two anti-

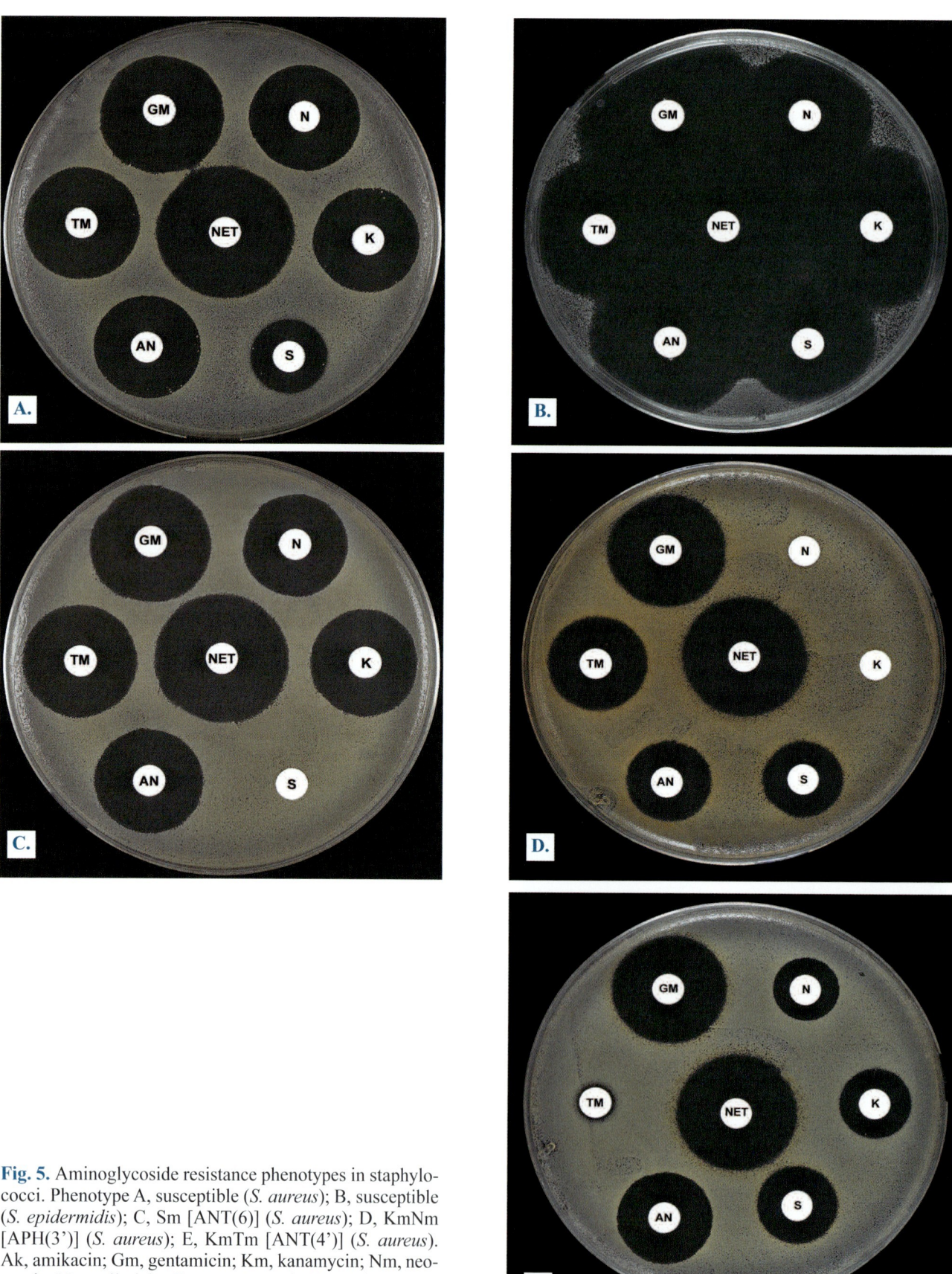

Fig. 5. Aminoglycoside resistance phenotypes in staphylococci. Phenotype A, susceptible (*S. aureus*); B, susceptible (*S. epidermidis*); C, Sm [ANT(6)] (*S. aureus*); D, KmNm [APH(3')] (*S. aureus*); E, KmTm [ANT(4')] (*S. aureus*). Ak, amikacin; Gm, gentamicin; Km, kanamycin; Nm, neomycin; Nt, netilmicin; Sm, streptomycin; Tm, tobramycin.

Table 3. Impact of modifying enzymes on the bacteriostatic activity of aminoglycosides against *S. aureus*

Enzyme (No. of strains)	MIC geometric mean (µg/ml)[a] (range of values)			
	Gentamicin	Tobramycin	Amikacin	Netilmicin
O (n=24)	0.2 (0.06-0.25)	0.12 (0.06-0.25)	1 (0.5-1)	0.1 (0.06-0.12)
APH(3') (n=24)	0.2 (0.06-0.5)	0.3 (0.12-1)	4 (1-16)	0.12 (0.06-0.25)
ANT(4') (n=24)	0.12 (0.06-0.5)	32 (8- ≥ 128)	4 (1-16)	0.12 (0.06-0.05)
AAC(6')-APH(2") (n=37)	16 (1- ≥ 128)	16 (2- ≥ 128)	4 (0.5-64)	1 (0.06-16)
APH(3')+AAC(6')-APH(2") (n=52)	28 (2- ≥ 128)	24 (4- ≥ 128)	12 (2-64)	2 (0.06-32)
ANT(4')+AAC(6')-APH(2") (n=4)	64 (32-128)	>128	12 (8-16)	7 (4-8)
APH(3')+ANT(4')+AAC(6')-APH(2") (n=3)	32	>128	16 (8-32)	2 (1-4)

[a] Determined by dilution in Mueller-Hinton agar.

Table 4. Impact of modifying enzymes on the bacteriostatic activity of aminoglycosides against coagulase-negative staphylococci

Enzyme (No. of strains)	Geometric mean MIC (µg/ml)[a]			
	Gentamicin	Tobramycin	Amikacin	Netilmicin
O (n=24)	0.07	0.08	0.37	0.08
APH(3') (n=10)	0.09	0.18	3	0.12
ANT(4') (n=19)	0.07	9.2	1	0.08
AAC(6')-APH(2") (n=15)	64	48	2	1
APH(3')+ANT(4') (n=1)	0.06	8	2	0.06
APH(3')+AAC(6')-APH(2") (n=15)	7	8	3.6	1.5
ANT(4')+AAC(6')-APH(2") (n=17)	29	77	9	3.1
ANT(4')+APH(3')+AAC(6')-APH(2") (n=10)	39	127	14	5.3

[a] Determined by dilution in Mueller-Hinton agar.

biotics as well as amikacin and isepamicin (Fig. 5D). MICs determined in agar and broth medium are presented in Tables 3 and 5. It can be seen that the MIC of amikacin for such strains is multiplied by a factor of 4. An examination of the bacteriostatic activity in broth medium shows that all the susceptible strains are inhibited by 8 µg/ml while only 70% of strains harboring APH(3')-III are inhibited by 16 µg/ml.

In coagulase-negative staphylococci, tests in agar (Table 7) and broth medium (Table 4) show that the MIC of amikacin for strains harboring APH(3')-III is ten-fold higher than that of susceptible strains.

KmTm phenotype [ANT(4')]

This phenotype confers high-level resistance to kanamycin and especially tobramycin. It is due to the presence of an ANT(4') which modifies these two antibiotics and also partially modifies neomycin, amikacin and isepamicin (Fig. 5E). The MIC of amikacin for *S. aureus* strains is four-fold higher in agar medium and seven-fold higher in broth medium (Tables 3 and 5). On the basis of the bacteriostatic activity determined in broth medium, it can be seen that only 45% of strains harboring an ANT(4') are inhibited by 16 µg/ml whereas all the susceptible strains are inhibited by 8 µg/ml. In coagulase-negative staphylococci, the MIC of amikacin is increased by a factor of four in strains harboring this enzyme (Tables 4 and 5).

KmGmTm phenotype [AAC(6')-APH(2")]

This phenotype confers high-level resistance to kanamycin, gentamicin and tobramycin. It is due to the presence of the bifunctional enzyme AAC(6')-APH(2"). This enzyme does not inactivate neomycin, which is why this antibiotic is useful to ascertain that the strain does harbor only this enzyme, since neomycin is a substrate of APH(3')-

Table 5. Impact of modifying enzymes on the bacteriostatic and bactericidal activity of aminoglycosides against *S. aureus*

Enzyme (No. of strains)	Geometric mean MIC (MBC) (µg/ml)[a]			
	Gentamicin	Tobramycin	Amikacin	Netilmicin
O (n=24)	0.6 (1)	0.6 (1)	5 (10)	0.4 (0.8)
APH(3') (n=24)	0.8 (2)	1 (2)	15 (30)	0.7 (0.9)
ANT(4') (n=24)	0.8 (1.2)	128 (> 128)	28 (56)	0.6 (1.2)
AAC(6')-APH(2") (n=37)	100 (> 128)	64 (> 128)	28 (60)	12 (34)
APH(3')+AAC(6')-APH(2") (n=52)	> 128 (> 128)	82 (> 128)	30 (100)	12 (34)
ANT(4')+AAC(6')-APH(2") (n=4)	> 128 (> 128)	> 128 (> 128)	56 (100)	8 (26)
ANT(4')+APH(3')+AAC(6')-APH(2") (n=3)	> 128 (> 128)	> 128 (> 128)	64 (100)	2 (12)

[a] Determined by dilution in Mueller-Hinton liquid medium.

III and ANT(4') (Fig. 6A). On the other hand, amikacin and netilmicin are partially modified.

The MIC of amikacin for *S. aureus* strains is increased four- to five-fold and that of netilmicin ten- to twenty-fold (Tables 3 and 5). On the basis of the bacteriostatic activity determined in broth medium, it can be seen that only 43% of strains harboring this enzyme are inhibited by 16 µg/ml amikacin whereas all the susceptible strains are inhibited by 8 µg/ml, and only 40% of strains are inhibited by 4 µg/ml netilmicin whereas all the susceptible strains are inhibited by 1 µg/ml.

In coagulase-negative staphylococci, the MICs of amikacin and netilmicin are increased ten-fold in strains harboring this enzyme (Tables 4 and 5).

Combined phenotypes

- The Sm phenotype ANT(6) can be found in combination with the phenotypes KmNm APH(3'), KmTm ANT(4'), or KmGmTm AAC(6')-APH(2") without modifying the activity of these aminoglycosides, apart from streptomycin (Fig. 6B and 6C).
- The most common combined phenotype (Sm)+KmGmTmNm can only be detected by testing neomycin (Fig. 6D and 6E).
- This phenotype can result from three different combinations of enzymes: APH(3')+AAC(6')-APH(2"), ANT(4')+AAC(6')-APH(2") and APH(3')+AAC(6')-APH(2")+ANT(4'). The fact that neomycin is modified can be due to the presence of an APH(3'), an ANT(4') or both enzymes.
- The most common enzyme combination is APH(3')+AAC(6')-APH(2"). In *S. aureus*, these two enzymes have an additive effect on the level of amikacin resistance.
- In coagulase-negative staphylococci, these two enzymes act synergistically on the level of resistance.

By determining the bacteriostatic activity of amikacin and netilmicin against *S. aureus* in agar or broth medium (Tables 3 and 5), it can be seen that the MICs of amikacin are increased five-fold in strains harboring one enzyme, ten-fold in strains harboring two enzymes and fifteen-fold when three enzymes are present. Similarly, the MICs of netilmicin are multiplied by a factor of ten or more in strains harboring an AAC(6')-APH(2") alone or in combination.

On the basis of the bacteriostatic activity determined in broth medium, only 35% of strains are inhibited by 16 µg/ml amikacin whereas all the susceptible strains are inhibited by 8 µg/ml.

For coagulase-negative staphylococci, the MICs of amikacin are multiplied by a factor of eight in strains harboring one enzyme, fifteen in those with two enzymes and thirty in strains harboring three enzymes (Tables 4 and 6).

IMPACT OF MODIFYING ENZYMES ON BACTERICIDAL ACTIVITY

Aminoglycoside-susceptible strains are killed by 2 µg/ml gentamicin, tobramycin or netilmicin and 16 µg/ml amikacin (Table 5). Amikacin has less bactericidal activity and the MBC is three-fold higher in strains harboring an APH(3'), six-fold higher in strains with an ANT(4') or AAC(6')-APH(2"), and ten-fold higher in strains harboring both enzymes (Tables 5 and 6). This loss of amikacin's bactericidal activity becomes even more apparent when one examines the percentage of strains killed by 16 µg/ml, the bactericidal concentration for all susceptible strains. This concentration kills only 40%, 20% and 20%

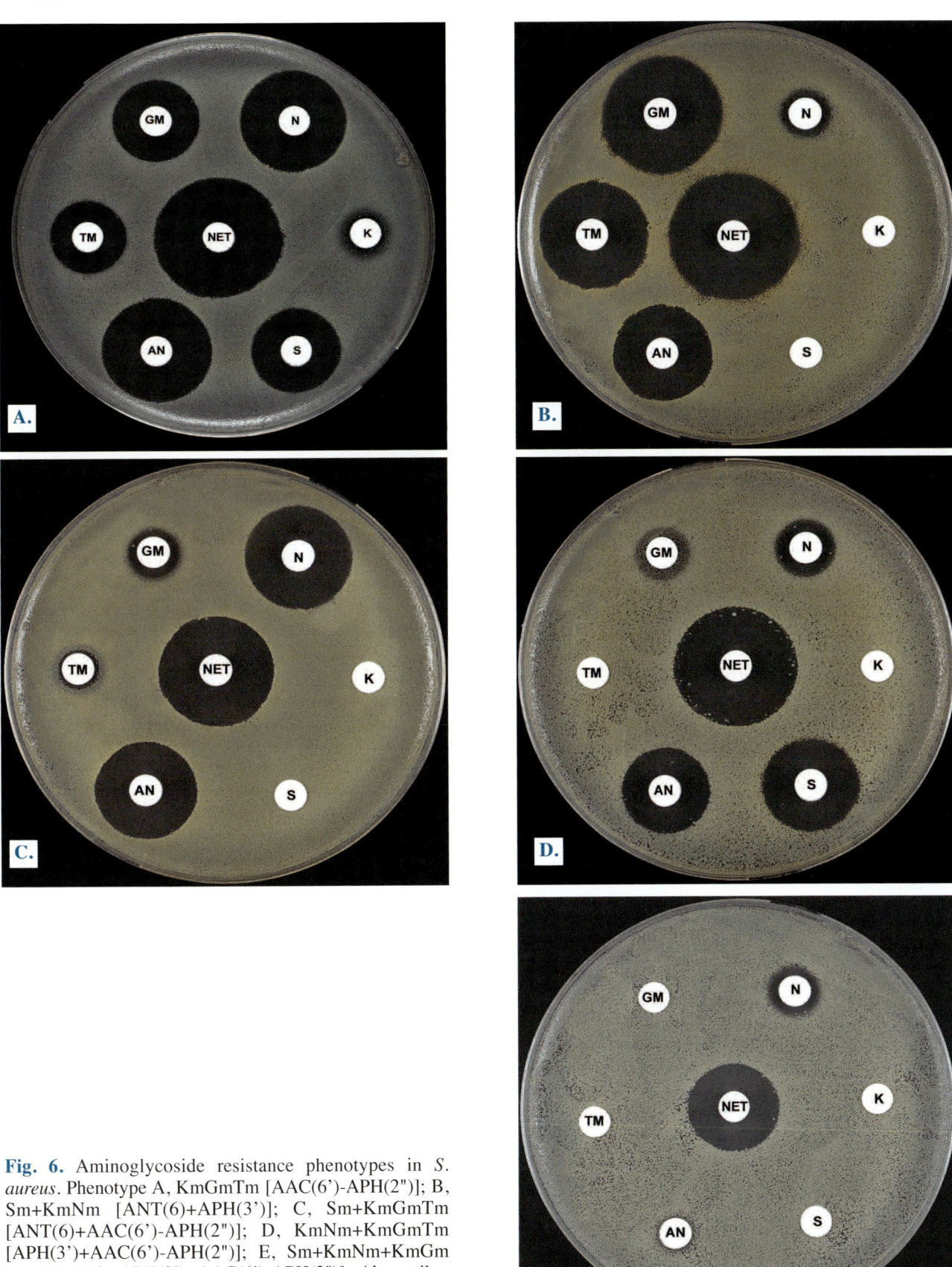

Fig. 6. Aminoglycoside resistance phenotypes in *S. aureus*. Phenotype A, KmGmTm [AAC(6')-APH(2")]; B, Sm+KmNm [ANT(6)+APH(3')]; C, Sm+KmGmTm [ANT(6)+AAC(6')-APH(2")]; D, KmNm+KmGmTm [APH(3')+AAC(6')-APH(2")]; E, Sm+KmNm+KmGmTm [ANT(6)+APH(3')+AAC(6')-APH(2")]; Ak, amikacin; Gm, gentamicin; Km, kanamycin; Nm, neomycin; Nt, netilmicin; Sm, streptomycin; Tm, tobramycin.

Table 6. Impact of modifying enzymes on the bacteriostatic and bactericidal activity of aminoglycosides against coagulase-negative staphylococci

Enzyme (No. of strains)	MIC (MBC) geometric mean (µg/ml)[a]			
	Gentamicin	Tobramycin	Amikacin	Netilmicin
O (n=20)	0.1 (0.18)	0.1 (0.22)	0.85 (1.4)	0.08 (0.15)
APH(3') (n=10)	0.12 (0.25)	0.25 (0.5)	8 (12)	0.09 (0.2)
ANT(4') (n=19)	0.1 (0.3)	23 (74)	4 (11.5)	0.15 (0.3)
AAC(6')-APH(2") (n=15)	48 (> 128)	32 (64)	12 (32)	16 (24)
APH(3')+ANT(4') (n=1)	0.25 (0.25)	32 (128)	8 (32)	0.06 (0.5)
APH(3")+AAC(6')-APH(2") (n=15)	25 (53)	16 (32)	8 (18.5)	2 (5)
ANT(4')+AAC(6')-APH(2") (n=17)	71 (100)	83 (> 128)	22 (> 128)	5 (22)
ANT(4')+APH(3')+AAC(6')-APH(2") (n=10)	64 (> 128)	114 (> 128)	32 (> 128)	21 (> 128)

[a] Determined by dilution in Mueller-Hinton liquid medium.

of strains harboring an APH(3'), ANT(4') or AAC(6')-APH(2"), respectively, and only 4% of strains harboring two enzymes. Similar results are seen with netilmicin in strains harboring an AAC(6')-APH(2"): the MBC is increased by a factor of 40 and only 5% of strains are killed by 4 µg/ml netilmicin, whereas all the susceptible strains are killed by 2 µg/ml. The bactericidal activity of netilmicin appears to be more affected by the bifunctional enzyme than that of amikacin. This is easily explained by the structural features of the two drugs: amikacin has more difficult access to the enzyme active site due to a hydroxyaminobutyric acid (HABA) substitution at position 1 of the DOS ring (Fig. 1) (13) and also by the fact that netilmicin is modified by both enzyme domains while amikacin is only modified by the AAC(6') domain (21). Similar but more pronounced results are seen in coagulase-negative staphylococci. Amikacin MBCs are increased by a factor of ten in strains harboring one enzyme and twenty or more in those with two or three enzymes. Netilmicin MBCs are thirty-fold higher in strains harboring an AAC(6')-APH(2") (Table 6).

ANTIBIOTICS TO BE TESTED

CLSI (8) mentions gentamicin in the group C of antibiotics to be tested against staphylococci. Group C antibiotics are supplemental agents to be tested and reported selectively in institutions that harbor endemic or epidemic strains resistant to one or more of the primary drugs. Breakpoints are available for amikacin, kanamycin, gentamicin, tobramycin, and netilmicin.

EUCAST provides recommendations for the report of aminoglycosides in case of resistance to kanamycin, tobramycin, or gentamicin on the basis of loss of synergism with cell-wall active agents. If resistant to kanamycin, report as resistant to kanamycin and amikacin. If resistant to gentamicin, report as resistant to all aminoglycosides (except streptomycin). If resistant to tobramycin, report as resistant to kanamycin, tobramycin, and amikacin. Although there is no current recommendation from EUCAST for aminoglycosides that should be routinely tested, it seems logical to test at least gentamicin, and possibly kanamycin to predict the activity of amikacin. Since clinical breakpoints are not available for kanamycin and staphylococci, epidemiological cut-off might be used.

RESISTANCE PHENOTYPES IN STREPTOCOCCI, PNEUMOCOCCI, AND ENTEROCOCCI

Streptococci, pneumococci and enterococci, which are oxygen-tolerant anerobes, are intrinsically resistant to low aminoglycoside concentrations (MICs ranging from 4-64 µg/ml). This low-level resistance is due to inefficient active transport across the cytoplasmic membrane resulting from the absence of respiratory chain enzymes. However these organisms are intrinsically susceptible to high aminoglycoside concentrations (≥ 1000 µg/ml). Combination with a penicillin, which acts by inhibiting cell wall synthesis, increases uptake of aminoglycosides and results in bactericidal synergy. The MICs of aminoglycosides for the main groups of streptococci are presented in Table 7.

Table 7. MIC (μg/ml) of aminoglycosides against low-level resistant enterococci and streptococci

Aminoglycoside	Streptococcus A	S. pneumoniae	Non-groupable streptococci	E. faecalis
Streptomycin	12-50	6-25	6-25	25-128
Kanamycin	12-50	6-25	12-50	64 - ≥ 128
Gentamicin	4-8	3-6	6-12	4-16

Some strains may become highly resistant (MIC > 1000 μg/ml) either by alteration of the target, or by acquisition of genes encoding modifying enzymes. The first mechanism is uncommon and is linked to a mutation of the ribosomal target. It has been described in clinical isolates of E. faecalis resistant to streptomycin and has not been found for other aminoglycosides. These mutants display very high streptomycin resistance (MIC ≥ 128,000 μg/ml) far above strains which produce a modifying enzyme. The presence of modifying enzymes is by far the most common resistance mechanism and concerns all the aminoglycosides.

E. faecium is a special case since all strains of this species intrinsically synthesize an AAC(6')-Ii encoded by a chromosomal gene (10). This resistance affects the bactericidal activity more than the bacteriostatic activity of aminoglycosides, explaining why it can be difficult to detect on an antibiogram. It abolishes the synergy between cell wall-active antibiotics such as penicillins and glycopeptides, and the aminoglycoside substrates of this enzyme: kanamycin, tobramycin, amikacin and netilmicin. Although amikacin is only weakly inactivated by AAC(6')-Ii of E. faecium, synergy is maintained when it is combined with penicillins or glycopeptides. Nonetheless it is preferable when treating severe E. faecium infections to use a penicillin + gentamicin combination, which is not a substrate of AAC(6')-Ii.

The same genes present in staphylococci can be acquired and expressed by streptococci and enterococci (22), as initially seen in S. pneumoniae and then in group A, B and C streptococci and other streptococci including S. bovis.

AAC(6')-APH(2") has been found in E. faecalis and E. faecium but only rarely in other species such as streptococci from group A (M. Galimand et al., submitted for publication), B (4, 18), G, and S. mitis. It has not yet been described in group C streptococci or S. pneumoniae.

ANT(4') has been detected in a few enterococcal strains (7).

In contrast to the staphylococci, APH(2") has been detected alone in a few strains of E. faecalis and E. faecium. Various APH(2") enzymes have been characterized in the US; they are rarely found in human enterococcal isolates but more frequently in strains isolated from animals. The APH(2") family includes the related enzymes APH(2")-Ib, -Ic and -Id.

APH(2")-Ib confers high-level resistance to kanamycin, tobramycin, gentamicin and netilmicin. It modifies amikacin to some extent. This enzyme has been found in vancomycin-resistant strains of E. faecium.

A plasmid-encoded APH(2")-Ic was first described in E. gallinarum, then in human and animal isolates of E. faecium and E. faecalis. The gene confers variable resistance to gentamicin (MICs range from 128-1024 μg/ml), tobramycin and kanamycin but not to amikacin or netilmicin. Penicillin-gentamicin synergy is abolished.

APH(2")-Id confers high-level resistance to kanamycin, tobramycin, gentamicin and netilmicin. The corresponding gene has been found in E. casseliflavus and subsequently in E. faecium (15).

IMPACT OF MODIFYING ENZYMES ON SYNERGISM OF AMINOGLYCOSIDES WITH CELL-WALL ACTIVE AGENTS AGAINST ENTEROCOCCI

In the case of a highly aminoglycoside-resistant strain, combination with a cell wall-active antibiotic (penicillin or glycopeptide) is no longer synergistic (7). Table 7 shows the increases in MICs of aminoglycosides related to the presence of one or more modifying enzymes in genetically characterized strains. MICs of amikacin and netilmicin for strains harboring AAC(6')-APH(2") show little change but synergy with penicillin is abolished; the same is true for amikacin in strains harboring an ANT(4') (7) or APH(3') (11). Amikacin has been shown to antagonize the effect of penicillin G against strains producing APH(3') (27). It is important to test for high-level resistance in streptococci and enterococci when these organisms are implicated in serious infections such as endocarditis, because in this case it is necessary to use a bactericidal combination such as amoxicillin or glycopeptide + aminoglycoside.

Table 8. Impact of modifying enzymes on aminoglycoside MICs against enterococci

Enzyme	MIC (µg/ml)					
	Sm[a]	Km	Gm	Tm	Ak	Nt
None	128	64	8	16	128	8
AAC(6')-APH(2")	256	>8192	8192	4 096	1024	64
ANT(6)+APH(3')	2048	>8192	16	32	128	8
ANT(6)+APH(3')+AAC(6')-APH(2")	>8192	>8192	8192	8192	2048	128
ANT(4')	32	>8192	4	>8192	128	4

[a] Ak, amikacin; Gm, gentamicin; Km, kanamycin; Nt, netilmicin; Sm, streptomycin; Tm, tobramycin.

DETECTION OF HIGH LEVEL RESISTANCE

High-level resistance is easy to detect by disk diffusion using highly loaded antibiotic disks. The Clinical and Laboratory Standards Institute (CLSI) recommends two disks: streptomycin 300 µg and gentamicin 120 µg, which for the latter corresponds to an MIC > 500 µg/ml (8). Mueller-Hinton agar is used for enterococci and supplemented with 5% horse blood for streptococci and pneumococci. According to the European Committee for Antimicrobial Susceptibility Testing (EUCAST) there is no synergistic effect in enterococci with high-level aminoglycoside resistance, i.e., with an MIC of gentamicin which is > 128 µg/ml (http://www.srga.org/eucastwt:MICTAB/).

The French committee CA-SFM (http://www.sfm.asso.fr/publi/general.php?pa=1) recommends the use of a kanamycin disk (1000 µg) in addition to that of gentamicin. In case of high level resistance to kanamycin, kanamycin and amikacin should not be used.

GRAM-POSITIVE BACTERIA

Virtually all *Bacillus* spp. are susceptible to aminoglycosides. An ANT(6) has been described in *B. subtilis* (21), an APH(3')-IVa in *B. circulans* (6) and a chromosomal and species-specific ANT(4') in *B. clausii* (1).

Corynebacteria, apart from *C. jeikum* and *C. urealyticum*, are susceptible to aminoglycosides. Plasmid-mediated kanamycin resistance has been described in *C. striatum* (26). *C. glutamicum* is resistant to many antibiotics including streptomycin, kanamycin and gentamicin (20, 25). Deletion of the structural gene results in reduced susceptibility to many antibiotics including aminoglycosides. *L. monocytogenes* is susceptible to aminoglycosides although kanamycin resistance conferred by an APH(3') has been described (16).

In contrast, the lactobacilli have intrinsic low-level resistance to aminoglycosides. Gram-positive bacteria with anerobic metabolism are also resistant.

REFERENCES

(1) **Bozdogan, B., S. Galopin, G. Gerbaud, P. Courvalin, and R. Leclercq**. 2003. Chromosomal *aad*D2 encodes an aminoglycoside nucleotidyltransferase in *Bacillus clausii*. **47**:1343-1346.

(2) **Bryan, L.E., S.K. Kowand, and H.M. Van den Elsen**. 1979. Mechanism of aminoglycoside antibiotic resistance in anaerobic bacteria : *Clostridium perfringens* and *Bacteroides fragilis*. Antimicrob. Agents Chemother. **15**:7-13.

(3) **Bryan, L.E., and H.M. Van den Elsen**. 1977. Effects of membrane-energy mutations and cations on streptomycin and gentamicin accumulation by bacteria: a model for entry of streptomycin and gentamicin in susceptible and resistant bacteria. Antimicrob. Agents Chemother. **12**:163-177.

(4) **Buu-Hoi, A., C. Le Bougenec, and T. Horaud**. 1990. High level chromosomal gentamicin resistance in *Streptococcus agalactiae* (group B). Antimicrob. Agents Chemother. **34**:995-998.

(5) **Caillaud, F., P. Trieu-Cuot, C. Carlier, and P. Courvalin**. 1987. Nucleotide sequence of the kanamycin resistance determinant of the pneumococcal transposon Tn*1545* : Evolutionary relationships and transcriptional analysis of *aphA-3* genes. Mol. Gen. Genet. **207**:509-513.

(6) **Carlier, C., and P. Courvalin**. 1982. A plasmid which does not encode the aminoglycoside phosphotransferase in the butirosin-producing strain of *Bacillus circulans*. J. Antibiotics **35**:629-634.

(7) **Carlier, C., and P. Courvalin**. 1990. Emergence of 4'-4" aminoglycoside nucleotidyltransferase in enterococci. Antimicrob. Agents Chemother. **34**:1565-1569.

(8) **Clinical and Laboratory Standards Institute**. Performance standards for antimicrobial susceptibility testing; nineteenth informational supplement. Standard M100-S19. CLSI. Wayne, PA, USA, 2009.

(9) **Collatz, E., C. Carlier, and P. Courvalin**. 1984. Characterization of high-level aminoglycoside resistance in a strain of *Streptococcus pneumoniae*. J. Gen. Microbiol. **130**:1665-1671.

(10) **Costa, Y., M. Gallimand., R. Leclercq, J. Duval, and P. Courvalin**. 1993. Characterization of the chromosomal *aac(6')-Ii* gene specific for *Enterococcus faecium*. Antimicrob. Agents Chemother. **25**:398-399.

(11) **Courvalin, P., and C. Carlier**. 1981. Resistance towards aminoglycoside-aminocyclitol antibiotics in bacteria. J. Antimicrob. Chemother. **8**:57-69.

(12) **Courvalin, P., and C. Carlier**. 1986. Transposable multiple antibiotic resistance in *Streptococcus pneumoniae*. Mol. Gen. Genet. **205**:291-297.

(13) **Courvalin, P., and J. Davies**. 1977. Plasmid-mediated aminoglycoside phosphotransferase of broad substrate range that phosphorylates amikacin. Antimicrob. Agents Chemother. **11**:619-624.

(14) **Davies, J**. 1987. Mechanism of bactericidal action of aminoglycosides. Microbiol. Rev. **51**:341-350.

(15) **Donabedian, S.M., L.A. Thal, E. Hershberger, M.B. Perri, J.W. Chow, P. Bartlett, R. Jones, K. Joyce, S. Rossiter, K. Gay, J. Johnson, C. Mackinson, E. Debess, J. Madden, F. Angulo, and M.J. Zervos**. 2003. Molecular characterization of gentamicin-resistant enterococci in the United States: evidence of spread from animals to humans through food. J. Clin. Microbiol. **41**:1109-1113.

(16) **Facinetti, B., E. Giovanetti, P.E. Varaldo, P. Casolari, and U. Fabio**. 1991. Antibiotic resistance in foodborne listeria. Lancet **338**:1272.

(17) **Ferretti, J.J., K.S. Gilmore, and P. Courvalin**. 1986. Nucleotide sequence analysis of gene specifying the bifunctionnal 6'-aminoglycoside acetyltransferase 2''-aminoside phosphotransferase enzyme in *Streptococcus faecalis* and identification and cloning of genes regions specifying the two activities. J. Bacteriol. **167**:631-638.

(18) **Kaufold, A., A. Poblielski, T. Horaud, and P. Ferrieri**. 1992. Identical genes confer high-level resistance to gentamicin upon *Enterococcus faecalis*, *Enterococcus faecium* and *Streptococcus agalactiae*. Antimicrob. Agents Chemother. **36**:1215-1218.

(19) **Le Goffic, F., B. Bacca, C.J. Soussy, A. Dublanchet, and J. Duval**. 1976. ANT(4')-I : une nouvelle nucléotidyl-transférase d'aminoglycosides isolée de *Staphylococcus aureus*. Ann. Microbiol. (Institut Pasteur) **127A**:391-399.

(20) **Nesvera, J., J. Hochmannová, and M. Pátek**. 1998. An integron of class 1 is present on the plasmid pCG4 from Gram-positive bacterium *Corynebacterium glutamicum*. FEMS Microbiol. Lett. **169**:391-395.

(21) **Noguchi, N., M. Sasatsu, and M. Komo**. 1993. Genetic mapping in *Bacillus subtilis* 168 of the *aadK* gene which encodes aminoglycoside 6-adenylyltransferase. FEMS Microbiol. Lett. **114**:47-52.

(22) **Ounissi, H., E. Derlot, C. Carlier, and P. Courvalin**. 1990. Gene homogeneity for aminoglycoside-modifying enzymes in Gram-positive cocci. Antimicrob. Agents Chemother. **34** : 2164-2168.

(23) **Shaw, K.J., P.N. Rather, R.S. Hare, and G.H. Miller**. 1993. Molecular genetics of aminoglycoside resistance genes and familial relationships of the aminoglycoside-modifying enzymes. Microbiol. Rev. **57**:138-163.

(24) **Taber, H.W., J.P. Mueller, P.F. Miller, and A.S. Arrow**. 1987. Bacterial uptake of aminoglycoside antibiotics. Microbiol. Rev. **51**:439-457.

(25) **Tauch, A., S. Götker, A. Pühler, J. Kalinowski, and G. Thierbach**. 2002. The 27.8-kb R-plasmid pTET3 from *Corynebacterium glutamicum* encodes the aminoglycoside adenyltransferase gene cassette *aadA9* and the regulated tetracycline efflux system Tet 33 flanked by active copies of the widespread insertion sequence IS*6100*. Plasmid **48**:117-129.

(26) **Tauch, A., S. Krieft, J. Kalinowski, and A. Pühler**. 2000. The 51,409-bp R-plasmid pTP10 from the multiresistant clinical isolate *Corynebacterium striatum* M82B is composed of DNA segments initially identified in soil bacteria and in plant, animal, and human pathogens. Mol. Gen. Genet. **263**:1-11.

(27) **Thauvin, C., G.M. Eliopoulos, C. Wennersten, and R.C. Moellering Jr**. 1985. Antagonistic effect of penicillin-amikacin combinations against enterococci. Antimicrob. Agents Chemother. **28**:78-83.

(28) **Trieu-Cuot, P., and P. Courvalin**. 1983. Nucleotide sequence of the *Streptococcus faecalis* plasmid gene encoding the 3'5' aminoglycoside phosphotansferase type III. Gene. **23**:331-341.

Chapter 17. AMINOGLYCOSIDES AND GRAM-NEGATIVE BACTERIA

Thierry LAMBERT

INTRODUCTION

After a certain fall from favor at the expense of third generation cephalosporins and fluoroquinolones, aminoglycosides have now regained their indispensable place in the hospital antibiotic armentarium. Aminoglycosides are composed of a 6-carbon aminocyclitol ring linked by glycosidic bonds to one or more sugar derivatives. The aminocyclitol may be streptidine or, more often, 2-deoxystreptamine (2-DOS) leading to a first classification into two subfamilies. The 2-DOS ring may be substituted at the 4 and 5 positions (4,5-substituted 2-DOS group: neomycin, paromomycin) or at the 4 and 6 positions (4,6-substituted 2-DOS group: amikacin, kanamycin, gentamicin, isepamicin, netilmicin, tobramycin). Aminoglycosides have a broad antibacterial spectrum which includes Gram-negative and Gram-positive bacteria; only strict anaerobic bacteria are naturally resistant to their activity. Aminoglycoside usage has improved with shorter treatments and optimized dosages with, in particular, once-daily regimens in order to benefit from their rapid and concentration-dependent bactericidal activity (34). For the treatment of nosocomial infections by Gram-negative bacilli, which mainly involve the enterobacteria, *Pseudomonas aeruginosa* and *Acinetobacter baumannii*, they are usually combined with a β-lactam or a fluoroquinolone. Their widespread use has contributed to the emergence of resistant strains which restrict their efficacy. This phenomenon has undoubtedly been amplified in the hospital setting through antibiotic selection pressure in intensive care units. A short summary of the mode of action of aminoglycosides is necessary to understand bacterial resistance mechanisms.

MODE OF ACTION

Aminoglycosides are protein synthesis inhibitors with pleiotropic effects on bacteria. They inhibit the initiation, elongation, and termination stages of translation. They also interfere with the respiratory chain electron transport system, induce ionic disorders, damage bacterial envelopes, and indirectly impact DNA replication. Their target is bacterial 16S ribosomal RNA (rRNA). It has been known for many years that the inhibitory effect of aminoglycosides is due to their binding to the 30S ribosomal subunit. Recent studies by (i) X-ray diffraction of crystallized complexes composed of RNA fragments carrying the A (aminoacyl) site and aminoglycosides and (ii) nuclear magnetic resonance have identified the bonds between aminoglycosides and certain 16S RNA bases (Fig. 1) (48). The A-Site is the binding site of 4,6-substituted 2-DOS derivatives which comprise most clinically used aminoglycosides (35). This site forms a pocket occupied by transfer RNAs (tRNA) during codon-anticodon recognition. The bases of the A-site which bind to aminoglycosides play an essential role in the activity of these antibiotics (21). This binding stabilizes non-canonical pairings normally eliminated by mismatch repair and consequently generates mistranslations. The comparison between bacterial and eukaryotic ribosomal RNA shows that adenine 1408 of 16S RNA is replaced by a guanine at an homologous position of 18S RNA, and this single change explains the natural resistance of the eukaryotic ribosome to 4,6-substituted 2-DOS derivatives (37). In addition, recent studies have shown that mistranslation and rearrangement of membrane proteins generated by aminoglycosides play an essential role in the induction of oxidative stress leading to cell death (20).

RESISTANCE MECHANISMS

The general mechanisms of antibiotic resistance which include target alterations, enzymatic detoxification, and reduction in intracellular antibiotic levels due to cellular impermeability or export are found with aminoglycosides.

Target alteration

The action mechanism of aminoglycosides suggests that a possible means of resistance would be mutation of 16S RNA; this mechanism, however, is limited by the existence of several copies of the

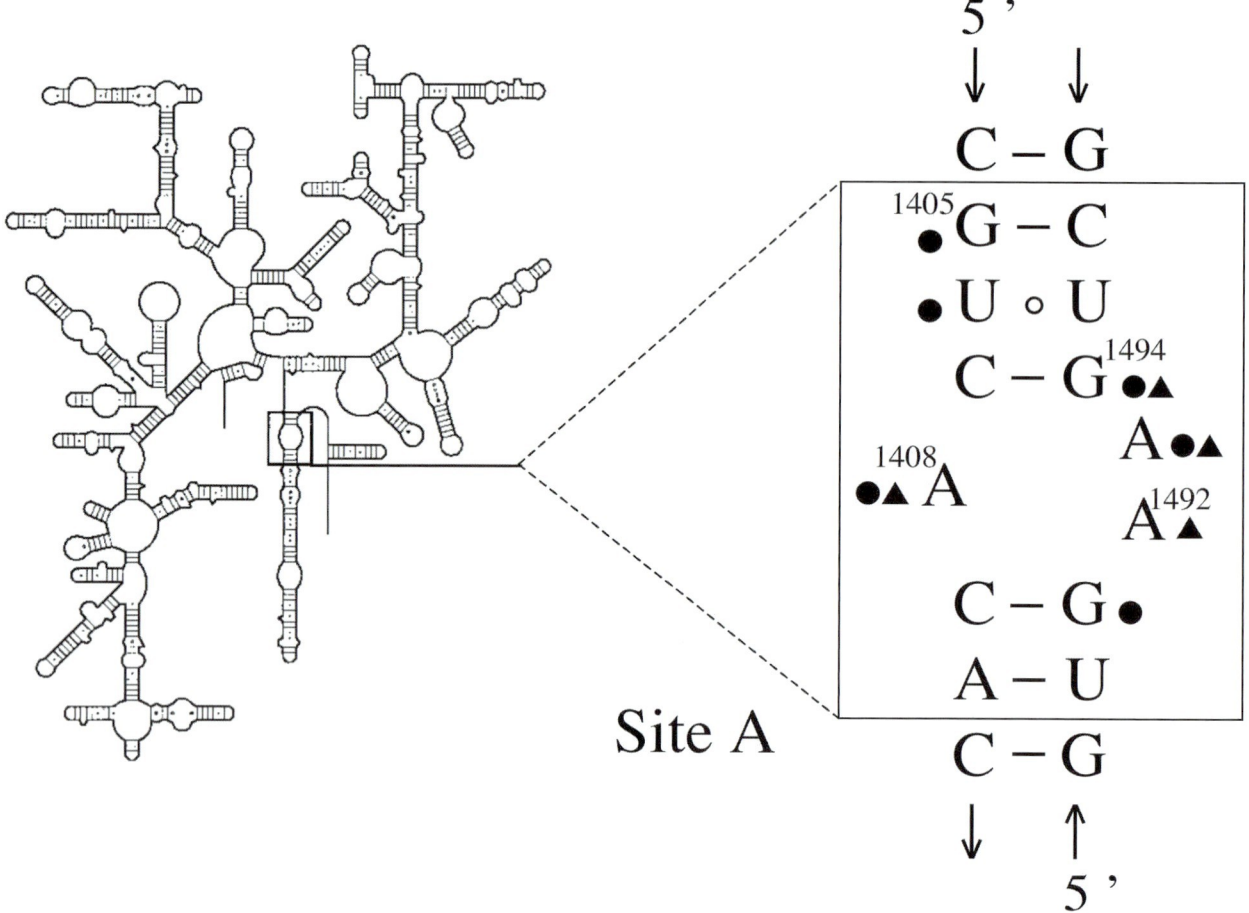

Fig. 1. Secondary structure of 16S RNA with details of the decoding A-site. ● Nucleotides involved in binding with aminoglycosides, ▲ nucleotides involved in interactions with tRNA.

ribosomal RNA operon. For example, *Escherichia coli* has seven copies of this operon and, as more than 50% of all ribosomes must be affected for resistance to be dominant, the probability of occurrence of concomitant mutations is very low. However, amplification may result from gene conversion. Although this mechanism has a limited distribution and mainly concerns bacteria with a small number of copies of the rARN operon such as *Mycobacterium tuberculosis* (a single copy), spectinomycin resistance has been observed (13) in *Neisseria meningitidis* and *Neisseria gonorrhoeae* due to G1064C and C1192U mutations, respectively, of 16S RNA (three 16S RNA copies in these species). In addition, certain mutations affecting ribosomal proteins are responsible for resistance to streptomycin and spectinomycin. The S5 and S12 proteins are in contact with rRNA and certain mutations generate conformational changes in the 16S RNA affecting the interaction with aminoglycosides. Finally, three 16S RNA methylation activities modify the A-site at positions G1405 (N7), A1408, and C1407 (N5) (1). As cytosine 1407 does not interact with aminoglycosides, its methylation, as expected, has no effect on resistance. The 7G1405 and 1A1408 methylations detected in actinomycetes are self-defence mechanisms implemented by bacteria producing antibiotics.

G1405 methylation of 16S rRNA has recently been reported in bacteria pathogenic for man. Five genes have been described *armA*, *rmtA*, *rmtB*, *rmtC*, and *rmtD* (9, 10, 12, 47). The first, *armA*, is carried by the composite transposon Tn*1548* (14). This transposon was detected on a broad-host-range plasmid of incompatibility group IncL/M capable of replicating in enterobacteria and which also confers resistance to cefotaxime by production of CTX-M3 ß-lactamase. The *armA* gene has been detected in France, in several other European countries, in Japan, and more recently in the USA. The *rmtA* and *rmtB* genes were demonstrated in *P. aeruginosa* and Gram-negative enterobacteria, respectively, *rmtC* in *Proteus mirabilis*, and *rmtD* in *Klebsiella pneumoniae* and *P. aeruginosa* (9, 47). G1405 methylation confers a high level of resistance to 4,6-substituted 2-DOS derivatives (amikacin, gentamicin, kanamycin, netilmicin, and tobramycin) but does not affect the activity of 4,5-substituted 2-DOS aminoglycosides (neomycin, paromomycin).

The enzyme which methylates A1408 was characterized in a clinical strain of *E. coli* in Japan (46). This mechanism encoded by a selftransferable plasmid affects the activity of both 4,6 and 4,5-substituted 2-DOS aminoglycosides and concerns neomycin and apramycin, unlike G1405 methylation.

Enzymatic modification

Likewise, when an aminoglycoside is modified by bacterial enzymes, its binding to 16S rRNA may be affected resulting in loss of activity. Knowledge about the genes involved in resistance has considerably increased and this has improved our understanding of the mechanisms involved. It has recently been shown that (i) the expression of the structural genes of certain aminoglycoside-modifying enzymes was regulated whereas, generally, these enzymes are produced constitutively, *i.e.* in the absence of the aminoglycoside; (ii) point mutations in structural genes may cause modifications of the substrate profiles of the enzymes (23, 42), and (iii) enzyme hyperproduction may lead to "trapping" of the antibiotic (30). It is conceptually interesting to note that genes for aminoglycoside-modifying enzymes may be inherited from antibiotic-producing microorganisms and fulfill their original detoxification role or be an integral part of the host bacterium where they have a different role so that the aminoglycoside is then an occasional substrate.

Aminoglycoside-modifying enzymes are divided into groups according to the reaction they catalyze: acetylation of an amino group [*N*-acetyltransferase (AAC)], phosphorylation or nucleotidylation of a hydroxyl group [*O*-phosphotransferase (APH), O-nucleotidyltransferase (ANT)] (Fig. 2). Subclasses are defined by the aminoglycoside-modifying site. Each enzyme recognizes a certain number of structurally related aminoglycosides which it modifies (in vitro substrate profile, Table 1) leading to an *in vivo* resistance phenotype. Many enzymes exist in various isozyme forms (or types) (Tables 2 and 3). Considering the overlapping of the enzyme substrate profiles, a same compound may be modified by different enzymes.

As the antibiotic is modified intracellularly, it is not completely destroyed in the culture medium (8). Enzymes are necessary and sufficient to confer resistance to the bacterial host (7). The level of resistance varies according to (i) the class of enzyme (phosphotransferases usually confer a high level resistance); (ii) the antibiotic (the MICs of amikacin, and in particular isepamicin, are markedly lower than those of netilmicin or tobramycin in strains producing a 6'-acetyltransferase); (iii) the host cell; an enzyme may confer a low resistance in one species and more easily detectable resistance in another (7).

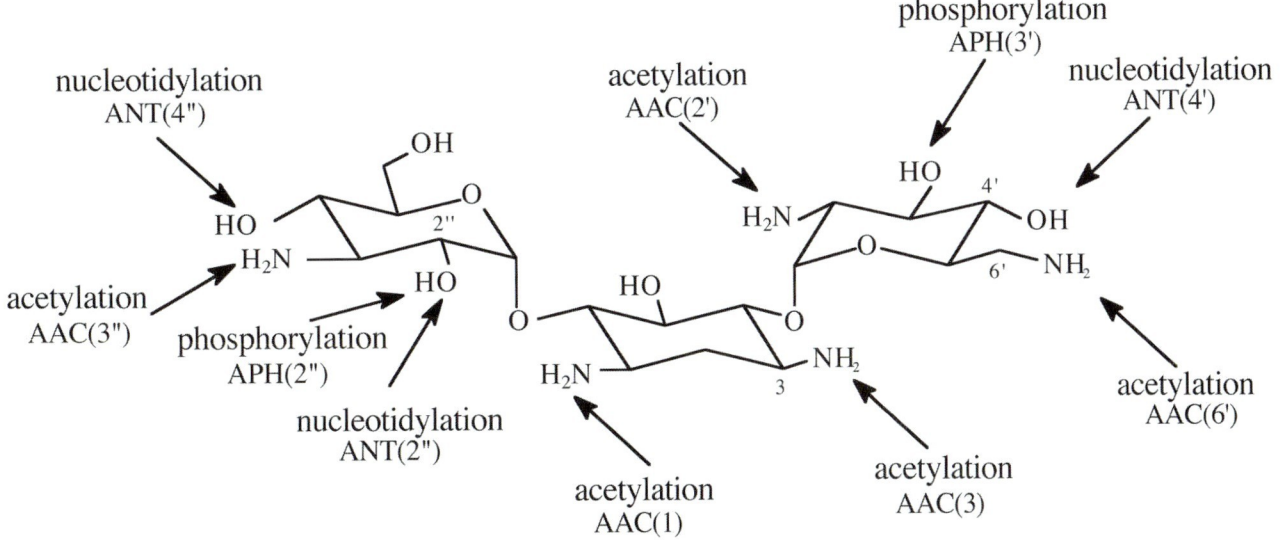

Fig. 2. Structure of kanamycin B. The arrows indicate the radicals modified by the enzymes. 3''-*N*-acetyltransferase activity was described in *Streptomyces* (23).

Table 1. Substrate profiles of aminoglycoside modifying enzymes[a].

Aminoglycoside	Phosphotransferase (APH)					Nucleotidyltransferase (ANT)					Acetyltransferase (AAC)			
	(6')	(3')	(2")	(3"')	(5")	(6)	(9)	(2")	(3")(9)	(4')(4")	(1)	(3)	(2')	(6')-I
Neomycin B	-	+	-	-	(+)	-	-	-	-	+	(+)	(+)	(+)	+
Paromomycin	-	+	-	-	(+)	-	-	-	-	+	+	-	(+)	+
Lividomycin A	-	(+)	-	-	(+)	-	-	-	-	+	+	-	(+)	+
Ribostamycin	-	+	-	-	+	-	-	-	-	+	+	+	(+)	+
Butirosin	-	(+)	-	-	(+)	-	-	-	-	+	(+)	(+)	-	+
Kanamycin A	-	+	(+)	-	-	-	-	+	-	+	-	+	(+)	+
Kanamycin B	-	+	(+)	-	-	-	-	+	-	+	-	+	(+)	+
Kanamycin C	-	+	(+)	-	-	-	-	+	-	+	-	-	(+)	+
Tobramycin	-	-	(+)	-	-	-	-	+	-	+	-	+	(+)	+
Dibekacin	-	-	(+)	-	-	-	-	+	-	(+)	-	+	(+)	+
Amikacin	-	(+)	(+)	-	-	-	-	-	-	+	-	-	-	+
Habekacin	-	-	(+)	-	-	-	-	-	-	-	-	-	+	+
Isepamicin	-	(+)	(+)	-	-	-	-	-	-	+	-	-	-	+
Gentamicin C1a	-	-	+	-	-	-	-	+	-	-	-	+	+	+
Gentamicin C1	-	-	+	-	-	-	-	+	-	-	-	(+)	+	-
Gentamicin C2	-	-	+	-	-	-	-	+	-	-	-	(+)	+	+
Sisomicin	-	-	+	-	-	-	-	-	-	-	-	(+)	+	+
5-episisomicin	-	-	-	-	-	-	-	-	-	-	-	(+)	-	+
Netilmicin	-	-	+	-	-	-	-	-	-	-	-	(+)	(+)	+
2-N-ethylnetilmicin	-	-	+	-	-	-	-	-	-	-	-	(+)	+	+
6'-N-ethylnetilmicin	-	-	+	-	-	-	-	-	-	-	-	(+)	+	-
Streptomycin	+	-	-	+	-	+	-	-	+	-	-	-	-	-
Spectinomycin	-	-	-	-	-	-	+	-	+	-	-	-	-	-
Apramycin	-	-	-	-	-	-	-	-	-	-	+	(+)	-	-
Fortimicin	-	-	-	-	-	-	-	-	-	-	-	(+)	-	-

[a] +, substrate; (+), substrate for certain isozymic forms of the enzyme; -, non substrate. The fact that an antibiotic is a substrate *in vitro* for an enzyme does not imply that strains producing that enzyme are necessarily resistant to this antibiotic.

Table 2. Substrate profiles of 3'-O-aminoglycoside phosphotransferases [APH(3')]

Aminoglycoside	Type of APH(3')						
	I	II	III	IV	V	VI	VII
Kanamycin	+	+	+	+	(+)[a]	+	+
Neomycin	+	+	+	+	+	+	+
Butirosin	−	+	+	+	−	+	−
Lividomicin	+	−	+	−	−	−	−
Amikacin	−	−	(+)	(+)	−	+	+

[a] Antibiotic with little or no change in MIC but with a decreased or abolished bactericidal activity and which no longer synergizes the effects of ß-lactams.

Type I and II enzymes are present in Gram-negative bacilli. The type III enzyme widely distributed in Gram-positive cocci exists also in *Campylobacter*. Type IV and V enzymes were found in *Bacillus circulans* and *Streptomyces fradiae*, respectively, which are non-pathogenic for humans. The type VI enzyme is mainly present in *Acinetobacter* but may be found in enterobacteria and *Pseudomonas*. The type VII enzyme was only described in *Campylobacter*.

Table 3. Substrate profiles of 3'-N-aminoglycoside acetyltransferases [AAC(3)]

Antibiotic	AAC(3)				
	I	II	III	IV	VI
Gentamicin	+	+	+	+	+
Tobramycin	−	+	+	+	−
Netilmicin	−	+	−	+	−
Amikacin	−	−	−	−	−
2'-N-ethylnetilmicin	−	+	−	+	−
6'-N-ethylnetilmicin	−	+	−	+	+
Fortimicin	+	−	−	−	−
Apramycin	−	−	−	+	−
5-episisomicin	−	(+)	+	−	−

The previously proposed AAC(3)-V profile is identical to that of AAC(3)-II.
The type III enzyme is specific to *Pseudomonas*.

The presence of a modifying enzyme does not necessarily lead to resistance (according to the clinical category criterion) to the modified aminoglycosides and the strain may sometimes be found to be susceptible in antibiotic susceptibility tests. A more precise analysis may then show a slight increase in the MICs of modified aminoglycosides, though these may remain lower than the lower critical concentration. The clinical significance of these low resistance levels is open to question and this problem may be solved by using animal models (11). A loss of the bactericidal effect of the aminoglycoside and/or the loss of synergy with ß-lactam antibiotics may occur. This was observed with APH(3)-III in Gram-positive cocci (6) but does not seem to be the rule in Gram-negative bacilli, at least with certain enzymes such as AAC (6') (6); there may also be an increase in the level of resistance, either by mutation of the regulatory region of the structural gene, by an increase in the number of gene copies per cell, secondary to an increase in the copy number of the plasmid carrying the gene, or by gene amplification (42). For example, *Serratia marcescens* carries the *aac*(6)-*Ic* gene in its chromosome (43) which is easily detectable from the slight reduction in the activity of tobramycin which is the best indicator of this enzymatic activity. However, most strains of *S. marcescens* are apparently susceptible to amikacin, netilmicin, and even tobramycin. Exposure of a netilmicin-susceptible strain to increasing concentrations of this antibiotic *in vitro* was found to select for highly resistant mutants (42). These mutants, also highly resistant to amikacin and tobramycin, synthesize detectable AAC(6') activity. In the rabbit endocarditis model induced by a susceptible strain of *S. marcescens*, tobramycin is not bactericidal, amikacin has a time dependant bactericidal action whereas gentamicin is the most effective aminoglycoside after bolus injection (34). However, it should be noted that, in practice, amikacin is often used with good results in combination with a ß-lactam antibiotic or a fluoroquinolone to treat *S. marcescens* septicemia. The risk of selection of a resistant mutant is therefore low but must be taken into account in certain situations, in particular infections on a prosthesis. A special situation was observed with *Salmonella enterica*, a species that carries the normally cryptic *aac (6')-Iy* gene in its chromosome. This gene, however, may confer resistance to tobramycin and netilmicin when it is controlled by a strong promoter provided, for example, by a transcriptional fusion (26). This event was observed in a clinically isolated strain of *Salmonella enteritidis* in which the *aac(6')-Iy* gene was under the control of the NmpC promoter after deletion of approximately 60 kb. Aminoglycosides are in fact poor substrates for the AAC(6')-Iy enzyme which is able to acetylate some histones and may interfere as transcriptional regulator (45). Aminoglycoside-*N*-acetyltransferases belong to the GCN5 acetyltransferase family which form a very large group of enzymes, universally distributed in nature, and which use acetyl-CoA as cofactor.

Taking into account the large number of modifying enzymes, the existence of isozymes with an expression depending on the host, their frequent coexistence in the same strain, and their possible association with other resistance mechanisms (7, 41), it may be difficult to deduce the genotype of a resistant bacterium from the observed phenotype.

The enzymatic contents may sometimes be deduced from the resistance phenotype if the latter includes a minimum number of aminoglycosides. However, this analysis may be difficult, in particular when there are several enzymes, and then requires the additional use of unmarketed molecules such as apramycin, fortimicin, 5-episosomicin, 2'-*N*-ethylnetilmicin, and 6'-*N*-ethylnetilmicin (42). Interpretation is based on the comparison of the activity of different antibiotics and requires a careful analysis taking into account all the enzyme substrate profiles.

It is essential to understand these resistance phenotypes in order to proceed to interpretative reading of the antibiotic susceptibility tests before choosing an adapted antibiotic therapy (6). This overcomes the pitfalls of antibiotic susceptibility testing and constitutes an epidemiological tool to detect the emergence and follow the spread of resistance characters in the hospital.

Enzymes inactivating aminoglycosides are widely distributed in species pathogenic for man (7, 8). There is a certain absolute or relative specificity in their distribution (Table 4). The presence of a resistance gene does not necessarily mean that it is phenotypically expressed (silent gene). This possibility is the rule for the *aac(3)-VI* gene in *E. coli* (42), relatively frequent for the *aac(6)-Ic* gene in *S. marcescens* and rare for the other resistance genes.

Point mutations in enzyme structural genes may be responsible for modifications in the resistance phenotype. Hence, it has been shown *in vitro* that the Leu119Ser substitution transformed the substrate profile of AAC(6')-I into AAC(6')-II (Table 5) (42). This substitution was also detected in clinical isolates (23).

Detection of genes by DNA-DNA hybridization or amplification has made it possible to analyze their distribution and to better understand the prevalence of different resistance mechanisms in bacterial species. The localization of certain genes on plasmids, mobile genetic elements or as part of integrons explains their mobility.

Table 4. Genus or species-specific inactivating enzymes in Gram-negative bacilli[a]

Enzyme	Gene	Organism
AAC(2')	*aac(2')-Ia*	*Providencia* spp.
AAC(3)-III	*aac(3)*	*Pseudomonas* spp.
AAC(6')-Ic	*aac(6')-Ic*	*Serratia marcescens*
AAC(6')-Ig	*aac(6')-Ig*	*A. haemolyticus*
AAC(6')-II	*aac(6')-IIa*	*Pseudomonas* spp.
	aac(6')-IIb	*Pseudomonas* spp.
APH(3')-VI	*aphA-6*	*Acinetobacter* spp.
APH(3')-VII	*aphA-7*	*Campylobacter* spp.

[a] Specificity is absolute for AAC(6')-Ic, AAC(6')-Ig, AAC(3)-III, APH(3')-VII, and AAC(2') and relative in the other cases.

Table 5. Substrate profiles of 6'-*N*-aminoglycoside acetyltransferases [AAC(6')]

Antibiotic	Type of AAC(6')	
	I	II
Gentamicin	–	+
Tobramycin	+	+
Netilmicin	+	+
Amikacin	+	–
Isepamicin	(+)	–
2'-*N*-ethylnetilmicin	+	+
6'-*N*-ethylnetilmicin	–	–
Fortimicin	–	–
Apramycin	–	–
5-episisomicin	+	+

Trapping

A modifying enzyme may sometimes neutralize the action of an aminoglycoside by binding without necessarily modifying its structure. Antibiotic trapping was proposed as the mechanism responsible for kanamycin and tobramycin resistance whereas gentamicin and netilmicin remain active. When bacteria produce a large quantity of type I 3'-*O*-phosphotransferase, which recognizes tobramycin (3'-deoxykanamycin B) without modifying it (absence of 3'-hydroxyl group), the antibiotic may be trapped in a functionally inactive enzyme-substrate complex (30). A similar mechanism was observed with 6'-*N*-acetyltransferase AacA29a (33). This protein truncated of the C-terminal end common to AAC(6')-I does not modify aminoglycosides but is able to trap them and confer resistance on the host bacterium (28). The conferred resistance is usually less than that observed after acetylation, in particular of amikacin and netilmicin.

Impermeability or efflux

There are several steps in the access of aminoglycosides to their target site. Due to their hydrophilic nature, aminoglycosides penetrate the outer membrane of Gram-negative bacteria by porins, though lipopolysaccharide transport was proposed in *P. aeruginosa* (9, 16). Transport by the lipophilic pathway is associated with their polycationic nature by substitution with the calcium or magnesium of the external membrane. Mutants of this bacterium which synthesize an increased quantity of OprH protein are in fact resistant to aminoglycosides (17). In *S. marcescens*, mutations affecting both porins and other structures of the external membrane cause cross-resistance between ß-lactams and aminoglycosides (15).

The second phase consists in crossing the hydrophobic cytoplasmic membrane and requires the energy of the proton motive force produced by the respiratory chain (8, 16). Susceptible bacteria accumulate aminoglycosides at impressive levels of up to 400 times the surrounding concentrations. On the contrary, strict anaerobic bacteria unable to synthesize quinones are resistant to aminoglycosides. The alteration of the respiratory chain by mutations may generate variants which develop in microcolonies and generally express low level resistance to all aminoglycosides. These have been observed clinically, in particular in *P. aeruginosa* (8) and *E. coli* (17).

Some bacteria may export aminoglycosides via efflux systems. Efflux pumps are ubiquitous and affect numerous compounds, though aminoglycosides are rarely substrates of these pumps. In Gram-negative bacteria, four resistance-nodulation-cell division-type (RND) efflux pumps were found to be capable of exporting aminoglycosides: these were the AmrAB-OprA and BpeAB-OprB systems in *Burkholderia pseudomallei* and AcrD, MexXY-OprM, and AdeABC in *E. coli*, *P. aeruginosa* and *Acinetobacter baumannii* respectively (4, 18, 27, 32, 36, 39). Efflux proteins may be associated with a fusion protein and an external membrane protein or act autonomously like AcrD (39). These efflux pumps are generally strictly regulated and naturally confer a low level of resistance. Mutations may lead to their overexpression and increase the level of resistance. Such a mechanism was observed in *A. baumannii* following mutations either in the sensor or the regulator of the AdeSR two-component system which controls expression of the AdeABC pump (29).

Certain concepts, apparently far from routine concerns, contribute to the understanding of aminoglycoside resistance mechanisms and are necessary to interpret the data of antibiotic susceptibility tests with this family of antibiotics.

RESISTANCE PHENOTYPES

Anaerobiosis, acidity, and high NaCl concentrations reduce the activity of aminoglycosides and the divalent cation content affects their antibacterial effect (17). The phenotypes described concern the four aminoglycosides which must be routinely studied: amikacin, gentamicin, netilmicin, and tobramycin. Isepamicin which is less affected by AAC(6') may also be studied; dibekacin, paromomycin, and sisomicin have been withdrawn from clinical use. Neomycin, which is still used locally, may contribute to the phenotypic analysis and deserves to be studied secondarily. Streptomycin and kanamycin, which are rarely used in clinical medicine, will be mentioned. Fortimicin and apramycin are used to detect AAC(3)-II and AAC(3)-IV respectively.

The "susceptible" phenotype of a genus or a species corresponds to that of its "main susceptible population". Both the MICs or inhibition zone diameters of the aminoglycosides studied must be simultaneously analyzed in order to determine the resistance phenotype of a strain. The critical concentrations, and in particular the MICs distribution of the main susceptible population, must be known for each aminoglycoside. This latter criterion is crucial for the detection of low level resistance and optimization of the interpretative reading of the results.

We will briefly summarize acquired resistance in *Neisseria spp.*, *Haemophilus spp.* (see the corresponding sections), and *Campylobacter spp.* as well as natural resistance in *Burkoldheria spp.* and *Stenotrophomonas* in order to focus on the analysis of phenotypes of the enterobacteria, *Acinetobacter spp.* and *Pseudomonas spp.*

Spectinomycin resistance has been reported in *Neisseria meningitidis* and *Neisseria gonorrhoeae* due to the G1064C and C1192U mutations, respectively (13). Kanamycin resistance has been observed in *Branhamella catarrhalis* and commensal species of *Neisseria* (38) and is associated with the *aph(3')-III* gene of Gram-positive bacteria (unpublished personal data).

In *Haemophilus influenzae*, streptomycin and kanamycin resistance have been known for many years and are assigned to a kinase, APH(3')-I for kanamycin. On the contrary, gentamicin resistance, which is very seldom observed, is not due to enzymatic modification.

The resistance of *Campylobacter jejuni* and *Campylobacter coli* to kanamycin and amikacin is due to production of APH(3')-III and APH(3')-VII (42). It is interesting to note that recently reported resistance to gentamicin and tobramycin in *Campylobacter* is due to the *aac(6')-Ib7* gene detected in a class 1 integron (25).

Burkholderia cepacia and *Stenotrophomonas maltophilia* are two species naturally resistant to aminoglycosides. The inactivity of aminoglycosides is explained by their natural impermeability, though an efflux system may be involved. In addition, in the case of *S. maltophilia*, inhibition zones may often be observed around aminoglycoside discs when the diffusion susceptibility tests are read after 18 to 24 h of incubation at 37°C. On the contrary, late reading of dishes left for 24 h or more at room temperature shows the presence of numerous colonies in the inhibition zones (Fig. 3). The latter finding suggests the absence of a bactericidal effect and the expression of resistance at a temperature below 37°C. This may be explained by regulation of external membrane protein synthesis or efflux pumps according to environmental conditions. Moreover, most strains of *S. maltophilia* carry AAC(6')-Iz (24).

Susceptible phenotypes

Nearly all the bacterial genera composing the *Enterobacteriaceae* family are naturally susceptible to aminoglycosides, except *Providencia* which produces an AAC(2') (7). The MICs of aminoglycosides for *E. coli* are summarized in Table 6.

Resistance phenotypes

As already mentioned, a strain may produce one or several aminoglycoside-modifying enzymes (Table 1). The *in vitro* substrate profile of each enzyme contributes to the phenotype of the host bacterium which is a result of the superposition of the resistance profiles. When a strain synthesize a single enzyme, it is often easy to deduce the biochemical mechanism of the observed resistance phenotype (7). However, when a bacterium synthesizes two or more enzymes, it is more difficult to deduce the enzymatic content, as analysis generally requires the use of more discriminating aminoglycosides which are unfortunately not routinely available (42).

For example, a high gentamicin activity compared to that of tobramycin suggests production of an AAC(6')-I or an ANT(4')-II activity. 2'-*N*-ethylnetilmicin, and 6'-*N*-ethylnetilmicin which are particularly useful to detect 2'- and 6'-*N*-acetyltransferase, may be used to determine which enzyme is responsible. 5-episisomicin is used to distinguish ANT(2") from AAC(3)-III and to detect the presence of an AAC(6') when this is associated with other enzymes. AAC(3)-I and AAC(3)-IV may be identified by studying fortimicin and apramycin, respectively. A high level of isepamicin resistance suggests the presence of an APH(3')-VI in particular if it is dissociated from that to gentamicin (42). A high level of resistance to 4,6-substituted 2-DOS suggests a m7G1405 16S

Table 6. Minimum inhibitory concentrations (μg/ml) of routinely used aminoglycosides on *E. coli* with a susceptible phenotype

Aminoglycoside[a]	Mean MIC[b]
Amikacin	0.5–2
Gentamicin	0.25–2
Kanamycin	1–4
Neomycin	1–4
Netilmicin	0.25–0.5
Streptomycin	4–16
Tobramyin	0.25–1

[a] These results are valid for enterobacteria except *Serratia* (tobramycin) and *Providencia* (gentamicin, tobramycin, and netilmicin).
[b] From reference 29.

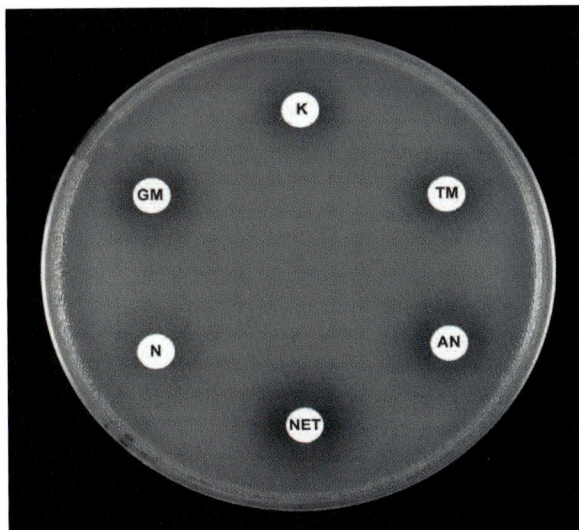

3.A. *S. maltophilia* multiresistance due to membrane impermeability and/or efflux.

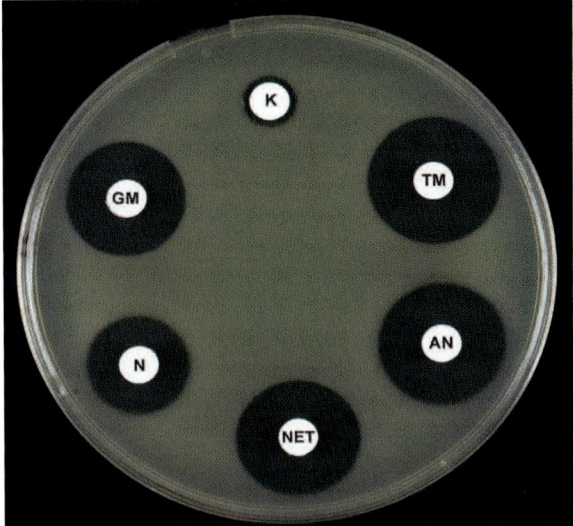

3.B. *P. aeruginosa* PAO1.

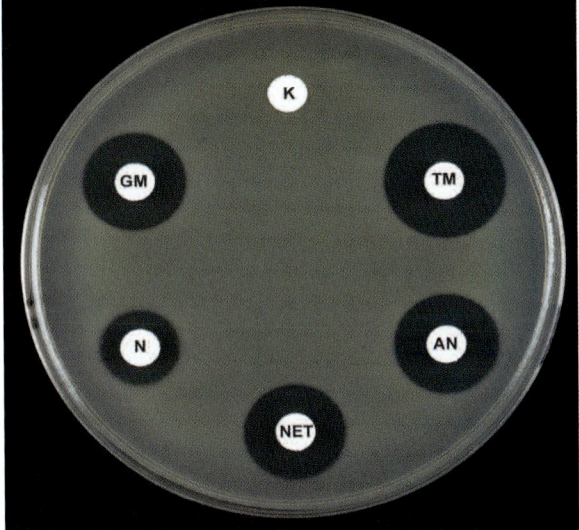

3.C. mutant of PAO1 overexpressing the MexXY efflux system.

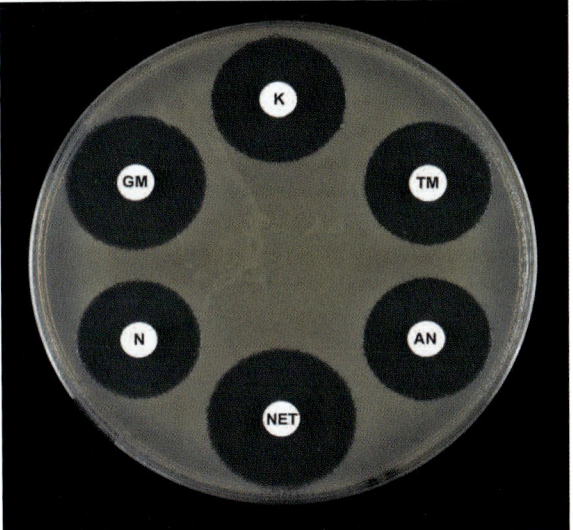

3.D. *A. baumannii* wild phenotype.

Fig. 3. Aminoglycoside resistance phenotypes of gram-negative bacteria. AN, amikacin; GM, gentamicin; K, kanamycin; N, neomycin; NET, netilmicin; TM, tobramycin.

RNA methyltransferase in particular if neomycin (4,5-substituted 2-DOS) is still active.

Routine analysis must be limited to the recognition of the phenotypes described below. Most of the observed resistances are due to the presence of modifying enzymes which may be detected both in enterobacteria and in *P. aeruginosa* and *A. baumannii*. Specific features are caused by intrinsic resistances in: (i) *P. aeruginosa* the presence of an APH(3')-I confers kanamycin resistance and the frequent expression of the MexXY-OprM efflux system leads to a reduction in the activity of all aminoglycosides (Fig. 3). The remarkable activity of tobramycin against this bacterial species should be pointed out. (ii) *A. baumannii*: the AdeABC system present in the species either in a cryptic state or overexpressed should be taken into account as it is responsible for global resistance to aminoglycosides but with different levels depending on the compound (Table 7) (Fig. 3). The MexXY-OprM efflux system plays a key role in the adaptive resistance of *P. aeruginosa* to aminoglycosides. This resistance, with a clinical impact that remains to be determined, facilitates the selection of recalcitrant subpopulations which express unstable resistance (adaptive) following exposure

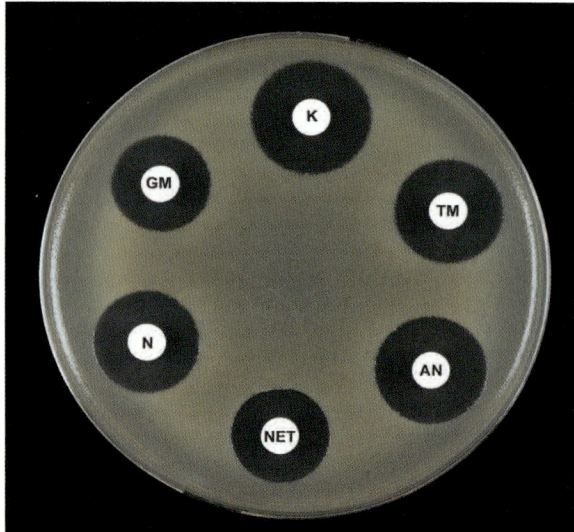

3.E. *A. baumannii* overexpressing the AdeABC efflux system.

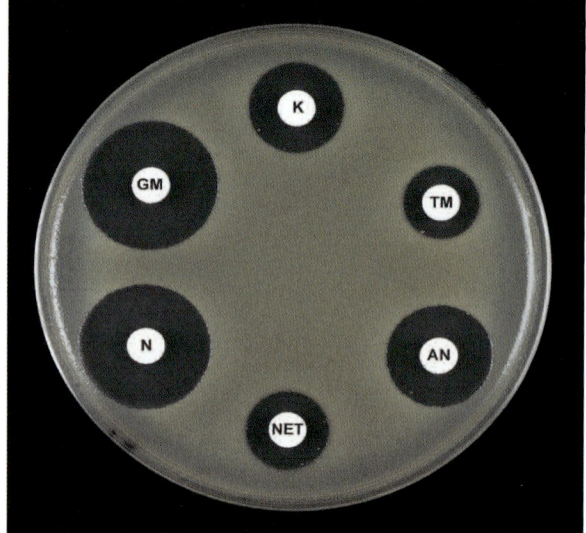

3.F. *A. haemolyticus* [AAC(6')-I].

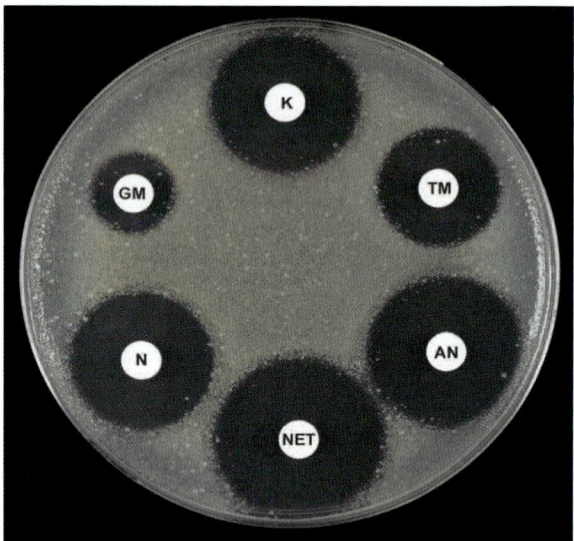

3.G. *S. marcescens* [AAC(3)-I] overlapping the species AAC(6')-I.

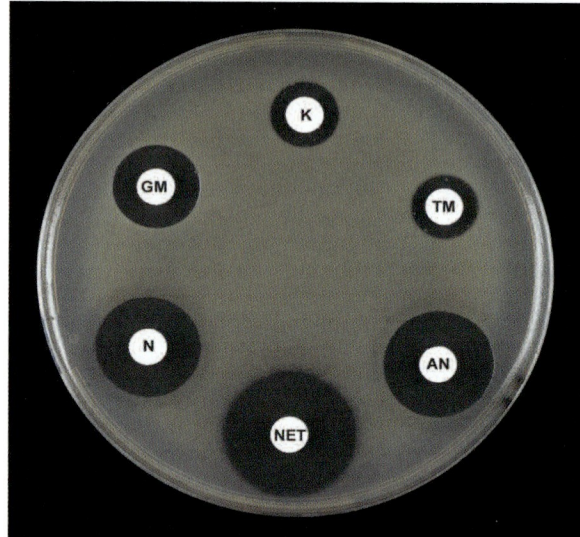

3.H. *E. coli* [ANT(2")].

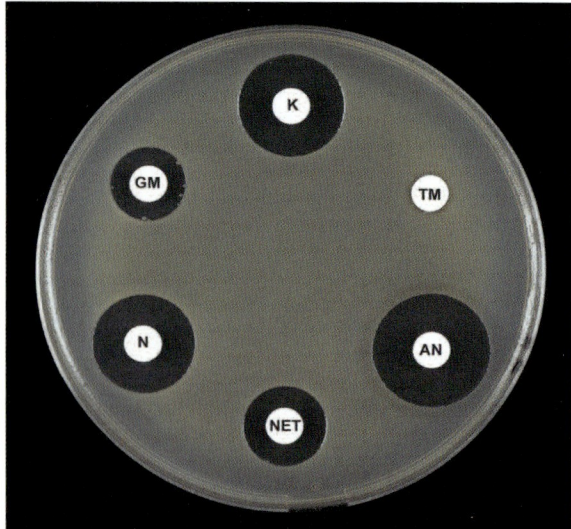

3.I. *E. coli* [AAC(3)-II].

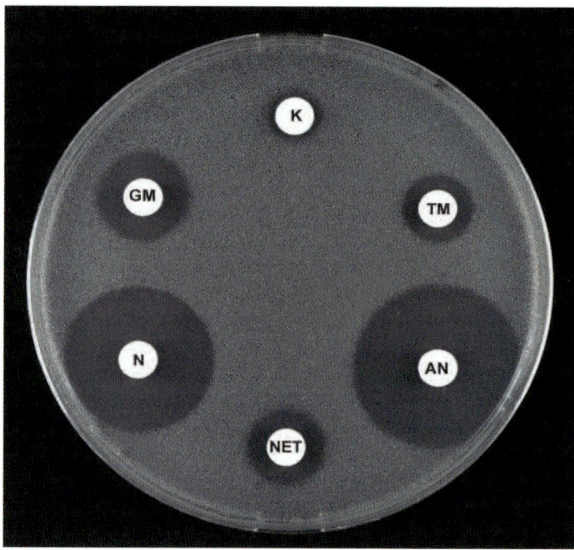

3.J. *P. aeruginosa* [AAC(6')-II].

Chapter 17. AMINOGLYCOSIDES AND GRAM-NEGATIVE BACTERIA

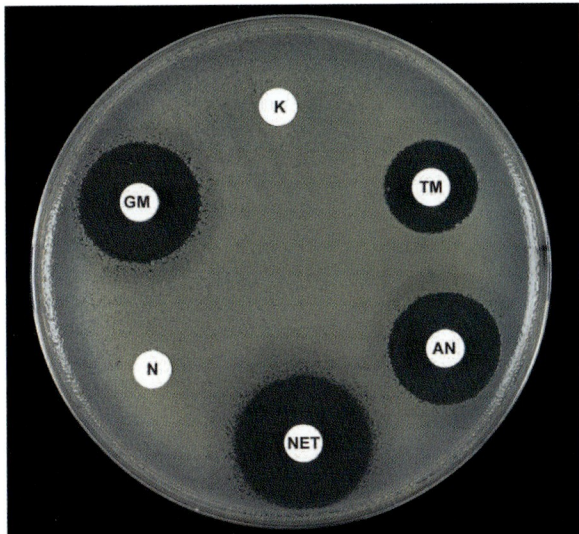

3.K. *E. coli* [APH(3')-I highly expressed].

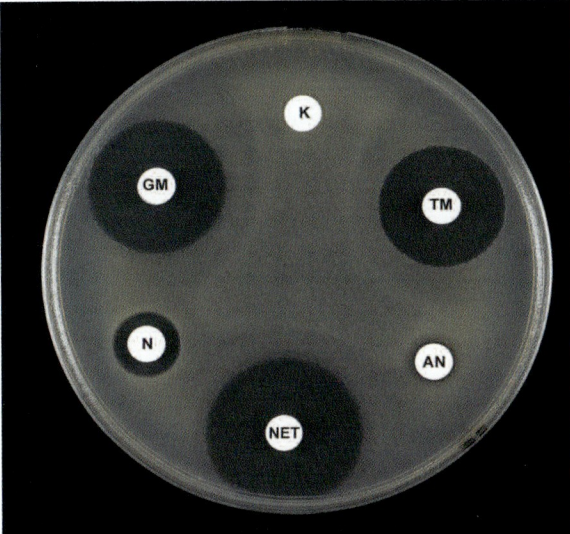

3.L. *E. coli* [APH(3')-VI].

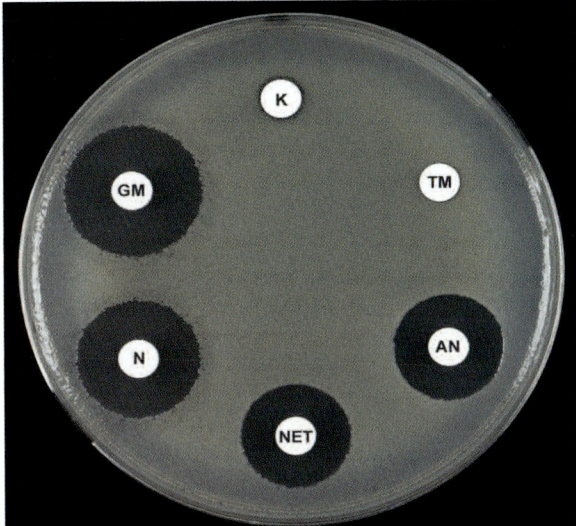

3.M. *E. coli* [AAC(6')-I + APH(3')-I].

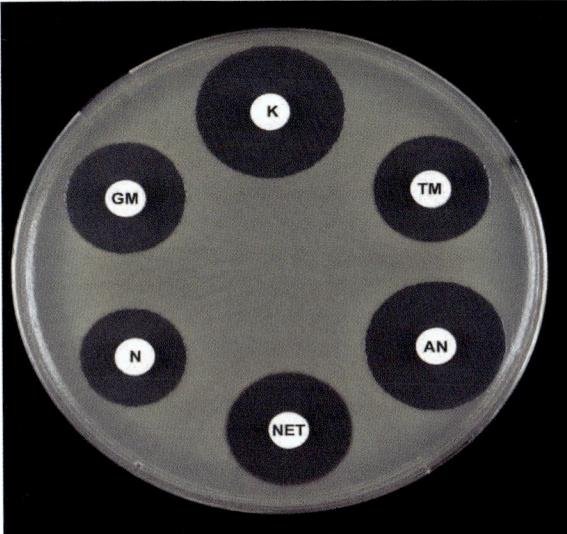

3.N. *P. stuartii* [AAC(2')].

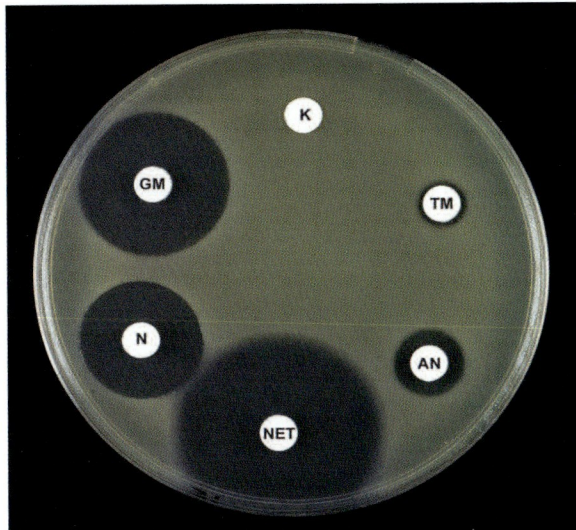

3.O. *P. aeruginosa* [ANT(4')].

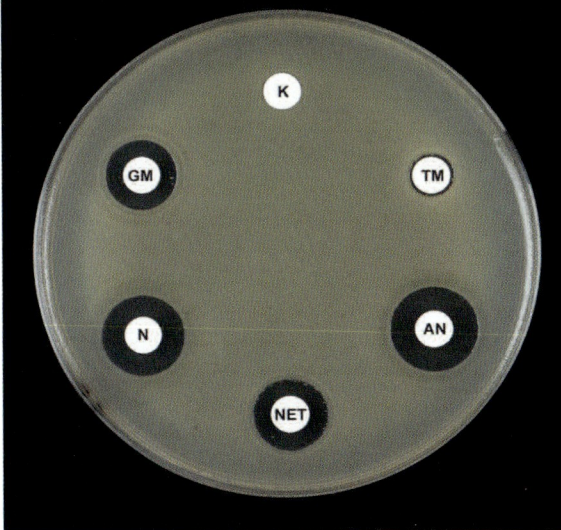

3.P. *E. coli* [AAC(6') affecting gentamicin and amikacin].

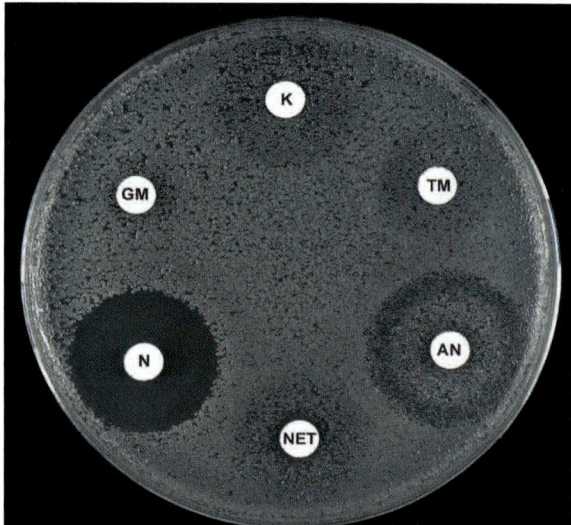

3.Q. *E. coli* [ArmA + AAC(3)-II].

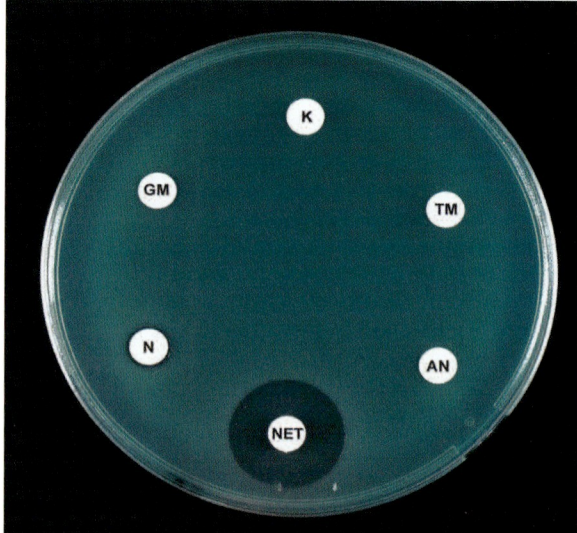

3.R. *P. aeruginosa* [ANT(4') + ANT(2")].

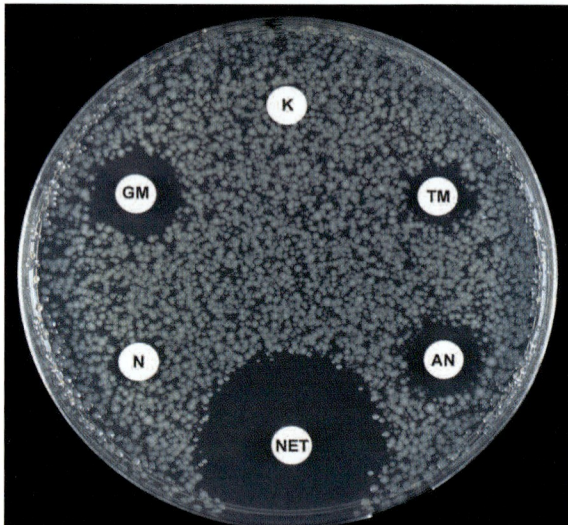

3.S. *C. freundii* [APH(3')-VI + ANT(2")].

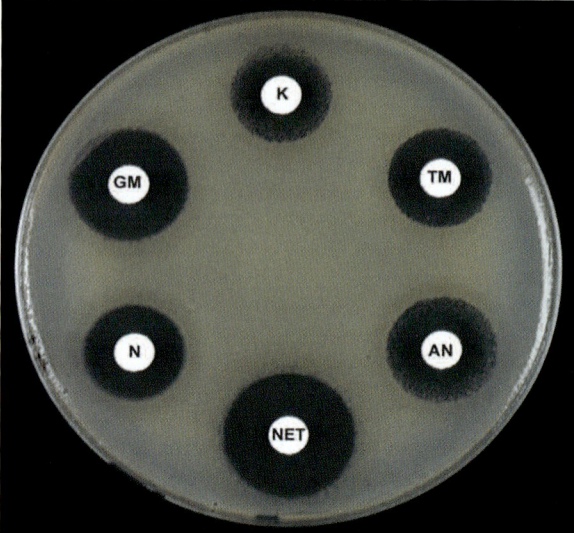

3.T. *E. coli* multiresistance due to membrane impermeability or efflux.

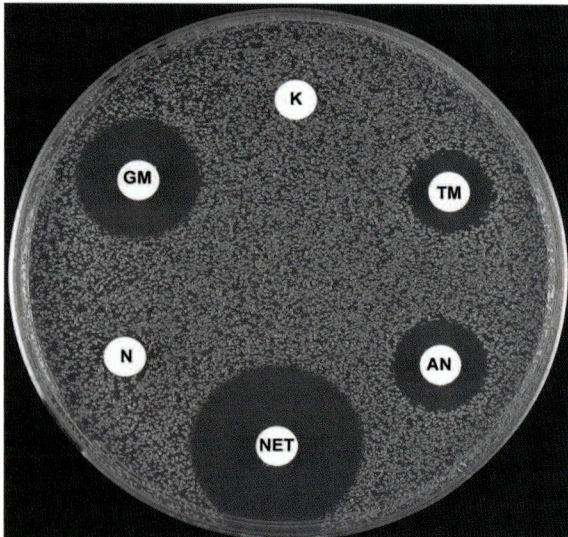

3.U. *E. coli* multiresistance due to membrane impermeability or efflux + APH(3').

to aminoglycosides (18). It nevertheless provides an additional argument for increasing the intervals between doses. Proteolytic *Acinetobacter* strains, such as *A. haemolyticus*, naturally carry AAC(6')-I genes which are often weakly expressed (Fig. 3) (22). The reduction in or the presence of isolated colonies at the edge the inhibition zone around the tobramycin disk are the best indicators of this enzymatic activity.

Presence of a single enzyme

Sm phenotype [APH(3") or ANT(3")(9)]

This phenotype consists in isolated resistance to streptomycin. This resistance is due to the production of either an APH(3"), or an ANT(3")(9) (42).

The study of spectinomycin makes it possible to discriminate these two enzymes; the second, with a high incidence (41), confers cross-resistance to the two antibiotics.

Gm (Km) phenotype [AAC(3)-I]

This phenotype consists in resistance to gentamicin and sisomicin by production of an AAC(3)-I (42). A major reduction in gentamicin activity is observed. On the contrary, there is a smaller reduction in kanamycin activity and the MICs may remain lower than the low critical concentration values (Table 8). Comparative analysis of the gentamicin (reduced) and tobramycin (unchanged) activity makes it possible to detect low phenotypic expression. Moreover, the presence of colonies of normal size at the edge of the gentamicin inhibition zone is an additional sign of enzymatic modification of this antibiotic. Confirmation may be obtained by studying fortimicin (MIC > 256 µg/ml).

Gm Tm (Km) phenotype [AAC(3)-I]

In *S. marcescens*, the superposition of gentamicin resistance conferred by AAC(3)-I with a low level of tobramycin resistance (MIC, 4 µg/ml) due to AAC(6')-Ic generates the Gm, Tm phenotype (Fig. 3). Fortimicin resistance (MIC > 256 µg/ml) confirms the enzymatic content.

Km Gm Tm phenotype [ANT(2")]

This phenotype is due to the synthesis of an ANT(2") (42). Gentamicin and tobramycin activities are strongly reduced (Fig. 3).

Km Gm Tm Nt phenotype [AAC(3)-II or AAC(3)-IV or AAC(6')-II, or AAC(3)-III]

At least four enzymes may confer this resistance phenotype.

Two genes have been characterized for AAC(3)-II: *aac(3)-IIa* (42) which is widespread and *aac(3)-IIb* (42) which is rare and only seen in *Serratia*. The effect on aminoglycoside activity is different with a particularly marked fall for gentamicin (Gm > Nt, Tm # Km) (Table 8, Fig. 3).

AAC(3)-IV (42) may be easily distinguished from AAC(3)-II by studying apramycin which is only inactivated by AAC(3)-IV. This enzyme is mainly encountered in enterobacteria isolated in animals because of the use of this antibiotic in veterinary medicine (42).

AAC(6')-II is clearly identified by the difference in activity of 6'-N-ethylnetilmicin (inactive) and 2'-N-ethylnetilmicin (active) and by resistance to 5-episisomicin (42). This phenotype is mainly due to the *aac(6')-IIa* and *aac(6')-IIb* genes in *P. aeruginosa* but may also be conferred by the *aac(6)-Ib* gene following a Leu119Ser (23, 42) point mutation (Fig. 3).

The AAC(3)-III identified in *P. aeruginosa* is rare and its presence is suggested by resistance to 5-episisomicin (42).

Km Tm phenotype [APH(3')-I]

This is low level resistance to tobramycin (MIC, 8 µg/ml) associated with high level resistance to kanamycin (MIC > 1000 µg/ml) is due to the synthesis of an APH(3')-I (Fig. 3). As already mentioned, a "trapping" mechanism was proposed to explain this resistance (31).

Km Ak phenotype [APH(3')-VI]

This phenotype, frequent in *Acinetobacter* and much rarer in enterobacteria and *P. aeruginosa*, is due to the synthesis of an APH(3')-VI (Fig. 3) (42). This resistance also concerns isepamicin and neomycin. In enterobacteria, the MICs of amikacin range from 16 to 128 µg/ml. This phenotype is all the rarer as the few strains of enterobacteria (*E. coli, E. cloacae, Providencia, Serratia*) that produce this enzyme also carry other inactivating enzymes.

Table 7. Impact of the AdeABC efflux system on aminoglycoside resistance of *A. baumannii*.

Aminoglycoside	MIC (µg/ml)		
	AdeABC overexpressed	AdeABC	AdeABC
Kanamycin	4	1	1
Amikacin	8	1	0.5
Gentamicin	8	0.5	0.25
Tobramycin	2	0.5	0.25
Netilmicin	16	0.5	0.25

Km Tm (Ak) Nt phenotype [AAC(6')-I]

This phenotype is due to the synthesis of an AAC(6')-I (Fig. 3). This enzyme confers different resistance levels according to the host bacterium and the number of copies of the corresponding gene (Table 8). It is frequent in *Serratia* and has been found in other enterobacteria, in particular *Klebsiella* and *Enterobacter*. Numerous AAC(6') have been identified. The AAC(6')-Ib enzyme is by far the most widely distributed (44). Amikacin resistance levels are variable and MICs corresponding to those of susceptible strains, according to EUCAST and CLSI criteria, are frequently observed in strains carrying an AAC(6')-I. Because of modification of amikacin it should be used with caution against such strains. These enzymes modify isepamicin *in vitro* although the MICs of this antibiotic often remain moderate. The AAC(6')-In detected in Venezuelan strains of enterobacteria confers resistance to this antibiotic (49).

Tm Gm Nt phenotype [AAC(2')]

Resistance to gentamicin-sisomicin, netilmicin and tobramycin is due to the chromosomal production by *Providencia* of an AAC(2') (Fig. 3) (42). Levels of resistance to gentamicin, netilmicin, and tobramycin are similar. Certain strains have a low level of resistance and the MICs of these three antibiotics are between 2 and 8 µg/ml.

A resistance profile suggesting production of an AAC(2') with MICs of 2-*N*-ethylnetilmicin lower than those of 6'-*N*-ethylnetilmicin was described in *Enterobacter* (42). HPLC studies showed that the aminoglycoside molecule was not modified on the C-2' amine group but on the C-3 group and the enzyme was named AAC(3)-VI. This confers gentamicin resistance and has only been detected in very rare strains.

Tm Ak phenotype [ANT(4')-II]

This phenotype, due to nucleotidylation of antibiotics, was observed in very rare strains of enterobacteria isolated in Czechoslovakia and then in the USA (Fig. 3) (44). Czech strains are also resistant to dibekacin (4'-deoxytobramycin) indicating that the 4' and 4"-hydroxyl groups may be modified [ANT(4', 4")]. US strains are susceptible to dibekacin [ANT(4')]. The enzymes were designated ANT(4')-I and ANT(4')-II, respectively. An ANT(4')-II activity was also reported in *P. aeruginosa* strains isolated in Bulgaria (40).

Km Tm Ak Gm Nt phenotype [AAC(6')-Im]

Variants of AAC(6')-Ib with Gln118Leu and Leu119Ser substitutions were found to simultaneously confer resistance to gentamicin and amikacin (2, 3) though the resistance levels were usually moderate (MICs of these compounds ≤ 64 µg/ml) (Fig. 3). Two adjacent genes *aph2"-Ib-aac(6')-Im* homologous to the gene specifying the bifunctional enzyme APH2"-AAC(6') in Gram-positive bacteria were identified both in enterobacteria and *Enterococcus* in Germany and in Slovakia (5). The AAC(6')-Im does not confer resistance to fortimicin unlike the AAC(6')-Ie activity of the bifunctional enzyme, whereas the five aminoglycosides defining this phenotype are all affected. As explained above, resistance to 4,6-substituted 2-DOS derivatives may be due to G1405 methylation of 16S rRNA, and it is then a high-level resistance (MICs of 4,6-substituted 2-DOS ≥ 128 µg/ml). Oddly, a heterogeneous zone is frequently observed around the disks of these aminoglycosides which, however, is not associated with an induction phenomenon (Fig. 3).

Presence of several enzymes

There is no overlapping between the substrate profiles of enzymes modifying streptomycin and/or spectinomycin on the one hand and other aminoglycosides (deoxystreptamines) on the other. The phenotype resulting from the coexistence of an enzyme belonging to each one of these two groups in the same strain simply results in the juxtaposition of the two phenotypes (Fig. 3). Accumulation of resistance mechanisms also occurs from the phenotypic point of view when different mechanisms are associated: modifying enzyme, efflux, 16S RNA methylation resistance pathways. Gene detection by DNA-DNA hybridization or by amplification is particularly useful because of this overlapping of substrate profiles due to different enzyme associations.

"Impermeability" phenotypes

As already mentioned, certain structural changes in the external membrane may alter aminoglycoside diffusion. In addition, mutations of the respiratory chain give rise to small colonies sometimes capable of dissociating and reverting to normal-sized colonies. The reduction in inhibition zone diameters varies with the mutation and the species considered, but is analogous for all aminoglycosides (the inhibition zones around netilmicin disks show the higher intrinsic activity of this antibiotic) (Fig. 3). The

Table 8. MIC of aminoglycosides on *Klebsiella* with or without modifying enzymes

Aminoglycoside	Critical concentration[a] (µg/ml) c	C	No enzyme[b]	AAD(2") UL[d]	AAD(2") LL	AAC(3)-I UL	AAC(3)-I LL	AAC(3)-II UL	AAC(3)-II LL	AAC(6')-I UL	AAC(6')-I LL
Tobramycin	≤4 (2)	>8 (4)	0.74	**16**[e]	**4**	0.5	1	16	4	**32**	**8**
Amikacin	≤16 (8)	>32 (16)	1.6	0.5	0.5	1	1	1	1	**32**	**2**
Isepamicin	ND[f]	ND	1.1	0.25	0.5	0.25	0.25	0.5	0.25	4	0,5
Gentamicin	≤4 (2)	>8 (4)	0.69	**32**	**4**	**32**	**8**	**64**	**16**	1	2
Netilmicin	≤8 (2)	>6 (4)	0.48	0.25	<0.125	1	1	**32**	**4**	**64**	**4**
2'-N-ethylnetilmicin	ND[f]	ND	4	1	1	8	8	**128**	**16**	**512**	**64**
6'-N-ethylnetilmicin	ND	ND	6	1	1	16	16	**256**	**16**	8	8
5-episisomicin	ND	ND	0.48	0.5	0.25	0.25	0.25	2	0,25	**16**	**2**
Fortimicin	ND	ND	3.4	2	2	>256	>256	2	2	8	2
Apramycin	ND	ND	3.8	2	1	2	2	2	2	2	2

[a] CLSI values and EUCAST values are indicated in parentheses.
[b] Modal MIC for 41 strains (Miller et al. 1980).
[c] From G. Miller et al., Schering-Plough multicenter study. Clinical isolates carrying a single enzyme.
[d] UL, usual level; LL, low level.
[e] The MICs of aminoglycosides substrates for the enzymes are indicated in bold type.
[f] ND, not determined.

enlarged susceptibility pattern confirms this mechanism: the reduction in diameters concerns apramycin, fortimicin and 5-episomicin imparting a phenotype that would result from an improbable association of enzymes. Like the efflux systems of *A. baumannii* and *P. aeruginosa*, the AcrD pump of *E. coli* may export aminoglycosides and it is probable that other as yet uncharacterized systems may exert a similar effect in other species and in particular in bacterial genera comprising strict aerobic bacteria giving a positive oxidase reaction. As it is almost impossible to routinely distinguish between these different mechanisms (excluding defective respiratory mutants) we propose the « miscellaneous » and criticizable term « impermeability ».

PREVALENCE OF RESISTANCE MECHANISMS

Globally, there does not seem to have been an unrelenting increase in aminoglycoside resistance (31). As these antibiotics are almost exclusively used in hospital, the problems of resistance are primarily associated with this healthcare setting and in particular the intensive care unit. Apart from naturally refractory species such as *B. cepacia* and *S. maltophilia*, resistance only reaches alarming levels in certain species and in particular *A. baumannii*, *P. aeruginosa*, and a moderate number of enterobacteria species *E. coli*, *Klebsiella*, *Enterobacter*, *Serratia* etc. The enzyme(s) responsible for the routinely observed resistance phenotypes are shown in Table 9.

Distribution of resistance to aminoglycosides

Surveys of the distribution of resistance are dependent on the representativity of sampling of strains, i.e. factors that are difficult to control:
- Sufficient number of strains of varied geographical origin from private practice and hospital sectors.
- Accounting of epidemic strains or those carrying an epidemic plasmid, specific for a given ecosystem (hospital).
- Variability of results according to susceptibility testing methods.
- Insufficient number of representative strains isolated in private practice.
- Possibility of correlating phenotypes with resistance mechanisms deduced from the genotype.

Table 9. Correlation between aminoglycoside resistance phenotype and genotype

Phenotype	Genotype		
Gm[a]	aac(3)-I		
Gm, Tm	ant(2") ± [aac(3)-I]		
Gm, Tm, Nt	aac(3)-V aac(3)-IV aac(2') aac(6')-II	±	aac(3)-I ant(2")
Ak, Tm, Nt	aac(6')-I		
Gm, Tm, Nt, Ak	aac(6')-I + aac(6')-I + armA		aac(3)-I aac(3)-IV aac(3)-V aac(2') ant(2") aph(2")[b]

[a] Ak, amikacin; Gm, gentamicin; Nt, netilmicin; Tm, tobramycin.
[b] Rare resistance in Gram-negative bacteria due to aac(6')-Im-aph(2")-Ib.

Because of these different problems, rather than list the global prevalence studies that are regularly conducted to monitor resistance in hospitals which are generally accessible on the Internet, we will restrict ourselves to reporting older studies based on a genetic approach.

From 1987 to 1991, the company Schering-Plough monitored bacterial aminoglycoside resistance mechanisms by comparing the minimum contents in modifying enzymes deduced from the phenotype with the genotype obtained by hybridization (41). Several international multicenter studies gave important information about the prevalence of the various resistance mechanisms (31, 41). Studies conducted in the USA, South America, Europe and in Japan (44) showed significant variations in the prevalence of enzymes according to time and geographical area. These differences could be partly explained by aminoglycoside prescription practices.

CONCLUSIONS

The purpose of interpretative reading of antibiotic susceptibility tests is to correct the results obtained by simply classifying bacteria into clinical categories. Resistance due to enzymatic inactivation of aminoglycosides confers a phenotype which may be used to deduce the biochemical resistance mechanism. This approach makes it possible to detect low level resistance. Our still limited understanding of the clinical consequences of this resistance, suggests that in enterobacteria, the MIC is predictive of therapeutic efficacy. However, the physician must bear in mind the existence of low-level resistance mechanisms. Taking into account the narrow therapeutic range of aminoglycosides, the increase in their dosage is limited but is more compatible with a single daily dose. An intermediate response only authorizes their use in combination with other antibiotics.

For a finer analysis, in particular in the presence of enzyme associations, the use of non-marketed aminoglycosides, completed by the detection of resistance genes is necessary but cannot be routinely performed.

Despite the large number of results obtained, certain aminoglycoside resistance genes still remain to be characterized. Moreover, it is currently impossible to evaluate the impact of point mutations in structural genes on the enzyme substrate profile. Caution is therefore required when reading the antibiotic susceptibility pattern and interpreting genotypes in the absence of any hybridization or gene amplification data.

REFERENCES

(1) **Beauclerk, A.A.D., and E. Cundliffe**. 1987. Sites of action of two ribosomal RNA methylases responsible for resistance to aminoglycosides. J. Mol. Biol. **193**:661-671.
(2) **Casin, I., F. Bordon, P. Bertin, A. Coutrot, I. Podglajen, R. Brasseur, and E. Collatz**. 1998. Aminoglycoside 6'-N-acetyltransferase variants of the Ib type with altered substrate profile in clinical isolates of *Enterobacter cloacae* and *Citrobacter freundii*. Antimicrob. Agents Chemother. **42**:209-215.
(3) **Casin, I., B. Hanau-Berçot, I. Podglajen, H. Vahaboglu, and E. Collatz**. 2003. *Salmonella enterica* serovar typhimurium bla_{PER-1}- carrying plasmid pSTI1 encodes an extended-spectrum aminoglycoside 6'-N-acetyltransferase of type Ib. Antimicrob. Agents Chemother. **47**:697-703.
(4) **Chan, Y.Y., T.M.C. Tan, Y.M. Ong, and K. L. Chua**. 2004. BpeAB-OprB, a multidrug efflux pump in *Burkholderia pseudomallei*. Antimicrob. Agents Chemother. **48**:1128-1135.
(5) **Chow, J.W., V. Kak, I. You, S.J. Kao, J. Petrin, D.B. Clewell, S.A. Lerner, G.H. Miller, and K.J. Shaw**. 2001. Aminoglycoside resistance genes

aph(2")-Ib and *aac(6')-Im* detected together in strains of both *Escherichia coli* and *Enterococcus faecium*. Antimicrob. Agents Chemother. **45**:2691-2694.

(6) **Courvalin, P**. 1992. Interpretive reading of antimicrobial susceptibility tests. ASM news **58**:368-375.

(7) **Davies, J.E**. 1991. Aminoglycoside-aminocyclitol antibiotics and their modifying enzymes p.691-713. In V. Lorian (ed.), Antibiotics in Laboratory Medecine; The Williams & Wilkins Co., Baltimore.

(8) **Davis, B.D**. 1987. Mechanism of bactericidal action of aminoglycosides. Microbiol. Rev. 51:341-350.

(9) **Doi, Y., D. de Oliviera Garcia, J. Adams, and D.L. Paterson**. 2007. Coproduction of novel 16S rRNA methylase RmtD and metallo-ß-lactamase SPM1 in a panresistant *Pseudomonas aeruginosa* isolate from Brazil. Antimicrob. Agents Chemother. **51**:852-856.

(10) **Doi, Y., K. Yokoyama, K. Yamane, J. Wachino, N. Shibata, T. Yagi, K. Shibayama, H. Kato, and Y. Arakawa**. 2004. Plasmid-mediated 16S rRNA methylase in *Serratia marcescens* conferring high-level resistance to aminoglycosides. Antimicrob. Agents Chemother. **48**:491-496.

(11) **Fantin, B., and C. Carbon**. 1992. In vivo antibiotic synergism: contribution of animal models. Antimicrob. Agents Chemother. **36**:907-912.

(12) **Galimand, M., P. Courvalin, and T. Lambert**. 2003. Plasmid-mediated high-level resistance to aminoglycosides in *Enterobacteriaceae* due to 16S rRNA methylation. Antimicrob. Agents Chemother. **47**:2565-2571.

(13) **Galimand, M., G. Gerbaud, and P. Courvalin**. 2000. Spectinomycin resistance in *Neisseria* spp. due to mutations in 16S rRNA. Antimicrob. Agents Chemother. **44**:1365-1366.

(14) **Galimand, M., S. Sabtcheva, P. Courvalin, and T. Lambert**. 2005. World-wide disseminated *armA* aminoglycoside resistance methylase gene is borne by composite transposon Tn*1548*. Antimicrob. Agents Chemother. **49**:2949-2953.

(15) **Goldstein, F.W., L. Gutmann, R. Williamson, E. Collatz, and J.F. Acar**. 1983. In vivo and in vitro emergence of simultaneous resistance to both ß-lactam and aminoglycoside antibiotics in a strain of *Serratia marcescens*. Ann. Microbiol. (Inst. Pasteur) **134A**:329-337.

(16) **Hancock, R.E.W**. 1981. Aminoglycoside uptake and mode of action with special reference to streptomycin and gentamicin. I. Antagonists and mutants. J. Antimicrob. Chemother. **8**:249-276.

(17) **Hancock, R.E.W., S.W. Fariner, Z. Li, and K. Poole**. 1991. Interaction of aminoglycosides with the outer membranes and purified lipopolysaccharide and OmpF porin of *Escherichia coli*. Antimicrob. Agents Chemother. **35**:1309-1314.

(18) **Hocquet, D., C. Vogne, F.E. Garch, A. Vejux, N. Gotoh, A. Lee, O. Lomovskaya, and P. Plésiat**. 2003. MexXY-OprM efflux pump is necessary for adaptive resistance of *Pseudomonas aeruginosa* to aminoglycosides. Antimicrob. Agents Chemother. **47**:1371-1375.

(19) **Hotta, K., A. Sunada, J. Ishikawa, J. Mizuno, Y. Ikeda, and S. Kondo**. 1998. The novel enzymatic 3"-*N*-acetylation of arbekacin by an aminoglycoside 3-*N*-acetyltransferase of *Streptomyces* origin and the resulting activity. J. Antibiot. **8**:735-742.

(20) **Kohanski, M.A., D.J. Dwyer, J. Wierzbowski, G. Cottarel, and J.J. Collins**. 2008. Mistranslation of membrane proteins and two-component system activation trigger antibiotic-mediated cell death. Cell **135**:679-690.

(21) **Kotra, L.P., J. Haddad, and S. Mobashery**. 2000. Aminoglycosides: perspectives on mechanisms of action and resistance and strategies to counter resistance. Antimicrob. Agents Chemother. **44**:3249-3256.

(22) **Lambert, T., G. Gerbaud, and P. Courvalin**. 1993. Characterization of *Acinetobacter haemolyticus aac(6)-Ig* gene encoding an aminoglycoside 6'-*N*-acetyltransferase which modifies amikacin. Antimicrob. Agents Chemother. **37**:2093-2100.

(23) **Lambert, T., M.C. Ploy, and P. Courvalin**. 1994. A spontaneous point mutation in the *aac(6) Ib* gene results in altered substrate specificity of aminoglycoside 6'-*N*-acetyltransferase of a *Pseudomonas fluorescens* strain. FEMS Microbiol. Lett. **115**:297-304.

(24) **Lambert, T., M.C. Ploy, F. Denis, and P. Courvalin**. 1999. Characterization of the chromosomal *aac(6')-Iz* gene of *Stenotrophomonas maltophilia*. Antimicrob. Agents Chemother. **43**:2366-2371.

(25) **Lee, M.D., S. Sanchez, M. Zimmer, U. Idris, M.E. Berrang, and P.F. McDermott**. 2002. Class 1 integron-associated tobramycin-gentamicin resistance in *Campylobacter* jejuni isolated from the broiler chicken house environment. Antimicrob. Agents Chemother. **46**:3660-3664.

(26) **Magnet, S., P. Courvalin, and T. Lambert**. 1999. Activation of the cryptic *aac(6')-Iy* aminoglycoside resistance gene of *Salmonella* by a chromosomal deletion generating a transcriptional fusion. J. Bacteriol. **181**:6650-6655.

(27) **Magnet, S., P. Courvalin, and T. Lambert**. 2001. Resistance-nodulation-cell division-type efflux pump involved in aminoglycoside resistance in *Acinetobacter baumannii* strain BM4454. Antimicrob. Agents Chemother. **45**:3375-3380.

(28) **Magnet, S., T.-A. Smith, R. Zheng, P. Nordmann, and J-S. Blanchard**. 2003. Aminoglycoside resistance resulting from tight drug binding to an altered aminoglycoside acetyltransferase. Antimicrob. Agents Chemother. **47**:1577-1583.

(29) **Marchand, I., L. Damier-Piolle, P. Courvalin, and T. Lambert**. 2004. Expression of the RND- type efflux pump AdeABC in *Acinetobacter baumannii* is regulated by the AdeRS two-component system. Antimicrob. Agents Chemother. **48**:3298-3304.

(30) **Menard, R., C. Molinas, M. Arthur, J. Duval, P. Courvalin, and R. Leclercq**. 1993. Overproduction of 3'-aminoglycoside phosphotransferase type I confers resistance to tobramycin in *Escherichia coli*. Antimicrob. Agents Chemother. **37**:78-83.

(31) **Miller, G.H., F.J. Sabatelli, R.S. Hare, Y. Glupczynski, P. Mackey, D. Schlaes, K. Shimizu, and K.J. Shaw**. 1997. The most frequent aminoglycoside resistance mechanisms-changes with time and geographic area: a reflection of aminoglycoside usage patterns ? Aminoglycoside Resistance Study Groups. Clin. Infect. Dis. **24**:S46-62.

(32) **Moore, R.A., D. DeShazer, S. Reckseidler, A. Weissman, and D.E. Woods**. 1999. Efflux-mediated aminoglycoside and macrolide resistance in *Burkholderia pseudomallei*. Antimicrob. Agents Chemother. **43**:465-470.

(33) **Poirel, L., T. Lambert, S. Türkoglü, E. Ronco, J-L. Gaillard, and P. Nordmann**. 2001. Characterization of class 1 integrons from *Pseudomonas aeruginosa* that contain the bla_{VIM-2} carbapenem-hydrolyzing ß-lactamase gene and of two novel aminoglycoside resistance gene cassettes. Antimicrob. Agents Chemother. **45**:546-552.

(34) **Potel, G., J. Caillon, F. Le Gallou, D. Bugnon, P. Le Conte, J. Raza, J.Y. Lepage, D. Baron, and H. Drugeon**. 1992. Identification of factors affecting in vivo aminoglycoside activity in an experimental model of Gram-negative endocarditis. Antimicrob. Agents Chemother. **36**:744-750.

(35) **Puglisi, J.D., S.C. Blanchard, K.D. Dahlquist, R.G. Eason, D. Fourmy, S.R. Lynch, M.I. Recht, and S. Yoshizawa**. 2000. Aminoglycoside antibiotics and decoding, p. 419-429. In R.A. Garrett, S.R. Douthwaite, A. Liljas, A.T. Matheson, P.B. Moore, and H.F. Noller (ed.), The ribosome: structure, function, antibiotics, and cellular interactions. American Society for Microbiology, Washington, D.C.

(36) **Ramos Aires, J., T. Köhler, H. Nikaido, and P. Plésiat**. 1999; Involvement of an active efflux system in the natural resistance of *Pseudomonas aeruginosa* to aminoglycosides. **43**:2624-2628.

(37) **Recht, M.I., S. Douthwaite, and J. D. Puglisi**. 1999. Basis for prokaryotic specificity of action of aminoglycoside antibiotics. EMBO J. **18**:3133-3138.

(38) **Robledano, l., M.J. Rivera, I. Otal, and R. Gomezlus**. 1987. Enzymatic modification of aminoglycoside antibiotics by *Branhamella catarrhalis* carrying an R factor. Drugs Exp. Clin. Res. **13**:137-143.

(39) **Rosenberg, E.Y., D. Ma, and H. Nikaido**. 2000. AcrD of *Escherichia coli* is an aminoglycoside efflux pump. J. Bacteriol. **182**:1754-1756.

(40) **Sabtcheva, S., M. Galimand, G. Gerbaud, P. Courvalin, and T. Lambert**. 2003. Aminoglycoside resistance gene *ant(4')-IIb* of *Pseudomonas aeruginosa* BM4492, a clinical isolate from Bulgaria. Antimicrob. Agents Chemother. **47**:1584-1588.

(41) **Shaw, K.J., R.S. Hare, F.J. Sabatelli, M. Rizzo, C.A. Cramer, L. Naples, S. Kocsi, H. Munayyer, P. Mann, G.H. Miller, L. Verbist, H. van Landùyt, Y. Glupczynski, M. Catalano, and M. Woloj**. 1991. Correlation between aminoglycoside resistance profiles and DNA hybridization of clinical isolates. Antimicrob. Agents Chemother. **35**:2253-2261.

(42) **Shaw, K.J., P.N. Rather, R.S. Hare, and G.H. Miller**. 1993. Molecular genetics of aminoglycoside resistance genes and familial relationships of the aminoglycoside-modifying enzymes. Microbiol. Rev. **57**:139-163.

(43) **Shaw, K.J., P.N. Rather, F.J. Sabatelli, P. Mann, H. Munayyer, R. Mierzwa, G.L. Petrikkos, R.S. Hare, G.H. Miller, P. Bennett, and P. Downey**. 1992. Characterization of the chromosomal *aac(6)-Ic* gene from *Serratia marcescens*. Antimicrob. Agents Chemother. **36**:1447-1455.

(44) **Shimizu, K., T. Kumada, W.C. Hsieh, H.Y. Chung, Y. Chong, R.S. Hare, G.H. Miller, F.J. Sabatelli, and L. Howard**. 1985. Comparison of aminoglycoside resistance patterns in Japan, Formosa, Korea, Chile, and the United States. Antimicrob. Agents Chemother. **28**:282-288.

(45) **Vetting, M-W., S. Magnet, E. Nieves, S-L. Roderick, and J-S. Blanchard**. 2004. A bacterial acetyltransferase capable of regioselective *N*-acetylation of antibiotics and histones. Chem. Biol. **11**:565-573.

(46) **Wachino, J., K. Shibayama, H. Kurokawa, K. Kimura, K. Yamane, S. Suzuki, N. Shibata, Y. Ike, and Y. Arakawa**. 2007. Novel plasmid-mediated 16S rRNA m1A1408 methyltransferase, NpmA, found in a clinically isolated *Escherichia coli* strain resistant to structurally diverse aminoglycosides. Antimicrob. Agents Chemother. **51**:4401-4409.

(47) **Wachino, J., K. Yamane, K. Shibayama, H. Kurokawa, N. Shibata, S. Suzuki, Y. Doi, K. Kimura, Y. Ike, and Y. Arakawa**. 2006. Novel plasmid-mediated 16S rRNA methylase, RmC, found in a *Proteus mirabilis* strain isolate demonstrating extraordinary high-level resistance against various aminoglycosides. Antimicrob. Agents Chemother. **50**:178-184.

(48) **Walter, F., Q. Vicens, and E. Westhof**. 1999. Aminoglycoside-RNA interactions. Curr. Opin. Chem. Biol. **3**:694-704.

(49) **Wu, H.Y., G.H. Miller, M. Guzman Blanco, R. S. Hare, and K.J. Shaw**. 1997. Cloning and characterization of an aminoglycoside 6'-*N*-acetyltransferase gene from *Citrobacter freundii* which confers an altered resistance profile. Antimicrob. **41**:2439-2447.

Chapter 18. QUINOLONES AND GRAM-POSITIVE BACTERIA

Emmanuelle VARON

INTRODUCTION

Gram-positive bacteria, with the exception of *Bacillus* species, are resistant to the "classical" quinolone antibiotics: nalidixic acid, pipemidic acid, oxolinic acid, and flumequine. Staphylococci were the first Gram-positive bacteria included in the spectrum of fluoroquinolones (pefloxacin, norfloxacin, ofloxacin, and ciprofloxacin). With the development of new fluoroquinolones that are active against pneumococci (levofloxacin and moxifloxacin), various other Gram-positive species are now part of the spectrum of activity of these drugs (Table 1). The use of fluoroquinolones, which has seen an overall increase in hospitals since the beginning of the 1990's, has increased relatively little in outpatient settings, especially in the treatment of community-acquired respiratory infections. Nonetheless, the emergence of pneumococcus strains with at least one acquired mechanism of resistance has occurred, albeit with a prevalence which remains low.

MODE OF ACTION

For the chemical structure and the mode of action, the reader should refer to the next chapter. The fluoroquinolones target essential enzymes, the type II topoisomerases, the gyrase composed of two GyrA and GyrB subunits, and the topoisomerase IV, which is composed of two ParC and ParE subunits. Their function is to regulate the topology of DNA in order to enable replication. By binding to the DNA-topoisomerase II complexes, fluoroquinolones induce a morphological change in the enzyme and block the cleavage-ligation process of the DNA strand. This blockage reversibly inhibits bacterial growth and has a bacteriostatic effect. The bactericidal effect of quinolones, which mechanism has not been completely clarified, may be related to the release of DNA fragments by the complex, as well as to the dissociation of the topoisomerase subunits, and may lead to complete inhibition of replication. The action of quinolones therefore results less in the inhibition of topoisomerase activity than in their transformation into replication-arrest agents (27).

The gyrase of Gram-positive bacteria (with the exception of *Bacillus*) is generally less susceptible to the quinolones than that of Gram-negative bacteria. The preferential target of the quinolones in Gram-negative bacteria is the gyrase, particularly its GyrA subunit. In Gram-positive bacteria, however, although the preferential target is usually topoisomerase IV, notably its ParC subunit, it depends in fact on both the species and the drug considered (Table 2). In *Staphylococcus aureus*, ParC is the preferential target of all fluoroquinolones, with the exception of garenoxacin; in *Streptococcus pneumoniae*, however, it is either ParC for ciprofloxacin and levofloxacin, or GyrA for sparfloxacin, moxifloxacin, gatifloxacin, and garenoxacin.

IN VITRO ACTIVITY ON SUSCEPTIBLE SPECIES

The "classical" quinolone antibiotics are not active against Gram-positive bacteria. Fluoroquinolones (pefloxacin, norfloxacin, ofloxa-

Table 1. Gram-positive bacteria (except mycobacteria) usually susceptible to fluoroquinolones

Enoxacin, Lomefloxacin, Norfloxacin, Pefloxacin	Ciprofloxacin, Ofloxacin	Levofloxacin	Moxifloxacin
Staphylococcus spp.	*Staphylococcus* spp. *B. anthracis*	*Staphylococcus* spp. *S. pneumoniae* *Streptococcus* spp. *B. anthracis*	*Staphylococcus* spp. *S. pneumoniae* *Streptococcus* spp.

cin, and ciprofloxacin) result from the addition of a fluorine atom in position 6 and substituents in position 7; these antibiotics are about one hundred times more active than the "classic" quinolones and have a spectrum which covers staphylococci. More recently, the modification of substituents in position 5, 7 and/or 8 resulted in quinolones that are even more active against Gram-positive bacteria, sometimes to the detriment of the activity against Gram-negative bacteria: 1) broad-spectrum fluoroquinolone antibiotics, since they also have very good activity against Gram-negative bacteria including *Pseudomonas* and strict anaerobes, such as temafloxacin, trovafloxacin, and clinafloxacin, which have had to be discontinued due to their toxicity ; 2) fluoroquinolone antibiotics that are active against the main respiratory pathogens, particularly *S. pneumoniae*, the other streptococci, and atypical bacteria: levofloxacin, sparfloxacin, grepafloxacin, gatifloxacin, moxifloxacin, garenoxacin, and gemifloxacin. The latter are also active against some Enterococcus species, particularly *Enterococcus faecalis*.

The bacteriostatic activity of most fluoroquinolones is shown in Table 3 for the main susceptible species. Moxifloxacin, gatifloxacin, garenoxacin, and gemifloxacin are the most active against staphylococci, streptococci, and *S. pneumoniae*. The distribution of the minimum inhibitory concentrations (MICs) of levofloxacin and moxifloxacin against *S. pneumoniae* is presented in Fig. 1. Their overall activity is still insufficient against susceptible strains of certain species such as *Enterococcus faecium* and most Gram-positive bacilli, except for *Bacillus*.

BACTERICIDAL ACTIVITY

The bactericidal activity of fluoroquinolones, which is concentration dependent, varies according to the drugs and the species involved. On susceptible *S. aureus*, ciprofloxacin, levofloxacin, moxifloxacin, and garenoxacin are bactericidal in 2 to 4 h at double concentrations of the MIC (21, 28). The bactericidal effect is slower against *S. pneumoniae* (from 10 to 16 h) for all fluoroquinolones, and equivalent to that of ciprofloxacin at a concentration four times the MIC (14).

MECHANISMS OF RESISTANCE

Resistance to fluoroquinolones is due to point mutations in either of the two targets (gyrase and topoisomerase IV) or to active efflux. In Gram-positive bacteria, resistance is determined at the chromosomal level.

In *S. aureus* and *S. pneumoniae*, the first step of resistance is modification of a single target, the preferential target, which confers a low-level of resistance and which, more or less, affects the activity of various fluoroquinolones. The next step, which is modification of the second target, confers a higher level of resistance. The mutations are generally found in a restricted area called QRDR (Quinolone Resistance-Determining Region) (9, 24). Amino acid substitutions in this region reduce the affinity of quinolones for the DNA-topoisomerase complex. Certain mutations, however, that are found outside of the QRDR may also play a role in resistance. Such mutations have been described in the N-terminal region of ParE and the

Table 2. Preferential targets of fluoroquinolones in Gram-positive bacteria

Quinolone	Preferential target (1st step mutant)		
	S. aureus (10, 19, 21, 28)[a]	S. pneumoniae (11, 16, 18, 31, 34, 35, 40)	B. anthracis (37)
Nalidixic acid	GyrA	ND[b]	GyrA
Pefloxacin	ParC	ParC	-
Norfloxacin	ParC	ParC	-
Ciprofloxacin	ParC	ParC	GyrA
Levofloxacin	ParC	ParC	-
Sparfloxacin	ParC	GyrA	-
Moxifloxacin	ParC	GyrA	GyrA
Gatifloxacin	ParC	GyrA	-
Garenoxacin	GyrA	GyrA	-

[a] References
[b] ND, not determined.

Table 3. *In vitro* activity of quinolones against susceptible Gram-positive bacteria (2, 5, 12, 29, 30, 41)

Species	Quinolone	MIC (µg/ml)		
		Range	MIC$_{50}$	MIC$_{90}$
S. aureus Methi^S	Ciprofloxacin	0.12 - > 16	0.25	0.5
	Ofloxacin	0.25 - > 64	0.5	0.5
	Levofloxacin	0.06 - > 16	0.12	0.25
	Gatifloxacin	0.03 - > 16	0.06	0.12
	Moxifloxacin	0.01 - 16	0.06	0.06
	Garenoxacin	< 0.01 - > 4	0.01	0.03
	Gemifloxacin	0.008 - 16	0.01	0.03
S. aureus Methi^R	Ciprofloxacin	0.12 - 128	16	128
	Ofloxacin	0.25 - 128	32	64
	Levofloxacin	0.12 - > 16	4	16
	Gatifloxacin	0.06 - 16	4	4
	Moxifloxacin	0.03 - 16	2	4
	Garenoxacin	< 0.01 - > 4	0.01	0.03
	Gemifloxacin	0.01 - 16	1	4
S. epidermidis	Ciprofloxacin	0.12 - > 16	8	> 16
	Ofloxacin	0.25 - > 64	8	32
	Levofloxacin	0.12 - 32	4	16
	Gatifloxacin	0.01 - 16	0.5	2
	Moxifloxacin	0.01 - 16	0.25	2
	Garenoxacin	< 0.01 - > 4	0.25	2
	Gemifloxacin	0.008 - 64	0.06	1
S. pyogenes	Ofloxacin	1 - 4	1	2
	Ciprofloxacin	0.12 - 4	0.5	1
	Levofloxacin	0.12 - 4	0.5	1
	Gatifloxacin	0.06 - 0.5	0.25	0.5
	Moxifloxacin	0.03 - 0.5	0.12	0.25
	Garenoxacin	< 0.03 - 0.25	0.06	0.12
	Gemifloxacin	0.008 - 0.06	0.01	0.03
S. agalactiae	Ofloxacin	1 - 64	2	2
	Ciprofloxacin	0.5 - 16	1	1
	Levofloxacin	0.5 - >16	0.5	1
	Gatifloxacin	0.06 - 1	0.25	0.5
	Moxifloxacin	0.03 - 0.12	0.06	0.12
	Garenoxacin	< 0.03 - 0.25	0.06	0.12
	Gemifloxacin	0.01 - 1	0.03	0.03
Oral streptococci	Ofloxacin	0.25 - 64	2	4
	Ciprofloxacin	0.12 - 64	1	4
	Levofloxacin	0.06 - 16	0.5	1
	Gatifloxacin	0.06 - 4	0.25	0.5
	Moxifloxacin	0.1 - 4	0.12	0.25
	Garenoxacin	0.06 - 1	0.06	0.12
	Gemifloxacin	0.01 - 1	0.03	0.12
S. pneumoniae	Ciprofloxacine	0.25 - 64	2	2
	Levofloxacin	0.25 - 64	1	1
	Sparfloxacin	0.06 - 64	0.25	0.5
	Gatifloxacin	0.06 - 16	0.25	0.5
	Moxifloxacin	0.06 - 8	0.12	0.12
	Garenoxacin	0.01 - 2	0.06	0.06
	Gemifloxacin	0.008 - 1	0.03	0.03
E. faecalis	Ofloxacin	1 - > 64	2	64
	Ciprofloxacin	0.5 - > 64	1	> 16
	Levofloxacin	0.25 - > 16	1	16

Table 3. *In vitro* activity of quinolones against susceptible Gram-positive bacteria (2, 5, 12, 29, 30, 41) (continued)

Species	Quinolone	MIC (µg/ml)		
		Range	MIC$_{50}$	MIC$_{90}$
E. faecalis	Gatifloxacin	0.12 - > 16	0.5	16
	Moxifloxacin	0.12 - > 16	0.25	8
	Garenoxacin	0.12 - 16	0.25	4
	Gemifloxacin	0.06 - 16	0.06	2
E. faecium	Ofloxacin	4 - > 64	> 64	> 64
	Ciprofloxacin	0.12 - > 16	4	> 16
	Levofloxacin	0.25 - > 16	4	> 16
	Gatifloxacin	0.12 - > 16	2	> 16
	Moxifloxacin	0.12 - > 16	2	> 16
	Garenoxacin	0.12 - > 16	> 4	> 4
	Gemifloxacin	0.12 - 64	4	> 16
Bacillus anthracis	Nalidixic acid	0.12 - 32	4	8
	Ofloxacin	0.06 - 2	0.25	0.25
	Pefloxacin	0.03 - 1	0.12	0.25
	Gatifloxacin	0.12	0.12	0.12
	Levofloxacin	0.03 - 1	0.12	0.25
	Ciprofloxacin	0.03 - 0.5	0.06	0.25

COOH terminal region of GyrA in *S. aureus* (19), as well as in the N-terminal region of ParE in *S. pneumoniae*. The latter mutation, found in the ATP-hydrolase region, only results in resistance when it is associated with a mutation in GyrA (23).

Efflux may or may not be associated with modification of one or several targets, thus contributing to the elevated level of resistance. This mechanism is linked to the activation of export pumps which, by reducing their cytoplasmic concentration, limit the access of certain fluoroquinolones, such as ciprofloxacin and norfloxacin, to their targets. Efflux, which to date does not concern other fluoroquinolones, has been described in staphylococci, pneumococci, *Bacillus* species, oral streptococci and enterococci. Its frequency in the latter organisms could explain in part their natural resistance to fluoroquinolones. It is a complex mechanism, poorly understood at the molecular level, which can involve one or several pumps present in the membrane of all bacteria. In *S. aureus*, a mutation in the *norA* gene promoter leads to overexpression of an inducible pump of the MultiDrug Resistance family, i.e., capable of exporting various compounds, including ciprofloxacin, norfloxacin, but also chloramphenicol and ethidium bromide, among others (26, 39). In *Bacillus subtilis*, Bmr is a pump that is homologous to NorA, which causes efflux of norfloxacin and ciprofloxacin, similarly to EmeA, recently described in *E. faecalis* (25). A related efflux mechanism has been described in *S. pneumoniae* (44) which could be dependent on the *pmrA* gene (12), but its genetic determinism has not been completely clarified. Other pumps may contribute to this phenotype since efflux persists after *pmrA* inactivation. These pumps are all inhibited by reserpine. Thus, a reduction of more than two dilutions of the MIC of norfloxacin or ciprofloxacin in the presence of reserpine (10 to 20 µg/ml) indicates the presence of efflux. The impact of the mechanisms of resistance on the activity of quinolones is summarized in Tables 4 to 8.

The bactericidal effect of fluoroquinolones is more or less affected by the mechanisms of resistance. In *S. aureus*, ciprofloxacin is bactericidal in 4 h on ParC mutants but not on ParC + GyrA mutants, even at a concentration four times higher than the MIC. Conversely, garenoxacin is bactericidal in 4 h at a concentration twice the MIC on ParC and ParC + GyrA mutants (21, 28). The bactericidal effect of fluoroquinolones in *S. pneumoniae* is not significantly modified on the different types of resistant mutants (14).

GENOTYPES AND PHENOTYPES OF RESISTANCE

Most *S. aureus* that are resistant to fluoroquinolones are strains that have a high level of resistance

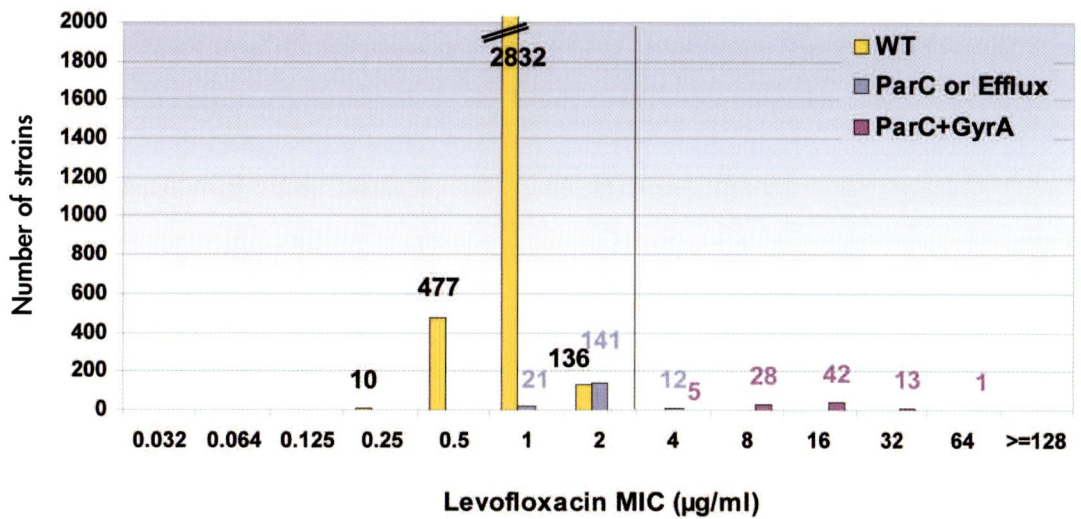

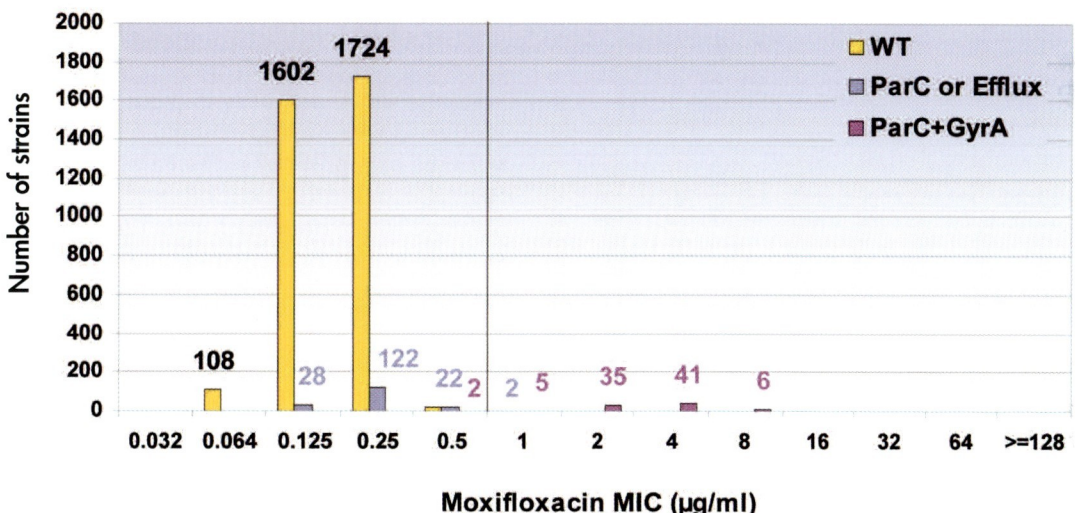

Fig. 1. Susceptibility to levofloxacin and moxifloxacin of 3718 strains of *S. pneumoniae* isolated between 2001 and 2004. The vertical line indicates the critical concentration recommended by the CA-SFM (http://www.sfm.asso.fr).

with one or several mutations in both ParC (or ParE) and GyrA targets, which confer cross-resistance to pefloxacin, ciprofloxacin, ofloxacin, levofloxacin, and moxifloxacin (MIC ≥ 4 µg/ml, Table 4). Strains with low levels of resistance are rare and have either an isolated mutation in ParC, efflux, or an association of the two mechanisms of resistance (Fig. 2 to 6).

In *S. pneumoniae*, as in oral streptococci, mutants with a low level of resistance display either active efflux or a mutation in the QRDR of ParC (8, 24), and more rarely a mutation in the QRDR of ParE (7, 34). Until now, with the exception of a single case (33), no mutants with GyrA as the only mutated target have been detected clinically (7, 36, 41). High level resistance mutants usually accumulate one or several mutations in ParC or GyrA, and more rarely in ParE and GyrA (Fig. 7 to 12).

It has been shown that for strains that have acquired a first mechanism of resistance to fluoroquinolones (low level), there was a risk of selection of high resistance mutants depending to the quinolone considered. This risk increases as the quinolone concentration approaches its MIC. The selection of fluoroquinolone-resistant pneumonia during treatment of *pneumonia* has been reported (6) and epidemics of resistant strains have

Table 4. Impact of resistance mechanisms on the activity of quinolones against S. aureus (19, 20, 21, 26, 28, 39)

Strain	Genotype	MIC (µg/ml)							
		NAL[a]	NOR	CIP	OFX	LVX	MXF	GAT	GRN
ISP794	Wild	64	0.5	0.25	0.25	0.12	0.06	0.06	0.032
MT5224c4	ParC (Ser$_{80}$Phe)	64	8	1 – 2	2	1	0.25	0.25	0.125
MT5224c3	ParC (Ala$_{116}$Glu)	-	-	1-2	-	0.5	0.25	0.5	0.06
P4	ParC (Arg$_{43}$Cys)	128	-	1	-	-	-	-	0.06
P21	ParC (Asp$_{69}$Tyr)	128	-	1	-	-	-	-	0.06
P10	ParC (Ala$_{176}$Thr)	128	-	1	-	-	-	-	0.06
MT5224c9	ParE (Asn$_{470}$Asp)	-	-	1 – 2	-	-	0.25	0.25	0.06
GB	ParE (Pro$_{25}$His)	-	-	1	-	-	-	-	0.01
SS1	GyrA (Ser$_{84}$Leu)	256	0.5	0.25	-	0.25	0.06	0.125	0.032
MT23142	Efflux NorA	>256	8 [2][b]	2 [0.5]	2	0.25	0.06 [0.06]	0.25	0.06
1199B	Efflux NorA + ParC (Ala$_{116}$Glu)	>256	128 [16]	16 [4]	4	-	-	-	-
EN8	ParC (Ser$_{80}$Phe) + GyrA (Ser$_{84}$Leu)	256	64	32	64	16	4	4	4
EN14	ParE (Asn$_{470}$Asp) + GyrA (Ser$_{84}$Leu)	128	8	4	-	4	1	1	1

[a] CIP, ciprofloxacin ; GAT, gatifloxacin ; GRN, garenoxacin ; LVX, levofloxacin ; MXF, moxifloxacin ; NAL, nalidixic acid; NOR, norfloxacin ; OFX, ofloxacin.
[b] [ ], MIC in the presence of reserpine.

occurred in institutions for the elderly (43). It is possible that, as for resistance to β-lactam antibiotics, other streptococci species are a gene reservoir for pneumococci and play a role in the spread of resistance. Mutation transfer is possible *in vitro* from different species of fluoroquinolone-resistant oral streptococci to *S. pneumoniae* and vice-versa. In addition, the genetic determinant of the oral streptococci efflux can be easily introduced in *S. pneumoniae* (13). Although occurring rarely, *parC* and *gyrA* mosaic genes have been found in clinical strains of pneumococci (2, 7).

FREQUENCY OF RESISTANCE

The prevalence of fluoroquinolone resistance is currently less than 10 % among methicillin-resistant *S. aureus* isolated from bacteraemia and reaches 90 % in the resistant strains (Onerba, http://www.onerba.org).

The prevalence of *S. pneumoniae* strains with decreased susceptibility to fluoroquinolones (ciprofloxacin MIC > 2 µg/ml) is even lower worldwide, estimated at about 5 % (1, 4, 7, 32, 36), with the exception of Hong Kong where, after having exceeded 15 % in 2001 (17), it was 7.5 % in 2005 (22). In France, 1.4 % (26/1794) of strains studied at the French National Reference Centre for pneumococci [Centre National de Référence des Pneumocoques (CNRP)] in 2007 had acquired at least one mechanism of resistance to fluoroquinolones, and this proportion remained stable since 2001. A slightly higher prevalence was seen among strains isolated from adult respiratory samples, being close to 3.6 % in 2007. The level of resistance was low in 70 % of cases, related to a mutation in ParC (2 out of 3 times) or efflux (41). The use of previous-generation fluoroquinolones which have ParC as a preferential target and had little activity on pneumococci and streptococci probably allowed the selection of such strains.

There are few data concerning in the prevalence of fluoroquinolone resistance enterococci. In *E. faecalis*, it progressed in France between 1987 and 1993 from less than 2 % to 14 % (38). It is more common among strains with a high level of resistance to gentamicin and among the vancomycin-resistant strains.

Resistance is rare in *Bacillus anthracis*. Out of 96 strains isolated in France between 1996 and 2000, 5.2 % had a low level of resistance (reduced susceptibility to nalidixic acid); the mechanism is not known and all the strains are susceptible to ciprofloxacin and levofloxacin (3).

Chapter 18. QUINOLONES AND GRAM-POSITIVE BACTERIA

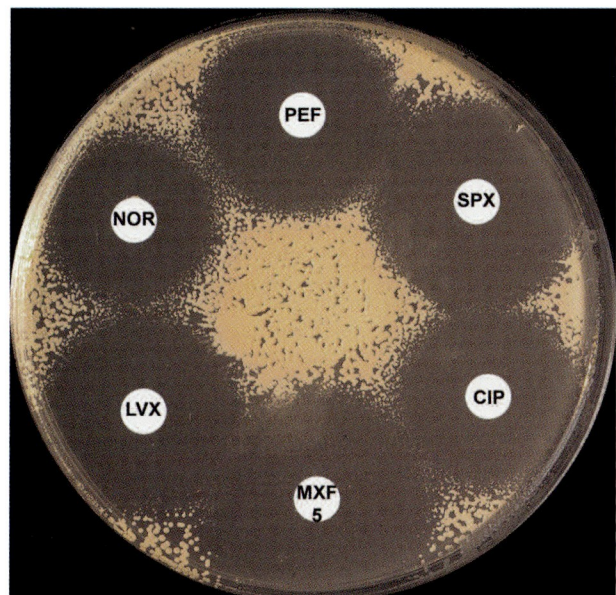

Fig. 2. *S. aureus* RN4220: WT phenotype (9). CIP, ciprofloxacin; LVX, levofloxacin; MXF, moxifloxacin; NOR, norfloxacin; PEF, pefloxacin; SPX, sparfloxacin.

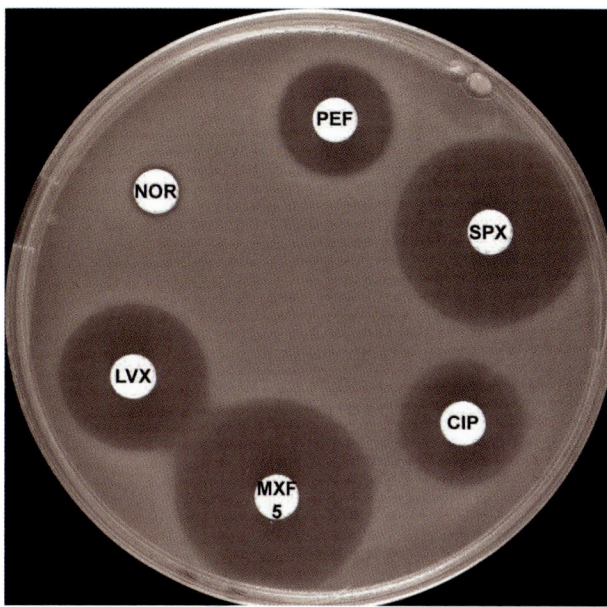

Fig. 3. *S. aureus* 2-2: ParC phenotype ($Ser_{80}Tyr$) (9). Only the inhibition diameters around SPX and MXF are maintained. CIP, ciprofloxacin; LVX, levofloxacin; MXF, moxifloxacin; NOR, norfloxacin; PEF, pefloxacin; SPX, sparfloxacin.

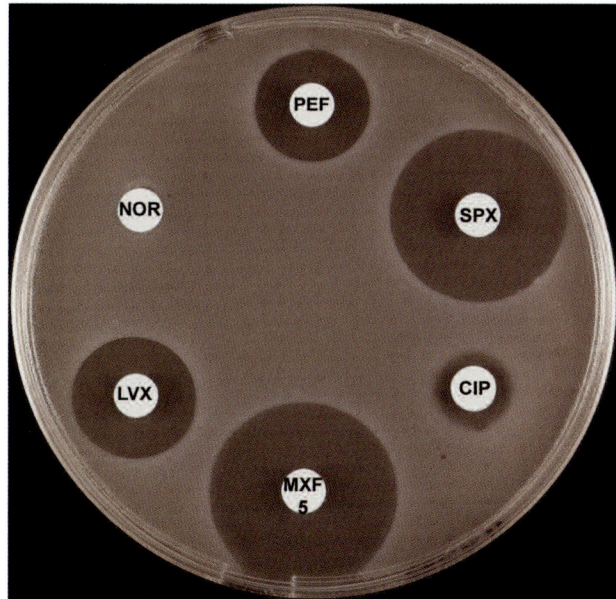

Fig. 4. *S. aureus* 1199B: Efflux (NorA) + ParC ($Ala_{116}Glu$) phenotype (26). The efflux results in a significant reduction of inhibition diameters around CIP and NOR; this phenotype superimposes to the ParC phenotype described in Fig. 3. CIP, ciprofloxacin; LVX, levofloxacin; MXF, moxifloxacin; NOR, norfloxacin; PEF, pefloxacin; SPX, sparfloxacin.

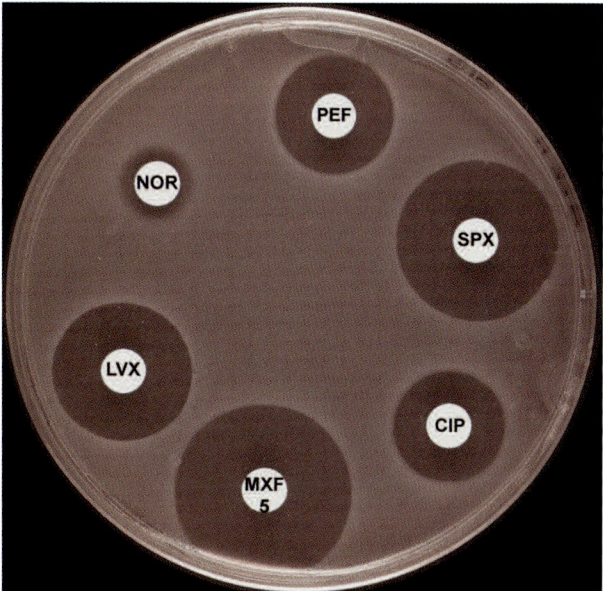

Fig. 5. *S. aureus* 1199B. Efflux (NorA) + ParC ($Ala_{116}Glu$) phenotype (26). Antibiotic susceptibility test done in the presence of reserpine (20 µg/ml): the efflux is inhibited, unmasking the ParC phenotype. CIP, ciprofloxacin; LVX, levofloxacin; MXF, moxifloxacin; NOR, norfloxacin; PEF, pefloxacin; SPX, sparfloxacin.

ANTIBIOTICS TO BE STUDIED

Whether for routine practice or for epidemiological purposes, it is necessary to detect not only the strains that are resistant to fluoroquinolones (high level) but also the low level resistant strains which are difficult to distinguish, in certain species, from the susceptible strains, and for which there is a risk of selection of mutants with a high level of resistance during treatment.

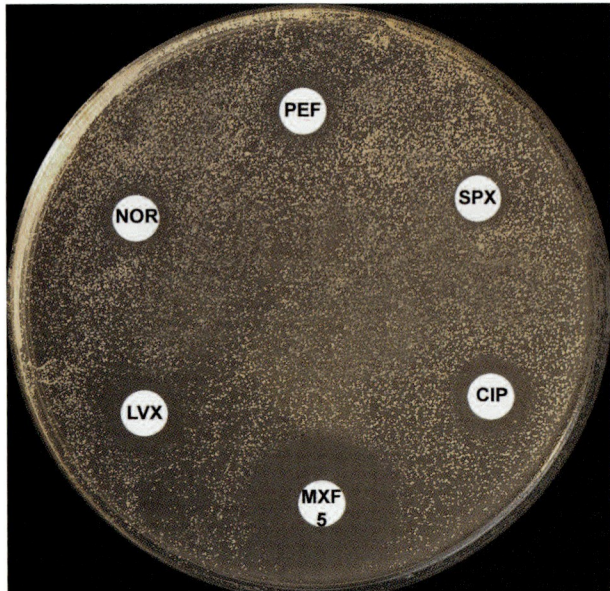

Fig. 6. *S. aureus* 2C32C128B: ParC (Ser$_{80}$Tyr) + GyrA (Ser$_{84}$Leu) phenotype (9). CIP, ciprofloxacin; LVX, levofloxacin; MXF, moxifloxacin; NOR, norfloxacin; PEF, pefloxacin; SPX, sparfloxacin.

Antibiotic susceptibility testing

The resistance phenotypes as studied by diffusion associated with the main mechanisms of resistance are illustrated in Fig. 2 to 6 for *S. aureus* and Fig. 7 to 12 for *S. pneumoniae*.
- Resistance in staphylococci, whether low or high level, is detected by the study of ofloxacin or levofloxacin. Ciprofloxacin or norfloxacin can be used since they are subtrates for efflux, but this phenotype is rare. The presence of efflux can be confirmed using a norfloxacin or a ciprofloxacin disk in the presence of 20 μg/ml of reserpine.
- High level resistance in *S. pneumoniae* is better detected by the study of levofloxacin activity than by that of moxifloxacin, as evidenced by the distribution of MICs and inhibition zone diameters in Fig. 13 A and B. This is not the case for low level resistance however, in which case there is little modification of anti-pneumococcal fluoroquinolone activity (Fig. 13 A and B). It is therefore necessary to study the activity of one or several previous generation fluoroquinolones which are affected more specifically, either by efflux (norfloxacin), or by the modification of topoisomerase (pefloxacin) or gyrase (sparfloxacin) (Table 5). The distribution of their MICs and their inhibition zone diameters are presented in Fig. 13 C, D, and E.

Minimum antibiotic susceptibility testing of *S. pneumoniae*

This is based on the study of two fluoroquinolones: norfloxacin and levofloxacin (Table 9).

Detection of topoisomerase IV and efflux mutants with a low level of resistance can be achieved using a norfloxacin disk (5μg), the inhibition zone being less than 10 mm (Fig. 8 and 10) (42). In this case the clinician should be warned of the risk of selection of mutants highly resistant to levofloxacin or moxifloxacin if event these drugs are used. The same type of reasoning may be used for antibiotic susceptibility testing in liquid medium, with the critical concentration of norfloxacin being 16 μg/ml (CA-SFM, 2005; http://www.sfm.asso.fr).

The detection of mutants with a high level of resistance (topoisomerase IV and gyrase) is done using a levofloxacin disk (5μg), with the zone of inhibition being less than 17 mm (Fig. 12) (42). For antibiotic susceptibility testing in liquid medium, the critical concentration of levofloxacin is 2 μg/ml.

Detection of resistance mechanisms to fluoroquinolones in *S. pneumoniae* by diffusion

This protocol proposes an approach for identifying the different mechanisms of resistance present in pneumococci and can be used for epidemiological purposes. It requires the use of five fluoroquinolones: norfloxacin, ciprofloxacin, sparfloxacin, levofloxacin, and pefloxacin (42). Table 9 shows the different mechanisms of resistance and the expected resistance profiles (see also Fig. 7 to 12). This method allows to identify the GyrA mutants by comparing the zones inhibition diameters that are centred by the sparfloxacin and ciprofloxacin disks (Fig. 11). In the absence of pefloxacin, as in the minimum antibiotic susceptibility test, efflux and ParC mutants cannot be distinguished. The presence of efflux can be demonstrated by the restoration of the activity of a norfloxacin disk in the presence of 10 μg/ml of reserpine (Fig. 9 and 10) (42).

Table 5. Impact of resistance mechanisms on the activity of quinolones against *S. pneumoniae* (14, 18, 40)

Strain	Phenotype	Mutation						MIC (µg/ml)							
		ParC		ParE	GyrA			PEF[a]	NOR	CIP	SPX	LVX	MXF	GRN	GEM
		79	83	435	81	85									
R6		S	D	D	S	E		8	4	1	0.25	0.5	0.125	0.032	0.016
R6Tr5929	Efflux	-	-	-	-	-		8	32 [8][b]	4 [8]	0.25	0.5	0.125	0.064	0.064
R6Tr1	ParC	Y	-	-	-	-		64	64	4	0.5	1	0.25	0.064	0.064
R6Tr2	ParC	F	-	-	-	-		64	64	4	0.5	1	0.25	0.064	0.064
R6Tr3	ParC	-	G	-	-	-		64	64	4	0.5	1	0.25	0.064	0.064
R6Lv2	ParC	-	N	-	-	-		32	64	4	1	2	0.5	0.125	0.064
R6Tr4	ParC	Y	Y	-	-	-		64	64	4	0.5	1	0.25	0.064	0.064
Tr2Fqf	ParC+efflux	F	-	-	-	-		32	64	16	0.5	2	0.25	0.064	0.064
SP003	ParE	-	-	N	-	-		32	32	8	1	2	0.25	0.125	0.125
R6Mx8	GyrA	-	-	-	A	-		8	4	1	0.5	1	0.5	0.064	0.064
R6Tr5	GyrA	-	-	-	Y	-		8	4	1-2	1	0.5	0.5	0.125	0.064
R6Tr6	GyrA	-	-	-	F	-		8	4	2	1	0.5	0.5	0.125	0.064
R6Tr7	GyrA	-	-	-	-	K		8	4	1-2	2	0.5	0.5	0.125	0.064
R6Tr8	GyrA	-	-	-	Y	K		8	4	1-2	2	0.5	0.5	0.125	0.064
R6Mx9Mx5	ParE+GyrA	-	-	N	F	-		64	128	16	4	8	2	0.5	0.25
R6Tr13	ParC+GyrA	-	G	-	Y	-		128	128	32	8	4	4	0.5	0.125
R6Tr12	ParC+GyrA	Y	-	-	-	K		128	128	32	32	8	4	1	0.5
R6Tr9	ParC+GyrA	Y	-	-	Y	-		128	128	32	16	8	4	1	0.25
R6Tr10	ParC+GyrA	Y	-	-	F	-		128	128	32	16	8	4	1	0.25
R6Tr11	ParC+GyrA	F	-	-	F	-		128	128	32	16	8	4	1	0.25
R6Tr17	ParC+GyrA	Y	Y	-	Y	-		128	128	64	16	16	4	1	0.5
R6Tr18	ParC+GyrA	Y	Y	-	F	-		128	128	32	16	32	8	1	0.5
R6Tr16	ParC+GyrA	Y	-	-	Y	K		128	128	32	64	32	8	2	1
R6Tr19	ParC+GyrA	Y	Y	-	-	K		128	128	32	64	32	8	2	1
R6Tr20	ParC+GyrA	Y	Y	-	Y	K		128	128	64	128	128	256	64	16

[a] CIP, ciprofloxacin ; GEM, gemifloxacin ; GRN, garenoxacin ; LVX, levofloxacin ; MXF, moxifloxacin ; PEF, pefloxacin ; SPX, sparfloxacin.
[b] Susceptible type strain.
[c] [ ], MIC in the presence of reserpine.

Table 6. Impact of resistance mechanisms on the activity of quinolones against oral streptococci (13, 14)

Strain	Efflux	Mutation ParC 79	ParC 83	GyrA 81	GyrA 85	ParE 435	ParE 474	MIC (μg/ml) PEF[a]	CIP	SPX	LVX	MXF	GRN	GEM
S. mitis 103335[Tb]	-	S	D	S	E	D	E	8	2 [1][c]	0.5	1	0.125	0.06	0.032
S. mitis B13	-	I	-	-	-	-	-	64	16 [4]	2	2	0.25	0.25	0.125
S. mitis B14	-	-	-	F	-	-	K	128	64 [8]	2	4	0.5	0.25	0.25
S. oralis 109922[Tb]	+	-	-	-	-	-	-	16	4 [1]	0.5	0.5	0.25	0.125	0.032
S. oralis B3	+	R	-	-	-	-	-	16	4 [1]	0.5	1	0.125	0.064	0.032
S. oralis B6	+	-	N	-	-	-	-	32	8 [2]	1	2	0.25	0.125	0.125
S. oralis B7	+	-	H	-	-	-	-	64	8 [4]	1	2	0.25	0.125	0.125
S. oralis B9	+	F	-	-	-	-	-	128	16 [4]	1	2	0.25	0.25	0.125
S. oralis B14	+	Y	-	-	-	-	-	>128	16 [4]	2	2	0.5	0.25	0.125-
S. oralis B11	-	F	-	-	G	-	-	128	128 [64]	64	8	2	1	1
S. oralis B12	-	F	-	Y	-	-	-	>128	128 [64]	32	8	2	1	0.5
S. oralis B13	-	-	N	Y	-	-	-	>128	128 [64]	64	8	4	1	1
S. sanguis 55128[Tb]	-	-	-	-	-	-	-	16	4 [2]	0.5	0.5	0.25	0.125	0.064
S. sanguis B1	+	-	Y	-	-	-	-	32	4 [1]	0.5	4	0.5	0.125	0.064
S. mitis B9	+	-	-	-	-	-	-	16	16 [1]	1	2	0.25	0.25	0.25
S. oralis B5	+	-	-	-	-	-	-	16	16 [2]	1	2	0.25	0.25	0.125
S. sanguis B2	+	-	-	-	-	-	-	16	16 [2]	0.5	4	0.5	0.125	0.064

[a] CIP, ciprofloxacin ; GEM, gemifloxacin ; GRN, garenoxacin ; LVX, levofloxacin ; MXF, moxifloxacin ; PEF, pefloxacin ; SPX, sparfloxacin.
[b] Susceptible type strain.
[c] [ ], MIC in the presence of reserpine.

Table 7. Impact of resistance mechanisms on the activity of quinolones against *E. faecalis* (14)

Strain	Efflux	Mutation ParC 80	ParC 84	GyrA 83	GyrA 87	ParE 453	MIC (µg/ml) PEF[a]	CIP	SPX	LVX	MXF	GRN	GEM
JH2-2[b]	-	S	E	S	E	P	4	2 [2][c]	0.5	1	0.25	0.25	0.125
EF12	-	I	-	-	-	-	32	4 [2]	1	2	0.5	0.25	0.12
EF13	-	-	K	-	-	-	32	4 [2]	1	2	0.5	0.5	0.12
EF14	-	I	-	-	G	-	256	32 [32]	8-32	16	2-4	1	0.5
EF16	-	I	-	Y	-	-	256	64 [64]	64	64	8	2	1
EF30	-	I	-	R	-	-	256	32 [32]	16	32	8	2	1
EF31	-	I	-	K	-	-	256	128 [128]	16	32	4	2	2
EF32	-	I	-	-	K	S	256	64 [64]	64	32	8	2	1
EF28	-	I	-	Y	-	-	256	128 [128]	64	64	8	4	2
EF33	-	I	-	I	-	-	256	256 [128]	128	128	132	8	8
EF 44	+	I	-	I	-	-	256	128 [32]	64	64	32	8	8

[a] CIP, ciprofloxacin ; GEM, gemifloxacin ; GRN, garenoxacin ; LVX, levofloxacin ; PEF, pefloxacin ; SPX, sparfloxacin.
[b] Susceptible strain.
[c] [ ], MIC in presence of reserpine.

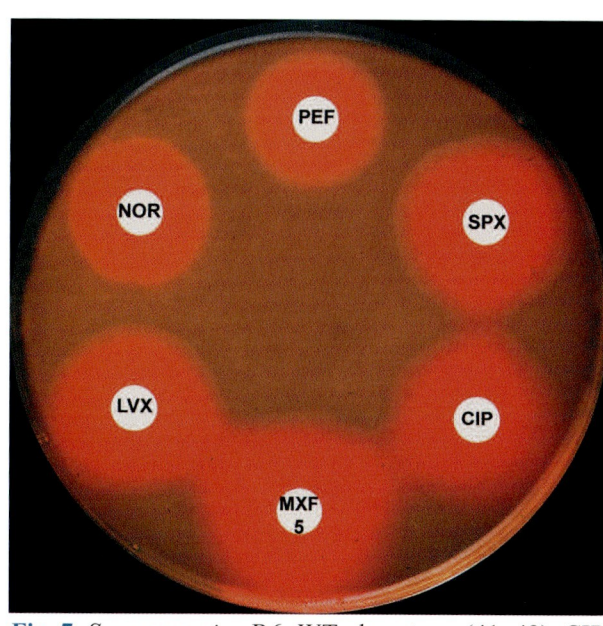

Fig. 7. *S. pneumoniae* R6: WT phenotype (41, 42). CIP, ciprofloxacin; LVX, levofloxacin; MXF, moxifloxacin; NOR, norfloxacin; PEF, pefloxacin; SPX, sparfloxacin.

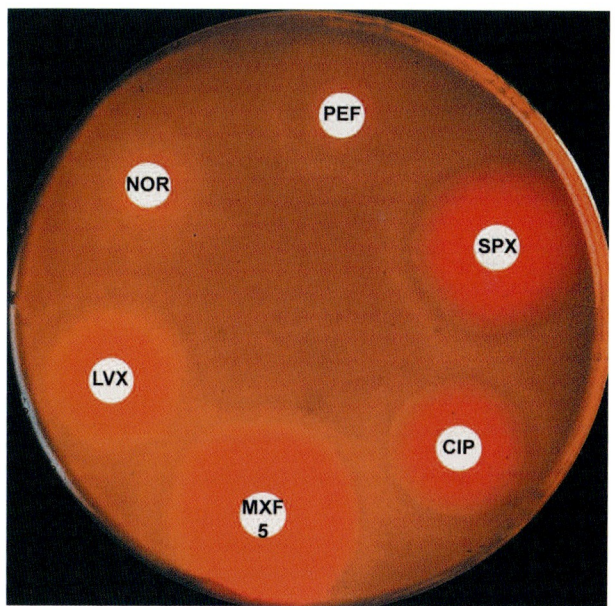

Fig. 8. *S. pneumoniae*: ParC (Ser$_{79}$Tyr) phenotype (41, 42). Significant reduction in diameter (< 10 mm) or absence of inhibition zone around the NOR and PEF disks. It also results a reduction of the inhibition diameter around CIP. The zones of inhibition around SPX, LVX and MXF remain unchanged. CIP, ciprofloxacin; LVX, levofloxacin; MXF, moxifloxacin; NOR, norfloxacin; PEF, pefloxacin; SPX, sparfloxacin.

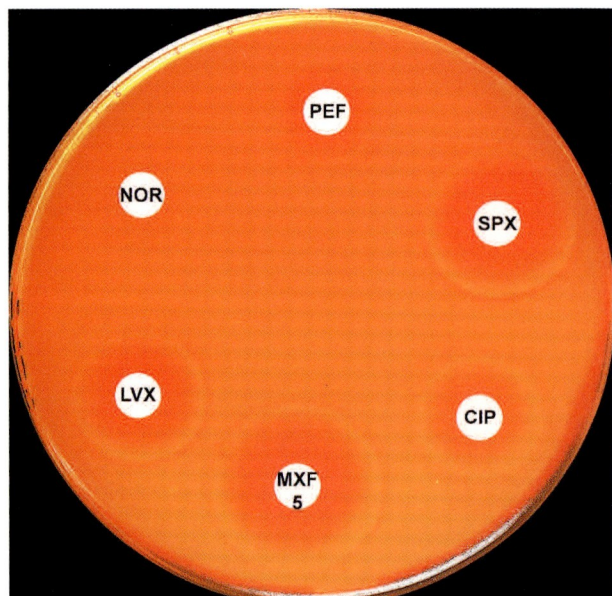

Fig. 9. *S. pneumoniae* CNRP-3: Efflux phenotype (41, 42). Significant reduction in the diameter (<10 mm), or absence of inhibition zone around NOR, and reduction of inhibition zone around CIP. The inhibition zones around the other fluoroquinolones remain unchanged. CIP, ciprofloxacin; LVX, levofloxacin; MXF, moxifloxacin; NOR, norfloxacin; PEF, pefloxacin; SPX, sparfloxacin.

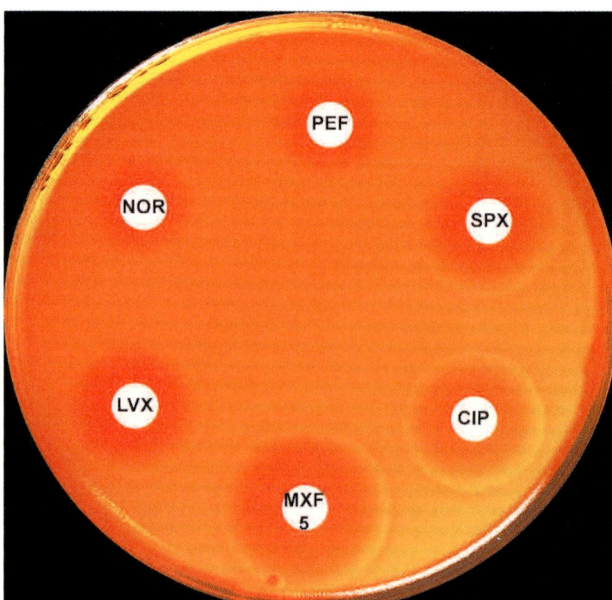

Fig. 10. *S. pneumoniae* CNRP-3: Efflux phenotype (41, 42). Antibiotic susceptibility test done in the presence of reserpine (10 µg/ml): inhibition of efflux results in the restoration of inhibition zone around NOR and CIP; the phenotype then is comparable to that of a wild strain. CIP, ciprofloxacin; LVX, levofloxacin; MXF, moxifloxacin; NOR, norfloxacin; PEF, pefloxacin; SPX, sparfloxacin.

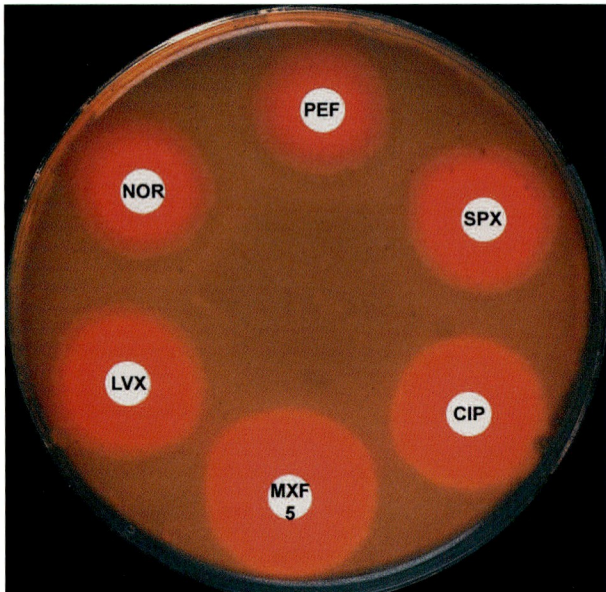

Fig. 11. *S. pneumoniae* CNRP-25: GyrA (Ser$_{81}$Phe) phenotype (41, 42). Only the inhibition zone around SPX is reduced and is smaller than that of CIP. The inhibition zones around the other fluoroquinolones remain unchanged. CIP, ciprofloxacin; LVX, levofloxacin; MXF, moxifloxacin; NOR, norfloxacin; PEF, pefloxacin; SPX, sparfloxacin.

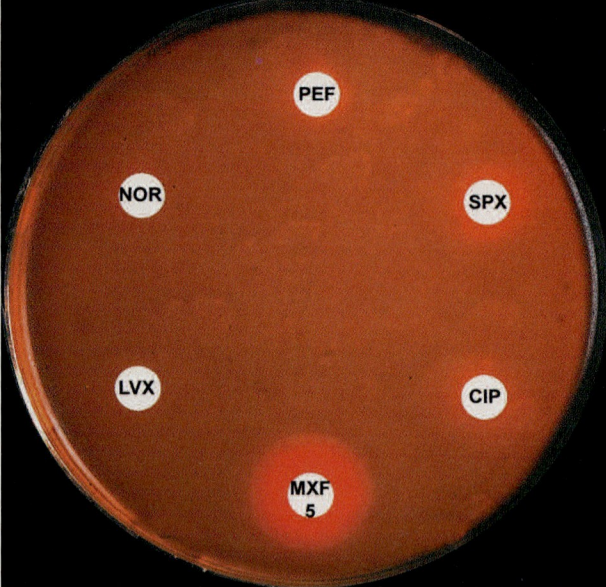

Fig. 12. *S. pneumoniae* CNRP-18: ParC (Ser$_{79}$Tyr) + GyrA (Ser$_{81}$Phe) phenotype (41, 42). This phenotype is characterised by the absence or the marked reduction of the inhibition zone around LVX, SPX, and MXF together with lack of inhibition zone around PEF, NOR, and CIP, ciprofloxacin; LVX, levofloxacin; MXF, moxifloxacin; NOR, norfloxacin; PEF, pefloxacin; SPX, sparfloxacin.

Chapter 18. QUINOLONES AND GRAM-POSITIVE BACTERIA

Table 8. Impact of resistance mechanisms on the activity of quinolones against *Bacillus anthracis* (15, 37)

Strain	Genotype	MIC (µg/ml)				
		Nalidixic acid	Ciprofloxacin	Levofloxacin	Moxifloxacin	Garenoxacin
Ames strain	WT	0.25	0.06-0.12	0.12	0.06	0.01
BA9131	gyrA Ser_{85}Leu	16-32	0.12	0.12	0.12	0.01
BAM3	gyrA Ser_{85}Leu + parC Ser_{81}Phe	>64	8	8	8	0.5
BAC3	gyrA Ser_{85}Leu + parC Ser_{82}Pro	>64	16	4	4	0.5
BAC15	gyrA Ser_{85}Leu + parC Ser_{81}Tyr +efflux	>64	256 [64][a]	32	16	2

[a] [ ], MIC in the presence of reserpine.

Table 9. Inhibition diameters of fluoroquinolones for the detection of resistance mechanisms (42)

Resistance mechanism	Interpretive values [a]			
	Norfloxacin	Levofloxacin	Pefloxacin	Sparfloxacin / ciprofloxacin
	R < 10 mm[b]	R < 17 mm[b]	R < 10 mm	_[c]
Topo IV	**R**	S	R	SPX > CIP
Efflux	**R**	S	S	SPX > CIP
Gyrase (GyrA)	S	S	S	**SPX < CIP**
Topo IV + Gyrase	**R**	**I or R**	R	SPX > CIP

[a] The minimum antibiotic susceptibility test and the mechanisms of resistance it allows to detect are indicated by the grey zone.
[b] Values recommended by CA-SFM [Antibiotic Susceptibility Testing Committee of the French Microbiology Society] since 2005 (Communique 2009, http://www.sfm.asso.fr/).
[c] Comparison of diameters suggests a GyrA phenotype when the inhibition zone diameter of sparfloxacin is smaller than that of ciprofloxacin.

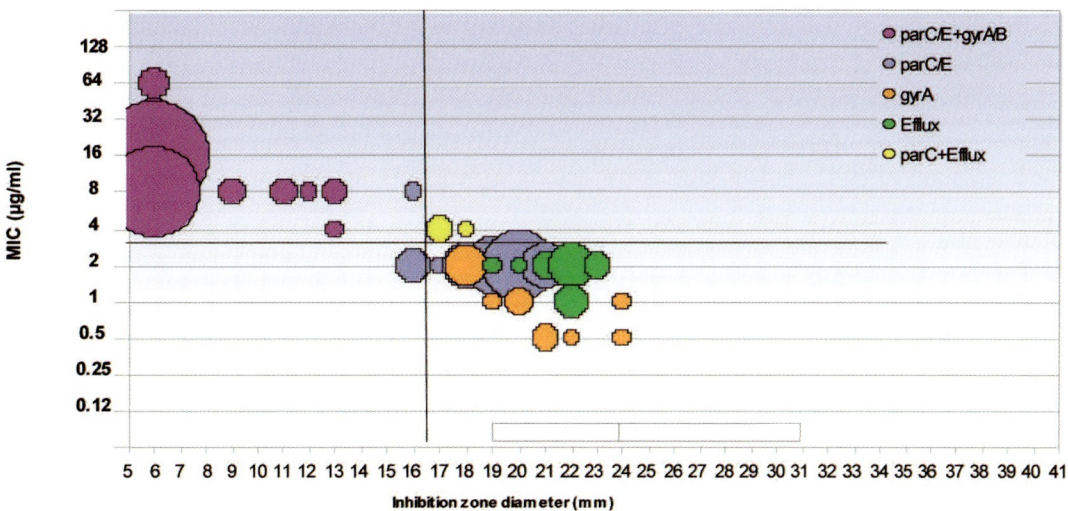

Fig. 13 A to E. Distribution of MICs and inhibition zone diameters according to genotype. The size of the disks is proportional to the number of strains. The distribution of diameters for the susceptible population is represented by the rectangle at the bottom the figure. The mean diameter is indicated by the vertical bar within the rectangle. The horizontal and vertical black lines indicate the critical concentrations and diameters or the threshold values used for the interpretation the tests described (42).

B - Moxifloxacin

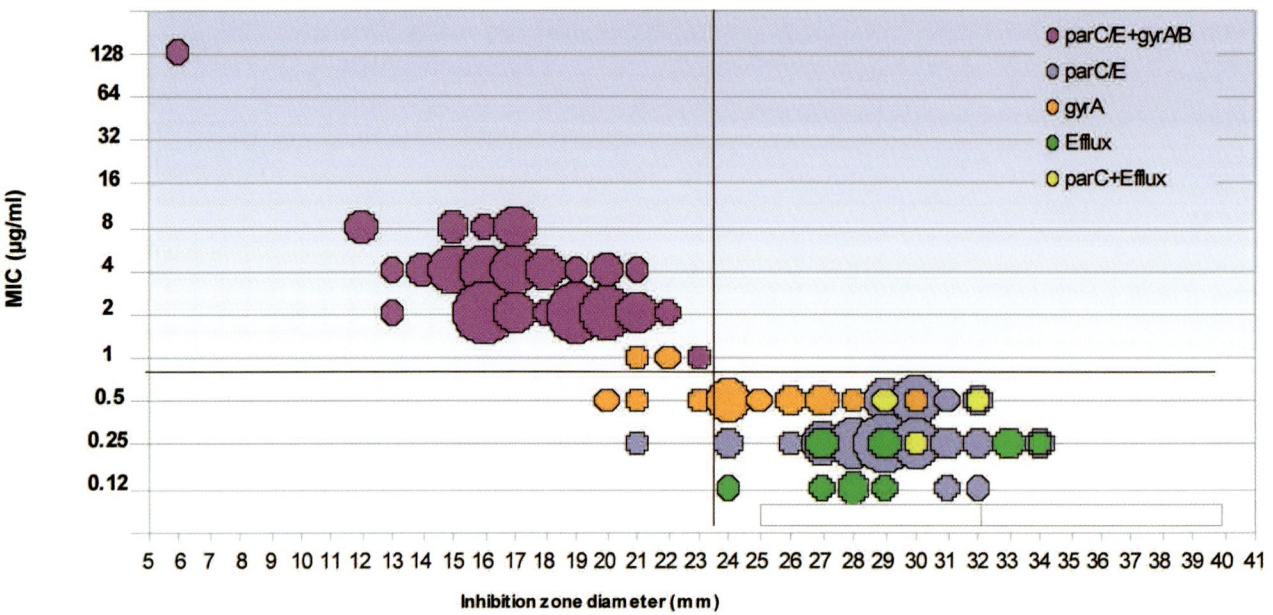

C - Norfloxacin

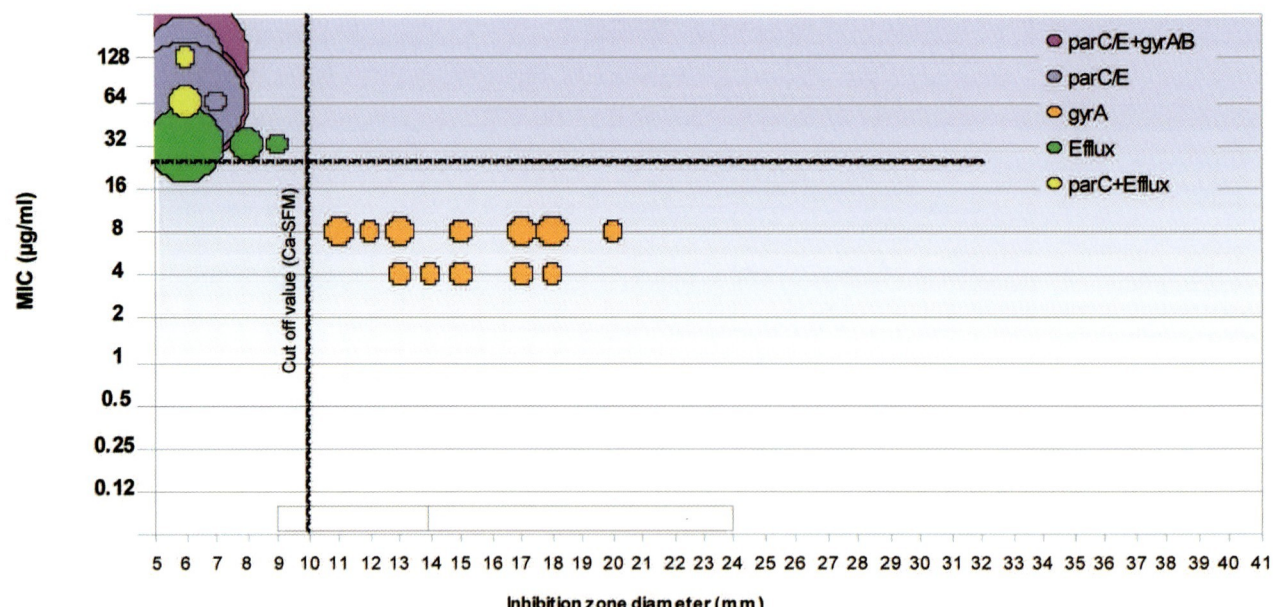

Chapter 18. QUINOLONES AND GRAM-POSITIVE BACTERIA

D- Pefloxacin

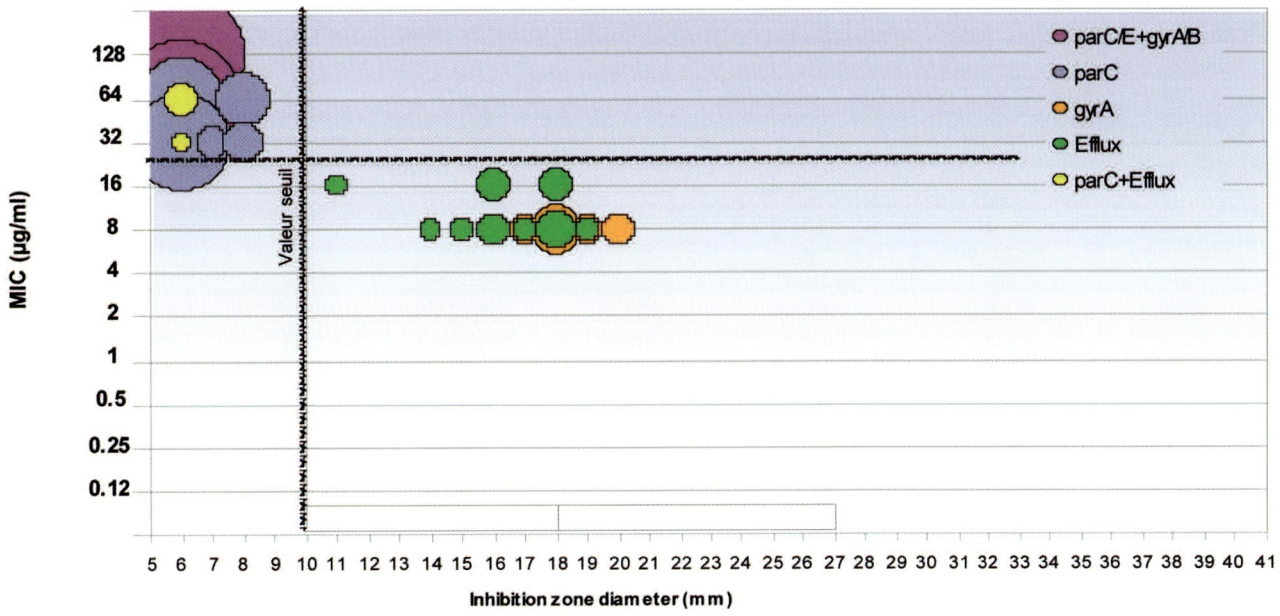

E- Sparfloxacin

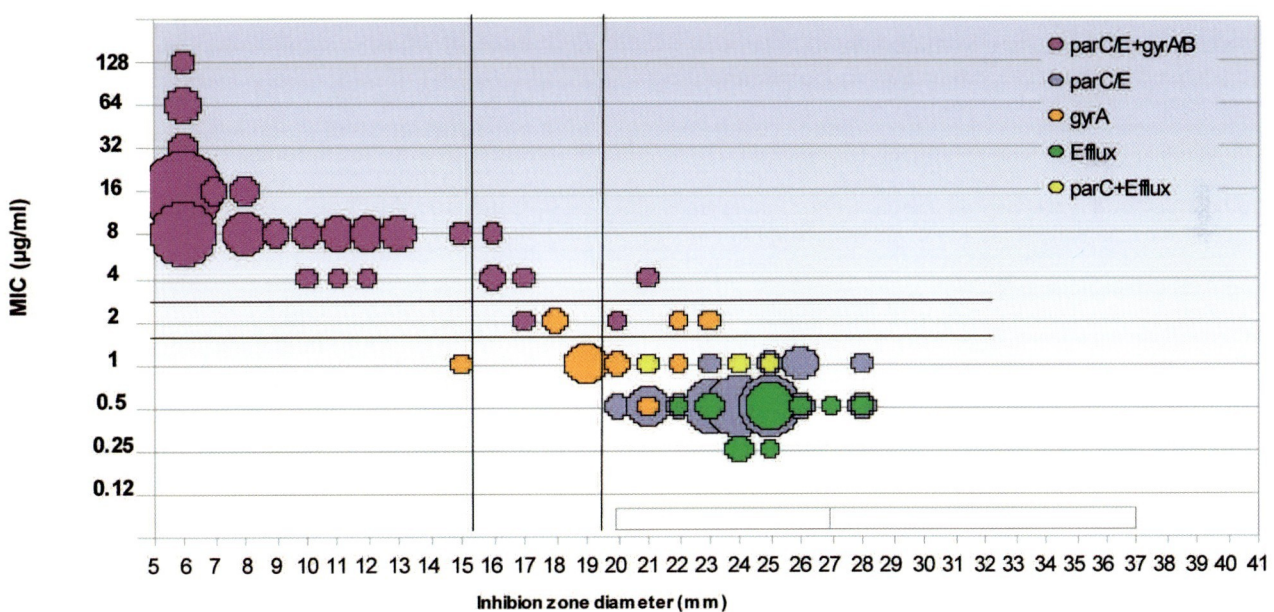

REFERENCES

(1) **Adam, H. J., D. J. Hoban, A. S. Gin, and G. G. Zhanel.** 2009. Association between fluoroquinolone usage and a dramatic rise in ciprofloxacin-resistant *Streptococcus pneumoniae* in Canada, 1997-2006. Int. J. Antimicrob. Agents. **34**:82-85.

(2) **Balsalobre, L., M. J. Ferrandiz, J. Linares, F. Tubau, and A. G. de la Campa.** 2003. Viridans group streptococci are donors in horizontal transfer of topoisomerase IV genes to *Streptococcus pneumoniae*. Antimicrob. Agents Chemother. **47**:2072-2081.

(3) **Cavallo, J. D., F. Ramisse, M. Girardet, J. Vaissaire, M. Mock, and E. Hernandez.** 2002. Antibiotic susceptibilities of 96 isolates of *Bacillus anthracis* isolated in France between 1994 and 2000. Antimicrob. Agents Chemother. **46**:2307-2309.

(4) **Chen, D. K., A. McGeer, J. C. de Azavedo, and D. E. Low.** 1999. Decreased susceptibility of *Streptococcus pneumoniae* to fluoroquinolones in Canada. Canadian Bacterial Surveillance Network. N. Engl. J. Med. **22**:233-239.

(5) **Christiansen, K. J., J. M. Bell, J. D. Turnidge, and R. N. Jones.** 2004. Antimicrobial activities of garenoxacin (BMS 284756) against Asia-Pacific region clinical isolates from the SENTRY program, 1999 to 2001. Antimicrob. Agents Chemother. **48**:2049-2055.

(6) **Davidson, R., R. Cavalcanti, J. L. Brunton, D. J. Bast, J. C. de Azavedo, P. Kibsey, C. Fleming, and D. E. Low.** 2002. Resistance to levofloxacin and failure of treatment of pneumococcal pneumonia. N. Engl. J. Med. **346**:747-750.

(7) **De la Campa, A. G., C. Ardanuy, L. Balsalobre, E. Pérez-Trallero, J. M. Marimón, A. Fenoll, and J. Liñares.** 2009. Changes in fluoroquinolone-resistant *Streptococcus pneumoniae* after 7-valent conjugate vaccination, Spain. Emerg. Infect. Dis. **15**:905-911.

(8) **Ferrandiz, M. J., J. Oteo, B. Aracil, J. L. Gomez-Garces, and A. G. De La Campa.** 1999. Drug efflux and *parC* mutations are involved in fluoroquinolone resistance in viridans group streptococci. Antimicrob. Agents Chemother. **43**:2520-2523.

(9) **Ferrero, L., B. Cameron, and J. Crouzet.** 1995. Analysis of *gyrA* and *grlA* mutations in stepwise-selected ciprofloxacin-resistant mutants of *Staphylococcus aureus*. Antimicrob. Agents Chemother. **39**:1554-1558.

(10) **Fournier, B., X. Zhao, T. Lu, K. Drlica, and D. C. Hooper.** 2000. Selective targeting of topoisomerase IV and DNA gyrase in *Staphylococcus aureus*: different patterns of quinolone-induced inhibition of DNA synthesis. Antimicrob. Agents Chemother. **44**:2160-2165.

(11) **Fukuda, H., and K. Hiramatsu.** 1999. Primary targets of fluoroquinolones in *Streptococcus pneumoniae*. Antimicrob. Agents Chemother. **43**:410-412.

(12) **Gill, M. J., N. P. Brenwald, and R. Wise.** 1999. Identification of an efflux pump gene, *pmrA*, associated with fluoroquinolone resistance in *Streptococcus pneumoniae*. Antimicrob. Agents Chemother. **43**:187-189.

(13) **Guerin, F., E. Varon, A. Buu-Hoï, L. Gutmann, and I. Podglajen.** 2000. Fluoroquinolone resistance associated with target mutations and active efflux in oropharyngeal colonizing isolates of viridans group streptococci. Antimicrob. Agents Chemother. **44**:2197-2200.

(14) **Grohs, P., S. Houssaye, A. Aubert, L. Gutmann, and E. Varon.** 2003. *In vitro* activities of garenoxacin (BMS-284756) against *Streptococcus pneumoniae*, viridans group streptococci, and *Enterococcus faecalis* compared to those of six other quinolones. Antimicrob. Agents Chemother. **47**:3542-3547.

(15) **Grohs, P., I. Podglajen, and L. Gutmann.** 2004. Activities of different fluoroquinolones against *Bacillus anthracis* mutants selected *in vitro* and harboring topoisomerase mutations. Antimicrob. Agents Chemother. **48**:3024-3027.

(16) **Hartman-Neumann, S., K. DenBleyker, L. A. Pelosi, L. E. Lawrence, J. F. Barrett, and T. J. Dougherty.** 2001. Selection and genetic characterization of *Streptococcus pneumoniae* mutants resistant to the Des-F(6) Quinolone BMS-284756. Antimicrob. Agents Chemother. **45**:2865-2870.

(17) **Ho, P. L., R. W. Yung, D. N. Tsang, T. L. Que, M. Ho, W. H. Seto, T. K. Ng, W. C. Yam, and W. W. Ng.** 2001. Increasing resistance of *Streptococcus pneumoniae* to fluoroquinolones: results of a Hong-Kong multicentre study in 2000. J. Antimicrob. Chemother. **48**:659-65.

(18) **Houssaye, S., L. Gutmann, and E. Varon.** 2002. Topoisomerase mutations associated with *in vitro* selection of resistance to moxifloxacin in *Streptococcus pneumoniae*. Antimicrob. Agents Chemother. **46**:2712-2715.

(19) **Ince, D., and D. C. Hooper.** 2000. Mechanisms and frequency of resistance to premafloxacin in *Staphylococcus aureus*: novel mutations suggest novel drug-target interactions. Antimicrob Agents Chemother. **44**:3344-3450.

(20) **Ince, D., X. Zhang, L. C. Silver, and D. C. Hooper.** 2002 Dual targeting of DNA gyrase and topoisomerase IV: target interactions of garenoxacin (BMS-284756, T-3811ME), a new desfluoroquinolone. Antimicrob. Agents Chemother. **46**:3370-3380.

(21) **Ince, D., X. Zhang, and D. C. Hooper.** 2003. Activity of and resistance to moxifloxacin in *Staphylococcus aureus*. Antimicrob. Agents Chemother. **47**:1410-1415.

(22) **Ip, M., S. S. Chau, F. Chi, E. S. Cheuk, H. Ma, R. W. Lai, and P. K. Chan.** 2007. Longitudinally tracking fluoroquinolone resistance and its determinants in penicillin-susceptible and -nonsusceptible *Streptococcus pneumoniae* isolates in Hong Kong, 2000 to 2005. Antimicrob. Agents Chemother. **51**.2192-2194.

(23) **Janoir, C., E. Varon, M. D. Kitzis, and L. Gutmann.** 2001. New mutation in ParE in a pneumococcal in vitro mutant resistant to fluoroquinolones. Antimicrob. Agents Chemother. **45**:952-955.

(24) **Janoir, C., V. Zeller, M. D. Kitzis, N. J. Moreau, and L. Gutmann.** 1996. High-level fluoroquinolone resistance in *Streptococcus pneumoniae* requires mutations in *parC* and *gyrA*. Antimicrob. Agents Chemother. **40**:2760-2764.

(25) **Jonas, B. M., B. E. Murray, and G. M. Weinstock.** 2001. Characterization of *emeA*, a NorA homolog and multidrug resistance efflux pump, in *Enterococcus faecalis*. Antimicrob. Agents Chemother. **45**:3574-3579.

(26) **Kaatz, G. W., V. V. Moudgal, S. M. Seo, and J. E. Kristiansen.** 2003. Phenothiazines and thioxanthenes

inhibit multidrug efflux pump activity in *Staphylococcus aureus*. Antimicrob Agents Chemother.**47**:719-726.

(27) **Khodursky, A. B., and N. R. Cozzarelli**. 1998. The mechanism of inhibition of topoisomerase IV by quinolone antibacterials. J. Biol. Chem. **273**:27668-27677.

(28) **Lawrence, L. E., M. Frosco, B. Ryan, S. Chaniewski, H. Yang, D. C. Hooper, and J. F. Barrett**. 2002. Bactericidal activities of BMS-284756, a novel Des-F(6)-quinolone, against *Staphylococcus aureus* strains with topoisomerase mutations. Antimicrob. Agents Chemother. **46**:191-195.

(29) **McCloskey, L., T. Moore, N. Niconovich, B. Donald, J. Broskey, C. Jakielaszek, S. Rittenhouse, and K. Coleman**. 2000. In vitro activity of gemifloxacin against a broad range of recent clinical isolates from the USA. J. Antimicrob. Chemother. **45** (Suppl 1):13-21.

(30) **Milatovic, D., F. J. Schmitz, S. Brisse, J. Verhoef, and A. C. Fluit**. 2000. *In vitro* activities of sitafloxacin (DU-6859a) and six other fluoroquinolones against 8,796 clinical bacterial isolates. Antimicrob. Agents Chemother. **44**:1102-1107.

(31) **Pan, X. S., J. Ambler, S. Mehtar, and L. M. Fisher**. 1996. Involvement of topoisomerase IV and DNA gyrase as ciprofloxacin targets in *Streptococcus pneumoniae*. Antimicrob. Agents Chemother. **40**:2321-2326.

(32) **Perez-Trallero, E., C. Garcia-Rey, A. M. Martin-Sanchez, L. Aguilar, J. Garcia-de-Lomas, J. Ruiz, and Spanish Surveillance Group for Respiratory Pathogens (SAUCE Program)**. 2002. Activities of six different quinolones against clinical respiratory isolates of *Streptococcus pneumoniae* with reduced susceptibility to ciprofloxacin in Spain. Antimicrob. Agents Chemother. **46**:2665-2667.

(33) **Pérez-Trallero, E., J. M. Marimon, L. Iglesias, and J. Larruskain**. 2003. Fluoroquinolone and macrolide treatment failure in pneumococcal pneumonia and selection of multidrug-resistant isolates. Emerg. Infect. Dis. **9**:1159-1162.

(34) **Perichon, B., Tankovic, J., and P. Courvalin**. 1997. Characterization of a mutation in the *parE* gene that confers fluoroquinolone resistance in *Streptococcus pneumoniae*. Antimicrob. Agents Chemother. **41**:1166-1167.

(35) **Pestova, E., J. J. Millichap, G. A. Noskin, and L. R. Peterson**. 2000. Intracellular targets of moxifloxacin: a comparison with other fluoroquinolones. J. Antimicrob. Chemother. **45**:583-590.

(36) **Pletz, M. W., L. McGee, J. Jorgensen, B. Beall, R. R. Facklam, C. G. Whitney, and K. P. Klugman**. 2004. Levofloxacin-resistant invasive *Streptococcus pneumoniae* in the United States: evidence for clonal spread and the impact of conjugate pneumococcal vaccine. Antimicrob. Agents Chemother. **48**:3491-3497.

(37) **Price, L. B., A. Vogler, T. Pearson, J. D. Busch, J. M. Schupp, and P. Keim**. 2003. In vitro selection and characterization of *Bacillus anthracis* mutants with high-level resistance to ciprofloxacin. Antimicrob. Agents Chemother. **47**:2362-2365.

(38) **Tankovic, J., F. Mahjoubi, P. Courvalin, J. Duval, and R. Leclercq**. 1996. Development of fluoroquinolone resistance in *Enterococcus faecalis* and role of mutations in the DNA gyrase gyrA gene. Antimicrob. Agents Chemother. **40**:2558-2561.

(39) **Truong-Bolduc, Q. C., X. Zhang, and D. C. Hooper**. 2003. Characterization of NorR protein, a multifunctional regulator of *norA* expression in *Staphylococcus aureus*. J. Bacteriol. **185**:3127-3138.

(40) **Varon, E., C. Janoir, M. D. Kitzis, and L. Gutmann**. 1999. ParC and GyrA may be interchangeable initial targets of some fluoroquinolones in *Streptococcus pneumoniae*. Antimicrob. Agents Chemother. **43**:302-306.

(41) **Varon, E., and L. Gutmann**. 2008. Rapport annuel d'activité du Centre National de Référence des Pneumocoques. http://www.invs.sante.fr/surveillance, rubrique Centres Nationaux de Référence.

(42) **Varon, E., S. Houssaye, S. Grondin, and L. Gutmann; Groupe des Observatoires Régionaux du Pneumocoque**. 2006. Nonmolecular test for detection of low-level resistance to fluoroquinolones in *Streptococcus pneumoniae*. Antimicrob Agents Chemother. **50**:572-579.

(43) **Weiss, K., C. Restieri, R. Gauthier, M. Laverdiere, A. McGeer, R. J. Davidson, L. Kilburn, D. J. Bast, J. de Azavedo, and D. E. Low**. 2001. A nosocomial outbreak of fluoroquinolone-resistant *Streptococcus pneumoniae*. Clin. Infect. Dis. **33**:517-522.

(44) **Zeller, V., C. Janoir, M. D. Kitzis, L. Gutmann, and N. J. Moreau**. 1997. Active efflux as a mechanism of resistance to ciprofloxacin in *Streptococcus pneumoniae*. Antimicrob. Agents Chemother. **41**:1973-1978.

Chapter 19. QUINOLONES AND GRAM-NEGATIVE BACTERIA

Claude-James SOUSSY

INTRODUCTION

Quinolones are a family of synthetic antimicrobial agents. The first quinolone, nalidixic acid, was discovered in 1962 by Lesher et al. (13). All quinolones possess a pyridine ring which can have various substituents on the nitrogen atom, as well as a ketone function at C-4 and a carboxylic acid at C-3. This ring is fused to another aromatic ring such as benzene, pyridine, or pyrimidine (Fig. 1).

Nalidixic acid was later joined by pipemidic acid, oxolinic acid, and flumequin, the first fluoroquinolone. Due to their narrow spectrum and their pharmacokinetic properties, these antibiotics are still used today to treat adult urinary tract infections caused by susceptible enterobacteria.

The 1980s saw the rise of the fluoroquinolone class strictly speaking, *i.e.*, distinguished by the addition of a fluorine atom at C-6 and a nitrogen ring, usually piperazine, at C-7. The fluoroquinolones include agents with specific activity in urinary tract infections, such as enoxacin, lomefloxacin, and norfloxacin, and systemically acting agents such as ciprofloxacin, ofloxacin, and pefloxacin, with higher intrinsic activity against enterobacteria but also active against staphylococci and to a certain extent, against *Pseudomonas aeruginosa*.

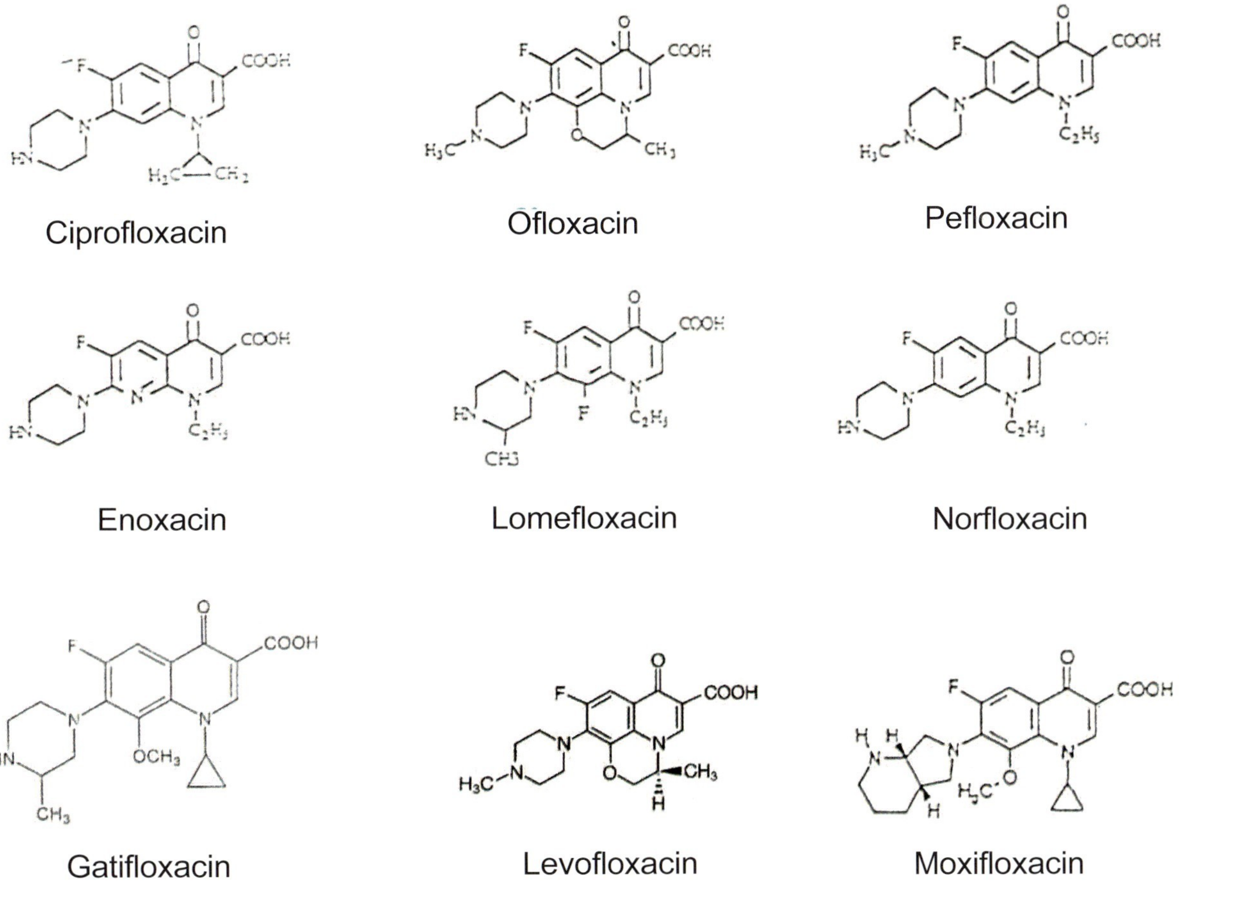

Fig. 1. Chemical structure of quinolones.

The introduction of newer molecules like levofloxacin, moxifloxacin and gatifloxacin further broadened the indications of the fluoroquinolones, mainly to include respiratory tract infections, in large part thanks to increased activity against pneumococci although with no improvement against enterobacteria and other Gram-negative organisms. All these molecules are composed of a pyridine ring variously substituted at the nitrogen atom and with a ketone at C-4 and a carboxylic acid at C-3. This ring is fused to another aromatic ring which can be benzene, pyridine, pyrimidine, etc.

Levofloxacin is the L-isomer of ofloxacin, while gatifloxacin and moxifloxacin are 8-methoxyfluoroquinolones.

MODES OF ACTION

Mechanism of action

The quinolones selectively interfere with bacterial DNA replication by inhibiting two enzymes involved in DNA synthesis: the type II DNA topoisomerase known as DNA gyrase, and DNA topoisomerase IV.

Inhibition of DNA gyrase

Following the discovery of DNA gyrase in 1976, extensive studies were carried out on this enzyme, enabling its characterization and its identification as the primary intracellular target of quinolone drugs (4). DNA gyrase is a type II topoisomerase that introduces negative supercoils into DNA during replication. The enzyme is composed of two subunits, A and B, each present in dimeric form in the active species. The A subunit, encoded by the *gyrA* gene, is a 100 kD protein of 875 amino acids. Its main role is to cut the DNA strands prior to supercoiling. The A subunit is the primary target of the quinolones in Gram-negative bacteria. The B subunit, encoded by the *gyrB* gene, is a 90 kD protein composed of 804 amino acids. It hydrolyzes ATP which provides the energy to drive enzymatic catalysis. It is the target of novobiocin and coumermycin and also at least an indirect target of quinolones (4).

Shen et al. (27) were the first to describe the interaction between quinolones and DNA gyrase: several quinolone molecules (at least four) cooperatively bind to DNA in a region where the two strands have been separated and cut by DNA gyrase, the A subunit itself being covalently bound to DNA via tyrosine-122. This results in the formation of an irreversible ternary complex between DNA, gyrase and the antibiotic, although the precise nature of the molecular interactions within this complex remains obscure. This locks up the enzyme on the DNA, preventing the progression of the bacterial DNA polymerase during replication and thereby inhibiting DNA synthesis and resultant bacterial growth. Since the quinolones are bactericidal, however, other mechanisms must also come into play. For instance, cuts in the double-stranded DNA stabilized by quinolones would act as irreparable DNA lesions capable of triggering the synthesis of certain proteins, leading to bacterial cell death (14).

However, it has since been shown that binding of quinolones to the DNA-DNA gyrase complex is possible even in the absence of DNA cleavage. Other evidence suggests that the DNA is only cut after quinolones have bound to the DNA-DNA gyrase complex (4).

A second model proposed by A. Maxwell (18) suggests that quinolones bind to both DNA and to DNA gyrase, which better explains the fact that mutations in both GyrA and GyrB contribute to resistance.

Other authors have speculated that quinolones bind to DNA via magnesium ions.

Inhibition of DNA topoisomerase IV

In 1990, it was discovered that another bacterial topoisomerase, DNA topoisomerase IV, is a second intracellular target of quinolones. This enzyme, which shares almost 40% homology with DNA gyrase, was first described in *Escherichia coli* (4) and subsequently found in other species. Like DNA gyrase, it has a tetrameric structure C^2E^2: two genes, *parC* and *parE*, respectively code for the subunits ParC (75 kD, homologous to GyrA) and ParE (70 kD, homologous to GyrB). Topoisomerase IV appears to have the specific role of decatenating the DNA strands following replication. Quinolones can inhibit the activity of this enzyme *in vitro* and *in vivo*.

The interaction between quinolones and topoisomerase IV is thought to stimulate DNA cleavage and inhibit religation. As in the case of DNA gyrase, it is likely that quinolones act on topoisomerase IV prior to DNA cleavage, even though in a later step they block religation of the cleaved DNA.

Bacterial penetration

In order to reach their targets in the cytoplasm, quinolones must cross the outer and cytoplasmic membranes of Gram-negative bacteria. This intracellular penetration depends on the hydrophobicity coefficient, ionic type, and molecular mass of the molecule. Hydrophobicity coefficients range from 0.007 for enoxacin, the most hydrophilic, to 13 for flumequin, the most hydrophobic. Apart from pipemidic acid and the fluoroquinolones, which are amphoteric, the other quinolone molecules are acidic. Molecular mass varies over a small range, from 232 for nalidixic acid to 360 for ofloxacin.

Porins located in the outer membrane of Gram-negative bacteria allow the diffusion of hydrophilic molecules with a molecular mass < 600. While small hydrophilic molecules like β-lactams can diffuse through porins OmpF and perhaps also OmpC of *E. coli*, it appears that the OmpC porin is only a very minor route of penetration for the quinolones. Thus, hydrophilic quinolones (pipemidic acid, ciprofloxacin, norfloxacin) diffuse mainly through the OmpF porin of *E. coli* and the OprD protein of *Pseudomonas aeruginosa*. The more hydrophobic compounds (nalidixic acid, flumequin, pefloxacin, sparfloxacin) bind via chelation of magnesium ions to the outer membrane thanks to their C-2 group and then diffuse through the OmpF porin but also penetrate through the phospholipid bilayer of the outer membrane. Nalidixic acid might even penetrate directly through the phospholipid bilayer without using the porin pathway. Data concerning the mechanism of penetration through the cytoplasmic membrane are conflicting, since both active and passive mechanisms have been proposed in different studies.

There are also systems which actively remove some of the antibiotic which entered the bacterial cell, as seen in both Gram-positive organisms like *Staphylococcus aureus* and Gram-negative bacteria like *E. coli* or *P. aeruginosa*. These efflux pumps are not specific for quinolones but extrude many compounds with vastly different chemical structures, including other antibiotics. They influence the level of intrinsic susceptibility to quinolones but can also be involved in acquired resistance.

Bacteriostatic activity against susceptible Gram-negative bacteria

The broadened activity spectrum of the quinolones is the result of successive modifications of the chemical structure of the parent molecule: substitutions at position 1 globally affect antibacterial activity, substitutions at position 5 affect Gram-positive activity, and a piperazine ring at position 7 affects Gram-negative while a pyrolidine ring at position 7 affects Gram-positive activity (36).

The antibacterial activity of the older quinolones can be summarized as follows: oxolinic acid, flumequin and pipemidic acid are respectively eight, four and two times more active than nalidixic acid against enterobacteria susceptible to the latter agent, while piromidic acid is two to four times less active.

The bacteriostatic activity of nine fluoroquinolones against Gram-negative organisms as compared to nalidixic acid is given in Tables 1 and 2. These nine fluoroquinolones include three "systemic" agents (pefloxacin, ofloxacin and ciprofloxacin), three "urinary tract" agents (enoxacin, lomefloxacin and norfloxacin) and three "respiratory tract" fluoroquinolones (levofloxacin, moxifloxacin and gatifloxacin). The comparison is based on the MIC_{50} for the different species since this value reflects the intrinsic activity of the antibiotic, as opposed to the MIC_{90} which can vary considerably over time and local epidemiology of resistance.

- Ciprofloxacin has the highest activity against enterobacteria, followed closely by levofloxacin and gatifloxacin. Ofloxacin and moxifloxacin are less active. MIC_{50} values are as follows:
  - The ciprofloxacin MIC_{50} for *E. coli, Klebsiella pneumoniae, Klebsiella oxytoca, Enterobacter cloacae, Citrobacter freundii,* and *Morganella morganii* ranges from 0.016-0.03 µg/ml, while those of levofloxacin and gatifloxacin are equivalent in some cases but usually two times higher. MICs of ofloxacin and moxifloxacin for these same species usually range from 0.06-0.12 µg/ml.
  - For *Proteus mirabilis*, the MIC_{50} of these five fluoroquinolones is generally two times higher than for the above species, generally comprised between 0.03-0.06 µg/ml for ciprofloxacin, 0.06-0.12 µg/ml for levofloxacin, 0.12-0.25 µg/ml for gatifloxacin, and 0.25-0.5 µg/ml for moxifloxacin.
  - For *Serratia marcescens*, the antibacterial activity of all these molecules is again at least two times higher (MIC_{50} of 0.06-0.12 and 0.12-0.25 µg/ml, respectively).
- Activity against *P. aeruginosa* is generally lower than against enterobacteria but far from negligible. Ciprofloxacin is the most active with an MIC_{50} of 0.12-0.5 µg/ml, followed by levofloxacin (0.12-1 µg/ml), gatifloxacin (0.5-2 µg/ml), ofloxacin (1-2 µg/ml), and moxifloxacin (2-4 µg/ml).

Table 1. MIC$_{50}$ of fluoroquinolones (FQ) for enterobacteria and non fermenters

Species	MIC$_{50}$ (µg/ml) of :								
	Urinary FQ			Systemic FQ			Respiratory FQ		
	NOR[a]	ENO	LOM	PEF	CIP	OFL	LEV	MOX	GAT
E. coli	0.06	0.12	0.12	0.12	0.016	0.12	0.03	0.06	0.03
K. pneumoniae	0.12	0.12	0.25	0.12	0.03	0.12	0.06	0.12	0.06
P. mirabilis	0.06	0.5	0.25	0.25	0.016	0.25	0.06	0.5	0.25
P. aeruginosa	0.5	2	2	1	0.25	2	1	4	2
Acinetobacter spp.	4	2	2	0.25	0.25	0.5	0.25	0.12	0.06
S. maltophilia	32	-	-	4	2	4	2	0.5	0.5

[a] CIP, ciprofloxacin; ENO, enoxacin; GAT, gatifloxacin; LEV, levofloxacin; LOM, lomefloxacin; MOX, moxifloxacin; NOR, norfloxacin; OFL, ofloxacin; PEF, pefloxacin.

Table 2. MIC$_{50}$ of fluoroquinolones (FQ) for Gram-negative bacteria (other than enterobacteria and non fermenters)

Species	MIC$_{50}$ (µg/L) of :				
	Systemic FQ		Respiratory FQ		
	OFL[a]	CIP	LEV	MOX	GAT
H. influenzae	0.03	0.03	0.06	0.03	0.016
M. catarrhalis	0.12	0.03	0.06	0.06	0.016
L. pneumophila	0.016	0.008	0.016	0.016	0.016
N. gonorrhoeae	0.03	0.008	0.016	0.016	0.016
C. jejuni	-	1	0.5	0.12	0.5
B. fragilis	4	2	1	0.25	0.5

[a] CIP, ciprofloxacin; GAT, gatifloxacin; LEV, levofloxacin; MOX, moxifloxacin; OFL, ofloxacin.

- For *Acinetobacter*, the systemic agents are more active than the urinary agents but equally or less active than the respiratory agents.
- The five fluoroquinolones have similar activity against *Stenotrophomonas maltophilia* with MICs usually around 0.5 µg/ml, although MICs of 2-4 µg/ml have been reported in some studies, particularly with ofloxacin and ciprofloxacin.
- *Haemophilus influenzae* is highly susceptible to fluoroquinolones. The MIC$_{50}$ is usually between 0.016-0.03 µg/ml for ciprofloxacin, levofloxacin, gatifloxacin, and moxifloxacin and 0.03-0.06 µg/ml for ofloxacin.
- The same is true for *Moraxella catarrhalis*, although the MIC$_{50}$ is generally double that seen for *H. influenzae*.
- The MIC$_{50}$ values for *Legionella pneumophila* and *Neisseria gonorrhoeae* are even lower: approximately 0.016 µg/ml.
- *Campylobacter jejuni* and *Bacteroides fragilis* appear to be more susceptible to the new fluoroquinolones.

Bactericidal activity

The quinolones display bactericidal activity against Gram-negative bacteria at concentrations close to the MIC.

With the older agents like nalidixic acid, bactericidal activity disappears at very high concentrations, characterizing a biphasic response. Bactericidal activity also disappears after addition of the RNA synthesis inhibitor rifampin or the protein synthesis inhibitor chloramphenicol, suggesting the synthesis of a cell death protein.

The bactericidal activity of the fluoroquinolones is more pronounced than that of nalidixic acid and addition of the aforementioned inhibitors only slows but does not abolish it.

These differences are due to the existence of several bactericidal mechanisms: mechanism A requires RNA and protein synthesis and concerns cells in the growth phase; mechanism B can cause cell death independently of RNA and protein synthesis; mechanism C requires RNA and protein synthesis and concerns cells in stationary phase (14).

RESISTANCE MECHANISMS

Acquired quinolone resistance in Gram-negative bacilli was believed to be due exclusively to chromosomal mutations, until the first report of plasmid-mediated resistance in 1998 (7). Early studies by Hane and Wood in *E. coli* revealed two types of mutants selected by nalidixic acid: *nalA*, conferring high-level resistance to nalidixic acid with MICs of 60 to > 100 µg/ml, and *nalB* conferring low-level resistance with MICs of 4-10 µg/ml, barely higher than the MIC of a susceptible strain. Dominance studies in partial diploids showed that the *nalA^s* gene (s = susceptible) is dominant over the *nalA^r* gene (r = resistant).

Today, the following resistance mechanisms can be distinguished:
- resistance due to chromosomal mutations resulting in:
1. decreased affinity of the intracellular targets: DNA gyrase and topoisomerase IV complexes,
2. reduced intracellular accumulation of the antibiotic due to decreased passive penetration and/or active efflux.
- plasmid-mediated resistance which is due to protection of DNA gyrase against quinolone binding, inactivation, or active efflux.

It should be noted that cross-resistance to the majority of quinolones is almost always observed, although the extent of increase in the MIC varies considerably according to the molecule.

Resistance by modification of DNA gyrase

Modification is due to a chromosomal mutation and can affect either the A subunit, the most common case, or the B subunit of the enzyme.

Modification of the A subunit

gyrA mutations affecting the A subunit are mostly situated between amino acids 67 and 106, that is to say, near the N-terminal domain and in the vicinity of tyrosine-122, the site of attachment of the A subunit to DNA in a region of the protein which is highly conserved between different species. This highly conserved region is known as the *quinolone resistance-determining region* (QRDR) and specifies the enzyme active site. Substitutions at position 83, particularly Ser$_{83}$Leu, are the most frequently found (Table 3).

These mutants usually confer high-level resistance to nalidixic acid and low-level resistance to fluoroquinolones. However, the level of resistance differs according to the site of the mutation: higher for substitutions at positions 83 and 87, lower for those at positions 67 and 106, and also according to the substituted amino acid. MICs associated with these mutations range from 12.5-400 µg/ml for nalidixic acid (4-128 times the MIC of a susceptible strain), 0.1-0.8 µg/ml for norfloxacin (2-16 times the "susceptible" MIC), and 0.05-0.4 µg/ml for ciprofloxacin (4-32 times higher).

The level of resistance conferred by the Asp$_{87}$Val substitution is four to eight-fold lower than for substitutions at position 83. On the other hand, the only known strain with a Gly$_{81}$Asp substitution had high-level fluoroquinolone resistance with an MIC of 16 µg/ml, whereas the nalidixic acid MIC was barely above that of a susceptible strain.

gyrA mutations in quinolone-resistant strains have been found in all species in which they have been sought. These mutations are very similar to those described in *E. coli*, both in terms of their position and in terms of the substituted amino acids. Two *gyrA* mutations may be present in a same strain, resulting in higher level resistance (12).

The recent discovery in *E. coli* and *Salmonella typhimurium* of mutations in codons 51 and 119 is an exception to the rule, since these mutations are slightly outside the QRDR.

Modification of the B subunit

The two known mutations in the B subunit, *nalC* and *nalD*, result in amino acid substitutions at positions 426 and 447 located in the central part of the molecule (Table 4).

The *nalD* mutation confers moderate resistance to nalidixic acid with an MIC of 50 µg/ml, or 16 times above that of a susceptible strain, and low-level resistance to fluoroquinolones, with MICs of 0.4 and 0.1 µg/ml for norfloxacin and ciprofloxacin, respectively, or eight times the MIC of a susceptible strain. On the other hand, the *nalC* mutation, which also confers moderate nalidixic acid resistance, is associated with hypersusceptibility (MICs four-fold lower) to hydrophilic quinolones with a piperazine ring at position 7, *i.e.*, the new fluoroquinolones as well as pipemidic acid. The following hypothesis has been advanced to explain this paradoxical observation: in a susceptible strain, the interaction between the negative charge of aspartic acid-426 and the positive charge of lysine-447 would create a favorable environment for high affinity binding of hydrophobic groups like the methyl group of nalidixic acid. Furthermore, the negative charge of aspartic acid-

426 would interact with the positive charge of the piperazine ring at position 7 of amphoteric quinolones. In the *nalD* mutant, where aspartic acid at position 426 is replaced by asparagine, the negative charge disappears and conformational changes alter the hydrophobicity of the region, making it more difficult to interact with a positive charge but also with a hydrophobic group such as a methyl. In the *nalC* mutant, where lysine-447 is replaced by glutamic acid, the electrical charge is altered but the hydrophobicity of the region is not, thereby favoring a more efficient interaction with positively charged groups at position 7, hence the hypersusceptibility to molecules possessing a piperazine nucleus.

gyrB mutations have also been detected in other species (Table 4), but only rarely in clinical isolates. The predominance of *gyrA* mutations *in vivo* can probably be explained by the fact that these mutations confer a higher level of resistance.

Resistance by modification of DNA topoisomerase IV

The discovery of mutations in the structural genes encoding DNA topoisomerase IV (*parC* and *parE*) was a major step forward in understanding the mechanisms of resistance to this class of antibiotics.

In *E. coli*, topoisomerase IV plays a role in quinolone resistance, but in this case as a secondary target. A *parC* mutation did not alter quinolone susceptibility of a wild-type strain but increased the level of resistance of a *gyrA* mutant (26). *parC* mutations have also been found in highly quinolone-resistant clinical isolates (Table 5). A *parE* mutation ($Leu_{445}His$ substitution) involved in quinolone resistance of a mutant *in vitro*, but again expressed only in the concomitant presence of a *gyrA* mutation, has also been described (Table 6) (7).

Similar observations to those in *E. coli* have also been reported in *N. gonorrhoeae*, *K. pneumoniae*, and *H. influenzae*.

Table 3. Quinolone resistance in *E. coli* [from (7)]. Mutations in GyrA subunit of DNA gyrase

Position	Wild-type aa[a]	Mutant aa	CIP[b] CMI (X)
51	Ala	Val	2
67	Ala	Ser	4
81	Gly	Cys, Asp	8
82	Asp	Gly	8
83	Ser, (Thr)	Leu, Trp, Ala	10 - 32
84	Ala, (Ser)	Pro	8
87	Asp, (Asn)	Asn, Val, Gly, Tyr	16
106	Gln	His, Arg	4 - 10
196	Ala	Gln	1.5

[a] aa, amino acid.
[b] CIP, ciprofloxacin.

Table 4. Quinolone resistance [from (7)]. Mutations in GyrB subunit of DNA gyrase

Species	Position	Wild-type aa[a]	Mutant aa	CIP[b] CMI (X)
E. coli	426 (*nalD*)	Asp	Asn	8
	447 (*nalC*)	Lys	Glu	0,25
Salmonella spp.	463	Ser	Tyr	ND[c]
P. mirabilis	466	Glu	Asp	ND
P. aeruginosa	464	Ser	Phe	ND
	466	Glu	Asp	ND
N. gonorrhoeae	426	Asp	Asn	ND

[a] aa, amino acid.
[b] CIP, ciprofloxacin.
[c] ND, not determined.

Resistance by reduced accumulation

Decreased permeability

Among the nonspecific mutations which alter the outer membrane, OmpF- causes only a two-fold increase in the quinolone MIC, perhaps due to a compensatory increase in intracellular penetration through the OmpC porin. Conversely, no changes in the MIC are observed in OmpC- mutants (Table 7). Permeability mutants that are selected by quinolones mainly show a quantitative decrease in OmpF.

These mutations are distinct from OmpF-. They confer low-level resistance to quinolones, increasing MICs four-fold, but also to other antibiotics such as tetracyclines, chloramphenicol, and some β-lactams. The *norC* mutant which additionally harbors an altered lipopolysaccharide, is hypersusceptible to nalidixic acid.

The precise mechanisms of quinolone resistance in some of these mutants are complex and still unclear. For instance, *nfxB* and *cfxB* mutants are two to four times more resistant than the OmpF- mutant, suggesting that other factors are involved.

Increased active efflux

One of the factors underlying quinolone resistance might be a saturable active efflux system. Indeed, it has been shown that the diminished accumulation of norfloxacin in *nfxB* or *cfxB* mutants is due in part to an energy-dependent system (7). Membrane energy transport inhibitors increase norfloxacin accumulation and abolish the differences between the mutants and the susceptible strain.

Active efflux systems in Gram-negative bacilli allow the bacterium to extrude molecules including antibiotics through the outer membrane. These efflux systems are composed of three proteins:
- an efflux pump located in the cytoplasmic membrane;
- a protein channel (equivalent to a porin) in the outer membrane;
- a periplasmic protein which acts as a bridge between the two membranes.

Examples of efflux systems include the AcrA-AcrB-TolC system in *E. coli* and the MexA-MexB-OprM and MexC-MexD-OprJ systems in *P. aeruginosa*. These systems also exist in susceptible strains, contributing to their level of intrinsic susceptibility to fluoroquinolones. In strains which are resistant due to an active efflux mechanism, a regulatory mutation can render one of these systems hyperactive. However, to date, no mutants have been identified in which active efflux is the sole mechanism of quinolone resistance.

Plasmid-mediated resistance

The first transferable quinolone resistance plasmid was described in 1998 (17). This plasmid from a clinical isolate of *K. pneumoniae* conferred low-level resistance in transconjugants with an eight-fold increase in the nalidixic acid MIC and a 32-fold increase in the MIC of ciprofloxacin. Transfer of this plasmid to porin-deficient strains

Table 5. Quinolone resistance in *E. coli* [from (7)]. Mutations in ParC subunit of topoisomerase IV

Position	Wild-type aa[a]	Mutant aa
78	Gly	Asp
80	Ser	Leu, Ile, Arg
84	Glu	Lys, Gly, Val

[a] aa, amino acid.

Table 6. Quinolone resistance [from (7)]. Mutations in ParE subunit of topoisomerase IV

Species	Position	Wild-type aa[a]	Mutant aa
E. coli	445	Leu	His
P. aeruginosa	473	Ala	Val
S. maltophilia	465	Ile	Val

[a] aa, amino acid.

Table 7. Quinolone resistance due to impermeability in *E. coli* [from (7)]

Mutation	Phenotype	MIC (µg/ml) Nalidixic acid	MIC (µg/ml) Norfloxacin
ompF	OmpF-OmpC+	8	0.16
ompC	OmpF+OmpC-	4	0.08
nfxB	OmpF-OmpC+	16	0.32
cfxB	OmpF-OmpC+	16	0.32
none (KL16)	OmpF+OmpC+	4	0.08

led to high-level resistance, increasing MICs as high as 32 µg/ml for ciprofloxacin. Moreover, higher-level fluoroquinolone-resistant mutants could be obtained from strains harboring this plasmid at more than 100 times the frequency of a plasmid-free strain. The plasmid was found to carry the *qnrA1* gene encoding the 218-amino acid QnrA1 protein, a member of the pentapeptide repeat protein (PRP) family, which acts by protecting DNA gyrase from quinolone binding.

Since this initial report, five other QnrA variants (QnrA2 to QnrA6) have been identified; they differ from QnrA1 by several amino acid substitutions (8, 10). Three other plasmid Qnr determinants have also been identified, all members of the same PRP biochemical family: QnrB, QnrC, and QnrS. QnrA1 shares 40, 60 and 59% identity with QnrB1, QnrC1 and QnrS1, respectively. To date, 19 QnrB variants (QnrB1 to QnrB19), a single QnrC variant (QnrC1) and three QnrS variants (QnrS1 to QnrS3) have been described.

The earliest publications reporting the isolation of strains harboring these qnr determinants are analyzed below:
- In 2003 in the US, 16 *Klebsiella* and 1 *E. coli* isolate were found in three studies involving a total of 885 Gram-negative strains (31).
- In a Shanghai hospital, 8% of ciprofloxacin-resistant *E. coli* isolates, which accounted for 50% of clinical isolates, harbored a *qnr* gene (30).
- In 2004 in the US, 14 strains (12 *E. cloacae* and 2 *K. pneumoniae*) out of 92 (23) and 19 strains (11 *Enterobacter* spp. and 8 *K. pneumoniae*) out of 103 (10) were identified. The latter strains harbored the *qnrB* gene, which was also found in three strains isolated in India (10).
- In Egypt, 4 *P. stuartii* strains were found among 30 enterobacterial isolates (33).
- In the Netherlands, a epidemic clone of 84 *E. cloacae* strains was identified in addition to 13 other enterobacterial isolates from the same patients, indicating intergeneric transfer of the gene (20).
- In Korea, 2 of 260 *E. coli* strains tested harbored the *qnr* gene (11).
- In a French multicenter study, 21 strains, including 18 *E. cloacae*, were isolated from 987 enterobacterial strains (6). In addition, an *E. coli* strain was isolated at the Bicêtre Hospital (16).

The strains described so far produce plasmid-encoded cephalosporinases or extended spectrum β-lactamases, but it is important to note that they may appear susceptible to fluoroquinolones if no other resistance mechanism is present.

The prevalence of the *qnr* genes ranges from 0.1% to almost 50%, according to the selection criteria for the strains, but it generally ranges from 1-5% (2, 18).

Lastly, two other plasmid-mediated quinolone resistance mechanisms have been identified to date: the aminoglycoside acetyltransferase AAC(6')-Ib-cr, and the QepA efflux pump. AAC(6')-Ib-cr decreases the activity of ciprofloxacin and norfloxacin by N-acetylating the piperazine ring (24). So far, 30 AAC(6')-Ib variants have been identified. The –Ib-cr variant, first described in 2003, differs from –Ib by only two substitutions, $Trp_{102}Arg$ and $Asp_{179}Tyr$, which are absent in the other variants. The capacity to acetylate the piperazine ring is due mainly to the $Asp_{179}Tyr$ mutation (29). This mutation alone doubles the MIC of ciprofloxacin whereas both mutations together cause a three to four-fold increase (24). Epidemiological studies indicate that the plasmid-encoded AAC(6')-Ib-cr is by far the most widely disseminated mechanism of quinolone resistance with a prevalence of 0.4 to > 34% (15).

The QepA efflux pump, related to the Major Facilitator Superfamily (MFS) systems found in environmental organisms such as actinomycetales, confers resistance to hydrophilic quinolones such as ciprofloxacin, enrofloxacin, and norfloxacin (22). The reduction in the activity of these quinolones is reflected by an 8-32 fold increase in their MICs according to the level of efflux pump expression. The *qepA* gene is carried by transposable elements located on IncF1 plasmids (21). About half the time, this resistance mechanism is associated with the RmtB methylase conferring multiresistance to aminoglycosides (34, 35). At present, the prevalence of this resistance mechanism appears to be low, although there have been reports of its presence on several continents and in different animal species including companion animals (1, 9, 15). The fact that the *qepA* genes are located on mobile genetic elements can contribute to its dissemination.

Interestingly, some strains have been found to harbor the three plasmid-mediated fluoroquinolone resistance determinants: Qnr, AAC(6')-Ib-cr and QepA (15).

SUSCEPTIBLE AND RESISTANT PHENOTYPES

Description

Figures 2a to 2h illustrate the phenotypes observed on the antibiogram of enterobacteria.

- Fig. 2a shows a strain susceptible to nalidixic acid, norfloxacin, pefloxacin, and ciprofloxacin. Fig. 2b shows a strain with reduced accumulation where the three inhibition zone diameters are slightly smaller, particularly around the nalidixic acid disk.

Strains harboring a single *gyrA* mutation appear resistant to nalidixic acid. These strains may remain susceptible to the two fluoroquinolones or have only intermediate susceptibility to pefloxacin or norfloxacin, as in Fig. 2c.

When both a *gyrA* mutation and a *parC* mutation are present, inhibition zone diameters are even further reduced, and the strains may appear ciprofloxacin-intermediate, as shown in Fig. 2d.

This is even more pronounced when a second *gyrA* mutation is associated with a *parC* mutation, as in Fig. 2e.

Finally, the highest level of resistance in which several mechanisms are present leads to a total absence of inhibition by the three molecules, as shown in Fig. 2f.

The high-level fluoroquinolone resistant *E. cloacae* strain HM477 isolated at Henri Mondor Hospital harbors the *qnr* gene (Fig. 2g). Plasmid transfer to *E. coli* decreases the inhibition zone diameters around the three disks but the transconjugant appears susceptible to fluoroquinolones, as shown in Fig. 2h.

Table 8 summarizes the different phenotypes observed, their probable mechanism and their approximate frequency. The RRR phenotype is currently found in 8-9% of enterobacterial isolates and the RIS phenotype in 3-4%, while the other phenotypes are only observed in less than 1-2% of strains.

Nalidixic acid resistance is associated with a slight increase in the MIC of the fluoroquinolones and, in strains categorized as "intermediate" (or even "resistant") to pefloxacin, the MICs of ofloxacin and ciprofloxacin are again increased 4-10 fold.

This increase in the MICs decreases the inhibitory quotient. It has been shown that when the inhibitory quotient is < 8, the risk of selecting resistant mutants is sharply increased. Thus, when treating severe infections and when the bacterial inoculum is large, it is advisable to use a combination of antibiotics (at least during the first few days of therapy) in order to avoid the emergence of such mutants (5, 12).

Prevalence of resistance

In *E. coli*, resistance to nalidixic acid and ciprofloxacin has increased over the past decade and

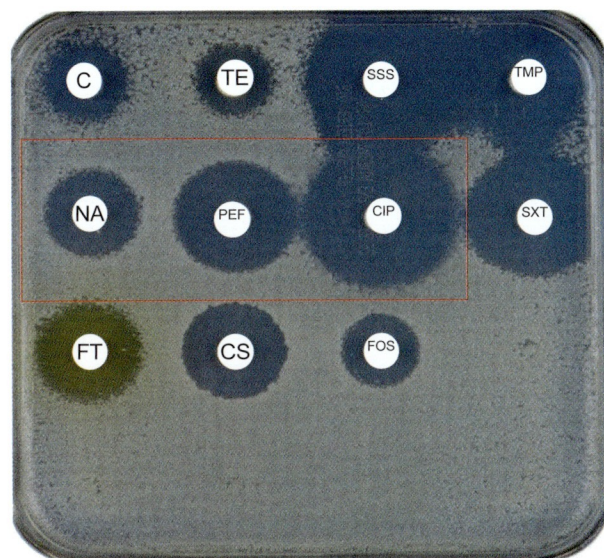

2a. Susceptible "wild-type" strain.   2b. Reduced accumulation

Fig. 2. Enterobacteria and quinolones. C, chloramphenicol; CIP, ciprofloxacin; CS, colistin; FOS, fosfomycin; FT, furans; NA, nalidixic acid; OFX, ofloxacin; PEF, pefloxacin; RA, rifampin; SSS, sulfonamides; SXT, sulfamethoxazole-trimethoprim; TE, tetracyclines; TMP, trimethoprim.

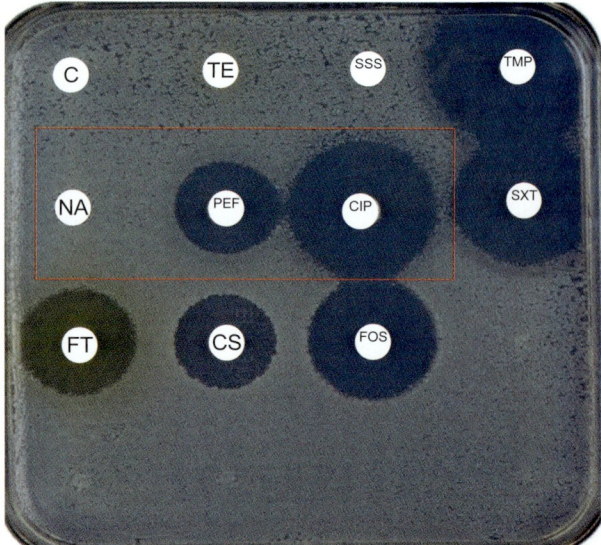

2c. One *gyrA* mutation.

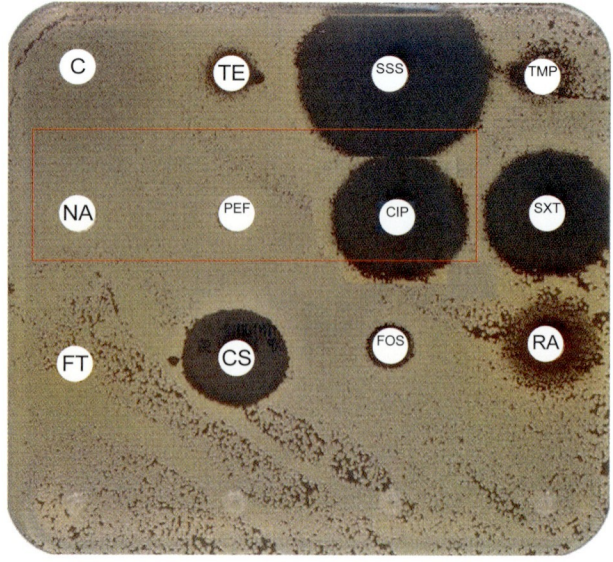

2d. One *gyrA* mutation + one *parC* mutation.

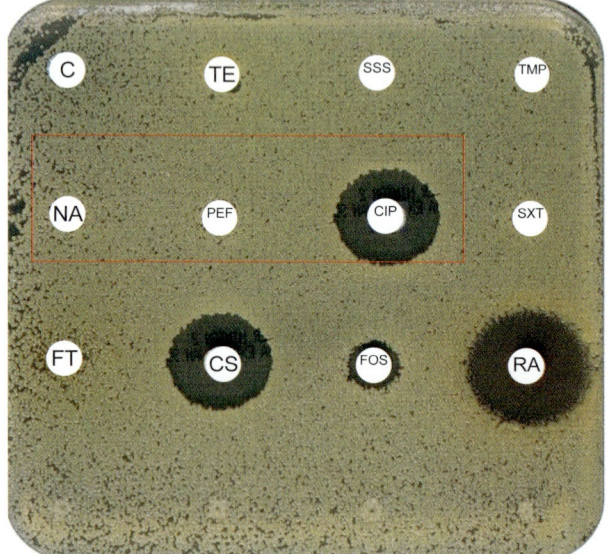

2e. Two *gyrA* mutations + one *parC* mutation.

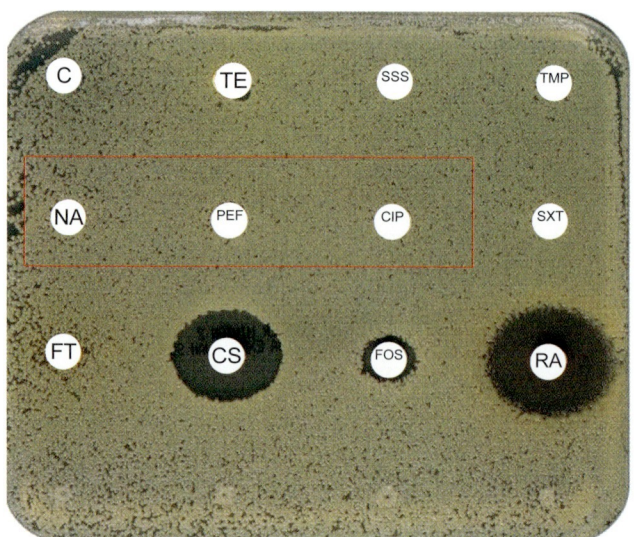

2f. Two *gyrA* mutations + one *parC* mutation (+/- reduced accumulation)

Fig. 2. Enterobacteria and quinolones (continued). C, chloramphenicol; CIP, ciprofloxacin; CS, colistin; FOS, fosfomycin; FT, furans; NA, nalidixic acid; OFX, ofloxacin; PEF, pefloxacin; RA, rifampin; SSS, sulfonamides; SXT, sulfamethoxazole-trimethoprim; TE, tetracyclines; TMP, trimethoprim.

currently exceeds 15% and 10%, respectively.

Data obtained by the EARSS surveillance network show large differences in fluoroquinolone resistance rates in *E. coli* according to the country:
- 5-10 % in France, Ireland, the Netherlands, Sweden, Finland, and Poland;
- 10-25 % in Spain, Belgium, Germany, Central Europe, and Greece;
- 25-50 % in Portugal and Italy.

In *P. mirabilis*, ciprofloxacin resistance has been rising steadily for the past fifteen years.

In *K. pneumoniae*, after a period of stability which lasted until 1985, resistance rates increased rapidly, reaching 50% for nalidixic acid and close to 35% for ciprofloxacin in the early 1990s. This situation reflected the emergence and dissemination of extended spectrum β-lactamase-producing strains. Subsequently, as these strains which were

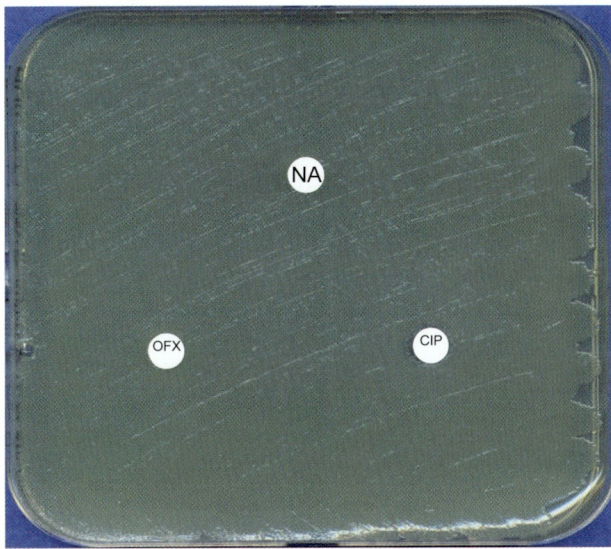

2g. *E. cloacae* with high level resistance and harboring a *qnr* gene

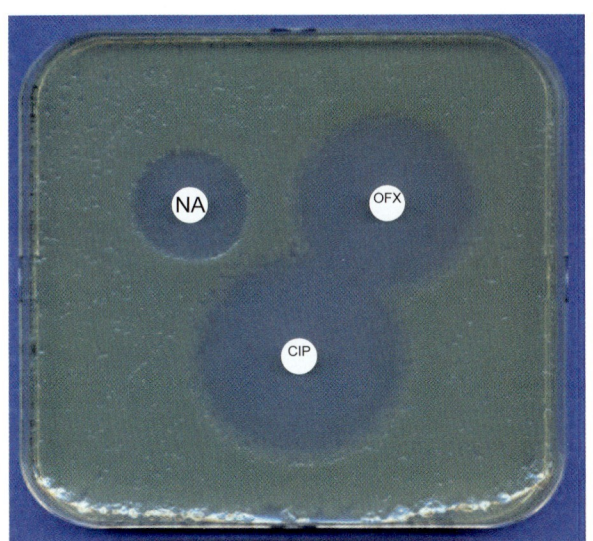 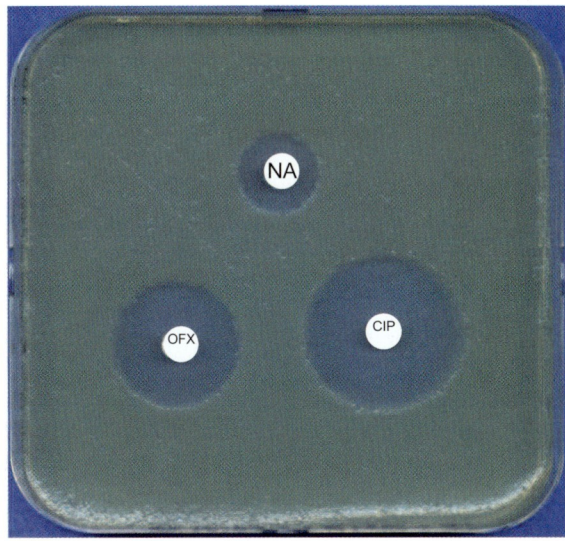

2h. Quinolone-susceptible *E. coli* recipient (left) and transconjugant harboring the *qnr* gene (right).

Fig. 2. Enterobacteria and quinolones (continued). CIP, ciprofloxacin; NA, nalidixic acid; OFX, ofloxacin

also quinolone-resistant began to be isolated less frequently, resistance rates also decreased steadily, although recently there has been a slight increase.

The prevalence of ciprofloxacin resistance in *P. aeruginosa* has remained stable at approximately 25-30% for the last several years.

In *Acinetobacter baumannii*, resistance rates have followed an irregular pattern. Despite a marked decrease in recent years between 40 and 50%, they are on the rise again, probably as a result of outbreaks.

Resistance rates are 26% in *Campylobacter*, 15% in *N. gonorrhoeae*, and 6-10% in *B. fragilis*.

On the other hand, fluoroquinolone resistance is rare in *H. influenzae* and *L. pneumophila*.

LABORATORY STUDIES

Susceptibility testing conditions

The pitfalls encountered when conducting and interpreting the quinolone antibiogram are related to the test conditions and the choice of antibiotics to be tested. Mueller-Hinton medium meets the requirements for the routine antibiogram. It should

Table 8. Quinolone resistance phenotypes in enterobacteria: probable mechanisms and approximate frequency

NAL[a]	NOR	CIP	Probable mechanism	Frequency (%)
S[b]	S	S	Wild-type	83 - 85
I	S	S	Reduced accumulation	< 1
R	S	S	1 gyrA mutation	< 1
R	I	S	1 gyrA mutation	3 - 4
R	R	S	1 gyrA mutation + 1 parC mutation	1 - 2
R	R	I	2 gyrA mutation + 1 parC mutation	1
R	R	R	2 gyrA mutation + 1 parC mutation (± permeability)	8 - 9
I	S	S	Plasmid-mediated resistance	1 - 2

[a] CIP, ciprofloxacin; NAL, nalidixic acid; NOR, norfloxacin.
[b] I, intermediate; R, resistant; S, susceptible.

Table 9. Quinolones to be studied according to the French Committee of Antibiogram (CA-SFM) (3)

Microorganism	Standard list[a]	Additional list
Enterobacteriaceae	NAL, NOR, CIP	Other fluoroquinolones
P. aeruginosa	CIP	Other fluoroquinolones
Other non-fermenting Gram-negative bacilli	CIP	
H. influenzae	NAL	If NAL diameter < 21 mm, determine MIC of a FQ
N. gonorrhoeae	NAL	If NAL diameter < 25 mm, determine MIC of CIP or OFL
Campylobacter	CIP	NAL (identification)
Anaerobes	-	OFL, MOX

[a] CIP, ciprofloxacin; MOX, moxifloxacin; NAL, nalidixic acid; NOR, norfloxacin; OFL, ofloxacin. Other proposals may be found in the documents of National Committees for Antimicrobial Susceptibility Testing

Table 10. Breakpoints (S ≤ / > R) (µg/ml)

Quinolone	Enterobacteriaceae		Pseudomonas-Acinetobacter		Non species related
	EUCAST[a]	CLSI	EUCAST	CLSI	EUCAST
Ciprofloxacin	0.5 / 1	1 / 2	0.5/1 - 1/1	1 / 2	0.5 / 1
Levofloxacin	1 / 2	2 / 4	1 / 2	2 / 4	1 / 2
Moxifloxacin	0.5 / 1	-	-	-	0.5 / 1
Norfloxacin	0.5 / 1	4 / 8	-	4 / 8	0.5 / 1
Ofloxacin	0.5 / 1	2 / 4	-	2 / 4	0.5 / 1

[a] CLSI, Clinical and Laboratory Standards Institute; EUCAST, European Committee on Antimicrobial Susceptibility Testing. For sake of comparison, the ≥ R of CLSI has been replaced by >, as EUCAST.

be borne in mind that different quinolones show different sensitivities to pH variations, whether more acidic or more basic.

Divalent cations (particularly magnesium) reduce the activity of quinolones. The usual concentration to be used for testing quinolones is 20-30 µg/ml in Mueller-Hinton medium.

Among the different supplements, blood does not alter the results. On the other hand, the charcoal present in Legionella BCYE medium increases MICs by a factor of 16-64.

Antibiotics to be studied and breakpoints

Table 9 shows a list of antibiotics that should be considered for testing according to the French Committee of Antibiogram (CA-SFM) (3). Other suggestions can be found in the recommendations of CLSI (document M100-S19, 2009).

For enterobacteria, it has been established that nalidixic acid is sufficient to predict the response of the other older quinolones. If not all the fluoroquinolones are tested, and excepting special cases, norfloxacin and ciprofloxacin should satisfy the

Table 11. Breakpoints (S ≤ / > R) (µg/ml)

Quinolone	H. influenzae-M. catarrhalis		N. gonorrhoeae	
	EUCAST	CLSI	EUCAST	CLSI
Ciprofloxacin	0.5 / 0.5	1 / 1	0.03 / 0.06	0.06 / 05
Levofloxacin	1 / 1	2 / 2	-	-
Moxifloxacin	0.5 / 0.5	1 / 1	-	-
Norfloxacin	-	-	-	-
Ofloxacin	0.5 / 0.5	2 / 2	0.12 / 0.25	0.25 / 2

CLSI, Clinical and Laboratory Standards Institute; EUCAST, European Committee on Antimicrobial Susceptibility Testing. For sake of comparison, the ≥ R of CLSI has been replaced by >, as EUCAST.

requirements of interpretation; the norfloxacin result predicts response of the other molecules. Several National committees, including the French Committee CA-SFM (3) and CLSI in the document M100-S19, provide a list of quinolones that should be considered for routine testing on nonfastidious organisms.

The CLSI and EUCAST breakpoints are shown in Tables 10 and 11. EUCAST non species related breakpoints and those for Gram-negative bacilli are generally lower than CLSI breakpoints.

For *H. influenzae*, *M. catarrhalis* and *N. gonorrhoeae*, the EUCAST breakpoints are 0.5 or 1 µg/ml, once again lower than the CLSI breakpoints.

CONCLUSION

- The mode of action of the quinolones has yet to be fully elucidated.
- Ciprofloxacin is the most active drug against Gram-negative bacteria, including with respect to the new fluoroquinolones.
- Plasmid-mediated resistance will probably become more prevalent in the future.
- Resistance rates appear to be increasing in certain species like *E. coli* and *N. gonorrhoeae*.

REFERENCES

(1) **Cattoir V., L. Poirel, and P. Nordmann**. 2008. Plasmid-mediated quinolone resistance QepA2 from *Escherichia coli* in France. Antimicrob. Agents Chemother. **10**:3801-3804.

(2) **Cattoir V., F.X. Weill, L. Poirel, L. Fabre, C.J. Soussy, and P. Nordmann**. 2007. Prevalence of *qnr* genes in *Salmonella* in France. J. Antimicrob. Chemother. **59**:751-754.

(3) **Comité de l'Antibiogramme de la Société Française de Microbiologie**. Recommandations 2009. http://www.sfm.asso.fr

(4) **Drlica, K., and D.C. Hooper**. 2003. Mechanisms of quinolone action, pp. 18-40. *In* D.C. Hooper and E. Rubinstein (ed.). Quinolone Antimicrobial Agents. American Society for Microbiology, Washington, D.C.

(5) **Goldstein, F.W., M. Meyran, J. Sirot, C.J. Soussy, et J. Duval**. 1993. Interprétation des tests de sensibilité aux fluoroquinolones systémiques. Lett. Infect. **VIII** : 581-582.

(6) **Honoré, S., C. Lascols, P. Legrand, C.J. Soussy, and E. Cambau**. 2004. Investigation of the new QNR-based mechanism of quinolone resistance and first description in *Enterobacter cloacae*. Int. J. Antimicrob. Agents **24**, **Suppl. 2**:S89

(7) **Hooper, D.C.** 2003. Mechanisms of quinolone resistance, pp. 41-67. *In* Hooper D.C. and E. Rubinstein (ed.). Quinolone Antimicrobial Agents. American Society for Microbiology, Washington, D.C.

(8) **Jacoby G.A., V. Cattoir, D. Hooper, L. Martinez-Martinez, P. Nordmann, A. Pascual, L. Poire, and M. Wang**. 2008. qnr gene nomenclature. Antimicrob. Agents Chemother. **52**:2297-2299.

(9) **Jacoby, G.A., N. Chow, and K.B. Waites**. 2003. Prevalence of plasmid-mediated quinolone resistance. Antimicrob. Agents Chemother. **2**:559-562.

(10) **Jacoby, G.A., K. Walsh, D. Mills, V. Walker, H. Oh, A. Robicsek, and D.C Hooper**. 2006. A new plasmid-mediated gene for quinolone resistance. Antimicrob. Agents Chemother. **50**:1178-1182

(11) **Kim, S.H., Y. Kwak, M. Lee, N. Kim, J. Jeong, and Y. Kim**. 2004. Plasmid-mediated quinolone resistance in clinical isolates of *E. coli* from Korea. 44th Interscience Conf. Antimicrob. Agents Chemother. Washington, DC. 2004, October 30 – November 2 : C2-1711

(12) **Komp Lindgren, P., A. Karlsson, and D. Hughes**. 2003. Mutation rate and evolution of fluoroquinolone resistance in *Escherichia coli* isolates from patients with urinary tract infections. Antimicrob. Agents Chemother. **10**:3222-3232

(13) **Lesher, G.Y., E.D. Forelich, M.D. Gruet, J.H. Bailey, and R.P. Brundage**. 1962. 1,8-Naphthyridine derivatives. A new class of chemotherapeutic agents. J. Med. Pharm. Chem. **5**:1063-1068.

(14) **Lewin, C., B. Howard, and J.T. Smith**. 1991. Protein- and RNA-synthesis independent bactericidal activity of ciprofloxacin that involves the A subunit of DNA gyrase. J. Med. Microbiol. **34**:19-22.

(15) **Ma, J., Z. Zeng, Z. Chen, X. Xu, X. Wang, Y. Deng, D. Lü, L. Huang, Y. Zhang, J. Liu, and M. Wang.** 2009 High prevalence of plasmid-mediated quinolone resistance determinants *qnr*, *aac(6')-Ib-cr*, and *qepA* among ceftiofur-resistant *Enterobacteriaceae* isolates from companion and food-producing animals. Antimicrob. Agents Chemother. **43**:519-524.

(16) **Mammeri, H., M. Van De Loo, L. Poirel, L. Martinez-Martinez, and P. Nordmann.** 2005. Emergence of plasmid-mediated quinolone resistance in *Escherichia coli* in Europe. Antimicrob. Agents Chemother. **49**:71-76.

(17) **Martinez-Martinez, L., A. Pascual, and G.A. Jaboby.** 1998. Quinolone resistance from a transferable plasmid. Lancet **351**:797-799.

(18) **Maxwell, A.** 1992. The molecular basis of quinolone action. J. Antimicrob. Chemother. **30**:409-414.

(19) **Minarini L.A., L. Poirel, V. Cattoir, A.L. Darini, and P. Nordmann.** 2008. Plasmid-mediated quinolone resistance determinants among enterobacterial isolates from outpatients in Brazil. J. Antimicrob. Chemother. **62**:474-478.

(20) **Paauw, A., A.C. Fluit, J. Verhoef, and M.A. Leverstein-Van Hall.** 2006. *Enterobacter cloacae* outbreak and emergence of quinolone resistance gene in Dutch hospital. Emerg. Infect. Dis. **12**:807-812.

(21) **Périchon, B., P. Bogaerts, T. Lambert, P. Courvalin, and M. Galimand.** 2008. Sequence of conjugative plasmid pIP1206 mediating resistance to aminoglycosides by rRNA methylation and to hydrophilic fluoroquinolones by efflux. Antimicrob. Agents Chemother. **52**: 2581-2592.

(22) **Périchon B., P. Courvalin, and M. Galimand.** 2007. Transferable resistance to aminoglycosides by methylation of G1405 in 16S rRNA and to hydrophilic fluoroquinolones by QepA-mediated efflux in *Escherichia coli*. Antimicrob. Agents Chemother. **51**:2464-2469.

(23) **Robicsek, A., D.F. Sahm, G.A. Jacoby, and D.C. Hooper.** 2005. Broader distribution of plasmid-mediated quinolone resistance in the United States. Antimicrob. Agents Chemother. **49**:3001-3003.

(24) **Robicsek, A., J. Strahilevitz, G.A. Jacoby, M. Macielag, D. Abbanat, C.H. Park, K. Bush, and D.C. Hooper.** 2006. Fluoroquinolone-modifying enzyme: a new adaptation of a common aminoglycoside acetyltransferase. Nat. Med. **12**:83-88.

(25) **Rodriguez-Martinez, J.M., A. Pascual, I. Garcia, and L. Martinez-Martinez.** 2003. Detection of the plasmid-mediated quinolone resistance determinant *qnr* among clinical isolates of *Klebsiella pneumoniae* producing AmpC-type ß-lactamase. J. Antimicrob. Chemother. **52**:703-706.

(26) **Ruiz, J**. 2003. Mechanisms of resistance to quinolones : target alterations, decreased accumulation and DNA gyrase protection. J. Antimicrob. Chemother. **51**:1109-1117.

(27) **Shen, L.L., J. Baranowski, and A.G. Pernet.** 1989. Mechanism of inhibition of DNA gyrase by quinolone antibacterials : specificity and cooperativity of drug binding to DNA. Biochemistry **28**:3879-3885.

(28) **Tran, J.H., and G.A. Jacoby.** 2002. Mechanism of plasmid-mediated quinolone resistance. Proc. Natl. Acad. Sci. USA **99**:5638-5642.

(29) **Vetting, M.W., C.H. Park, S.S. Hegde, G.A. Jacoby, D.C. Hooper, and J.S. Blanchard.** 2008. Mechanistic and structural analysis of aminoglycoside *N*-acetyltransferase AAC(6')-Ib and its bifunctional, fluoroquinolone-active AAC(6')-Ib-cr variant. Biochemistry **47**:9825-9835.

(30) **Wang, M., J.H. Tran, G.A. Jacoby, and Y. Zhang**. 2003. Plasmid-mediated quinolone resistance in clinical isolates of *Escherichia coli* from Shanghai, China. Antimicrob. Agents Chemother. **7**:2242-2248.

(31) **Wang, M., D.F. Sahm, G.A. Jacoby, and D.C. Hooper.** 2004. Emerging plasmid-mediated quinolone resistance associated with the *qnr* gene in *Klebsiella pneumoniae* clinical isolates in the United States. Antimicrob. Agents Chemother. **4**:1295-1299.

(32) **Weigel, L.M., G.J. Anderson, and F.C. Tenover.** 2002. DNA gyrase and topoisomerase IV mutations associated with fluoroquinolone resistance in *Proteus mirabilis*. Antimicrob. Agents Chemother. **8**:2582-2587.

(33) **Wiegand, I., N. Khalaf, M.H.M. Al-Agamy, and B. Wiedemann.** First detection of the transferable quinolone resistance determinant in clinical *Providencia stuartii* strains in Egypt. 44th Interscience Conf. Antimicrob. Agents Chemother. Washington, D.C., Abstr.: 0347.

(34) **Yamane, K., J. Wachino, S. Suzuki, K. Kimura, N. Shibata, H. Kato, K. Shibayama, T. Konda, and Y. Arakawa.** 2007. New plasmid-mediated fluoroquinolone efflux pump, QepA, found in an *Escherichia coli* clinical isolate. Antimicrob. Agents Chemother. **51**:3354-3360.

(35) **Yamane, K., J. Wachino, S. Suzuki, and Y. Arakawa.** 2008. Plamid-mediated *qepA* gene among *Escherichia coli* clinical isolates from Japan. Antimicrob. Agents Chemother. **52**:1564-1566.

(36) **Zhanel, G.G., A. Walkty, L. Vercaigne, J.A. Karlowsky, J. Embil, A.S. Gin, and D.J. Hoban**. 1999. The new fluoroquinolones : A critical review. Can. J. Infect. Dis. **10**:207-238.

Chapter 20. GLYCOPEPTIDES AND STAPHYLOCOCCI

Roland LECLERCQ

INTRODUCTION

Development studies on vancomycin in 1956 revealed that vancomycin resistance in staphylococci was difficult to induce *in vitro*, requiring about a hundred serial passages in vancomycin-containing liquid medium and resulting in only a slight increase in the vancomycin MIC. This *in vitro* finding was confirmed by the long period during which no vancomycin-resistant staphylococcal clinical isolates were reported. It was during the development of another glycopeptide, teicoplanin, in the mid-1980s that teicoplanin-intermediate or resistant (MIC > 4 µg/ml) but vancomycin-susceptible coagulase-negative staphylococci were described (3). The first vancomycin-intermediate (MIC = 8 µg/ml) and teicoplanin-resistant strain of *Staphylococcus haemolyticus* (25), as well as the first teicoplanin-intermediate clinical isolate of *Staphylococcus aureus*, were reported in 1987 (17). These observations remained anecdotal until the mid-1990s, when *S. aureus* strains with reduced glycopeptide susceptibility were isolated in a number of countries, although their prevalence seemed to be low (12, 13, 20). The discovery of these strains opened a still ongoing debate as to their definition and the methods of their detection. It therefore comes as no surprise that there are wide discrepancies in the prevalence, methodology and categorization of these strains reported in the literature. More recently, vancomycin- and teicoplanin-resistant *S. aureus* isolates having acquired the *vanA* resistance operon were reported in the United States. This has been a cause of great concern, even if for the moment these strains appear to be confined to the United States and are still rare. The structure and mode of action of the two glycopeptides currently on the market – vancomycin and teicoplanin – are described in Chapter 21.

METHODS

Mueller-Hinton is the reference medium for susceptibility testing of antibiotics, including glycopeptides, in staphylococci. Regardless of the method used, the incubation time should be 24 hours.

The MICs of vancomycin for *S. aureus* and coagulase-negative staphylococci determined by broth microdilution, agar or broth dilution or E-test® show essential agreement (± 1 dilution) (26). In some cases MICs were one dilution lower in broth medium.

Good essential agreement was also observed with respect to the MICs of teicoplanin for *S. aureus*. No significant differences were found between teicoplanin MICs for coagulase-negative staphylococci determined in broth or agar medium (18). However, there can be notable differences in teicoplanin MICs for some coagulase-negative staphylococci according to the medium and the method used. For these strains, teicoplanin MICs are 4-32 fold lower in broth than in agar medium. Furthermore, the results can differ considerably according to the lot and supplier of the Mueller-Hinton medium (19). Table 1 shows the results of glycopeptide susceptibility tests in 263 coagulase-negative staphylococci isolates recovered from 35 French hospitals. MICs were determined identically by the agar dilution method as recommended by the Comité de l'Antibiogramme de la Société Française de Microbiologie (CA-SFM; www.sfm.asso.fr). Essential accordance between the three media was good (98%) for vancomycin but poor (58%) for teicoplanin, leading to different results in terms of clinical categorization. These differences were due to the particular behavior, for unknown reasons, of a subgroup of 25 strains belonging to various species and isolated in different laboratories. There is no evidence to argue for one method, medium or supplier over another. However, the broth microdilution method yields the lowest and least different MICs.

There is a larger inoculum effect for teicoplanin than for vancomycin in both *S. aureus* and coagulase-negative staphylococci, with MICs increased by a factor of 4-8 for each 100-fold increase in the inoculum. The presence of human serum has little effect on MICs. Increasing the pH lowers the MICs of teicoplanin.

Since glycopeptides are very large molecules which diffuse poorly in agar, the diffusion method cannot reliably distinguish vancomycin-susceptible from vancomycin-intermediate strains of *S. aureus*. The same is true for coagulase-negative staphylococci. For this reason, the Clinical and Laboratory Standards Institute (CLSI) does not recommend the disk method but rather MIC determination for testing vancomycin susceptibility in staphylococci (7). Other national committees like the CA-SFM (www.sfm.asso.fr) propose critical diameters but also consider that the diffusion method is not efficient for glycopeptides.

However, the diffusion method does allow the detection of *S. aureus* strains which have acquired the *vanA* glycopeptide resistance gene (VRSA), because such strains express high-level resistance which is visible as the growth of colonies in contact with the disks. The identification of such strains must be verified and their resistance confirmed by MIC determination.

CLINICAL CATEGORIZATION AND GLYCOPEPTIDE ACTIVITY

The breakpoints recommended by the European Committee on Antimicrobial Susceptibility Testing (EUCAST) (http://www.srga.org/eucastwt/MICTAB/MICglycopeptides.html; 2006/06/20, V 1.3), and the CLSI are summarized in Table 2. The values differ between the two committees, in particular because the CLSI has recently revised its breakpoints whereas EUCAST is in the process of doing so. However, it should be noted that the CLSI did not change the breakpoints for teicoplanin which, in rare cases, might yield a paradoxically "susceptible" response for a vancomycin-intermediate strain.

The MICs of vancomycin for *S. aureus* usually range from 0.12-4 µg/ml (Fig. 1) whereas there is wider dispersion for teicoplanin MICs (0.12-16 µg/ml) (9). Depending on the method, the MIC_{50} of teicoplanin is 0.5 or 1 µg/ml and that of vancomycin is 1 µg/ml. The MIC_{90} of both drugs is

Table 1. MIC (µg/ml) of vancomycin and teicoplanin for 263 strains of coagulase-negative[a] staphylococci according to the batch of Mueller-Hinton medium

Mueller-Hinton	Vancomycin		Teicoplanin		Clinical categorization of teioplanin (% of strains)[b]	
	MIC_{50}	MIC_{90}	MIC_{50}	MIC_{90}	Intermediate	Resistant
Difco	1	1	1	4	2	0.4
bioMérieux	1	2	1	4	4.6	0.4
Bio-Rad	2	2	4	8	22	1

[a] *S. epidermidis*, 123; *S. haemolyticus*, 13; *S. saprophyticus*, 8; *S. capitis*, 6; *S. hominis*, 7; *S. warneri*, 6; *S. lugdunensis*, 4; *S. xylsus*, 1; not identified, 95 (from 18).
[b] Breakpoints from CA-SFM. S ≤ 4µg/ml R > 8µg/ml.

Table 2. Breakpoints recommended by the Clinical Laboratory Standards Institute (CLSI) and the European Committee on Antimicrobial Susceptibility Testing (EUCAST)

Clinical categorization	Vancomycin		Teicoplanin	
	CLSI (2009)	EUCAST (2006)	CLSI (2009)	EUCAST (2006)
S. aureus				
Susceptible	≤ 2	≤ 4	≤ 8	≤ 4
Intermediate	4-8	8	16	8
Resistant	≥ 16	> 8	≥ 32	> 8
Coagulase-negative staphylococci				
Susceptible	≤ 4	≤ 4	≤ 8	≤ 4
Intermediate	8-16	8	16	8
Resistant	≥ 32	> 8	≥ 32	> 8

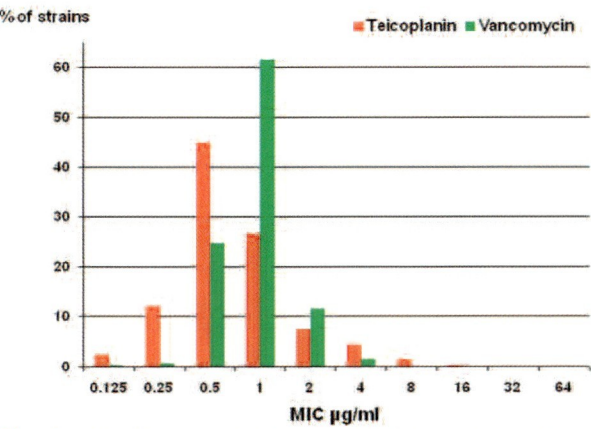

Fig. 1. Distribution of glycopeptide MICs for 2852 *S. aureus* strains isolated in Europe (9).

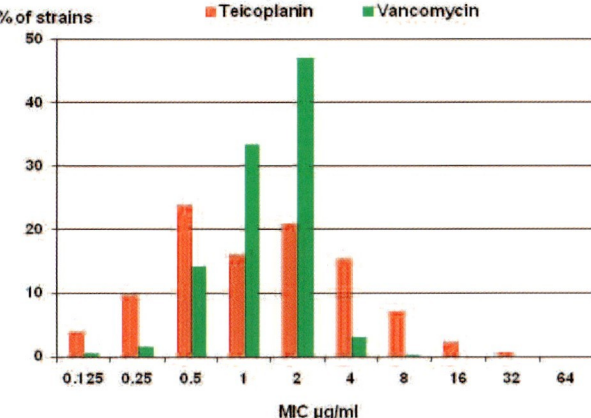

Fig. 2. Distribution of glycopeptide MICs for 1,444 coagulase-negative staphylococcus strains isolated in Europe (9).

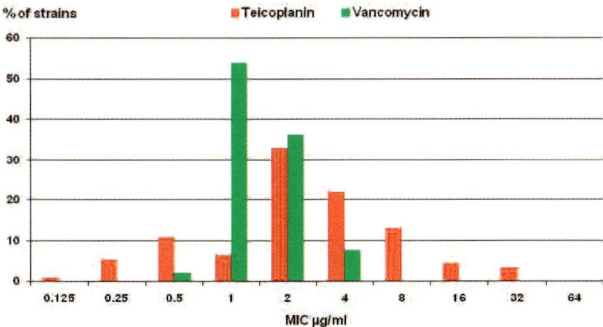

Fig. 3. Distribution of glycopeptide MICs for 91 S. haemolyticus strains isolated in Europe (9).

usually 1-2 µg/ml. In several studies, the MIC_{50} of teicoplanin was one or two dilutions higher for methicillin-resistant *S. aureus* (MRSA), a trend also seen for vancomycin.

The MIC_{50} and MIC_{90} of both vancomycin and teicoplanin are generally one dilution higher for coagulase-negative staphylococci than for *S. aureus*. Teicoplanin MICs show a wider dispersion (Fig. 2), even more so for the species *S. haemolyticus* (Fig. 3) which comprises a considerable number of vancomycin-intermediate and especially teicoplanin-intermediate or resistant strains.

The bactericidal activity of vancomycin and teicoplanin against staphylococci is time-dependent. The MBC/MIC ratios range from 2 to 8, but cell killing is slow, generally not observable at 18 h but occurring instead at 24 or 48 h. This is what is meant by "tolerance" of staphylococci to glycopeptides, which is a natural state of these bacteria. Human serum has virtually no effect on the bactericidal activity of vancomycin but slightly diminishes that of teicoplanin (27).

DEFINITIONS OF RESISTANCE

Different terms and acronyms are used to define *S. aureus* strains with reduced glycopeptide susceptibility: VISA, GISA, hetero-VISA and VRSA. VRSA (Vancomycin Resistant *S. aureus*) must be discussed separately because of their different resistance determinants and expression and the particular problems they pose. The other strains can be grouped under the term "reduced glycopeptide susceptibility".

VRSA

VRSA are strains for which the MIC of vancomycin is > 16 µg/ml and which have acquired the enterococcal *vanA* operon via a transposon carried on transferable conjugative plasmids. These strains are also resistant to teicoplanin.

Strains with reduced susceptibility

Reduced glycopeptide susceptibility strains are isolated at a low frequency throughout the world. Most of them are MRSA, although some methicillin-susceptible *S. aureus* (MSSA) also display this trait (4).

VISA and GISA

VISA (Vancomycin Intermediate *S. aureus*) was the term originally used because the strains so-named, with intermediate susceptibility to vancomycin (MIC = 8 µg/ml), were isolated in countries (Japan and then the United States) where vancomycin was the only glycopeptide in use (12, 13). Subsequently, the term GISA (Glycopeptide Intermediate *S. aureus*) was introduced to account for cross-resistance to teicoplanin.

Hetero-VISA

The definition of hetero-VISA is not based on clinical categorization (S/I/R) as in the previous case. Rather, this term was coined by K. Hiramatsu et al. (14) to describe S. aureus strains initially isolated in Japan which were susceptible to vancomycin (MIC 2-4 µg/ml) but contained vancomycin-intermediate subpopulations (MIC 6-8 µg/ml) occurring at a low frequency of roughly 10^{-5} to 10^{-7} (Fig. 4).

The hetero-VISA trait cannot be detected by simple determination of MICs because the test inoculum is approximately 10^4 CFU and the frequency of the vancomycin-intermediate subpopulation is below this threshold. For most of these strains, the MIC of teicoplanin is 8 µg/ml (CLSI category: S; EUCAST category: I) or higher. Lowering the vancomycin breakpoint from 4 to 2 µg/ml allows the majority of these strains to be categorized as "vancomycin intermediate" since the MIC of vancomycin is usually 4 µg/ml.

The hetero-VISA definition is imprecise and there is no molecular method to serve as a reference. Furthermore, the clinical significance of these strains is debatable. Some authors question their very existence and feel that too much time and money are spent looking for them (2), while others claim that one has only to look, and one shall find, and that these strains are clinically important (15). Nonetheless, many believe that hetero-VISA strains form the reservoir of VISA/GISA strains, the group as a whole simply comprising a continuum of strains with different glycopeptide susceptibilities.

RESISTANCE MECHANISMS

VISA, GISA, and hetero-VISA

Strains with the VISA/GISA phenotype appear to be mutants which have accumulated several determinants of glycopeptide resistance (12). These strains have a cell wall that is about twofold thicker; they also have increased autolytic activity, expel peptidoglycan debris, produce more monomeric precursors, have fewer peptidoglycan side chains, have an inactive PBP4, show less amidation of the muropeptide, and have a more disorganized cell wall. This results in complex alterations of peptidoglycan metabolism, probably related to mutations in the many genes that regulate this metabolism or to changes in the expression of these genes. This reorganization might prevent vancomycin from reaching its target. Another, non-exclusive hypothesis is the hyperproduction of peptidoglycan precursors, which then act as traps to sequester the glycopeptide. Hetero-VISA strains also have a thicker cell wall. Thickness varies according to whether or not the strain is cultivated in the presence of vancomycin.

VRSA

As noted earlier, the mechanism of resistance in VRSA strains is completely different. These strains have acquired the enterococcal vanA operon and glycopeptide resistance is conferred by the same mechanism as in enterococci (6) (see also Chapter 21).

DETECTION OF RESISTANCE

There are a number of difficulties inherent to the study of glycopeptide activity *in vitro* and detection of resistance:
- As indicated earlier, glycopeptides diffuse poorly into agar and so the agar diffusion method is unsatisfactory.
- Rapid automated methods are not suitable because long incubation times are necessary for resistance to be expressed.
- The large inoculum effect for teicoplanin can lead to an overestimation of resistance.
- For VISA/GISA strains, there is no molecular method that can serve as reference.

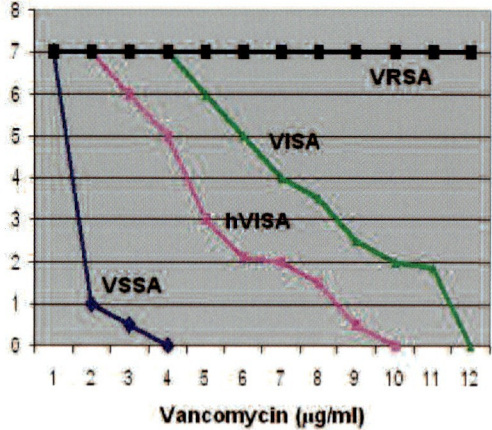

Fig. 4. Population analysis in the presence of vancomycin. Four strains were tested: VSSA (vancomycin-susceptible S. aureus), VRSA, VISA and hetero-VISA (h-VISA). 10^8 CFU of each strain were inoculated on BHI agar containing increasing vancomycin concentrations. Colonies that grew after a 48-h incubation were counted and their relative frequency calculated

- Strains with reduced glycopeptide susceptibility do not form a population that is clearly distinguishable from susceptible strains. In particular, the MICs of vancomycin for hetero-VISA strains place these strains in the susceptible category.
- As a general rule, agar-based methods (agar dilution and E-test®) are preferable, considering the heterogeneity of the subpopulations with reduced glycopeptide susceptibility.

It is important to be able to detect strains with only moderate glycopeptide resistance, since the use of vancomycin or teicoplanin in infections caused by strains classified as I (or even more so, as R) is frequently associated with treatment failures.

Reduced glycopeptide susceptibility can be suspected during routine testing on the basis of certain alert criteria, or else by specific screening. If reduced susceptibility is suspected, the clinical categorization (S/I/R) of the strains should be carried out by MIC determination under standard conditions.

Presumptive criteria for reduced glycopeptide susceptibility

Routine methods

The CLSI does not recommend the **diffusion** method to test glycopeptide activity, since this method underestimates resistance to vancomycin and teicoplanin in *S. aureus* and either under- or over-estimates resistance to both drugs in coagulase-negative staphylococci. For example, the vancomycin-intermediate (MIC = 8 µg/ml) and teicoplanin-resistant (MIC = 16 µg/ml) strain *Staphylococcus epidermidis* WHO6 was tested by 96 laboratories in the WHONET network as part of a quality control using the agar diffusion method (26). Ninety-two of these laboratories reported the strain as vancomycin-susceptible, with inhibition zone diameters ranging from 15-34 mm. The results of the four laboratories which reported resistance can be called into question by the abnormally small inhibition zone diameters of vancomycin, ranging from 6-14 mm. Out of 41 laboratories which tested teicoplanin by the diffusion method, 30 reported susceptibility. Several other studies have yielded less discordant albeit mediocre results.

Although they consider this method unacceptable, some national committees have proposed critical diameters. After a full 24-h incubation, reduced glycopeptide susceptibility can be suspected in the presence of an abnormally small inhibition zone diameter for vancomycin or teicoplanin, or if colonies are present in the inhibition zone of a glycopeptide.

With **automated systems**, an I or R result for vancomycin or teicoplanin should also be considered an alert. Automated systems have not been extensively evaluated. The VITEK 7.01 software upgrade improved system performance but it still remains imperfect (22). ATB expression galleries tend to produce false intermediate (or false resistant) results for teicoplanin in coagulase-negative staphylococci due to the large inoculum used (equivalent to a 2 McFarland standard). In a series of staphylococcal strains tested on the Phoenix system, three vancomycin-I or R coagulase-negative strains were correctly reported (8). The performance of the VITEK2 also appears satisfactory, with teicoplanin MICs for coagulase-negative staphylococci that are one to two dilutions higher than those determined by agar dilution, thus generating false intermediates (personal data). A more methodical evaluation of the performance of the newest generation of automated systems with respect to reduced susceptibility strains would be a worthwhile undertaking.

In the case of an I or R result for vancomycin or teicoplanin on an automated system or in the presence of one of the presumptive criteria noted above, it is necessary to determine the MIC of vancomycin (and teicoplanin in countries where it is marketed) by a validated method (agar dilution, broth microdilution or E-test®). Even better, MICs can be determined straightaway.

It is especially important to use a validated method of glycopeptide susceptibility testing in the case of severe infections.

Specific tests

As routine testing methods can be flawed with respect to the detection of GISA, and since they do not detect hetero-VISA strains, several screening methods have been proposed.
- The Vancomycin Agar Screen Test is recommended by the CLSI (7). Briefly, Brain-Heart Infusion (BHI) agar containing 6 µg/ml vancomycin is inoculated with 10 µl of a 0.5 McFarland suspension or with the aid of a swab immersed in the suspension and spread or streaked on an area of 10-15 mm. After a full 24-h incubation at 35°C, the test is positive if at least two colonies are present. *S. aureus* ATCC 25923 and *E. faecalis* ATCC 51299 are used as negative and positive control, respectively. One

criticism of this test is its lack of reproducibility, especially if the agar is prepared in the laboratory (16). Other authors recommend media containing 4 µg/ml vancomycin, but these media have poor specificity. One study found that Mueller-Hinton medium supplemented with 5 µg/ml vancomycin had better reproducibility (16).

- The CA-SFM recommends Mueller-Hinton medium supplemented with 5 µg/ml teicoplanin, inoculated with 10 µl of a 2 McFarland suspension, and incubated at 35-37°C for 24 and 48 h. The test is positive if at least four colonies are present. *S. aureus* ATCC 25923 and *S. haemolyticus* CIP 107204 can be used as negative and positive controls, respectively. This method has the advantage of being highly sensitive, as teicoplanin is the better resistance marker, but it lacks specificity. This method was used in a study of 2,066 methicillin-resistant *S. aureus* isolates recovered from 165 institutions, among which 254 isolates tested positive, 45 of which had confirmed reduced glycopeptide susceptibility (hetero-VISA strains) (Report 2001 RAISIN/CCLIN/InVS: ACTU_DIVERS/gisa2004.pdf).

- The E-test® can be used for screening purposes. To this end, BHI agar should be inoculated by swabbing 200 µl of a heavy 2 McFarland suspension. Plates are read after 24 h and confirmed at 48 h. If vancomycin and teicoplanin MICs are greater than or equal to 8 µg/ml (a MIC of 6 µg/ml should not be converted to 8 µg/ml), or else if only the MIC of teicoplanin is greater than or equal to 12 µg/ml, the strain probably has reduced glycopeptide susceptibility (31).

A positive result in one or more of the above tests is not grounds to report the strain as having reduced glycopeptide susceptibility, since these tests lack specificity and the level of resistance must be determined (Table 3). It is necessary to determine the MIC which allows categorization of the strain.

Categorization of strains

MIC determination

Glycopeptide MICs are determined by agar dilution in Mueller-Hinton medium (10^4 CFU per spot) or by microdilution in Mueller-Hinton broth. MIC determination by E-test® in Mueller-Hinton (and not BHI) agar with a 0.5 McFarland (and not a 2 McFarland) inoculum is a good alternative since it correlates well with the previous methods, as noted above. Plates should be read after a full 24 hours of incubation.

It should be kept in mind that the "I" categorization for a glycopeptide is associated with frequent treatment failures. Taking inhibitory quotients into account (serum concentration/MIC ratio) is one of the ways by which to monitor glycopeptide therapy in staphylococcal infections. Fig. 5 presents an example of a teicoplanin-intermediate strain. A decision algorithm is given in Fig. 6.

Case of hetero-VISA

The determination of vancomycin MICs does not enable identification of hetero-VISA strains because it does not detect vancomycin-intermediate subpopulations. The only currently available way to identify a hetero-VISA strain is to perform a population analysis. However, these techniques are exploratory and no consensus exists for a particular method or for the subpopulation thresholds that define hetero-VISA. Furthermore, the hypothesis that there is a higher risk of vancomycin failure in hetero-VISA infections as compared with infections due to susceptible strains remains to be demonstrated. The following methods may be used to establish a correlation with treatment failures.

The population analysis method described by Wootton *et al.* (32) allows the strain to be classified by comparison with the hetero-VISA refe-

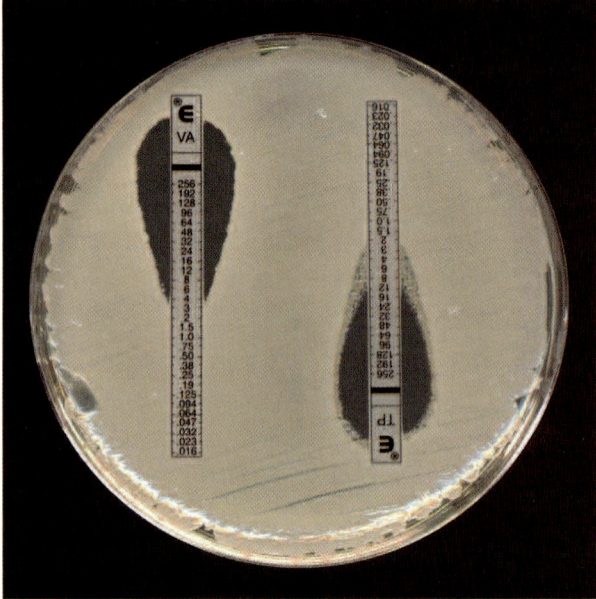

Fig. 5. Glycopeptide MICs determined by E-test® of a strain with intermediate susceptibility to teicoplanin (MIC = 12 µg/ml) and vancomycin (MIC = 4 µg/ml).

Table 3. Sensitivity and specificity of screening tests for identification of GISA and hetero-VISA (characterized by population analysis)

Reference Screening medium[a]	Sensitivity (%)		Specificity (%)
	GISA	Hetero-VISA	GISA + Hetero-VISA
Wootton et al. (33)			
BHI + vancomycin 6 µg/ml	58	11	97
M-H + teicoplanin 5 µg/ml	92	79	75
E-test® BHI	94	69	89
Voss et al. (30)			
BHI + vancomycin 6 µg/ml	44	4,5	68
M-H + vancomycin 6 µg/ml	25	14	58
M-H + teicoplanin 5 µg/ml	90	85	92
E-test® BHI	99	98	93
Yusof et al. (34)			
BHI + vancomycin 6 µg/ml	27		100
M-H + teicoplanin 5 µg/ml	65		95
E-test® BHI	80 (48 h incubation: 94)		87 (48 h incubation: 96)

[a] BHI, brain heart infusion; M-H, Mueller-Hinton.

rence strain *S. aureus* Mu3. Cultures of the test strain and strain Mu3 are diluted 10^{-3} to 10^{-6} and 100 µl are inoculated on BHI agar containing 0.5, 1, 2, 2.5 and 4 µg/ml vancomycin. Colonies which grow on these media are counted after a 48-h incubation and the percentage of bacteria that grow at the different concentrations is calculated. The area under the curve (AUC) for each concentration and for each strain is measured and the AUC ratio for the test/Mu3 strain is calculated. The test strain is hetero-VISA if the ratio is not less than 0.9. Other authors have simplified this method by eliminating the Mu3 control and testing only the 2, 3 and 4 µg/ml vancomycin concentrations. In this case, hetero-VISA strains are recognized by the detection of subpopulations as in Fig. 4. Still other authors inoculate 10^8 CFU on BHI agar containing 4 µg/ml vancomycin (5). Colonies are counted at 48 h and strains that produce colonies at a frequency of 10^{-7} to 10^{-6} are considered hetero-VISA.

If a population analysis is not performed, the following criteria are grounds to suspect a hetero-VISA strain:

- A strain which is teicoplanin-intermediate (MIC = 8 µg/ml) and vancomycin-susceptible (MIC = 2 µg/ml) by E-test®.
- A positive screening test. Table 3 shows the sensitivity and specificity of screening methods for the detection of GISA and hetero-GISA. The Vancomycin Agar Screen Test has low sensitivity for detection of hetero-VISA whereas the other tests, including the modified E-test® (2 McFarland inoculum) and Mueller-Hinton agar with 5 µg/ml teicoplanin are sensitive methods (30, 33, 34).

It should be kept in mind that the clinical importance of screening for hetero-VISA strains has not been clearly established. The CLSI does not propose methods for the detection of such strains.

Case of VRSA

Resistance may be difficult to detect in these strains. A specific example concerns the strain isolated in Pennsylvania, which tested susceptible on the Microscan, VITEK and VITEK2 (Phoenix not tested) (29). Glycopeptide susceptibility of three VRSA isolates from the United States, including the Pennsylvania strain, was recently tested by different methods (10). The screening method of the CLSI (6 µg/ml vancomycin) and CA-SFM (5 µg/ml teicoplanin), the vancomycin disk test and the ATB STAPH gallery performed well. In contrast to VISA/GISA strains, vancomycin was more effective than teicoplanin at identifying glycopeptide resistance. It appears that some of the difficulty of glycopeptide susceptibility testing in these strains lies in the spontaneous loss of plasmids, generating mixtures of susceptible and resistant populations and/or prolongation of the latency period required for induction of resistance.

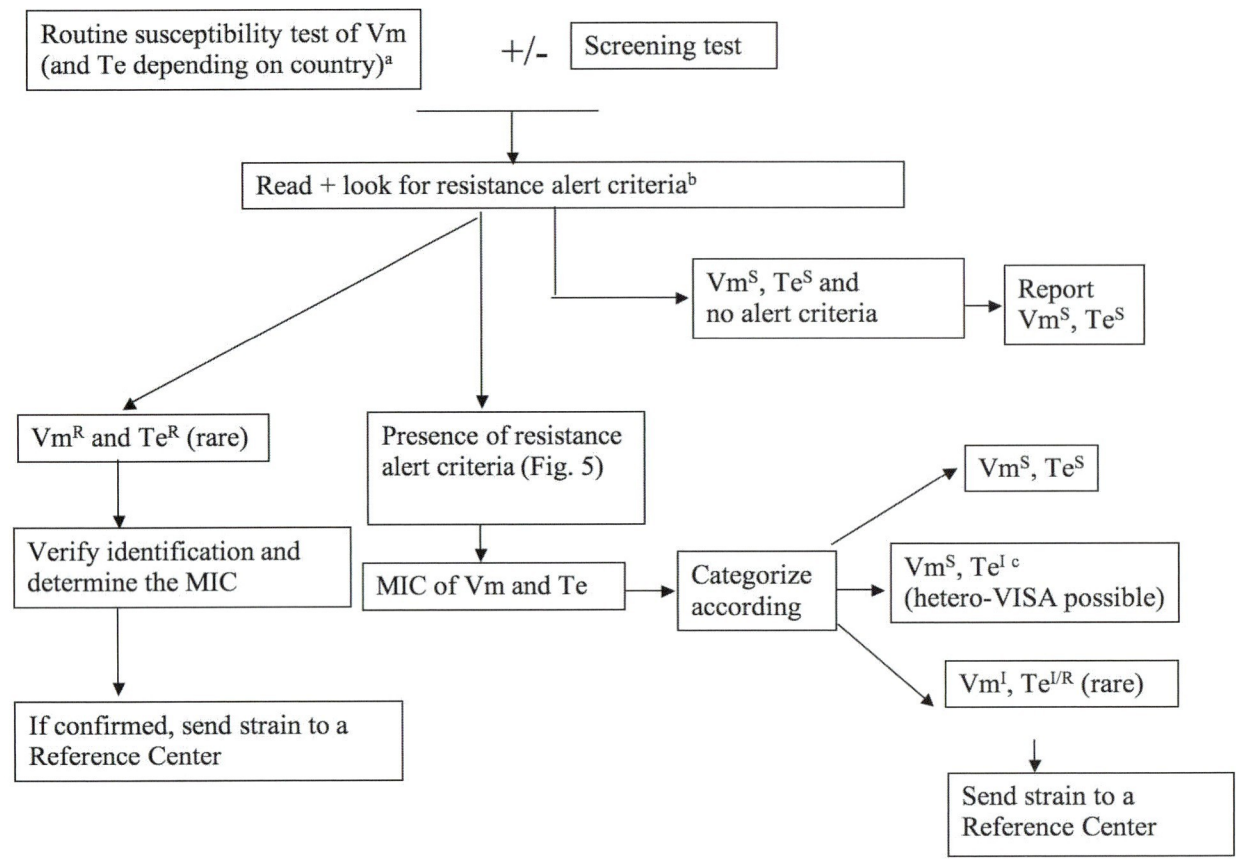

Fig. 6. Decision algorithm for glycopeptide susceptibility testing in staphylococci.

[a] Te, teicoplanin; Vm, vancomycin.
[b] For reduced susceptibility presumptive criteria, see text.
[c] hetero-VISA, see text.

PREVALENCE OF RESISTANCE

Vancomycin-I and teicoplanin I/R strains of *S. aureus* are rare (23). With respect to coagulase-negative staphylococci, a European study carried out in 1995 revealed that vancomycin resistance is rare (9). Excluding *S. haemolyticus*, approximately 15% of strains had a teicoplanin MIC > 4 µg/ml. Among *S. haemolyticus* strains, 23% had a teicoplanin MIC > 4 µg/ml.

VRSA strains are very rare. Between 2002 and 2009, only nine VRSA isolates were reported in the United States, particularly in Michigan, and recent publications reported one strain in India and one in Iran (1, 6, 24).

REFERENCES

(1) **Aligholi M., M. Emaneini, F. Jabalameli, S. Shahsavan, H. Dabiri, and H. Sedaght**. 2008. Emergence of high-level vancomycin-resistant *Staphylococcus aureus* in the Imam Khomeini Hospital in Tehran. Med. Princ. Pract. **17**:432-434.

(2) **Arakawa, Y., Y. Ike, and M. Nagasawa**. 2004. Where has vancomycin-heterogeneously resistant *Staphylococcus aureus* gone ? Lancet **363**:1401.

(3) **Arioli, V., and R. Pallanza**. 1987. Teicoplanin-resistant coagulase-negative staphylococci. Lancet **1**:39.

(4) **Bobin-Dubreux, S., M.E. Reverdy, C. Nervi, M. Rougier, A. Bolmstrom, F. Vandenesch, and J. Etienne**. 2001. Clinical isolate of vancomycin-heterointermediate *Staphylococcus aureus* susceptible to methicillin and in vitro selection of a vancomycin-resistant derivative. Antimicrob. Agents Chemother. **45**:349-352.

(5) **Chesneau, O., A. Morvan, and N.E. Solh**. 2000. Retrospective screening for heterogeneous vancomycin resistance in diverse *Staphylococcus aureus* clones disseminated in French hospitals. J. Antimicrob. Chemother. **45**:887-890.

(6) **Clark, N.C., L.M. Weigel, J.B. Patel, and F.C. Tenover**. 2005. Comparison of Tn*1546*-like elements in vancomycin-resistant *Staphylococcus aureus* iso-

lates from Michigan and Pennsylvania. Antimicrob. Agents Chemother. **49**:470-472.

(7) **Clinical and Laboratory Standards Institute.** 2009. Methods for dilution antimicrobial susceptibility tests for bacteria that grow aerobically; approved standard-eighth edition & performance standards for antimicrobial susceptibiliy testing; nineteenth informational supplement, M07A8, M100S19.

(8) **Fahr, A.M., U. Eigner, M. Armbrust, A. Caganic, G. Dettori, C. Chezzi, L. Bertoncini, M. Benecchi, and M.G. Menozzi.** 2003. Two-center collaborative evaluation of the performance of the BD Phoenix automated microbiology system for identification and antimicrobial susceptibility testing of *Enterococcus* spp. and *Staphylococcus* spp. J. Clin. Microbiol. **41**:1135-1142.

(9) **Felmingham, D., D.F. Brown, and C.J. Soussy.** 1998. European glycopeptide susceptibility survey of gram-positive bacteria for 1995. European glycopeptide resistance survey study group. Diagn. Microbiol. Infect. Dis. **31**:563-571.

(10) **Girard-Blanc, C., and P. Courvalin.** 2005. Evaluation of non-automated techniques for phenotypic detection of VanA-type *Staphylococcus aureus*. Eur. J. Clin. Microbiol. Infect. Dis. **24**:562-565.

(11) **Guerin, F., A. Buu-Hoi, J.L. Mainardi, G. Kac, N. Colardelle, S. Vaupre, L. Gutmann, and I. Podglajen.** 2000. Outbreak of methicillin-resistant *Staphylococcus aureus* with reduced susceptibility to glycopeptides in a Parisian hospital. J. Clin. Microbiol. **38**:2985-2988.

(12) **Hiramatsu, K.** 2001. Vancomycin-resistant *Staphylococcus aureus*: a new model of antibiotic resistance. Lancet Infect. Dis. **1**:147-155.

(13) **Hiramatsu, K., H. Hanaki, T. Ino, K. Yabuta, T. Oguri, and F.C. Tenover.** 1997. Methicillin-resistant *Staphylococcus aureus* clinical strain with reduced vancomycin susceptibility. J. Antimicrob. Chemother. **40**:135-136.

(14) **Hiramatsu, K., N. Aritaka, H. Hanaki, S. Kawasaki, Y. Hosoda, S. Hori, Y. Fukuchi, and I. Kobayashi.** 1997. Dissemination in Japanese hospitals of strains of *Staphylococcus aureus* heterogeneously resistant to vancomycin. Lancet **350**:1670-1673.

(15) **Howe, R.A., and T.R. Walsh.** 2004. hGISA: seek and ye shall find. Lancet **364**:500-501.

(16) **Hubert, S.K., J.M. Mohammed, S.K. Fridkin, R.P. Gaynes, J.E. McGowan Jr, and F.C. Tenover.** 1999. Glycopeptide-intermediate *Staphylococcus aureus*: evaluation of a novel screening method and results of a survey of selected U.S. hospitals. J. Clin. Microbiol. **37**:3590-3593.

(17) **Kaatz, G.W., S.M. Seo, N.J. Dorman, and S.A. Lerner.** 1990. Emergence of teicoplanin resistance during therapy of *Staphylococcus aureus* endocarditis. J. Infect. Dis. **162**:103-108.

(18) **Kenny, M.T., J.K. Dulworth, and M.A. Brackman.** 1989. Comparison of the agar dilution, tube dilution, and broth microdilution susceptibility tests for determination of teicoplanin MICs. J. Clin. Microbiol. **27**:1409-1410.

(19) **Leclercq, R., C.J. Soussy, H.B. Drugeon, M. Auzou, and N. Moniot-Ville.** 2001. Influence majeure des lots de milieu de Mueller-Hinton sur les CMI de la téicoplanine vis-à-vis des staphyloques à coagulase negative (SCN). 21ème Réunion Interdisciplinaire de Chimiothérapie Anti-Infectieuse (RICAI), Paris, 6-7 Décembre. Résumé 200/C17.

(20) **Mainardi, J.L., D.M. Shlaes, R.V. Goering, J.H. Shlaes, J.F. Acar, and F.W. Goldstein.** 1995. Decreased teicoplanin susceptibility of methicillin-resistant strains of *Staphylococcus aureus*. J. Infect. Dis. **171**:1646-1650.

(21) **Ploy, M.C., C. Grelaud, C. Martin, L. de Lumley, and F. Denis.** 1998. First clinical isolate of vancomycin-intermediate *Staphylococcus aureus* in a French hospital. Lancet **351**:1212.

(22) **Raney, P.M., P.P. Williams, J.E. McGowan, and F.C. Tenover.** 2002. Validation of Vitek version 7.01 software for testing staphylococci against vancomycin. Diagn. Microbiol. Infect. Dis. **43**:135-140.

(23) **Reverdy, M.E., S. Jarraud, S. Bobin-Dubreux, E. Burel, P. Girardo, G. Lina, F. Vandenesc, and J. Etienne.** 2001. Incidence of *Staphylococcus aureus* with reduced susceptibility to glycopeptides in two French hospitals. Clin. Microbiol. Infect. **7**:267-272.

(24) **Saha, B., A.K. Singh, A. Ghosh A, and M. Bal.** 2008. Identification and characterization of a vancomycin-resistant *Staphylococcus aureus* isolated from Kolkata (South Asia). J. Med. Microbiol. **57**:72-79.

(25) **Schwalbe, R.S., J.T. Stapleton, and P.H. Gilligan.** 1987. Emergence of vancomycin resistance in coagulase-negative staphylococci. N. Engl. J. Med. **316**:927-931.

(26) **Smith, J.A., D.A. Henry, A.M. Bourgault, L. Bryan, G.J. Harding, D.J. Hoban, G.B. Horsman, T. Marrie, and P. Turgeon.** 1987. Comparison of agar disk diffusion, microdilution broth, and agar dilution for testing antimicrobial susceptibility of coagulase-negative staphylococci. J. Clin. Microbiol. **29**:1741-1746.

(27) **Stanley, D., B.J. McGrath, K.C. Lamp, and M.J. Rybak.** 1994. Effect of human serum on killing activity of vancomycin and teicoplanin against *Staphylococcus aureus*. Pharmacotherapy **14**:35-39.

(28) **Tenover, F.C., M.J. Mohammed, J. Stelling, T. O'Brien, and R. Williams.** 2001. Ability of laboratories to detect emerging antimicrobial resistance: proficiency testing and quality control results from the World Health Organization's external quality assurance system for antimicrobial susceptibility testing. J. Clin. Microbiol. **39**:241-250.

(29) **Tenover, F.C., L.M. Weigel, P.C. Appelbaum, L.K. McDougal, J. Chaitram, S. McAllister, N. Clark, G. Killgore, C.M. O'Hara, L. Jevitt, J.B. Patel, and B. Bozdogan.** 2004. Vancomycin-resistant *Staphylococcus aureus* isolate from a patient in Pennsylvania. Antimicrob. Agents Chemother. **48**:275-280.

(30) **Voss, A., J.W. Mouton, E.P. van Elzakker, R.G. Hendrix, W. Goessens, J.A. Kluytmans, P.F. Krabbe, H.J. de Neeling, J.H. Sloos, N. Oztoprak, R.A. Howe, and T.R. Walsh.** 2007. A multi-center blinded study on the efficiency of phenotypic screening methods to detect glycopeptide intermediately susceptible *Staphylococcus aureus* (GISA) and heterogeneous GISA (h-GISA). Ann. Clin. Microbiol. Antimicrob.;**6**:9.

(31) **Walsh, T.R., A. Bolmström, A. Qwärnström, P. Ho, M. Wootton, R.A. Howe, A.P. MacGowan, and D. Diekema.** 2001. Evaluation of current methods for

detection of staphylococci with reduced susceptibility to glycopeptides. J. Clin. Microbiol. **39**:2439-2444.

(32) **Wootton, M., R.A. Howe, R. Hillman, T.R. Walsh, P.M. Bennett, and A.P. MacGowan.** 2001. A modified population analysis profile (PAP) method to detect hetero-resistance to vancomycin in *Staphylococcus aureus* in a UK hospital. J. Antimicrob. Chemother. **47**:399-403.

(33) **Wootton, M., A.P. MacGowan, T.R. Walsh, and R.A. Howe**. 2007. A multicenter study evaluating the current strategies for isolating *Staphylococcus aureus* strains with reduced susceptibility to glycopeptides. J. Clin. Microbiol. **45**:329-232.

(34) **Yusof, A., A. Engelhardt, A. Karlsson, L. Bylund, P. Vidh, K. Mills, M. Wootton, and T.R. Walsh**. 2008. Evaluation of a new E-test vancomycin-teicoplanin strip for detection of glycopeptide-intermediate *Staphylococcus aureus* (GISA), in particular, heterogeneous GISA. J. Clin. Microbiol. **46**:3042-3047.

Chapter 21. GLYCOPEPTIDES AND ENTEROCOCCI

Patrice COURVALIN

INTRODUCTION

Only two of the twelve species of *Enterococcus* described are responsible for the majority of infections: *Enterococcus faecalis* which represents 80 to 90% of clinical isolates and *Enterococcus faecium* which represents 5 to 15%. Other species (*E. gallinarum, E. casseliflavus, E. durans, E. avium,* and *E. raffinosus*) are isolated in about 5% of cases. Since the mid-1970s, enterococci have become one of the leading causes of nosocomial infections, at least partly due to the increasing use of third generation cephalosporins to which these bacteria are not susceptible (13). Enterococci present a natural low-level resistance to many antibiotic classes, including β-lactams and aminoglycosides. The treatment of systemic infections due to these bacteria is based on a combination of a cell wall-active antibiotic, a β-lactam or glycopeptide, and an aminoglycoside based on the bactericidal synergy observed both *in vitro* and *in vivo* between these two classes of molecules.

Two glycopeptides, vancomycin and teicoplanin, are used in Europe and only vancomycin is used in the USA. The first glycopeptide-resistant strains of enterococci were isolated in 1986 (10, 19) and have subsequently spread all over the world, especially in the hospital setting. Glycopeptide resistance is frequently part of multidrug resistance for which no treatment options may be available.

MODE OF ACTION

The synthesis of peptidoglycan comprises several steps (Fig. 1). A cytoplasmic racemase converts L-alanine (L-Ala) into D-alanine (D-Ala). Two molecules of D-Ala are then linked by the D-Ala:D-Ala ligase (Ddl) to form the dipeptide D-Ala-D-Ala which is added to UDP-*N*-acetylmuramyl-tripeptide to generate UDP-*N*-acetylmuramyl-pentapeptide. UDP-*N*-acetylmuramyl-pentapeptide is then bound to the undecaprenol lipid carrier, which, after addition of *N*-acetylglucosamine from UDP-*N*-acetylglucosamine, allows the translocation of precursors onto the surface of the cytoplasmic membrane. Incorporation of *N*-acetylmuramyl-pentapeptide into the nascent peptidoglycan by transglycosylation then allows the formation of cross-links by transpeptidation (15).

The structure of glycopeptides comprises a heptapeptide domain in which five amino acids are conserved (15). These antibiotics do not enter the cytoplasm and the interaction with the target can therefore only occur after translocation of the precursors across the bacterial membrane. Glycopeptides bind with high affinity via five hydrogen bonds to the terminal D-Ala-D-Ala of pentapeptide precursors (Fig. 1) thereby blocking the addition of precursors by transglycosylation to the nascent peptidoglycan chain and preventing the subsequent polymerization steps catalysed by D,D-transpeptidases, resulting in cytoplasmic accumulation of precursors.

MECHANISMS OF RESISTANCE

Glycopeptides do not interact with cell wall biosynthesis enzymes, but form complexes with peptidoglycan precursors and prevent their incorporation in the cell wall (Fig. 1). The activity of glycopeptides is therefore not determined by their affinity for target enzymes but by the substrate specificity of the enzymes which determine the structure of peptidoglycan precursors. Glycopeptide resistance is due to the presence of operons which specify enzymes for i) synthesis of low affinity precursors in which the C-terminal D-Ala is replaced by D-lactate (D-Lac) (1) or D-serine (D-Ser) (16) and ii) elimination of high affinity precursors produced for the host bacterium.

Target modification

VanA-type resistance, characterized by high-level, inducible resistance to vancomycin and teicoplanin (Table 1), was the first type of resistance to be described and is the most widespread. The *vanA* operon codes for a dehydrogenase (VanH) which reduces pyruvate to D-Lac and a

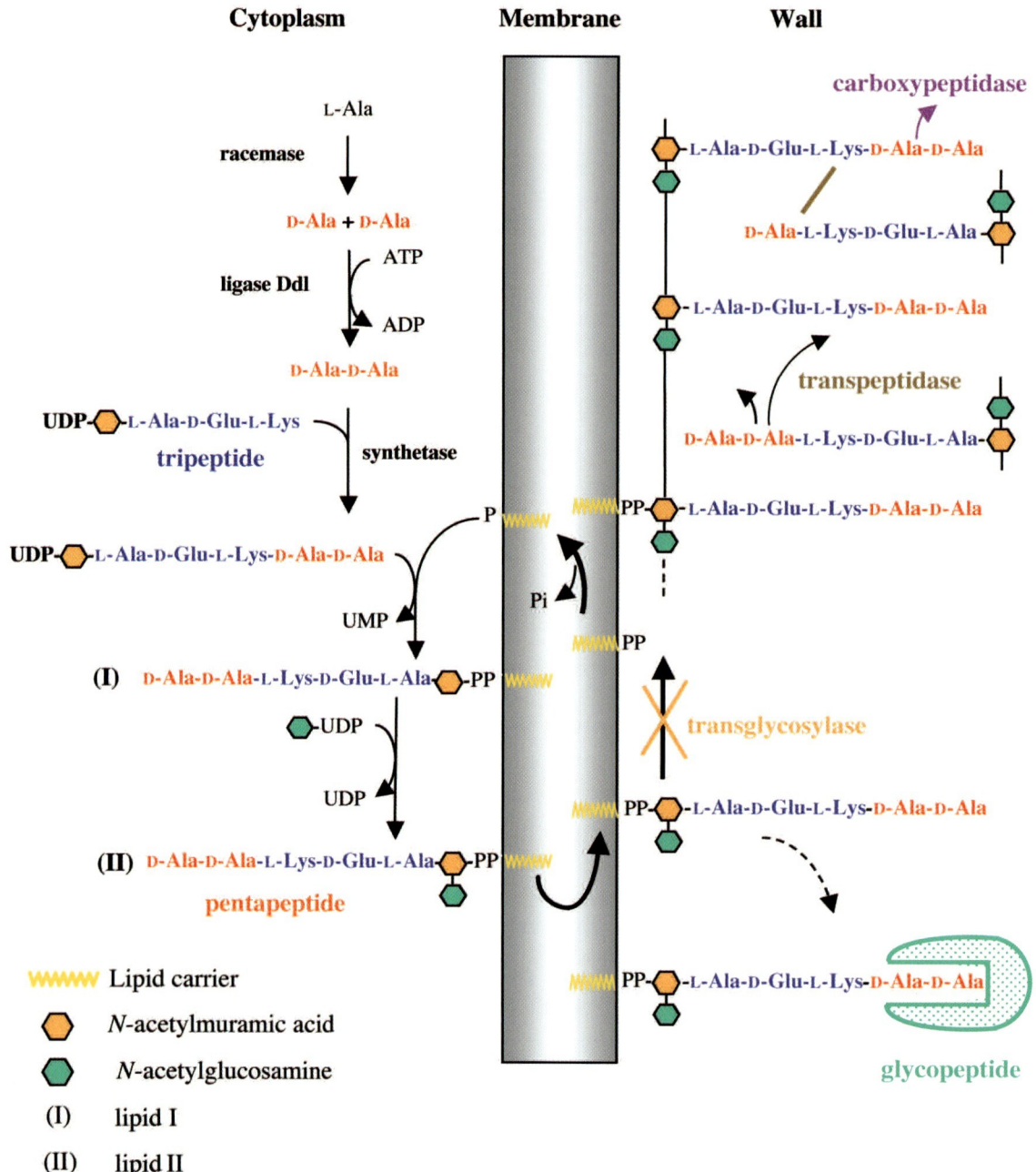

Fig. 1. Peptidoglycan biosynthetic pathway and mechanism of action of vancomycin. The formation of complexes between the antibiotic and the terminal D-ananyl-D-alanine dipeptide in the peptidoglycan precursors prevents the transfer of precursors from the lipid carrier to the peptidoglycan by transglycosylation. The reactions catalyzed by transpeptidases and D,D-carboxypeptidases are also inhibited.

ligase (VanA) which catalyses the formation of an ester bond between D-Ala and D-Lac. The depsipeptide D-Ala-D-Lac replaces the dipeptide D-Ala-D-Ala in the peptidoglycan synthesis pathway. This substitution eliminates a hydrogen bond essential for the binding of antibiotics and considerably reduces the affinity for glycopeptides.

VanC-type glycopeptide resistance is found in *E. gallinarum* and *E. casseliflavus*. Low-level vancomycin resistance but teicoplanin susceptibility is an intrinsic property of these species (Table 1). The *vanC* operon encodes a serine racemase (VanT) which produces D-serine, and a ligase (VanC) which catalyses formation of the

Table 1. Glycopeptide resistance in enterococci

Resistance Level	Acquired						Intrinsic
	High	Variable	Intermediate		Low		Low
Type	VanA	VanB	VanD	VanG	VanE	Van L	VanC1/C2/C3
MIC (µg/ml)							
Vancomycin	64 - 1000	4 - 1000	64 - 128	16	8 - 32	8	2 - 32
Teicoplanin	16 - 512	0.5 - 1	4 - 64	0.5	0.5	0.5	0.5 - 1
Conjugative transfer	+	+	-		+	-	-
Transposon	Tn1546	Tn1547 Tn1549 - Tn5382					
Bacterial species	E. faecium E. faecalis E. gallinarum E. casseliflavus E. avium E. durans E. mundtii E. raffinosus	E. faecium E. faecalis	E. faecium E. faecalis	E. faecalis	E. faecalis	E. faecalis	E. gallinarum E. casseliflavus
Expression	Inducible	Inducible	Constitutive	Inducible	Inducible Constitutive	Inducible	Constitutive Inducible
Location of resistance genes	Plasmid (Chromosome)		Chromosome (Plasmid)	Chromosome	Chromosome		Chromosome
Precursors terminating in:	D-Ala-D-Lac ⇨				D-Ala-D-Ser ⇨		

dipeptide D-Ala-D-Ser. Substitution of the terminal D-Ala-D-Ala by the D-Ala-D-Ser dipeptide in peptidoglycan precursors, leading to a terminal D-Ser in place of a D-Ala residue, results in reduced affinity for vancomycin due to steric hindrance (Fig. 3).

Elimination of the target

Interaction of a glycopeptide with its target is prevented by eliminating precursors with a terminal D-Ala residue. Two enzymes are involved in this process: a D,D-dipeptidase (VanX) which hydrolyses the dipeptide D-Ala-D-Ala synthesized by the host Ddl ligase, and a D,D-carboxypeptidase (VanY) which cleaves the C-terminal D-Ala residue from the precursors when elimination of D-Ala-D-Ala by VanX is incomplete.

As opposed to VanA-type resistance where VanX and VanY activities are encoded by two genes (Fig. 2), VanXY$_C$ possesses both the D,D-peptidase and D,D-carboxypeptidase activities and therefore catalyses hydrolysis of the D-Ala-D-Ala dipeptide and cleavage of the terminal D-Ala residue from the pentapeptide [D-Ala] (Fig. 3).

TYPES OF RESISTANCE

Seven types of glycopeptide-resistant enterococci have been identified on the basis of phenotypic and genotypic criteria (Table 1). Five result from acquired resistance (VanA, VanB, VanD, VanE, VanG, and VanL) and one (VanC) is an intrinsic property of *E. gallinarum* and *E. casseliflavus*. The classification of glycopeptide resistance is now based on the primary sequence of the structural genes encoding the ligases responsible for resistance, rather than on the levels of glycopeptide resistance, in so far as the MIC values of vancomycin and teicoplanin among the various types of resistance show some overlap (Table 1). VanA-type strains have inducible, high-level resistance to vancomycin and teicoplanin while VanB-type strains show inducible and variable resistance to vancomycin only, since teicoplanin is not an inducer (3). In both cases, induction of resistance requires a certain period of time. This explains why rapid automated systems may underestimate vancomycin resistance and the requirement for a full 24-h incubation to detect resistance. Induction of VanD-type strains display constitutive, intermediate-level resistance to both glycopeptides. VanC-, VanE-, VanG-, and VanL-type strains show

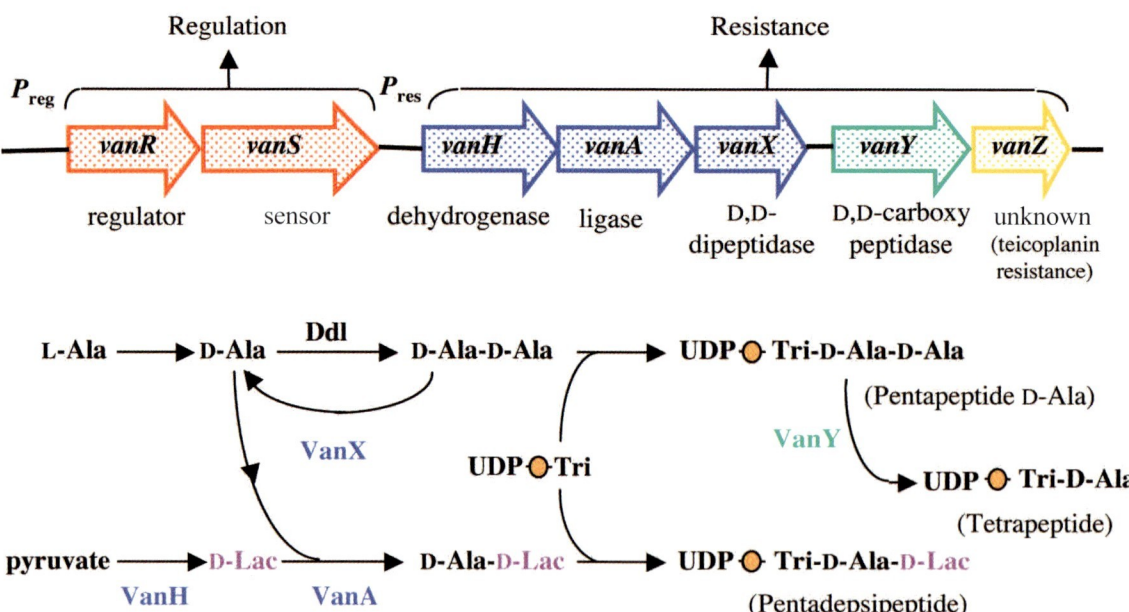

Fig. 2. VanA-type resistance. Top: map of the *vanA* operon. Arrows indicate genes and direction of transcription. Bottom: peptidoglycan precursor synthesis after induction by a glycopeptide. Ddl, D-Ala:D-Ala ligase; ◯-, *N*-acetylmuramic acid; Ala, alanine; Ddl, D-Ala : D-Ala ligase; D, dextrogyre; Lac, lactate; L, levogyre; P_{reg}, promoter for regulatory genes; P_{res}, promoter for resistance genes; Tri, L-Ala-γ-D-Glu-L-Lys.

low-level vancomycin resistance but are susceptible to teicoplanin.

GLYCOPEPTIDE-DEPENDENT STRAINS

Such strains are not only resistant to vancomycin and teicoplanin but also require the presence of these glycopeptides for growth. VanA- or VanB-type *E. faecalis* and *E. faecium* have been isolated from patients receiving prolonged treatment with vancomycin. They harbor a D-Ala:D-Ala ligase (Ddl) which is nonfunctional due to various mutations in the *ddl* gene. Therefore, for cell wall synthesis to occur, they depend entirely on the resistance operon which is only expressed after induction (20). Considering the particular growth requirements of these strains, their prevalence is probably underestimated by routine testing laboratories.

SUSCEPTIBLE PHENOTYPE

Minimum inhibitory concentrations (MIC) of vancomycin and teicoplanin range from 0.25 to 4 μg/ml for *E. faecalis* and *E. faecium* with a modal value of 2 μg/ml. Due to the intrinsic VanC resistance in *E. gallinarum* and *E. casseliflavus*, these species show higher MIC values of vancomycin, ranging from 1 to 16 μg/ml with a modal value of 8 μg/ml for *E. gallinarum* and 4 μg/ml for *E. casseliflavus*.

RESISTANCE PHENOTYPES

The different types of glycopeptide resistance have a dual impact on therapy: they lead to a reduction in the bactericidal activity of glycopeptide antibiotics and they can result in the selection of (more highly) resistant mutants during treatment. These phenomena have mainly been studied in the rabbit endocarditis model (11).

VanA type

In strains with this type of resistance, vancomycin and teicoplanin alone are inactive and their synergy with gentamicin is abolished. These drug combinations are therefore ineffective.

VanB type

This type of resistance is characterized by a reduction in the activity of vancomycin and a loss of synergy with gentamicin and also with streptomycin. On the other hand, teicoplanin alone remains active but, in monotherapy, leads to the

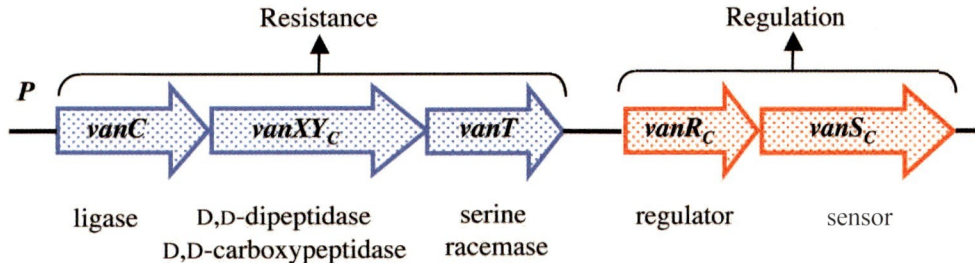

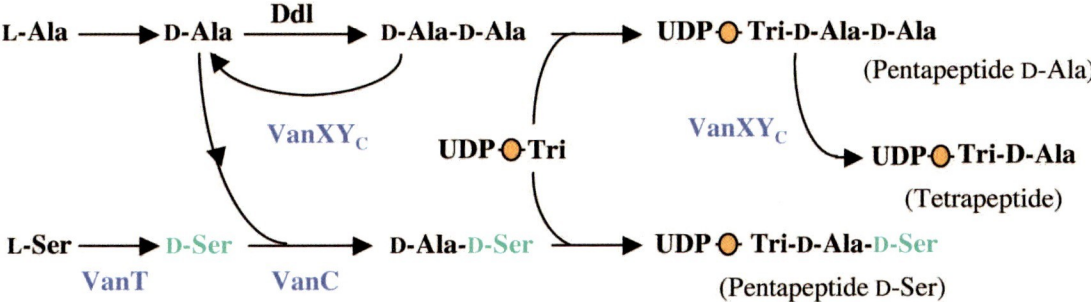

Fig. 3. VanC resistance. Top: map of the *vanC* operon. Arrows indicate genes and direction of transcription. Bottom: peptidoglycan precursor synthesis after induction by vancomycin. O, *N*-acetylmuramic acid; Tri, L-Ala-γ-D-Glu-L-Lys.

selection of mutants with higher resistance to both glycopeptides (3). Such mutants have also been isolated in humans. Combining teicoplanin with gentamicin or streptomycin results in synergistic bactericidal activity and prevents the emergence of resistant mutants, indicating that the teicoplanin-gentamicin combination might be used for infections caused by VanB-type enterococci.

VanC type

Theoretically, this type of resistance should only affect the activity of glycopeptides when the latter are used at suboptimal doses. However, failure of vancomycin treatment in *E. gallinarum* endocarditis has been reported in one study (2). Identification of enterococci with intermediate susceptibility to vancomycin should be carefully checked since commercial galleries have difficulties to differentiate *E. gallinarum* from *E. faecium*.

VanD type

VanD resistance abolishes vancomycin and teicoplanin activity *in vivo* although these strains show susceptibility *in vitro*. Both antibiotics select mutants with high level glycopeptide resistance.

VanE type

As with VanC resistance, which is similar, the activity of vancomycin is reduced against VanE-type strains, particularly when used at suboptimal doses. The use of vancomycin should be discouraged or, if there is no alternative, it should be used at optimal doses, in combination with an aminoglycoside whenever possible.

VanG and VanL types

The impact of these types of resistance on therapy has not yet been studied.

ANTIBIOTICS TO BE STUDIED

The two glycopeptides currently on the market, vancomycin and teicoplanin (in countries where it is available), should be used for antibiotic susceptibility testing. No alternative or additional molecules exist.

PHENOTYPIC DETECTION OF RESISTANCE

CLSI and EUCAST guidelines

The criteria for clinical categorization of both committees are shown in Table 2.

MIC

MIC values of glycopeptides can be determined by dilution in solid or broth medium in the usual conditions. Results should be interpreted after a full 24-hour incubation at 37°C.

Diffusion

Disk diffusion methods show a good correlation with the genotype for VanA-type resistance but not for VanB (Table 3). The E-test correlates well with the reference methods (Table 4) and is therefore a good alternative. Again, plates should

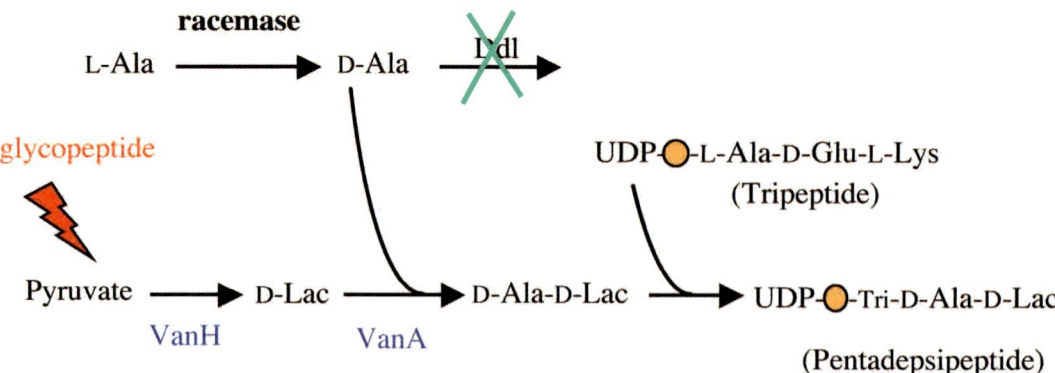

Fig. 4. Peptidoglycan precursor synthesis in a vancomycin-dependent VanA-type strain. Presence of the glycopeptide is required to induce the synthesis of peptidoglycan precursors terminating in D-Ala-D-Lac and allow bacterial growth, ⊙, N-acetylmuramic acid.

Chapter 21. GLYCOPEPTIDES AND ENTEROCOCCI

Table 2. Glycopeptide critical concentrations and diameters (30 µg disks) for Gram-positive cocci

	Critical concentrations (µg/ml)		Critical diameters (mm)	
	Susceptible	Resistant	Susceptible	Resistant
CLSI				
S. aureus				
Vancomycin	≤ 2	≥ 16	-	-
Teicoplanin	≤ 8	≥ 32	≥ 14	≤ 10
Enterococcus				
Vancomycin	≤ 4	≥ 32	≥ 17	≤ 14
Teicoplanin	≤ 8	≥ 32	≥ 14	≤ 10
EUCAST				
Staphylococcus				
Vancomycin	≤ 2	> 8	-	-
Teicoplanin[c]	≤ 2	> 8	-	-
Enterococcus				
Vancomycin	≤ 4	> 8	-	-
Teicoplanin	≤ 4	> 8	-	-

[c] ≤4 >8 for coagulase negative staphylococci.

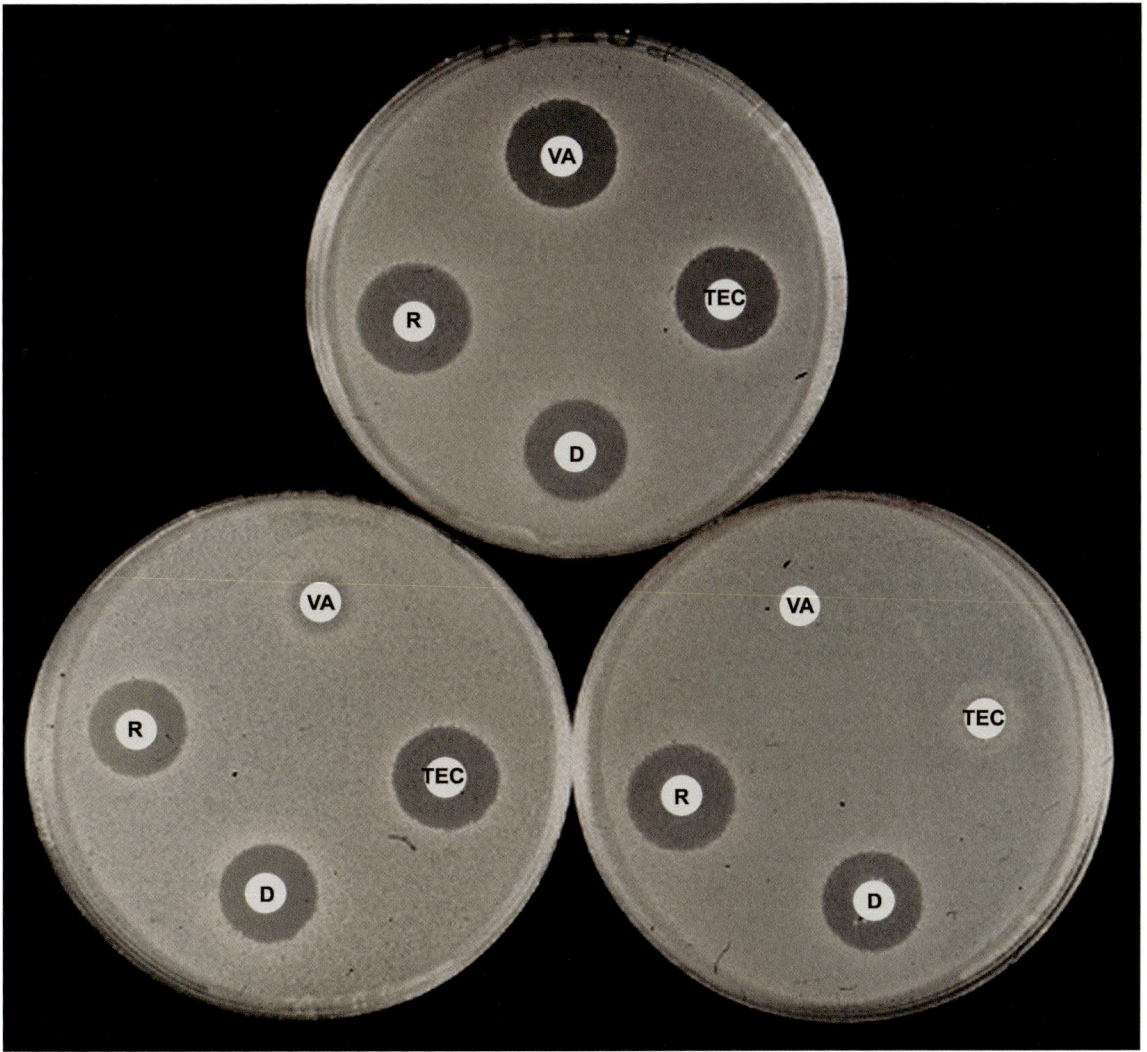

Fig. 5. Study of Van type enterococci by diffusion. Top: VanB-type strain; Bottom right: VanA-type strain; Bottom left: vancomycin-dependent strain. D, daptomycin; R, ramoplanin; Tec, teicoplanin; Va, vancomycin.

Table 3. Detection of glycopeptide resistance in enterococci by diffusion methods and automated systems

System (reference method)		No. of strains	Level of agreement (%)		Reference
			Vancomycin	Teicoplanin	
Diffusion (genotype)	vanA	45	96	93	
	vanB	45	56	100	7
	Susceptible	45	100	96	
API (genotype)	vanA	32	100	100	
	vanB	32	91	94	7
	Susceptible	32	100	100	
VITEK 1 (genotype)	vanA	17	94	88	
	vanB	17	47	100	7
	Susceptible	17	100	100	
Microscan (genotype)	vanA	7	100	100	
	vanB	7	100	100	7
	Susceptible	7	100	100	
VITEK 2 (agar dilution and microdilution)	vanA	57			
	vanB	16	95	97	6
	vanC	26			
	Susceptible	51			
(agar dilution)	vanA	50	100		
	vanB	15	93		
	vanC1	50	88		21
	vanC2	30	93		
	Susceptible	50	100		
(agar dilution)	Resistant	22			
	Intermediate	0	99	91	12
	Susceptible	67			
Phoenix (microdilution)	Resistant	28			
	Intermediate	4	99	99	5
	Susceptible	131			

Table 4. Detection of glycopeptide resistance in enterococci by E-test®

Reference method	No. of strains				Results	Reference
Agar dilution	36 susceptible				100 % agreement	9
	4 resistant				(± 1 dilution)	
Microdilution	25 E. faecium				100 % agreement (± 1 dilution)	16
Agar dilution	MIC (µg/ml)	C.C.[a]	No		100 % agreement	
	< 4	S	14			
	8 - 16	I	14			21
	32 -128	R	8			
	≥ 256	R	6			
Microdilution	vanA 10				0	
	vanB 20				2 minor errors	22
	vanC 10				1	
	Susceptible 10				0	
Microdilution	vanA 11				0	
	vanB 32				0	11
	vanC 20				5 minor errors	
	Susceptible 37				0	
Agar dilution	vanA 50				0	
	vanB 15				13 minor errors	5
	vanC 80				2	

[a] C.C., clinical categorization.

be incubated a full 24 hours for detection of resistance. CLSI recommends examination of inhibition zones using transmitted light: the presence of a haze or of any growth within the zone of inhibition indicates resistance. MIC should be determined for organisms with intermediate zones.

Automated systems

Table 3 presents the behavior of automated systems with respect to genotype or to reference methods. The degree of correlation varies according to the system, particularly for the oldest automats, although there has been some improvement over time as new expert systems and instruments are developed.

CLSI screening

The CLSI recommends the following method for vancomycin-resistance screening in enterococci:

Medium: brain-heart infusion agar
Antibiotic concentration: 6 µg/ml
Inoculum: 1-10 µl of broth or colony suspension adjusted to obtain a turbidity equivalent to 0.5 McFarland standard.
Incubation: 35°C in ambient atmosphere for 24 h.
Interpretation of results: growth of > 1 colony indicates resistance.

CONCLUSION

Glycopeptide antibiotics, alone or in combination with aminoglycosides, are often the only treatment option for infections caused by multi-resistant enterococci. The prevalence of glycopeptide-resistant enterococci has been on a sharp rise and, over the past few decades, enterococci have become a leading cause of nosocomial infections and serve as reservoirs of resistance genes. The transfer of glycopeptide resistance to more highly pathogenic organisms such as *Staphylococcus aureus* has already occurred. For all of these various reasons, the detection of glycopeptide resistance in Gram-positive bacteria should be carried out under optimal technical conditions.

REFERENCES

(1) **Arthur, M., P. Reynolds, and P. Courvalin.** 1996. Glycopeptide resistance in enterococci. Trends Microbiol. **4**:401-407.

(2) **Dargere, S., M. Vergnaud, R. Verdon, E. Saloux, O. Le Page, R. Leclercq, and C. Bazin.** 2002. *Enterococcus gallinarum* endocarditis occurring on native heart valves. J. Clin. Microbiol. **40**:2308-2310.

(3) **Depardieu, F., I. Podglajen, R. Leclercq, E. Collatz, and P. Courvalin.** 2007. Modes and modulations of antibiotic resistance gene expression. Clin. Microbiol. Rev. **20**:79-114.

(4) **Endtz, H.P., N. Van Den Braak, A. Van Belkum, W. H. Goessens, D. Kreft, A. Barnard Stroebel, and H.A. Verbrugh.** 1998. Comparison of eight methods to detect vancomycin resistance in enterococci. J. Clin. Microbiol. 1998. **36**:592-594.

(5) **Fahr, A.M., U. Eigner, M. Armbrust, A. Caganic, G. Dettori, C. Chezzi, L. Bertoncini, M. Benecchi, and M.G. Menozzi.** 2003. Two-center collaborative evaluation of the performance of the BD Phoenix automated microbiology system for identification and antimicrobial susceptibility testing of *Enterococcus* spp. and *Staphylococcus* spp. J. Clin. Microbiol. **41**:1135-1142.

(6) **Garcia-Garrote, F., E. Cercenado, and E. Bouza.** 2000. Evaluation of a new system, VITEK 2, for identification and antimicrobial susceptibility testing of enterococci. J. Clin. Microbiol. **38**:2108-2111.

(7) **Gazagne, L., P. Pina, A. Boisivon, H. Chardon, P. Allouch, B. Pangon, et al. B.V.H.** 1998. Antibiogramme des entérocoques : résultats d'un contrôle de qualité. 5ème Congrès Société Française de Microbiologie. Lille, France. Abstract No. 14.

(8) **Huang, M.B., C.N. Baker, S. Banerjee, and F.C. Tenover.** 1992. Accuracy of the E test for determining antimicrobial susceptibilities of staphylococci, enterococci, *Campylobacteur jejuni*, and Gram-negative bacteria resistant to antimicrobial agents. J. Clin. Microbiol. **30**:3243-3248.

(9) **Kohner, P.C., R. Patel, J.R. Uhl, K.M. Garin, M.K. Hopkins, L.T. Wegener, and F.R. Cockerill.** 1997. Comparison of agar dilution, broth microdilution, E-test, disk diffusion, and automated Vitek methods for testing susceptibilities of *Enterococcus* spp. to vancomycin. J. Clin. Microbiol. **35**:3258-3263.

(10) **Leclercq, R., E. Derlot, J. Duval, and P. Courvalin.** 1988. Plasmid-mediated resistance to vancomycin and teicoplanin in *Enterococcus faecium*. N. Engl. J. Med. **319**:157-161.

(11) **Lefort, A., M. Baptista, B. Fantin, F. Depardieu, M. Arthur, C. Carbon, and P. Courvalin.** 1999. Two-step acquisition of resistance to the teicoplanin-gentamicin combination by VanB-type *Enterococcus faecalis* in vitro and in experimental endocarditis. Antimicrob Agents Chemother. **43**:476-482.

(12) **Ligozzi, M., C. Bernini, M.G. Bonora, M. de Fatima, J. Zuliani, and R. Fontana.** 2002. Evaluation of the VITEK 2 system for identification and antimicrobial susceptibility testing of medically relevant gram-positive cocci. J. Clin. Microbiol. **40**:1681-1686.

(13) **Low, D. E., N. Keller, A. Barth, and R. N. Jones.** 2001. Clinical prevalence, antimicrobial susceptibility, and geographic resistance patterns of enterococci: results from the SENTRY Antimicrobial Surveillance Program, 1997-1999. Clin. Infect. Dis. **32 Suppl 2**:S133-145.

(14) **Ngui-Yen, J.H., E.A. Bryce, C. Porter, and J.A. Smith.** 1992. Evaluation of the E test by using selec-

ted Gram-positive bacteria. J. Clin. Microbiol. **30**:2150-2152.
(15) **Reynolds, P. E.** 1989. Structure, biochemistry and mechanism of action of glycopeptide antibiotics. Eur. J. Clin. Microbiol. Infect. Dis. **8**:943-950.
(16) **Reynolds, P.E., and P. Courvalin.** 2005. Vancomycin resistance in enterococci due to synthesis of precursors terminating in D-alanyl-D-serine. Antimicrob. Agents Chemother. **49**:21-25.
(17) **Schulz, J.E., and D.F. Sahm**. 1993. Reliability of the E test for detection of ampicillin, vancomycin, and high-level aminoglycoside resistance in *Enterococcus* spp. J. Clin. Microbiol. **31**:3336-3339.
(18) **Tenover, F.C., J.M. Swenson, C.M. O'Hara, and S.A. Stocker**. 1995. Ability of commercial and reference antimicrobial susceptibility testing methods to detect vancomycin resistance in enterococci. J. Clin. Microbiol. **33**:1524-1527.
(19) **Uttley, A.H., C.H. Collins, J. Naidoo, and R.C. Georges**. 1988. Vancomycin resistant enterococci. Lancet **i**:57-58.
(20) **Van Bambeke, F., M. Chauvel, P.E. Reynolds, H.S. Fraimow, and P. Courvalin**. 1999. Vancomycin-dependent *Enterococcus faecalis* clinical isolates and revertant mutants. Antimicrob Agents Chemother. **43**:41-47.
(21) **Van Den Braak, N., W. Goessens, A. Van Belkum, H. A. Verbrugh, and H. P. Endtz**. 2001. Accuracy of the Vitek 2 system to detect glycopeptide resistance in enterococci. J. Clin. Microbiol. **39**:351-353.

Chapter 22. LIPOPEPTIDES, LIPOGLYCOPEPTIDES, AND GLYCOLIPODEPSIPEPTIDES

Henry S. FRAIMOW

INTRODUCTION

The emergence and spread of highly resistant organisms including methicillin resistant *S. aureus* (MRSA), glycopeptide-resistant enterococci (GRE), glycopeptide-intermediately-resistant *S. aureus* (GISA) and vancomycin-resistant *S. aureus* (VRSA) during the 1990's has spurred the development of several novel classes of antimicrobial agents specifically targeting resistant Gram-positive pathogens. Among these novel classes are the lipopeptides, lipoglycopeptides, and glycolipodepsipeptides. The lipopeptide daptomycin and the lipodepsipeptide ramoplanin are each members of novel drug classes with mechanisms of activity distinct from currently available agents and with little or no evidence of cross-resistance. The newer lipoglycopeptides in advanced stage development include dalbavancin, oritavancin, and telavancin. These all contain synthetic modifications of the basic glycopeptide structure, but result in agents with sufficiently distinct pharmacokinetics, mechanisms of activity and/or resistance profiles as to be considered separately from the older glycopeptides vancomycin and teicoplanin discussed in Chapters 20 and 21.

LIPOPEPTIDES: DAPTOMYCIN

Daptomycin (Fig. 1) is a member of the 10-member cyclic lipopeptide family of antibiotics and is a semi-synthetic derivative of a natural product of *Streptomyces roseosporus*. Features of the structure include a 13-amino acid peptide portion, 10 amino acids of which comprise the cyclic portion of the molecule, and a C_{10} fatty acid tail. Daptomycin has broad *in vitro* activity against a wide variety of Gram-positive organisms including anaerobic bacteria, but has no activity against Gram-negative organisms. Daptomycin was initially developed in the 1970's and first introduced into clinical trials in the 1980's by Eli Lilly and Co. The development of daptomycin as a potential therapeutic agent for MRSA and GRE was revitalized a decade later after acquisition of the drug by Cubist Pharmaceuticals, Inc. Daptomycin was initially approved in the US in 2003 for treatment of *S. aureus* infections, and in Europe in 2006 for treatment of skin and soft tissue infections. Approved indications have subsequently been expanded as additional trials have been completed.

Mechanisms of action

Daptomycin exhibits rapid bactericidal activity against methicillin-susceptible and methicillin-resistant staphylococci including most glycopeptide-resistant strains, and is also active against enterococci including GRE. The proposed mechanism of activity involves binding of daptomycin to and disruption of the bacterial cytoplasmic membrane, resulting in membrane depolarization and ultimately in cell death (5). Activity first requires binding of the anionic daptomycin molecule to calcium and formation of a daptomycin-calcium complex. Thus, *in vivo* activity is dependent on serum calcium, and optimized calcium concentrations are a critical variable in the performance of *in vitro* susceptibility testing. The cationically charged calcium-daptomycin complex functions essentially as a cationic antimicrobial peptide at the level of the bacterial cell membrane. However, evidence from transcriptional profiling of daptomycin exposed cells and from electron microscopy images suggests that some of daptomycin's mechanism of lethality may also be due to direct cell wall synthesis inhibition (18).

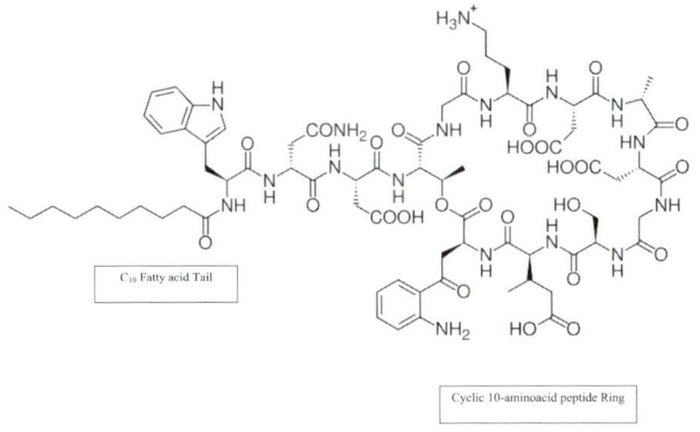

Fig. 1. Structure of Daptomycin

Mechanisms of resistance

Current understanding of the specific mechanisms of resistance to daptomycin remains incomplete. Spontaneous daptomycin resistant mutants are extremely difficult to select *in vitro*, (frequency $< 1 \times 10^{-10}$) but can be generated more easily with serial passaging in sub-inhibitory daptomycin concentrations (5, 13). Several studies have looked for specific mutations in laboratory-generated resistant mutants as well as in strains with higher daptomycin MICs isolated from patients failing daptomycin therapy. In staphylococci, attention has been focused particularly on mutations in three classes of genes: those important in regulation of cell-surface charge such as *mprF*, those associated with fatty acid biosynthesis such as *yyfG*, and on the *rpoB* and *rpoC* RNA polymerases. Functional alteration in each of these genes has been observed in laboratory-generated resistant strains, although some of these may be hyperfuctioning rather than deletion mutants (13). Mutations in *mprF*, which is involved in phospholipid production and insertion into the lipid membrane, appear to be the most common early mutations that develop in the course of serial passaging of strains *in vitro*. However, there is as yet no single mutation or collection of mutations that reliably predicts decreased susceptibility to daptomycin. Mutations also differ between clinical and laboratory-generated resistant strains, and some resistant strains have had none of the above described mutations. In the absence of any clearly defined genetic mutations that correlate highly with daptomycin resistance, there are no simple genotypic screens to aid in detection of daptomycin resistance though several studies have used PCR methods to amplify and sequence these proposed "resistance" genes. At the cellular level, acquired daptomycin resistance is usually associated with distinct changes in membrane fluidity and membrane surface charge as well as decreased daptomycin binding by the bacterial cell membrane and decreased daptomycin-induced membrane depolarization (16). However, none of these reported phenotypic changes are traits that are readily adaptable to simple screening methods. Techniques for measurement of membrane potential using flow cytometry and for assessment of membrane fluidity in daptomycin-resistant strains have been described (16). Daptomycin resistance in clinical isolates of *E. faecium* and *E. faecalis* is even less well characterized than in *S. aureus*, but in several isolates studied has not been associated with mutations in homologues of the proposed staphylococcal daptomycin "resistance" genes (17). *Bacillus subtilis* has also been used as a model for assessing the genetics of daptomycin resistance. Daptomycin inactivation by soil bacteria can occur *in vitro*, but this mechanism has not been observed in clinical resistant isolates.

The risk of emergence of resistance to daptomycin in treated patients remains poorly quantified, but higher risk has been associated with prolonged usage in patients with a variety of co-morbidities (5). Most of the available information on emergence of resistance comes from use of daptomycin as salvage therapy or in difficult to eradicate infections such as complicated bacteremia, endocarditis, and osteomyelitis. In one study 6 of 67 patients treated for persistent *S. aureus* bacteremia relapsed and had *S. aureus* isolates with daptomycin MICs of 2 µg/ml. In another randomized trial of *S. aureus* bacteremia and endocarditis, post treatment isolates with increased daptomycin resistance (MIC > 1 µg/ml) were found in 5.8% of 120 patients (5). The primary clinical implication of these findings is that serial isolates from patients with persistent bacteremia or other non-eradicated foci must be monitored for evolution of decreased susceptibility to daptomycin. A linkage between decreased glycopeptide susceptibility and decreased daptomycin susceptibility has been observed in clinical isolates and laboratory mutants, but the clinical relevance and specific mechanisms underlying this linkage remain uncertain (5). Glycopeptide exposure and resulting increased glycopeptide MIC's in staphylococci are associated with induction and expression of numerous stress response pathways and result in a wide array of phenotypic changes in the bacterial cell wall and membrane, and some of these global responses may also have a role in mediating resistance to daptomycin. Current understanding of prevalence and mechanisms of daptomycin resistance are summarized in Table 1.

Susceptibility breakpoints and reporting of non-susceptible isolates

The FDA and the Clinical Laboratory Standards Institute (CLSI) have established concordant criteria for testing and reporting of daptomycin susceptibility for *S. aureus*, ß–hemolytic streptococci and *E. faecalis* (7, 8). Currently isolates are reported as susceptible or non-susceptible only, as there are as yet no CLSI defined breakpoints for either intermediate or resistant categories for these organisms. *S. aureus* and ß-hemolytic streptococci with MIC's of ≤ 1 µg/ml and *E. faecalis* isolates with MIC's of ≤ 4 µg/ml

Table 1. Clinical and laboratory features of daptomycin resistance

Organism	Resistant phenotype (µg/ml)	Selection of resistance in vitro	Frequency of resistance in vivo	Genetic Associations	Physiologic changes associated with resistant in clinical or laboratory strains
S. aureus	> 1 µg/ml Some strains heteroresistant	Spontaneous resistant mutants: <10^{-10} Selectable by serial passaging	Prevalence in resistance surveys: < 0.1% Resistance more common in GISA including de novo resistance: > 50%? Emergence on therapy: multiple reports	mprF yycG rpoB rpoC Other/ unknown	Enhanced membrane fluidity Increase in synthesis of phospholipid lysylphosphotidylglycerol and translocation to the outer membrane leaflet Increased expression of mprF and dlt operons Increased net positive surface charge Lower surface binding of daptomycin Resistance to daptomycin-induced depolarization and autolysis Cross resistance to cationic antimicrobial host defense peptides Increased cell wall thickness Loss of 81 kd membrane protein
E. faecium E. faecalis E. durans	> 4 µg/ml (usually > 12 µg/ml)	Spontaneous resistant mutants: < 10^{-9} Selectable by serial passaging	Prevalence in resistance surveys: < 0.2% Emergence on therapy: multiple case reports De novo resistance reported	unknown	Not reported

are reported as susceptible. Interpretive criteria are not yet established for other Gram-positive organisms including *S. pneumoniae*, *E. faecium* and other enterococci, or for the coagulase negative staphylococci. EUCAST provides organism specific daptomycin breakpoints of ≤ 1 µg/ml for susceptibility reporting of staphylococci and ß-hemolytic streptococci, but has not yet established susceptibility breakpoints for *Enterococcus* species (11). The epidemiologic cut-off values for *E. faecium* and *E. faecalis* from the EUCAST database, each derived from more than 10,000 isolates, are both 4 µg/ml. The mean MIC's for *E. faecium* are approximately one dilution higher than for *E. faecalis* (11). The CLSI currently includes daptomycin in Test Group B for reporting purposes for staphylococci and enterococci, and recommends that any isolate that tests as non-susceptible in a clinical laboratory be saved for confirmation of results in a reference laboratory using the reference broth microdilution method (8). Daptomycin susceptibility ranges for common Gram-positive organisms are shown in Table 2.

Methods

Daptomycin susceptibility testing is complicated by the requirement for standardized calcium supplementation of test medium to produce concentrations that mimic physiologic levels. A practical limitation to this is the lack of optimal standardization of calcium in agar and broth formulations of commercial media, which results in variability of calcium concentrations between different formulations of media, different brands, and even batches of media. Daptomycin also diffuses poorly in agar, and the combination of poor diffusion and difficulty of standardizing calcium has severely hindered development of agar based test methods. Thus there is no approved disk diffusion method for daptomycin, and agar dilution methods are also not recommended (7, 8). Currently approved daptomycin test methods include E-test®, commercially prepared broth micro dilution test panels employing Mueller-Hinton broth and a standardized calcium concentration of 50 µg/ml, and some (but not all) of the major automated susceptibility test systems (9). The daptomycin E-test® (AB Biodisk) overcomes the calcium problem by providing a unique test strip configuration that includes a daptomycin gradient strip overlaid with a constant concentration of Ca^{+2}, designed to achieve a constant Ca^{+2} concentration of 40 µg/ml. This permits use of the E-test® strips on standard commercial Mueller-Hinton agar

Table 2. *In vitro* activity of daptomycin against representative clinical isolates of important Gram-positive bacteria (Data from reference 11 except as noted by*, other data from multiple published studies)

Organism	Range	MIC$_{50}$ (µg/ml)	MIC$_{90}$ (µg/ml)	%Susceptible or below epidemiologic cutoff	Breakpoint (epidemiologic cutoff)
S. aureus (n = 35965)	0.64 – 2	0.25	0.5	99.97	1 (1)
MRSA* (n=1247)	<0.12-1	0.25	0.5	100	1 (1)
hGISA* (n=88)	0.25-1	0.5	1	100	1 (1)
GISA* (n=17)	0.5-4	1	4	47	1 (1)
GISA* (n=70)	Up to ≥ 2	≥ 2	≥ 2	16	1 (1)
VRSA* (n= 5)	≤ 1	-	-	100	1 (1)
Coagulase negative staphylococci (n = 9059)	0.64 – 2	0.25	0.5	99.9	1 (1)
Methicillin-resistant* (n=699)	<0.12-2	0.25	0.5	99.9	1 (1)
E. faecalis (n = 9695)	0.125 – 8	1	2	99.97	4 (4)
E. faecium (n = 12497)	0.64 – 8	2	2	99.8	- (4)
GREF* (n = 55)	0.5-4	2	4	100	- (4)
S. pneumoniae (n = 8108)	0.032 – 1	0.125	0.25	99.7	- (0.5)
S. pyogenes (n = 982)	0.016 – 0.25	0.064	0.064	100	1 (0.25)
S. agalactine (n = 1860)	0.016 – 1	0.125	0.25	100	1 (0.5)
Viridans group *Streptococcus* (n = 987)	0.032 – 4	0.5	1	99	- (1)
Listeria monocytogenes (n = 78)	0.25 – 4	2	4	100	- (4)
Clostridium difficile (n = 206)	0.032 – 4	1	2	–	–

plates. Due to variability of calcium concentrations even between different brands of standard Mueller-Hinton plates, only BBL Mueller-Hinton agar plates are recommended. For performing broth microdilution MIC's, pre-prepared lyophilized and frozen daptomycin MIC panels are currently available from Trek Diagnostic Systems and PML Microbiologicals. Automated susceptibility panels that incorporate daptomycin and have FDA approval include Sensititre® (Trek Diagnostic Systems), Phoenix™ (BD Diagnostic Systems), and MicroScan® (Dade Behring). Efforts to incorporate daptomycin into Vitek®2 panels (bioMérieux) are in progress (9). When preparing daptomycin stock solutions for susceptibility testing, the antibiotic should be dissolved and diluted in sterile water (8).

LIPOGLYCOPEPTIDES: ORITAVANCIN, TELAVANCIN, AND DALBAVANCIN

Recent development of the glycopeptide class of antimicrobials has focused on semi-synthetic derivatives with hydrophobic side chains on the 4th sugar moiety of the heptapeptide structure. A lipid side-chain is also a feature of the older glycopeptide teicoplanin. The presence of the hydrophobic side chain is postulated to facilitate anchoring of the glycopeptide in the cellular membrane and may also affect dimerization of the glycopeptide molecule, both of which are proposed to be important in facilitating interactions between glycopeptides and peptidoglycan precursors (20). However, these agents may be much more rapidly bactericidal than the older glycopeptides vancomycin and teicoplanin, and may maintain activity even against glycopeptide-resistant organisms, suggesting that there are additional, incompletely understood mechanisms of activity for these newer agents. Three lipoglycopeptides are in advanced stages of clinical development including the vancomycin-like derivatives oritavancin and telavancin, and dalbavancin, a semi-synthetic derivative of the teicoplanin-like glycopeptide MDL 62476 (20).

Oritavancin

Oritavancin (formerly LY333328) is a semi-synthetic derivative of the naturally occurring vancomycin-like glycopeptide chloroeremomycin and was initially discovered by Eli Lilly and Co. but is now being developed by the Medicines Company.

Oritavancin possesses potent, rapidly bactericidal activity against a broad range of Gram-positive organisms including drug-resistant pathogens. Oritavancin has activity similar to or better than vancomycin against staphylococci but is active against most GISA strains, and demonstrates enhanced activity against enterococci compared to vancomycin and teicoplanin and is active against most GRE strains including VanA-type strains. Oritavancin is currently under review by the FDA and EMEA.

Mechanisms of action and resistance

Oritavancin differs from older glycopeptides in that it is rapidly, rather than slowly, bactericidal against staphylococci *in vitro*. The rapid cidal action (1/2 to 2 h *in vitro* compared to 24 h for vancomycin) is postulated to result from the activity of oritavancin against the bacterial cell membrane in addition to the typical glycopeptide cell wall synthesis inhibitory effects (2). Oritavancin exposure in staphylococci results in disruption of membrane potential and increased bacterial cell permeability, and ultrastructural studies show distortion of the cell septum in oritavancin-treated staphylococci and enterococci (2). Oritavancin also causes inhibition of RNA synthesis, but the importance of this is unclear (2). Unlike older glycopeptides and other drugs primarily targeting the cell wall, oritavancin maintains bactericidal activity against staphylococci in stationary growth phase as well as in biofilms, which may be related to it's membrane-disrupting mode of action.

MIC's of oritavancin reported in the literature for staphylococci are similar to those of vancomycin for both methicillin-susceptible and methicillin-resistant *S. aureus* and for coagulase negative staphylococci, though many published studies may have significantly underestimated the potency of oritavancin due to recently identified methodological issues (1). Oritavancin is also more active than vancomycin against most GISA strains. This drug is much more bactericidal than vancomycin against staphylococci, as oritavancin MBC's are only 1 to 8 fold higher than the corresponding MICs. Oritavancin also has enhanced activity against both vancomycin-susceptible and vancomycin-resistant enterococci, including VanA-, VanB-, and VanC-type strains, with MIC's of ≤ 1 µg/ml, and is bactericidal against most strains, though not as rapidly bactericidal as against staphylococci. Spontaneous oritavancin resistance or emergence of resistance to oritavancin has not been reported in serially passaged *S. aureus* isolates, including GISA. However, selection of low level resistant VanA- and VanB-type strains with MIC's of 8-16 µg/ml has occurred *in vitro* and in animal endocarditis models. Oritavancin-resistant mutants were selectable from *vanA* and *vanB* strains at a frequency of 1×10^{-7}. Spontaneous low level oritavancin resistance was also observed in laboratory constructs with mutations in one of several genes in the *van* cluster or mutations in the host D-Ala: D-Ala ligase (3).

In vitro susceptibility testing

Susceptibility breakpoints for oritavancin against staphylococci and enterococci have not yet been established by CLSI or EUCLAST. The standard reference method for oritavancin susceptibility testing is broth microdilution MIC (7, 8). However, current CLSI standards incorporate recent observations that addition of the surfactant polysorbate-80 is necessary for optimal determination of broth dilution MICs for staphylococci and enterococci (8). This is presumed to be due to significant binding of oritavancin to plastic and glass, which is eliminated with addition of the surfactant. The effect of polysorbate-80 is not seen in susceptibility testing with the older glycopeptides

Table 3. Effects of 0.002% polysorbate-80 on oritavancin MICs for important Gram-positive organisms[a]

Organism	Oritavancin MIC (range, µg/ml)	Oritavancin + Polysorbate-80 MIC (range, µg/ml)	Ratio of MIC90 without/with polysorbate-80
S. aureus (n = 76)	1 – 8	0.015 – 0.25	32
CoNS[b] (n = 26)	0.12 – 8	0.015 – 0.25	16
E. faecalis (n = 70)	0.12 – 8	0.008 – 0.5	16
E. faecium (n = 30)	0.12 – 4	0.004 – 0.5	16
S. pneumoniae (n =19)	0.00025 – 0.004	0.0005 – 0.004	1
S. pyogenes (n = 29)	0.015 – 0.5	0.015 – 0.5	1

[a] From reference 1.
[b] Coagulase negative staphylococci.

vancomycin and teicoplanin. Addition of polysorbate-80 does not change oritavancin susceptibility results for streptococci when testing is performed in 2% lysed horse blood. All of the older published susceptibility data for oritavancin was generated without polysorbate-80 supplementation, so these data must be reinterpreted in view of these new observations. As shown in Table 3, MICs for staphylococci and enterococci obtained when polysorbate-80 is present (at a final concentration of 0.002%) throughout all phases of the testing, including preparation of drug stocks, are 16-32 fold lower than corresponding MIC's without any polysorbate-80 supplementation (1). Recent testing performed according to the new standards with polysorbate-80 supplementation indicates that MIC's of oritavancin are 0.015-0.25 µg/ml for *S. aureus* and ≤ 0.5 µg/ml for coagulase negative staphylococci, and will be in the range of 0.004 to 0.5 µg/ml for *E. faecium* and *E. faecalis* (Table 4). There are no approved agar dilution, disk diffusion, or E-test® methods currently available for oritavancin, and these methods may be difficult to develop due oritavancin's poor diffusion in agar. Oritavancin stocks and dilutions should be prepared in 0.002% polysorbate-80 in water (8).

Telavancin

Telavancin is a semi-synthetic derivative of vancomycin containing a hydrophobic decyclaminoethyl side chain on the vancosamine sugar, as well as a negatively charged phosphonomethyl aminomethyl substituent on the 4' position of amino acid 7 of the cyclic peptide core (20). Similar to oritavancin, telavancin demonstrates enhanced cidality against staphylococci and enterococci compared to older glycopeptides, and it is active against many glycopeptide-resistant strains. Telavancin is currently being developed by Theravance, Inc. Phase III clinical trials have been completed for treatment of skin and soft tissue infections as well as for more complicated infections including nosocomial pneumonia. Telavancin was approved in September 2009 by the FDA for treatment of skin and soft tissue infection. Telavancin was recently withdrawn from consideration by the EMEA for approval for skin and soft tissue infection, pending completion of additional clinical trials.

Mechanisms of action and resistance

Like other glycopeptides, telavancin causes disruption of cell wall synthesis by binding to D-Ala-D-Ala-containing peptidoglycan precursors, but is approximately 10-fold more potent as a cell wall synthesis inhibitor than vancomycin (15). Similar to oritavancin, telavancin also demonstrates effects on the bacterial cell membrane that likely contribute to telavancin's rapidly cidal mode of action. Effects of telavancin on MRSA membranes include concentration-dependent, rapid depolarization of the membrane, increased permeability, and leakage of K^+ and ATP (15). The membrane effects of telavancin appear to be different from the membrane actions of cationic peptides such as daptomycin. Telavancin has potent bactericidal activity against a broad array of Gram-positive pathogens comprising methicillin-susceptible and methicillin-resistant *S. aureus* including most GISA strains, as well as coagulase negative staphylococci, streptococci, and *S. pneumonia*. Telavancin is active against vancomycin-susceptible and VanB-type *E. faecalis* and *E. faecium*, but its MIC's are increased for VanA type vancomycin-resistant enterococci. Telavancin is also active against *Corynebacterium* and anaerobic Gram-positive organisms, including *C. difficile*. In resistance selection studies, no spontaneous telavancin-resistant mutants of *S. aureus*, coagulase negative staphylococci or vancomycin-susceptible enterococci were detected at inoculums of up to 10^{10} to 10^{11} cells; after serial passage, resistant derivatives were selectable only from a VanA-type GRE strain (19). Little additional information on telavancin resistance has been reported

In vitro susceptibility testing

The reference standard for *in vitro* susceptibility testing of telavancin is broth microdilution although disk diffusion can also be used. Telavancin stock solutions are prepared in DMSO with water as the diluent (8). Unlike for the other new lipoglycopeptides oritavancin and dalbavancin, there is no requirement for addition of polysorbate-80 or other surfactants to test media. The FDA has established susceptibility interpretive criteria for telavancin. *S. aureus* (including MRSA) and vancomycin-susceptible *E. faecalis* isolates with MIC's of ≤ 1 µg/ml are considered susceptible (21). Susceptibility breakpoints are ≤ 0.12 µg/ml for *S. pyogenes*, *S. agalactiae* and the *S. angiosus* group (21). Isolates are to be categorized as susceptible or non-susceptible only. Telavancin susceptibility breakpoints have not yet been established by CLSI or EUCLAST. Recent susceptibility surveys of large collections of *S. aureus* isolates from the US and Europe found that

Table 4. Comparison of MICs (μg/ml) of lipoglycopeptides oritavancin, telavancin and dalbavancin with vancomycin against Gram-positive organisms (from references 1,4,10,19,20)

Organism	Vancomycin[a] MIC	Vancomycin[a] MIC$_{90}$	Oritavancin[b] MIC	Oritavancin[b] MIC$_{90}$	Telavancin MIC	Telavancin MIC$_{90}$	Dalbavancin MIC	Dalbavancin MIC$_{90}$
S. aureus								
Methicillin-susceptible	≤0.12-4	1	0.015-0.25	0.12	0.03-1	0.25	≤0.03-0.25	0.06
MRSA	0.5-4	1-2	0.015-0.5	0.25	0.06-1	0.25	≤0.03-0.5	0.06
GISA	4-8	8	≤1	-	0.125-1	1	0.06-16	1-2
VRSA	32->128	>128	≤1	-	2-4	-	-	-
CoNS								
Methicillin-susceptible	≤0.12-4	2	0.008-1	0.25	0.06-1	0.5	≤0.03-1	0.06
Methicillin-resistant	≤0.12-8	2	≤0.004-1	0.25	0.12-1	1	≤0.03-2	0.12
Enterococcus faecalis								
Vancomycin-susceptible	<0.5-4	2	0.008-0.5	0.12	0.12-1	0.5	≤0.03-0.5	0.06
Vancomycin-resistant								
VanA	128->512	>512	-	-	4-32	16	≤0.03->4	>4
VanB	32-256	128	-	-	0.25-1	1	-	-
Enterococcus faecium								
Vancomycin susceptible	≤0.5-4	1	0.004-0.5	0.25	≤0.015-0.5	0.25	≤0.03-2	0.12
Vancomycin resistant								
VanA	64->512	>512	0.004-0.5[c]	-	2-16	16	≤0.03->4	>4
VanB	32->512	128	0.004-0.25[c]	-	0.12-4	2	-	-
S. pneumoniae	≤0.6-1	0.5	0.0005-0.004	0.004	≤0.002-0.06	0.03	0.004-0.125	0.03-0.06
S. pyogenes	0.25-1	0.5	0.015-0.5	0.25	0.015-0.12	0.06	≤0.002-0.06	0.015
S. agalactiae	0.25-0.5	0.5	0.03-0.5	0.25	0.03-0.12	0.06	0.008-0.06	0.015
Viridans Group Streptococci	0.12-1	0.5-1	0.004-2	1	≤0.001-1	0.12	≤0.03-0.12	≤0.03
C. difficile	0.25-2	1	0.25-1	1	0.125-0.5	0.25	0.125-0.5	0.25
C. perfringens	0.25-0.5	0.5	0.25-1	1	0.06-0.25	0.125	0.03-0.125	0.125

[a] Data from multiple studies.
[b] Oritavancin data performed with polysorbate-80, except as noted.
[c] Estimated from older studies performed without polysorbate-80 supplementation, using adjustments as suggested by reference 1.

MIC's for all isolates tested fell in the range of < 0.015 to 1 µg/ml, and there were no differences in susceptibility profiles for methicillin-susceptible and MRSA strains (10). MIC's of telavancin for all GISA strains tested were ≤ 1 µg/ml and telavancin was bactericidal against these at concentrations of 4 x the MIC (19). The three VRSA strains tested had telavancin MIC's in the range of 1-4 µg/ml. Telavancin MIC's for *S. pneumoniae* are ≤ 0.3 µg/ml. MIC's for vancomycin-susceptible *E. faecalis* were in the range of 0.06 to 4 µg/ml and were typically one dilution lower than the corresponding vancomycin MIC's; for vancomycin susceptible *E. faecium* the range was 0.15 to 2 µg/ml. MIC's for GRE were higher, though all strains had MIC's of ≤ 16 µg/ml. The FDA also gives guidelines for agar disk diffusion testing using a 30 µg telavancin disk. Isolates with zone sizes of ≥ 15 mm are interpreted as susceptible, but there are as yet no criteria for interpretation of either intermediate or resistant isolates (21). A telavancin E-test® has been developed and in preliminary testing E-test® results compared favorably to the reference broth microdilution method.

Dalbavancin

Dalbavancin (formerly BI397) is a novel, semi-synthetic 3,3-dimethylaminoprophyl amide- substituted derivative of the naturally produced teicoplanin-like glycopeptide MDL 62461 (20). Dalbavancin has enhanced potency compared to vancomycin and teicoplanin against *S. aureus*, coagulase negative staphylococci and ß-hemolytic streptococci, and is more rapidly bactericidal. Dalbavancin is also active against anaerobic Gram-positive organisms but has no activity against Gram-negative organisms. Dalbavancin is also distinguished by some unique pharmacokinetic properties including a very prolonged serum half life of 5-7 days, permitting a proposed weekly dosing schedule. Dalbavancin is currently being developed by Vicuron Pharmaceuticals. Several large clinical trials in skin and soft tissue infections and bacteremia have already been completed, but further consideration for approval by the FDA and EMEA is currently on hold pending availability of data from additional clinical studies.

Mechanisms of action and resistance

Like the older glycopeptides, dalbavancin is a cell wall synthesis inhibitor whose primary mechanism of action is related to binding to D-Ala-D-Ala terminal residues of peptidoglycan precursors. The enhanced potency of dalbavancin compared to vancomycin has been attributed to it's ability to dimerize and more efficiently insert into the bacterial membrane (20). Comparative MIC's for *S. aureus* including MRSA and for coagulase negative staphylococci from testing of several large collections of isolates are typically 8-16 fold lower than of vancomycin. Dalbavancin remains active against GISA strains, but MIC's for these are higher than for other *S. aureus*. Dalbavancin is bactericidal against most *S. aureus*, including GISA, with MBC's generally within one dilution of the MIC (14). Spontaneous dalbavancin resistant staphylococcal mutants were not selectable (frequency < 10^{-10}) and were also not readily selectable by serial passage on sub-inhibitory concentrations of dalbavancin (14). Dalbavancin is very active against vancomycin-susceptible *E. faecalis* and *E. faecium*. Like teicoplanin, dalbavancin is active against VanB-type but not against VanA-type GRE. MIC's for the majority of VanA type *E. faecium* and *E. faecalis* are ≥ 32 µg/ml, though many VanB-type strains remain susceptible (4).

In vitro susceptibility testing

Dalbavancin breakpoints have not yet been proposed or accepted by CLSI or EUCAST, though extensive pharmacodynamic modeling data taking into consideration the unique pharmacokinetic properties of this agent suggests that breakpoints of 0.5 or 1 µg/ml for staphylococci may be appropriate. Broth microdilution remains the standard reference method for susceptibility testing. However, due to binding of dalbavancin to plastic and glass surfaces, addition of 0.002% of the surfactant polysorbate-80 is required when performing *in vitro* susceptibility tests. Dalbavancin testing differs from oritavancin susceptibility testing, where polysorbate-80 must be included in all phases of the MIC including preparation of drug stocks. For dalbavancin, addition of the surfactant only needs to occur at the point of addition of bacteria to the test wells. This requirement has been incorporated into recent CLSI guidelines (7, 8). Dalbavancin stocks should be prepared and diluted in DMSO. The MIC's of dalbavancin for *S. aureus* (Table 4) from several large isolate collections have been in the range of 0.03-0.5 µg/ml, with MIC_{90} for both methicillin susceptible and MRSA strains of 0.06 µg/ml (4). MIC's for GISA are typically higher than for other *S. aureus*, at 1-2 µg/ml, but MIC's as high as 4 µg/ml have been reported. Vancomycin-susceptible *E. faecalis* and *E. faecium* are uniformly susceptible to dalbavancin with MIC_{90} of 0.06 µg/ml and 0.12 µg/ml, respectively. Dalbavancin was also very active against ß-hemolytic streptococci and viridians group streptococci. Agar dilution testing with dalbavancin has not performed as well as broth microdilution, with trend towards higher MIC results, and is not currently recommended. Preliminary published data suggest that E-test® results will likely correlate well with reference broth microdilution testing.

Glycolipodepsipeptides: Ramoplanin

The only clinical agent of the glycolipodepsipeptide class that has reached advanced stages of clinical development is ramoplanin. Ramoplanin is actually a family of similar large molecular weight compounds derived from the *Actinoplanus* spp. ATTC 33076. These compounds have a 17 amino-acid core structure different from other established classes of antimicrobial agents. The most abundant and potent of the constituents of ramoplanin is ramoplanin A2. Ramoplanin is a cell wall synthesis inhibitor with potent bactericidal activity against Gram-positive aerobic and anaerobic organisms. Ramoplanin has poor oral bioavailability and is rapidly hydrolyzed when given intravenously, thus it has been primarily developed as a topical agent and as an oral agent for eradication of intestinal GRE colonization and treatment of *C. difficile* infections (20).

Mechanisms of action and resistance

Ramoplanin affects two steps in peptidoglycan biosynthesis including the Mur-G catalyzed conversion of Lipid I to Lipid II and the transglycosylation of Lipid II molecules (12). Ramoplanin binds more strongly to Lipid II than Lipid I, suggesting that this may be the primary mode of action (12). Ramoplanin is highly active against Gram-positive organisms including GRE. To date, no laboratory or clinical resistant isolates have been reported and no cross resistance with other agents has been demonstrated.

In vitro susceptibility testing

Studies have demonstrated that broth microdilution MICs of ramoplanin for aerobic Gram-positive organisms are considerably higher than those obtained by agar dilution and dilution in glass tubes when using unsupplemented media, but that addition of 0.02% BSA eliminated the discordance in susceptibility results. These findings have been attributed to binding of ramoplanin to plastic surfaces that is eliminated with albumin supplementation, although not by supplementation with lysed blood cells. Thus either agar dilution, tube dilution in glass tubes only, or broth micro-dilution with addition of BSA are all acceptable methods for susceptibility testing. Ramoplanin stock solutions should be prepared in 0.1 M potassium phosphate, pH 4.5, and must be stored in glass rather than plastic. Typical susceptibility test ranges for staphylococci are 0.25-1 µg/ml and for enterococci are 0.125-1 µg/ml. Standards for agar dilution testing of *C. difficile* isolates using Brucella agar have been established (6).

REFERENCES:

(1) **Arhin, F. F., I. Sarmiento, A. Belley, G. A. McKay, D. C. Draghi, P. Grover, D. Sahm, T. R. Parr, Jr., and G. Moeck.** 2008. Effect of polysorbate 80 on oritavancin binding to plastic surfaces—implications for susceptibility testing. Antimicrob. Agents Chemother. **52**:1597-1603.

(2) **Arhin, F. F., I. Sarmiento, T. R. Parr, Jr., and G. Moeck.** 2007. Mechanisms of action of oritavancin in *Staphylococcus aureus*,. Abstr. 47th Intersci. Conf. Antimicrob. Agents Chemother., abstr. C1-1471, Chicago, IL.

(3) **Arthur, M., F. Depardieu, P. Reynolds, and P. Courvalin.** 1999. Moderate-level resistance to glycopeptide LY333328 mediated by genes of the *vanA* and *vanB* clusters in enterococci. Antimicrob. Agents Chemother. **43**:1875-1880.

(4) **Biedenbach, D. J., J. M. Bell, H. S. Sader, J. D. Turnidge, and R. N. Jones.** 2009. Activities of dalbavancin against a worldwide collection of 81,673 Gram-positive bacterial isolates. Antimicrob. Agents Chemother. **53**:1260-1263.

(5) **Boucher, H. W., and G. Sakoulas.** 2007. Perspectives on daptomycin resistance, with emphasis on resistance in *Staphylococcus aureus*. Clin. Infect. Dis. **45**:601-608.

(6) **Clinical and Laboratory Standards Institute**. 2007. Methods for antimicrobial susceptibility testing of anaerobic bacteria; approved standard 7th ed. CLSI document M11-A7. Clinical Laboratory and Standards Institute, Wayne, PA.

(7) **Clinical and Laboratory Standards Institute**. 2009. Methods for dilution antimicrobial susceptibility tests for bacteria that grow aerobically; approved standard, 8th ed. CLSI document M07-A8. Clinical and Laboratory Standards Institute, Wayne, PA.

(8) **Clinical and Laboratory Standards Institute**. 2009. Performance standards for antimicrobial susceptibility testing; Nineteenth informational supplement. CLSI document M100-S19. Clinical and Laboratory Standards Institute, Wayne, PA.

(9) **Cubist Pharmaecuticals**. Cubicin susceptibility test systems. Cubicin web site, last accessed 22 06 2009.

(10) **Draghi, D. C., B. M. Benton, K. M. Krause, C. Thornsberry, C. Pillar, and D. F. Sahm.** 2008. Comparative surveillance study of telavancin activity

against recently collected Gram-positive clinical isolates from across the United States. Antimicrob. Agents Chemother. **52**:2383-2388.

(11) **European Committee on Antimicrobial Susceptibility Testing**. Data from the EUCAST MIC distribution website for Daptomycin, last accessed 16 06 2009.

(12) **Fang, X., K. Tiyanont, Y. Zhang, J. Wanner, D. Boger, and S. Walker.** 2006. The mechanism of action of ramoplanin and enduracidin. Mol. BioSyst. **2**:69-76

(13) **Friedman, L., J. D. Adler, and J. A. Silverman.** 2006. Genetic changes that correlate with reduced susceptibility to daptomycin in *Staphylococcus aureus*. Antimicrob. Agents Chemother. **50**:2137-2145

(14) **Goldstein, B.P., D. C. Draghi, D. J. Sheehan, P. Hogan and D. F. Sahm.** 2007. Bactericidal activity and resistance development profiling of dalbavancin. Antimicrob. Agents Chemother. **51**:1150-1154

(15) **Higgins, D. L., R. Chang, D. V. Debabov, J. Leung, T. Wu, K. M. Krause, E. Sandvik, J. M. Hubbard, K. Kaniga, D. E. Schmidt, Jr., Q. Gao, R. T. Cass, D. E. Karr, B. M. Benton, and P. P. Humphrey.** 2005. Telavancin, a multifunctional lipoglycopeptide, disrupts both cell wall synthesis and cell membrane integrity in methicillin-resistant *Staphylococcus aureus*. Antimicrob. Agents Chemother. **49**:1127-1134.

(16) **Jones, T., M. R. Yeaman, G. Sakoulas, S.-J. Yang, R. A. Proctor, H.-G. Sahl, J. Schrenzel, Y. Q. Xiong, and A. S. Bayer.** 2008. Failures in clinical treatment of *Staphylococcus aureus* infection with daptomycin are associated with alterations in surface charge, membrane phospholipid asymmetry, and drug binding. Antimicrob. Agents Chemother. **52**:269-278.

(17) **Montero, C. I., F. Stock, and P. R. Murray.** 2008. Mechanisms of resistance to daptomycin in *Enterococcus faecium*. Antimicrob. Agents Chemother. **52**:1167–1170.

(18) **Muthaiyan, A., J. A. Silverman, R. K. Jayaswal, and B. J. Wilkinson.** 2008. Transcriptional profiling reveals that daptomycin induces the *Staphylococcus aureus* cell wall stress stimulon and genes responsive to membrane depolarization. Antimicrob. Agents Chemother. **52**:980-990

(19) **Sahm, D. F., B. M. Benton, M. E. Jones, K. M. Krause, C. Thornsberry, and D. C. Draghi.** 2006. Telavancin demonstrates a low potential for in vitro selection of resistance among key target Gram-positive species. Abstr. 46th Intersci. Conf. Antimicrob. Agents Chemother., abstr. C1-681. San Francisco, CA

(20) **Van Bambeke, F.** 2006. Glycopeptides and glycodepsipeptides in clinical development: a comparative review of their antibacterial spectrum, pharmacokinetics and clinical efficacy. Curr. Opin. Investig. Drugs **7**:740-749.

(21) **Vibativ™** (telavancin) for injection, initial US approval 2009, full prescribing information; http://www.astellas.us/docs/us/VIBATIV_PI_Final.pdf: last accessed 21 09 2009.

Chapter 23. MACROLIDES, LINCOSAMIDES, AND STREPTOGRAMINS

Roland LECLERCQ

INTRODUCTION

Macrolides, lincosamides, and streptogramins (MLS) are chemically distinct antibiotics but are classified in the same group. This is partly justified by the similar mechanisms of action of inhibition of protein synthesis and by the cross-resistance due to target modification which, for a long time, was the only identified resistance mechanism. However, MLS differ in terms of their mechanisms of action and many other resistance mechanisms have now been described which do not induce cross-resistance. For antibiotic susceptibility testing, it is therefore important to consider the various classes in the MLS group, which can have a different behaviour according to the resistance mechanism acquired by the bacterial strain.

The oldest commercially available macrolide is erythromycin. Resistance to this antibiotic was described in staphylococci soon after its release onto the market. Emergence of resistance was then reported in β-haemolytic streptococci and pneumococci and resistance to macrolides has subsequently emerged and spread to almost all species of Gram-positive bacteria with variable frequencies, with diversification of resistance mechanisms.

Many semisynthetic derivatives of erythromycin A have been developed over the last decade. They present improvements in terms of their pharmacokinetic properties and have provided a progress in the ease of administration and safety of this class of antibiotics, but they are still subject to cross-resistance with erythromycin A. Ketolides have been recently shown to be active on macrolide-resistant pneumococci, leading to renewed interest in these antibiotics.

STRUCTURE

MLS are presented in Table 1. Marketed macrolides are composed of at least two amino or neutral sugars attached to a large lactone ring of variable size according to the compound. Macrolides used in clinical therapeutics have a 14-atom lactone ring (clarithromycin, dirithromycin, erythromycin, oleandomycin, and roxithromycin) or a 15-atom lactone ring (sometimes called azalides) (azithromycin). Ketolides, erythromycin A derivatives, have been recently developed. Telithromycin, a ketolide derived from clarithromycin, comprises a keto group instead of the L-cladinose sugar of erythromycin A and an 11-12-carbamate chain substituted by an arylalkyl chain. Macrolides with a 16-atom lactone ring (josamycin, midecamycin, spiramycin, and tylosin) are used in some countries or in veterinary practice.

Table 1. Macrolides, lincosamides and streptogramins

Antibiotic class	Antibiotic
Macrolide	
14-membered ring	Clarithromycin, dirithromycin, erythromycin, oleandomycin, roxithromycin
14-membered ring, ketolide subgroup	Telithromycin
15-membered ring	Azithromycin
16-membered ring	Josamycin, miokamycin, midecamycin, rokitamycin, spiramycin, tylosin
Lincosamide	Lincomycin, clindamycin
Streptogramin	
Streptogramin A	Pristinamycin IIA, dalfopristin, virginiamycin M
Streptogramin B	Pristinamycin IA, quinupristin, virginiamycin S
Streptogramin A+B	Pristinamycin, quinupristin-dalfopristin, virginiamycin

Lincosamides are alkyl derivatives of prolines. Clindamycin is the 7-chloro-7-deoxy derivative of lincomycin.

Streptogramins are mixtures of at least two compounds that can be classified into two groups, A (pristinamycin IA, dalfopristin and virginiamycin M) and B (pristinamycin IIA, quinupristin and virginiamycin S). Streptogramins used in therapy are: quinupristin-dalfopristin, a parenteral streptogramin, pristinamycin, an oral streptogramin used in only a few countries (including France), and virginiamycin, an oral veterinary streptogramin.

MECHANISM OF ACTION

MLS inhibit protein synthesis by binding to the bacterial ribosome. The ribosome is composed of a small 30S subunit and a large 50S subunit, comprising 23S and 5S RNA and at least 30 proteins designated by the letter L ("large") and numbered. The secondary structure of 23S RNA is folded due to the formation of complementary base pairs and forms 6 domains numbered from I to VI. Complex contacts between RNA and proteins ensure the three dimensional conformation of the molecule (tertiary structure). The stability of this conformation is ensured by interactions with various proteins. The structure of the ribosome is globally conserved in all bacterial species.

Erythromycin binds to the 50S subunit of the bacterial ribosome. Binding of a single molecule to the ribosome blocks protein synthesis. The erythromycin binding site is situated adjacent to the base of the cavity that contains the peptidyl transferase centre, in domain V of 23S rRNA, the site of synthesis of the peptide and the entry of the peptide exit tunnel. The surface of this tunnel is formed by domains I to V of 23S RNA, globular parts of proteins L22 and L4 and a β chain of L22. The critical bases for binding of erythromycin are adenines in positions 2058, 2059 and 2062, guanine 2505 and uridine 2609 (domain V). Erythromycin blocks extension of the peptide chain by steric hindrance and stimulates dissociation of peptidyl-tRNA as soon as the peptide has reached a length of 6 to 8 amino acids. It also prevents assembly of the ribosome at the time of initiation of protein synthesis. Natural resistance of enterobacteria to macrolides is not due to insensitivity of ribosomes but to a physiological active efflux mechanism associated with a certain degree of impermeability of the external membrane of these bacteria to these antibiotics.

The binding site of clindamycin and lincomycin, like that of erythromycin, is adenine 2058.

Streptogramins A and B act via a synergistic interaction in the binding of the two antibiotics to the ribosome. Binding of streptogramin A to the wall of the peptide exit tunnel (A_{2451}, G_{2061}, A_{2503}) induces a change of conformation of adenine 2062. This repositioning allows high affinity binding of streptogramin B in an adjacent site to that of streptogramin A; it occupies a part of the lumen of the peptide exit tunnel.

SUSCEPTIBLE PHENOTYPE AND NATURAL RESISTANCE

The activity spectrum of macrolides essentially comprises Gram-positive bacteria (streptococci, staphylococci) but also Gram-negative cocci, certain anaerobes and Gram-negative bacilli (*Bordetella pertussis*, *Campylobacter*, *Helicobacter*, *Legionella*, *Moraxella catarrhalis*), intracellular bacteria (*Chlamydia* and *Rickettsia*) and *Mycobacterium avium* (clarithromycin). Only rare non-pathogenic species of Gram-positive bacteria present natural resistance, such as macrolide-producing bacteria and certain species of bacillus (*Bacillus clausii*, *B. licheniformis*) which possess ribosomal methylase *erm* genes. Several species of mycobacteria also possess specific *erm* genes.

Some species of Gram-positive bacteria present natural resistance to lincosamides and streptogramins due to resistance to streptogramin A (LS_A phenotype) providing an aid to identification of these bacteria. This is the case for *Enterococcus faecalis* in which this natural resistance is associated with the species-specific *lsa* gene which encodes a protein related to an efflux pump. Rare clinical strains of *E. faecalis* susceptible to lincosamides and streptogramins A do not express the Lsa protein. This type of natural resistance is also observed for other *Enterococcus* species such as *E. avium*, *E. gallinarum* and *E. casseliflavus*. In contrast, *E. faecium*, *E. durans* and *E. hirae* are naturally susceptible to LS_A.

The staphylococcus species *S. cohnii*, *S. xylosus* and *S. sciuri* also present the LS_A phenotype although the mechanism of resistance remains unknown

BACTERICIDAL ACTIVITY

Macrolides are reputed to be non-bactericidal. Although this is true for *S. aureus*, these antibiotics are bactericidal on streptococci, including pneumococci.

Streptogramins are bactericidal on staphylococci, pneumococci and streptococci and are effective by the 3rd hour for MLS-susceptible staphylococci and very rapidly effective for pneumococci. The bactericidal effect on staphylococci is slightly greater than 3 $\log_{10}$ at 18 hours. Quinupristin-dalfopristin is not bactericidal on *E. faecium*.

METHODS

Macrolide susceptibility testing of the usual bacteria does not raise any particular problems and is performed according to the recommendations of the CLSI or other national committees. However, the spectrum of macrolides also comprises Gram-positive bacteria that may require particular *in vitro* culture conditions, such as addition of blood to the culture medium and incubation in a CO_2-enriched atmosphere, conditions which can alter their activity (27).

The acidity of culture media has an important effect. At pH 6, macrolides are 4 to 16 times less active than at pH 7. This effect is particularly marked for azithromycin (MIC increased 16- to 32-fold) and then, in decreasing order, erythromycin (MIC increased 16-fold), clarithromycin (16-fold), roxithromycin (8-fold), and josamycin (4-fold). Macrolides, except for josamycin, are 2 to 8 times more active at pH 8. This pH effect appears to be dependent on the pKa of the basic group of the macrolide (8.6 for erythromycin, 8.4 for azithromycin, and 9.2 for roxithromycin), so that, at pH 8, the nonionized macrolide is more easily able to cross the cytoplasmic membrane than the ionized macrolide at pH 6. This largely explains the effect of incubation in CO_2 which results in acidification of the culture medium and reduction of the activity of macrolides regardless of the method used. The increase of minimum inhibitory concentrations (MIC) of macrolides is then 2- to 32-fold with the same order as that indicated above. This effect is also observed for telithromycin.

The addition of blood to culture media only slightly affects the activity of macrolides, inducing a one-dilution reduction of the MIC due to slight alkalinization of the medium. The addition of horse or foal serum has a similar effect (4- to 8-fold reduction of the MIC of erythromycin in the presence of 50% horse serum).

The inoculum effect is moderate with a twofold increase of the MIC of macrolides for a 2 $\log_{10}$ increase of the number of bacteria per mL.

The Clinical and Standard Laboratory Institute (CLSI) (9) and the Comité de l'Antibiogramme of the Société Française de Microbiologie (CA-SFM) (www.sfm.asso.fr) recommend Mueller-Hinton agar medium with 5% sheep blood for the study of streptococci by the agar diffusion method. Incubation in a CO_2-enriched atmosphere is recommended by the CLSI but not by the French committee (except for CO_2-requiring strains).

According to the CLSI, MIC must be determined for streptococci in Mueller-Hinton broth supplemented with 2-5% of lysed horse blood or in Mueller-Hinton agar medium supplemented with 5% of sheep blood. The CA-SFM proposes similar recommendations.

RESISTANCE MECHANISMS

Three main types of mechanisms are responsible for acquired resistance to MLS (16).

Target modification

Modification of the ribosomal target of macrolides induces resistance due to reduction of the affinity of MLS for their target. Bacteria can modify the ribosome either by the production of methylases encoded in clinical strains by plasmidic or transposable genes (Tn*1545*, Tn*551*, Tn*554*, Tn*917*, etc.) or by mutation of RNA or ribosomal proteins.

Ribosomal methylation

The resistance phenotype due to this mechanism was first described in 1956 in staphylococci by Y.A. Chabbert and the mechanism responsible for resistance was elucidated over the following years by Weisblum *et al*. This resistance is due to methylation of a single adenine in position 2058 of 23S ribosomal RNA. Methylation of this adenine, which plays a key role in the binding of macrolides, prevents the binding of these molecules to their target. As adenine 2058 is a common binding site for macrolides, lincosamides and streptogramins B, cross-resistance is observed between these three groups of antibiotics, and this resistance phenotype is therefore called MLS_B. The MLS_B phenotype was subsequently reported in a large number of bacterial species. This resistance is encoded by *erm* genes (erythromycin ribosome methylase). Several classes of *erm* genes have been described and classified according to the similarity of the deduced peptide sequence. Only Erm classes that differ by more than 20% are given distinct names. There are currently more than thirty of classes of *erm* genes corresponding to as many classes of Erm proteins (see the web site managed by M.C. Roberts: http://faculty.washington.edu/marilynr/); those described in Gram-positive bacteria are listed in Table 2. Each class is relatively specific for a bacterial genus, although not strictly confined to this genus. Most bacteria producing macrolides and related antibiotics intrinsically harbour an *erm* gene to resist the antibiotic that they produce. In pathogenic bacteria, *erm* genes are carried by plasmids or transposons.

Although the various *erm* genes globally confer cross-resistance between MLS_B, various levels of resistance can be observed according to whether the gene is responsible for monomethylation (low level of resistance to erythromycin) or dimethylation (high level of resistance to erythromycin). In staphylococci, *erm*(A) and *erm*(C) genes are responsible for dimethylation while the *erm*(B) gene appears to be responsible for mono- or dimethylation according to the host that harbours it (11).

The expression of *erm* genes can be inducible or constitutive. In the case of inducible resistance, the methylase is only fully synthesized in the presence of certain inducing MLS. In the case of constitutive resistance, the methylase is produced throughout bacterial growth without the need for an inducer.

The mechanism of induction is translational for the *erm*(C) gene and can be described schematically as follows. The *erm*(C) gene is preceded by a translational attenuator which comprises a gene encoding a short peptide called leader peptide. The *erm*(C) gene and the leader peptide gene are co-transcribed into a single messenger RNA. In the absence of erythromycin, this RNA forms a hairpin secondary structure by base pairing (inverted repeats) which sequesters the initiation sequence of methylase synthesis (ribosomal binding site and start codon of the *erm* gene). These initiation sequences are therefore masked for ribosomes which are consequently unable to translate the methylase. However, translation of the leader peptide occurs normally but is not directly responsible for resistance. Although the strain possesses the erythromycin resistance gene, it does not produce the resistance protein to this antibiotic. In the presence of low concentrations of erythromycin, binding of the antibiotic to ribosomes in the process of translating the leader peptide blocks translation. The presence of blocked ribosome induces downstream destabilization of the hairpin structure and the subsequent release of methylase translation initiation sequences. This enzyme is then translated by ribosomes that have not yet bound erythromycin and then by methylated ribosomes due to initiation of methylase synthesis. The strain then expresses resistance to the inducer macrolide. Non-inducer macrolides do not exert this effect, probably because they do not allow a ribosomal

Table 2. Distribution of *erm* genes in Gram-positive bacteria (excluding antibiotic-producing actinomycetes and anaerobic bacteria) (Adapted from MC Roberts)

Gene class	Usual host	Other bacterial hosts
erm(A)	*Staphylococcus aureus* *Streptococcus pyogenes*[a]	*Streptococcus, Enterococcus,* group B, C, G streptococci
erm(B)	*Streptococcus, Enterococcus*	*Staphylococcus*
erm(C)	*Staphylococcus*	*Bacillus, Lactobacillus, Streptococcus*
erm(D)	*Bacillus*	
erm(F)	*Bacteroides*	*Lactobacillus, Staphylococcus, Streptococcus*
erm(G)	*Bacillus*	*Lactobacillus*
erm(Q)	*Clostridium*	*Staphylococcus, Streptococcus*
erm(T)	*Lactobacillus*	
erm(X)	*Corynebacterium*	
erm(Y)	*Staphylococcus*	
erm(33)	*Staphylococcus*	
erm(34)	*Bacillus clausii*	
erm(36)	*Micrococcus*	

[a] *S. pyogenes* harbors the *ermTR* gene which is a subclass of *erm*(A).

pause in the correct position to induce the necessary structural rearrangements.

The inducing capacity of an antibiotic depends on its structure and the structure of the *erm* gene attenuator. The attenuators of the various *erm* genes have different structures: for example, *erm*(C) has a short leader peptide, *erm*(B) has a longer leader peptide and *erm*(A) has two leader peptides (16). This explains why a given macrolide may or may not be an inducer according to the genes: tylosin is not an inducer for staphylococci harbouring *erm*(C) but is an inducer for streptococci or staphylococci harbouring *erm*(B). In staphylococci, the inducing nature of the macrolide is usually correlated to the number of atoms in its lactone ring (14, 15 or 16). Although this was true for macrolides marketed up until recently, it is no longer strictly exact, as it is the global structure of the macrolide rather than the number of atoms of the lactone ring that determines whether or not the molecule is an inducer. For example, erythromycin and telithromycin both have a 14-atom ring, but erythromycin is an inducer for MLS_B resistance while telithromycin is not.

Clinical strains with constitutive expression of *erm* genes possess various mutations in the attenuator, especially large deletions. In the presence of non-inducing MLS, constitutive mutants can be selected *in vitro* in a strain with inducible expression of an *erm*(A) or *erm*(C) gene at frequencies of the order of 10^{-7}. These mutants also present alterations of attenuator structures.

Mutation of the ribosomal target

MLS-resistant mutants have been recently reported in clinical strains of Gram-positive bacteria. The first mutations to be detected concerned adenines in positions 2058, 2059 or 2062 of 23S ribosomal RNA. These mutations were initially described in bacteria such as *Mycobacterium avium* and *Helicobacter pylori* possessing only one or two copies of ribosomal RNA (*rrn*) operons, often with each copy carrying the mutation. The preferential distribution of this mechanism in these bacteria is explained by the fact that at least one half of the *rrn* operon copy number probably needs to be mutated in order to express significant macrolide resistance. The rarity of macrolide resistance in staphylococci and streptococci could be explained by the presence of several *rrn* copies in these bacterial species (4 in pneumococcus, 5 or 6 in *S. aureus*).

Mutations in ribosomal proteins L4 and L22 lining the exit tunnel of the polypeptides synthesized by the ribosome are also responsible for resistance. L22 mutations induce an enlargement of the tunnel, allowing the synthesis and exit of proteins in the presence of erythromycin.

Enzymatic modification

Several enzymes are able to inactivate MLS. The synthesis of a given enzyme only affects molecules with a related structure within the MLS group due to its specificity and is responsible for a dissociated resistance profile between various MLS.

Erythromycin can be inactivated by various enzymes including esterases (*ere* class of genes) or phosphotransferases (*mph* class of genes). These genes are essentially present in enterobacteria but have sometimes been reported in staphylococci. Lincosamides are inactivated by nucleotidyltransferases (*lnu* class of genes)

Streptogramin resistance is frequently explained by a combination of *vat* and *vgb* class genes encoding streptogramin A acetylases and streptogramin B lyases, respectively.

Efflux

The acquisition of resistance by active efflux in Gram-positive bacteria is due to two classes of efflux pumps, members of the ATP-binding cassette (ABC) transporter family and the Major Facilitator Superfamily (MFS).

An ABC transporter encoded by the plasmidic *msr(A)* gene has been reported in staphylococci. ABC transporters use ATP as energy source and are usually composed of a channel with two cytoplasmic membrane-associated domains and two ATP-binding domains situated on the internal surface of the membrane. The *msr(A)* gene encodes a protein possessing the two ATP-binding domains characteristic of ABC-transporters. However, the nature of the transmembrane component of the pump is unknown. It is probably recruited from the proteins encoded by staphylococcal chromosomal genes.

Other efflux genes have also been reported; *msr(C)* (enterococci) and *msr(D)*.

Efflux of streptogramins A is related to a Vga protein of the same family but whose efflux function is only hypothetical.

The *mef(A)* gene, essentially found in streptococci, encodes an MFS family efflux pump, which derives its energy from the proton motive force.

STAPHYLOCOCCI

The phenotypes and genotypes described below are reported in *S. aureus* and in coagulase-negative staphylococci; only their frequency differs according to the species (16).

MLS$_B$ phenotype (*erm* genotype)

The MLS$_B$ phenotype in staphylococci results from the expression of *erm*(A) or *erm*(C) genes, or more rarely *erm*(B) and exceptionally *erm*(Y) and *erm*(33) genes [hybrids of *erm*(A) and *erm*(C)]. *erm*(A) genes are essentially found in methicillin-resistant strains of *S. aureus* where they are carried by Tn*554* transposons, while *erm*(C) genes are mainly observed in methicillin-susceptible strains where they are generally carried by plasmids.

The phenotypes conferred by inducible expression of *erm*(A) and *erm*(C) are similar and characterized by dissociated MLS$_B$ resistance. Resistance is expressed in relation to macrolides which induce methylase production, i.e. 14- and 15-membered macrolides (erythromycin, roxithromycin, clarithromycin, dirithromycin, and azithromycin), except for telithromycin (non-inducer). 16-membered macrolides, lincosamides, and streptogramins A and B are not inducers and therefore remain active (Tables 3 and 4). This phenotype is characterized, on agar diffusion, by flattening of the inhibition zone around lincomycin, clindamycin, spiramycin, or josamycin disks compared to the erythromycin disk (D-shaped zone) (Fig. 1). It is due to the decreasing diffusion gradient of erythromycin in the agar; the subinhibitory concentration of erythromycin situated away from the disk is sufficient to induce methylase production and resistance to non-inducing MLS.

Constitutive expression is characterized by resistance to all macrolides (including telithromycin), lincosamides, and streptogramins B (Fig. 2). The marker of this phenotype is the high level of resistance to clindamycin or lincomycin (associated with resistance to erythromycin). As the synergy between streptogramins A and B is preserved, pristinamycin and quinupristin-dalfopristin are active with similar MIC or MIC generally increased by one dilution compared to those of susceptible strains. However, the bactericidal activity of streptogramins is affected: the early bactericidal activity is essentially eliminated. The log reduction of the number of surviving bacteria per mL is situated between 2 and 3 after 18-24 hours.

Automated methods accurately identify MLS$_B$ resistance. The concordance between the Phoenix automat and the diffusion method is 100% for *S. aureus* (10). A number of *S. aureus* strains with intermediate susceptibility to erythromycin on VITEK1 are actually inducible MLS$_B$-resistant strains; the resistance of these staphylococci is accurately identified by Phoenix (100%) and VITEK2 (96%) (28).

Interpretation and reporting of the results

The 16-membered macrolides and lincosamides are active in the presence of inducible MLS$_B$ resistance, but, as mentioned above, there is

Table 3. Main MLS resistance phenotypes in staphylococci

Mechanism	Gene class	Phenotype	Resistance phenotype[a]			
			14-, 15-M	16-M	L	S
Ribosomal methylation	*erm*(A), *erm*(C)	Inducible MLS$_B$	R	S[b]	S[b]	S
		Constitutive MLS$_B$	R	R	R	S[c]
Efflux	*msr*(A)	MS$_B$	R	S	S	S
Enzymatic modification	*lnu*(A)	L	S	S	R[d]	S
Efflux?	*vga*(A), *vga*(Av), *lsa*(B), unknown determinants	LS$_A$	S	S	I	S/I
Enzymatic modification of factors A or B +/- efflux of factor A	*vat*(A), *vat*(B), *vat*(C), *vga*(A), *vga*(Av), *vga*(B), *vgb*(A), *vgb*(B) in various combinations	S or LS [e]	S	S	S or I [e]	R

[a] 14-, 15-M ; 14- and 15-membered macrolides ; L, lincosamide ; S, streptogramms.
[b] Risk of selection of resistant mutants.
[c] Reduced bactericidal activity.
[d] Resistance to lincomycin and susceptibility to clindamycin (interpret as "I").
[e] Possibility of lincomycin and clindamycin resistance in the presence of *vga*(A) or *vga*(Av) genes.

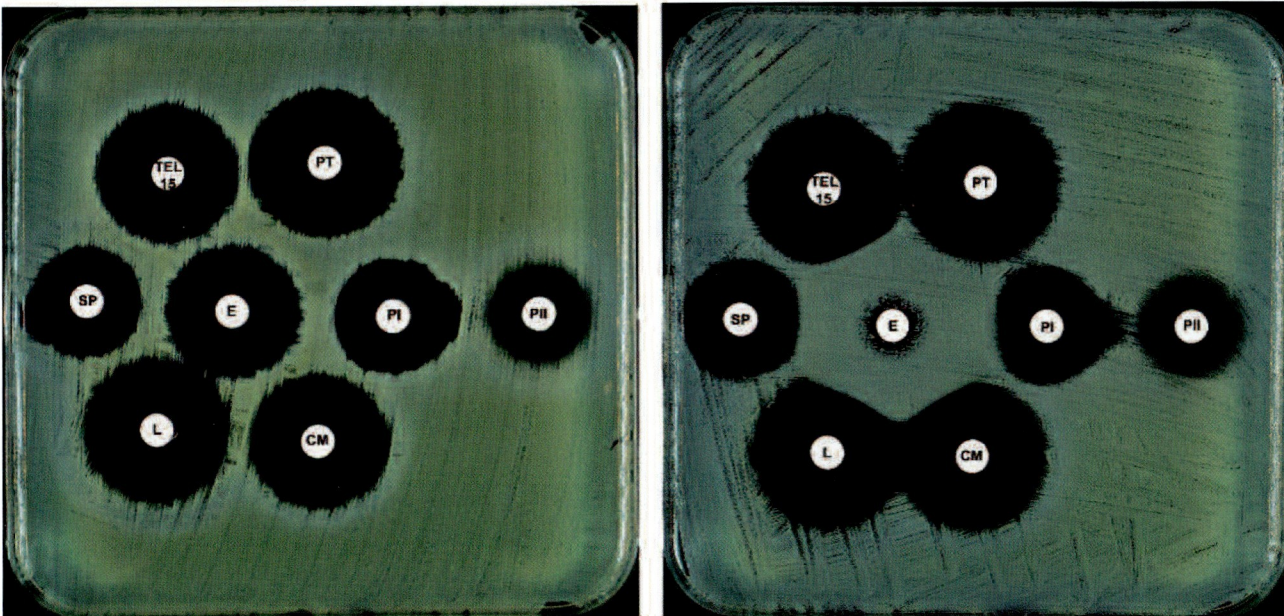

Fig. 1. Inducible MLS$_B$ phenotype *S. aureus*. Left, susceptible strain. Right, inducible MLS$_B$ phenotype strain. CM, clindamycin; E, erythromycin; L, lincomycin; SP, spiramycin; PI, pristinamycin IA (streptogramin factor B); PII, pristinamycin IIA; PT, pristinamycin; TEL, telithromycin.

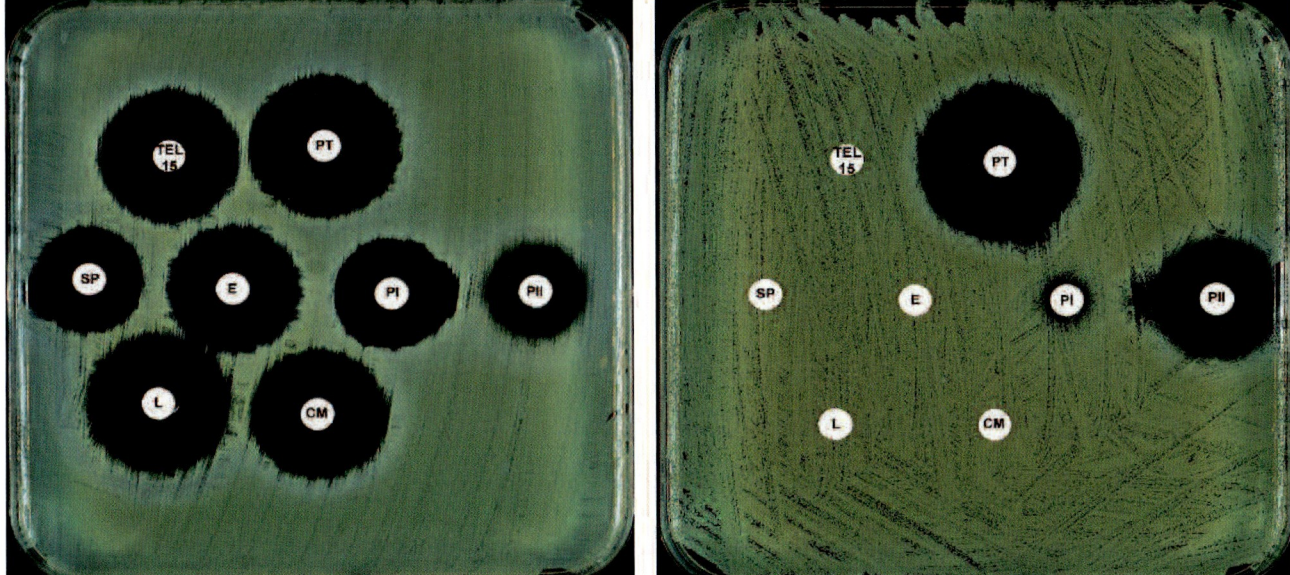

Fig. 2. Constitutive MLS$_B$ phenotype *S. aureus*. Left, susceptible strain. Right, constitutive MLS$_B$ phenotype strain. CM, clindamycin; E, erythromycin; L, lincomycin; SP, spiramycin; PI, pristinamycin IA (streptogramin factor B); PII, pristinamycin IIA; PT, pristinamycin; TEL, telithromycin. Synergy is maintained between the two streptogramin factors.

a risk of clinical failure due to selection of constitutive mutants during treatment with these antibiotics. Failures have been reported but are not constant. The numbers of treated patients included in published series are too small to allow analysis of the risk of failure. The way in which the results should be reported to the clinician is therefore a matter of debate.

The CLSI recommends the search for signs of antagonism by using a clindamycin disk (2 μg) and an erythromycin disk (15 μg) separated by an interval of 15 to 26 mm (9). If a D-shaped inhibition zone is observed around the clindamycin disk, the strain should be reported as resistant to erythromycin and clindamycin. The CLSI considers it acceptable to indicate on the report that clin-

Table 4. MIC of the main MLS on staphylococci according to the resistance mechanism

Resistance mechanism	Phenotype	Main resistance genes	Modal MIC (µg/ml)[a]					
			ERY	SPI	LIN	CLI	PRI I	PRI II	PRI
None	Susceptible	Aucun	0.5	4	1	0.12	4	2	0.25
Ribosomal methylation	Inducible MLS$_B$	erm(A), erm(C)	32->128	4-8	1	0.12	4	2	0.25
	Constitutive MLS$_B$		>128	>128	>128	>128	>128	2	0.25-0.5
Efflux	MS$_B$	msr(A)	32	4	1	0.12	4	2	0.25
Modification lincosamides	L	lnu(A)	0.5	4	32-64	0.12	4	2	0.25
Efflux ?	LS$_A$	vga(A), vga(Av), lsa(B)	0.5	4	8	**2**	4	32-64	**0,5-1**
Enzymatic modification	S	vat(A), vat(B), vat(C), vga(B), vgb(A), vgb(B)	0.5	4	1	0.12	64	32-64	**4**
Ribosomal mutation	M	Mutant rplD	4-8	16	1	0.12	4	2	0.25
Ribosomal mutation	MS$_B$	Mutant rplV	4-8	ND	0.5	0.06	16	2	**2-4**
Ribosomal mutation	MLS$_B$	Mutant A$_{2058}$	>128	8->128	ND	**0.5-16**	8-64	0.5-2	0.25
Ribosomal mutation	ML	Mutant A$_{2059}$	>128	128	ND	**1**	2	2	0.25

[a] CLI, clindamycin; ERY, erythromycin; LIN, lincomycin; PRI I, pristinamycin IA (factor B); PRI II, pristinamycin IIA (factor A); PRI, pristinamycin; SPI, spiramycin. Higher MIC than those observed for susceptible strains are shown in bold type. ND, not determined.

damycin may be effective in some patients. A well containing clindamycin and an inducing concentration of erythromycin in broth microdilution methods, including automated methods, can be used to detect the inducible phenotype. BAA-976 and BAA-977 strains of *S. aureus* are used as positive and negative quality controls.

EUCAST recommends reporting these strains as being resistant to clindamycin and lincomycin or informing the clinician about the risk of selection of resistant mutants and to avoid the use of lincosamides in severe infections (http://www.eucast.org/expert_rules/).

The risk of selection must be taken into account in the context of safe use of antibiotics. The level of risk depends on several factors including the bacterial inoculum, as the risk is higher with a heavier inoculum at the site of infection (mediastinitis, certain respiratory tract infections).

In the case of constitutive MLS$_B$ resistance, pristinamycin and quinupristin-dalfopristin are active but the response to the clinician must be modulated due to alteration of their bactericidal activity. No definitive conclusions on a possible alteration of their *in vivo* activity can be drawn due to the insufficient clinical data concerning these two antibiotics. *In vivo* data for quinupristin-dalfopristin have been obtained in experimental models of rabbit or rat endocarditis. The results are contradictory with decreased activity of streptogramin during infection by a strain with a constitutive MLS$_B$ phenotype in two cases (12, 13) and not decreased in one case (2). The failure of the combination was attributed, in the rat endocarditis mode, to a shorter half-life for factor A (dalfopristin) than for factor B (quinupristin), resulting in periods during which only factor B, to which the strain is resistant, is present (12). EUCAST recommends adding a comment on the decreased bactericidal activity of quinupristin-dalfopristin to the report. The activity of pristinamycin is probably sufficient for common infections in which a bactericidal activity is not required, but data concerning the efficacy of this oral antibiotic in more severe infections, for quinupristin-dalfopristin and for or oral pristinamycin (bone infections) are insufficient. Recommendations can only be based on well conducted clinical trials.

MS$_B$ phenotype [*msr*(A) genotype]

The MS$_B$ phenotype in staphylococci is due to active efflux of the antibiotic related to the *msr(A)* gene. The only known substrates of this ATP-dependent pump are 14-membered macrolides (except for telithromycin which is a poor substrate) and 15-membered macrolides and streptogramins B. MS$_B$ resistance is inducible, mediated by a transcriptional or translational attenuation mechanism. As only 14-membered (except for telithromycin) and 15-membered macrolides are inducers, MS$_B$ resistance is only expressed in relation to these antibiotics and not in relation to streptogramins B (Fig. 3) (Table 3). The level of resistance to erythromycin is moderate (Table 4). Resistance to streptogramins B is expressed after induction by an inducing macrolide: flattening of the streptogramin B inhibition zone over the erythromycin disk is visible when the disks are placed sufficiently close together (there is no visible antagonism with a streptogramin-disk due to the preserved synergy between the two factors). No antagonism is observed with the other macrolides (16-member) and lincosamides. Constitutive mutant resistant to 14-member macrolides and streptogramins B have been obtained *in vitro* but have not been reported in the clinical setting. These variants remain susceptible to 16-membered macrolides and lincosamides.

Overall, this phenotype is identified by moderate erythromycin resistance that can be distinguished from the inducible MLS$_B$ phenotype by the absence of antagonism images (no D-shaped zone) between erythromycin and clindamycin or lincomycin by agar diffusion.

Interpretation and reporting of the results

In the case of MS$_B$ resistance, the search for antagonism, as indicated above, between erythromycin (or azithromycin or clarithromycin) and clindamycin is negative. Tests for clindamycin and 16-membered macrolides must be reported as observed because acquisition of the MsrA pump by the bacterium has no effect on the selection of resistant mutants to these antibiotics.

Streptogramins remain fully active and there is no reason to modify the interpretation.

L phenotype [*lnu*(A) genotype]

The L phenotype is related to acquisition by staphylococci of genes of the *lnu*(A) class encoding 3-lincomycin, 4-clindamycin *O*-nucleotidyltransferases, which only inactivate lincosamides. Two closely related plasmidic genes, *linA* and *linA'*, reported in coagulase-negative staphylococci and *Staphylococcus aureus*, were initially described, but are now grouped in the same class renamed *lnu*(A).

These strains are resistant to lincomycin (MIC: 32 to 64 μg/ml) but remain susceptible to clindamycin with a one- or two-fold higher MIC compared to the susceptible phenotype (MIC: 0.12 to 0.25 μg/ml), although *in vitro* the LnuA enzyme inactivates this antibiotic more rapidly than lin-

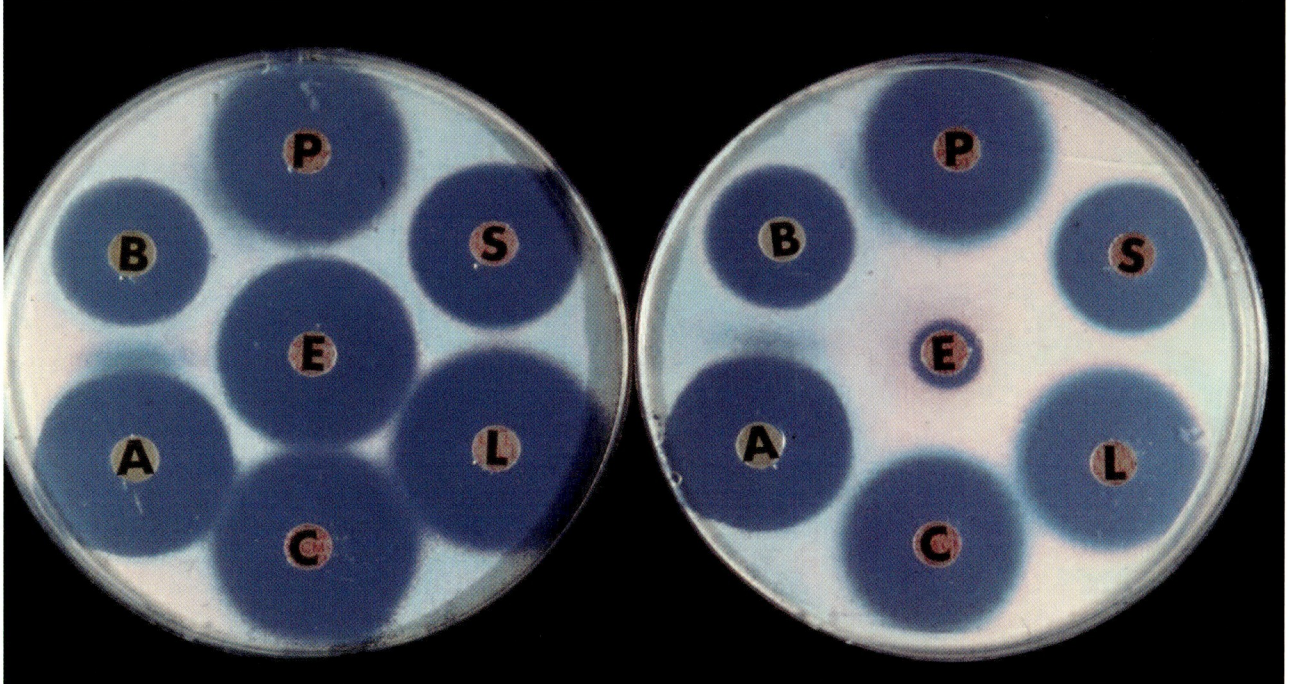

Fig. 3. MS$_B$ phenotype *S. aureus*. Left, susceptible strain. Right, MS$_B$ phenotype strain. C, clindamycin; E, erythromycin; L, lincomycin; S, spiramycin; B, pristinamycin IA (streptogramin factor B); A, pristinamycin IIA; PT, pristinamycin. Antagonism between pristinamycin IA and erythromycin is not visible, as the disks are too far apart.

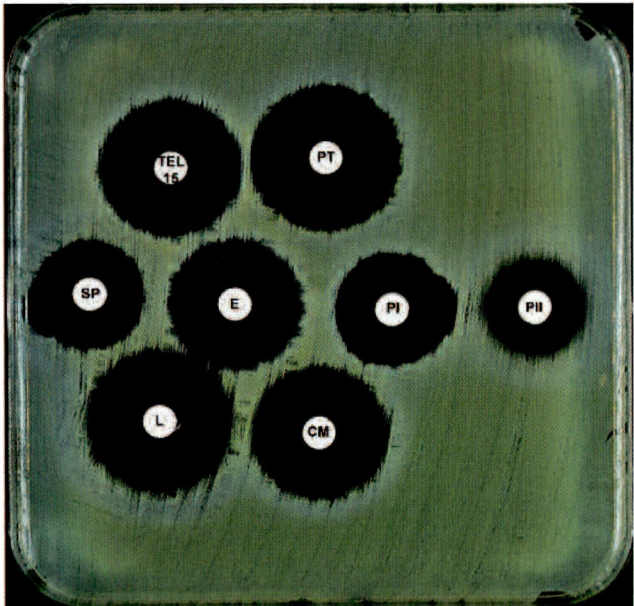 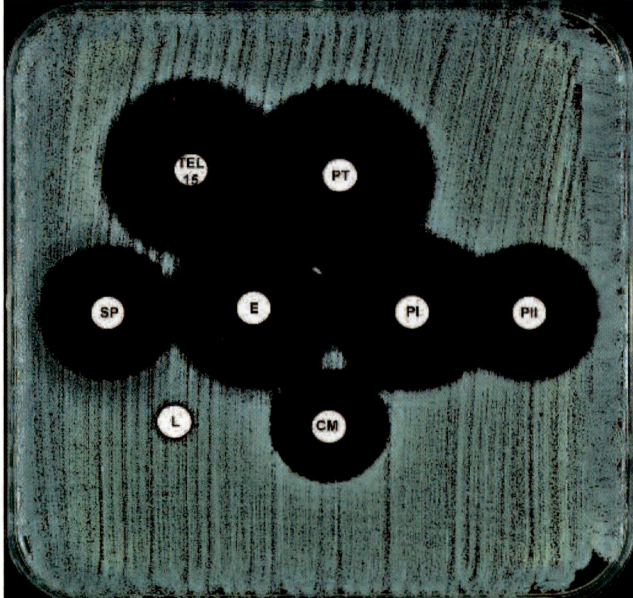

Fig. 4. L phenotype *S. aureus*. Left, susceptible strain. Right, L phenotype strain. CM, clindamycin; E, erythromycin; L, lincomycin; SP, spiramycin; PI, pristinamycin IA (streptogramin factor B); PII, pristinamycin IIA; PT, pristinamycin; TEL, telithromycin. Note the difference in diameter between lincomycin and clindamycin and the presence of large colonies at the edge of the clindamycin inhibition zone characteristic of this phenotype.

comycin (Tables 3 and 4). However, the MBC of clindamycin, already poorly bactericidal, are increased (> 128 µg/ml).

This phenotype is only identified when lincomycin is studied and cannot be identified by clindamycin alone. After detecting resistance to lincomycin, the L phenotype can be easily identified by studying lincomycin and clindamycin in parallel: the very marked difference in MIC or inhibition zone diameter between the two antibiotics is characteristic. Furthermore, on disk diffusion, the clindamycin inhibition zone is delineated by sudden arrest of growth and is lined by large colonies reflecting inactivation of the antibiotic (Fig. 4).

Interpretation and reporting of the results

As macrolides and streptogramins remain active, no correction needs to be made to their interpretation. Lincomycin is affected by L resistance but clindamycin often appears to be active. Although there are no national committee recommendations, or any conclusive clinical or experimental data, it may be wise to classify clindamycin as "I" rather than "S".

LS_A phenotype

The mechanisms and genetic determinants of the LS_A resistance have not been fully elucidated. Plasmid genes *vga*(A) and *vga*(Av) confer low-level resistance to lincomycin, clindamycin and streptogramins A. The deduced amino acid sequence homology with ABC-transporters suggests that LS_A resistance is due to efflux (8). Another plasmidic gene, *lsa*(B), encoding a protein similar to an ABC-transporter and conferring the same phenotype, has been reported in *S. sciuri* (15). However, these genes do not fully account for the LS_A phenotype in all clinical strains. In particular, mutants may have this phenotype (31).

These strains are classified as "I" due to the moderately increased MIC of lincomycin and clindamycin (Tables 3 and 4). The MIC of streptogramins A are high (MIC of pristinamycin IIA: 32 to 64 µg/ml) with an impact on the activity of the combination with factor B, which is only moderately effective, resulting in MIC of pristinamycin equal to 0.5 or 1 µg/ml (instead of usual values of 0.25 µg/ml) and classification as "I" or "S" (Fig. 5, Table 4).

The LS_A phenotype is recognized on antibiotic susceptibility testing by the "I" or "R" classification of clindamycin or lincomycin, more than by the slight reduction of the inhibition zone diameter or the increased MIC of streptogramins, which often remain classified as "S" or sometimes "I". As a streptogramin A cannot be studied specifically, this phenotype can therefore be confused with the L phenotype. On the agar diffusion, the edge of the clindamycin inhibition zone has a different appearance, without any large colonies at the rim.

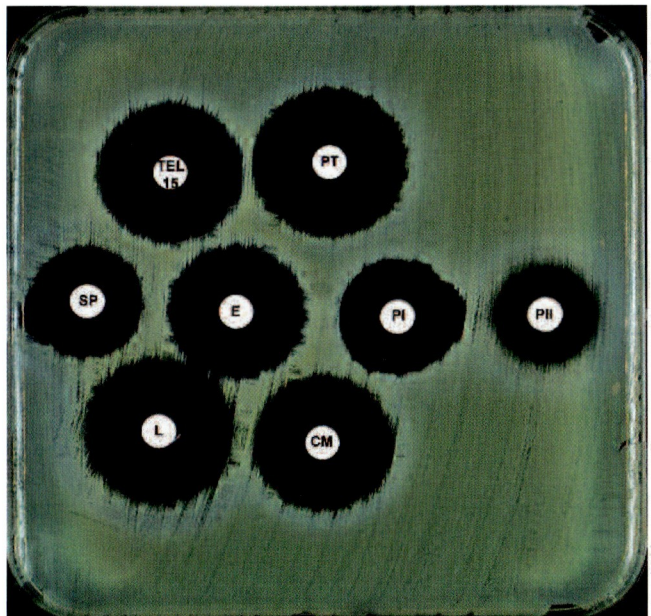 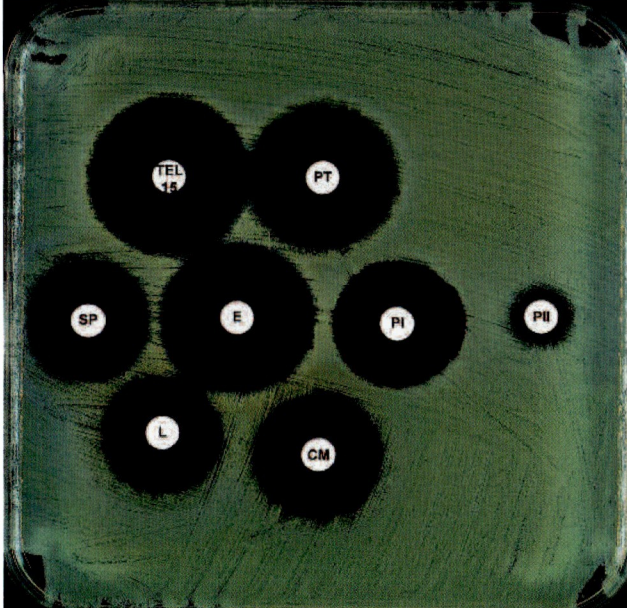

Fig. 5. LS$_A$ phenotype *S. aureus*. Left, susceptible strain. Right, LS$_A$ phenotype strain. CM, clindamycin; E, erythromycin; L, lincomycin; SP, spiramycin; PI, pristinamycin IA (streptogramin factor B); PII, pristinamycin IIA; PT, pristinamycin; TEL, telithromycin.

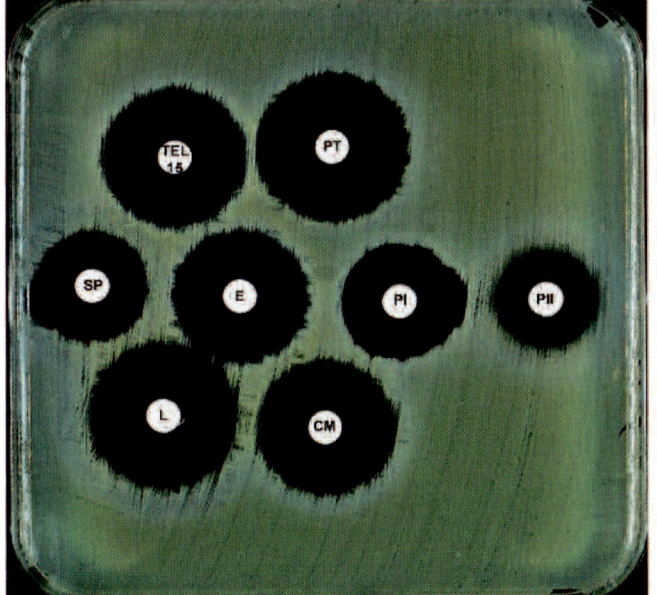 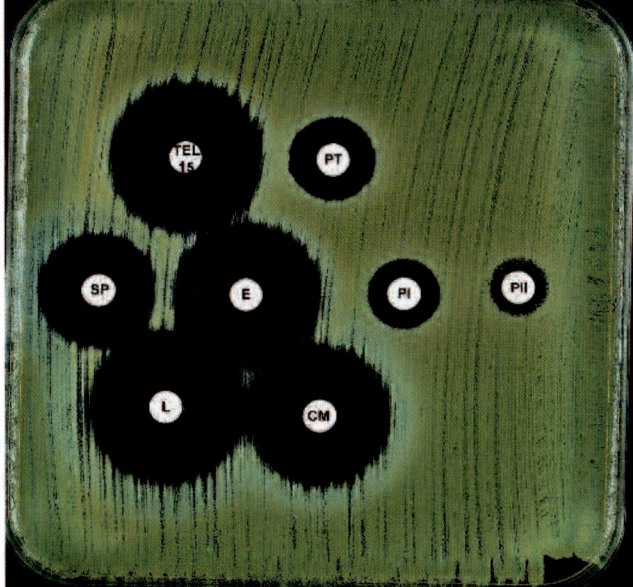

Fig. 6. S phenotype *S. aureus*. Left, susceptible strain. Right, S phenotype strain. CM, clindamycin; E, erythromycin; L, lincomycin; SP, spiramycin; PI, pristinamycin IA (streptogramin factor B); PII, pristinamycin IIA; PT, pristinamycin; TEL, telithromycin.

The VITEK2 automat frequently reports LS$_A$ phenotype strains as falsely susceptible to lincomycin (but the MIC are higher than normal) and falsely intermediate or resistant to pristinamycin (4b).

Interpretation and reporting of the results

Although strains with the LS$_A$ phenotype are often classified as "S" to pristinamycin or quinupristin-dalfopristin, these antibiotics may have a decreased activity due to resistance to factor A. Quinupristin-dalfopristin has been shown to be bactericidal *in vitro* and *in vivo* in an experimental model of rabbit endocarditis in which two *S. aureus* strains with an LS$_A$ phenotype (MIC of streptogramin = 0.5 and 1 µg/ml) were studied (31). However, for one of the two strains, resistant mutants were selected with a low frequency. No data are available for pristinamycin. No recommendation has been issued by national committees. On the basis of favourable *in vitro* and experimental results, there does not appear to be any reason to modify the "S" interpretation for streptogramins, but no definitive conclusion can be drawn in the absence of clinical evaluation.

S phenotype

This phenotype is responsible for isolated resistance to streptogramins (Fig. 6, Tables 3 and 4). Several resistance genes to streptogramin factors A or B have been reported. Apart from the *erm* genes described above, *vgb*(A) and *vgb*(B) genes encoding lyases confer resistance to streptogramins B. *vat*(A), *vat*(B) and *vat*(C) genes encoding streptogramin A acetylases and *vga*(A), *vga*(Av) and *vga*(B) genes possibly encoding an ATP-dependent efflux pump, are responsible for resistance to streptogramin factor B. These genes are frequently associated in strains of staphylococci resistant to pristinamycin or quinupristin-dalfopristin (14). They are individually more or less effective to confer resistance to combinations of streptogramins due to the synergy between factors. For example, the *vga*(A) and *vga*(Av) determinants alone do not confer resistance to pristinamycin, while *vga*(B) significantly increases the MIC of pristinamycin (9). The levels of resistance to pristinamycin vary due to the various combinations of genotypes. The most frequent gene combinations are *vat*(A) + *vgb*(A) and *vga*(Av) + *vga*(B) + *vat*(B) (14). When the *vga*(A) and *vga*(Av) determinants are present, they add a decreased susceptibility to lincomycin and clindamycin to the S phenotype.

The VITEK2 automat accurately detects pristinamycin resistance (4). No published data are available for the other automats.

Rare phenotypes

Ribosomal mutations

Rare MLS resistance phenotypes due to ribosomal mutations have been recently described. Mutant strains have been essentially isolated in the context of cystic fibrosis. Mutations affect ribosomal protein L4 or L22 and adenines 2058 and 2059 in 23S rRNA. These mutations sometimes confer characteristic phenotypes. For example, the $R_{168}S$, $G_{69}A$ and $T_{70}P$ mutations of protein L4 (encoded by the *rplD* gene) are responsible for moderate resistance of erythromycin and spiramycin with no alteration of the activity of clindamycin, lincomycin and streptogramins. The decreased activity of spiramycin distinguishes this phenotype from the MLS_B and MS_B phenotypes (Table 4). There are no signs of antagonism between erythromycin and clindamycin (26) (Fig. 7). Protein

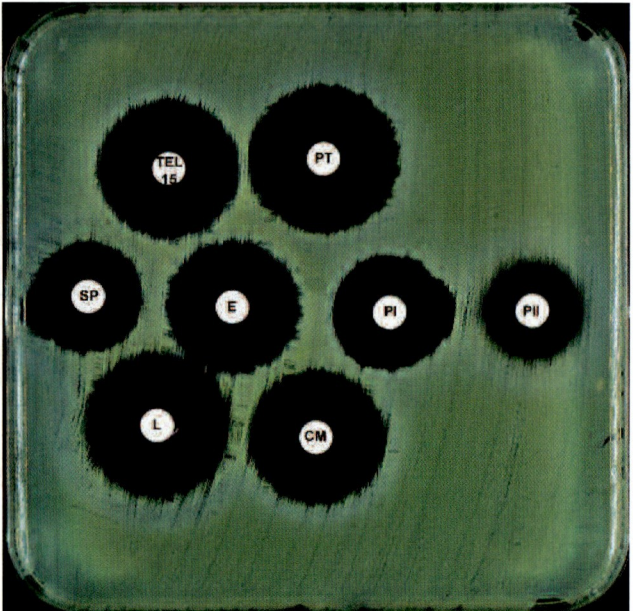
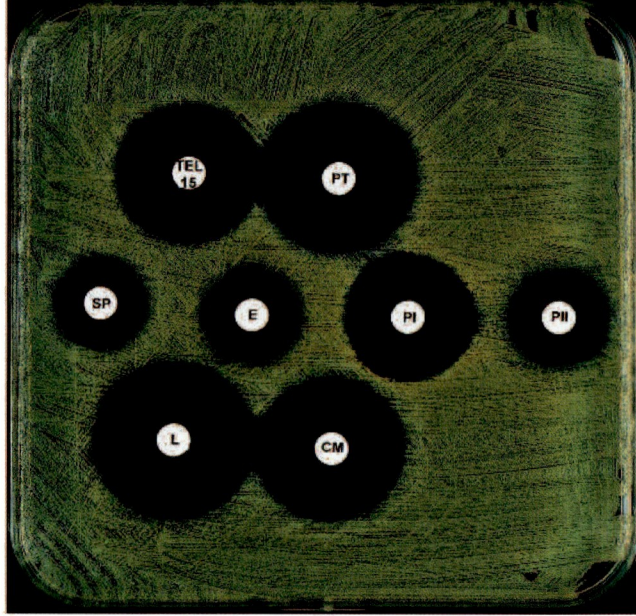

Fig. 7. *S. aureus* with protein L4 mutation. Left, susceptible strain. Right, protein L4 mutant strain. CM, clindamycin; E, erythromycin; L, lincomycin; SP, spiramycin; PI, pristinamycin IA (streptogramin factor B); PII, pristinamycin IIA; PT, pristinamycin; TEL, telithromycin.

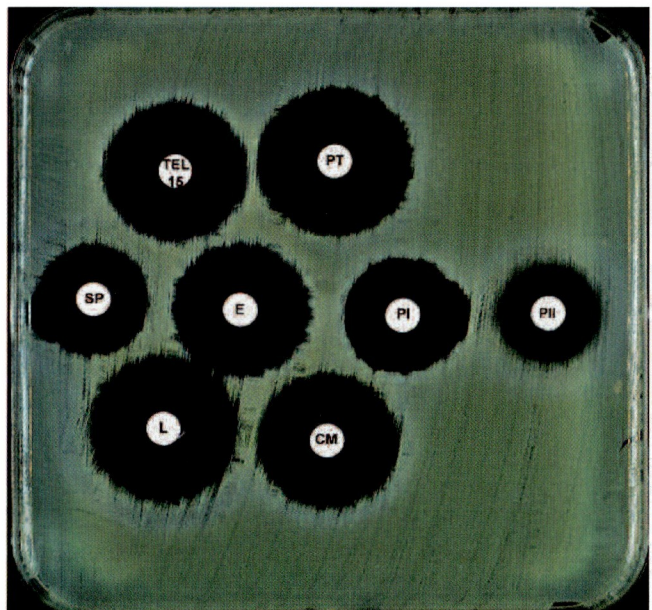 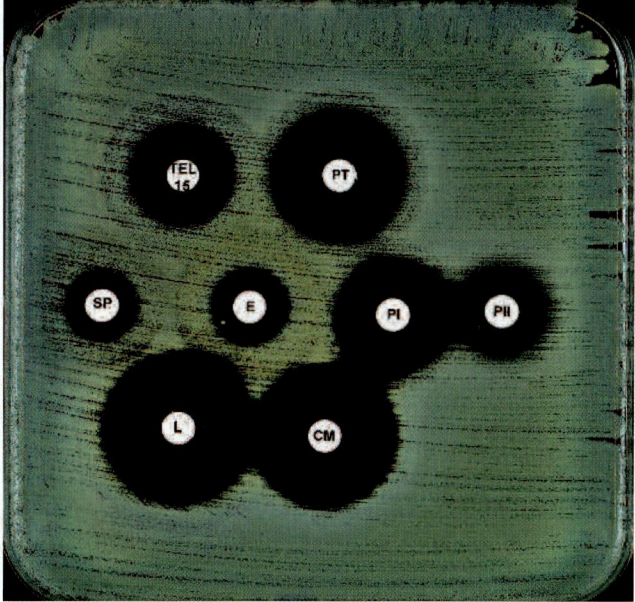

Fig. 8. *S. aureus* with protein L22 mutation. Left, susceptible strain. Right, protein L22 mutant strain. CM, clindamycin; E, erythromycin; L, lincomycin; SP, spiramycin; PI, pristinamycin IA (streptogramin factor B); PII, pristinamycin IIA; PT, pristinamycin; TEL, telithromycin. The presence of a double zone around certain disks is related to the presence of spontaneous susceptible revertants.

L22 mutations have been isolated in cystic fibrosis patients or have been selected during failure of treatment with quinupristin-dalfopristin (19). These mutations affect 14- and 15-membered macrolides, including ketolides, as well as streptogramins B and combinations of streptogramins A + B due to suppression of the synergy between the two factors. This phenotype is identified by a moderate degree of resistance to erythromycin and pristinamycin associated with susceptibility (or even hypersusceptibility) to clindamycin (Fig. 8, Table 4).

$A_{2058}G/U$ mutations confer a MLS_B phenotype similar to that conferred by constitutively expressed *erm* genes but with slightly lower levels of clindamycin resistance (MIC: 2 to 32 µg/ml) (26) (Fig. 9, Table 4). The $A_{2059}G$ mutation affects macrolides and lincosamides but does not appear to affect streptogramins B.

Enzymatic modification of erythromycin

The presence of macrolide-inactivating enzymes (esterases and phosphotransferases) is mainly reported in enterobacteria. However, the *mph*(C) gene encoding an erythromycin phosphotransferase has been reported in a strain of *S. aureus* in which it was associated with a *msr*(A) gene and an *erm*(Y) gene on the same plasmid (22).

Composite phenotypes

All of the phenotypes described above can be associated, which can complicate identification of the resulting composite phenotype. For example, Fig. 10 shows a combination of an inducible MLS_B phenotype and L phenotype. Some combinations are more frequent than others, such as the combination of constitutive MLS_B phenotype and S phenotype (Fig. 11).

ANTIBIOTICS TO BE TESTED

The study of erythromycin (or azithromycin, or clarithromycin) and clindamycin (or lincomycin) is sufficient for standard antibiotic susceptibility testing. The choice of lincomycin rather than clindamycin would be useful to identify the L phenotype and to more clearly identify the LS_A phenotype. Pristinamycin should be tested in the countries in which it is used, together with quinupristin-dalfopristin. Telithromycin must be tested separately, if necessary.

The response for one of the 14- or 15-membered macrolides is valid for the other macrolides of the same class (except for telithromycin). The response for lincomycin is valid for 16-membered macrolides and telithromycin in the case of MLS_B and MS_B phenotypes, which are the most common.

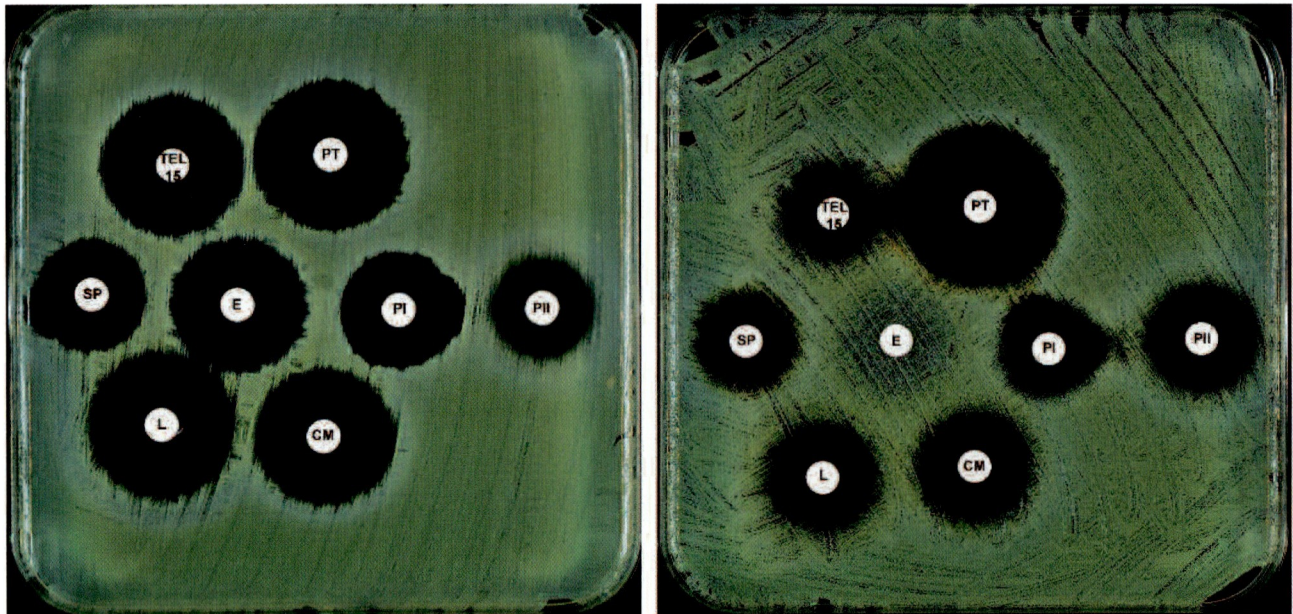

Fig. 9. *S. aureus* with A2058G mutation. Left, susceptible strain. Right, A2058G mutant strain. CM, clindamycin; E, erythromycin; L, lincomycin; SP, spiramycin; PI, pristinamycin IA (streptogramin factor B); PII, pristinamycin IIA; PT, pristinamycin; TEL, telithromycin.

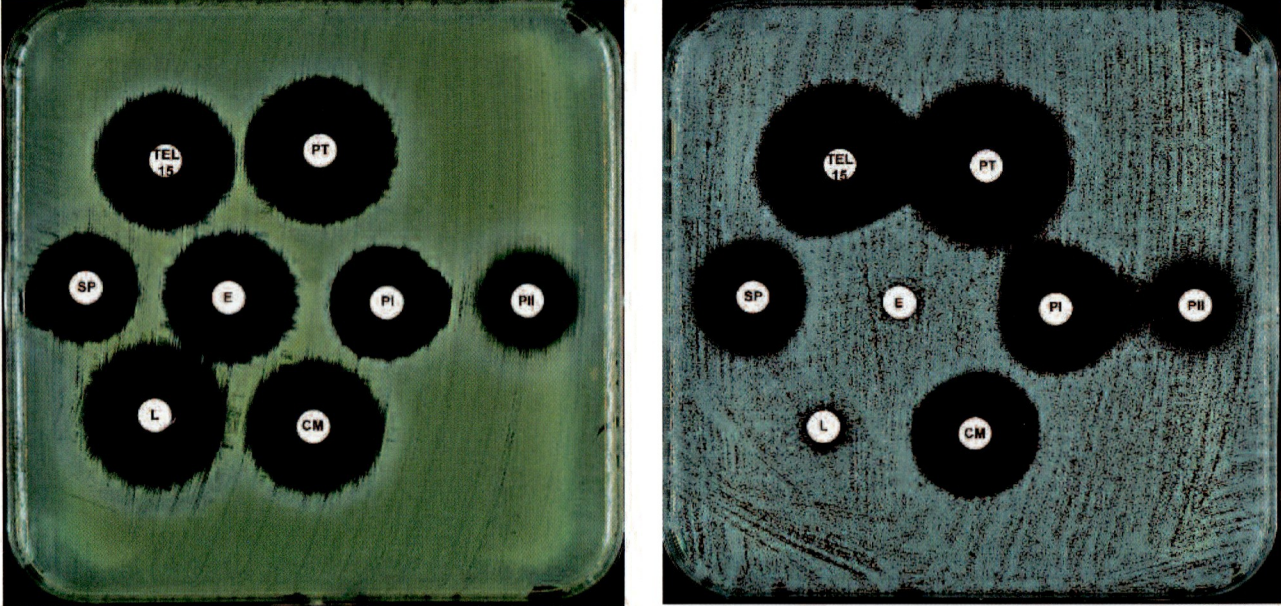

Fig. 10. Composite phenotype *S. aureus*. Left, susceptible strain. Right, strain comprising L phenotype and inducible MLS$_B$ phenotype. CM, clindamycin; E, erythromycin; L, lincomycin; SP, spiramycin; PI, pristinamycin IA (streptogramin factor B); PII, pristinamycin IIA; PT, pristinamycin; TEL, telithromycin.

On the other hand, the response for lincomycin is not valid for 16-membered macrolides in the case of the uncommon L and LS$_A$ phenotypes or some rare ribosomal mutation phenotypes. In countries in which these antibiotics are used, spiramycin (or josamycin) should therefore be added in a complementary antibiotic susceptibility test.

PNEUMOCOCCI AND β-HAEMOLYTIC STREPTOCOCCI

As for staphylococci, various phenotypes are due to similar mechanisms but are conferred by different classes of genes.

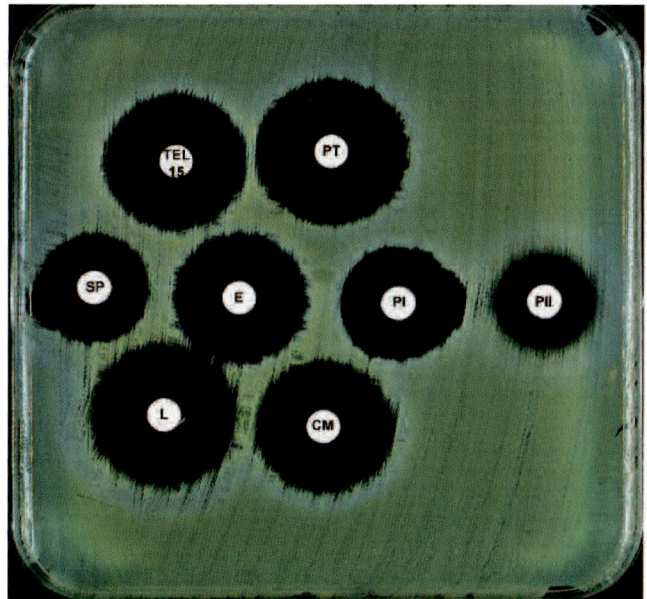 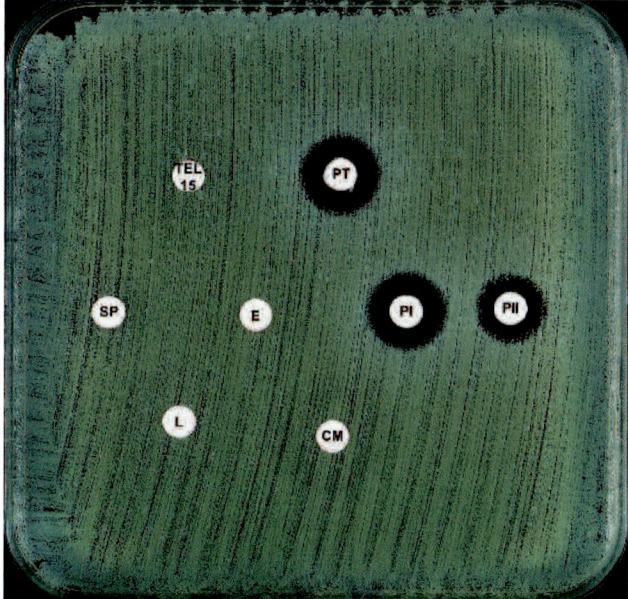

Fig. 11. Composite phenotype *S. aureus*. Left, susceptible strain. Right, strain comprising S phenotype and constitutive MLS$_B$ phenotype. CM, clindamycin; E, erythromycin; L, lincomycin; SP, spiramycin; PI, pristinamycin IA (streptogramin factor B); PII, pristinamycin IIA; PT, pristinamycin; TEL, telithromycin.

MLS$_B$ phenotype (*erm* genotype)

The dissemination of *erm* genes belonging to the *erm*(B) class and to a subgroup of the *erm*(A) class, *ermTR*, is responsible for MLS$_B$ resistance in streptococci. The phenotypes and their correlation with the *erm* genotype and the mode of expression of the gene have not been fully elucidated.

erm(B) genes with inducible expression are present in many species of *Streptococcus*, including β-haemolytic streptococci, pneumococci and streptococci of the oral flora. In general, this phenotype corresponds to high-level cross-resistance between macrolides, lincosamides and streptogramins B, as, unlike *erm*(A) and *erm*(C) genes in staphylococci, the various macrolides, including the 16-membered macrolides, induce the production of ErmB methylase. Induction studies, particularly including fusions of the attenuator with a reporter gene, have shown that the MLS$_B$ phenotype characterized by high-level cross-resistance between macrolides and lincosamides, commonly observed in pneumococci, is very frequently inducible (Fig. 12). In *Streptococcus pneumoniae*, this characteristic associated with the production of various baseline levels of enzyme due to decreased control of methylase synthesis by the *erm*(B) attenuator can explain the complexity of the phenotypes observed. Some strains of *S. pneumoniae* can present lower MIC for clindamycin or may even appear to be falsely susceptible to clindamycin (Fig. 13). In this case, MLS$_B$ phenotype is recognized by the spiramycin resistance expressed by these strains and by the visible antagonism between erythromycin and clindamycin on the disk diffusion method, indicating the production of methylase. A longer incubation period often reveals microcolonies in the clindamycin inhibition zone indicating that this antibiotic is not truly active and should therefore not be recommended to the clinician. The high frequency of inducible resistance in *S. pneumoniae* partly explains the activity of telithromycin, a non-inducing antibiotic, in relation to erythromycin-resistant pneumococci. More than 30% of pneumococcus strains harbouring *erm*(B) are falsely intermediate-susceptible to telithromycin when they are incubated in CO_2 (Fig. 14) (3).

Similar phenotypes are conferred by *erm(B)* in *Streptococcus pyogenes* and *Streptococcus agalactiae*. Some erythromycin-resistant strains apparently susceptible to clindamycin express double zone resistance on disk diffusion antibiotic susceptibility tests, characterized by regrowth close to the clindamycin disk after a prolonged incubation period. It should be noted that telithromycin is much less frequently active on *erm*(B) *S. pyogenes* strains than on *erm*(B) pneumococci. This could be related to the dimethylation activity of ErmB in *S. pyogenes*, which more effectively confers telithromycin resistance than the monomethylation activity exerted by this enzyme in *S. pneumoniae* (8).

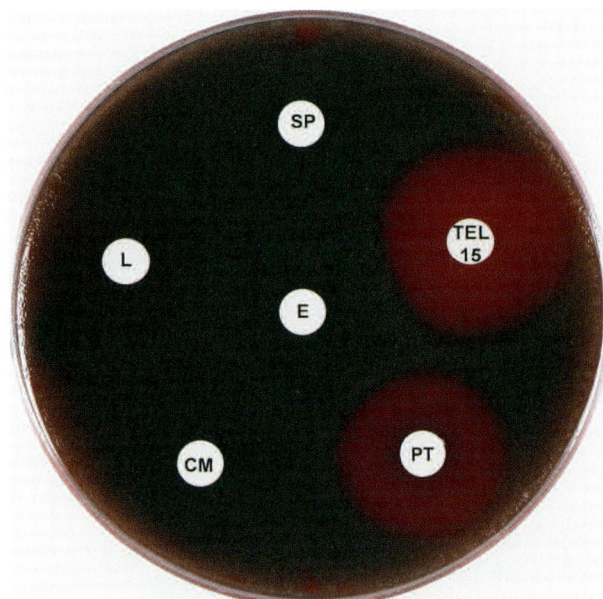

Fig. 12. *S. pneumoniae* harbouring the *erm*(B) gene (MLS$_B$ phenotype). CM, clindamycin; E, erythromycin; L, lincomycin; SP, spiramycin; PT, pristinamycin; TEL, telithromycin.

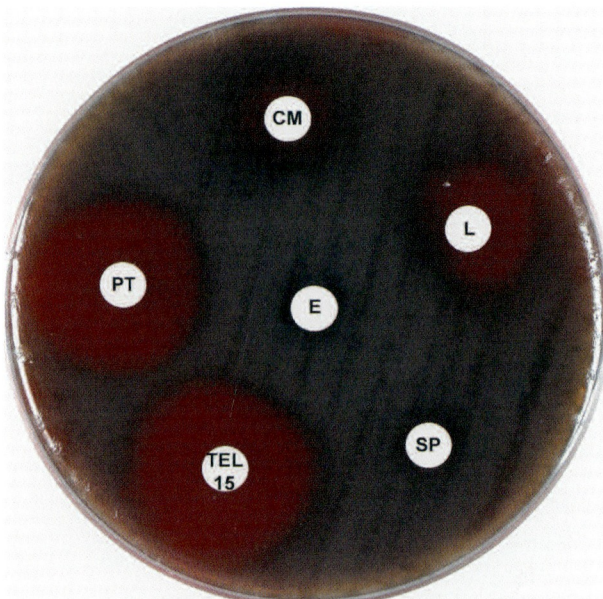

Fig. 13. *S. pneumoniae* harbouring the *erm*(B) gene (MLS$_B$ phenotype) apparently susceptible to lincomycin. CM, clindamycin; E, erythromycin; L, lincomycin; SP, spiramycin; PT, pristinamycin; TEL, telithromycin.

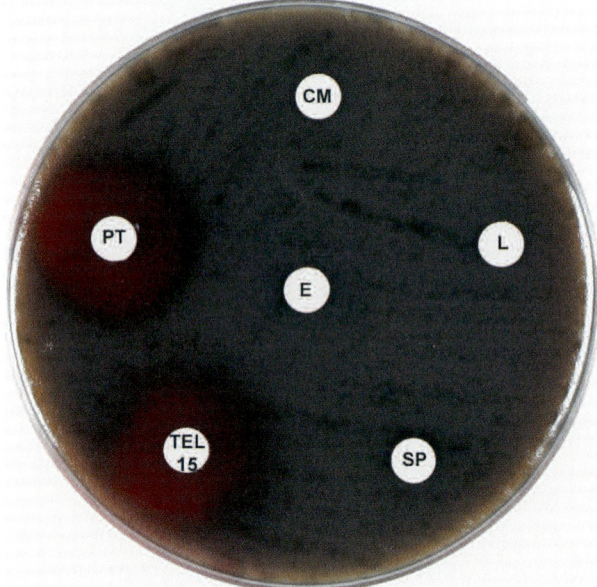

Fig. 14. *S. pneumoniae* harboring the *erm*(B) gene (MLS$_B$ phenotype) incubated in CO_2. The strain appears to be falsely intermediate to telithromycin. CM, clindamycin; E, erythromycin; L, lincomycin; SP, spiramycin; PT, pristinamycin; TEL, telithromycin.

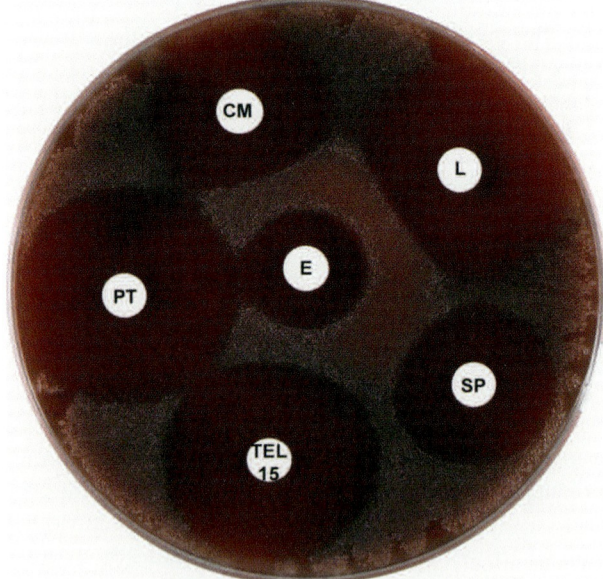

Fig. 15. S. pneumoniae harboring the *erm*(A) gene (MLSB phenotype). CM, clindamycin; E, erythromycin; L, lincomycin; SP, spiramycin; PT, pristinamycin; TEL, telithromycin.

Streptogramins remain rapidly bactericidal on *S. pyogenes* and *S. pneumoniae* strains with an MLS$_B$ phenotype.

The constitutive expression of *erm*(B) leads to high-level MLS$_B$ cross-resistance; telithromycin is not active on strains presenting this phenotype (rare in pneumococcus).

The *ermTR* gene [subclass of the *erm(A)* class] is mainly present in β-haemolytic streptococci, but has also been found in several strains of *S. pneumoniae*. This gene very often confers inducible resistance to 14-membered macrolides (except for telithromycin) with a low expression (MIC: 1 to 8 μg/ml) or more rarely a high expression (MIC > 128 μg/ml), while 16-membered macrolides and clindamycin remain active. Antagonism is observed between erythromycin and clindamycin (Fig. 15). This phenotype therefore resembles the inducible phenotype due to *erm*(A) described above for staphylococci. Constitutive resistant strains have been reported; they are highly resistant to clindamycin but often preserve MIC for erythromycin similar to those of inducible strains.

Interpretation and reporting of the results

The CLSI recommends looking for signs of antagonism by using a clindamycin disk (2 μg) and an erythromycin disk (15 μg) separated by an interval of 12 mm. If a D-shaped inhibition zone is observed around the clindamycin disk, the strain should be reported as resistant to erythromycin and clindamycin, possibly with a comment that clindamycin may be effective in some patients.

The EUCAST recommends that strains with a positive antagonism test should be reported as resistant to erythromycin and clindamycin, but without mentioning the possible efficacy of clindamycin in some patients, as false susceptibility to clindamycin may be observed in cases of inducible MLS_B phenotype due to the *erm*(B) gene with delayed expression of resistance.

As the bactericidal activity of pristinamycin and quinupristin-dalfopristin is not altered in strains with an MLS_B phenotype, the "S" interpretation does not need to be changed to "I".

M phenotype [*mef*(A) genotype]

The M phenotype in streptococci is due to active efflux encoded by genes initially called *mefA* in *S. pyogenes* and *mefE* in *S. pneumoniae*. Due to the high degree of deduced amino acid sequence homology, these two genes have been grouped into a single class *mef*(A). The only known substrates of this MFS efflux pump are 14-membered macrolides (except for telithromycin which is a poor substrate) and 15-membered macrolides. M resistance is inducible with a moderate level of resistance to erythromycin (Tables 5 and 6). The MIC for telithromycin are slightly increased in *S. pyogenes* and *S. pneumoniae*, but do not justify classification of these strains as intermediate strains. No antagonism is observed between erythromycin and clindamycin or lincomycin on disk diffusion. The *mef*(A) gene is transferable by conjugation in *S. pyogenes* and *S. pneumoniae*. It is carried by a large transposon in *S. pneumoniae*.

Interpretation and reporting of the results

As indicated above, the search for antagonism between erythromycin (or azithromycin or clarithromycin) and clindamycin is negative in the case of type M resistance. Tests for clindamycin and 16-membered macrolides must be reported as observed, as acquisition of the Mef pump by the strain has no effect on selection of mutants resistant to these antibiotics.

L phenotype [*lnu*(B) and *lnu*(C) genotypes]

The L phenotype is a rare phenotype only reported in *S. agalactiae* and *S. uberis* and is related to the acquisition of genes belonging to classes *lnu*(B), *lnu*(C) and *lnu*(D) (1, 5, 24). These distinct classes, but related to *lnu*(A) described above for staphylococci, encode lincosamide O-nucleotidyltransferases that only inactivate lincosamides [modification of the hydroxyl in position 3 of clindamycin and lincomycin in the case of *lnu*(B)]. The *lnu*(C) gene is carried by a transposon.

These strains are resistant to lincomycin (MIC: 16 to 32 μg/ml) but are intermediate or remain susceptible to clindamycin with MIC one to two dilutions higher than for the susceptible phenotype (MIC: 0.12 to 0.5 μg/ml). A 100-fold increase of the inoculum leads to a threefold increase of the MIC in relation to the strain harbouring the *lnu*(C) gene, while this inoculum effect is not observed for susceptible strains.

This lincosamide resistance is more clearly identified by the lincomycin test. On disk diffusion, the clindamycin inhibition zone is delineated by sudden growth arrest and is lined by large colonies reflecting inactivation of the antibiotic.

LS_A phenotype

This rare phenotype was reported in *S. agalactiae*, but is also observed in streptococci of the oral flora (20). Clindamycin, lincomycin and streptogramins A present decreased activity, as for the LSA phenotype of staphylococci. The mechanism and genetic basis for this resistance are unknown.

Phenotypes due to ribosomal mutations

Mutants of clinical strains have only been reported in recent years. Fig. 17 shows the mutations identified in pneumococci and the phenotypes conferred. Table 7 presents the MIC of MLS for various clinical isolates of mutant pneumococci. The first mutants to be identified were those

Table 5. MIC and clinical classification of *S. pneumoniae* in relation to the main MLS according to the most frequent resistance mechanisms

Resistance mechanism	Main resistance genes	Phenotype	MIC$_{50}$ – MIC$_{90}$ (µg/ml) (clinical classification)[a]				
			ERY	SPI	TEL	CLI	PRI
None	None	Susceptible	0.03 - 0.06 (S)	0.25 - 0.5 (S)	0.008 - 0.03 (S)	0.06 - 0.12 (S)	0.06 - 0.25 (S)
Ribosomal Methylation	*erm*(B)	MLS$_B$	>128 - >128 (R)	>128 - >128 (R)	0.03 - 0.25 (S)	>128 - >128 (R)	0.06 - 0.25 (S)
Efflux	*mef*(A)	M	4 - 16 (I/R)	0.25 - 0.5 (S)	0.12 - 0.5 (S)	0.06 - 0.12 (S)	0.06 - 0.25 (S)

[a] CLI, clindamycin; ERY, erythromycin; PRI, pristinamycin; SPI, spiramycin; TEL, telithromycin.

Table 6. MIC and clinical classification of *S. pyogenes* in relation to the main MLS according to the most frequent resistance mechanisms (personal results and according to 4 and 6)

Resistance mechanism	Main resistance genes	Phenotype	MIC$_{50}$ – MIC$_{90}$ (µg/ml)[a]				
			ERY	SPI	TEL	CLI	PRI
None	None	Susceptible	0.03 - 0.06 (S)	0.5 - 1 (S)	0.008 - 0.016 (S)	0.06 - 0.12 (S)	0.06 - 0.25 (S)
Ribosomal methylation	*erm*(A) *ermTR* subclass	Inducible MLS$_B$	2 - >128 (I/R)	1 - 32 (S/R)	0.008 - 0.03 (S)	0.06 - 0.25 (S)	0.06 - 0.25 (S)
	erm(B)	MLS$_B$	>128 - >128 (R)	>128 - >128 (R)	4 - 8 (R)	>128 - >128 (R)	0.06 - 0.25 (S)
Efflux	*mef*(A)	M	8 - 16 (R)	0.5 - 1 (S)	0.25 - 0.5 (S)	0.06 - 0.12 (S)	0.06 - 0.25 (S)

[a] CLI, clindamycin; ERY, erythromycin; PRI, pristinamycin; SPI, spiramycin; TEL, telithromycin.

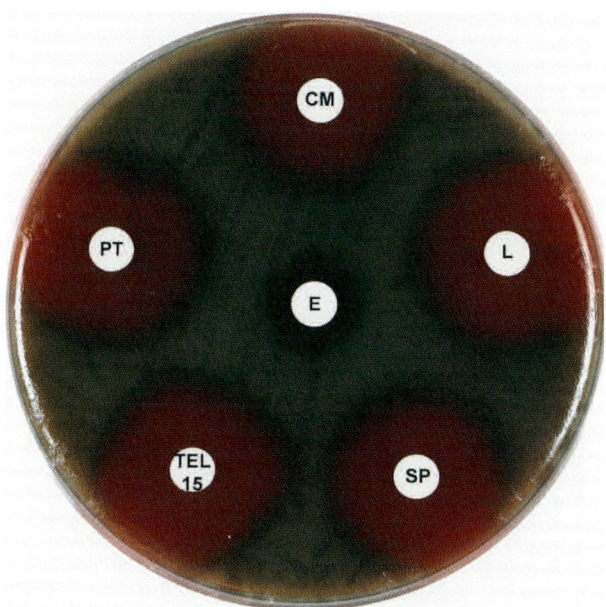

Fig. 16. *S. pneumoniae* harboring the *mef(A)* gene (M phenotype). CM, clindamycin; E, erythromycin; L, lincomycin; SP, spiramycin; PT, pristinamycin; TEL, telithromycin.

affecting adenine 2058 of 23S ribosomal RNA, which plays an important role in binding macrolides to the target, and adenine 2059 (17). At least two of the four copies of ribosomal RNA genes present in pneumococcus are mutant. These mutations confer MLS_B and MLS phenotypes, respectively. Other ribosomal RNA mutations have also been described in pneumococci. Mutation of adenine 2062 confers resistance to 16-membered macrolides and pristinamycin (17).

L4 and L22 ribosomal protein mutations are detected in clinical strains of pneumococci (17). L4 mutations are located in a highly preserved region of the protein and confer moderate resistance to macrolides but not to clindamycin. The L22 mutation confers low-level resistance to erythromycin and streptogramins and also affects telithromycin.

Various mutations have been described in β-haemolytic streptococci (4a, 21), for example the $C_{2611}U$ mutation of 23S rRNA and ribosomal protein L4 mutations ($_{69}KG$, $_{72}RA$ insertions, $_{63}WR$, $_{68}TG$ deletions) in *S. pyogenes* and the $_{71}EGTGR$ insertion in protein L4 in a group G streptococcus. Oral streptococci are also affected with a $_{70}RREKGTG$ insertion in L4 in *S. oralis* (4a, 21).

These mutants are rarely isolated, their clinical significance remains unclear and their frequency is possibly underestimated. However, their corresponding characteristic phenotypic profiles are starting to be identified and the possible presence

Table 7. MIC of MLS on clinical strains of *S. pneumoniae* harbouring ribosomal mutations (17)

Mutant structure	Mutation	Number of strains	MIC (µg/ml)[a]							
			AZM	CLR	ERY	SPI	JOS	TEL	CLI	QUI	PRI ou Q-D
23S rRNA domain V (mutant copy number)	$A_{2059}G$ (2 or 3)	5	>100 - >512	12.5 - >512	50 - >100	512	>100	0.01 - 0.25	0.78 - 2	3.12 - 32	2 - 4
	$A_{2059}C$ (2 to 4)	7	128 - 512	512 - >512	256 - >512	512 - >512	ND	0.06 - 0.12	1 - 2	16 - 32	1 - 2
	$A_{2062}C$ (4)	1	0.5	ND	<0.25	512	64	<0.0075	<0.015	32	2
	$C_{2611}G$ (4)	1	128	>512	>512	16	ND	0.5	1	>64	2
Protein L4	69TPS71	17	>100 - >512	12.5 - >512	100 - >512	64	100	0.03 - 0.2	0.05 - 0.2	12.5 - 25	2
	Insertion (71GREKGTGR72)[b]	1	12.5	12.5	6.25	ND	6.25	3.12	0.05	25	ND
Protein L22	Duplication (102KRTAHITRTAHITVA116)[b]	1	>1	ND	>1	ND	ND	ND	ND	ND	>1

[a] AZM, azithromycin; CLI, clindamycin; CLR, clarithromycin; ERY, erythromycin; JOS, josamycin; PRI, pristinamycin; Q-D, quinupristin-dalfopristin; QUI, quinupristin; SPI, spiramycin; TEL, telithromycin; ND, not determined.
[b] The mutation is underlined.

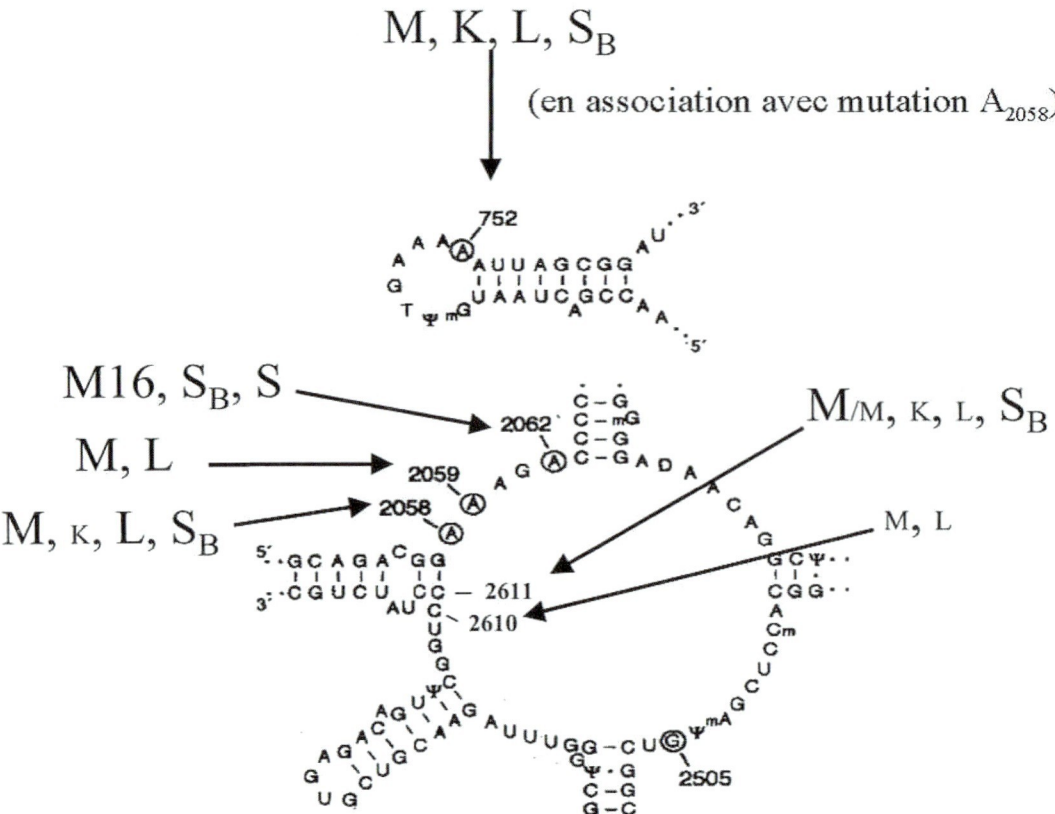

Fig. 17. Secondary structure of hairpin 35 (domain II) (above) and domain V (below) of *E. coli* 23S rRNA (16). Nucleotides protected by erythromycin are circled. Arrows indicate mutations conferring macrolide resistance in *S. pneumoniae*. The corresponding phenotype is indicated (K, ketolides; L, lincosamides; M, macrolides; M16, 16-member macrolides; S_B, streptogramin B; S, streptogramins A and B). Small capital letters correspond to low-level resistance.

of a mutation must be considered in the presence of any of these phenotypes or another unusual phenotype.

Antibiotics to be tested

Erythromycin (or azithromycin or clarithromycin), clindamycin or lincomycin are sufficient for standard antibiotic susceptibility testing. Pristinamycin should be tested in countries in which it is used. Spiramycin (or josamycin) and quinupristin-dalfopristin can also be added as complementary tests. Telithromycin must be studied specifically because its response cannot be deduced from those of the other MLS. Note that testing of telithromycin in CO_2 in relation to pneumococci harbouring *erm*(B) can lead to false-intermediate results which must be verified without CO_2.

The response for 14- or 15-membered macrolides tested by erythromycin applies to the other members of the same class (except telithromycin).

The response for clindamycin or lincomycin is valid for 16-membered macrolides in the case of MLS_B and M phenotypes, which are the most frequent, but not in the case of L and LS_A phenotypes or certain rare phenotypes due to ribosomal mutation.

ENTEROCOCCI

The MLS_B and M phenotypes, due to *erm*(B) and *mef*(A) genes respectively, are identified in erythromycin-resistant strains of *E. faecalis*, *E. faecium* and streptococci. The MLS_B phenotype is very frequent (more than 50-60% of strains) and is added to the natural LS_A resistance observed in *E. faecalis*. Some *E. faecium* strains possess the *lnu*(B) gene and therefore appear to be exclusively resistant to lincomycin (5). Streptogramins are active on *E. faecium* which does not express any natural LS_A resistance. However, many *E. faecium* strains acquire an LS_A phenotype although the resistance mechanism has not been identified (5). Most of these strains are intermediate to quinupristin-dalfopristin and some strains present frank resistance to quinupristin-dalfopristin (MIC: 8 or 16 µg/ml). They harbour *vat*(D) or *vat*(E) genes encoding streptogramin A acetyltransferases. These genes can be associated with the *vgb*(A) gene encoding a streptogramin B lyase.

OTHER GRAM-POSITIVE BACTERIA

Many other Gram-positive bacteria are resistant to macrolides. Streptococci other than pneumococci and β-haemolytic streptococci frequently express macrolide resistance and the various concepts described above also apply to these organisms. In a series of 128 strains of *Streptococcus gallolyticus*, 76 (59.4%) were resistant to erythromycin, 75 had a MLS_B phenotype and harboured *erm*(B) (n = 73) and two harboured an *erm*(B)-*mef*(A) combination (18). Only one strain expressed an M phenotype and harboured the *mef*(A) gene. Lactic bacteria (*Lactococcus, Lactobacillus, Pediococcus*) and *Corynebacterium* species also express macrolide resistance (see the chapters concerning these bacteria). *Nocardia* are very frequently resistant to macrolides; some strains can inactivate various macrolides by phosphorylation, glycosylation, reduction, or deacylation.

REFERENCES

(1) **Achard, A., C. Villers, V. Pichereau, and R. Leclercq**. 2005. New *lnu*(C) gene conferring resistance to lincomycin by nucleotidylation in *Streptococcus agalactiae* UCN36. Antimicrob. Agents Chemother. **49**:2716-2719.

(2) **Batard, E., C. Jacqueline, D. Boutoille, A. Hamel, H. B. Drugeon, N. Asseray, R. Leclercq, J. Caillon, G. Potel, and D. Bugnon**. 2002. Combination of quinupristin-dalfopristin and gentamicin against methicillin-resistant *Staphylococcus aureus*: experimental rabbit endocarditis study. Antimicrob. Agents Chemother. **46**:2174-2178.

(3) **Batard, E., M.E. Juvin, C. Jacqueline, D. Bugnon, J. Caillon, G. Potel, and H.B. Drugeon**. 2005. Influence of carbon dioxide on the MIC of telithromycin for *Streptococcus pneumoniae*: an in vitro-in vivo study. Antimicrob. Agents Chemother. **49**:464-466.

(4a) **Bingen, E., P. Bidet, L. Mihaila-Amrouche, C. Doit, S. Forcet, N. Brahimi, A. Bouvet, and R. Cohen**. 2004. Emergence of macrolide-resistant *Streptococcus pyogenes* strains in French children. Antimicrob. Agents Chemother. **48**:3559-3562.

(4b) **Bemer, P., M.E. Juvin, S. Corvec, A. Ros, and H. Drugeon**. 2005. Correlation of agar dilution and VITEK2 system for detection of resistance to macrolides, lincosamides and pristinamycin among *Staphylococcus aureus* and *Staphylococcus epidermidis* : association with genotypes. Clin. Microbial. Infect. **11**:656-661

(5) **Bozdogan, B., L. Berrezouga, M. Kuo, D. Yurek, K. Farley, B. Stockman, and R. Leclercq**. 1999. A new resistance gene, *linB*, conferring resistance to lincosamides by nucleotidylation in *Enterococcus faecium* HM1025. Antimicrob. Agents Chemother. **43**:925-929.

(6) **Canton, R., A. Mazzariol, M.I. Morosini, F. Baquero, and G. Cornaglia**. 2005. Telithromycin activity is reduced by efflux in *Streptococcus pyogenes*. J. Antimicrob. Chemother. **55**:489-495.

(7) **Canu, A., B. Malbruny, M. Coquemont, T. A. Davies, P. C. Appelbaum, and R. Leclercq**. 2002. Diversity of ribosomal mutations conferring resistance to macrolides, clindamycin, streptogramin, and telithromycin in *Streptococcus pneumoniae*. Antimicrob. Agents Chemother. **46**:125-13.

(8) **Chesneau, O., H. Ligeret, N. Hosan-Aghaie, A. Morvan, and E. Dassa**. 2005. Molecular analysis of resistance to streptogramin A compounds conferred by the Vga proteins of staphylococci. Antimicrob. Agents Chemother. **49**:973-980.

(9) **CLSI**. 2009. Performance standards for antimicrobial susceptibility testing: 19th informational supplement. NCCLS document M100–S19. CLSI, Wayne, PA.

(10) **Donay, J.L., D. Mathieu, P. Fernandes, C. Pregermain, P. Bruel, A. Wargnier, I. Casin, F.X. Weill, P.H. Lagrange, and J.L. Herrmann**. 2004. Evaluation of the automated phoenix system for potential routine use in the clinical microbiology laboratory. J. Clin. Microbiol. **42**:1542-1546.

(11) **Douthwaite, S., J. Jalava, and L. Jakobsen**. 2005. Ketolide resistance in *Streptococcus pyogenes* correlates with the degree of rRNA dimethylation by Erm. Mol. Microbiol. **58**:613-622.

(12) **Entenza, J. M., H. Drugeon, M. P. Glauser, and P. Moreillon**. 1995. Treatment of experimental endocarditis due to erythromycin-susceptible or -resistant methicillin-resistant *Staphylococcus aureus* with RP 59500. Antimicrob. Agents Chemother. **39**:1419-1424.

(13) **Fantin, B., R. Leclercq, Y. Merlé, L. Saint-Julien, C. Veyrat, J. Duval, and C. Carbon**. 1995. Critical influence of resistance to streptogramin B-type antibiotics on activity of RP 59500 (quinupristin-dalfopristin) in experimental endocarditis due to *Staphylococcus aureus*. Antimicrob. Agents Chemother. **39**:400-405.

(14) **Haroche, J., A. Morvan, M. Davi, J. Allignet, F. Bimet, and N. El Solh**. 2003. Clonal diversity among streptogramin A-resistant *Staphylococcus aureus* isolates collected in French hospitals. J. Clin. Microbiol. **41**:586-591.

(15) **Kehrenberg, C., K.K. Ojo, and S. Schwarz**. 2004. Nucleotide sequence and organization of the multiresistance plasmid pSCFS1 from *Staphylococcus sciuri*. J. Antimicrob. Chemother. **54**:936-939.

(16) **Leclercq, R**. 2002. Mechanisms of resistance to macrolides and lincosamides: nature of the resistance

elements and their clinical implications. Clin. Infect. Dis. **15**:482-492.

(17) **Leclercq, R., and P. Courvalin.** 2002. Resistance to macrolides and related antibiotics in *Streptococcus pneumoniae.* Antimicrob. Agents Chemother. **46**:2727-2734.

(18) **Leclercq, R., C. Huet, M. Picherot, P. Trieu-Cuot, and C. Poyart.** 2005. Genetic basis of antibiotic resistance in clinical isolates of *Streptococcus gallolyticus* (*Streptococcus bovis*). Antimicrob. Agents Chemother. **49**:1646-1648.

(19) **Malbruny, B., A. Canu, B. Bozdogan, V. Zarrouk, B. Fantin, and R. Leclercq.** 2002. Resistance to quinupristin-dalfopristin due to mutation of L22 ribosomal protein in *Staphylococcus aureus.* Antimicrob. Agents Chemother. **46**:2200-2207.

(20) **Malbruny, B., A. M. Werno, T. P. Anderson, D. R. Murdoch, and R. Leclercq.** 2004. A new phenotype of resistance to lincosamide and streptogramin A-type antibiotics in *Streptococcus agalactiae* in New Zealand. J. Antimicrob. Chemother. **54**:1040-1044.

(21) **Malbruny, B., K. Nagai, M. Coquemont, B. Bozdogan, A. T. Andrasevic, H. Hupkova, R. Leclercq, and P. C. Appelbaum.** 2002. Resistance to macrolides in clinical isolates of *Streptococcus pyogenes* due to ribosomal mutations. J. Antimicrob. Chemother. **49**:935-939.

(22) **Matsuoka, M., K. Endou, H. Kobayashi, M. Inoue, and Y. Nakajima.** 1998. A plasmid that encodes three genes for resistance to macrolide antibiotics in *Staphylococcus aureus.* FEMS Microbiol. Lett. **167**:221–227.

(23) **Mihaila-Amrouche, L., A. Bouvet, and J. Loubinoux.** 2004. Clonal spread of emm type 28 isolates of *Streptococcus pyogenes* that are multiresistant to antibiotics. J. Clin. Microbiol. **42**:3844-3846.

(24) **Petinaki, E., V. Guérin-Faublée, V. Pichereau, C. Villers, A. Achard, B. Malbruny, and R. Leclercq.** 2008 Lincomycin resistance gene *lnu*(D) in *Streptococcus uberis*. Antimicrob Agents Chemother. **52**:626-630.

(25) **Prunier, A. L., B. Malbruny, D. Tande, B. Picard, and R. Leclercq.** 2002. Clinical isolates of *Staphylococcus aureus* with ribosomal mutations conferring resistance to macrolides. Antimicrob. Agents Chemother. **46**:3054-3056.

(26) **Prunier, A.L, H.N. Trong, D. Tande, C. Segond, and R. Leclercq.** 2005. Mutation of L4 ribosomal protein conferring unusual macrolide resistance in two independent clinical isolates of *Staphylococcus aureus*. Microb. Drug Resist.**11**:18-20.

(27) **Siebor, E, and A. Kazmierczak.** 1993. Factors influencing the activity of macrolides antibiotics *in vitro*, pp. 197-203. *In* A.J. Bryskier, J.P. Butzler, H.C. Neu, and P.M. Tulkens (ed.), Macrolides: chemistry, pharmacology and clinical uses. Arnette-Blackwell, Paris.

(28) **Tang, P., D.E. Low, S. Atkinson, K. Pike, A. Ashi-Sulaiman, A. Simor, S. Richardson, and B.M. Willey.** 2003. Investigation of *Staphylococcus aureus* isolates identified as erythromycin intermediate by the Vitek-1 System: comparison with results obtained with the Vitek-2 and Phoenix systems. J. Clin. Microbiol. **41**:4823-4825.

(29) **Weisblum, B.** 1995. Insights into erythromycin action from studies of its activity as inducer of resistance. Antimicrob. Agents Chemother. **39**:797-805

(30) **Wondrack, L., M. Massa, B. V. Yang, and J. Sutcliffe.** 1996. Clinical strain of *Staphylococcus aureus* inactivates and causes efflux of macrolides. Antimicrob. Agents Chemother. **40**:992-998.

(31) **Zarrouk, V., B. Bozdogan, R. Leclercq, L. Garry, C. Carbon, and B. Fantin.** 2000. Influence of resistance to streptogramin A type antibiotics on the activity of quinupristin-dalfopristin in vitro and in experimental endocarditis due to *Staphylococcus aureus.* Antimicrob. Agents Chemother. **44**:1168-1173.

Chapter 24. TETRACYCLINES

Claire POYART

INTRODUCTION

Discovered more than 60 years ago, tetracyclines are bacterial protein synthesis inhibitors. They are wide spectrum bacteriostatic antibiotics that are active against Gram positive and Gram negative bacteria and also against other microorganisms such as *Chlamydia*, mycoplasma, rickettsia and certain protozoa. These molecules have long been prescribed for human and veterinary treatment and are also used in sub-therapeutic doses as growth promoters in animals. Their massive use has become uncontrollable and has been the cause of the selection and the dissemination of resistant bacteria leading over the years to the limitation of their use. Meanwhile, new molecules have appeared, the glycylcyclines, a new generation in this family.

STRUCTURE

The oldest molecules, chlortetracycline and oxytetracycline, are natural antibiotics, produced by *Streptomyces aureofaciens* and *Streptomyces rimosus*. The other molecules are, in some cases produced by other bacterial species, and in others hemisynthetic products such as doxocycline and minocycline. In recent years, in the mid 1990s, new hemisynthetic compounds have appeared, third generation cyclins or glycylcyclines, such as tigecycline (6). The basic chemical structure of cyclines can be seen in Figure 1. They are formed by four cycles (A, B, C, D). Carbons 1, 10, 11 and 12 are always substituted by oxygenated compounds, Carbon 14 always by a dimethylamine, and Carbons C5, C6 and C7 are replaced by diverse substitutes. The structures of doxycycline, minocycline and tigecycline is represented in Figure 2. The configuration of available molecules is depicted in Table 1.

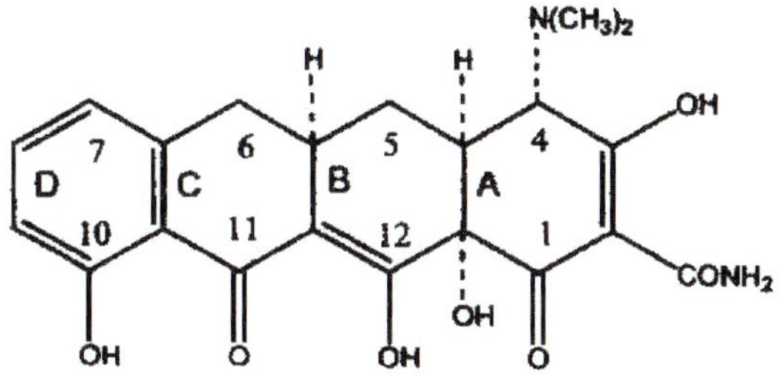

Fig. 1. The common skeleton of tetracyclines. The cycles are indicated by a letter and the carbon atoms by a number.

Table 1. Main tetracyclines

International nonproprietary name	Chemical name	Commercial name
Doxycycline	6-Deoxy-5-hydroxytetracycline	Doxy ; Doxycycline Arrow ; Doxycycline Biogaran ; Doxycycline G Gam ; Doxycycline GNR ; Doxycycline MERCK ; Doxycycline Ratiopharm ; Doxygram ; Granudoxy ; Spanor ; Tolexine ; Vibramycine
Lymecycline	2-*N*-lysinomethyltetracycline	Tetralysal
Methacycline	6-Methylene-5-hydroxytetracycline	Lysocycline ; Physiomycine
Minocycline	7-Dimethylamino-6-demethyl-6-deoxytetracycline	Logryx ; Mestacine ; Minocycline Biogaran ; Minocycline EG ; Minocycline GNR ; Minocycline IREX ; Minocycline IVAX ; Minocycline MERCK ; Minocycline TEVA ; Minolis ; Mynocine ; Yelnac ; Zacnan
Tigecycline	9-(tbutylglycylamido)-minocycline	Tygacil

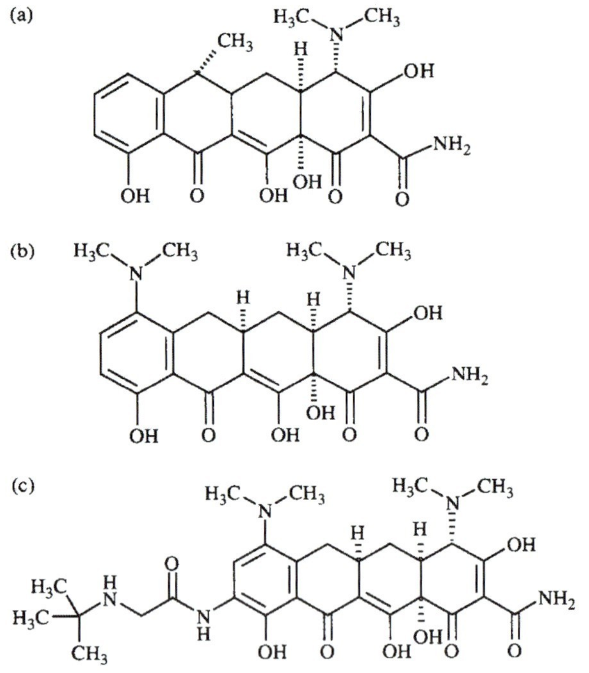

Fig. 2. Structure of doxycycline (a), minocycline (b), and tigecycline (c).

MECHANISM OF ACTION

Bacterial penetration

Two processes occur during bacterial penetration: passive diffusion through the wall which is different in Gram positive and Gram negative bacteria and active absorption at cytoplasmic membrane level that is specific for tetracyclines and is present in all prokaryotes. In the case of Gram negative bacteria, tetracyclines cross the outer membrane through the OmpF and OmpC porins as a chelation complex with a Mg^{2+} ion. The Mg^{2+}-tetracycline complex becomes disassociated in the bacterial periplasm and the antibiotic crosses the cytoplasmic membrane by means of an energy process driven by protomotrice force. In the cytoplasm, the tetracyclines once more chelate Mg^{2+} ions so that they can attach to their ribosomal target. Maintenance of a significant concentration of antibiotic is absolutely essential for antibacterial action (23,31).

Action at ribosome level

Tetracyclines are inhibitors of the elongation phase of protein synthesis. They attach to the 30S ribosome subunit and especially to protein S7 of the nucleotides G693, A892, U1052, C1054, G1300 and G1338 of rRNA 16S to prevent the attachment of tRNA aminoacyl. These molecules have little activity in eukaryote cells because they possess only low affinity for 80s ribosomes. On the other hand, they can interact with 70S ribosomes of the mitochondria which accounts for their use in the treatment of infections caused by parasites such as *Plasmodium falciparum*, *Entamoeba histolytica*, *Giardia lamblia*, *Leshmania major*, *Trichomonas vaginalis* and *Toxoplasma gondii*.

ANTIBACTERIAL ACTIVITY AND MAIN THERAPEUTICAL INDICATIONS

Minimum inhibitory concentrations (MIC) of tetracycline for the main bacterial species are detailed in Tables 2 and 3. There are currently few therapeutic indications for use of these antibiotics in humans (Table 4). The main ones are treatment of atypical community pneumonia caused by

Table 2. Tetracycline activity against the main bacterial species against Gram negative species (3, 4, 24)

Species	MIC (µg/ml)		
	MIC_{50}	MIC_{90}	Limit values
Escherichia coli			
Tetracycline	< 2	> 8	0.06 - 8
Minocycline	1	8	< 0.5 - > 1
Tigecycline	0.12	0.25	0.03 - 16
Enterobacter spp.			
Tetracycline	< 2	> 8	0.06 - 8
Minocycline	2	16	≤ 2 - > 8
Tigecycline	0.5	1	0.06 - 16
Klebsiella spp.			
Tetracycline	< 2	> 8	0.06 - 8
Minocycline	2	16	< 0.5 - > 16
Tigecycline	0.5	0.25	0.12 - 8
Proteus mirabilis			
Tetracycline	< 2	> 8	0.25 - 16
Minocycline	2	16	< 0.5 - > 16
Tigecycline	4	4	0.12 - 8
Serratia spp.			
Tetracycline	> 8	> 8	< 2 - > 8
Minocycline	4	> 8	< 0.5 - > 16
Tigecycline	1	2	0.12 - 8
P. aeruginosa			
Tetracycline	> 8	> 8	< 2 - > 8
Minocycline	> 16	> 16	< 0.5 - > 16
Tigecycline	8	16	0.25 - > 32
Acinetobacter spp.			
Tetracycline	1	8	< 2 - > 8
Minocycline	> 16	> 16	< 0.5 - > 16
Tigecycline	1	2	0.06 - 8
S. maltophilia			
Tetracycline	> 8	> 8	< 2 - > 8
Minocycline	> 16	> 16	< 0.5 - > 16
Tigecycline	1	2	0.12 - 8

Table 3. Tetracycline activity against the main bacterial Gram positive species (3, 4, 24)

Bacteria[a]	MIC (µg/ml)		
	MIC$_{50}$	MIC$_{90}$	Limit values
Staphylococcus aureus methicilin^S			
Tetracycline	< 2	> 8	<0.2 - > 8
Minocycline	< 0.25	< 0.25	< 0.25 - > 8
Tigecycline	0.12	0.25	0.016 - 1
Staphylococcus aureus methicilin^R			
Tetracycline	< 2	> 8	0.06 - 32
Minocycline	< 0.25	0.5	< 0.25 - > 8
Tigecycline	0.12	0.25	0.016 - 1
Staphylococcus negative coagulase			
Tetracycline	< 2	> 8	0.03 - 1
Minocycline	2	16	< 0.5 - > 16
Tigecycline	0.25	0.5	0.12 - 8
Streptococcus pneumoniae			
Tetracycline	< 4	> 8	< 4 - > 8
Tigecycline	< 0.12	< 0.12	<0.12 - 1
Streptococcus β-hemolytic (A, B, C, G)			
Tetracycline	> 8	> 8	< 2 - > 8
Tigecycline	< 0.12	< 0.12	< 0.12 - 0.5
Streptococcus "viridans" group			
Tetracycline	> 8	> 8	< 2 - > 8
Tigecycline	< 0.12	< 0.12	< 0.12 - 5
Enterococcus spp.			
Tetracycline	> 8	> 8	≤ 2 - > 8
Tigecycline	0.12	0.25	≤ 0.016 - 2

[a] R, resistant; S, susceptible.

Mycoplasma pneumoniae, *Chlamydophila pneumoniae* and *Chlamydophila psittaci*, genitourinary infections (non-gonococcal urethritis, lymphogranuloma venereum), infections caused by *Rickettsia* infections (Rocky Mountain spotted fever), *Coxiella* (Q fever), *Borrelia* (Lyme disease, relapsing fever), *Brucella* (brucellosis), *Leptospira* (leptospirosis), *Pasteurella* (tularemia) and specific infections such as periodontitis or acne and gastritis caused by *Helicobacter pylori* in association with other antibiotics. Furthermore, these molecules are part of the prophylaxis or treatment of infections caused by biological weapons such as *Bacillus anthracis*, *Francisella tularensis* and *Yersinia pestis*.

PHARMACOKINETICS, PHARMACODYNAMICS, CONTRA-INDICATIONS AND SIDE-EFFECTS

The digestive tract absorption of tetracyclines, such as doxycycline and minocycline, is close to 100% and is better on an empty stomach than in post-prandial conditions. Ingestion of minerals salts, aluminum, calcium, magnesium, iron or bismuth in their diverse forms, reduces digestive tract absorption of tetracyclines since it binds to them forming insoluble chelates. Tetracyclines bind to plasma proteins (80 to 90%) and have good diffusion into most body cell compartments.

Their passage across the blood-brain barrier increases if there is inflammation of the meninges. Tetracyclines cross the placental barrier and are also secreted in milk. Their half-life is variable depending on the molecule, from 16 to 22 hours, and is not modified by renal failure.

On the other hand, it is markedly reduced by the administration of barbiturates, diphenylhydantoin and carbamazepine. Tetracyclines are not metabolized but when administered orally form complexes with different cations in the intestine. They are eliminated by the kidneys, 35 to 50% of the dose administered is eliminated in urine in an active form. A small fraction of the dose administered is also excreted in the bile. Tetracyclines, that have a great affinity for bone tissue, if administered to children less than eight years of age with developing teeth may cause permanent staining (dental dyschromies) or enamel hypoplasia.

Table 4. Main therapeutic indications for tetracyclines in humans

First Intention	Alternative
Bacillus anthracis (curative)	*Bacillus anthracis* (prophylaxis)
Bartonella quintana	*Burkholderia* spp.
Bartonella henselae	*Donovania granulomatis*
Borrelia burgdoferi	*Francisella tularensis*
Brucella spp.	*Helicobacter pylori*
Chlamydophila pneumoniae	*Leptospira* spp.
Chlamydophila psittaci	*Mycobacterium abcessus*
Chlamydophila trachomatis	*Mycobacterium fortuitum*
Francisella tularensis (curative)	*Yersinia pestis* (curative)
Mycoplasma pneumoniae	*P. falciparum*
Mycoplasma hominis	
Ureaplasma	
Pasteurella spp.	
Plasmodium falciparum mefloquine resistant	
Rickttesia spp.	
Yersinia pestis (prophylaxis)	
Perionditite	
Cutanous acne	

Tetracyclines may also cause hematological problems (thrombopenia, neutropenia), phototoxic reactions and digestive alterations (diarrhea, sometimes due to *Clostridium difficile,* hepatitis). Tetracyclines are contraindicated in pregnant women during the last part of pregnancy and also in women who breast-feed due to the risk of dental anomalies in infants.

DETERMINATION OF SUSCEPTIBILITY AND DETECTION OF RESISTANCE

To determine susceptibility to tetracycline it is advisable to use the techniques recommended by the European Committee on Antimicrobial Susceptibility Testing (EUCAST) and the Clinical and Laboratory Standards Institute (CLSI). In Table 5 shows the critical concentrations for the main molecules and the main pathogens for which these are indicated. The determination of susceptibility using liquid media techniques furnishes results that are in perfect concordance with those obtained in solid media. Recent studies of susceptibility to tigecycline in liquid media show that the accumulation of oxygen dissolved in the Mueller-Hinton medium over the course of time inhibits tigecycline action by oxidation. Therefore, it is advisable to use media batches of less than one week or to supplement them with Oxyrase®, a biocatalytic oxygen-reducing agent (5).

Susceptibility to tetracycline (Tc) and to minocycline (Mn) makes it possible to distinguish between the two main mechanisms of resistance, efflux type of resistance (Tc^R, Mn^S), or ribosome protection type of resistance (Tc^R Mn^R). The genotype detection of the resistance genes by PCR by using specific or degenerated oligonuceotides has made it possible to determine the prevalence of the different determinants, especially among streptococci and staphylococci, and also to characterize new resistance genes.

RESISTANCE MECHANISMS AND GENETIC BASIS

Resistance to tetracyclines is one of the most frequent type of resistance, both in Gram negative and Gram positive bacteria. Sequence analyses of tetracycline resistance gene enable a genetic nomenclature. Therefore, determinants are considered identical if their deduced peptide sequences share more than 80% of identical amino-acids (18). More than thirty resistance genes have been described and are designated by *tet* or *otr* followed by a letter or a number. The list of these different genes and their distribution is described in Tables 6 to 8. Three main acquired resistance mechanisms

Chapter 24. TETRACYCLINES

have been described: efflux, ribosome protection and, very rarely, enzyme inactivation (6, 31). Resistance acquired by chromosome gene mutation is rare and affects few bacterial species. Mutations are located in the genes coding for rRNA 16S or in the genes encoding membrane transport proteins.

Efflux

This is the main mechanism of resistance in Gram negative bacteria. The corresponding *tet* genes code for the membrane proteins that allow antibiotic efflux out of the cell preventing its intracellular accumulation and ribosome binding (Table 6). These proteins, of approximately 46 kDa, also share structural homologis with other efflux proteins such as MDR systems (multidrug resistance) are responsible for resistance to quarternary ammonium, chloramphenicol or quinolones. These determinants cause bacterial resistance to tetracycline, but not to minocycline with the exception of the determinant *tet*(B) that causes resistance to both antibiotics.

In the case of Gram negative bacteria, these genes are often located on mobile genetic elements, such as plasmids, frequently conjugative, or transposable elements such as Tn*10* that contains the *tet*(B) gene.

Tetracycline induces the expression of resistance. In the case of Gram negative bacteria, this regulation mechanism is linked to the presence of a gene that codes for a transcriptional repressor, usually located upstream from the corresponding *tet* gene and transcribed in opposite orientation. The inter-gene region contains a promotor sequence and an operator sequence. In absence of tetracycline, the repressor that is in the form of a homodimer binds to the operator and begins transcription whereas that of the *tet* gene codes for the

Table 6. Resistance mechanisms conferred by *tet* or *otr* genes (6, 27)

Efflux
tet(A), *tet*(B), *tet*(C), *tet*(D), *tet*(D), *tet*(E), *tet*(G), *tet*(H), *tet*(I), *tet*(J), *tet*(K), *tet*(L), *tet*(V), *tet*(Y), *tet*(Z), *tet*(30), *tet*(31), *tet*(33), *tet*(35), *tet*(38), *tet*(39), *tet*P(A), *ort*(B), *ort*(C), *tcr*3

Ribosome protection
tet(M), *tet*(O), *tet*(S), *tet*(Q), *tet*(T), *tet*(W), *ort*(A), *tet*P(B), *tet*(32), *tet*(36), *tet*

Enzyme inactivation
tet(X), *tet*(34), *tet*(37)

Unknown
tet(U)

Table 5. Critical concentrations of tetracyclines for the main bacterial species according to the recommendations of EUCAST and CLSI (µg/ml; S </R >)

EUCAST	Enterobacteriaceae	Pseudomonas	Acinetobacter	Staphylococcus	Enterococcus	Streptococcus	S. pneumoniae	H. influenzae	N. gonorrhoeae	N. meningitidis
Tetracycline	--[a]	--	--	1/2	--	1/2	1/2	1/2	0.5/1	1/2
Doxycycline	--	--	--	0.5/1	--	1/2	1/2	1/2	IE	--
Minocycline	--	--	IE[b]	1/2	--	0.5/1	0.5/1	1/2	1/2	1/2
Tigecycline	1/2	--	IE	0.5/0.5	0.25/0.5	0.25/0.5	IE	IE	IE	IE
CLSI										
Tetracycline	4/16	8/16	--	4/16	4/16	2/8[c]	2/8[c]	2/8[c]	0.25/2	2
Doxycycline	4/16	8/16	--	4/16	4/16					
Minocycline	4/16	8/16	--	4/16	4/16					
Tigecycline	2	ND	2	0.5	0.25	0.25	0.25	2	2	2

[a] --, Susceptbility testing not recommended as the species is a poor target for therapy with the drug.
[b] IE, There is insufficient evidence that the species in question is a good target for for therapy with the drug.
[c] Organisms that are susceptible to tetracycline are also considered susceptible to doxycycline and minocycline.

Table 7. Distribution of *tet* resistance genes in Gram negative bacteria (6, 27)

Genus	Efflux	Ribosome protection	Enzyme inactivation
Acinetobacter	*tet*(A), *tet*(B), *tet*(H), *tet*(39)	*tet*(M)	
Actinobacillus	*tet*(B), *tet*(L), *tet*(H)		
Afipia		*tet*(M)	
Aeromonas	*tet*(A), *tet*(B), *tet*(C), *tet*(D), *tet*(E)		
Agrobacterium	*tet*(30)		
Alcaligenes	*tet*(E)		
Alteromonas	*tet*(D)		
Bacteroides		*tet*(M), *tet*(Q), *tet*(36)	*tet*(X)
Brevundimonas	*tet*(B)		
Butyrivibrio		*tet*(Q), *tet*(W)	
Campylobacter		*tet*(O)	
Capnocytophaga		*tet*(Q)	
Citrobacter	*tet*(A), *tet*(B), *tet*(C), *tet*(D)		
Edwarsiella	*tet*(A), *tet*(D)		
Eikenella		*tet*(M)	
Enterobacter	*tet*(B), *tet*(C), *tet*(D)	*tet*(M)	
Erwinia	*tet*(B)		
Escherichia	*tet*(A), *tet*(B), *tet*(C), *tet*(D), *tet*(E), *tet*(G), *tet*(I), *tet*(Y)	*tet*(M)	
Eubacterium	*tet*(K)		
Fusobacterium	*tet*(L)	*tet*(M), *tet*(W)	
Klebsiella	*tet*(A), *tet*(B), *tet*(C), *tet*(D)	*tet*(M)	
Haemophilus	*tet*(A), *tet*(B), *tet*(K)	*tet*(M)	
Mannheimia	*tet*(B), *tet*(G), *tet*(H)		
Mitsuokella		*tet*(M), *tet*(Q), *tet*(W)	
Moraxella	*tet*(B), *tet*(H)		
Neisseria	*tet*(B)	*tet*(M), *tet*(O), *tet*(Q), *tet*(W)	
Pantoea	*tet*(B)		
Pasteurella	*tet*(B), *tet*(D), *tet*(G), *tet*(H)	*tet*(M)	
Photobacterium	*tet*(B)		
Pleisiomonas	*tet*(A), *tet*(B), *tet*(D)		
Porphyromonas		*tet*(M), *tet*(Q) *tet*(W)	
Prevotella		*tet*(Q)	
Proteus	*tet*(A), *tet*(B), *tet*(C), *tet*(J), *tet*(L)		
Providencia	*tet*(B), *tet*(E), *tet*(I), *tet*(G)		
Pseudomonas	*tet*(A), *tet*(B), *tet*(C), *tet*(E), *tet*(G) *tet*(34)	*tet*(M)	
Salmonella	*tet*(A), *tet*(B), *tet*(C), *tet*(D), *tet*(G), *tet*(L)		
Selenomonas		*tet*(M), *tet*(Q), *tet*(W)	
Serratia	*tet*(A), *tet*(B), *tet*(C), *tet*(E), *tet*(34)		
Shigella	*tet*(A), *tet*(B), *tet*(C), *tet*(D)		
Stenotrophomonas	*tet*(35)		
Treponema	*tet*(B		
Veillonella	*tet*(L)	*tet*(M), *tet*(Q), *tet*(S), *tet*(W)	
Vibrio	*tet*(A), *tet*(B), *tet*(C), *tet*(D), *tet*(E), *tet*(G), *tet*(35)	*tet*(M)	*tet*(34)
Yersinia	*tet*(D)		
Unknown			*tet*(37)

Table 8. Distribution of tetracycline resistance genes in Gram positive bacteria, *Mycobacterium*, *Mycoplasma*, *Ureaplasma*, *Nocardia*, *Streptomyces*, and *Chlamydophila* (6, 27)

Genus	Efflux	Ribosome protection
Abiotrophia		tet(M)
Actinomyces	tet(L)	tet(M), tet(W)
Aerococcus		tet(M), tet(O)
Arcanobacterium		tet(W)
Bacillus	tet(K), tet(L),	tet(M), tet(W)
Bacterionema		tet(M)
Bifidobacterium		tet(M), tet(W)
Clostridium	tet(K), tet(L),	tet(M), tet(P), tet(Q), tet(32), tet(36)
Corynebacterium		tet(M), tet(Z)
Enterococcus	tet(K), tet(L),	tet(M), tet(O), tet(S),
Erysipelothrix		tet(M)
Eubacterium	tet(K)	tet(M), tet(Q)
Gardnerella		tet(M), tet(Q)
Gemella		tet(M)
Lactobacillus		tet(M), tet(Q), tet(S) tet(W), tet(36)
Lactococcus		tet(M), tet(S)
Listeria	tet(K), tet(L)	tet(M), tet(S)
Mobilincus		tet(O), tet(Q)
Mycobacterium	tet(K), tet(L), tet(V), otr(B)	tet(M), otr(A)
Mycoplasma		tet(M)
Nocardia	tet(K)	
Peptostreptococcus	tet(K), tet(L)	tet(M), tet(O), tet(Q)
Staphylococcus	tet(K), tet(L)	tet(M), tet(O), tet(W)
Streptococcus	tet(K), tet(L)	tet(M), tet(O), tet(Q), tet(T), tet(W)
Streptomyces	tet(K), tet(L), tet(V), otr(B), otr(C)	tet(M), tet(W), otr(A)
Ureaplasma		tet(M)
Chlamydophila	tet(C)	

efflux protein. In the presence of tetracycline, the repressor adopts a form that does not allow it to bind to the operator and this allows transcription of the resistance gene. This regulation system is present in almost all the efflux systems described in Gram negative bacteria (1).

In the case of Gram positive bacteria, and especially in the genus *Staphylococcus*, efflux genes are usually located in the small rolling circle replicating plasmids, the prototype of which is pT181 that carries the tet(K) gene. The expression of these determinants is also regulated by a transcriptional attenuation mechanism different from the above and similar to that described for inducible resistance to macrolides of the *erm* type in streptococci and enterococci (30).

With regard to Gram negative bacteria, as well as the previously described *tet* genera, the chromosome genes for transport membrane proteins can also be responsible for resistance to tetracyclines (19). We will only mention the most relevant. In *Escherichia coli*, the *mar* (multiple antibiotic resistance) system increases its level of resistance to many antibiotics, including tetracyclines. It is formed by two genes *marA* and *marR*. The *marA* gene codes for a transcriptional activator which acts at the level of many promoters, where synthesis is repressed in the absence of the antibiotic by a repressor, which is a product of gene *marR*. The overexpression of MarA causes a decrease in the expression of OmpF porin and the overexpression of the AcrAB efflux pump and resistance to tetracyclines. In other enterobacteria derivatives resistant to tetracyclines by mutation, other AcrAB homologous efflux systems have been described (6). In *Pseudomonas aeruginosa*, the membrane proteins of the efflux systems belonging to the RND family (resistance-nodulation-cell-division) such as MexAB-OprM are also involved in multiresistance to antibiotics and affect the sensitivity to tetracyclines. Finally, in *Acinetobacter baumannii*, the AdeIJK efflux system contributes to the intrinsic resistance of this species to many antibiotics including tetracyclines (10). The AdeABC system, cryptic in approximately 80% of the strains of *A. baumannii*, confers, when overexpressed, resistance to several classes of antibiotics including tetracyclines (22). This overexpression is a consequence of a mutation in the regulation system of two AdeRS components adjacent to *adeABC* operon (21) or the transposition of a copy of IS*Aba*1 upstream to *adeABC* (29.

Ribosome protection

Eleven genes code for cytoplasmic proteins which, when they attach to the ribosome at the level of protein h34, cause the attached antibiotic to be cast off and allow the ribosome to return to its original configuration(Table 6). These proteins are homologous to elongation factors EF-Tu and EF-G and experimental studies suggest that they possess GTPase activity. These determinants confer resistance to tetracycline and minocycline (6). These genes, with the exception of *tet*(W) and those of *Streptomyces* have a G+C content below 50 % which suggests an origin in Gram positive bacteria with a low G+C %. Furthermore, the *tet*(M) and *tet*(O) determinants have been those most studied. These genes are most often located on mobile genetic elements, *tet*(M) on conjugative transposons of which the prototype is Tn*916* and *tet*(O) on conjugative plasmids. Recently, it has been demonstrated that *tet*(O) and *mef*(A), that confer resistance by efflux to erythromycine, are located on the conjugative transposon Tn*2009* in *Streptococcus pyogenes* . These determinants, initially described in *Streptococcus* and *Enterococcus,* have been found in almost all Gram positive bacteria with a low G+C % and also in Gram negative bacteria (Tables 7 and 8). The expression of resistance by ribosome protection is also regulated by the presence of tetracycline. Results suggest that, in the case of Tn*916*, the expression of *tet*(M) is controlled by a mechanism of transcriptional attenuation .

Enzyme inactivation

The *tet*(X) determinant that confers low level resistance to tetracycline by means of enzyme inactivation has been found only in the *Bacteroides* genus. This gene codes for a cytoplasmic protein of 44 kDa that is activated in the presence of oxygen and NADH and that has similarities to other bacterial NADH oxidases. The enzyme activity of this protein has been demonstrated after cloning with *E. coli* since in this *Bacteroides* its importance and significance are poorly assessed. Two other determinants, *tet*(34) and *tet*(37), have been recently found in *Vibrio cholerae* and in non-identified bacteria of the oral cavity.

EPIDEMIOLOGY OF RESISTANCE

We will only mention data related to bacteria for which tetracycline constitutes an epidemiological marker and infection causing bacteria which may benefit from treatment with said antibiotics.

Staphylococci

There is little recent national data available on the incidence of resistance to tetracyclines in Staphylococcus. The analysis of data collected during a recent 4 year period (2000-2004) in a Paris hospital centre with 1200 beds reveals that out of 800 strains of *S. aureus* isolated on average each year, the incidence of resistance is stable and affects 18% of the isolates. In 60 % of cases, these strains are resistant to tetracycline and susceptible to minocycline which suggests an efflux mechanisms due to the presence of the determinants *tet*(K) or *tet*(L). The incidence of resistance is much higher in those isolates that are resistant to methicillin and affects an average of 35% of these strains.

Streptococci and enterococci

The data published in the National Reference Centre for Pneumococci show that the incidence of resistance to tetracyclines is of about 30% with comparable levels for invasive strains isolated from blood cultures or from cerebrospinal fluid and for strains isolated from acute otitis media in children.

With *Streptococcus pyogenes*, the incidence to resistance is about 35 %. With *Streptococcus agalactiae*, this is very high since, in studies published recently, it affects more than 80 % of strains .

In enterococci, all species without distinction, data collected over a 4 year period (2000-2004) in a Paris hospital centre with 1200 beds reveals that of an average 970 strains of enterococci per year, the incidence of resistance was stable and affected 75 % of the strains. In streptococci and enterococci, in more than 99 % of cases, strains are resistant to tetracycline and to minocycline due to the presence of a *tet*(M) determinant.

Chlamydia and *Mycoplasma*

In *C. trachomatis* and *C. psittacci* resistance to tetracycline is exceptional and no resistance mechanism has been characterized. Resistance to tetracycline, by acquisition of the *tet*(C) determinant, in *Chlamydophila suis*, a swine pathogen, has been found in herds where tetracyclines are used as growth promoters (27).

In mycoplasma, the data on incidence of resistance to tetracyclines are very few. Studies published in 1990 have described the presence of the *tet*(M) determinant in certain strains of *Mycoplasma* and of *Ureaplasma* resistant to tetracyclines. It would seem that lately resistance to tetracyclines is increasing (see Chapter on Mycoplasma).

GLYCYLCYCLINES

Tigecycline is the first and the only glycylcycline used in human medicine. It is a derivative of minocycline with a long lateral chain (9-t-butyl-glycylamide) linked to the C9 position at cycle D level (Fig. 1 and 2). This structural characteristic allows it, by means of steric hindrance, to remain active against bacteria that have become resistant to tetracyclines by ribosome protection and/or active efflux (24). As in the case of other tetracyclines, tigecycline inhibits protein synthesis after reversible attachment to the 30S ribosome subunit blocking the attachment of amino acyl tRNA at site A. Meanwhile, tigecycline attaches to the ribosome target with an affinity five times greater than that of other tetracyclines, which explains its significant *in vitro* activity (2).

Tigecycline is a bacteriostatic antibiotic that possesses a wide antibacterial spectrum of activity (24).

It is markedly active against cocci and Gram positive bacteria. staphylococci, streptococci also pneumococci, enterococci and Gram negative bacteria: *Campylobacter* spp., *Haemophilus influenzae*, *Neisseria gonorrhoeae*, *Moraxella catarrhalis* and *Pasteurella* spp. It is active against enterobacteria but this activity is limited to strains of *Proteus* spp., *Providencia* spp. and *Morganella morganii* with a MIC_{90} of 4 to 8 µg/ml. It is active against *Acinetobacter* spp. and *Stenotrophomonas maltophilia* but not against *P. aeruginosa* with a CIM_{90} of 16 µg/ml. This antibiotic is also active against anaerobic bacteria, both Gram positive and negative (*Bacteroides* of the *fragilis* group, *Clostridium perfringens* and *Clostridium difficile*, *Propionibacterium acnes*, *Peptostreptococcus* spp., *Fusobacterium* spp., *Prevotella* spp., *Porphyromonas* spp.). Finally, tigecycline has a good level of activity against atypical bacteria such as *C. trachomatis* and *C. psittaci* as also against *M. pneumoniae* and *M. hominis*, against rapid growing mycobacteria such as the *fortuitum* group, especially *Mycobacterium chelonae* and *Mycobacterium abcessus*, and the *smegmatis* group. On the other hand, it is inactive against mycobacteria of the *tuberculosis* group, the *avium* group and against *Mycobacterium xenopi*, *Mycobacterium marinum*, *Mycobacterium kansasii*. The MIC values of tigecycline for certain species can be seen in Tables 2 and 3.

Tigecycline is an antibiotic that is only available for parenteral IV use. It diffuses widely throughout the body's tissues (especially the gall bladder, lungs and colon) and is excreted in the bile (59%) and through the kidneys (33%) (24). It is indicated for the treatment of complicated skin infections, soft tissue infections and complicated intra-abdominal infections. Finally, tigecycline should be approved in the United States for the treatment of community pneumonias and diabetic foot infections.

The advantage of tigecycline lies in the fact that it escapes the two main resistance mechanisms to classical tetracyclines: ribosome protection and active efflux (see above).

Furthermore, the respective MICs of tetracycline, of minocycline and of tigecycline against a strain of wild-type *E. coli* are generally 2, 1 and 0.25 µg/ml and change to 8, 2 and 0.5 µg/ml in the presence of *tet*(M) and to > 64, 8 and 0.25 µg/ml in the presence of *tet*(E) (33). Certain chromosomal efflux systems of the Resistance-Nodulation-cell Division (RND) type which are however responsible for resistance to tigecycline, and are intrinsic with MexXY-OprM in *P. aeruginosa* and AcrAB-TolC in *P. mirabilis* and *M. morganii* (Table 9) (11, 28, 34), are acquired.

It has been demonstrated *in vitro* that tigecycline is a substrate that is undermined by the efflux pump systems AcrAB-TolC and AcrEF-TolC in *E. coli* (13). Although it is very difficult to select for tigecycline resistance caused by *in vitro* mutation (frequency of 10^{-8} to 10^{-9}), many cases of acquired resistance have been reported in strains of enterobacteria selected by treatment, such as *E. coli*, *K. pneumoniae* and *Enterobacter* spp. (Table 9) (14, 15, 30). In *E. coli*, overexpression of the AcrAB-TolC system is due to overexpression of the MarA (15) global regulator whereas in *K. pneumoniae* and *Enterobacter* spp. it is due to overexpression of another global regulator, RamA (not present in *E. coli*) (14, 30).

Table 9. Contribution of RND pumps to resistance to tigecycline (10, 11, 14, 15, 28-30, 34)

Species	Genotype[a]	Tigecycline MIC (µg/ml)
A. baumannii	adeABC +, adeIJK +	1.5
	adeABC ++, adeIJK +	4
	adeABC –, adeIJK +	0.5
	adeABC +, adeIJK –	1.5
	adeABC –, adeIJK –	0.05
E. coli	acrAB +	0.5
	acrAB ++	0.5-1
	acrAB –	0.25
E. cloacae	acrAB +	0.5-1
	acrAB ++	16
K. pneumoniae	acrAB +	0.25
	acrAB ++	4-16
M. morganii	acrAB +	1
	acrAB ++	4-8
P. mirabilis	acrAB +	4
	acrAB ++	16
	acrAB –	0.25
P. aeruginosa	mexXY +	8
	mexXY –	0.5

[a] +, efflux system present (wild-type phenotype); ++, overexpression of efflux system; –, efflux system absent.

In *A. baumannii*, tigecycline is a substrate for AdeABC and AdeIJK pumps that, overexpressed, confer a decrease in sensitivity (Table 9) (10, 29). Both systems contribute synergistically to the resistance to tigecycline (10).

In Gram positive bacteria, studies of resistance by successive passages in subinhibitory concentrations have made it possible to obtain mutants of *S. aureus* (MIC of 4 and 16 µg/ml) that have an overexpression of the MepRAB efflux system (20); whereas no clinical strain of *S. aureus* with decreased sensitivity to tigecycline has so far been described.

Finally, the presence of resistance determinants to β-lactamines (ex. *mecA*) or to glycopeptides (ex. *vanA*) in Gram positive bacteria, as also the presence of BLSE, of cephalosporinases, or a decrease of sensitivity to carbapenems in Gram negative bacteria, do not alter or only slightly alter the activity of tigecycline (24).

REFERENCES

(1) **Berens, C., and W. Hillen.** 2004. Gene regulation by tetracyclines. Genet. Eng. **26**:255-277.

(2) **Bouchillon, S. K., D. J. Hoban, B. M. Johnson, J. L. Johnson, A. Hsiung, and M. J. Dowzicky.** 2005. *In vitro* activity of tigecycline against 3989 Gram negative and Gram positive clinical isolates from the United States. Tigecycline Evaluation and Surveillance Trial (TEST Program; 2004). Diagn. Microbiol. Infect. Dis. **52**:173-179.

(3) **Bouchillon, S. K., D. J. Hoban, B. M. Johnson, T. M. Stevens, M. J. Dowzicky, D. H. Wu, and P. A. Bradford.** 2005. *In vitro* evaluation of tigecycline and comparative agents in 3049 clinical isolates: 2001 to 2002. Diagn. Microbiol. Infect. Dis. **51**:291-295.

(4) **Bradford, P. A., P. J. Petersen, M. Young, C. H. Jones, M. Tischler, and J. O'Connell.** 2005. Tigecycline MIC testing by broth dilution requires use of fresh medium or addition of the biocatalytic oxygen-reducing reagent oxyrase to standardize the test method. Antimicrob. Agents Chemother. **49**:3903-3909.

(5) **Chopra, I., and M.C. Roberts.** 2001. Tetracycline antibiotics: mode of action, applications, molecular biology, and epidemiology of bacterial resistance. Microbiol. Mol. Biol. Rev. **65**:232-260.

(6) **Clermont, D., O. Chesneau, G. De Cespedes, and T. Horaud.** 1997. New tetracycline resistance determinants coding for ribosomal protection in streptococci and nucleotide sequence of *tet*(T) isolated from *Streptococcus pyogenes* A498. Antimicrob. Agents Chemother. **41**:112-116.

(7) **Clewell, D. B., S. E. Flannagan, and D. D. Jaworski.** 1995. Unconstrained bacterial promiscuity: the Tn*916*-Tn*1545* family of conjugative transposons. Trends Microbiol. **2**:229-236.

(8) **Comité de l'Antibiogramme de la Société Française de Microbiologie.** Communiqué 2006. http://www.sfm.asso.fr.

(9) **Khan, S. A., and R. P. Novick.** 1983. Complete nucleotide sequence of pT181, a tetracycline-resistance plasmid from *Staphylococcus aureus*. Plasmid **10:**251-259.

(10) **Levy, S. B.** 1992. Active efflux mechanisms for antimicrobial resistance. Antimicrob. Agents Chemother. **36:**695-703.

(11) **Levy, S. B., L. M. McMurry, T. M. Barbosa, V. Burdett, P. Courvalin, W. Hillen, M. C. Roberts, J. I. Rood, and D. E. Taylor.** 1999. Nomenclature for new tetracycline resistance determinants. Antimicrob. Agents Chemother. **43:**1523-1524.

(12) **Li, X. Z., and H. Nikaido.** 2004. Efflux-mediated drug resistance in bacteria. Drugs **64:**159-204.

(13) **Livermore, D. M.** 2005. Tigecycline: what is it, and where should it be used? J. Antimicrob. Chemother. **56:**611-614.

(14) **Nikaido, H., and D. G. Thanassi.** 1993. Penetration of lipophilic agents with multiple protonation sites into bacterial cells: tetracyclines and fluoroquinolones as examples. Antimicrob. Agents Chemother. **37:**1393-1399.

(15) **Pankey, G. A.** 2005. Tigecycline. J. Antimicrob. Chemother. **56:**470-480.

(16) **Poyart, C., L. Jardy, G. Quesne, P. Berche, and P. Trieu-Cuot.** 2003. Genetic basis of antibiotic resistance in *Streptococcus agalactiae* strains isolated in a French hospital. Antimicrob. Agents Chemother. **47:**794-797.

(17) **Roberts, M. C.** 2003. Tetracycline therapy: update. Clin. Infect. Dis. **36:**462-467.

(18) **Roberts, M. C.** 2005. Update on acquired tetracycline resistance genes. FEMS Microbiol. Lett. **245:**195-203.

(19) **Schnappinger, D., and W. Hillen.** 1996. Tetracyclines: antibiotic action, uptake, and resistance mechanisms. Arch. Microbiol. **165:**359-369.

(20) **Schwarz, S., M. Cardoso, and H. C. Wegener.** 1992. Nucleotide sequence and phylogeny of the *tet*(L) tetracycline resistance determinant encoded by plasmid pSTE1 from *Staphylococcus hyicus*. Antimicrob. Agents Chemother. **36:**580-588

(21) **Magnet, S., P. Courvalin, and T. Lambert.** 2001. Resistance-nodulation-cell division type efflux pump involved in aminoglycoside resistance in *Acinetobacter baumanii* strain BM4454. Antimicrob. Agents Chemother. **45:**3375-3380.

(22) **Marchand, I., L. Damier-Piolle, P. Courvalin, and T. Lambert.** 2004. Expression of the RND-type efflux pump AdeABC in *Acinetobacter baumannii* is regulated by the AdeRS two-component system. Antimicrob. Agents Chemother. **48:**3298-3304.

(23) **Nikaido, H., and D. G. Thanassi.** 1993. Penetration of lipophilic agents with multiple protonation sites into bacterial cells: tetracyclines and fluoroquinolones as examples. Antimicrob. Agents Chemother. **37:**1393-1399.

(24) **Pankey, G. A.** 2005. Tigecycline. J. Antimicrob. Chemother. **56:**470-480.

(25) **Poyart, C., L. Jardy, G. Quesne, P. Berche, and P. Trieu-Cuot.** 2003. Genetic basis of antibiotic resistance in *Streptococcus agalactiae* strains isolated in a French hospital. Antimicrob. Agents Chemother. **47:**794-797.

(26) **Roberts, M. C.** 2003. Tetracycline therapy: update. Clin. Infect. Dis. **36:**462-467.

(27) **Roberts, M. C.** 2005. Update on acquired tetracycline resistance genes. FEMS Microbiol. Lett. **245:**195-203.

(28) **Ruzin, A., D. Keeney, and P. A. Bradford.** 2005. AcrAB efflux pump plays a role in decreased susceptibility to tigecycline in *Morganella morganii*. Antimicrob. Agents Chemother. **49:**791-793.

(29) **Ruzin, A., D. Keeney, and P. A. Bradford.** 2007. AdeABC multidrug efflux pump is associated with decreased susceptibility to tigecycline in *Acinetobacter calcoaceticus-Acinetobacter baumannii* complex. J. Antimicrob. Chemother. **59:**1001-1004.

(30) **Ruzin, A., M. A. Visalli, D. Keeney, and P. A. Bradford.** 2005. Influence of transcriptional activator RamA on expression of multidrug efflux pump AcrAB and tigecycline susceptibility in *Klebsiella pneumoniae*. Antimicrob. Agents Chemother. **49:**1017-1022.

(31) **Schnappinger, D., and W. Hillen.** 1996. Tetracyclines: antibiotic action, uptake, and resistance mechanisms. Arch. Microbiol. **165:**359-369.

(32) **Schwarz, S., M. Cardoso, and H. C. Wegener.** 1992. Nucleotide sequence and phylogeny of the *tet*(L) tetracycline resistance determinant encoded by plasmid pSTE1 from *Staphylococcus hyicus*. Antimicrob. Agents Chemother. **36:**580-8.

(33) **Tuckman, M., P. J. Petersen, A. Y. Howe, M. Orlowski, S. Mullen, K. Chan, P. A. Bradford, and C. H. Jones.** 2007. Occurrence of tetracycline resistance genes among *Escherichia coli* isolates from the phase 3 clinical trials for tigecycline. Antimicrob. Agents Chemother. **51:**3205-3211.

(34) **Visalli, M. A., E. Murphy, S. J. Projan, and P. A. Bradford.** 2003. AcrAB multidrug efflux pump is associated with reduced levels of susceptibility to tigecycline (GAR-936) in *Proteus mirabilis*. Antimicrob. Agents Chemother. **47:**665-669.

Chapter 25. OXAZOLIDINONES

Roland LECLERCQ

INTRODUCTION

Oxazolidinones are synthetic antibiotics first discovered by researchers at DuPont Pharmaceuticals. They were initially studied as monoamine oxidase inhibitor antidepressants but, in 1978, were found to be active against tomato plant pathogens and, in the 1980s, against certain human pathogens (DuP 105 and DuP 721). Yet it was not until the 1990s that the first drug from this class was brought to market by the Upjohn Corporation. Oxazolidinones are unrelated to other classes of antibiotics. Linezolid is the only commercially available oxazolidinone; it is used in the treatment of nosocomial and community-acquired pneumonia and in complicated skin and soft tissue infections caused by susceptible organisms.

STRUCTURE AND MECHANISM OF ACTION

Oxazolidinones are cyclic molecules possessing a 2-oxazeneca-olidinyl nucleus with an acetamide chain at position 5 and a phenyl moiety at position 3 of the 2-oxazolidinone nucleus. Linezolid is 3-(fluorophenyl)-2-oxazolidinone, or more precisely, (S)-N-[[3-(3-fluoro-4-morpholinylphenyl)-2-oxo-5-oxazolidinyl]methyl]acetamide (Fig. 1). The acylaminomethyl substituent at C5 and the presence of a fluorine at position 3 of the phenyl moiety confer improved antibacterial activity relative to the progenitor compounds.

Oxazolidinones inhibit protein synthesis by interacting with the 50S ribosomal subunit. They have an original mechanism of action which has not yet been fully elucidated. Linezolid targets the early step of protein synthesis: initiation (35). By binding to the P-site in the peptidyltransferase center in 23S ribosomal RNA, linezolid prevents the binding of N-formylmethionyl-tRNA and the formation of the 70S initiation complex (formed from the 30S and 50S subunits, N-formylmethionyl-tRNA, messenger RNA and various proteins). This makes translation impossible. The ribosomes of Gram-negative bacteria are susceptible to the action of linezolid but membrane efflux pumps make this drug inactive in these bacteria.

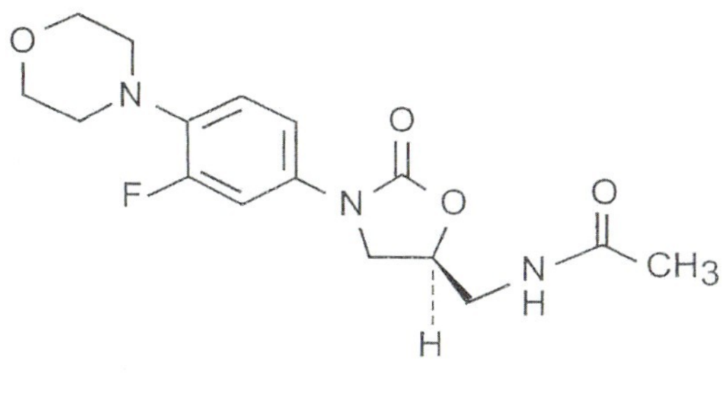

Several groups have attempted to identify the binding site(s) of linezolid. While linezolid competes for binding with chloramphenicol and lincomycin, it does not inhibit peptidyltransferase activity like the latter antibiotics. Although the interaction with the peptidyltransferase center has been clearly established, the nucleic bases involved in these interactions have proved more difficult to identify. Initially, nucleotides (E. coli numbering) A2062, U2113, A2114, U2118, A2119, C2153, C2452, A2453, C2499, U2500, U2504, G2608 and also A864, a 16S RNA nucleotide (30S ribosomal subunit), were each implicated in turn according to the bacteria under study (*Haloarcula marismortui*, an archaebacterium, or *E. coli*). The results were sometimes conflicting depending on the method used, and some of these nucleotides were located far from the peptidyltransferase center (35). More recent studies in *S. aureus* indicate that oxazolidinones bind to nucleotide A2602 in the 23S rRNA V domain, to transfer RNA, and to riboprotein L27 (11). *E. coli* ribosomal resistance mutants obtained *in vitro* harbor mutations G2032 and G2447 while enterococcus and staphylococcus mutants carry mutations at G2447 and G2576 (31, 40). These nucleotides are located in the 23S rRNA V domain. Some mutations, such as the one at position 2032, confer cross-resistance to chloramphenicol.

The binding site of linezolid therefore still needs to be clearly defined. It should be noted that adenine 2058, an essential binding site for macrolides, does not appear to be implicated, which is consistent with the fact that strains car-

Fig. 1. Structure of linezolid.

rying an *erm* gene encoding a methylase that acts on this adenine do not show cross-resistance to linezolid.

SPECTRUM OF ACTIVITY

Linezolid is active against Gram-positive bacteria incriminated in the infections that correspond to its clinical indications, including multiresistant strains (Table 1): *Enterococcus faecalis*, *Enterococcus faecium*, *Staphylococcus aureus*, coagulase-negative staphylococci, *Streptococcus agalactiae*, *Streptococcus pneumoniae*, *Streptococcus pyogenes*, group C and G streptococci. It also provides anaerobic coverage, with higher activity against Gram-positive anaerobes, *Clostridium* spp., *Peptostreptococcus* spp., and *Fusobacterium* than against *Bacteroides*.

Linezolid also shows notable activity *in vitro* against other less common but significant bacteria, for which its clinical effectiveness has not been evaluated (Table 2). This is the case for *Legionella* and particularly for certain mycobacteria including *Mycobacterium tuberculosis* and *Mycobacterium kansasii*, whereas in most cases higher MICs are seen with *Mycobacterium avium*, *Mycobacterium fortuitum*, *Mycobacterium abcessus*, and *Mycobacterium cheloneae*. Linezolid has been successfully used to treat *Nocardia* brain abscesses (27) as well as multiresistant corynebacterial infections.

Linezolid has no effect on aerobic Gram-negative bacteria including enterobacteria, *Pseudomonas*, and *Neisseria*. *Haemophilus influenzae* shows slightly lower resistance with MICs usually on the order of 16 µg/ml (41). MICs for *Moraxella catarrhalis* isolates are fairly low (4-8 µg/ml) but these strains are not classified as susceptible. Linezolid is also active against *Bordetella pertussis*, *Pasteurella multocida*, *Chryseobacterium* (*Flavobacterium*) *meningosepticum* (renamed *Elizabethkingia meningoseptica*), with MIC_{90} = 4 µg/ml.

It is ineffective against *Mycoplasma pneumoniae* and *Ureaplasma* and has only marginal activity against *Mycoplasma hominis*.

BACTERICIDAL ACTIVITY

In time-kill studies linezolid was shown to be bacteriostatic against staphylococci and enterococci with a time-dependent effect (32). At four times the MIC there was < 2 log10 reduction in survival in the enterococcal and staphylococcal strains tested. Additive effects are seen when linezolid is combined with gentamicin, vancomycin, rifampicin, ciprofloxacin, fusidic acid, or fosfomycin (16). However, bactericidal synergy has been described between linezolid and subinhibitory concentrations of imipenem *in vitro* and in an animal model (20).

METHODS

Susceptibility testing methods may be found in CLSI and EUCAST documents. CLSI breakpoints are as follows: for enterococci, susceptible ≤ 2 µg/ml and resistant ≥ 8 µg/ml; for staphylococci, susceptible ≤ 4 µg/ml; for streptococci (viridans, pneumococci and beta-hemolytic), susceptible ≤ 2 µg/ml. EUCAST breakpoints are slightly higher so as to avoid dividing up the susceptible populations among the principal species: for enterococci, staphylococci and pneumococci, susceptible ≤ 4 µg/ml and resistant > 4 µg/ml; for beta-hemolytic streptococci, susceptible ≤ 2 µg/ml and resistant > 4 µg/ml; non species-specific breakpoints: susceptible ≤ 2 µg/ml and resistant > 4 µg/ml. In genera other than enterococci, resistance to linezolid is very uncommon or has not been described. After ruling out the possibility of a technical error, the result should be confirmed by a reference laboratory. For enterococci, resistance should also be confirmed in countries where linezolid resistance has not been reported.

Agar diffusion and automated methods can slightly overestimate resistance rates (8). Note that for the agar diffusion method, the CLSI recommends that inhibition zones be read by transillumination. Any visible growth in the inhibition zone indicates resistance. In any case, I or R results should be checked by determining the MICs.

MICs obtained by agar dilution are frequently one dilution lower than those obtained by broth microdilution, particularly for *E. faecalis* and staphylococci (28). For routine testing, the MICs can be determined by the E test which, according to some authors, is well correlated with broth microdilution for staphylococci and enterococci (1), while others report values lower by one or two dilutions for staphylococci, streptococci and enterococci (12, 37). Where pneumococci are concerned, E test values are also sometimes one dilution lower than those obtained by agar dilution (28). It should also be added that differences in interpretation may occur due to the bacterio-

Table 1. Activity of linezolid against common Gram-positive cocci pathogens and against anaerobic bacteria

Species	MIC (µg/ml)			Reference
	Range	MIC$_{50}$	MIC$_{90}$	
S. aureus	0.12-4	2	2-4	4, 7, 19, 21, 28, 37
S. aureus methicillin-susceptible	1-4	2	2-4	7, 21, 28, 37
S. aureus methicillin-resistant	0.5-4	2	2-4	7, 21, 28, 37
Coagulase-negative staphylococci	0.06-4	1-2	1-4	4, 21, 28, 37
Enterococcus spp.	0.06->8	1-2	2-4	4, 37
E. faecalis	2-4	2	2	21, 28
E. faecium	2-4	2	2-4	21, 28
S. bovis	0.5-2		1	36
ß-hemolytic streptococci	≤ 0.06-2	0.5-1	1-2	4, 21, 28
S. agalactiae	0.5-2	1-2	2	21, 37
Streptococcus pyogenes	0.25-2	0.5	2	37
S. pneumoniae	≤ 0.03-4	≤ 0.5-2	1-2	4, 7, 19, 28, 40
S. mitis	≤ 0.12-2	1	1	36
S. anginosus	0.25-2	1	1	36
S. constellatus	≤ 0.12-1	1	1	36
S. intermedius	≤ 0.12-2	1	1	36
S. mutans	≤ 0.12-2	1	1	36
S. oralis	0.25-16	1	1	36
S. salivarius	0.25-2	1	1	36
S. sanguis	0.25-2	1	1	36
S. anginosus	0.25-2	1	1	36
Streptococcus viridans	≤ 0.06-2	1	1-2	4, 21
Bacteroides fragilis	2-4	4	4	6
Bacteroides group fragilis other than B. fragilis	0.5-4	4	4	6
Prevotella	≤ 0.06-8	2	4	6
Fusobacterium spp.	≤ 0.06-2	0.5	1	6
Porphyromonas spp.	≤ 0.06-1	NA[1]	NA	6
Veillonella spp.	≤ 0.06-0.5	NA	NA	6
Actinomyces israelii	0.12-16	0,5	16	14, 15
Actinomyces meyeri/turicensis	0.12-1	0.5	0.5	15
Actinomyces odontolyticus	0.5-1	0.5	0.5	15
Actinomyces viscosus	0.5	0.5	0.5	15
Actinomyces spp	0.25-1		1	14
Clostridium clostridioforme	2-8	2	4-8	14, 15
Clostridium difficile	1-16	2	2-8	2, 14, 15, 30
Clostridium innocuum	2-4	2	4	14
Clostridium perfringens	1-2	2	2	14, 15
Clostridium ramosum	4-8	8	8	14, 15
Clostridium spp.	≤ 0.06-4	2	4	5
Eubacterium spp.	0.25-8	2	2-4	14, 15
Eubacterium lentum	0.5-2	2	2	14
Eubacterium limosum	1-4	2	4	15
Propionibacterium spp.	0.25-1	0.5	0.5-1	6, 14
Propionibacterium acnes	0.25-0.5	0.5	0.5	6
Propionibacterium avidum	≤ 0.5	≤ 0.5	≤ 0.5	6
Propionibacterium granulosum	0.25-0.5	0.25	0.25	6
Peptostreptococcus anaerobius	0.5-8	0.5	8	6
Peptoniphilus asaccharolyticus	0.5-1	0.5	1	6
Finegoldia magna	0.5-2	1	2	6
Micromonas micros	0.05-1	0.5	0.5	6
Anaerococcus prevotii	≤ 0.03-2	0.5	1	6

[1] NA, not applicable (fewer than 10 strains tested).

Table 2. Activity of linezolid against different Gram-positive bacteria, mycobacteria, *Moraxella* spp., *Haemophilus* spp. and intracellular bacteria

Species	MIC (µg/ml)			Reference
	Range	MIC_{50}	MIC_{90}	
Micrococcus spp.	0.5-1	1	1	22
Stomatococcus sp.	0.5-1	NA[1]	NA	22
Aerococcus sp.	1	NA	NA	22
Dermabacter hominis	0.5	NA	NA	22
Lactobacillus spp.	0.5-8	4	8	14, 15
Lactobacillus plantarum	4-8	8	8	15
Lactobacillus casei	4	NA	NA	15
Leuconostoc sp.	2	NA	NA	22
Bacillus spp.	0.25-2	1	2	21, 22
Listeria spp.	2	2	2	24
Corynebacterium spp.	0.12-4	0.25	0.5-4	15, 21
Corynebacterium amycolatum	≤ 0.06-2	0.25-0.5	0.5-2	15, 33
Corynebacterium jeikeium	0.25-1	0.5-1	0.5-1	15, 33
Corynebacterium urealyticum	0.5-1	0.5	1	33
Rhodococcus sp.	1	NA	NA	22
Nocardia asteroides	1-4	2	4	10
Nocardia farcinica	1-8	4	4	10
Nocardia nova	0.5-2	2	2	10
Nocardia brasiliensis	1-8	2	4	10
Other *Nocardia*	1-4	4	4	10
Moraxella catarrhalis	4-8	8	8	38
Haemophilus influenzae	2-32	16	16	36
Mycobacterium tuberculosis	≤ 0.12-1		1	3
Mycobacterium kansasii	0.12-4	≤ 2	1-≤ 2	9, 17
Mycobacterium avium complex	≤ 0.2- > 32	32	64	9
Mycobacterium. szulgai	≤ 0.2-4	≤ 2	4	9
Mycobacterium marinum	1-2	≤ 2	2	9
Mycobacterium fortuitum (group)	1-32	4	16	38
Mycobacterium abscessus	0.5-128	32	64	38
Mycobacterium chelonae	1-64	8	16	38
Mycobacterium smegmatis (group)	0.5-4	NA	NA	38
Mycoplasma hominis	2-8	8	8	23
Ureaplasma urealyticum	> 64	> 64	> 64	23
Mycoplasma pneumoniae	> 64	> 64	> 64	23
Coxiella burnetii	2-4	4	4	13
Legionella spp.	1-8	2-4	4-8	32

[1] NA, not applicable (fewer than 10 strains tested).

static activity of the antibiotic which, according to whether solid or broth medium is used, respectively manifests as the presence of microcolonies on agar, or as slight cloudiness at the MIC for certain strains. Likewise, in difficult cases and as with other bacteriostatic antibiotics, the manufacturer of the E test recommends reading the result at 80-90% inhibition based on the reader's evaluation of significant growth arrest, ignoring any microcolonies.

RESISTANCE MECHANISMS AND PHENOTYPES

Ribosomal mutation

As noted earlier, different linezolid-resistant ribosomal mutants have been selected in the laboratory, particularly among *E. coli*, *S. aureus* and *E. faecalis*. In enterococci, mutations have been identified at different positions but mainly at positions 2505, 2447, or 2576 (25, 31).

In a similar manner, the development of resistance in clinical isolates is due to mutations in the ribosome. In enterococci and staphylococci, two independent mutations $G_{2447}U$ and $G_{2576}U$ in the 23S rRNA, already observed *in vitro*, have been reported. Recently, mutation $T_{2500}A$, also in the 23S rRNA V domain, has been implicated in *S. aureus* (26).

The frequency of selection of resistance *in vitro* is low (10^{-9}-10^{-11}) in enterococci and staphylococci and *in vivo* resistance develops slowly. This is probably related to the fact that these bacteria contain multiple copies of the *rrl* gene encoding the 23S rRNA (4 copies in *S. pneumoniae*, 6 in *E. faecium*, 4 in *E. faecalis*, 5 or 6 in *S. aureus*) and that several copies need to be mutated for resistance to occur. Resistance can emerge through successive mutation of these copies or instead through homologous recombination following mutation of one copy (25). These characteristics probably explain why mutations which emerged during therapy occurred in patients with prolonged exposure and who often carried prosthetic or other foreign material. Epidemics of linezolid-resistant enterococci have been reported (18).

MICs for resistant mutants range from 16 (or sometimes 8) µg/ml to 128 µg/ml. Two pneumococcal isolates cross-resistant to macrolides and chloramphenicol were recently reported (39). These strains harbor a mutation in the *rplD* gene encoding riboprotein L4. The MIC of linezolid in these strains is borderline susceptible (4 µg/ml). Transformation of a susceptible pneumococcus by the mutated *rplD* gene results in an increase in the MIC from 1 to 4 µg/ml (39).

Ribosomal methylation

Ribosomal methylation by the product of the *cfr* gene has recently been identified as a mechanism of resistance in *Staphylococcus sciuri* (24). The *cfr* gene encodes an RNA methylase which adds a methyl group to adenine 2503 of the 23S RNA and perturbs the ribosomal binding of five different classes of antibiotics: phenicols, lincosamides, oxazolidinones, pleuromutilins, and streptogramin A. *cfr* is the first gene reported to confer transferable resistance to oxazolidinones. It has mainly been identified in veterinary strains of *Staphylococcus* spp. and to date, only rarely in human isolates of coagulase-negative staphylococcus and *S. aureus*. In the latter strains, resistance may be difficult to detect due to a double halo of inhibition, requiring careful examination of the inhibition zone when the E test is used (5).

PREVALENCE OF RESISTANCE

Preclinical susceptibility studies did not detect linezolid resistance in any strains tested. Such strains emerged when the antibiotic came into clinical use. Nevertheless, resistance remains sporadic and has been reported mainly in the US, and less frequently in Europe (United Kingdom, Germany, Austria). Resistance has been described primarily in *E. faecium* and *E. faecalis*, and rarely in *S. aureus*, *Staphylococcus epidermidis*, or *Streptococcus oralis* (29).

CONCLUSION

Linezolid is a recent addition to the arsenal of antibiotics used in particular to treat infections caused by multiresistant Gram-positive bacteria. Other oxazolidinones will undoubtedly be developed in the future. After this antibiotic came to market in the US, the first resistant mutants appeared in enterococci and then in staphylococci. Yet these resistant strains have remained rare and their detection does not appear to pose a problem in the laboratory, except plasmid-mediated resistance due to the *cfr* gene. Nonetheless, the first hospital epidemic of vancomycin- and linezolid-resistant enterococci has already been reported (18). The emergence of transferable linezolid resistance in *S. aureus* is worrisome.

REFERENCES

(1) **Abb, J.** 2002. In vitro activity of linezolid, quinupristin-dalfopristin, vancomycin, teicoplanin, moxifloxacin and mupirocin against methicillin-resistant *Staphylococcus aureus*: comparative evaluation by the E test and a broth microdilution method. Diagn. Microbiol. Infect. Dis. **43**:319-321.

(2) **Ackermann, G., D. Adler, and A.C. Rodloff.** 2003. In vitro activity of linezolid against *Clostridium difficile*. J. Antimicrob. Chemother. **51**:743-745.

(3) **Alcala, L., M.J. Ruiz-Serrano, C. Perez-Fernandez Turegan, D. Garcia De Viedma, M. Diaz-Infantes, M. Marin-Arriaza, and E. Bouza.** 2003. In vitro activities of linezolid against clinical isolates of *Mycobacterium tuberculosis* that are susceptible or resistant to first-line antituberculous drugs. Antimicrob. Agents Chemother. **47**:416-417.

(4) **Anderegg, T.R., H.S. Sader, T.R. Fritsche, J.E. Ross, and R.N. Jones.** 2005. Trends in linezolid susceptibility patterns: report from the 2002-2003 worldwide Zyvox Annual Appraisal of Potency and Spectrum (ZAAPS) Program. Int. J. Antimicrob. Agents. **26**:13-21.

(5) **Arias, C.A., M. Vallejo, J. Reyes, D. Panesso, J. Moreno, E. Castañeda, M.V. Villegas, B.E. Murray, J.P. Quinn.** 2008. Clinical and microbio-

logical aspects of linezolid resistance mediated by the cfr gene encoding a 23S rRNA methyltransferase. J. Clin. Microbiol. **46**:892-896.

(6) **Behra-Miellet, J., L. Calvet, and L. Dubreuil.** 2003. Activity of linezolid against anaerobic bacteria. Int. J. Antimicrob. Agents. **22**:28-34.

(7) **Bouchillon, S.K., D.J. Hoban, B.M. Johnson, J.L. Johnson, A. Hsiung, and M.J. Dowzicky.** 2005. Tigecycline Evaluation and Surveillance Trial (TEST) Group. In vitro activity of tigecycline against 3989 Gram-negative and Gram-positive clinical isolates from the United States Tigecycline Evaluation and Surveillance Trial (TEST Program; 2004). Diagn. Microbiol. Infect. Dis. **52**:173-179.

(8) **Brauers, J., M. Kresken, D. Hafner, and P.M. Shah.** 2005. German Linezolid Resistance Study Group. Surveillance of linezolid resistance in Germany, 2001-2002. Clin. Microbiol. Infect. **11**:39-46.

(9) **Brown-Elliott, B.A., C.J. Crist, L.B. Mann, R.W. Wilson, and R.J. Wallace Jr.** 2003. In vitro activity of linezolid against slowly growing nontuberculous mycobacteria. Antimicrob. Agents Chemother. **47**:1736-1738.

(10) **Brown-Elliott, B.A., S.C. Ward, C.J. Crist, L.B. Mann, R.W. Wilson, and R.J. Wallace Jr.** 2001. In vitro activities of linezolid against multiple *Nocardia* species. Antimicrob. Agents Chemother. **45**:1295-1297.

(11) **Colca, J.R., W.G. McDonald, D.J. Waldon, L.M. Thomasco, R.C. Gadwood, E.T. Lund, G.S. Cavey, W.R. Mathews, L.D. Adams, E.T. Cecil, J.D. Pearson, J.H. Bock, J.E. Mott, D.L. Shinabarger, L. Xiong, and A.S. Mankin.** 2003. Cross-linking in the living cell locates the site of action of oxazolidinone antibiotics. J. Biol. Chem. **278**:21972-21979.

(12) **Gemmell C.G.** 2001. Susceptibility of a variety of clinical isolates to linezolid: a European inter-country comparison. J. Antimicrob. Chemother. **48**:47-52.

(13) **Gikas, A., I. Spyridaki, E. Scoulica, A. Psaroulaki, and Y. Tselentis.** 2001. In vitro susceptibility of *Coxiella burnetii* to linezolid in comparison with its susceptibilities to quinolones, doxycycline, and clarithromycin. Antimicrob. Agents Chemother. **45**:3276-3278.

(14) **Goldstein, E.J., D.M. Citron, C.V. Merriam, Y. Warren, K. Tyrrell, and H.T. Fernandez.** 2003. In vitro activities of dalbavancin and nine comparator agents against anaerobic gram-positive species and corynebacteria. Antimicrob. Agents Chemother. **47**:1968-1971.

(15) **Goldstein, E.J., D.M. Citron, C.V. Merriam, Y.A. Warren, K.L. Tyrrell, H.T. Fernandez, and A. Bryskier.** 2005. Comparative in vitro activities of XRP 2868, pristinamycin, quinupristin-dalfopristin, vancomycin, daptomycin, linezolid, clarithromycin, telithromycin, clindamycin, and ampicillin against anaerobic gram-positive species, actinomycetes, and lactobacilli. Antimicrob. Agents Chemother. **49**:408-413.

(16) **Grohs, P., M.D. Kitzis, and L. Gutmann.** 2003. In vitro bactericidal activities of linezolid in combination with vancomycin, gentamicin, ciprofloxacin, fusidic acid, and rifampin against *Staphylococcus aureus*. Antimicrob. Agents Chemother. **31**:533-541.

(17) **Guna, R., C. Munoz, V. Dominguez, A. Garcia-Garcia, J. Galvez, J.V. de Julian-Ortiz, and R. Borras.** 2005. In vitro activity of linezolid, clarithromycin and moxifloxacin against clinical isolates of *Mycobacterium kansasii*. J. Antimicrob. Chemother. **55**:950-953.

(18) **Herrero, I.A., N.C. Issa, and R. Patel.** 2002. Nosocomial spread of linezolid-resistant vancomycin-resistant *Enterococcus faecium*. N. Engl. J. Med. **346**:867-869.

(19) **Hoellman, D.B., G. Lin, L.M. Ednie, A. Rattan, M.R. Jacobs, and P.C. Appelbaum.** 2003. Antipneumococcal and antistaphylococcal activities of ranbezolid (RBX 7644), a new oxazolidinone, compared to those of other agents. Antimicrob. Agents Chemother. **47**:1148–1150.

(20) **Jacqueline, C., D. Navas, E. Batard, A.F. Miegeville, V. Le Mabecque, M.F. Kergueris, D. Bugnon, G. Potel, and J. Caillon.** 2005. In vitro and in vivo synergistic activities of linezolid combined with subinhibitory concentrations of imipenem against methicillin-resistant *Staphylococcus aureus*. Antimicrob. Agents Chemother. **49**:45-51.

(21) **Johnson, A.P., C. Henwood, S. Mushtaq, D. James, M. Warner, D.M. Livermore, and ICU Study Group.** 2003. Susceptibility of Gram-positive bacteria from ICU patients in UK hospitals to antimicrobial agents. J. Hosp. Infect. **54**:179-187.

(22) **Jones, R.N., D.J. Biedenbach, and T.R. Anderegg.** 2002. In vitro evaluation of AZD2563, a new oxazolidinone, tested against unusual gram-positive species. Diagn. Microbiol. Infect. Dis. **42**:119-122.

(23) **Kenny, G.E., and F.D. Cartwright.** 2001. Susceptibilities of *Mycoplasma hominis*, *M. pneumoniae*, and *Ureaplasma urealyticum* to GAR-936, dalfopristin, dirithromycin, evernimicin, gatifloxacin, linezolid, moxifloxacin, quinupristin-dalfopristin, and telithromycin compared to their susceptibilities to reference macrolides, tetracyclines, and quinolones. Antimicrob. Agents Chemother. **45**:2604-2608.

(24) **Kehrenberg C., S. Schwarz, L. Jacobsen, L.H. Hansen, and B. Vester.** 2005. A new mechanism for chloramphenicol, florfenicol and clindamycin resistance: methylation of 23S ribosomal RNA at A2503. Mol. Microbiol. **57**:1064-1073.

(25) **Lobritz, M., R. Hutton-Thomas, S. Marshall S, and L.B. Rice.** 2003. Recombination proficiency influences frequency and locus of mutational resistance to linezolid in *Enterococcus faecalis*. Antimicrob. Agents Chemother. **47**:3318-3320.

(26) **Meka, V.G., S.K. Pillai, G. Sakoulas, C. Wennersten, L. Venkataraman, P.C. DeGirolami, G.M. Eliopoulos, R.C. Moellering Jr, and H.S. Gold.** 2004. Linezolid resistance in sequential *Staphylococcus aureus* isolates associated with a T2500A mutation in the 23S rRNA gene and loss of a single copy of rRNA. J. Infect. Dis. **190**:311-317.

(27) **Moylett, E.H., S.E. Pacheco, B.A. Brown-Elliott, T.R. Perry, E.S. Buescher, M.C. Birmingham, J.J. Schentag, J.F. Gimbel, A. Apodaca, M.A. Schwartz, R.M. Rakita, and R.J. Wallace Jr.** 2003. Clinical experience with linezolid for the treatment of *Nocardia* infection. Clin. Infect. Dis. **36**:313-318.

(28) **Muller-Serieys, C., H.B. Drugeon, J. Etienne, C. Lascols, R. Leclercq, J. Nguyen, and C.J. Soussy.**

2004. Activity of linezolid against Gram-positive cocci isolated in French hospitals as determined by three in-vitro susceptibility testing methods. Clin. Microbiol. Infect. **10**:242-246.

(29) **Mutnick, A.H., V. Enne, and R.N. Jones.** 2003. Linezolid resistance since 2001: SENTRY Antimicrobial Surveillance Program. Ann. Pharmacother. **37**:769-774.

(30) **Pelaez, T., R. Alonso, C. Perez, L. Alcala, O. Cuevas, and E. Bouza.** 2002. In vitro activity of linezolid against *Clostridium difficile*. Antimicrob. Agents Chemother. **46**:1617-1718.

(31) **Prystowsky, J., F. Siddiqui, J. Chosay, D.L. Shinabarger, J. Millichap, L.R. Peterson, and A. Noskin.** 2001. Resistance to linezolid: characterization of mutations in rRNA and comparison of their occurrences in vancomycin-resistant enterococci. Antimicrob. Agents Chemother. **45**:2154-2156.

(32) **Rybak, M.J., D.M. Cappelletty, T. Moldovan, J.R. Aeschlimann, and G.W. Kaatz.** 1998. Comparative in vitro activities and postantibiotic effects of the oxazolidinone compounds eperezolid (PNU-100592) and linezolid (PNU-100766) versus vancomycin against *Staphylococcus aureus*, coagulase-negative staphylococci, *Enterococcus faecalis*, and *Enterococcus faecium*. Antimicrob. Agents Chemother. **42**:721-724.

(33) **Sanchez Hernandez, J., B. Mora Peris, G. Yague Guirao, N. Gutierrez Zufiaurre, J.L. Munoz Bellido, M. Segovia Hernandez, and J.A. Garcia Rodriguez.** 2003. In vitro activity of newer antibiotics against *Corynebacterium jeikeium*, *Corynebacterium amycolatum* and *Corynebacterium urealyticum*. Int. J. Antimicrob. Agents. **22**:492-496.

(34) **Schulin, T., C.B. Wennersten, M.J. Ferraro, R.C. Moellering Jr, and G.M. Eliopoulos.** 1998. Susceptibilities of *Legionella* spp. to newer antimicrobials in vitro. Antimicrob. Agents Chemother. **42**:1520-1523.

(35) **Shinabarger, D.** 1999. Mechanism of action of the oxazolidinone antibacterial agents. Expert Opin. Investig. Drugs. **8**:1195-1202.

(36) **Streit, J.M., J.N. Steenbergen, G.M. Thorne, J. Alder, and R.N. Jones.** 2005. Daptomycin tested against 915 bloodstream isolates of viridans group streptococci (eight species) and *Streptococcus bovis*. J. Antimicrob. Chemother. **55**:574-578.

(37) **Tubau, F., R. Fernandez-Roblas, J. Linares, R. Martin, and F. Soriano.** 2001. In vitro activity of linezolid and 11 other antimicrobials against 566 clinical isolates and comparison between NCCLS microdilution and E-test methods. J. Antimicrob. Chemother. **47**:675-680.

(38) **Wallace, R.J. Jr, B.A. Brown-Elliott, S.C. Ward, C.J. Crist, L.B. Mann, and R.W. Wilson.** 2001. Activities of linezolid against rapidly growing mycobacteria. Antimicrob. Agents Chemother. **45**:764-467.

(39) **Wolter, N., A.M. Smith, D.J. Farrell, W. Schaffner, M. Moore, C.G. Whitney, J.H. Jorgensen, and K.P. Klugman.** 2005. Novel mechanism of resistance to oxazolidinones, macrolides, and chloramphenicol in ribosomal protein L4 of the pneumococcus. Antimicrob. Agents Chemother. **49**:3554-3557.

(40) **Xiong, L., P. Kloss, S. Douthwaite, N.M. Andersen, S. Swaney, D.L. Shinabarger, and A.S. Mankin.** 2000. Oxazolidinone resistance mutations in 23S rRNA of *Escherichia coli* reveal the central region of domain V as the primary site of drug action. J. Bacteriol. **182**:5325-5331.

(41) **Zurenko, G.E., B.H. Yagi, R.D. Schaadt, J.W. Allison, J.O. Kilburn, S.E. Glickman, D.K. Hutchinson, M.R. Barbachyn, and S.J. Brickner.** 1996. In vitro activities of U-100592 and U-100766, novel oxazolidinone antibacterial agents. Antimicrob. Agents Chemother. **40**:839-845.

Chapter 26. SULFONAMIDES AND TRIMETHOPRIM

Fred W. GOLDSTEIN

INTRODUCTION

Sulfonamide-trimethoprim combinations and co-trimoxazole have been marketed and used for nearly forty years to be the most widely prescribed antibiotics in the world until the advent of the fluoroquinolones. This global success is related to their very broad spectrum of activity which not only comprises virtually all pathogenic bacteria but also fungi and parasites, from the smallest to the biggest: *Pneumocystis*, coccidioides and paracocciodioides, *Histoplasma*, *Phycomycosis*, *Plasmodium*, *Toxoplasma*, *Isospora*, *Cyclospora*, and all the way to lice! Taken together with the excellent clinical outcomes obtained in a wide variety of infections and a very low cost, it is easy to understand why these drugs are still widely used today. Yet the price to be paid for this widespread use is the emergence of resistance which has been described in every species (1-4, 6, 11, 14, 15, 19, 20, 32, 34, 36, 39).

The sulfonamides (Fig. 1) ushered in the antibiotic era with the discovery by Domagk in 1932 that a red dye known as prontosil had antibacterial properties. Tréfouel later showed this compound to be active against streptococcal infections in rodents. The first clinical use came in 1933 when a young child was treated and cured of *Staphylococcus aureus* septicemia.

As time went on, many other molecules were synthesized, all showing similar activity but differing in their pharmacokinetic and toxicological properties. Some of the metabolic activities of sulfonamides have also been used in the synthesis of drugs such as diuretics (furosemide) and hypoglycemic agents (tolbutamide) in particular.

Trimethoprim (Fig. 1) was first synthesized in 1961 by Hitchings and Bushby. It is structurally similar to other diaminopyrimidines such as pyrimethamine, azathioprim, and methotrexate. This is why the latter agents should never be given concomitantly with trimethoprim since this may cause cumulative toxicity. The antibacterial activity of the other compounds may also explain certain "miraculous" cures in patients treated with other diaminopyrimidines for other reasons. While occasionally used alone, trimethoprim should be combined with a sulfonamide, except in case of

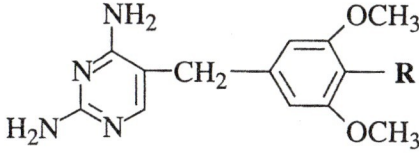

Fig. 1. Structure of some sulfonamides and trimethoprim analogs.

allergy. It would be foolish not to take advantage of the very potent synergy between these two drugs (1, 12, 15, 33) including in sulfonamide-resistant strains.

Many trimethoprim analogs with similar activity have been synthesized, including brodimoprim, metioprim, tetroxoprim, epiroprim, aditoprim, etc. Newer molecules like iclaprim, which are active against trimethoprim-resistant strains, are currently under investigation (5, 34).

MODE OF ACTION

Sulfonamides and trimethoprim interfere with nucleic acid and protein synthesis (11, 17, 20, 24).

Sulfonamides

The sulfonamides are structural analogs of para-aminobenzoic acid (PABA) and compete with the latter in the synthesis of dihydropteroic acid, the first step in dihydrofolic acid (DHF) synthesis (Fig. 2). Sulfonamides bind in place of PABA to dihydropteroate synthetase (DHPS), an enzyme which catalyzes the formation of dihydropteroic acid from PABA and pteridine. In the next step, dihydropteroic acid and glutamic acid are used to form dihydrofolic acid (DHF), commonly called folic acid (2, 11, 16, 17, 24, 28, 29, 33).

It was long speculated that another sulfonamide target existed. Indeed, very recently it was shown that DHPS could convert sulfonamides into sulfa-dihydropteroate, which competes with dihydrofolate reductase (DHFR), the target of trimethoprim (26).

Some bacteria such as enterococci or lactobacilli are incapable of synthesizing DHF; these DHF auxotrophs are therefore intrinsically resistant to sulfonamides (Table 1).

Trimethoprim

Trimethoprim acts at a second step of nucleic acid synthesis (Fig. 2). As a structural analog of DHF, it binds to DHFR, an enzyme which converts DHF to tetrahydrofolic acid (THF) or folinic acid, required for nucleic acid synthesis. This synthesis is catalyzed by thymidylate synthetase starting from several precursors. Bacteria lacking this enzyme become auxotrophic for thymidine. Thus, strains which are thymine-negative are resistant to the activity of trimethoprim (1, 2, 11, 13, 17, 20,

Table 1. Intrinsic resistance to sulfonamides and trimethoprim

Sulfonamides	Trimethoprim
Enterococcus faecalis	*Pseudomonas*
Lactobacilli	*Stenotrophomonas*
	Burkholderia
	Acinetobacter
	Campylobacter
	Legionella
	Brucella
	Helicobacter
	Neisseria
	Bacillus
	Nocardia
	Actinomyces
	Mycobactéries
	Bacteroïdes
	Chlamydia
	Coxiella
	Rickettsia
	Ehrlichia
	Bartonella
	Borrelia
	Treponemes

28, 29, 31, 33, 34). Other synthetic pathways not involving DHPS and DHFR are also possible (11, 13, 24).

In contrast to the sulfonamides, many bacteria are intrinsically resistant to trimethoprim, but this resistance is generally low-level and the synergy between trimethoprim and sulfonamides is conserved (Table 1). This is true in particular for Mycobacteria, *Nocardia* and *Stenotrophomonas*, where co-trimoxazole remains a first-choice antibiotic. It is also true for fungi and parasites susceptible to this combination. Intrinsic resistance results from low affinity of the drug for DHFR, weak bacterial permeability, or active efflux. These mechanisms often co-exist in the same organism, such as in *Pseudomonas*. More rarely, resistance in some genera is due to an absence of DHFR (*Rickettsia, Helicobacter, Bartonella, Treponema, Campylobacter*) (24).

New diaminopyrimidines

In spite of more than thirty years of research, few new molecules have been developed, since most have turned out to be too toxic or not significantly more active than trimethoprim itself. The molecule which has incited the most interest is iclaprim. This compound is active even against Gram-positive bacteria with intermediate trimethoprim resistance and has an MIC of 0.06 µg/ml versus 8-16 µg/ml for trimethoprim.

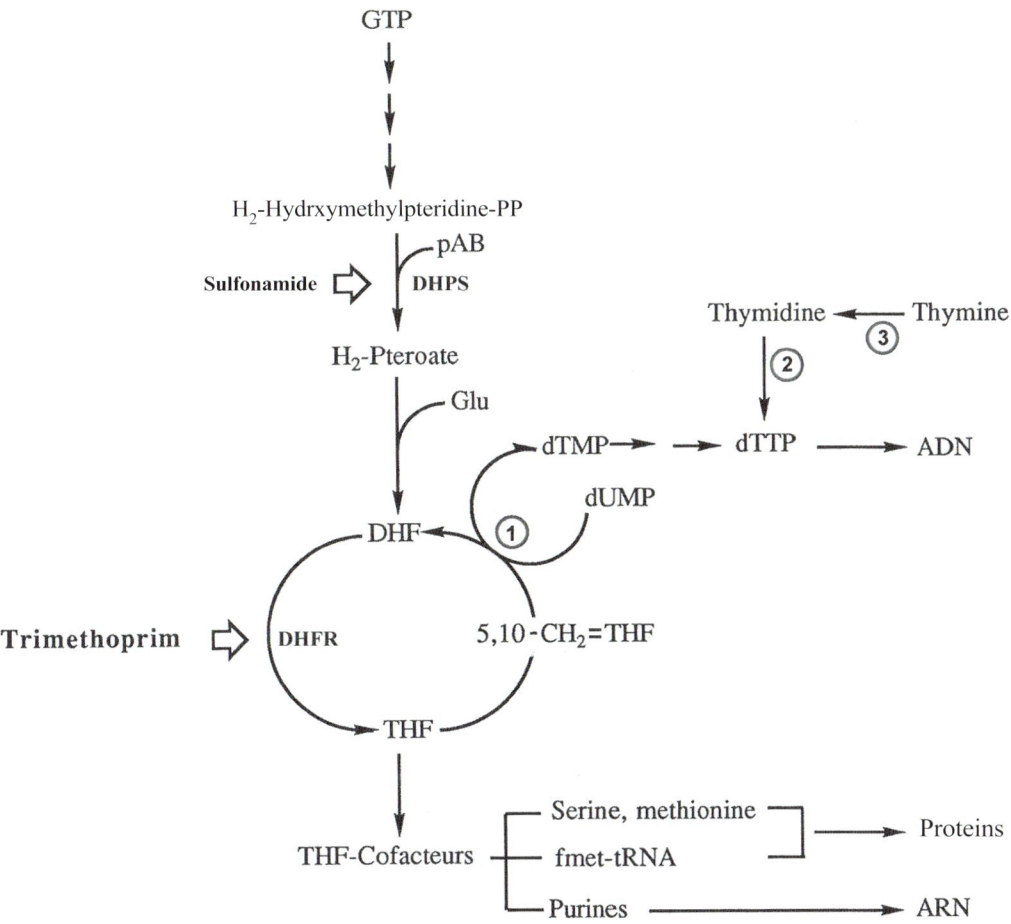

Fig. 2. Mechanism of action of sulfonamides and trimethoprim. 1, thymidilate synthetase; 2, thymidine kinase; 3, thymidine phosphorylase.

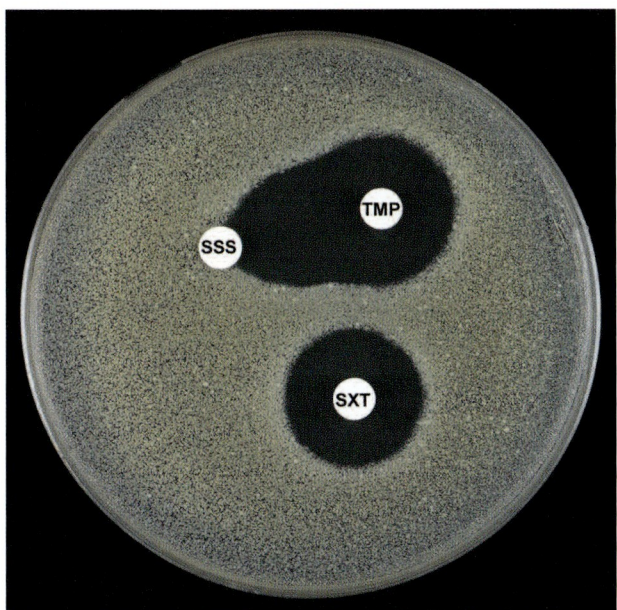

Fig. 3. Methicillin-resistant *S. aureus*. Sulfonamide-trimethoprim synergy despite high-level sulfonamide resistance (MIC > 1000 µg/ml). SSS, sulfonamides; SXT, sulfamethoxazole-trimethoprim; TMP, trimethoprim.

However, in pneumococci with high-level trimethoprim resistance (which account for over 90% of pneumococci "resistant" to penicillin G), the MIC of iclaprim is approximately 4 µg/ml. Brodimoprim and epiroprim are not widely used because their presumed pharmacokinetic advantages are not apparent. Their main targets are the mycobacteria against which they are more active than trimethoprim (22, 27).

More noteworthy is the search for new molecules active against trimethoprim- and/or sulfonamide-resistant bacteria, such as *Bacillus anthracis*. The fact that this species has intrinsic or acquired resistance to many antibiotics has sped up research efforts. New derivatives with a dihydrodiphthalazine side chain have lowered the MICs of trimethoprim from 1024 to 16-128 µg/ml (5).

Culture media

The difficulties associated with the composition of culture media arise from the antimetabolic activity of sulfonamides and trimethoprim: too much PABA antagonizes the activity of sulfonamides while too much thymidine has an antagonistic effect on trimethoprim. Culture media can be improved by supplementation with 5% hemolyzed **horse** blood containing thymidine phosphorylase, which converts thymidine to thymine, the latter being less well assimilated by the bacteria (11, 13, 32).

Synergism sulfonamide – trimethoprim

The remarkable synergy of this combination results from the sequential activity of the two drugs (Fig. 3).

Optimum synergy is obtained by using a 20:1 ratio of the MICs of sulfonamide-trimethoprim. This lowers the MIC of each drug 4 to 32-fold, which is considerable (1, 2, 11, 13, 16, 26, 28, 32). The goal, then, is to achieve this 20:1 ratio in serum. This can be done by administering a 5:1 ratio, taking into account the pharmacokinetic properties of each drug. The 20:1 ratio is valid for enterobacteria, staphylococci, streptococci, *Listeria*, etc. However, for bacteria with intrinsic low-level trimethoprim resistance, a ratio of 5:1 to 2:1 should be used, as in the case of *Neisseria*, *Branhamella*, *Nocardia*, or nonfermenting Gram-negative bacilli, where appropriate. In order to achieve this optimal ratio for the above-mentioned bacteria, treatment with co-trimoxazole should be optimized by adding trimethoprim to the combination.

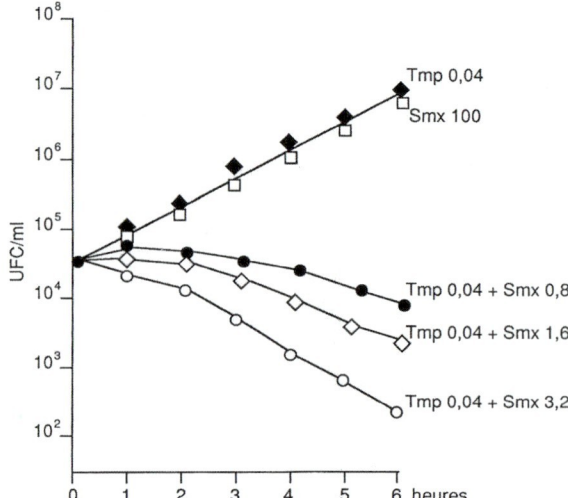

Fig. 4. Activity of sulfamethoxazole (SMX) + trimethoprim (TMP) against *E. coli* harboring a plasmid conferring high-level sulfonamide resistance (MIC > 2000 µg/ml). Synergy is observed at very low sulfonamide concentrations (≤ 1/500 MIC).

Table 2. MICs (µg/ml) of sulfonamides and trimethoprim

Microorganism	Sulfonamides	Trimethoprim
Streptococci	4 - 32	0.5 - 4
Staphylococci	2 - 4	0.25
Corynebacteria	2 - 4	0.5
Listeria	1 - 2	0.12
Nocardia	2 - 4	16 - 32
Mycobacterium tuberculosis	256 - 512	128
Mycobacterium fortuitium	8 - 16	64
Clostridium perfringens	16	64
Neisseria	1	16
Enterobacteria	2 - 8	0.1 - 1
P. mirabilis	8	4
P. aeruginosa	32	128
S. maltophilia	4	32
Acinetobacter	4	16
H. influenzae	4	0.5
Legionella	2	32
Pasteurella	1	0.1
Brucella	2	16
Campylobacter	1	16
Helicobacter	2	32
Bacteroïdes	4	32
Chlamydia	4	64
Bartonella	4	64
Rickettsia	16	8
Coxiella	2	32
Tropheryma whippeli	2	0.5

The MICs of sulfonamides and trimethoprim, alone and in combination, are given in Table 2.

Another remarkable feature of this combination is that synergy is conserved against the majority of sulfonamide-resistant strains (Fig. 3) (11, 13, 16, 29, 33). The mechanism for this remains obscure but, as noted above, it might be related to a second sulfonamide target on DHFR (26).

Sulfonamides are primarily bacteriostatic against all susceptible organisms, but in the presence of trimethoprim they potentiate the bactericidal activity of the latter (Fig. 4).

RESISTANCE MECHANISMS

Out of all the different classes of antibiotics, sulfonamides-trimethoprim undeniably have the widest diversity of acquired resistance mechanisms and their genetic determinants. These include altered permeability, activation of efflux pumps, quantitative or qualitative modification of targets, metabolic bypass, overproduction of precursors, absence of certain enzymes as well as a wide variety of exogenous genes acquired by the bacteria (2, 7, 9, 11, 16, 17, 20, 34).

Resistance to sulfonamide

Sulfonamide resistance emerged shortly after these drugs came into clinical use, initially in streptococci and staphylococci and then in other species.

Streptococcus

Sulfonamides have truly performed miracles in certain *Streptococcus* group A (erysipelas, septicemia) and group B infections. It is therefore absurd to claim, as do most Anglosaxon publications (and French publications which have not verified these data), that group A and B streptococci are intrinsically resistant to sulfonamides (and to trimethoprim). There are even selective media containing trimethoprim used to isolate group A streptococci. Luckily, there are also poor culture media which inhibit trimethoprim activity, thereby allowing the isolation of group A streptococci!

So far, acquired resistance rates in streptococci have remained low, usually < 20% with the notable exception of so-called penicillin G "resistant" pneumococci where sulfonamide resistance rates are very close to those for penicillin G. Resistance has been more closely studied in pneumococci, where it has been shown to be due to amino acid duplications between positions 61 and 64 of DHPS, leading to high-level resistance at a very low biological cost (2, 9, 13, 30). Other resistance mechanisms have been described, most notably overproduction of PABA (11).

Staphylococcus

In contrast to streptococci, sulfonamide resistance is much more prevalent in staphylococci, occurring in 30-50% of methicillin-susceptible strains and 80-95% of methicillin-resistant strains. As early as 1965, qualitative modifications of DHPS were found *in vitro* in staphylococcal clinical isolates (11).

Neisseria

In meningococci, gonococci, and saprophytic *Neisseria*, it has been shown that, like streptococci, an amino acid duplication at position 68 results in reduced sulfonamide affinity for DHPS and high-level resistance. This resistance can be transmitted by transformation, particularly among meningococci, a naturally competent species, thus explaining the high prevalence of sulfonamide resistance (30-80%).

Another mechanism has also been described in which two amino acids are inserted in the DHPS active site, resulting in lower affinity for sulfonamides.

Gram-negative bacilli

While mutations in DHPS are also found in Gram-negative bacilli, what has made sulfonamide resistance so "successful" has been the fact that it is plasmid-mediated. The first plasmid described, in 1955 in *Escherichia coli* and *Shigella*, conferred resistance to sulfonamides (2, 11, 17, 20).

Plasmid-borne sulfonamide resistance is due to a DHPS gene displaying lower affinity for sulfonamides. The bacterium therefore harbors two DHPS genes: the susceptible DHPS gene carried on the chromosome, inhibited by sulfonamides, and a resistant DHPS permissive for folic acid synthesis in the presence of high sulfonamide concentrations. The MICs of sulfonamides for these bacteria are generally in excess of 1,000 µg/ml. At least three different genes have been identified: *sul1*, *sul2*, and, more recently, *sul3*; the latter has been found in *E. coli* and *Salmonella* isolates from human or animal sources (18). Plasmid determinism explains the very large variations in sulfonamide susceptibility according to the epidemic, ranging from 10 to 90% for *Shigella* and *Salmonella*.

Other microorganisms

Acquired resistance resulting from a modification of DHPS poses very serious problems in the treatment of infections due to *Plasmodium* and especially *Pneumocystis jirovecii* (formerly *P. carinii*) for which co-trimoxazole has always been the reference treatment. Given that these organisms are intrinsically resistant to trimethoprim, they are no longer susceptible to the drug combination (32, 39).

Resistance to trimethoprim

Resistance to trimethoprim has been the focus of intensive research which is equalled solely by the number and variety of resistance mechanisms (1, 2, 9, 11-17, 19-22, 24-26, 28-31, 34, 38).

Chromosomal resistance

Qualitative and quantitative target alteration

Different resistance mechanisms observed in clinical isolates or mutants selected *in vitro* have been described:
- Qualitative modification of DHFR: this has been observed in staphylococci and Gram-negative bacilli and is due to amino acid substitutions in DHFR which reduce its affinity for trimethoprim. This usually results in low-level resistance (MIC 8-64 µg/ml) (11, 13, 20). The same mechanism predominates in pneumococci. In a recent study of fifty trimethoprim-resistant pneumococcus strains from different sources, all harbored the same $Ile_{100}Leu$ substitution, associated with other mutations (30).
- Quantitative modification of DHFR: in this case, the bacterium overproduces DHFR, thus requiring more trimethoprim to inhibit it. This very common mechanism is often associated with the previous one in enterobacteria and *H. influenzae*.
The presence of both of these resistance mechanisms can lead to high-level resistance (MIC ≥ 1000 µg/ml) (2, 11, 13, 20).

Decreased bacterial permeability

K. pneumoniae, *Enterobacter*, *Serratia*, and *Salmonella* mutants can be easily selected *in vitro* on trimethoprim-containing media *via* decreased production of certain porins (17, 19). The MIC is increased approximately four to sixteen-fold, four-fold for chloramphenicol and two-fold for tetracyclines and β-lactams. Interestingly, in *K. pneumoniae* the quinolones select approximately five to ten times more mutants of this type than gyrase mutants (M.D. Kitzis, personal communication).

Overexpression of efflux pumps

Efflux pumps are found in all Gram-negative bacilli and can be either constitutively or inducibly expressed (34). In the former case, as in *Pseudomonas*, the bacterium will display intrinsic, generally low-level resistance. Three efflux pumps have been identified in *P. aeruginosa*: MexAB-OprM, MexCD-OprJ, and MexEF-OprN. These efflux systems also confer resistance to β-lactams, chloramphenicol, macrolides, tetracyclines, and to many antiseptics including triclosan in particular (35). They are also associated with decreased permeability of *P. aeruginosa* to trimethoprim, explaining the fairly high-level resistance (MIC 128-256 µg/ml).

In some bacteria, efflux pumps can be induced by salicylates and induction is amplified by iron depletion, as in the case of bronchial secretions in cystic fibrosis. This has been observed in *Burkholderia cenocepacia* (25). The *ceoABopcM* operon of *B. cenocepacia* is similar to *mexEF-OprN* of *P. aeruginosa*. In *E. coli* and *S. dysenteriae*, efflux systems conferring resistance to quinolones, chloramphenicol, macrolides, tetracyclines, aminoglycosides, β-lactams and trimethoprim have been described. They belong to the superfamilies MATE (YdhE) or MFS (Ycel, YebQ, SetA, Fsr or AcrB) (35).

Acquisition of exogenous genes

As with the sulfonamides, what has made trimethoprim resistance so "successful" is the variety of exogenous resistance genes. Plasmids encoding trimethoprim resistance were first described in 1972 (2, 11, 20). In 1974, Amyes and Smith showed that resistance is conferred by a novel trimethoprim-resistant DHFR gene, a mechanism similar to that seen with the sulfonamides. Thus, the bacterium possesses two DHFR genes: the chromosomally-encoded enzyme which is susceptible, and an additional, plasmid-encoded

DHFR. The latter trimethoprim-resistant DHFR gene is 20,000 times less susceptible than the chromosomal enzyme, allowing bacterial nucleic acid synthesis to occur in the presence of trimethoprim (2, 11, 13, 16, 20, 28). In France, the first trimethoprim-resistance plasmids in *E. coli* were isolated in 1974 (2, 11).

In 1977, we identified a second enzyme named DHFR II. This enzyme was found to be 10,000 times more resistant than the previous enzyme, henceforth named DHFR I (2, 11, 17). Unlike DHFR I, DHFR II shows no similarities with DHFRs isolated in animals or man. Since 1977, at least twenty-five DHFR genes have been identified in Gram-negative bacilli. These genes are much less different from each other than the first two described (4, 20, 38). DHFRs are specified by two groups of genes, *dfrA* and *dfrB*, part of integron cassettes (23). These DHFRs are encoded mainly in enterobacteria by integron cassettes (17, 20). There are at least nine trimethoprim-resistance cassettes which are often associated with other resistance cassettes, in particular to streptomycin/spectinomycin or sulfonamides. These integrons can be part of transposons (14, 20). The most common is transposon Tn7 coding for resistance to trimethoprim and streptomycin/spectinomycin.

Trimethoprim resistance genes generally confer high-level resistance. In rare cases, DHFR synthesis can be inducible, as for example DHFR IV (20).

Anecdotally, plasmid genes conferring high-level resistance have been described in bacteria intrinsically resistant to trimethoprim, such as *P. aeruginosa*, *Acinetobacter*, and *Campylobacter jejuni* (12, 20).

In staphylococci, at least eleven different DHFR genes have been identified to date. The most recent one, *dfrK*, is from a methicillin-resistant strain isolated in pigs (21).

IN VIVO ACTIVITY

There is an excellent correlation between *in vitro* and *in vivo* activity.

Some failures, which are seen mainly with *Enterococci* spp., are due to the presence of large amounts of thymine or thymidine in certain body compartments (including urine). These failures are explained by the ease with which these bacteria incorporate thymine. However, this phenomenon is not always observed and it would be inappropriate to think that all enterococci are resistant to sulfonamides-trimethoprim, especially since there is synergy between these two drugs (despite intrinsic sulfonamide resistance).

ANTIBIOTICS TO BE STUDIED

For epidemiological reasons, it is interesting to study sulfonamides and trimethoprim separately.

CULTURE MEDIA

Culture media for sulfonamide and trimethoprim susceptibility testing should be low in thymine and thymidine. In practice, this can be ensured by frequent, routine quality controls in each laboratory with the aid of reference strains such as *E. coli* ATCC 25922, *S. aureus* ATCC 25923 or *E. faecalis* ATCC 29212. With *E. coli* and *S. aureus*, sulfonamides and trimethoprim produce "clean" inhibition zones with diameters > 25 mm and containing no microcolonies. A poor medium can be improved by adding 5% hemolyzed horse blood but the use of an appropriate medium is preferable. As for other antibiotics, Mueller-Hinton medium is recommended although other media have been satisfactorily used in other countries. Regardless of the medium and the bacteria under study, the inoculum must not be too high.

Streptococci

Mueller-Hinton medium containing 5% hemolyzed horse blood is recommended.

Haemophilus

HTM or Fildes media give excellent results. For agar diffusion, disks should be placed about three centimeters apart so as to detect synergy between the two drugs. The use of separate disks aids in identification, considering the number of bacteria intrinsically resistant to trimethoprim (Table 1).

CONCLUSIONS

In the twenty-first century, will co-trimoxazole, an "antibiotic of the past", still be one of the most widely prescribed antibiotics in the world? It seems that in all likelihood it will, considering the almost daily discovery of new, hitherto unsuspected uses. Co-trimoxazole is the most effective way to get rid of head lice and fleas, to say nothing of body lice, and is very widely used in India in these indications. In November 2004 a WHO report enthusiastically described the successful use of co-trimoxazole as prophylaxis in HIV-infected Zambian children (8). This success is not explained by an antibacterial, antiparasitic, or antifungal action and the article did not advance any hypotheses. It is tempting to speculate: could co-trimoxazole also have antiviral activity? This possibility cannot be ruled out, considering that the drug acts by interfering with several steps of nucleic acid synthesis. It should be recalled that azidothymidine (AZT), the first antiviral drug active against HIV, has excellent antibacterial activity with a spectrum similar to that of trimethoprim (10). Here again this explains the miraculous cures of bacterial infections with AZT in HIV-infected patients; the opposite is therefore not impossible. One might also imagine that since co-trimoxazole is active in all cells of the organism (hence its relative toxicity), there may be an inhibition of viral replication in these cells.

REFERENCES

(1) **Acar, J.F., F. Goldstein, and Y.A. Chabbert.** 1973. Synergistic activity of trimethoprim-sulfamethoxazole on Gram negative bacilli: observations *in vitro* and *in vivo*. J. Infect. Dis. **128**: Suppl:470-477.

(2) **Acar, J.F., and F.W. Goldstein.** 1982. Genetic aspects and epidemiologic implications of resistance to trimethoprim. Rev. Infect. Dis. **4**:270-275.

(3) **Afeltra, J., and P.E. Verweij.** 2003. Antifungal activity of nonantifungal drugs. European J. Clin. Microbiol. Infect. Dis. **22**:397-407.

(4) **Agerso,Y., G. Peirano, and F.M. Aarestrup.** 2006. *dfrA25*, a novel trimethoprim resistance gene from *Salmonela* Agona isolated from a human urine sample in Brazil. J. Antimirob. Chemother. **58**:1044-1047.

(5) **Barrow, E.W., J. Dreier, S. Reinelt, P.C. Bourne, and W.W. Barrow.** 2007. In vitro efficacy of new antifolates against trimethoprim-resistant *Bacillus anthracis*. Antimicrob. Agents Chemother. **51**:4447-4452.

(6) **Brummer, E., E. Castenada, and A. Restrepo.** 1993. Paracoccidioides. An update. Clin Microbiol. Rev. **6**:89-117.

(7) **Chang, L.L., H.F. Chen, C.Y. Chang, T.M. Lee, and W.J. Wu.** 2004. Contribution of integrons, and SmeABC and SmeDEF efflux pumps to multidrug resistance in clinical isolates of *Stenotrophomonas maltophilia*. J. Antimicrob. Chemother. **53**:518-521.

(8) **Chintu, C., G.J. Bhat, A.S. Walker, V. Mulenga, F. Sinyinza, L. Farrelly, N. Kagangson, A. Zumla, S.H. Gillespie, A. Nunn, and D.M. Gibb.** 2004. Cotrimoxazole as prophylaxis against opportunistic infections in HIV-infected Zambian children (CHAP): a double-blind randomised placebo-controlled trial. Lancet **364**:1865-1871.

(9) **Coque, T.M., K.V. Singh, G.M. Weinstock, and B.E. Murray.** 1999. Characterization of dihydrofolate reductase genes from trimethoprim-susceptible and trimethoprim-resistant strains of *Enterococcus faecalis*. Antimicrob. Agents Chemother. **43**:141-147.

(10) **Elwell, L.P., R. Ferone, G.A. Freeman, J.A. Fyfe, J.A. Hill, P.H. Ray, C.A. Richards, S.C. Singer, V.B. Knick, and J.L. Rideout.** 1987. Antibacterial activity and mechanism of action of 3'-azido-3'-deoxythymidine. Antimicrob. Agents Chemother. **31**:274-280.

(11) **Gerbaud, G., and F. Goldstein**. Triméthoprime et sulfamides, pp. 65-72 In: P. Courvalin, F. Goldstein, A. Philippon, and J. Sirot (ed.) L'antibiogramme.MPC-Videom, Paris, Brussels.

(12) **Goldstein, F.W., A. Labigne-Roussel, G. Gerbaud, C. Carlier, E. Collatz, and P. Courvalin.** 1983. Transferable plasmid-mediated antibiotic resistance in *Acinetobacter*. Plasmid **10**:138-147.

(13) **Goldstein, F.W.** 1977. Mécanismes de résistance aux sulfamides et au triméthoprime. Bull. Institut Pasteur. **75**:109-139.

(14) **Goldstein, F., G. Gerbaud, and P. Courvalin.** 1986. Transposable resistance to trimethoprim and 0/129 in *Vibrio cholerae*. J. Antimicrob. Chemother. **17**:559-569.

(15) **Goldstein, F.W., J.C. Chumpitaz, J.M. Guevara, B. Papadopoulou, J.F. Acar, and J.F. Vieu.** 1986. Plasmid-mediated resistance to multiple antibiotics in *Salmonella typhi*. J. Infect. Dis. **153**:261-266.

(16) **Goldstein, F.** 1990. Entérobactéries, pp. 241-260 In: P. Courvalin, H. Drugeon, J.P. Flandrois, and F. Goldstein (ed.) Bactéricidie. Maloine, Paris.

(17) **Goldstein, F.W., and G.E. Stein.** 1990. Trimethoprim and trimethoprim-sulfamethoxazole. Pp. 995-1006 In: V.L. Yu, C.M. Thomas, Jr and S.L. Barriere (ed.), Antimicrobial therapy and vaccines. Williams & Wilkins, Baltimore, MD.

(18) **Grape, M., L. Sundström, and G. Kronvall.** 2003. Sulphonamide resistance gene *sul3* found in *Escherichia coli* isolates from human sources. J. Antimicrob. Chemother. **52**:1022-1024.

(19) **Gutmann, L., D. Billot-Klein, R. Williamson, F.W. Goldstein, J. Mounier, J.F. Acar, and E. Collatz.** 1988. Mutation of *Salmonella paratyphi A* conferring cross-resistance to several groups of antibiotics by decreased permeability and loss of invasiveness. Antimicrob. Agents Chemother. **32**:195-201.

(20) **Huovinen, P., L. Sundström, G. Swedberg, and O. Sköld.** 1995. Trimethoprim and sulphonamide resistance. Antimicrob. Agents Chemother. **39**:279-289.

(21) **Kadlec K., and S. Schwarz.** 2009. Identification of a novel trimethoprim resistance gene, *dfrK*, in a methicillin-resistant *Staphylococcus aureus* ST 398 and its physical linkage to the tetracycline resistance gene *tet*(L). Antimicrob. Agents Chemother. (in press).

(22) **Levings, R.S., D. Lightfoot, L.D.H. Elbourne, S.P. Djordjevic, and R.M. Hall.** 2006. New integron-associated gene cassette encoding a trimethoprim-resistant DfrB-type dihydrofolate reductase. Antimicrob. Agents Chemother. **50**:2863-2865.

(23) **Locher, H.H., H. Schlunegger, P.G. Hartman, P. Angehrn, and R.L. Then.** 1996. Antibacterial activities of epiroprim, a new dihydrofolate reductase inhibitor, alone and in combination with dapsone. Antimicrob. Agents Chemother. **40**:1376-1381.

(24) **Myllykallio, H., D. Leduc, J. Filee, and U. Liebl.** 2003. Life without dihydrofolate reductase FoIA. Trends Microbiol. **11**:220-223.

(25) **Nair B.M., K.J. Cheung, Jr, A. Griffith, and J.L. Burns.** 2004. Salicylate induces an antibiotic efflux pump in *Burkholderia cepacia* complex genomovar III (*B. cenocepacia*). J. Clin. Invest. **113**:464-473.

(26) **Patel, O., K. Karnik, and I.G. Macreadie.** 2004. Over-production of dihydrofolate reductase leads to sulfadihydropteroate resistance in yeast. FEMS Microbiol. Lett. **236**:301-305.

(27) **Periti, P.** 1995. Brodimoprim, a new bacterial dihydrofolate reductase inhibitor: a minireview. J. Chemother. **7**:221-223.

(28) **Quinlivan, E.P., J. McPartlin, D.G. Weir, and J. Scott.** 2000. Mechanism of the antimicrobial drug trimethoprim revisited. FASEB J.. **14**:2519-2524.

(28) **Richards, R.M., R.B. Taylor, and Z.Y. Zhu.** 1996. Mechanism for synergism between sulphonamides and trimethoprim clarified. J. Pharm. Pharmacol. **48**:981-984.

(30) **Schmitz, F.J., M. Perdikouli, A. Beeck, J. Verhoef, Ad C. Fluit, and for the European SENTRY participants.** 2001. Resistance to trimethoprim-sulfamethoxazole and modifications in genes coding for dihydrofolate reductase and dihydropteroate synthase in European *Streptococcus pneumoniae* isolates. J. Antimicrob. Chemother. **48**:935-936.

(31) **Tai, N., J.C. Schmitz, J. Liu, X. Lin, M. Bailly, T.M. Chen, and E. Chu.** 2004. Translational autoregulation of thymidylate synthase and dihydrofolate reductase. Front. Biosci. **9**:2521-2526.

(32) **Talisuna, A.O., A. Nalunkuma-Kazibwe, P. Langi, T.K. Mutabingwa, W.W. Watkins, E. Van Marck, T.G. Egwang, and U. D'Alessandro.** 2004. Two mutations in dihydrofolate reductase combined with one dihydropteroate synthase gene predict sulphadoxine-pyrimethamine parasitological failure in Ugandan children with uncomplicated falciparum malaria. Infect. Genet. Evol. **4**:321-327.

(33) **Then, R.** 1990. Sulfamides et triméthoprime. pp. 89-100 *In*: P. Courvalin, H. Drugeon, J.P. Flandrois, and F. Goldstein (ed.) Bactéricidie. Maloine, Paris.

(34) **Then, R.L.** 2004. Antimicrobial dihydrofolate reductase inhibitors: Achievements and future options. J. Chemother. **16**:3-12.

(35) **Van Bambeke, F., Y. Glupczynski, P. Plésiat, J.C. Pechère, and P.M. Tulkens.** 2003. Antibiotic efflux pumps in prokaryotic cells: occurrence, impact on resistance and strategies for the future of antimicrobial therapy. J. Antimicrob. Chemother. **51**:1055-1065.

(36) **Verdier, R.I., D.W. Fitzgerald, W.D. Johnson Jr, and J.W. Pape.** 2000. Trimethoprim-sulfamethoxazole compared with ciprofloxacin treatment and prophylaxis of *Isospora belli* and *Cyclospora cayetenensis* infection in HIV-infected patients. A randomized controlled trial. Ann. Intern. Med. **132**:885-888.

(37) **Wallace Jr, R.J., K. Wiss, M.B. Bushby, and D.C. Hollowell.** 1982. In vitro activity of trimethoprim and sulfamethoxazole against nontuberculous mycobacteria. Rev. Infect. Dis. **4**:326-31.

(38) **Yu, S.H., J.C. Lee, H.Y. Kang, Y.S. Jeong, E.Y. Lee, C.H. Choi, S.H. Tae, Y.C. Lee, S.Y. Seol, and D.T. Cho.** 2004. Prevalence of *dfr* genes associated with integrons and dissemination of *dfrA17* among urinary isolates of *Escherichia coli* in Korea. J. Antimicrob. Chemother. **53**:445-450.

(39) **Zar, H.J., M.J. Alvarez-Martinez, A. Harrison, and S.R. Meshnick.** 2004. Prevalence of dihydropteroate synthase mutants in HIV-infected South African children with *Pneumocystis jiroveci* pneumonia. Clin. Infect. Dis. **39**:1047-1051.

Chapter 27. CHLORAMPHENICOL, FOSFOMYCIN, FUSIDIC ACID, AND POLYMYXINS

Vincent CATTOIR

CHLORAMPHENICOL

Introduction

Isolated from *Streptomyces venezuelae* in 1947 and introduced into clinical practice in 1949, chloramphenicol (originally called chloromycetin) was the first broad spectrum antibiotic since the development of the sulfa drugs. By 1950 it had been synthesized thanks to its simple structure (Fig. 1). The molecule is composed of an aromatic nucleus with a para-nitro group, an aminopropanediol chain (containing two asymmetric carbons) and an acyl side chain (22). Of the four possible diastereoisomers, only the D-threo form has antibacterial activity. The two main derivatives are thiamphenicol, used in human medicine, and florfenicol for veterinary use (Fig. 1). These small, nonpolar, lipophilic molecules diffuse very easily across the cell membrane.

Usage

Because it is inexpensive and highly effective, chloramphenicol is still used in developing countries: the palmitate ester for oral administration and the succinate ester by the parenteral route (24). However, its potent myelotoxicity has sharply restricted its use in the industrialized world. The main indication of chloramphenicol was the treatment of pneumococcal, meningococcal or *Haemophilus influenzae* meningitis in patients with penicillin allergy or in case of resistance to aminopenicillins (29). It was also a reference treatment for typhoid and a second-line treatment for brain abscesses, rickettsiosis (when cyclins are contraindicated), psittacosis (caused by *Chlamydia psittaci*), glanders (caused by *Burkholderia mallei*, in combination with streptomycin), melioidosis (caused by *Burkholderia pseudomallei* in combination with doxycycline) and other infections (listeriosis, brucellosis, plague). The usual dosage is 50-100 mg/kg/day in three or four divided doses (serum levels 10-20 µg/ml); dosage adjustment is necessary in neonates (24).

In France, the use of chloramphenicol is limited to eye drops for local treatment of eye infections. Only thiamphenicol is available in oral or parenteral formulations; the adult dosage is 1.5-3 g per day. In the US, chloramphenicol has been used with success to treat vancomycin-resistant enterococci infections (29).

Chloramphenicol is completely absorbed by the gastrointestinal tract. Tissue diffusion is excellent (particularly CSF, synovial, pleural and peritoneal fluid, and aqueous humor) and it effectively penetrates into cells. Glucuronidated in liver, a reaction with high interindividual variability, it is excreted in the urine as an inactive metabolite.

Chloramphenicol is a highly toxic drug which can cause cytopenia, aplastic anemia and gray baby syndrome (29). Cytopenia is a common, dose-related (serum levels > 25 µg/ml), early (5-7 days) side effect which is reversible within 2-3 weeks after stopping treatment. It results from inhibition of mitochondrial protein synthesis. In contrast, aplastic anemia, while rare (affecting 1 in 40,000 and with a possible genetic predisposition), is independent of dose, irreversible, can occur up to 12 months after stopping treatment, and is often fatal. The risk is higher with oral chloramphenicol but has also been described for parenteral formulations and eye drops. Gray baby syndrome is an early (onset after 3-4 days of treatment) and reversible effect which is the result of chloramphenicol overdose (serum levels > 50 µg/ml). It should be noted that thiamphenicol is less toxic and has not been associated with fatal aplastic anemia (29).

Mode of action

The phenicols are inhibitors of protein synthesis. By reversibly binding to the 23S rRNA of the 50S ribosomal subunit, they block the progression of the growing peptide (22). They function by inhibiting the catalytic activity of peptidyltransferase. Chloramphenicol binds to the ribosomal A-site, even if a peptidyl-tRNA is present. Several ribosomal proteins are also involved in binding: L16 at the A-site, and L2 and L27 at the P-site. This site of action is very close to that of the macrolides and related compounds and a competitive effect is seen (29). There is also a second, low-

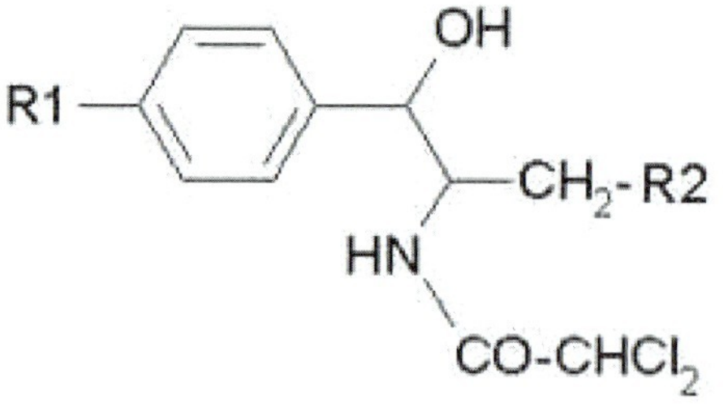

Phenicols[a]

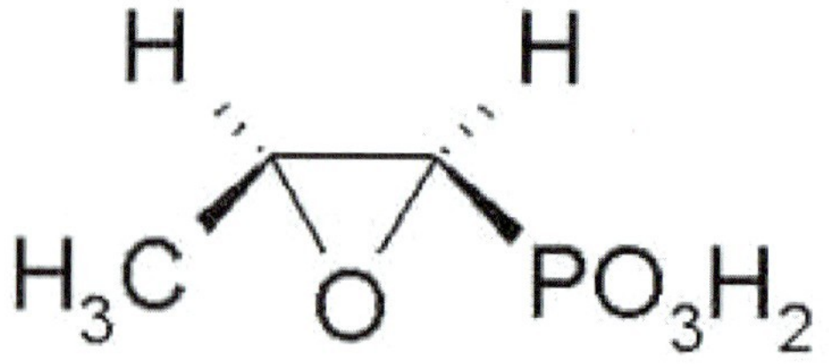

Fosfomycin

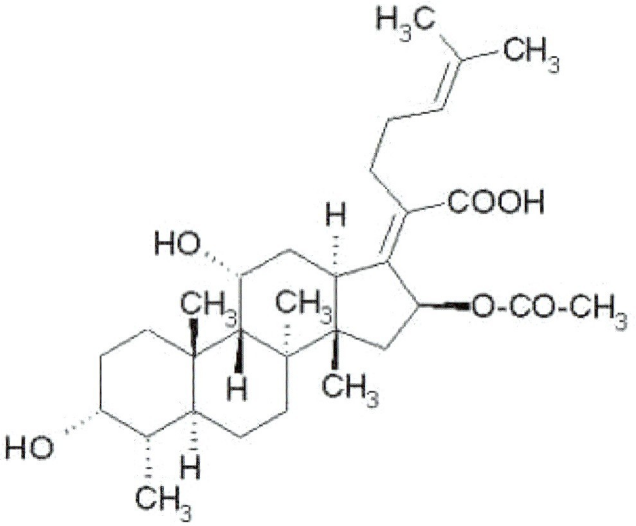

Fusidic acid

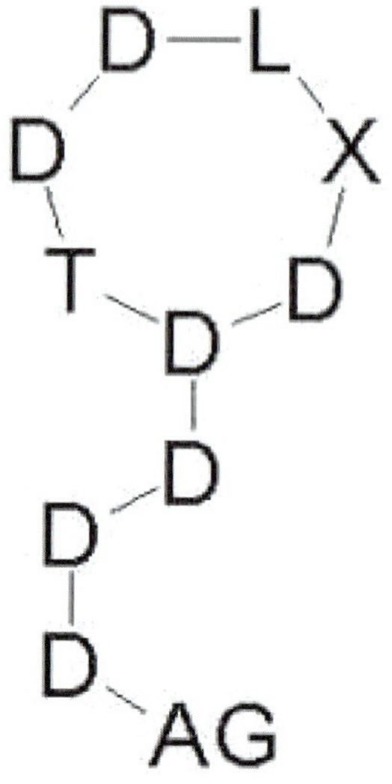

Polymyxins[b]

Fig. 1. Chemical structures of the phenicols, fosfomycin, and fusidic acid, and primary structure of polymyxins. a, Chloramphenicol (R1 = $-NO_2$; R2 = -OH), thiamphenicol (R1 = $-SO_2-CH_3$; R2 = -OH), florfenicol (R1 = $-SO_2-CH_3$; R2 = -F); b, FA: fatty acid (= 6-methyloctanoic acid), D: L-2,4-diaminobutyric acid; L: L-leucine; T: L-threonine, X = D-phenylalanine (polymyxin B) or X = D-Leucine (polymyxin E or colistin).

affinity binding site on the 30S subunit involving the S14 protein.

Spectrum of activity

Thiamphenicol has a very broad spectrum of activity similar to that of chloramphenicol, but its intrinsic activity is lower (Tables 1 and 2). The phenicols are bacteriostatic against most aerobic and anaerobic microorganisms but exert bactericidal activity against the species that cause meningitis: *H. influenzae*, *Streptococcus pneumoniae* and *Neisseria meningitidis* (29). They are effective against aerobic Gram-positive cocci ($MIC_{90} \leq 12.5$ μg/ml) and most enterobacteria, although activity varies according to strain in *Proteus* and related species, *Serratia*, and *Enterobacter*. It should be noted that *Providencia stuartii* are resistant and only one-third of *Proteus mirabilis* isolates are susceptible. Chloramphenicol also shows excellent activity against anaerobic bacteria (MIC usually < 8 μg/ml) and is one of the most active drugs against *Bacteroides* of the *fragilis* group. It is also active against spirochetes, *Chlamydiae*, mycoplasma, and *Rickettsiae* (including *Coxiella burnetii*). Some species such as *Pseudomonas aeruginosa*, *Acinetobacter* spp., *Nocardia asteroides*, and *Mycobacterium tuberculosis* are intrinsically resistant (24, 29).

Resistance mechanisms

Chloramphenicol resistance is mainly due to acquisition of the *cat* gene encoding the enzyme

Table 1. Chloramphenicol susceptibility of the main medically relevant bacteria

Organism	% susceptible strains
Streptococcus pneumoniae	100
S. pneumoniae with reduced penicillin G susceptibility	100
Staphylococcus aureus	94.4
S. aureus methicillin-resistant	82.4
Staphylococci coagulase-negative methicillin-resistant	73.9
Streptococcus agalactiae	99
Enterococcus spp.	68
Enterococcus spp. vancomycin-resistant	68
Neisseria meningitidis	100
Haemophilus influenzae	99.2
Moraxella catarrhalis	100
Escherichia coli	75
Salmonella Typhi	95
Shigella spp.	90
Clostridium spp.	100
Bacteroides fragilis	98

chloramphenicol acetyltransferase (CAT) (22). This enzyme catalyses the transfer of two acetyl groups, derived from acetylCoA, to the antiobiotic molecule, in a three-step reaction (Fig. 2). The mono- and di-acetylated derivatives are inactive because they cannot bind to the ribosome. The CAT enzymes can be divided into two groups according to structure: classical CAT (type A) and the new CAT (type B) (22). CAT-A are found in a wide variety of bacteria. These 24-26 kDa polypeptides exist as homotrimers. To date, 16 different CAT-A protein groups (A1 to A16) have been identified, encoded by either a gene part of the chromosome, a plasmid, or another genetic element (transposon, integron). The first CAT enzymes, described in enterobacteria, were named CAT_I, CAT_{II}, and CAT_{III} and have recently been renamed CAT-A1, CAT-A2, and CAT-A3, respectively (22). CAT-A1 from Escherichia coli confers resistance to fusidic acid (cf. infra) (27). These enzymes confer high-level resistance to chloramphenicol and thiamphenicol (MIC >128 µg/ml) but do not affect florfenicol (Table 2). CAT-B, also known as xenobiotic acetyltransferases (XAT), catalyse the transfer of one acetyl group but display lower affinity for their target and cannot diacetylate 3-acetyl-chloramphenicol. There are at least five groups of CAT-B enzymes - B1 to B5 - which also function in homotrimeric form (22). They are structurally similar to the streptogramin acetyltransferases described in staphylococci and enterococci (Vat proteins).

The second mechanism of resistance is active efflux mediated by membrane transporters known as efflux pumps, of which there are two types: drug-specific efflux pumps which expulse only phenicols, and multidrug pumps which expulse compounds with vastly different structures and thereby contribute to multidrug resistance (MDR) (22). There are at least eight groups of drug-specific pumps (E-1 to E-8). In Gram-negative bacteria they are encoded by the *cml* genes in Enterobacteriaceae and P. aeruginosa, and by the *flo* and *floR* genes in Salmonella Typhimurium, E. coli, and Vibrio cholerae. In Gram-positive organisms, these pumps are encoded by the plasmid gene *fexA* in Staphylococcus lentus, the *cmr* genes in coryneform bacteria and the chromosomal *cml*

Table 2. MICs of chloramphenicol, thiamphenicol, and florfenicol against E. coli and S. aureus according to the mechanism of resistance

Organism	Mechanism of resistance[a]	MIC (µg/ml)		
		Chloramphenicol	Thiamphenicol	Florfenicol
E. coli	Wild type	2	32	4
	Impermeability	32	128	32
	Ribosomal mutation	32	512	32
	CAT_I	256	1 024	4
	CAT_{II}	256	512	4
	CAT_{III}	512	1 024	8
S. aureus	Wild type	4	8	2
	CAT	64	512	2
	cfr	64	NA[b]	32

[a] CAT, Chloramphenicol acetyltransferase.
[b] -, not determined.

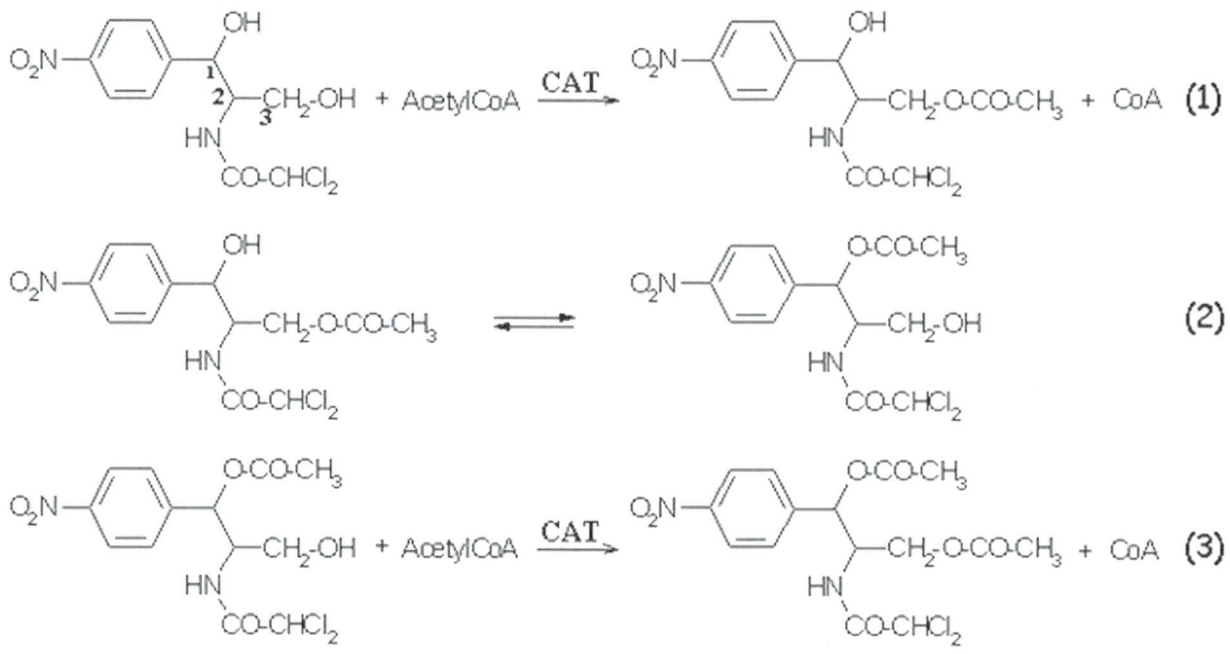

Fig. 2. Inactivation of chloramphenicol (Cm) by chloramphenicol acetyltransferase (CAT). The antibiotic is first acetylated on the hydroxyl group at position C-3 to form 3-acetyl-Cm (1), followed by slow, non-enzymatic rearrangement to 1-acetyl-Cm (2), and a second acetylation (approximately 150 times less efficient) to give 1,3-diacetyl-Cm (3).

and *cmlv* genes in *Streptomyces lividans* and *S. venezuelae*, respectively.

Resistance conferred by MDR efflux pumps is usually low-level and variable depending on the level of overexpression of the efflux machinery. In Gram-negative bacteria, several RND (Resistance-Nodulation-Division) pumps are involved in chloramphenicol efflux, such as AcrAB-TolC in *E. coli* with MIC values of 4 μg/ml for normal expression levels and 16-32 μg/ml in case of overexpression. The MexAB-OprM, MexCD-OprJ, and MexEF-OprN have been described in *P. aeruginosa* as well as CeoAB-OpcM in *Burkholderia cepacia*, ArpABC and TtgABC in *Pseudomonas putida*, AdeABC in *Acinetobacter baumannii* and CmeABC in *Campylobacter jejuni*. In Gram-positive bacteria, the MFS pumps (Major Facilitator Superfamily) NorA and Bmr have been described in *Staphylococcus aureus* and *Bacillus subtilis*, respectively (22).

Other, much less common resistance mechanisms include phosphorylation by a phosphotransferase (a reaction easily reversible by extracellular phosphatases) and hydrolytic degradation to p-nitrophenylserinol as described in *S. venezuelae* (22). Nitroreductase-mediated resistance has been described in *B. fragilis*. A membrane permeability barrier with loss of porins has also been described (e.g., OmpF in *Salmonella* Typhi). Resistance may also be due to mutations in the 23S rRNA binding site (at positions A2057, 2504 in *E. coli*) with cross-resistance to macrolides containing 14 but not 16 atoms (22). Lastly, the *cfr* gene, which confers chloramphenicol and florfenicol resistance, was recently identified in *Staphylococcus sciuri* (22). This gene encodes a methyltransferase which methylates the 23S RNA at position A2503. This interferes with the binding of various classes of antibiotics including phenicols, lincosamides, pleuromutilins, streptogramins A, and oxazolidinones, thereby conferring a MDR phenotype. The *cfr* gene has primarily been identified in *Staphylococcus* spp. of animal origin and, to date, has been found in only three human isolates (two *S. aureus* and one *Staphylococcus epidermidis*).

In vitro susceptibility testing

Chloramphenicol susceptibility testing *in vitro* is straightforward. The CLSI breakpoints differ according to species: for streptococci (including pneumococci), susceptibility is defined as MIC ≤ 4 μg/ml, for *Haemophilus* and *N. meningitidis*, MIC ≤ 2 μg/ml, and for other species (*Enterobacteriaceae, Staphylococcus, Enterococcus, Stenotrophomonas maltophilia, B. cepacia, V. cholerae, Yersinia pestis,* and *Francisella tularensis*), MIC ≤ 8 μg/ml (Table 3). The EUCAST defines susceptibility as MIC ≤ 8 μg/ml and resistance as MIC ≤ 8 μg/ml, breakpoints which are valid for enterobacteria,

Table 3. CLSI breakpoints and critical diameters for chloramphenicol, fosfomycin and, colistin

Antibiotic (disk content) Breakpoint		Chloramphenicol[a] (30 µg)					Fosfomycin[b] (200 µg)	Colistin[c] (10 µg)	
		Hpi	Nm	Spn	Str	Others		Aci	Pse
Critical Concentrations (µg/ml)	S	≤ 2	≤ 2	≤ 4	≤ 4	≤ 8	≤ 64	≤ 2	≤ 2
	R	≥ 8	≥ 8	≥ 8	≥ 16	≥ 16	≥ 256	≥ 4	≥ 8
Critical diameter (mm)	S	≥ 29	≥ 26	≥ 21	≥ 21	≥ 21	≥ 16	-	≥ 11
	R	≤ 25	≤ 19	≤ 20	≤ 17	≤ 17	≤ 12	-	≤ 10

[a] Specific recommendations exist for *Haemophilus influenzae/Haemophilus parainfluenzae* (*Hpi*), *Neisseria meningitidis* (*Nm*), *Streptococcus pneumoniae* (*Spn*), *Streptococcus* spp. other than *S. pneumoniae* (*Str*); The other values are valid for *Enterobacteriaceae*, *Staphylococcus*, *Enterococcus*, *Stenotrophomonas maltophilia**, *Burkholderia cepacia**, *Vibrio cholerae*, *Yersinia pestis**, and *Francisella tularensis** (* no recommendations for critical diameters).
[b] The recommendations for fosfomycin are valid for urine isolates of *Enterococcus* and *Enterobacteriaceae*. The 200-µg fosfomycin disk contains 50 µg glucose-6-phosphate.
[c] The recommendations for colistin are valid for *Acinetobacter* spp. (*Aci*) and *Pseudomonas aeruginosa* (*Pse*).

staphylococci, streptococci and anaerobes. Specific values exist for *H. influenzae* (susceptible, MIC ≤ 1 µg/ml; resistant, MIC ≤ 2 µg/ml) and *N. meningitidis* (susceptible, MIC ≤ 2 µg/ml; resistant, MIC > 4 µg/ml).

Combinations with other antibiotics

Chloramphenicol is a potent antagonist of the bactericidal activity of β-lactams; it acts by delaying the synthesis of autolysins and the peptidoglycan (emergence of "tolerant" bacteria). It partially or totally antagonises the bactericidal effect of quinolones (inhibition of exonuclease synthesis?) and aminoglycosides (24).

Prevalence of resistance

Resistance to chloramphenicol is rare (Table 1) and has mainly been investigated in the species that cause community-acquired meningitis. For example, in a series of 1,533 *H. influenzae* clinical isolates recovered in 1986 in Wales, only 19 (1.2%) were resistant. At Henri Mondor Hospital in Paris, France, only 10 (2.25%) of 446 *H. influenzae* strains isolated between 2002 and 2004 were resistant. Of approximately 1,400 clinical isolates of *N. meningitidis* serogroup B isolated in Australia between 1994 and 1997, only 2 were resistant (25). For *S. pneumoniae*, 85% of 562 isolates from Henri Mondor Hospital in Paris, collected between 2002 and 2004, were susceptible.

Resistance is also rare among anaerobic bacteria, although a few *Bacteroides* strains with MIC values above 25 µg/ml have been described. With respect to Gram-positive organisms, in a series of 3,589 *S. aureus* strains isolated at Henri Mondor Hospital between 2002 and 2004, all hospital departments combined, 3.3% tested as intermediate or resistant (6.9% of MRSA and 1.4% of MSSA). The emergence of a multiresistant *S*. Typhimurium clone, lysotype DT104, characterised by chromosomally-encoded resistance (after acquiring an integron) to ampicillin (A), chloramphenicol (C), streptomycin (S), sulfonamides (Su) and tetracycline (T) (ACSSuT resistance) has been described (2). In 1995, in a series of 3,903 strains of *Salmonella* from the CDC, 976 (25%) were serovar Typhimurium and 28% of these showed ACSSuT resistance, as compared to only 7% in 1990. In France, out of the 992 *S*. Typhimurium strains sent to the National Reference Center in 1997, 56% were resistant to chloramphenicol versus only 4% and 0% for serovars Enteritidis (n = 800) and Hadar (n = 141), respectively.

FOSFOMYCIN

Introduction

Fosfomycin (formerly known as phosphonomycin) is an antibiotic originally isolated in 1969 from cultures of *Streptomyces fradiae*. It is also produced by other strains of *Streptomyces* (*S. viridochromogenes*, *S. wedmorensis*) and *Pseudomonas* (*P. syringae*, *P. viridiflava*), but currently it is obtained by chemical synthesis. The chemical name is L-cis-1,2-epoxypropylphosphonic acid. The molecule has two structural features which are unusual for an antibiotic: an epoxide ring and a carbon-phosphorus bond (Fig. 1).

Notable physicochemical characteristics include a low molecular weight (MW 138.1) and high water solubility.

Usage

Incompletely absorbed by the gastrointestinal tract, fosfomycin diffuses well into tissues, particularly CSF, bone, and lung, and is excreted in the urine as the active drug. Tolerability is very good due to the absence of the target enzyme in human cells (20).

In some countries, the disodium salt of fosfomycin is used for intravenous administration at a daily dosage of 100-200 mg/kg divided into three doses, but it must always be used in combination therapy. In this context, it is mainly indicated in meningeal and bone/joint infections due to staphylococci, particularly methicillin-resistant strains (in combination with cefotaxime or imipenem, for example), and in *P. aeruginosa* infections (with a β-lactam or a fluoroquinolone). In a recent review of 62 studies describing the use of fosfomycin as monotherapy or in combination therapy for the treatment of infections other than those of the urinary or gastrointestinal tract, the cure rate was 81.1% (6). A few recent publications have highlighted the effectiveness of fosfomycin in soft tissue infections (cellulitis, diabetic foot) and in infections due to vancomycin-resistant enterococci or extended spectrum β-lactamase-producing *Enterobacteriaceae*.

The main indication of fosfomycin is the single-dose treatment of uncomplicated acute cystitis in young women, in the form of fosfomycin-trometamol, an oral formulation with superior bioavailability (ca. 40%) (20).

Mode of action

As with β-lactam and glycopeptide antibiotics, fosfomycin acts by inhibiting bacterial wall synthesis (formation of spheroplasts), but it does so at an earlier stage. It acts by specifically and irreversibly inhibiting the action of UDP-N-acetyl-glucosamine enolpyruvyltransferase (MurA). This enzyme catalyses the first step in peptidoglycan biosynthesis by transferring an enolpyruvyl residue derived from phosphoenol pyruvate (PEP) to the 3-hydroxyl group of UDP-N-acetyl-glucosamine (16). Being a structural analogue of PEP, fosfomycin covalently binds to cysteine-115 (*E. coli* numbering) in the active site of MurA. As this enzyme is present in the cytoplasm, the antibiotic must penetrate into the bacterial cell, which it accomplishes through two active transport mechanisms: the GlpT system, which is partially constitutive, and the UhpT system, inducible by glucose-6-phosphate (G6P). These two systems regulate the physiological transport of L-α-glycerophosphate and hexose phosphates, respectively (18).

Table 4. Bacteria with intrinsic fosfomycin resistance

Fosfomycin-resistant species
Acinetobacter baumannii
Stenotrophomonas maltophilia
Burkholderia cepacia
Morganella morganii
Vibrio cholerae
Staphylococcus saprophyticus
Staphylococcus capitis
Enterococcus spp. [a]
Corynebacterium
Erysipelothrix rhusiopathiae spp.
Listeria monocytogenes
Bacteroides fragilis
Prevotella spp.
Porphyromonas spp.
Clostridium spp.
Eubacterium spp.
Peptostreptococcus spp.
Chlamydia spp.
Mycoplasma spp.
Mycobacterium spp.

[a] Low-level resistance.

Spectrum of activity

Fosfomycin is a broad spectrum antibiotic (20). It exerts a slow bactericidal effect by disrupting the bacterial membrane, with MBC values similar to MIC values. Among Gram-positive bacteria, both methicillin-resistant and -susceptible staphylococci (except *Staphylococcus saprophyticus* and *Staphylococcus capitis*) as well as pneumococci, are inherently susceptible (Tables 4 and 5). On the other hand, fosfomycin is less effective against streptococci and enterococci (Table 5). Gram-positive bacilli such as *Corynebacterium*, *Arcanobacterium*, *Rhodococcus*, *Listeria monocytogenes*, and *Erysipelothrix rhusiopathiae* show intrinsic high-level resistance (MIC >256 μg/ml) (Table 4). Among Gram-negative organisms, the spectrum of activity encompasses the enterobacteria (except *Morganella morganii*), *N. meningitidis*, and *Pasteurella* spp. (Table 5). Most non-fermentative Gram-negative bacilli, with the exception of *P. aeruginosa*, are resistant (Tables 4 and 5).

Table 5. MICs of fosfomycin on agar containing 25 µg/ml glucose-6-phosphate

Species[a] (no. of strains)	MIC (µg/ml)		
	50 %	90 %	Range
Staphylococcus aureus (265)	3	13.4	0.125 - 128
Staphylococcus epidermidis (25)[b]	1.7	38	1 - > 256
Enterococcus faecalis (73)	13.9	40.8	0.25 - > 256
Streptococcus pyogenes (50)[b]	27.9	53.8	2 - 64
Streptococcus agalactiae (20)[b]	12.5	45.2	2 - 64
Streptococcus pneumoniae (7)	5.3	9.8	4 - 16
Escherichia coli (234)	0.4	8	0.125 - 64
Shigella spp. (72)	< 0.125	0.3	0.125 - 2
Citrobacter spp. (29)	< 0.125	0.5	0.125 - 2
Salmonella spp. (39)	0.45	2.6	0.125 - 16
Klebsiella spp. (157)	1	30.9	0.125 - > 256
Enterobacter spp. (98)	1.3	10.6	0.125 - > 256
Serratia spp. (56)	0.8	5.9	0.125 - 32
Proteus spp. (132)	0.4	1.9	0.125 - > 256
Morganella morganii (26)	24.2	115.4	8 - > 256
Providencia spp. (34)	1.7	6.5	0.125 - 32
Pseudomonas spp. (167)	5.1	14.4	0.125 - > 256
Acinetobacter spp. (46)	53.8	> 128	0.25 - > 256
Haemophilus spp. (9)	0.7	2.7	0.125 - 16

[a] Clinical strains isolated in the early 1980s.
[b] MIC determined on Mueller-Hinton agar supplemented with 50 µg/ml of glucose-6-phosphate.

Anaerobes, except for the genus *Fusobacterium*, show intrinsic resistance (Table 4).

Resistance mechanisms

Different mechanisms of natural resistance have been described, particularly in fosfomycin-producing microorganisms. This is the case for *P. syringae*, where the FosC protein catalyses ATP-dependent phosphorylation of fosfomycin. In *S. wedmorensis*, the *fomA* and *fomB* gene products inactivate by phosphorylation fosfomycin and fosfomycin monophosphate, respectively. In *M. tuberculosis* and *Chlamydia*, the presence of an aspartate in place of the cysteine at position 115 in the MurA active site (corresponding to residue 117 and 119, respectively), appears to render these two species inherently resistant (16).

Acquired resistance to fosfomycin is mainly carried by the chromosome but can also be plasmid-mediated (18). It is noteworthy that there is no cross-resistance with other antibiotics, with the exception of a similar compound, fosmidomycin.

Chromosomally-encoded resistance is often due to a defect in antibiotic transport by the GlpT and/or UhpT systems. Expression of the *gplT* and *uhpT* genes is upregulated by the cyclic AMP-cyclic AMP receptor protein complex (products of the *cyaA* and *ptsI* genes, respectively). High level expression of the *uhpT* gene depends on the local regulatory genes *uhpA*, *uhpB*, and *uhpC*. Mutations in the structural genes *uhpT* and *glpT* or in the regulatory genes are therefore responsible for fosfomycin resistance. It should also be noted that fosfomycin resistance considerably impairs the fitness of the bacterial cell (18). Indeed, both the growth rate and virulence of mutants is reduced (decreased adhesion to urinary tract epithelial cells, for example). Mutations which decrease the affinity of fosfomycin for its target, as well as increased *murA* transcription, have also been described.

Plasmid-mediated resistance involves inactivation of the antibiotic by a glutathione-S-transferase which catalyses the opening of the epoxide ring, leading to formation of an inactive compound (26). FosA, initially described in *Serratia marcescens*, is a homodimeric metalloenzyme (two 16 kDa subunits) which catalyses manganese-dependent covalent addition of a glutathione residue to C_1 of fosfomycin. Originally described in *S. epidermidis* and then in other staphylococcal species, FosB shares 38% amino acid identity with its FosA homolog. It is also a metallothiol-transferase, but it preferentially uses L-cysteine and magnesium as cofactors and has much lower catalytic activity than FosA. In *L. monocytogenes*, the product of the chromosomal gene *lmo1702*, FosX, shares 30% identity with FosA and 35% with FosB. This protein inactivates fosfomycin by opening the epoxide ring *via* addition of a water molecule, using magnesium as cofactor, and thereby confers natural resistance.

In vitro susceptibility testing

In vitro susceptibility testing of fosfomycin is difficult because different external factors as well as the test conditions can influence the results (20). For example, fosfomycin activity is antagonised by the presence of glucose, phosphates, or NaCl, but is increased at low pH, in the presence of human blood or by adding G6P. Activity also depends on the medium, the incubation atmosphere, and the inoculum. These problems explain the different susceptibility breakpoints which have been proposed, which range from ≤ 8 µg/ml to ≤ 128 µg/ml. EUCAST defines susceptibility/resistance as ≤ 32 µg/ml and > 32 µg/ml for *Enterobacteriaceae*, *Pseudomonas*, and *Staphylococcus*. In contrast, CLSI breakpoints are very different and have been validated only for enterococcal and enterobacterial urine isolates: ≤ 64 µg/ml, 128 µg/ml and ≥ 256 µg/ml for susceptible, intermediate, and resistant, respectively (Table 3). MIC values should also be interpreted by taking into account the concentrations that can be attained at the site of infection. For instance, urine concentrations after a single dose of 3 g fosfomycin-trometamol are very high, ranging from 1000 to 4000 µg/ml during the first 12 to concentrations in excess of 128 µg/ml at 48 (20). As fosfomycin has higher activity when the medium is supplemented with G6P (*via* induction of the UhpT transport system), the G6P concentration in MH medium has been standardized to 25 µg/ml. For the CLSI disk diffusion method, disks are loaded with 200 µg fosfomycin and 50 µg G6P; inhibition zone diameters ≥ 16 mm and ≤ 12 mm are respectively defined as the susceptibility and resistance breakpoints (Table 3). Finally, it is important that fosfomycin resistance is homogeneous: the presence of colonies in the inhibition zone should not be taken into account when interpreting the results (mutants selected *in vitro*).

Combinations with other antibiotics

Because the mutation rate is high (10^{-6}-10^{-9}), fosfomycin is not recommended for use as monotherapy (except for urinary tract infections). Synergy with other antibiotics is almost always observed, with the exception of rifampin. The fosfomycin-rifampin combination shows additive bacteriostatic activity and antagonistic bactericidal activity. Good synergy is observed against staphylococci when fosfomycin is combined with cloxacillin, cefotaxime, ceftriaxone, or imipenem. The synergy of a β-lactam and fosfomycin on methicillin-resistant staphylococci is due to a reduction in the synthesis of PLP2a induced by fosfomycin. Synergy is observed against *P. aeruginosa* when fosfomycin is combined with piperacillin, ceftazidime, or cefsulodine.

Prevalence of resistance

Recent studies have focused more specifically on the *in vitro* activity of fosfomycin on urinary tract pathogens. However, susceptibility rates show some variability due to differences in the breakpoints used. In 1998, a study in the US of 1,097 *E. coli* and 157 *Enterococcus faecalis* urinary tract isolates showed 100% and 97.5% susceptibility to fosfomycin, respectively (according to CLSI criteria) (7). The ECO-SENS study conducted in 16 European countries and in Canada between 1999 and 2000 determined *E. coli* resistance rates in uncomplicated lower urinary tract infections in women aged 18-65. Among 2,478 isolates, only 0.7% were classified as resistant (MIC ≥ 64 µg/ml) (10). In an Italian study conducted in 2000, 99%, 87.5%, 53%, 60%, 100%, 0% and 0% of *E. coli*, *P. mirabilis*, *Klebsiella pneumoniae*, *Enterobacter cloacae*, *Citrobacter freundii*, *M. morganii*, and *S. marcescens* strains were susceptible to fosfomycin, respectively (using CLSI criteria) (15).

With respect to staphylococci, the data are from the 1970s, but it appears that the prevalence of resistance in *S. aureus* remains low (<10%). More recent data collected between 2002 and 2004 at Henri Mondor Hospital in Paris, in a series of 3,589 *S. aureus* isolates, all hospital departments combined, showed a resistance rate of 1.7% (4.7% for MRSA and 0.4% for MSSA). For *S. pneumoniae*, a 1999 study of 35 strains isolated from CSF found that only 6.9% were resistant to fosfomycin. Lastly, for *P. aeruginosa*, a 1998 French study in a series of 735 strains found that 61% of those isolated from cystic fibrosis patients (n = 70) and 56% of the remaining strains were susceptible to fosfomycin. In a review of several publications comprising a total of 360 patients, overall fosfomycin resistance was 10.8% among isolates of *Staphylococcus* spp., *P. aeruginosa*, *Klebsiella* spp., and *Enterobacter* spp. (6).

Aid to bacterial identification

Natural resistance to an antibiotic in a bacterial species can sometimes be used as an indicator for species identification. For example, various susceptibilities to fosfomycin distinguish the corynebacteria (no inhibition zone) from *Actinomyces* (small inhibition zone of 10-12 mm). Among coagulase-negative staphylococci, a few clinical isolates are generally resistant, including *S. capitis* and *S. saprophyticus* (a species also resistant to novobiocin). Less medically relevant species are often found to be resistant, including *Staphylococcus auricularis*, *Staphylococcus warneri* and *Staphylococcus haemolyticus*. The enterobacteria *M. morganii*, *Leclercia adecarboxylata* and *Ewingella americana* harbor natural resistance to fosfomycin. Among *Pseudomonas*, *P. putida* and *P. fluorescens* have similar antibiotypes but contact resistance to a fosfomycin disk for *P. putida* can help differentiate between the two species.

FUSIDIC ACID

Introduction

Fusidic acid, introduced into clinical practice in 1962, is a natural antibiotic isolated from the micromycete *Fusidium coccineum*. This fusidane compound is chemically related to helvolic acid and cephalosporin P_1 (4). In spite of its sterol structure, fusidic acid does not possess any physiological properties common to corticosteroids or bile acids. Its antibacterial activity appears to derive from the conformation of the side chain at the C_{17}-C_{20} double bond and the carboxyl group at carbon C_{20} (4). Fusidic acid also exhibits immunosuppressive properties similar to those of cyclosporine A.

Usage

Sodium fusidate is rapidly absorbed after an oral dose and bioavailability is >90%. Therapeutic concentrations are reached in bone, synovial fluid, skin, bronchial secretions, and heart but the drug does not diffuse well into brain or CSF (even in case of meningitis). The drug is highly bound to serum albumin (91-98%) and is excreted as inactive metabolites in the bile. It is generally well tolerated at the usual doses (1-1.5 g/day in two or three divided doses), but hepatotoxicity can occur at high doses.

In some countries, this antibiotic is available for intravenous or oral administration, and ophthalmic and topical formulations are also available. The main indications are staphylococcal infections such as acute or chronic osteomyelitis, septic arthritis, infections on prosthetic joints, bacteremia and endocarditis, skin and soft tissue infections (including burns), and respiratory tract infections in cystic fibrosis patients (5, 9). It has also been used with success to eradicate nasal carriage of *S. aureus* and corynebacterial endocarditis. The ophthalmic gel is used for external infections of the eye and its appendages while topical preparations are indicated for superficial skin infections such as impetigo, infected eczema, or erythrasma due to *Corynebacterium minutissimum* (5). Recent studies report the use of fusidic acid *per os* (250 mg tid) for diarrhea where the incriminated organism is *Clostridium difficile*. Fusidic acid may also be of interest in the multidrug therapy of leprosy.

Mode of action

Fusidic acid inhibits bacterial protein synthesis by interfering with elongation factor G (EF-G) (4), a GTPase essential for translocation of the peptidyl-tRNA from the ribosomal A-site to the P-site. After hydrolysis of GTP, the EF-G/GDP complex is normally released from the ribosome for recycling. In the presence of fusidic acid, EF-G/GDP remains on the ribosome, thereby blocking elongation of the growing polypeptide chain. Fusidic acid must prevent the complex from adopting the conformation required for release of GDP. At high concentrations, fusidic acid also inhibits aminoacyl-tRNA binding to the P-site (4).

Spectrum of activity

Fusidic acid is considered to be a bacteriostatic antibiotic, although at high doses it is bactericidal (MBC/MIC ratio = 8 to 32 for staphylococci, with MBC values of 0.5-8 µg/ml). This hydrophobic molecule has a narrow spectrum of activity and is mainly effective against Gram-positive bacteria.

It is very active against *S. aureus*, including methicillin-resistant strains, generally with MIC values ranging from 0.03 to 0.25 µg/ml (4), and also against coagulase-negative staphylococci (particularly *S. epidermidis*), with the exception of *S. saprophyticus* (Table 6). Corynebacteria, including *C. jeikeium* which is often multiresistant, are generally highly susceptible. On the other hand, only marginal activity is seen against streptococci and enterococci (Table 6). Fusidic acid shows good *in vitro* activity against Gram-positive anaerobes (*Clostridium*, *Peptococcus*, *Peptostreptococcus*, and *Propionibacterium*) with MIC_{90} usually below 1 µg/ml; only *Actinomyces israelii* always appears to be resistant (4).

Table 6. MICs of fusidic acid

Species	MIC (µg/ml)[a]		
	50 %	90 %	Range
Staphylococcus aureus MS[b]	0.03 - 0.25	0.06 - 1	0.03 - 4
S. aureus MR[b]	0.03 - 2	0.06 - 4	0.03 - 64
Staphylocoques à coagulase négative (MS + MR)	0.03 - 0.25	0.06 - 0.5	0.03 - 32
Staphylococcus epidermidis	0.12 - 0.25	0.25 - 0.5	0.03 - 8
Staphylococcus saprophyticus	2 - 4	4	0.06 - 8
Streptococcus spp.	2 - 8	4 - 8	1 - 16
Enterococcus spp.	2 - 16	4 - 16	1 - 32
Corynebacterium spp.	0.04	2	0.04 - 12.5
Enterobacteriaceae, Pseudomonas	> 100	-	-
Bordetella pertussis	0.1	0.2	0.03 - 0.5
Moraxella catarrhalis	0.12	0.12	0.06 - 0.12
Neisseria meningitidis	0.03	0.12	0.016 - 0.5
Neisseria gonorrheae	0.6	2	0.25 - 2
Mycobacterium spp. (autre que M. leprae)	8 - 64	16 - >128	1 - >128
Mycobacterium leprae	-	-	0.16 - 20
Bacteroides spp.	0.5 - 2	2 - 16	0.12 - 16
Prevotella spp., Porphyromonas spp.	0.25 - 2	0.5 - 4	0.12 - 4
Fusobacterium spp.	1 - 16	32 - 64	< 0.25 - >128
Clostridium spp.	0.12 - 2	0.25 - 2	< 0.06 - 64
Peptococcus spp., Peptostreptococcus spp.	0.12 - 0,25	0.25 - 1	< 0.06 - 2

[a] Mean MIC values for the main medically relevant bacteria.
[b] Methicillin-susceptible.
[c] Methicillin-resistant.

The majority of Gram-negative bacilli including enterobacteria, *Pseudomonas* spp., and other non-fermentative bacilli show high-level resistance (MIC_{50} >100 µg/ml). However, *Moraxella catarrhalis*, *Bordetella pertussis*, *N. gonorrhoeae* and *N. meningitidis* are susceptible (Table 6). Fusidic acid shows modest activity against Gram-negative anaerobes (MIC_{90} = 2-16 µg/ml for *B. fragilis*), although *Fusobacterium* are resistant (4).

Weak *in vitro* activity is observed against mycobacteria, *Nocardia*, and *Borrelia burgdorferi* but fusidic acid is potentially active against *C. burnetii* and *Mycobacterium leprae* (9). Several studies have also demonstrated antiparasitic activity *in vitro* against *Plasmodium* and *Giardia*.

Resistance mechanisms

There is no cross-resistance with other antibiotics in clinical use. Two types of resistance have been described in *S. aureus* (1). The first mechanism involves alteration of the target by chromosomal mutations in the *fusA* gene encoding factor EF-G (27). Chromosomal resistance rates range from 10^{-6} to 10^{-8}. Resistant mutants therefore emerge easily, but their growth is slower and their pathogenicity is attenuated (1). Furthermore, spontaneous reversion in the absence of fusidic acid renders them fully susceptible. It should be noted that compensatory mutations in *fusA* have been described which improve mutant fitness. The second mechanism of resistance results from horizontal transfer of a plasmid determinant (*fusB*) described in several *Staphylococcus* species and encoding a protein which binds to factor EF-G, thereby protecting it from the action of fusidic acid (27, 28). Two homologs of the *fusB* gene have recently been identified: *fusC* in *S. aureus* and *S. intermedius*, and *fusD* in *S. saprophyticus*, the latter explaining the low-level intrinsic fusidic acid resistance in this species (19).

In other species, several mechanisms involving enzymatic inactivation have been described. First of all, in the enterobacteria, CAT_I (or CAT-A1) can inhibit the action of fusidic acid by sequestration without acetylation, whereas CAT_{II} (or CAT-A2) and CAT_{III} (or CAT-A3) have no effect. Another mechanism described in *S. lividans* involves secretion of FusH, a 50 kDa extracellular esterase which converts the antibiotic to an inactive product. This chromosomally-encoded protein, also found in *Streptomyces coelicolor*, deacetylates fusidic acid at position C_{16}. The final mechanism has been described in Gram-negative bacteria and is based on active efflux pumps involving RND transporters (Resistance-Nodulation-Division) such as AcrAB-TolC in *E. coli* (27).

In vitro susceptibility testing

Although the inoculum effect is modest, *in vitro* susceptibility testing of fusidic acid is affected by several factors including the presence of blood or serum and the alkalinity of the medium, which reduces antibacterial activity. Results should be interpreted by keeping in mind that fusidic acid is highly protein bound. In fact, *in vitro* tests overestimate antibacterial activity when one considers that only the unbound fraction of antibiotic is active *in vivo*. The usual breakpoints for susceptibility and resistance are ≤ 1 μg/ml and >1 μg/ml according to EUCAST; the CLSI has not issued any recommendations (4).

Combinations with other antibiotics

As with fosfomycin and rifampin, fusidic acid should always be used in combination therapy, to avoid the emergence of resistant mutants. Data from studies of fusidic acid combinations are conflicting (4). For example, combination with β-lactams has been reported to be additive, indifferent or antagonistic. For vancomycin (the most frequent combination), indifference is usually observed whereas modest synergy is seen with aminoglycosides and erythromycin. Interaction with fosfomycin has been found to be additive or indifferent, and no synergy is observed with linezolid. An antagonistic effect (or in some cases indifferent) is often seen with rifampin and with quinolones.

Prevalence of resistance

Mutants which are resistant to fusidic acid grow more slowly than susceptible strains, which might explain the low prevalence of chromosomal resistance *in vivo*. Resistance rates in *S. aureus* are generally low and constant, ranging from 1 to 3% for MSSA and from 2 to 12% for MRSA (27). A large multicenter study conducted in 1996 among a collection of 4,065 *S. aureus* isolates found that resistance rates varied widely from one country to another, ranging from 0 to 49%, with an average of 5% (9). At Henri Mondor Hospital in Paris, in a serie of 3,589 isolates recovered from all hospital departments between 2002 and 2004, approximately 5.1% were intermediate or resistant (8.1% of MRSA and 3.8% of MSSA). Resistance rates are higher among coagulase-negative staphylococci, ranging from 4 to 30%. However, several European countries have reported a recent rise in fusidic acid resistance among community-acquired *S. aureus* strains incriminated in skin infections (9, 28). In the United Kingdom, resistance rates increased 2-5 fold between 1992 and 2001. For example, in a study conducted in 2001 on isolates obtained from dermatology patients, 50% were resistant as compared to 9.6% of isolates obtained from patients in other departments (23). Similar increases have also been observed recently in Scandinavia and the Netherlands. In Norway, resistance rates rose from 3% in 1992 to 36% in 2001 among the causative strains of bullous impetigo (28). Although this increase appears to be related to prescription rates for topical fusidic acid formulations, this high prevalence is probably a reflection of epidemic dissemination of a resistant clone in northern Europe. Moreover, this epidemic clone harbors the *fusB* determinant whereas *fusA* mutations are prevalent in other non-epidemic isolates (28). Lastly, community-associated Panton-Valentine leucocidin-positive *S. aureus* has a characteristic resistance phenotype. These strains are classically resistant to oxacillin, kanamycin, tetracycline, fusidic acid, and susceptible to other antibiotics, including fluoroquinolones.

POLYMYXINS

Introduction

Polymyxins are naturally occurring cyclic antibiotics originally isolated from strains of *Bacillus*. These high molecular weight (ca. 1,200 Da) cationic polypeptides are composed of a ring of seven amino acids and a tripeptide side chain to which a fatty acid is covalently bound (Fig. 1). This structure confers both hydrophobicity and basic properties to these molecules, explaining their amphoteric nature. The polymyxin family is composed of five chemical classes: A, B, C, D, and E. Only two compounds are used therapeutically: polymyxin B isolated from *Paenibacillus* (*Bacillus*) *polymyxa* in 1947, and polymyxin E (also termed colistin) isolated from *P. polymyxa* var. *colistinus* in 1950.

Usage

Introduced into clinical practice in the early 1960s, the polymyxins quickly fell out of favour due to their nephrotoxicity, neurotoxicity, and the risk of neuromuscular blockade. However, more recent studies indicate a lower frequency of this toxicity which is dose-related, cumulative, and reversible when treatment is stopped (12). In the late 1990s, the emergence of multiresistant Gram-negative bacilli together with an absence of development of new antibiotics led to a renewed interest in these "old" antibiotics (12, 14). Unfortunately, recent pharmacodynamic, pharmacokinetic, and clinical data are lacking (12).

Polymyxin B sulfate is used in topical formulations (ear, eye, skin preparations, and vaginal pessaries) or parenterally (12). Colistin is available as two salts: the sulfate for topical and oral preparations and the methane-sulfonate (also known as colistimethate) for parenteral use (12, 14). Polymyxins can also be aerosolized for administration by inhalation, or given by the intrathecal or ventricular route or by bladder irrigation. Polymyxin B sulfate is more active than colistin sulfate, which in turn is more active than colistimethate, and the associated toxicities follow the same trend. Several IV formulations of colistimethate are on the market, and it should be kept in mind that 1 μg colistin base is equivalent to 1.5 μg colistin sulfate, 2.4 μg colistimethate and 30 IU of antibiotic activity (12). Also, 1 mg polymyxin B sulfate is equivalent to 10,000 IU of antibiotic activity (12).

Polymyxins are poorly absorbed by the gastrointestinal tract and tissue distribution is low (especially in CSF and pleural and synovial fluid). Approximately 50% is protein bound. Active drug is rapidly excreted in the urine and dosage adjustment is required in case of renal insufficiency.

In several countries including France, colistin sulfate is used orally for noninvasive infectious diarrhea and gastrointestinal tract decontamination in neutropenic patients, at doses of 100,000-250,000 IU/kg/day in three or four divided doses. For the past few years, colistimethate and polymyxin B sulfate IV formulations have offered an interesting treatment option for severe infections due to multiresistant *P. aeruginosa*, *A. baumannii*, or *K. pneumoniae*. However, these were mainly small studies or isolated case reports of septicemia, urinary tract infection, pneumonia, meningitis, endocarditis, peritonitis, or osteomyelitis (12, 14). The daily dosage of colistimethate IV is 50,000-100,000 IU/kg/day in two or three divided doses and that for polymyxin B sulfate IV is 15,000-25,000 IU/kg/day in two or three divided doses (12). There have been a few reports of successful use of intrathecal or intraventricular administration in CNS infections (meningitis, ventriculitis). The main use of polymyxins over the past twenty years has been in aerosolized form for the treatment of *P. aeruginosa* infections in cystic fibrosis patients. In addition, by virtue of its high affinity for LPS, polymyxin B-immobilized therapy has shown encouraging results as an adjuvant treatment of septic shock.

Mode of action

Polymyxins have a unique mechanism of action: these detergent-like compounds display high affinity for bacterial membranes, disrupting the morphology of the bacterial cell and producing blebs on the cell wall. The polycationic peptide ring binds to the negatively charged phosphate groups of LPS (core-lipid A region), competitively displacing Mg^{2+} and Ca^{2+} ions which normally stabilise LPS (14). Note that this initial binding can be antagonized by high concentrations of divalent cations, and that interaction with LPS is facilitated by hydrophobic interactions in the lipid A region. The antibiotic then promotes its own penetration into the cell by inducing the formation of pores which disrupt the integrity of the cytoplasmic membrane. This leads to cell death from rupture of the osmotic barrier, leakage of essential cytoplasmic components and release of lytic enzymes.

Spectrum of activity

Polymyxins have a narrow antibacterial spectrum comprising the majority of Gram-negative bacilli (Table 7) (14). They are bacteriostatic at low doses and become bactericidal at high doses. Enterobacterial species of the genus *Proteus*, *Providencia* as well as the species *M. morganii*, *S. marcescens* and *Edwardsiella tarda* show intrinsic resistance with $MIC_{50} > 128$ μg/ml (Table 8). Most *Yersinia pseudotuberculosis* strains are resistant and MIC values increase from 30°C to 37°C. *Aeromonas*, apart from *A. jandaei*, are susceptible whereas *A. hydrophila* has inducible resistance. Among non-fermentative Gram-negative bacilli, *B. cepacia* and *B. pseudomallei* are also naturally resistant, as are approximately 30-40% of *S. maltophilia* isolates (Table 9). Polymyxins are also effective against *H. influenzae*, *B. pertussis*, and *Pasteurella multocida*; on the other hand, *Neisseria*, *M. catarrhalis*, *Campylobacter*, *Helicobacter pylori*, *Legionella pneumophila*, and *Brucella* are intrinsiclly resistant. Among *V.*

Table 7. Activity of colistimethate against Gram-negative bacilli (clinical isolates collected in 1997)

Species (no. of strains)	Colistimethate (µg/ml)		
	MIC$_{50}$	MIC$_{90}$	Range
P. aeruginosa (80)	2	4	0.5 - 32
Providencia spp. (23)	> 128	> 128	> 128
Enterobacter spp. (47)	1	> 128	0.5 - > 128
Acinetobacter spp. (23)	1	2	1 - 128
Shigella spp. (12)	0.5	0.5	0.06 - 0.5
Serratia spp. (24)	> 128	> 128	16 - > 128
Salmonella spp. (12)	1	1	1 - 2
Citrobacter spp. (19)	1	1	0.5 - 1
Klebsiella spp. (50)	1	8	0.5 - 16
E. coli (50)	0.5	1	0.5 - 1

Table 8. Susceptibility and intrinsic resistance of *Enterobacteriaceae* species to polymyxins

Enterobacteriaceae	Susceptible to colistin	Resistant to colistin
Frequently isolated in human disease	Escherchia coli, E. hermanii Shigella spp. Salmonella enterica Citrobacter freundii, C. koseri Klebsiella pneumoniae, K. oxytoca Enterobacter cloacae, E. aerogenes Hafnia alvei Pantoea agglomerans, P. dispersa Yersinia enterocolitica	Proteus mirabilis, P. vulgaris, P. penneri Providencia stuartii, P. rettgerii Morganella morganii Serratia marcescens[a] Yersinia pseudotuberculosis[b]
Rarely isolated in human disease	Erwinia amylovora Ewingella americana Rahnella aquatilis Buttiauxella agrestis Kluyvera cryocrescens, K. ascorbata Lerclercia adecarboxylata Levinea malonatica Tatumella ptyseos[c] Trabulsiella guamensis Leminorella grimontii, L. richardii	Cedecea davisae, C. lapagei, C. neteri Moellerella wisconsensis Yokenella regensburgei Edwardsiella tarda, E. hoshinae

[a] Heterogeneous appearance with cocarde growth.
[b] Strains generally show a small inhibition zone diameter (10-12 mm).
[c] Species with high *in vitro* susceptibility to antibiotics, including penicillin G.

cholerae serotype O:1, the *El tor* biotype but not the classic biotype is resistant to polymyxin (50 IU). Among anaerobes, *Bacteroides* of the *fragilis* group, *Porphyromonas* and *Gardnerella vaginalis* are resistant (Table 10). Most Gram-positive bacteria including mycobacteria are intrinsically resistant, although certain *Bacillus* and *Staphylococcus* strains (other than *S. aureus* and *S. epidermidis*) have marginal susceptibility to polymyxins.

Resistance mechanisms

Natural resistance appears to be due to an outer membrane architecture which prevents polymyxin from interacting with the target phosphate groups on LPS in the lipid A region (e.g., *P. mirabilis*). As far as acquired resistance is concerned, the emergence of mutants during treatment is very rare and no resistance plasmids have been described (14). Due to the high molecular weight of polymyxins, membrane impermeability or active efflux phenomena probably do not exist. On the other hand, there is complete cross-resistance between colistin and polymyxin B. In *P. aeruginosa*, two types of resistance have been described: low-level resistance resulting from mutation or from culture in magnesium-depleted medium, and high-level (but unstable) resistance due to adaptation in the presence of antibiotic (17). At the molecular level, low-level resistance is related to overproduction of the basic H1 protein (or OprH porin) involving the two-component system PhoP-PhoQ. This protein replaces the Mg^{2+} ions at LPS sites, thereby inhibiting binding of the antibiotic. This mechanism also induces resistance to aminoglycosides and EDTA (17). Adaptive resistance is thought to result from the activation of another two-component system, PmrA-PmrB, involved in chemically modifying LPS as described in *S.* Typhimurium. In this enterobacterial species, PmrA-PmrB, which is activated directly or through the PhoP-PhoQ system, upregulates the loci involved in modifying LPS *via* addition of 4-amino-4-deoxy-L-arabinose (*pagA*, *ugd*, and *pbgP* genes) or phosphoethanolamine (*pmrC* gene) to lipid A phosphates and the LPS core. These structural changes reduce the negative charges on LPS, decreasing polymyxin affinity and binding to the outer membrane (13).

Table 9. Colistin susceptibility of non-fermentative Gram-negative bacilli as an indicator for bacterial identification

Species (no. of strains)	Susceptible[a]
Achromobacter (Alcaligenes) xylosoxidans subsp. *denitrificans* (14)	100
Achromobacter (Alcaligenes) xylosoxidans subsp. *xylosoxidans* (29)	69
Achromobacter (Alcaligenes) piechaudii (14)	86
Acinetobacter calcoaceticus / baumannii (221)[b]	98
Alcaligenes faecalis (21)	100
Bergeyella zoohelcum (3)[c]	0
Bordetella bronchiseptica (14)	100
Bordetella hinzii (5)	100
Brevundimonas diminuta (25)	0
Brevundimonas vesicularis (10)	0
Burkholderia cepacia (23)	0
Burkholderia pseudomallei (3)	0
Chryseobacterium indologenes (24)[c]	0
Chryseobacterium meningosepticum (16)[c]	0
Comamonas terrigena (34)	100
Comamonas testoroni (15)	100
Delftia (Comamonas) acidovorans (28)	0[d]
Empedobacter brevis (2)[c]	0
Myroides odoratus / odoratimimus (12)	0
Ochrobactrum anthropi / intermedium (31)	93
Pseudomonas (Chryseomonas) luteola (10)[b]	100
Pseudomonas (Flavimonas) oryzihabitans (17)[b]	100
Pseudomonas aeruginosa (35)	100
Pseudomonas fluorescens (21)	100
Pseudomonas putida (20)	100
Pseudomonas stutzeri (27)	100
Pseudomonas mendocina (3)	100
Pseudomonas alcaligenes / pseudoalcaligenes (17)	100
Ralstonia pickettii (22)	0
Ralstonia mannitolytica (4)	0
Ralstonia paucula (9)	100
Ralstonia gilardii (5)	100
Rhizobium (Agrobacterium) radiobacter (19)	53
Shewanella putrefaciens (6)	100
Sphingobacterium multivorum (10)	0
Sphingomonas paucimobilis (16)	19
Stenotrophomonas maltophilia (31)[b]	38
Weeksella virosa (13)[c]	100

[a] Percentage of strains with inhibition zone diameter > 6 mm (10-μg colistin disk on Muller-Hinton medium).
[b] Species with a negative oxidase reaction.
[c] Indole-producing species (formerly *Flavobacterium*).
[d] Typical ring-like resistance aspect.

Table 10. Identification of the main anaerobic Gram-negative bacilli with the aid of five indicators including colistin susceptibility

Species		Indicator[a]				
		Bile (20%)	BG (100 mg)	CS (10 µg)	K (1 mg)	VA (5 µg)
Common	*Bacteroides* group *fragilis*	R	S	R	R	R
	Bacteroides spp.	V	S	V	R	R
	Prevotella spp.	S	S	V	R	R
	Porphyromonas spp.	S	S	R	R	S
	Fusobacterium spp.	V	R	S	S	R
Rare	*Bilophila wadsworthia*	R	-	S	S	R
	Sutterella spp.	R	-	S	S	R
	Desulfovibrio spp.	V	-	R	S	R
	Dialister pneumosintes	S	-	R	S	R

[a] BG, susceptible to brilliant green; CS, colistin; K, kanamycin; R, resistant; S, susceptible to bile; VA, vancomycin; V, variable.

In vitro susceptibility testing

Polymyxin susceptibility testing in the laboratory should be carried out by determining MIC values either by agar dilution (reference method) or by microdilution (8). Indeed, there is an excellent correlation between these two methods. The E-test® also shows good agreement with the reference method. However, disk diffusion, though widely used, is not recommended because polymyxins diffuse poorly in agar medium and the inhibition zones are highly dependent on inoculum size. This has led to very major errors (false susceptibility) for colistin (5%) and polymyxin B (6%), especially with *S. maltophilia* and *Acinetobacter* spp. (8). It is therefore recommended that any strain with squatter colonies in the inhibition zone be classified as resistant. Thus, susceptibility should be checked by MIC determination when polymyxin is used to treat severe infections. It should be kept in mind that it is colistin sulfate which is used as a reagent in susceptibility testing, whereas colistimethate, which is 4-8 fold less active, is used therapeutically (14). The presence of serum reduces polymyxin activity by half, probably due to protein binding. There is also a need to harmonise the breakpoints for colistin, which vary according to country (12, 21):
- United States (CLSI): susceptible MIC ≤ 2 μg/ml; resistant MIC ≥ 4 μg/ml (*Acinetobacter* spp.) or ≥ 8 μg/ml (*P. aeruginosa*) (Table 3);
- Europe (EUCAST): susceptible MIC ≤ 2 μg/ml; resistant MIC > 2 μg/ml.

According to the CLSI guidelines, the colistin breakpoints are valid for polymyxin B and no recommendations exist for *Enterobacteriaceae*.

Combinations with other antibiotics

Synergy with rifampin has been described with respect to *P. aeruginosa*, *A. baumannii*, *S. maltophilia*, and *S. marcescens*. A lower degree of synergy has also been reported with cotrimoxazole. Colistin and ceftazidime have shown synergy on *P. aeruginosa* (leakage of periplasmic -lactamases due to polymyxin-induced membrane damage) whereas no synergy has been observed with ciprofloxacin (12).

Prevalence of resistance

The emergence of resistance under treatment is unusual and there is no cross-resistance with other antibiotic families. Recent studies indicate that the polymyxins continue to show activity against contemporary strains of *P. aeruginosa* and *A. baumannii* (resistance rates generally under 5%) (3). However, resistance rates appear to be higher for Gram-negative bacilli isolated from cystic fibrosis patients (14). As an example, in Germany, only 35% and 52% of *P. aeruginosa* strains were classified as susceptible out of 229 non-mucosal and 156 mucosal strains, respectively (according to German DIN committee criteria) (21). Finally, 90-95% of *K. pneumoniae* isolates are susceptible to polymyxins, although susceptibility rates are lower among multiresistant strains and particularly those that are carbapenemase-producers (12).

Aid to bacterial identification

Colistin is an excellent selective agent that can be added to different culture media to isolate certain bacteria including Gram-positive organisms, pathogenic *Neisseria*, *Legionella*, *Brucella*,

Campylobacter, or *H. pylori*. Colistin resistance is also a valuable indicator for the presumptive identification of certain enterobacterial species (Table 8) or non-fermentative Gram-negative bacilli (Table 9) (11). It is also one of the antibiotics to be tested, along with vancomycin and kanamycin, for rapid identification of Gram-negative anaerobes (Table 10).

REFERENCES

(1) **Besier, S., A. Ludwig, V. Brade, and T. A. Wichelhaus.** 2003. Molecular analysis of fusidic acid resistance in *Staphylococcus aureus*. Mol. Microbiol. **47**:463-469.

(2) **Bolton, L. F., L. C. Kelley, M. D. Lee, P. J. Fedorka-Cray, and J. J. Maurer.** 1999. Detection of multidrug-resistant *Salmonella enterica* serotype typhimurium DT104 based on a gene which confers cross-resistance to florfenicol and chloramphenicol. J. Clin. Microbiol. **37**:1348-1351.

(3) **Catchpole, C. R., J. M. Andrews, N. Brenwald, and R. Wise.** 1997. A reassessment of the *in-vitro* activity of colistin sulphomethate sodium. J. Antimicrob. Chemother. **39**:255-260.

(4) **Collignon, P., and J. Turnidge.** 1999. Fusidic acid *in vitro* activity. Int. J. Antimicrob. Agents **12 Suppl 2**:S45-S58.

(5) **Dobie, D., and J. Gray.** 2004. Fusidic acid resistance in *Staphylococcus aureus*. Arch. Dis. Child. **89**:74-77.

(6) **Falagas, M. E., K. P. Giannopoulou, G. N. Kokolakis, and P. I. Rafailidis.** 2008. Fosfomycin: use beyond urinary tract and gastrointestinal infections. Clin. Infect. Dis. **46**:1069-1077.

(7) **Fuchs, P. C., A. L. Barry, and S. D. Brown.** 1999. Fosfomycin tromethamine susceptibility of outpatient urine isolates of *Escherichia coli* and *Enterococcus faecalis* from ten North American medical centres by three methods. J. Antimicrob. Chemother. **43**:137-140.

(8) **Gales, A. C., A. O. Reis, and R. N. Jones.** 2001. Contemporary assessment of antimicrobial susceptibility testing methods for polymyxin B and colistin: review of available interpretative criteria and quality control guidelines. J. Clin. Microbiol. **39**:183-190.

(9) **Howden, B. P., and M. L. Grayson.** 2006. Dumb and dumber – the potential waste of a useful antistaphylococcal agent: emerging fusidic acid resistance in *Staphylococcus aureus*. Clin. Infect. Dis. **42**:394-400.

(10) **Kahlmeter, G.** 2003. Prevalence and antimicrobial susceptibility of pathogens in uncomplicated cystitis in Europe. The ECO.SENS study. Int. J. Antimicrob. Agents **22 Suppl 2**:49-52.

(11) **Laffineur, K., M. Janssens, J. Charlier, V. Avesani, G. Wauters, and M. Delmee.** 2002. Biochemical and susceptibility tests useful for identification of non-fermentative gram-negative rods. J. Clin. Microbiol. **40**:1085-1087.

(12) **Landman, D., C. Georgescu, D. A. Martin, J. Quale.** Polymyxins revisited. Clin. Microbiol. Rev. **21**:449-465.

(13) **Lee, H., F. F. Hsu, J. Turk, and E. A. Groisman.** 2004. The PmrA-regulated pmrC gene mediates phosphoethanolamine modification of lipid A and polymyxin resistance in *Salmonella enterica*. J. Bacteriol. **186**:4124-4133.

(14) **Li, J., R. L. Nation, R. W. Milne, J. D. Turnidge, and K. Coulthard.** 2005. Evaluation of colistin as an agent against multi-resistant Gram-negative bacteria. Int. J. Antimicrob. Agents **25**:11-25.

(15) **Marchese, A., L. Gualco, E. A. Debbia, G. C. Schito, and A. M. Schito.** 2003. In vitro activity of fosfomycin against gram-negative urinary pathogens and the biological cost of fosfomycin resistance. Int. J. Antimicrob. Agents **22 Suppl 2**:53-59.

(16) **McCoy, A. J., R. C. Sandlin, and A. T. Maurelli.** 2003. In vitro and in vivo functional activity of *Chlamydia* MurA, a UDP-N-acetylglucosamine enolpyruvyl transferase involved in peptidoglycan synthesis and fosfomycin resistance. J. Bacteriol. **185**:1218-1228.

(17) **Moore, R. A., L. Chan, and R. E. Hancock.** 1984. Evidence for two distinct mechanisms of resistance to polymyxin B in *Pseudomonas aeruginosa*. Antimicrob. Agents Chemother. **26**:539-545.

(18) **Nilsson, A. I., O. G. Berg, O. Aspevall, G. Kahlmeter, and D. I. Andersson.** 2003. Biological costs and mechanisms of fosfomycin resistance in *Escherichia coli*. Antimicrob. Agents Chemother. **47**:2850-2858.

(19) **O'Neill, A. J., F. McLaws, G. Kahlmeter, A. S. Henriksen, and I. Chopra.** 2007. Genetic basis of resistance to fusidic acid in staphylococci. Antimicrob. Agents Chemother. **51**:1737-1740.

(20) **Patel, S. S., J. A. Balfour, and H. M. Bryson.** 1997. Fosfomycin tromethamine. A review of its antibacterial activity, pharmacokinetic properties and therapeutic efficacy as a single-dose oral treatment for acute uncomplicated lower urinary tract infections. Drugs **53**:637-656.

(21) **Schulin, T.** 2002. *In vitro* activity of the aerosolized agents colistin and tobramycin and five intravenous agents against *Pseudomonas aeruginosa* isolated from cystic fibrosis patients in southwestern Germany. J. Antimicrob. Chemother. **49**:403-406.

(22) **Schwarz, S., C. Kehrenberg, B. Doublet, and A. Cloeckaert.** 2004. Molecular basis of bacterial resistance to chloramphenicol and florfenicol. FEMS Microbiol. Rev. **28**:519-542.

(23) **Shah, M., and M. Mohanraj.** 2003. High levels of fusidic acid-resistant *Staphylococcus aureus* in dermatology patients. Br. J. Dermatol. **148**:1018-20.

(24) **Shalit, I., and M. I. Marks.** 1984. Chloramphenicol in the 1980s. Drugs **28**:281-291.

(25) **Shultz, T. R., J. W. Tapsall, P. A. White, C. S. Ryan, D. Lyras, J. I. Rood, E. Binotto, and C. J. Richardson.** 2003. Chloramphenicol-resistant *Neisseria meningitidis* containing catP isolated in Australia. J. Antimicrob. Chemother. **52**:856-859.

(26) **Suarez, J. E., and M. C. Mendoza.** 1991. Plasmid-encoded fosfomycin resistance. Antimicrob. Agents Chemother. **35**:791-795.

(27) **Turnidge, J., and P. Collignon.** 1999. Resistance to fusidic acid. Int. J. Antimicrob. Agents **12 Suppl 2**:S35-S44.

(28) **Tveten, Y., A. Jenkins, and B. E. Kristiansen.** 2002. A fusidic acid-resistant clone of *Staphylococcus aureus* associated with *impetigo bullosa* is spreading in Norway. J. Antimicrob. Chemother. **50**:873-876.

(29) **Wareham, D. W., and P. Wilson.** 2002. Chloramphenicol in the 21st century. Hosp. Med. **63**:157-161.

Chapter 28. *LISTERIA MONOCYTOGENES*

Olivier F. JOIN-LAMBERT and Samer KAYAL

INTRODUCTION

Listeria monocytogenes is a non-spore-forming facultative anaerobic Gram-positive rod. This saprophytic bacterium is widespread in the environment and has been isolated from soil, decaying vegetable matter, water, animal and human faeces. It is estimated that 10-30% of sheep, cattle and goat naturally harbor *L. monocytogenes* in the digestive tract. Infections can be sporadic (more than 90% of clinical isolates) or occur during epidemic outbreaks (11). Both, in humans and animals, *L. monocytogenes* is able to cause systemic infections and shows a particular propensity to reach the central nervous system and the placenta. The ability of *L. monocytogenes* to survive in the host and to disseminate is due to many virulence factors that allow the bacterium to invade and survive within the cytoplasm of various cell types including enterocytes, hepatocytes and mononuclear phagocytes.

Human listeriosis is a rare disease since approximately 2,500 and 250 cases are reported yearly in the US and in France respectively. However, except for pregnant women, the mortality rate of systemic listeriosis is high, ranging from 20 to 30%. At the age of antibiotics, this high mortality rate is probably due to the fact that 60 to 80% of CNS infections occur in debilitated patients including cirrhosis, hemodialysis or kidney transplantation, solid organ or hematopoietic malignancies, patients under immunosuppressive treatments, HIV infection, and in the elderly. However, 20-40% of systemic listeriosis occur in patients without noteworthy debilitating conditions (11).

L. monocytogenes is predictable susceptible to penicillin and ampicillin and to synergy between these penicillins and gentamicin while it is intrinsically resistant to cephalosporin. Resistance to other antibiotics is still rare in *L. monocytogenes* isolates responsible for human disease but its prevalence is higher in strains of animal origin, highlighting the need to remain vigilant with respect to the emergence of resistance in clinical isolates.

Listeria monocytogenes is the only human pathogen of the genus Listeria. Six other species have been described including *L. innocua*, *L. ivanovii*, *L. seeligeri*, *L. welshimeri*, *L. grayi* and *L. murrayi*. Although *L. ivanovii* is pathogenic to animals, this species has been rarely found associated with human infections.

METHOD

CLSI document M45 provides recommendations for testing *L. monocytogenes* limited to determination of MICs by broth microdilution. The medium that should be used is cation-adjusted Mueller-Hinton broth supplemented with 2.5%-5% lysed horse blood. However, breakpoints used for determination of clinical categories are derived from general breakpoints used for common species. Although there is no specific recommendation for agar diffusion, antibiotic susceptibility testing *in vitro* may be carried out by the agar diffusion method using plain or 5% blood-supplemented Mueller-Hinton medium. The inoculum suspension is adjusted to a 0.5 McFarland standard in saline (0.9% NaCl). Agar plates should be incubated in ambient air for 18h at 37°C.

The following antibiotics should be tested:
- penicillin G, amoxicillin or ampicillin
- gentamicin
- tetracycline
- erythromycin
- chloramphenicol
- trimethoprim and sulfonamide
- rifampin
- vancomycin (and teicoplanin in countries where it is used).

Microbial identification can be facilitated by testing the following antibiotics that are inactive against *L. monocytogenes*:
- ceftriaxone (or cefotaxime)
- aztreonam
- clindamycin
- nalidixic acid
- fosfomycin.

INTRINSIC ANTIBIOTIC SUSCEPTIBILITY AND RESISTANCE

L. monocytogenes is intrinsically susceptible to a broad range of antibiotics active against Gram-positive bacteria (Table 1). Identification of *Listeria* can be facilitated by their intrinsic resistance phenotype comprising extended spectrum cephalosporins, mecillinam, aztreonam, fosfomycin and clindamycin. In contrast to *L. monocytogenes* and *L. innocua*, *L. ivanovii* is susceptible to fosfomycin (18). *L. grayi* is intrinsically resistant to trimethoprim.

Cephalosporins are inactive against *L. monocytogenes*, mainly due to their low affinity for penicillin binding protein 3 (PBP3), a PBP that is a transpeptidase essential for peptidoglycan biosynthesis. As opposed to cephalosporins, penicillin G and moreover, ampicillin and amoxicillin, show a high affinity for PBP3. Cephalosporin resistance in *L. monocytogenes* may also be due to an efflux system encoded by the *mdrL* gene that shows a high degree of similarity with multidrug efflux transporters of the major facilitator superfamily (13).

L. monocytogenes is intrinsically resistant to the older fluoroquinolones like nalidixic acid, which is used in some selective media. D-ofloxacin is inactive against *L. monocytogenes* whereas the *L*-isomer, levofloxacin, has moderate activity. Ciprofloxacin has variable activity and the newer fluoroquinolones, moxifloxacin, gatifloxacin, and clinafloxacin are active and display bactericidal activity *in vitro*. Chloramphenicol and clindamycin have low activity against *L. monocytogenes* (8).

BACTERICIDAL ACTIVITY OF ANTIBIOTICS

The majority of antibiotics that are active against Gram-positive organisms are also effective against *L. monocytogenes*. However, very few of them show a bactericidal activity (Table 1). Particularly, penicillins are only bacteriostatic against most clinical isolates, with minimum bactericidal concentrations (MBCs) far higher than their minimum inhibitory concentrations (MICs). *L. monocytogenes* is thus naturally tolerant to penicillins and imipenem.

Only the aminoglycosides are rapidly bactericidal, usually within 2 hours. Trimethoprim/sulfamethoxazole and glycopeptides act more slowly, with a bactericidal effect at 6-24 h (3). Although the new fluoroquinolones moxifloxacin, and gatifloxacin are active, no clinical data are currently available to recommend their use in the treatment of listeriosis.

As a general rule, antibiotics considered to be bacteriostatic such as macrolides, tetracyclines, and chloramphenicol are also bacteriostatic for *L. monocytogenes* (8). Telithromycin and linezolid are only bacteriostatic (10,17). The MIC_{90} of tigecycline is higher than that of tertracycline and similar to that of tetracycline and equivalent to that of minocycline and doxycycline (4).

ANTIBIOTIC COMBINATIONS

The combination of penicillin G, ampicillin, amoxicillin or imipenem with gentamicin is synergistic and shows a rapid bactericidal effect (8, 14). *In vitro*, ampicillin/rifampin combination has only an additive or agonist effect, while ampicillin/erythromycin and ampicillin/chloramphenicol are antagonistic.

ACQUIRED RESISTANCE

Incidence

The incidence of acquired antibiotic resistance among *L. monocytogenes* clinical isolates is still very low – less than 1% - and appears to be stable in comparison to the years 1970-1980. Out of 400 clinical strains of *L. monocytogenes* isolated in France between 2002 and 2003, three were resistant to tetracycline-minocycline and two of these were also resistant to trimethoprim. Three strains had high-level fluoroquinolone resistance (ciprofloxacin MIC $\geq$ 32 µg/ml).

Antimicrobial resistance appears to be more frequent in animal or environmental isolates probably as a result of the widespread use of antibiotics in veterinary medecine and of a poor controlled indications. Acquired resistance appears to have some species-specificity. In a study of 1,000 *Listeria* strains isolated from retail foods, acquired resistance to at least one antibiotic was found in 0.6% of *L. monocytogenes* versus 19.5% of *L. innocua* isolates. On the other hand, no resistance was detected in *L. seeligeri* or *L. welshimeri* (21). The reasons for these differences are not known. Studies have shown that genetic elements harboring resistance genes could be transferred between different *Listeria* species *in vitro*, suggesting that such phenomena may also take place *in vivo* (5). These data suggest that acquired resis-

Table 1. Susceptibility of *L. monocytogenes* to antibiotics[a]

Antibiotic	MIC (µg/ml)	Clinical Category[b] (EUCAST)	Bactericidal activity
β-lactams			
Penicillin G	0.06 - 2	S	weak
Ampicillin-Amoxicillin	0.06 - 2	S	weak
Azlocillin	0.5 - 2	ND[c]	weak
Cefalotin	0.25 - 16	ND	No
Cefotaxime	4 - ≥ 128	R	No
Cefepime	4 - > 64	R	No
Imipenem	0.03 - 0.25	S	weak
Meropenem	0.03 - 0.25	S	weak
Aminoglycosides			
Gentamicin	0.06 - 4	S	Yes
Sisomicin	0.01 - 0.12	ND	Yes
Netilmicin	0.06 - 32	S	Yes
Amikacin	< 0.06 - 32	S	Yes
Kanamycin	0.5 - 2	ND	Yes
Streptomycin	0.5 - 4	ND	Yes
Quinolones			
Nalidixic acid	> 128	R	No
Ofloxacin	> 64	R	No
Levofloxacin	1 - 4	I	No
Ciprofloxacin	0.5 - 2	I	No
Moxifloxacin	0.12 - 1	S	Yes
Gatifloxacin	0.25 - 1	ND	ND
Clinafloxacin	0.03 - 0.125	ND	Yes
Macrolides, lincosamides, and streptogramins			
Erythromycin	0.06 - 1	ND	No
Clarithromycin	0.06 - 0.125	ND	No
Azithromycin	0.125 - 2	ND	No
Telithromycin	0.06 - 1	ND	No
Clindamycin	0.25 - 4	ND	No
Quinupristin-dalfopristin	0.4 - 1.6	ND	No
Oxazolidinone			
Linezolid	0.38 - 2	S	No
Tetracyclines			
Tetracycline	0.12 - 4	S	No
Doxycycline	0.06 - 0.125	S	No
Tigecycline	0.25 - 0.5	S	No
Glycopeptides			
Vancomycin	0.12 - 2	S	Yes
Teicoplanin	0.12 - 0.5	S	Yes
Others			
Co-trimoxazole	0.03 - 0.6	S	Yes
Rifampin	0.04 - 0.25	S	No
Chloramphenicol	2 - 8	I	No
Fosfomycin	4 - 2048	R	No

[a] From references 4, 8, 9, 17.
[b] I, intermediate; R, resistant; S, susceptible.
[c] ND, not determined (no available breakpoint).

Table 2. Molecular basis of antibiotic resistance in *L. monocytogenes*[a]

Resistance	Gene	Localisation
Tetracycline + minocycline	*tet*(M)	Transposon
	tet(S)	Plasmid
Tetracycline	*tet*(L)	Plasmid
Erythromycin	*erm*(C)	Not plasmidic tranferable
	erm(B)	Plasmid
Chloramphenicol	*cat221/cat223*	Plasmid
	cat221	Plasmid
Streptomycin	*aad6*	Plasmid
Trimethoprim	*dfr*D	Plasmid
Fluoroquinolones	*lde*	Chromosome

[a] From references 5-7, 15.

tance may emerge in clinical isolates of *L. monocytogenes*.

Antimicrobial resistance

Although antimicrobial resistance in *L. monocytogenes* is not yet a significant issue in clinical practice, the emergence of resistance in *L. monocytogenes* is a real concern. Since the first multiresistante strain was isolated in 1988 (15), there have been many published reports showing that strains resistant to one or more antibiotics have been isolated from human or animal samples and their molecular mechanisms of resistance have been elucidated (Table 2). A growing number of antibiotic classes are concerned, mainly the tetracyclines and macrolides but also the quinolones, aminoglycosides, and trimethoprim. Antimicrobial resistance to antibiotics commonly used to treat listeriosis in humans may therefore emerge in the next future.

β-lactams

Resistance to penicillins, the major class of antibiotics used to treat listeriosis has not been reported (ampicillin MICs range : 0.06-2 µg/ml).

Aminoglycosides

Aminoglycoside resistance in human isolates has been described mainly for streptomycin (5). Two resistance mechanisms have been demonstrated: enzymatic inactivation (high level resistance, MIC=512µg/ml) or ribosomal mutation (low level resistance, MIC:32-64 µg/ml) when no enzymatic activity is detected (5). A clinical isolate with multidrug resistance to streptomycin (MIC > 1000 µg/ml), gentamicin (MIC ≥ 8 µg/ml) and tobramycin (MIC = 8 µg/ml) has been reported in Greece (1).

Trimethoprim

A *L. monocytogenes* isolate with high level resistance to trimethoprim has been studied. This strain harboured a dihydrofolate reductase gene (dfrD), that was identical to that of *Staphylococcus haemolyticus* MUR313, suggesting that horizontal gene transfer has occurred (5). This strain was susceptible to sulfamethoxazole, but trimethoprim resistance abolished the synergy normally observed between these two antimicrobial agents. Dissemination of trimethoprim resistance in *L. monocytogenes* could have a significant clinical impact since trimethoprim/sulfamethoxazole is one of the major alternatives to the reference treatment (β-lactam + aminoglycoside). In the Microbiology Laboratory, the importance of detecting resistance to both compounds of the trimethoprim /sulfamethoxazole combination calls for separate testing of each component, and strains showing acquired resistance to trimethoprim should be categorized as intermediate susceptibility to trimethoprim /sulfamethoxazole.

Glycopeptides

Glycopeptide resistance has not yet been observed although an *in vitro* study showed that *vanA* genes could be transferred from enterococci to *L. monocytogenes* but also from enterococci not only to *L. monocytogenes*, but also to *L. innocua* and *L. seeligeri* (2).

Fluoroquinolones

A recent French study of 488 clinical isolates reported five strains resistant to ciprofloxacin (MIC 6-16 µg/ml). Resistance was due to an efflux system encoded by the *lde* gene (Listeria drug efflux) (6). The transmembrane protein Lde is a member of the Major Facilitator Superfamily (MFS) of proton-motive pumps. Lde shares 44% similarity with the Pmra efflux system of *Streptococcus pneumoniae*, and has little activity on moxifloxacin.

Tetracyclines

Acquired resistance in clinical isolates mainly concerns the tetracyclines. Tetracycline was the most frequent resistance trait (7.3%) in a study of 41 strains isolated from the brains of sheep with *L. monocytogenes* meningoencephalitis between 1992 and 1996 (19).

The first tetracycline-resistant human isolate was described in 1988 (14). This was a strain with multidrug resistance to tetracycline and minocycline but also erythromycin, streptomycin, and chloramphenicol. All these determinants were harbored on a plasmid structurally analogous to a broad host range resistance plasmid found in *Enterococcus*. Several lines of experimental evidence suggest that this plasmid was acquired *in vivo* through conjugative transfer from enterococci (5).

Two tetracycline resistance mechanisms have been described in *L. monocytogenes*: efflux [*tet*(L) gene] and ribosomal protection [*tet*(M) and *tet*(S) genes]. These genes can be carried on different mobile genetic elements such as conjugative plasmids or transposons (5).

Macrolides

Acquired resistance to macrolides has been observed *in vivo* and is due to acquisition of the *erm*(B) or *erm*(C) genes encoding a ribosomal RNA methylase (5).

Rifampin

Rifampin resistance is rare: only one such human isolate has been reported, in 2000.

CONCLUSION

L. monocytogenes is a facultative intracellular bacterium which can cause serious illness due to its predilection for the central nervous system and placenta. It is intrinsically resistant to third generation cephalosporins, clindamycin and fosfomycin. Most clinical isolates are susceptible to the main antibiotics active against this pathogen, but the gradual emergence of resistance calls for close surveillance by microbiologists in order to prevent treatment failures.

REFERENCES

(1) **Abrahim, A., A. Papa, N. Soultos, I. Ambrosiadis, and A. Antoniadis.** 1998. Antibiotic resistance of *Salmonella spp.* and *Listeria spp.* isolates from traditionally made fresh sausages in Greece. J. Food. Prot. **61:**1378-1380.

(2) **Biavasco, F., E. Giovanetti, A. Miele, C. Vignaroli, B. Facinelli, and P. E. Varaldo.** 1996. In vitro conjugative transfer of VanA vancomycin resistance between Enterococci and Listeriae of different species. Eur. J. Clin. Microbiol. Infect. Dis. **15:**50-59.

(3) **Boisivon, A., C. Guiomar, and C. Carbon.** 1990. In vitro bactericidal activity of amoxicillin, gentamicin, rifampicin, ciprofloxacin and trimethoprim-sulfamethoxazole alone or in combination against *Listeria monocytogenes*. Eur. J. Clin. Microbiol. Infect. Dis. **9:**206-209.

(4) **Boucher, H. W., C. B. Wennersten, and G. M. Eliopoulos.** 2000. In vitro activities of the glycylcycline GAR-936 against gram-positive bacteria. Antimicrob. Agents Chemother. **44:**2225-2229.

(5) **Charpentier, E., and P. Courvalin.** 1999. Antibiotic resistance in *Listeria spp.* Antimicrob. Agents Chemother. **43:**2103-2108.

(6) **Godreuil, S., M. Galimand, G. Gerbaud, C. Jacquet, and P. Courvalin.** 2003. Efflux pump Lde is associated with fluoroquinolone resistance in *Listeria monocytogenes*. Antimicrob. Agents Chemother. **47:**704-708.

(7) **Hadorn, K., H. Hachler, A. Schaffner, and F. H. Kayser.** 1993. Genetic characterization of plasmid-encoded multiple antibiotic resistance in a strain of *Listeria monocytogenes* causing endocarditis. Eur. J. Clin. Microbiol. Infect. Dis. **12:**928-937.

(8) **Hof, H.** 1991. Therapeutic activities of antibiotics in listeriosis. Infection **19 Suppl 4:**S229-233.

(9) **Hoogkamp-Korstanje, J. A., and J. Roelofs-Willemse.** 2000. Comparative in vitro activity of moxifloxacin against Gram-positive clinical isolates. J. Antimicrob. Chemother. **45:**31-39.

(10) **Jones, R. N., D. J. Biedenbach, and T. R. Anderegg.** 2002. In vitro evaluation of AZD2563, a new oxazolidinone, tested against unusual gram-positive species. Diagn. Microbiol. Infect. Dis. **42:**119-122.

(11) **Lorber, B.** 1997. Listeriosis. Clin. Infect. Dis. **24:**1-9; quiz 10-1.

(12) **Martinez-Martinez, L., M. C. Ortega, and A. I. Suarez.** 1995. Comparison of E-test with broth microdilution and disk diffusion for susceptibility testing of coryneform bacteria. J. Clin. Microbiol. **33:**1318-1321.

(13) **Mata, M. T., F. Baquero, and J. C. Perez-Diaz.** 2000. A multidrug efflux transporter in *Listeria monocytogenes*. FEMS Microbiol. Lett. **187:**185-188.

(14) **Moellering, R. C., Jr., G. Medoff, I. Leech, C. Wennersten, and L. J. Kunz.** 1972. Antibiotic synergism against *Listeria monocytogenes*. Antimicrob. Agents Chemother. **1**:30-34.

(15) **Poyart-Salmeron, C., C. Carlier, P. Trieu-Cuot, A. L. Courtieu, and P. Courvalin.** 1990. Transferable plasmid-mediated antibiotic resistance in *Listeria monocytogenes*. Lancet **335**:1422-1426.

(16) **Poyart-Salmeron, C., P. Trieu-Cuot, C. Carlier, A. MacGowan, J. McLauchlin, and P. Courvalin.** 1992. Genetic basis of tetracycline resistance in clinical isolates of *Listeria monocytogenes*. Antimicrob. Agents Chemother. **36**:463-466.

(17) **Schulin, T., C. B. Wennersten, R. C. Moellering, Jr., and G. M. Eliopoulos.** 1998. In-vitro activity of the new ketolide antibiotic HMR 3647 against gram-positive bacteria. J. Antimicrob. Chemother. **42**:297-301.

(18) **Soriano, F., J. Zapardiel, and E. Nieto.** 1995. Antimicrobial susceptibilities of Corynebacterium species and other non-spore-forming gram-positive bacilli to 18 antimicrobial agents. Antimicrob. Agents Chemother. **39**:208-214.

(19) **Troxler, R., A. von Graevenitz, G. Funke, B. Wiedemann, and I. Stock.** 2000. Natural antibiotic susceptibility of Listeria species: L. *grayi, L. innocua, L. ivanovii, L. monocytogenes, L. seeligeri and L. welshimeri* strains. Clin. Microbiol. Infect. **6**:525-535.

(20) **Vela, A. I., J. F. Fernandez-Garayzabal, M. V. Latre, A. A. Rodriguez, L. Dominguez, and M. A. Moreno.** 2001. Antimicrobial susceptibility of *Listeria monocytogenes* isolated from meningoencephalitis in sheep. Int. J. Antimicrob. Agents **17**:215-220.

(21) **Vicente, M. F., J. C. Perez-Daz, F. Baquero, M. Angel de Pedro, and J. Berenguer.** 1990. Penicillin-binding protein 3 of *Listeria monocytogenes* as the primary lethal target for b-lactams. Antimicrob. Agents Chemother. **34**:539-542.

(22) **Walsh, D., G. Duffy, J. J. Sheridan, I. S. Blair, and D. A. McDowell.** 2001. Antibiotic resistance among Listeria, including *Listeria monocytogenes*, in retail foods. J. Appl. Microbiol. **90**:517-522.

Chapter 29. CORYNEBACTERIA

Philippe RIEGEL

INTRODUCTION

The corynebacteria comprise some highly pathogenic species like *Corynebacterium diphtheriae*, *Corynebacterium ulcerans,* and *Arcanobacterium haemolyticum* but the majority of these bacteria are part of normal human skin and mucosal flora. Some of these saprophytic species have the capacity to become resistant to antibiotics, causing opportunistic infections in frail patients. The molecular mechanisms of antibiotic resistance in corynebacteria are poorly understood and often do not allow determination of a particular resistance phenotype. *In vitro* susceptibility testing methods have not been extensively evaluated in corynebacteria. Moreover, the susceptible, intermediate and resistant breakpoints have not for the most part been validated by clinical studies demonstrating a correlation between *in vitro* susceptibility and clinical efficacy.

The *in vitro* activity of antibiotics against corynebacteria is only known for the species commonly encountered in clinical specimens. Some recently described species, or species defined from only a few strains, will not be discussed in this chapter.

METHODS

In 2005, the Clinical and Laboratory Standards Institute (CLSI) published guidelines for *in vitro* susceptibility testing of infrequently isolated or fastidious bacteria (17). For the corynebacteria, only the genus *Corynebacterium* is concerned. Minimal inhibitory concentrations (MICs) should be determined by the broth dilution method using Mueller-Hinton medium supplemented with 2.5-5% lysed horse blood. MIC breakpoints are given for the main antibiotics in each class, but no critical inhibition zone diameters are given for the diffusion method.

Most clinical bacteriology laboratories use the agar diffusion method with Mueller-Hinton agar containing 5% sheep blood for routine testing. There is a good correlation between the dilution method and disk diffusion or E-test® when the CLSI guidelines for *Listeria* or streptococci are used (1, 21, 41). However, there are more major discordances with the *Listeria* spp. guidelines than with those for streptococci. Erythromycin gives the most discordances.

Plates are incubated for 18-24 h at 35-37°C in an aerobic atmosphere. Standard techniques can be used for non-lipophilic species from the genus *Corynebacterium* (*C. diphtheriae*, *C. amycolatum*, *C. minutissimum*, *C. striatum*, *C. pseudodiphtheriticum*, *C. glucuronolyticum*, *C. ulcerans* to name the most common) and for species from the genera *Arthrobacter*, *Brevibacterium*, *Microbacterium*, *Cellulomonas*, *Rothia*, *Turicella*, and *Dermabacter*.

Lipophilic corynebacteria

These strains require lipids for growth and grow very slowly on blood agar. For optimal isolation of these strains, it is recommended to use media supplemented with 0.1-1% Tween 80 or to apply a droplet of Tween 80 on nutrient agar, in which case well-formed colonies develop around the point of application. Horse or rabbit serum (5%) can also be used to supply lipids. The diffusion method is difficult to read in the case of highly susceptible strains because the diffusion of the antibiotic is faster than the growth of the bacteria, so no growth can appear, even if the plate contains only a small number of disks. In such cases, an inoculum containing 1% Tween 80 can be used; three drops of this medium are spread on Mueller-Hinton agar supplemented with 5% sheep blood. Where appropriate, it is also possible to use agar containing 0.1% Tween 80, although the diffusion of the antibiotic may be altered in the presence of Tween. These difficulties are encountered for most *Corynebacterium* group G strains and for the species *C. tuberculostearicum*, *C. macginleyi*, *C. kroppenstedtii*, *C.* group F-1, and *C. accolens*. The diffusion antibiogram is easier to read in the case of resistant strains, particularly those of the species *C. jeikeium* and *C. urealyticum*.

SUSCEPTIBLE PHENOTYPES

Corynebacteria are generally susceptible to the main antibiotics. Some species including *C. urealyticum* and *C. jeikeium* exhibit a strong tendency to acquire a multiresistant phenotype under antibiotic pressure, explaining why they are sometimes described as intrinsically resistant.

All species are resistant to imidazoles and most are resistant to fosfomycin, with the exception of *Rothia dentocariosa* and *Dermabacter hominis*. Virtually all species are susceptible to glycopeptides.

β-lactams

The level of β-lactam susceptibility among corynebacteria is generally the same for all agents in this class with a few exceptions (Table 1). β-lactam susceptibility is usually evaluated by testing penicillin G and amoxicillin or ampicillin. MICs of ceftazidime, aztreonam and oxacillin are at least four dilutions higher than those of other β-lactams. Two groups of corynebacterial species can be distinguished according to their intrinsic β-lactam susceptibility and their ability to become resistant.

Group with intrinsic high-level susceptibility

The main species in this group are *Arcanobacterium* spp., *Rothia dentocariosa*, *Turicella otitidis*, *Arthrobacter cumminsii*, *C. pseudodiphtheriticum*, *C. glucuronolyticum* (*C. seminale*), *C. macginleyi*, *C. accolens,* and lipophilic strains from CDC groups G and F-1. The MIC_{50} of penicillin G is < 0.03 µg/ml and no strains belonging to known species have been found to be penicillin-resistant when streptococci criteria are used.

Group with moderate intrinsic susceptibility

For strains in this group, the penicillin G MIC is > 0.03 µg/ml and the MIC_{50} ranges from 0.25 to > 64 µg/ml according to species. Species with moderate *in vitro* susceptibility to penicillin G include *C. diphtheriae, C. afermentans, C. striatum, C. minutissimum, C. auris, C. aurimucosum,*

Table 1. MIC and MIC_{50} (µg/ml) of β-lactams for *Corynebacterium* spp. and related bacteria

Species	Penicillin G		Amoxicillin		Cefotaxime/ceftriaxone		Reference
	MIC	MIC_{50}	MIC	MIC_{50}	MIC	MIC_{50}	
C. diphtheriae	0.12-0.5	0.25	0.25 - 1	0.50	0.75 - 1.50	1	6
C. afermentans	ND[a]	ND	0.12 - 4	2	ND	ND	18
C. auris	0.5 - 2	1	1 - 4	2	4 - 16	8	11
C. macginleyi	≤ 0.01 - 0.125	0.03	≤ 0.06 - 0.25	0.06	≤ 0.06 - 0.25	0.125	9
C. aurimucosum	0.03 - 0.5	0.25	0.25 - 1	0.5	ND	ND	3
C. urealyticum	0.12 - > 64	> 64	0.03 - > 64	>64	0.5 - 128	128	13
C. jeikeium	0.1 - > 64	> 64	0.12 - > 64	>64	1 - 128	64	35
C. striatum	0.25 - 4	1	0.5 - 4	2	0.03 - 32	2	22
C. minutissimum	0.12 - 32	0.25	0.03 - 32	0.25	0.01 - 16	0.25	18.35
C. pseudodiphtheriticum	≤ 0.03	0.03	0.01 - 0.25	0.03	ND	ND	35
C. amycolatum	0.06 - >64	0.25	0.06 - > 64	4	0.125 - > 64	1	11
C. glucuronolyticum	≤ 0.03 - 0.2	0.06	< 0.03 - 0.2	0.06	≤ 0.03 - 4	0.25	11
Arcanobacterium haemolyticum	0.01 - 0.06	0.03	0.03 - 0.25	0.06	0.01-0.25	0.06	1.35
Turicella otitidis	≤ 0.06	< 0.06	< 0.06	< 0.06	≤ 0.03 - 0.25	≤ 0.125	11
Dermabacter hominis	0.06 - 4	0.25	≤ 0.03 - 4	0.5	≤ 0.03 - 8	≤ 0.5	11
Rothia dentocariosa	0.03 - 0.12	0.06	ND	0.05	ND	ND	4
Brevibacterium spp	1 - 4	1	4 - 16	8	0.5 - 32	4	11
Microbacterium spp	0.06 - 4	0.50	ND	ND	ND	ND	12.14
Leifsonia aquatica	1 - 16	8	ND	ND	ND	ND	12
Arthrobacter cumminsii	≤ 0.01 - 0.5	< 0.01	≤ 0.06 - 2	< 0.06	ND	ND	10

[a] ND, not determined.

C. resistens, *Arthrobacter woluwensis*, *Brevibacterium* spp., *Dermabacter hominis*, *Leifsonia aquatica*, *Microbacterium* spp. The species *C. jeikeium*, *C. urealyticum*, *C. amycolatum*, *C. resistens* and CDC group G strains are often highly penicillin resistant (MIC > 64 µg/ml). Resistance rates vary according to species and antibiotics received by the patients furnishing the specimens. Penicillin resistance is frequent in *C. jeikeium* and *C. urealyticum* and this can be exploited for selective media, particularly in the case of *C. urealyticum* urinary tract infections. However, the presence of susceptible strains must not be ruled out.

The bactericidal activity of these antibiotics has been evaluated in only a few species. *C. diphtheriae* is tolerant to penicillin G and the MBCs are often high (MBC/MIC ≥ 32 for 71% of 24 strains tested). Penicillin G tolerance has also been described for *Arcanobacterium haemolyticum*.

Aminoglycosides

Aminoglycoside MICs are usually low for species from the genus *Corynebacterium* (Table 2), but higher for other coryneform genera, except *Turicella otitidis* which has a very close phylogenetic relationship to the genus *Corynebacterium*. The genera exhibiting intrinsic aminoglycoside resistance are mostly environmental species which are rarely implicated in infection. There appears to be little difference in the activity of the aminoglycosides used therapeutically to treat corynebacterial infections. Gentamicin, neomycin, and kanamycin have similar activity against *C. diphtheriae*. *C. urealyticum* has the same intrinsic susceptibility to gentamicin, tobramycin, amikacin, and netilmicin, while neomycin appears less active (13). *C. striatum* and *C. macginleyi* were found to be susceptible to the different aminoglycosides tested (9, 22). Gentamicin, nétilmicine, and tobramycin have equivalent activity against *Turicella otitidis*, whereas amikacin, kanamycine, and streptomycin are less active. The principal aminoglycosides have similar activity against *Brevibacterium casei* and *Dermabacter hominis*.

Fluoroquinolones

The majority of species from the genus *Corynebacterium* as well as *Turicella otitidis* are intrinsically susceptible to ciprofloxacin which has an MIC < 0.12 µg/ml for the most susceptible strains (Table 2). Environmental corynebacteria (*Arthrobacter*, *Brevibacterium*, *Microbacterium*, *Leifsonia*) are less susceptible, as is *Dermabacter hominis*, a species frequently encountered in clinical specimens (ciprofloxacin MIC > 0.25 µg/ml). For susceptible strains, the activity of sparfloxacin, levofloxacin, trovafloxacin and gemifloxacin is similar to that of ciprofloxacin, while the MICs of norfloxacin, ofloxacin and pefloxacin are approximately two to three dilutions higher (8, 9, 13, 22). Fluoroquinolone resistance is common and mainly concerns the species *C. jeikeium* and *C. urealyticum*. Levofloxacin and moxifloxacin may remain active against strains which are resistant to ciprofloxacin due to a single *gyrA* mutation. Ciprofloxacin has good bactericidal activity against susceptible strains of *C. jeikeium*, with a MBC_{90} of 2 µg/ml and a MIC_{90} of 1 µg/ml. Ciprofloxacin and moxifloxacin are bactericidal against *C. urealyticum* but this activity is lower in the presence of a biofilm (33).

Rifampin

Corynebacteria are intrinsically susceptible to rifampin (MIC_{50} < 0.03 µg/ml for species of the genus *Corynebacterium* and 0.125 µg/ml for other genera) (Table 2). However, acquired resistance has been described in many species.

Macrolides and lincosamides

Most corynebacteria are intrinsically susceptible to erythromycin (MIC < 0.03 µg/ml for susceptible strains) (Table 3). High level resistance has been described in all species but at different frequencies. As compared to erythromycin, clarithromycin has similar activity but azithromycin MICs are an average of two dilutions higher. Azithromycin MIC50 values are generally low (< 0.06 µg/ml) but some species such as *Arthrobacter* spp. (MIC_{50} = 0.125 µg/ml), *C. diphtheriae* (0.044 µg/ml), *C. jeikeium* (> 128 µg/ml), *C. amycolatum* (> 128 µg/ml), *C. striatum* (> 64 µg/ml) and *C. glucuronolyticum* (128 µg/ml) are less susceptible (6, 25). Josamycin is less active against the majority of corynebacteria.

Clindamycin and lincomycin are slightly less active than erythromycin against most coryneform species (Table 3).

Telithromycin

The activity of telithromycin is at least equivalent to that of erythromycin against the species *C. urealyticum* (telithromycin MIC_{50} 0.25 to > 64 µg/ml according to the studies, *C. jeikeium* (0.12-

Table 2. MIC and MIC$_{50}$ (µg/ml) of antibiotics for *Corynebacterium* spp. and related bacteria

Species	Gentamicin		Ciprofloxacin		Rifampin		Reference
	MIC	MIC$_{50}$	MIC	MIC$_{50}$	MIC	MIC$_{50}$	
C. diphtheriae	≤ 0.12 - 0.50	0.18	0.12	0.12	≤ 0.06 - > 2	≤ 0.06	4
C. afermentans	0.06 - 1	0.12	0.12 - 8 (OFX)[a]	0.25	0.01	0.01	18
C. auris	≤ 0.03 - 1	0.125	≤ 0.03 - 0.25	0.06	≤ 0.03 - 0.06	≤ 0.03	11
C. macginleyi	≤ 0.06 - 0.50	0.125	0.06 - 0.125	0.06	≤ 0.01 - 0.125	0.03	5.9
C. aurimucosum	ND[b]	ND	≤ 0.12 (LEV)	< 0.12	ND	ND	3
C. urealyticum	0.25 - > 128	> 128	0.06 - >128	16	≤ 0.01 - > 128	≤ 0.01	13
C. jeikeium	0.06 - > 256	> 256	0.03 - 128	2	≤ 0.01 - > 256	≤ 0.01	35
C. striatum	≤ 0.06 - 128	1	≤ 0.015 - >16	4	≤ 0.06 - > 128	>128	22
C. minutissimum	0.01 - 2	0.06	0.12 - ≥ 32 (OFX)	0.25	0.01	0.01	18
C. pseudodiphtheriticum	0.03 - 1	0.06	≤ 0.015 - 0.5	0.25	≤ 0.03	≤ 0.03	35
C. amycolatum	0.06 - > 64	0,25	≤ 0.03 - >64	4	≤ 0.03 - > 64	≤ 0.03	11
C. glucuronolyticum	≤ 0.03 - 8	0.06	0.06 - 16	0.25	≤ 0.03	≤ 0.03	11
Arcanobacterium haemolyticum	0.06 - 1	0.5	0.125 - 0.5	0.25	≤ 0.01	≤ 0.01	35
Turicella otitidis	≤ 0.03	≤ 0.03	0.06 - 0.25	0.125	≤ 0.03	≤ 0.03	11
Dermabacter hominis	0.5 - 64	1	0.25 - 64	2	≤ 0.03 - 32	≤ 0.03	11
Rothia dentocariosa	ND	ND	ND	ND	ND	ND	
Brevibacterium spp	0.25 - 4	0.5	0.5 - 4	2	≤ 0.03	≤ 0.03	11
Microbacterium spp	2 - 64	16	0.5 - 32	2	≤ 0.03 - 32	1	12-14
Leifsonia aquatica	4 - 16	4	1 - 8	2	≤ 0.125 - 8	1	12
Arthrobacter cumminsii	2 - > 128	8	0.5 - >32	2	≤ 0.01	≤ 0.01	10
Arthrobacter woluwensis	32	32	16	16	32	32	8

[a] LEV, levofloxacin ; OFX, ofloxacin.
[b] ND, not determined.

1 µg/ml), *C. amycolatum* (0.12-0.25 µg/ml), *C. striatum* (≤ 0.03-16 µg/ml), *C. minutissimum* (≤ 0.015 - ≤ 0,030 µg/ml). *C. diphtheriae* is susceptible to telithromycin (MIC 0.002-0.12 µg/ml, MIC$_{50}$ 0.004 µg/ml) (6, 30, 34). The presence of a methylase confers high level resistance to macrolides and telithromycin. Like the macrolides, telithromycin is primarily bacteriostatic.

Streptogramins

The oral streptogramin (available only in certain countries), pristinamycin, is very active against the genus *Corynebacterium*. MIC$_{50}$ values are: *C. urealyticum* (≤ 1 µg/ml), *C. jeikeium* (≤ 1 µg/ml), *C. amycolatum* (0.25 µg/ml), *C. pseudodiphtheriticum* (0.06 µg/ml), *C. striatum* (0.38 µg/ml). MICs for *C. jeikeium* are higher (8 µg/ml) but are < 1 µg/ml for other species. Data for quinupristin-dalfopristin are similar. The latter molecule shows good activity against *Dermabacter hominis* and *Turicella otitidis* (MIC 0.03-1 µg/ml) but is less active against *Brevibacterium casei* (MIC 0.13-4 µg/ml). It only has bactericidal activity against *C. jeikeium*

Tetracyclines

Corynebacteria are intrinsically susceptible to tetracyclines. The MIC of oxytetracycline is < 1 µg/ml for susceptible strains (Table 3). Doxycycline is slightly more active than tetracycline: *C. urealyticum* (doxycycline MIC$_{50}$ = 0.25 µg/ml), *C. striatum* (0.125 µg/ml), *C. pseudodiphtheriticum* (≤ 0.06 µg/ml), *C. minutissimum* (0.25 µg/ml), *C. jeikeium* (0.125 µg/ml), *C. amycolatum* (≤ 0.06 µg/ml). *C. macginleyi* has comparable susceptibility to both drugs (MIC$_{50}$ = 0.5 and 0.25 µg/ml for tetracycline and doxycycline, respectively) (9). Nonetheless, resistance to these antibiotics is frequent. Tigecycline is more active than doxycycline against *Corynebacterium* spp. with

Table 3. MIC and MIC$_{50}$ (µg/ml) of antibiotics for *Corynebacterium* spp. and related bacteria

Species	Erythromycin		Clindamycin		Tetracycline		Reference
	MIC	MIC$_{50}$	MIC	MIC$_{50}$	MIC	MIC$_{50}$	
C. diphtheriae	0.016 - ≥ 4	0.015	0.125 - > 512	0.19	0.19 - ≥ 32	0.5	6.28
C. afermentans	1 - 32	16	32	32	0.12 - 1 (DOX)	0.25	18
C. auris	≤ 0.03 - > 64	0.5	≤ 0.06 - > 64	0.5	0.125 - 1	0.5	11
C. macginleyi	≤ 0.03 - > 64	0.06	0.006 - > 32	0.25	0.25 - 2	0.5	9
C. aurimucosum	0.03 - > 2	0.06	1 - > 2	2	0.25 - > 8	0.5	3
C. urealyticum	0.06 - > 128	> 128	0.06 - > 128	> 128	0.50 - > 128	64	13
C. jeikeium	0.030 - > 256	> 256	0.125 - > 256	> 256	0.50 - > 256	2	35
C. striatum	≤ 0.06 - > 128	4	1 - > 256	> 256	≤ 0.06 - > 64	16	22.35
C. minutissimum	0.030 - > 256	0.5	0.250 - > 256	4	0.125 - 64	4	35
C. pseudodiphtheriticum	≤ 0.015 - > 128	0.030	0.03 - > 256	0.125	1 - 2	1	35
C. amycolatum	≤ 0.03 - > 64	> 64	0.125 - > 64	> 64	0.25 - > 64	0.5	11
C. glucuronolyticum	≤ 0.03 - > 64	0.25	≤ 0.03 - > 64	2	0.5 - 64	32	11
Arcanobacterium haemolyticum	≤ 0.015 - > 256	0.03	0.03 - > 256	0.06	0.12 - 16	0.25	1.35
Turicella otitidis	≤ 0.03 - > 64	≤ 0.03	≤ 0.03 - > 64	0.125	≤ 0.03 - > 1	0.25	11
Dermabacter hominis	≤ 0.03 - > 64	1	≤ 0.03 - > 64	0.25	0.5 - 32	2	11
Rhodococcus equi	0.25 - 0.50	0.50	2 - 8	4	4 - 16	8	35
Rothia dentocariosa	ND[a]	0.050	ND	2	ND	0.06	4
Brevibacterium spp	0.125 - 16	2	0.06 - 8	4	0.125 - 1	0.5	11
Microbacterium spp	≤ 0.03 - >16	0.06	≤ 0.03 - > 8	0.06	0.13 - 2	0.25	12.14
Leifsonia aquatica	≤ 0.125	≤ 0.125	1 - 8	4	0.5 - 4	1	12
Arthrobacter cumminsii	≤ 0.03 - >1	≤ 0.03	0.03 - 1	0.125	1 - 64	1	10
Arthrobacter woluwensis	2	2	4	4	2	2	8

[a] ND, not determined.

MIC$_{50}$ values at least two dilutions lower (7). No strains have been described for which the MIC of tigecycline is above 2 µg/ml.

Chloramphenicol

Most corynebacteria are susceptible to chloramphenicol. MICs range from 0.5-2 µg/ml for the most highly susceptible strains (8, 9, 13, 20). *C. urealyticum* is the least susceptible species: MIC 16 -> 128 µg/ml, MIC$_{50}$ = 64 µg/ml (13). MICs for *Dermabacter hominis* range from 0.25-64 µg/ml.

Cotrimoxazole

Corynebacteria have low intrinsic susceptibility to this antibiotic. MICs are > 128 µg/ml for *C. urealyticum*, > 64 µg/ml for *C. amycolatum*, 8-64 µg/ml for *C. macginleyi*, and 0.015 -> 16 µg/ml for *C. striatum* (9, 13, 22). MICs are also high for the majority of *Dermabacter hominis* and *Turicella otitidis* strains.

Fusidic acid

Fusidic acid exhibits good activity against corynebacteria. *C. jeikeium* is the least susceptible species (MIC$_{50}$ ≥ 32 µg/ml). MICs for other species are lower: *C. amycolatum* (MIC$_{50}$ = 0.25 µg/ml), *C. striatum* (0.50 µg/ml), *C. minutissimum* (0.50 µg/ml), *C. urealyticum* (0.125 µg/ml), *C. pseudodiphtheriticum* (≤ 0.015 µg/ml) and *C. macginleyi* (0.03 µg/ml) (9, 18, 35). *Brevibacterium casei* has low susceptibility (MIC 4-32 µg/ml) whereas *Dermabacter hominis* and *Turicella otitidis* are susceptible (MIC 0.13-2 µg/ml).

Linezolid

MICs of linezolid for all strains of the species *C. amycolatum*, *C. jeikeium*, *C. pseudodiphtheriticum*, *C. striatum*, *C. minutissimum,* and *C. urealyticum* range from 0.125-2 µg/ml. Strains from the genera *Brevibacterium* and *Dermabacter* are also susceptible (≤ 2 µg/ml) (7, 15, 30).

Glycopeptides

With the exception of one *A. haemolyticum* strain and one *Oerskovia turbata* strain, the corynebacteria are consistently susceptible to vancomycin and teicoplanin. The first two strains show high-level resistance (vancomycin MIC = 1024 μg/ml; teicoplanin MIC = 32 and 64 μg/ml). MICs range from 0.125 to 1 μg/ml for the majority of corynebacteria, although vancomycin MICs of 4 μg/ml for strains of *Microbacterium* spp. and 8 μg/ml for strains of *Leifsonia aquatica* have been reported (12). Dalbavancin is as active as vancomycin with MICs of 0.015-1 μg/ml for strains in which the MICs range from 0.25-4 μg/ml for vancomycin and 0.02-8 μg/ml for daptomycin.

RESISTANCE MECHANISMS

β-lactams

High-level penicillin resistance (amoxicillin MIC > 128 μg/ml) concerns the species *C. urealyticum*, *C. jeikeium* and *C. amycolatum* and a minority of *C.* group G strains among which the species *C. resistens* was distinguished. Lower level resistance is seen in other species (MIC 32 μg/ml). The mechanism of β-lactam resistance in corynebacteria has not been widely studied. β-lactamases have only been found in strains from the genus *Brevibacterium* (25). It is generally thought that resistance is due to decreased permeability or affinity of the outer membrane for these antibiotics. Corynebacteria are less susceptible to molecules with a high molecular mass, such as certain cephalosporins, and cross-resistance to other antibiotics is often observed. Plasmids were only detected in 17 of 62 strains of *C. jeikeium* and there was no correlation with ampicillin susceptibility. On the other hand, resistance to penicillin G and cetrimide in strains of *C. jeikeium* appears to correlate with the existence of different genomic groups within this species (26). Porins allowing passage of hydrophilic molecules through the outer membrane have been detected in strains of *C. glutamicum*. Porin-deficient mutants obtained *in vitro* were found to have significantly decreased susceptibility to ampicillin, tetracycline, and aminoglycosides (2). The virtually constant oxacillin resistance among the corynebacteria might be explained in part by the presence of the PT10 plasmid harboring the *tet*AB gene which confers resistance to tetracycline and oxacillin.

Macrolides, lincosamides

Resistance of *C. diphtheriae* to these antibiotics is due to the presence of the plasmid pNG2 carrying the *erm*Cd gene, now included in the *erm*(X) class, which encodes a 23S rRNA methylase (31). The expression of MLS$_B$ resistance is inducible by erythromycin; the MICs of this antibiotic range from 32-256 μg/ml in the absence of induction and 500 μg/ml after induction. A plasmid *erm*Cx gene also encoding a methylase conferring MLS$_B$ resistance has been detected in a strain originally designated as *C. xerosis* but later identified as *C. striatum*. This plasmid, pTP10, harbors a transposon which also confers resistance to chloramphenicol. An *erm*Cj gene sharing > 93 % identity with other class X genes has been detected in the *C. jeikeium* chromosome (37). *C. jeikeium* strains displaying high-level resistance to macrolides, lincomycin and ketolides harbor this *erm*(X) class gene which is absent in susceptible strains. This resistance is inducible and all strains, regardless of their macrolide susceptibility, were highly resistant to ampicillin (29). The *mef* gene encoding an efflux system has been detected in a strain of *C. jeikeium* (19). The plasmid *Imr*B gene conferring resistance to lincosamides only (lincomycin MIC = 230 μg/ml) was detected in a *C. glutamicum* isolate and codes for a protein similar to those involved in efflux systems in other species (16). In a study of environmental corynebacteria, the *erm* gene was not detected in macrolide-resistant species (23). It therefore appears that strains harboring an integron carrying the methylase-encoding *erm*X gene display high-level resistance (inducible or constitutive) to macrolides and ketolides. In strains with variable resistance to 14- or 16-membered macrolides but susceptible to ketolides, other resistance mechanisms are involved (efflux, ribosomal mutations, other inactivating enzymes).

Tetracyclines

The plasmid pTP10 harboring two genes, *tet*(A) and *tet*(B), whose products are related to the ABC transporter superfamily, has been detected in a strain of *C. striatum*. These genes confer resistance to tetracycline and oxacillin, increasing the MIC by at least a factor of eight (38). The plasmids pAG1 and pTET3 present in *C. glutamicum* carry a gene encoding a protein related to those involved in transmembrane efflux of these drugs (36). Modification of a porin of *C. glutamicum* leads to resistance to several antibiotics including tetracycline.

Aminoglycosides

The plasmids pTET3 (*C. glutamicum*) and pTP10 (*C. striatum*) harbor aminoglycoside inactivating enzymes of the type 3'-phosphotransferase. The plasmid pTP10 also harbors a gene encoding an efflux protein (40). The *C. urealyticum* genome (39) contains an *aph*(3')Ia gene carried in a Tn *5715*-like transposon which confers kanamycin resistance. It also contains *strA-strB* genes carried in a Tn *5393*-like transposon which codes for a 3''-phosphotransferase and a 6-phosphotransferase conferring streptomycin resistance. The porin-deficient *C. glutamicum* mutant strain is resistant to aminoglycosides.

Fluoroquinolones

High-level fluoroquinolone resistance is due to a double mutation in the *gyrA* gene resulting in two amino acid substitutions. In *C. amycolatum* the substitutions are at positions 87 and 91 or 87 and 88, while in *C. striatum* only positions 87 and 91 are affected (32). For both species, a single mutation causes reduced susceptibility or resistance to ciprofloxacin and levofloxacin, but moxifloxacin remains very active *in vitro*. A study of fluoroquinolone-resistant *C. macginleyi* isolates revealed the presence of a double mutation at positions 83 and 87 conferring high-level resistance to all fluoroquinolones. A single substitution at position 83 was detected in a strain resistant to norfloxacin but susceptible to ciprofloxacin and levofloxacin (5).

Glycopeptides

A strain of *Arcanobacterium haemolyticum* and a strain of *Oerskovia turbata* highly resistant to vancomycin were found to harbor the *vanA* operon (24).

RESISTANCE PHENOTYPES

Some species display a typical resistance profile to the main antibiotics, but not all of the underlying mechanisms have been elucidated.

C. jeikeium, *C. urealyticum*, and *C. amycolatum*

Most clinical isolates of *C. urealyticum* and *C. jeikeium* are resistant to β-lactams, macrolides, fluoroquinolones, and aminoglycosides. This profile is not systematic and therefore it cannot be ascribed to a single mechanism or a single genetic support. No penicillinases or cephalosporinases have been detected in these species. Thus, there is no interpretative criterion for β-lactam resistance phenotypes, although cross-resistance to all β-lactams is often observed. No more than 20% of *C. jeikeium* and *C. urealyticum* clinical isolates are susceptible to penicillins, macrolides, and fluoroquinolones, whereas a higher percentage is susceptible to gentamicin, rifampin, and tetracyclines, although this varies widely in different studies. *C. urealyticum* often appears to be more macrolide susceptible than *C. jeikeium*. Most *C. jeikeium* and *C. urealyticum* strains are susceptible to pristinamycin.

β-lactam resistance in *C. amycolatum* varies widely in different studies. This species is quite difficult to identify and it may be misidentified as *C. xerosis*, *C. striatum*, or *C. minutissimum*. Resistance is present in 20-90% of clinical isolates but largely depends on the source of the strain and the breakpoints used for clinical categorization. Resistance to fluoroquinolones, macrolides and aminoglycosides is also detected frequently, but the resistance phenotypes cannot be determined. *C. amycolatum* is relatively susceptible to tetracyclines and fusidic acid and always susceptible to glycopeptides.

C. diphtheriae

Antibiotic resistance is uncommon in *C. diphtheriae*, although β-lactam susceptibility is only moderate, with MICs of 0.5 μg/ml for amoxicillin and 1 μg/ml for cefotaxime. Macrolide resistance is generally rare and appears to vary according to the source of the strain. Out of 59 non-toxigenic strains isolated from non-diphtheric infections in France between 1987 and 1993, only one strain was resistant. Erythromycin resistance was not detected in a study of 83 strains isolated in Russia prior to 1994, although 11% of isolates were resistant in another Russian study carried out in 1999. Among strains isolated from diphtheria cases in Vietnam between 1995 and 1996, 27% were resistant to macrolides. Tetracycline resistance was described for the first time in Jakarta in 1982 (28) and later found in one of 15 Vietnamese isolates. Cotrimoxazole and rifampin resistance is infrequent.

Other species

Other species usually do not display high-level β-lactam resistance, although isolated resistance to another antibiotic class, particularly macrolides or tetracyclines, is often seen (18, 27). Macrolide resistance rates among corynebacteria differ according to species. For instance, most *C. glucuronolyticum* strains are resistant to erythromycin whereas this is less frequent for *C. striatum*, and both species show similar susceptibility to telithromycin. Resistance to macrolides is generally found for both 14 and 16 carbon molecules and for lincosamides, in relation to the presence of *erm* genes in the corynebacteria. One study showed that 98% of erythromycin-resistant *Corynebacterium* spp. strains were also resistant to josamycin and lincomycin, whereas two strains were josamycin-susceptible but erythromycin- and lincomycin-resistant, suggesting another resistance mechanism of the efflux type (34). Resistance to lincosamides only is also possible.

Tetracycline susceptibility is variable. *C. glucuronolyticum* is the most resistant species (60% resistant strains). Tetracycline and doxycycline have about the same activity against this species (25).

ANTIBIOTICS TO BE STUDIED

Standard list

Ampicillin (or amoxicillin), ciprofloxacin (or levofloxacin), erythromycin, clindamycin (or lincomycin, disk close to the erythromycin disk), quinupristin-dalfopristin, gentamicin, vancomycin.

Additional list

Cefotaxime, rifampin (for *C. diphtheriae*), fusidic acid, linezolid, cotrimoxazole (for *C. glucuronolyticum*), telithromycin.

REFERENCES

(1) **Carlson, P**. 2000. Comparison of the E-test and agar dilution methods for susceptibility testing of *Arcanobacterium haemolyticum*. Eur. J. Clin. Microbiol. Infect. Dis. **19**:891-893.

(2) **Costa-Riu, N., A. Burkovski, R. Krämer, and R. Benz**. 2003. PorA represents the major cell wall channel of the gram-positive bacterium *Corynebacterium glutamicum*. J. Bacteriol. **185**:4779-4786.

(3) **Daneshvar, M.I., D.G. Hollis, R.S. Weyant, J.G. Jordan, J.P. MacGregor, R.E. Morey, A.M. Whitney, D.J. Brenner, A.G. Steigerwalt, L.O. Helsel, P.M. Raney, J.B. Patel, P.N. Levett, and J.M. Brown**. 2004. Identification of some charcoal-black-pigmented CDC fermentative coryneform group 4 isolates as *Rothia dentocariosa* and some as *Corynebacterium aurimucosum*: proposal of *Rothia dentocariosa* emend. Georg and Brown 1967, *Corynebacterium aurimucosum* emend. Yassin et al. 2002, and *Corynebacterium nigricans* Shukla et al. 2003 pro synon. *Corynebacterium aurimucosum*. J. Clin. Microbiol. **42**:4189-4198.

(4) **Dzierzanowska, D., R. Miksza-Zytkiewicz, M. Czerniawska, H. Linda, and J. Borowski**. 1978. Sensitivity of *Rothia dentocariosa*. J. Antimicrob. Chemother. **4**:469-471.

(5) **Eguchi, H., T. Kuwahara, T. Miyamoto, H. Nakayama-Imaohji, M. Ichimura, T. Hayashi, and H. Shiota**. 2008. High-level fluoroquinolone resistance in ophthalmic clinical isolates belonging to the species *Corynebacterium macginleyi*. J. Clin. Microbiol. **46**:527-532.

(6) **Engler, K.H., M. Warner, and R.C. George**. 2001. In vitro activity of ketolides HMR 3004 and HMR 3647 and seven other antimicrobial agents against *Corynebacterium diphtheriae*. J. Antimicrob. Chemother. **47**:27-31.

(7) **Fernandez-Roblas, R., H. Adames, N.Z. Martín-de-Hijas, D. Garcia Almeida, I. Gadea, J. Esteban**. 2009. In vitro activity of tigecycline and 10 other antimicrobials against clinical isolates of the genus *Corynebacterium*. Int. J. Antimicrob. Agents. **33**:453-455.

(8) **Funke, G., R.A. Hutson, K.A. Bernard, G.E. Pfiffer, G. Wauters, and M.D. Collins**. 1996. Isolation of *Arthrobacter* spp. from clinical specimens and description of *Arthrobacter cumminsii* sp. nov. and *Arthrobacter woluwensis* sp. nov. J. Clin. Microbiol. **34**:2356-2363.

(9) **Funke, G., M. Pagano-Niederer, and W. Bernauer**. 1998. *Corynebacterium macginleyi* has to date been isolated exclusively from conjunctival swabs. J. Clin. Microbiol. **36**:3670-3673.

(10) **Funke, G., M. Pagano-Niederer, B. Sjödén, and E. Falsen**. 1998. Characteristics of *Arthrobacter cumminsii*, the most frequently encountered *Arthrobacter* species in human clinical specimens. J. Clin. Microbiol. **36**:1539-1543.

(11) **Funke, G., V. Pünter, and A. von Graevenitz**. 1996. Antimicrobial susceptibility patterns of some recently established coryneform bacteria. Antimicrob. Agents Chemother. **40**:2874-2878.

(12) **Funke, G., A. von Graevenitz, and N. Weiss**. 1994. Primary identification of *Aureobacterium* spp. isolated from clinical specimens as "*Corynebacterium aquaticum*". J. Clin. Microbiol. **32**:2686-2691.

(13) **Garcia-Rodriguez, J.A., J.E. Garcia Sanchez, J.L. Munoz Bellido, T. Nebreda Mayoral, E. Garcia Sanchez, and I. Garcia Garcia**. 1991. In vitro activity of 79 antimicrobial agents against *Corynebacterium* group D2. Antimicrob. Agents Chemother. **35**:2140-2143.

(14) **Gneiding K., R. Frodl, and G. Funke**. 2008. Identities of *Microbacterium* spp. encountered in human clinical specimens. J. Clin. Microbiol. **46**:3646-3652.

(15) **Gomez-Garcés, J.L., J.I. Alos, and J. Tamayo**. 2007. In vitro activity of linezolid and 12 other antimicrobials against coryneform bacteria. Int. J. Antimicrob. Agents. **29**: 688-692.

(16) **Kim, H.J., Y. Kim, M.S. Lee, and H.S. Lee**. 2001. Gene *lmrB* of *Corynebacterium glutamicum* confers

efflux-mediated resistance to lincomycin. Mol. Cells **12**:112-116.

(17) **Jorgensen, J.H., J. Hindler, D.M. Citron, F.R. Cockerill, T.R. Fritsche, G. Funke, J.B. Patel, P.C. Schreckenberger, J.D. Turnidge, R.D. Walker, D.F. Welsch.** 2005. Methods for antimicrobial dilution and disk susceptibility testing of infrequently isolated or fastidious bacteria; proposed guideline. Clinical and Laboratory Standards Institute document M45-P. Vol. 25, No. 26: 18-19.

(18) **Lagrou, K., J. Verhaegen, M. Janssens, G. Wauters, and L. Verbist.** 1998. Prospective study of catalase-positive coryneform organisms in clinical specimens: Identification, clinical relevance, and antibiotic susceptibility. Diagn. Microbiol. Infect. Dis. **30**:7-15.

(19) **Luna, V.A., P. Coates, E.A. Eady, J.H. Cove, T.T.H. Nguyen, and M.C. Roberts.** 1999. A variety of Gram-positive bacteria carry mobile *mef* genes. J. Antimicrob. Chemother. **44**:19-25.

(20) **Maple, P.A.C., A. Efstratiou, G. Tseneva, Y. Rikushin, S. Deshevoi, M. Jahkola, and J. Vuopio-Varkila, and R.C. George.** 1994. The *in-vitro* susceptibilities of toxigenic strains of *Corynebacterium diphtheriae* isolated in Northwestern Russia and surrounding areas to ten antibiotics. J. Antimicrob. Chemother. **34**:1037-1040.

(21) **Martinez-Martinez, L., M.C. Ortega, and A.L. Suarez.** 1995. Comparison of E-test with broth microdilution and disk diffusion for susceptibility testing of coryneform bacteria. J. Clin. Microbiol. **33**:1318-1321.

(22) **Martinez-Martinez, L., A. Pascual, K. Bernard, and A.I. Suarez.** 1996. Antimicrobial susceptibility pattern of *Corynebacterium striatum*. Antimicrob. Agents Chemother. **40**:2671-2672.

(23) **Perrin-Guyomard, A., C. Soumet, R. Leclercq, F. Doucet-Populaire, and P. Sanders.** 2005. Antibiotic susceptibility of bacteria isolated from pasteurized milk and characterisation of macrolide-lincosamide-streptogramin resistance genes. J. Food. Prot. **68**:347-352

(24) **Power E.G.M.P., Y.H. Abdulla, H.G. Talsania, W. Spice, S. Aathithan, and G.L. French.** 1995. *vanA* genes in vancomycin-resistant clinical isolates of *Oerskovia turbata* and *Arcanobacterium (Corynebacterium) haemolyticum*. J. Antimicrob. Chemother. **36**:595-606.

(25) **Riegel, P**. Personal data.

(26) **Riegel, P., D. de Briel, G. Prévost, F. Jehl, and H. Monteil.** 1994. Genomic diversity among *Corynebacterium jeikeium* strains and comparison with biochemical characteristics and antimicrobial susceptibilities. J. Clin. Microbiol. **32**:1860-1865.

(27) **Riegel, P., R. Ruimy, R. Christen, and H. Monteil.** 1996. Species identities and antimicrobial susceptibilities of corynebacteria isolated from various clinical sources. Eur. J. Clin. Microbiol. Infect. Dis. **15**:657-662.

(28) **Rockhill, R., C. Umarmo, H. Hadiputranto, S.P. Siregar, and B. Muslihun.** 1982. Tetracycline resistance of *Corynebacterium diphtheriae* isolated from diphtheria patients in Jakarta, Indonesia. Antimicrob. Agents Chemother. **21**:842-843.

(29) **Rosato, A.E., B.S. Lee, and K.A. Nash.** 2001. Inducible macrolide resistance in *Corynebacterium jeikeium*. Antimicrob. Agents Chemother. **45**:1982-1989.

(30) **Sánchez-Hernández, J., B. Mora-Peris, G. Yagüe-Guirao, N. Gutiérrez-Zufiaurre, J.L. Muñoz-Bellido, M. Segovia-Hernandez, and J.A. García-Rodriguez.** 2003. In vitro activity of newer antibiotics against *Corynebacterium jeikeium, Corynebacterium amycolatum* and *Corynebacterium urealyticum*. Int. J. Antimicrob. Agents. **22**:492-496.

(31) **Serwold-Davis, T.M., and N.B. Groman.** 1988. Identification of a methylase gene for erythromycin resistance within the sequence of a spontaneously deleting fragment of *Corynebacterium diphtheriae* plasmid pNG2. FEMS Microbiol. Lett. **56**:7-14.

(32) **Sierra, J.M., L. Martinez-Martinez, F. Vazquez, E. Giralt, and Jordi Vila.** 2005. Relationship between mutations in the *gyrA* gene and quinolone resistance in clinical isolates of *Corynebacterium striatum* and *Corynebacterium amycolatum*. Antimicrob. Agents Chemother; **49**:1714-1719.

(33) **Soriano, F., L. Huelves, P. Naves, V. Rodriguez-Cerrato, G. del Prado, V. Ruiz, and C. Ponte.** 2009. *In-vitro* activity of ciprofloxacin, moxifloxacin, vancomycin and erythromycin against planktonic and biofilm forms of *Corynebacterium urealyticum*. J. Antimicrob. Chemother. **63**:353-356.

(34) **Soriano, F., R. Fernandez-Roblas, R. Calvo, G. Garcia-Calvo, M. Pardeiro, and A. Bryskier.** 1998. *In-vitro* antimicrobial activity of HMR 3004 (RU 64004) against erythromycin A-sensitive and –resistant *Corynebacterium* spp. isolated from clinical specimens. J. Antimicrob. Chemother. **42**:647-649.

(35) **Soriano, F., J. Zapardiel, and E. Nieto.** 1995. Antimicrobial susceptibilities of *Corynebacterium* species and other non-spore-forming gram-positive bacilli to 18 antimicrobial agents. Antimicrob. Agents Chemother. **39**:208-214.

(36) **Tauch, A., S. Gotker, A. Puhler, J. Kalinowski, and G. Thierbach.** 2002. The 27.8-kb R-plasmid pTET3 from *Corynebacterium glutamicum* encodes the aminoglycoside adenylyltransferase gene cassette *aadA9* and the regulated tetracycline efflux system *Tet* 33 flanked by active copies of the widespread insertion sequence IS6100. Plasmid **48**:117-129.

(37) **Tauch A, O. Kaiser, T. Hain, A. Goesmann, B. Weisshaar, A. Albersmeier, T. Bekel, N. Bischoff, I. Brune, T. Chakraborty, J. Kalinowski, F. Meyer, O. Rupp, S. Schneiker, P. Viehoever, and A. Pühler.** 2005. Complete genome sequence and analysis of the multiresistant nosocomial pathogen *Corynebacterium jeikeium* K111, a lipid-requiring bacterium of the human skin flora. J. Bacteriol. **187**:4671-82.

(38) **Tauch, A., S. Krieft, A. Pühler, and J. Kalinowski.** 1999. The *tetAB* genes of the *Corynebacterium striatum* R-plasmid pTP10 encode an ABC transporter and confer tetracycline, oxytetracycline and oxacillin resistance in *Corynebacterium glutamicum*. FEMS Microbiol. Lett. **173**:203-209.

(39) **Tauch A, E. Trost, A. Tilker, U. Ludewig, S. Schneiker, A. Goesmann, W. Arnold, T. Bekel, K. Brinkrolf, I. Brune, S. Götker, J. Kalinowski, P.B. Kamp, F.P. Lobo, P. Viehoever, B. Weisshaar, F.**

Soriano, M. Dröge, and A. Pühler. 2008. The lifestyle of *Corynebacterium urealyticum* derived from its complete genome sequence established by pyrosequencing. J. Biotechnol. **31**;136(1-2):11-21.

(40) **Tauch, A., Z. Zheng, A. Puhler, and J. Kalinowski**. 1998. *Corynebacterium striatum* chloramphenicol resistance transposon Tn*5564*: genetic organization and transposition in *Corynebacterium glutamicum*. Plasmid **40**:126-139.

(41) **Weiss, K., M. Laverdière, and R. Rivest**. 1996. Comparison of antimicrobial susceptibilities of *Corynebacterium* species by broth microdilution and disk diffusion methods. Antimicrob. Agents Chemother. **40**:930-933.

Chapter 30. *BACILLUS*

Eric HERNÀNDEZ-GUINÀT

INTRODUCTION

The genus *Bacillus* comprises a large number of Gram-positive, endospore-forming, facultative anaerobic bacilli, most of which are motile with the exception of *B. anthracis* which is always immotile.
- *B. anthracis* is the etiological agent of anthrax (23), a zoonosis which affects herbivorous animals with incidental transmission to humans. The most common form of the disease in humans is cutaneous anthrax, characterized by the formation of one or more vesicular lesions which develop over the course of a few days into necrotic ulcers always associated with severe edema. Inoculation occurs through direct contact with infected animals or when handling contaminated animal products such as hair, bones or wool (hence the name woolsorters' disease). In the majority of cases, prompt initiation of antibiotic therapy is curative. Gastrointestinal (8) and inhalation anthrax are less common but the latter is to be feared as a potential agent of bioterrorism (27). The gastrointestinal and inhalational forms result from ingestion or inhalation of spores and are always fatal in the absence of treatment. The Centers for Disease Control and Prevention (CDC) classifies anthrax as a Category A bioterrorism agent. The bacterium has already been used as a bioweapon or bioterrorism agent. In 1979, accidental release of anthrax spores from a military facility in Sverdlovsk, in the former Soviet Union, caused a fatal outbreak in the area surrounding a military research center (1). In 2001 in the United States, *B. anthracis* was deliberately placed in pieces of mail, resulting in the infection of 22 people. The main problem following inhalation or ingestion is the long survival time of spores within macrophages, which necessitates prolonged chemoprophylaxis to avoid occurrence of disease (Fig. 1).
- *B. cereus* causes food poisoning but also more serious infections such as septicemia, meningitis, and pulmonary infections in frail or immunocompromised individuals (20). This species can also infect wounds and cause osteomyelitis or necrotic damage to muscle and soft tissues, particularly after a trauma or war injury. Ocular infections have also been described.
- *B. thuringiensis* is an insect pathogen widely used around the world as a biopesticide. This species has been incriminated in gastroenteritis and infection following a burn or war injury, although its pathogenic potential for humans is a topic of debate.
- The other *Bacillus* species are opportunistic bacteria, but *B. subtilis*, *B. licheniformis,* and *B. sphaericus* have also been known to cause food poisoning.

Recent evidence indicates that *B. cereus*, *B. anthracis* and *B. thuringiensis* belong to one and the same species (25).

METHODS

The *B. anthracis* antibiogram must be carried out in a biosafety level BSL-3 laboratory, since this bacterium belongs to biosafety risk group 3. Moreover, the antibiogram for this species should not be performed outside of national centers in Europe and the United States. Routine antibiotic susceptibility testing of other *Bacillus* species does not pose any particular problems for hospital laboratories. In case of severe infection in humans, the isolate should systematically be sent to a reference laboratory to allow centralization and publication of MICs data on the isolated species. Antibiotic susceptibility testing of *Bacillus* ssp. should be carried out according to the guidance issued by the Clinical and Laboratory Standards Institute (CLSI) or the European Committee on Antimicrobial Susceptibility Testing (EUCAST), certain noteworthy aspects of which will be reviewed in this chapter.

Liquid medium

This is the reference method for determination of MICs. Mueller-Hinton medium is used, since all clinical isolates of *Bacillus* spp., including *B. anthracis*, grow easily and rapidly in this medium.

Inoculum

Strict standardization is essential since there is a large inoculum effect, especially with β-lactams antibiotics. If the inoculum is too small, some penicillin G-resistant strains of *B. anthracis* may appear susceptible due to slow induction of β-lactamase bla1. If the inoculum is too heavy, plates may be difficult to read due to turbidity. In practice, the inoculum should be prepared from colonies grown for 16-20 h on chocolate agar plates or from a 4-6 h exponentially growing shaking culture in Mueller-Hinton medium. An inoculum adjusted to a turbidity of a 0.5 McFarland standard provides good conditions for carrying out the *Bacillus* spp. antibiogram.

Microdilution

The antibiotics should be dissolved in the manufacturer-recommended solvent to a concentration ten-fold higher than the final test concentration. Great care should be taken since serial dilutions performed manually are common sources of error. Commercial microtiter plates are reliable but quality should always be checked by using at least two quality controls. Concentration ranges suitable for *Bacillus* are comprised between 0.06 and 128 μg/ml. An antibiotic-free well should be used as a growth control. Microtiter plates prepared in the laboratory can be stored at 4°C for 48 h or at –80°C for several months without affecting the quality of the results.

Incubation

The incubation time before reading the plates is critical to avoid errors. Ideally, incubation times range from 16-20 h; any longer, and plates may be difficult to read because the medium becomes turbid (2). A broth microdilution antibiogram is commercially available. MICs are read by detecting the fluorescence released by bacterial enzymes which cleave a chromogenic substrate contained in the medium. So far there is not enough experience to consider this technique validated for the *Bacillus* or even more so for the *B. anthracis* spp. antibiogram.

Quality control

It is essential to include reference strains in each series, such as *S. aureus* ATCC 29213 for validation of results obtained with antibiotics, and *E. coli* ATCC 25922.

SOLID MEDIUM

Diffusion

Disks

The agar disk diffusion method has not been validated for *Bacillus* and so to avoid any errors it should not be used as a routine method.

E-test®

MIC determination by E-test® is based on diffusion from antibiotic gradient strips. The manufacturer recommends an inoculum adjusted to the optical density of a 0.5 McFarland standard, prepared in sterile distilled water. The inoculum should be swabbed on the agar surface which should be allowed to dry for 10 min at 37°C before application of the strips. Results can be read after an 18-h incubation. For *B. anthracis*, this method shows good agreement with the reference method (32, 38). Difficulties with reading the MICs of penicillin G have been reported (33), probably due to very low-level expression of the β-lactamase bla1. The results may unreadable and, in about 10% of cases, the MIC value is falsified by the presence of an irregular ellipse or tiny colonies at the base of the ellipse (2). In such cases, the MIC should be read by taking the value on the strip at the intersection of two inhibition ellipses, ignoring any tiny colonies. If plates are difficult to read due to the presence of macrocolonies or changes in morphology, the result should always be read at the point of inhibition. Other authors have noted that, with this method, trimethoprim-sulfamethoxazole resistance was detectable in *B. anthracis* isolates at 30°C but not at 35°C (30).

Agar dilution

Dilution in Mueller-Hinton agar has already been used for antibiotic susceptibility testing of *B. anthracis* (14, 18). The main advantage of this method is its ease of implementation and good readability of results, especially when working at a biosafety workstation or biosafety cabinet. The antibiotics are prepared immediately before use from commercially available antibiotic powders, then incorporated into the agar by surfusion so as to obtain geometric doubling dilutions. Like the broth microdilution method, the concentration range is 0.06 to 128 μg/ml. Once prepared, media can be stored at 4°C for 3-5 days in hermetically sealed plastic bags to avoid desiccation.

Molecular biology

Molecular biology techniques have been developed to detect resistance to the main antibiotics used for the prophylaxis and treatment of *B. anthracis* infections, but they can only detect known and acquired mutations or genes (3).

β-lactamase production

The test using chromogenic cephalosporinase is unable to detect β-lactamases in *B. anthracis* because the production of these enzymes is slow and there is poor agreement of the results (2). However, β-lactamase production can be detected during routine testing by a modified chromogenic test which should be carried out in liquid medium (26). A colony obtained after 24 h of growth on trypticase-soy agar is diluted in 0.5 ml distilled water and the test disk added to the medium, which is then incubated for 30 min at 37°C. A pink coloration indicates a positive result (Fig. 2). The results of this test are in agreement with those of the agar dilution method.

RESISTANCE

Spores

Bacillus spores remain fully resistant to antibiotics.

Intrinsic

B. anthracis is intrinsically resistant to sulfonamides, trimethoprim, cotrimoxazole, and second and third generation cephalosporins (Table 1), but susceptible to cefalotin although this agent has very low activity *in vivo* (18).

B. cereus and *B. thuringiensis* are intrinsically resistant to penicillin G, aminopenicillins and carboxypenicillins (MICs of 8-16 μg/ml), and to second and third generation cephalosporins (Table 1). Some strains of *B. thuringiensis* may be susceptible to penicillin G. Among the penicillins, piperacillin is the poorest substrate of the enzymes detected in the *cereus* group, and all strains are susceptible to imipenem.

Apart from the *cereus* group, other *Bacillus* species are generally susceptible to penicillin G.

β-lactams

β-lactamase production is the predominant mechanism of resistance in *Bacillus* from the *cereus* group. Three β-lactamases have been iden-

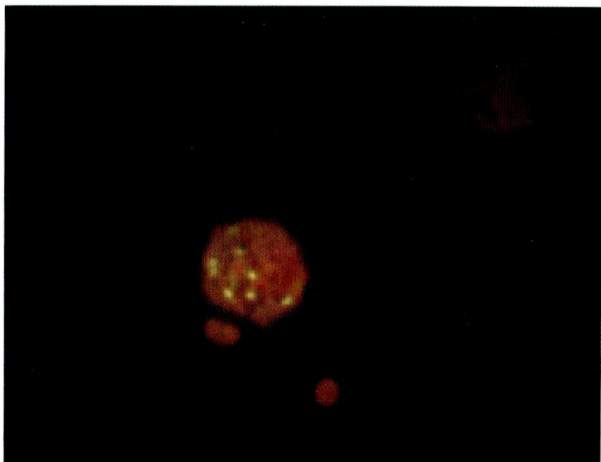

Fig. 1 : Spores of *B. anthracis* after aerosol infection of Balb/c mice (author collection)

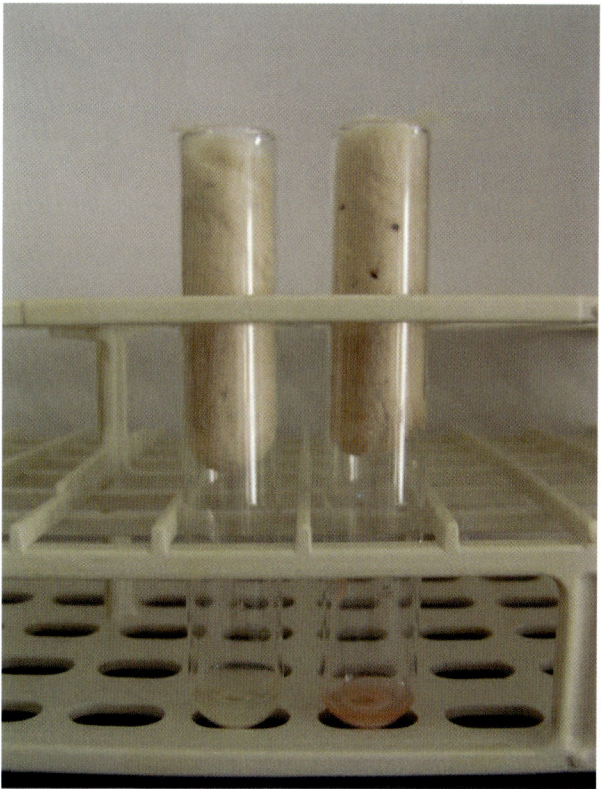

Fig. 2. Rapid detection of β-lactamase production by *B. anthracis*. Incubation 35 min at 37°C. Left, negative test ; right, positive test with pink colour

tified in this group: bla1, bla2, and bla3, but only the first two are found in *B. anthracis* (15).
- β-lactamase I (bla1) is an extracellular enzyme encoded by a chromosomal gene which mainly hydrolyzes benzylpenicillin, ampicillin, amoxicillin, and piperacillin (31). It is inhibited by clavulanic acid but not by EDTA. It is a 27.8 kDa protein with an isoelectric point of 8.6.

This β-lactamase is five times more active against penicillin G and ampicillin than against carbenicillin. Cephalosporins are poor substrates (31). The enzyme has been detected in *B. cereus*, *B. thuringiensis* and *B. anthracis* (15). It is produced constitutively in the first two species but in only 2-10% of *B. anthracis* isolates in which it is usually silent. In *B. anthracis* it confers penicillin G and ampicillin resistance when expressed (16).

- β-lactamase II (bla2) is an inducible metalloenzyme encoded by a chromosomal gene. Since it requires zinc as cofactor, it is strongly inhibited by EDTA (31). It belongs to functional group 3 in the Bush classification scheme (13). It has a molecular mass of 25 kDa and an isoelectric point of 8.3. This enzyme hydrolyzes cephalosporins in *B. cereus*, *B. thuringiensis*, and *B. anthracis* and also hydrolyzes imipenem (15, 31).
- β-lactamase III (bla3) is a chromosomally encoded lipoprotein which binds to the bacterial membrane. This 31.5 kDa protein has an isoelectric point of 6.8 and a substrate profile similar to that of bla1 but is approximately ten-fold less active. Bla3 has been detected in *B. cereus* and *B. thuringiensis* (9) but sequencing studies have shown that it is not present in the *B. anthracis* genome.

Penicillin G

B. cereus and *B. thuringiensis* are consistently resistant to penicillin G while wild type strains of *B. anthracis* and other *Bacillus* species are usually susceptible. A low penicillin G MIC_{50} of approximately 0.125 μg/ml has been reported in wild type strains of *B. anthracis* (Table 1). However, both penicillin G and amoxicillin have low bactericidal activity against *B. anthracis* (19).

Penicillin G susceptibility has long been considered the hallmark trait of *B. anthracis*, but this must now be put into perspective because resistance rates ranging from 0-10% of isolates have been reported in different series (14, 18, 21, 28,

Table 1. Minimal inhibitory concentrations (MIC, μg/ml) of antibiotics against *Bacillus*[a]

Antibiotic	*B. cereus*[b] (n=56)		*B. anthracis* (n=96)		Other species (n=35)	
	MIC_{50}	MIC_{90}	MIC_{50}	MIC_{90}	MIC_{50}	MIC_{90}
Penicillin G	8	16	0.125	8	0.03	2
Amoxicillin	8	16	0.125	4	ND[c]	ND
Piperacillin	1	2	1	1	ND	ND
Cefalotin	16	32	0.5	16	ND	ND
Cefoxitin	32	32	8	32	ND	ND
Ceftriaxone	64	128	32	32	1	128
Aztreonam	64	128	128	> 128	ND	ND
Imipenem	0.063	1	0.125	0.125	0.25	2
Chloramphenicol	2	4	2	4	4	16
Rifampin	0.125	0.5	0.06	1	ND	ND
Vancomycin	1	1	1	1	< 0.25	1
Erythromycin	1	1	0.06	1	ND	ND
Azithromycin	1 - 8	1 - 8	ND	ND	ND	ND
Clarithromycin	0.125 - 0.5	0.125 - 1	ND	ND	ND	ND
Telithromycin	0.06	0.25	ND	ND	ND	ND
Clindamycin	0.12 - 1	0.25 - 1	0.5	0.5	1	> 16
Co-trimoxazole	8	8	8	8	ND	ND
Levofloxacin	0.125	0.125	0.25	0.5	ND	ND
Pefloxacin	0.125	0.5 - 5	0.5	1	ND	ND
Ofloxacin	0.25	0.25	0.25	0.5	ND	ND
Ciprofloxacin	0.06	1	0.125	0.25	0.25	16
Doxycycline	0.125	0.25	0.25	0.25	ND	ND
Kanamycin	0.5	0.5	0.5	0.5	ND	ND
Gentamicin	0.125	0.5	0.06	0.25	ND	ND
Daptomycin	1	1	ND	ND	0.125	1

a From 5, 14, 17, 22, 39.
b Valid also for *B. thuringiensis*.
c ND, not determined.

34). However, typing data are not always available for all strains, leaving open the possibility that resistant strains spread via local outbreaks. The first penicillinase was described by a Russian group in 1971 (12). In intermediate or resistant strains the MICs of penicillin G or amoxicillin are 2-8 and 4-8 µg/ml, respectively. This penicillinase is expressed at a low level and so is difficult to detect (26). Resistant strains have been obtained by culture in the presence of subinhibitory concentrations of penicillin G (10). This resistance has also been described in other *Bacillus* spp. such as *B. circulans* and *B. polymyxa* (39).

Cephalosporins and carbapenems

All strains of *Bacillus* are resistant to third generation cephalosporins, but may appear susceptible to first or second generation cephalosporins *in vitro* (Table 1). Imipenem is consistently active, with low MICs for all strains. However, *in vivo* efficacy remains to be demonstrated because bla2 is a metalloenzyme which can weakly hydrolyze carbapenems.

Fluoroquinolones

Fluoroquinolones are active against all species from the genus *Bacillus* and are recommended for the prophylaxis of anthrax following exposure. Acquired resistance has been obtained experimentally by serial passages of *B. anthracis* in the presence of subinhibitory concentrations of ciprofloxacin (37). The mutations affect type II topoisomerases (7, 24). The first mutations to appear are located in the *gyrA* gene with a mutation rate of approximately 5.3×10^{10}. In this case the MICs of ciprofloxacin range from 0.06-0.5 µg/ml. Additional mutations in the *parC* gene raise the MICs to 8-16 µg/ml. *gyrB* mutations are less frequent but when combined with the previous mutations can raise the MICs to > 64 µg/ml. There have been some anecdotal reports of an efflux resistance mechanism at work in *B. anthracis*.

Tetracyclines

Tetracyclines show good activity against *Bacillus*. The MIC_{50} and MIC_{90} of doxycycline are 0.06 and 0.25 µg/ml. Doxycycline is currently recommended for prophylaxis following inhalational exposure. As in the case of the fluoroquinolones, resistant mutants can be obtained (35). The *tet*(M) gene in *B. anthracis* confers high-level cross-resistance to tetracyclines-minocyclines.

Aminoglycosides

MICs of aminoglycosides are low and acquired resistance has not been reported. Gentamicin is one of the most rapidly bactericidal antibiotics against *B. anthracis* and *B. cereus*; cell killing occurs within 24-48 hours.

Macrolides

Macrolides are only moderately active *in vitro*. Acquired resistance due to the presence of the methylase *erm*(D) gene has been described (29). Culture in the presence of subinhibitory antibiotic concentrations can induce acquired resistance. Clindamycin and telithromycin are more active *in vitro* against *B. anthracis* than macrolides.

Trimethoprim

B. anthracis is intrinsically resistant to trimethoprim and MICs are high. The resistance determinant is a dihydrofolate reductase with no affinity for trimethoprim. Newer antifolates may, however, be active against *B. anthracis* (6).

Other antibiotics

Bacillus are susceptible to rifampin (Table 1) but this drug must never be used alone, because spontaneous resistance occurs at a rate of 1.5×10^{-9} to 10^{-8} per generation. High-level rifampin resistance (> 128 µg/ml) has been obtained experimentally in *B. anthracis* and a mutation rate of 1×10^{-8} has been observed in the Sterne strain (36). Resistance mutations map to the *rpoB* gene of the RNA polymerase beta subunit.

Resistance to glycopeptides has not been reported.

Daptomycin is a lipopeptide with rapid bactericidal activity against Gram-positive organisms which is also active against *Bacillus* spp. (17). MICs for *B. cereus*, *B. thuringiensis*, *B. mycoides*, and *B. subtilis* range from 0.06-2 µg/ml with MIC_{90} of 1 µg/ml. Currently no reliable data are available for *B. anthracis*.

ANTIBIOTICS TO BE STUDIED

The choice of antibiotics to be tested in the antibiogram of *B. anthracis* and other species from the genus *Bacillus* depends primarily on treatment considerations and the need to seek a possible alternative to the recommended treatments. The antibiogram should always include penicillin G,

Table 2. Critical concentrations (μg/ml) of the Clinical and Laboratory Standards Institute (CLSI) for B.anthracis

Antibiotic	Susceptible	Resistant
Penicillin G	≤ 0.12	≥ 0.25
Tetracycline	≤ 1	-
Doxycycline	≤ 1	-
Ciprofloxacin	≤ 0.25	-
Levofloxacin	≤ 0.25	-

doxycycline, tetracycline, and ciprofloxacin. In our opinion, gentamicin, clindamycin, rifampin, chloramphenicol, and vancomycin should also be tested. Nalidixic acid is useful for detecting first level resistance to fluoroquinolones. Macrolides are not appropriate for the treatment of severe infections due to *Bacillus* spp. The usefulness of testing other anti-Gram-positive antibiotics, such as linezolid, fusidic acid or fosfomycin, remains to be established.

INTERPRETATION

Proposed breakpoints are based on the MIC distribution in wild-type strains and on pharmacokinetic/pharmacodynamic data which vary in a time- or concentration-dependent manner. The correlation between MICs and clinical and microbiological success, when it is known, helps validate the relevance of the guidelines proposed on the basis of the *in vitro* data. Such clinical experience is lacking for *Bacillus*.
- For *B. anthracis*, the CLSI recommends specific interpretive criteria for antibiotic susceptibility based on observed MIC distributions, pharmacokinetic/pharmacodynamic data and results obtained in animal models (Table 2).
- There are no specific interpretive criteria for antibiotic susceptibility of other *Bacillus* species in either the United States or Europe. This absence of interpretive criteria makes it necessary to refer to general guidelines which are not always appropriate. In some studies, breakpoints were similar to those of staphylococci. We propose some critical breakpoints for *B. cereus* and *B. thuringiensis* in Table 3.

The main risk associated with *B. anthracis* is the selection of resistant strains to be used as bioweapons. It has already been shown that serial passage in media containing subinhibitory concentrations of antibiotics can induce resistance *in vitro* (4, 11). In this indication, the ability to obtain a reliable antibiogram is of utmost epidemiological

Table 3. Proposed low critical breakpoints (μg/ml) for B. cereus and B. thuringiensis

Antibiotic	MIC$_{50}$ B. cereus / B. thuringiensis	Daily dose	Serum peak (μg/ml)	Half-life (h)	Inhibitory quotient[a]	Time over MIC (%)	Low critical concentration
Amoxicillin[b]	0.125 / 8	1 g 3x	15 - 25	1	ND[c]	90	≤ 0.25[c]
Ciprofloxacin	0.06 / 0.125	0.5 g 2x	2 - 3	4	33	100	≤ 0.25
Doxycycline	0.125 / 0.25	100 mg 2x	4 - 5	16	ND	100	≤ 0.25
Vancomycin	1 / 1	1 g 2x infusions	20 - 30	6	ND	100	≤ 2
Rifampicin	0.125 / 0.06	450 mg 2x	15 - 20	3	ND	100	≤ 0.5

[a] Calculated for concentration-dependent antibiotics.
[b] High critical concentration for penicillin G deduced from PK/PD = 1 μg/ml.
[c] ND, not determined.

and prophylactic urgency. Molecular methods for detecting mutations, based on real-time PCR, have a bright future in this regard.

REFERENCES

(1) **Abramova, F.A., L.M. Grinberg, O.V. Yampolskaya, and D.H. Walker.** 1993. Pathology of inhalational anthrax in 42 cases from the Sverdlovsk outbreak of 1979. Proc. Natl. Acad. Sci. USA **90**:2291-2294.

(2) **Andrews, J.M., and R. Wise.** 2002. Susceptibility testing of *Bacillus* species. J. Antimicrob. Chemother. **49**:1040-1042.

(3) **Antwerpen, M.H., M. Schellhase, E. Ehrentreich-Forster, F. Bier, W. Witte, and U. Nubel.** 2007. DNA microarray for detection of antibiotic resistance determinants in *Bacillus anthracis* and closely related *Bacillus cereus*. Mol. Cell Probes **21**:152-160.

(4) **Athamna, A., M. Athamna, N. Abu-Rashed, B. Medlej, D.J. Bast, and E. Rubinstein.** 2004. Selection of *Bacillus anthracis* isolates resistant to antibiotics. J. Antimicrob. Chemother. **54**:424-428.

(5) **Athamna, A., M. Massalha, M. Athamna, A. Nura, B. Medlej, I. Ofek, D. Bast, and E. Rubinstein.** 2004. In-vitro susceptibility of *Bacillus anthracis* to various antibacterial agents and their time-kill activity. J. Antimicrob. Chemother. **53**:247-251.

(6) **Barrow, E.W., J. Dreier, S. Reinelt, P.C. Bourne, and W.W. Barrow.** 2007. In vitro efficacy of new antifolates against trimethoprim-resistant *Bacillus anthracis*. Antimicrob. Agents Chemother. **51**:4447-4452.

(7) **Bast, D.J., A. Athamna, C.L. Duncan, J.C. de Azavedo, D.E. Low, G. Rahav, D. Farrell, and E. Rubinstein.** 2004. Type II topoisomerase mutations in *Bacillus anthracis* associated with high-level fluoroquinolone resistance. J. Antimicrob. Chemother. **54**:90-94.

(8) **Beatty, M.E., D.A. Ashford, P.M. Griffin, R.V. Tauxe, and J. Sobel.** 2003. Gastrointestinal anthrax: review of the literature. Arch. Intern. Med. **163**:2527-2531.

(9) **Boni, M., J.D. Cavallo, and E. Hernandez.** 2002. Sequence of bla3 of *B. thuringiensis*. Genbank access No. AY376064.

(10) **Brook, I., T.B. Elliott, H.I. Pryor, 2nd, T.E. Sautter, B.T. Gnade, J.H. Thakar, and G.B. Knudson.** 2001. In vitro resistance of *Bacillus anthracis* Sterne to doxycycline, macrolides and quinolones. Int. J. Antimicrob. Agents **18**:559-562.

(11) **Brouillard, J.E., C.M. Terriff, A. Tofan, and M.W. Garrison.** 2006. Antibiotic selection and resistance issues with fluoroquinolones and doxycycline against bioterrorism agents. Pharmacotherapy **26**:3-14.

(12) **Buravtseva, N.P.** 1971. Role of penicillinase in the mechanism of resistance of *Bacillus anthracis* to benzylpenicillin. Antibiotiki **16**:168-173.

(13) **Bush, K., G.A. Jacoby, and A.A. Medeiros.** 1995. A functional classification scheme for beta-lactamases and its correlation with molecular structure. Antimicrob. Agents Chemother. **39**:1211-1233.

(14) **Cavallo, J.D., F. Ramisse, M. Girardet, J. Vaissaire, M. Mock, and E. Hernandez.** 2002. Antibiotic susceptibilities of 96 isolates of *Bacillus anthracis* isolated in France between 1994 and 2000. Antimicrob. Agents Chemother. **46**:2307-2309.

(15) **Chen, Y., J. Succi, F.C. Tenover, and T.M. Koehler.** 2003. Beta-lactamase genes of the penicillin-susceptible *Bacillus anthracis* Sterne strain. J. Bacteriol. **185**:823-830.

(16) **Chen, Y., F.C. Tenover, and T.M. Koehler.** 2004. Beta-lactamase gene expression in a penicillin-resistant *Bacillus anthracis* strain. Antimicrob. Agents Chemother. **48**:4873-4877.

(17) **Citron, D.M., and M.D. Appleman.** 2006. In vitro activities of daptomycin, ciprofloxacin, and other antimicrobial agents against the cells and spores of clinical isolates of *Bacillus* species. J. Clin. Microbiol. **44**:3814-3818.

(18) **Doganay, M., and N. Aydin.** 1991. Antimicrobial susceptibility of *Bacillus anthracis*. Scand. J. Infect. Dis. **23**:333-335.

(19) **Drago, L., E. De Vecchi, A. Lombardi, L. Nicola, M. Valli, and M.R. Gismondo.** 2002. Bactericidal activity of levofloxacin, gatifloxacin, penicillin, meropenem and rokitamycin against *Bacillus anthracis* clinical isolates. J. Antimicrob. Chemother. **50**:1059-1063.

(20) **Drobniewski, F.A.** 1993. *Bacillus cereus* and related species. Clin. Microbiol. Rev. **6**:324-338.

(21) **Esel, D., M. Doganay, and B. Sumerkan.** 2003. Antimicrobial susceptibilities of 40 isolates of *Bacillus anthracis* isolated in Turkey. Int. J. Antimicrob. Agents **22**:70-72.

(22) **Frean, J., K.P. Klugman, L. Arntzen, and S. Bukofzer.** 2003. Susceptibility of *Bacillus anthracis* to eleven antimicrobial agents including novel fluoroquinolones and a ketolide. J. Antimicrob. Chemother. **52**:297-299.

(23) **Friedlander, A.M.** 2000. Anthrax: clinical features, pathogenesis, and potential biological warfare threat. Curr. Clin. Top. Infect. Dis. **20**:335-349.

(24) **Grohs, P., I. Podglajen, and L. Gutmann.** 2004. Activities of different fluoroquinolones against *Bacillus anthracis* mutants selected in vitro and harboring topoisomerase mutations. Antimicrob. Agents Chemother. **48**:3024-3027.

(25) **Helgason, E., O.A. Okstad, D.A. Caugant, H.A. Johansen, A. Fouet, M. Mock, I. Hegna, and A.B. Kolsto.** 2000. *Bacillus anthracis*, *Bacillus cereus*, and *Bacillus thuringiensis*-one species on the basis of genetic evidence. Appl. Environ. Microbiol. **66**:2627-2730.

(26) **Hernandez, E., F. Ramisse, and J.D. Cavallo.** 2003. A fast method for the detection of penicillin resistance in *Bacillus anthracis*. Clin. Microbiol. Infect. **9**:1153-1154.

(27) **Jernigan, J.A., D.S. Stephens, D.A. Ashford, C. Omenaca, M.S. Topiel, M. Galbraith, M. Tapper, T.L. Fisk, S. Zaki, T. Popovic, R.F. Meyer, C.P. Quinn, S.A. Harper, S.K. Fridkin, J.J. Sejvar, C.W. Shepard, M. McConnell, J. Guarner, W.J. Shieh, J.M. Malecki, J.L. Gerberding, J.M. Hughes, and B.A. Perkins.** 2001. Bioterrorism-related inhalational anthrax: the first 10 cases reported in the United States. Emerg. Infect. Dis. **7**:933-944.

(28) **Jones, M.E., J. Goguen, I.A. Critchley, D.C. Draghi, J.A. Karlowsky, D.F. Sahm, R. Porschen,**

G. Patra, and V.G. DelVecchio. 2003. Antibiotic susceptibility of isolates of *Bacillus anthracis*, a bacterial pathogen with the potential to be used in biowarfare. Clin. Microbiol. Infect. **9**:984-986.

(29) **Kim, H.S., E.C. Choi, and B.K. Kim.** 1993. A macrolide-lincosamide-streptogramin B resistance determinant from *Bacillus anthracis* 590: cloning and expression of *ermJ*. J. Gen. Microbiol. **139**:601-607.

(30) **Luna, V.A., D.S. King, J. Gulledge, A.C. Cannons, P.T. Amuso, and J. Cattani.** 2007. Susceptibility of *Bacillus anthracis*, *Bacillus cereus*, *Bacillus mycoides*, *Bacillus pseudomycoides* and *Bacillus thuringiensis* to 24 antimicrobials using Sensititre automated microbroth dilution and E-test agar gradient diffusion methods. J. Antimicrob. Chemother. **60**:555-567.

(31) **Materon, I.C., A.M. Queenan, T.M. Koehler, K. Bush, and T. Palzkill.** 2003. Biochemical characterization of beta-lactamases Bla1 and Bla2 from *Bacillus anthracis*. Antimicrob. Agents Chemother. **47**:2040-2042.

(32) **Merens, A., J. Vaissaire, J.D. Cavallo, C. Le Doujet, C. Gros, C. Bigaillon, J.C. Paucod, F. Berger, E. Valade, and D. Vidal.** 2008. E-test for antibiotic susceptibility testing of *Bacillus anthracis*, *Bacillus cereus* and *Bacillus thuringiensis*: evaluation of a French collection. Int. J. Antimicrob. Agents **31**:490-492.

(33) **Mohammed, M.J., C.K. Marston, T. Popovic, R.S. Weyant, and F.C. Tenover.** 2002. Antimicrobial susceptibility testing of *Bacillus anthracis*: comparison of results obtained by using the National Committee for Clinical Laboratory Standards broth microdilution reference and E-test agar gradient diffusion methods. J. Clin. Microbiol. **40**:1902-1907.

(34) **Odendaal, M.W., P.M. Pieterson, V. de Vos, and A.D. Botha.** 1991. The antibiotic sensitivity patterns of *Bacillus anthracis* isolated from the Kruger National Park. Onderstepoort J. Vet. Res. **58**:17-19.

(35) **Pomerantsev, A.P., N.A. Shishkova, and L.I. Marinin.** 1992. Comparison of therapeutic effects of antibiotics of the tetracycline group in the treatment of anthrax caused by a strain inheriting *tet*-gene of plasmid pBC16. Antibiot. Khimioter. **37**:31-34.

(36) **Pomerantsev, A.P., L.V. Sukovatova, and L.I. Marinin.** 1993. Characterization of a Rif-R population of *Bacillus anthracis*. Antibiot. Khimioter. **38**:34-38.

(37) **Price, L.B., A. Vogler, T. Pearson, J.D. Busch, J.M. Schupp, and P. Keim.** 2003. In vitro selection and characterization of *Bacillus anthracis* mutants with high-level resistance to ciprofloxacin. Antimicrob. Agents Chemother. **47**:2362-2365.

(38) **Turnbull, P.C., N.M. Sirianni, C.I. LeBron, M.N. Samaan, F.N. Sutton, A.E. Reyes, and L.F. Peruski, Jr.** 2004. MICs of selected antibiotics for *Bacillus anthracis*, *Bacillus cereus*, *Bacillus thuringiensis*, and *Bacillus mycoides* from a range of clinical and environmental sources as determined by the E-test. J. Clin. Microbiol. **42**:3626-3634.

(39) **Weber, D.J., S.M. Saviteer, W.A. Rutala, and C.A. Thomann.** 1988. In vitro susceptibility of *Bacillus* spp. to selected antimicrobial agents. Antimicrob. Agents Chemother. **32**:642-645.

Chapter 31. LACTIC ACID BACTERIA AND *ERYSIPELOTHRIX*

Jacques TANKOVIC

INTRODUCTION

Lactic acid bacteria are Gram-positive facultative anaerobes which use carbohydrates as a principal energy source with lactic acid as the main end-product. Lactic acid bacteria comprise the different *Streptococcaceae* genera including *Pediococcus*, *Leuconostoc* and the genus *Lactobacillus*. This chapter will focus exclusively on the lactobacilli, *Pediococcus* and *Leuconostoc*. The lactobacilli can be divided into three subgenera according to physiological differences, more specifically according to the fermentation pathways they use. The three subgenera are *Thermobacterium*, *Betabacterium* and *Streptobacterium*. Species in the subgenus *Thermobacterium* are obligate homofermenters, meaning that they catabolize glucose exclusively through a homofermentative pathway with lactic acid accounting for 85% of the fermentation products. Species in the subgenus *Betabacterium* are obligate heterofermenters since they catabolize glucose exclusively by a heterofermentative pathway with carbon dioxide as an abundant end-product. Species in the subgenus *Streptobacterium* are facultative heterofermenters since they catabolize glucose by the homofermentative pathway but can also catabolize pentoses by the heterofermentative pathway.

Lactobacilli, *Pediococcus* and *Leuconostoc* are widespread in the environment, mainly in plants, plant products and foods. In addition, lactobacilli in particular are part of the commensal oral, gut and genital flora. Some species are widely used in the food industry while others can diminish the quality of foods and beverages. Lactobacilli from the obligate homofermentative subgenus *Thermobacterium* are the most common strains employed as probiotics in humans.

Rarely, these bacteria, which admittedly have low virulence, can act as opportunistic pathogens. In particular, they are known to cause bacteremia with or without endocarditis, as well as abscesses, which may be polymicrobial in nature. The lactobacillus species most commonly incriminated in human infections usually belong to the heterofermentative subgenera, *Streptobacterium* (especially *Lactobacillus rhamnosus* but also *Lactobacillus casei*, *Lactobacillus paracasei* and *Lactobacillus plantarum*) and *Betabacterium* (*Lactobacillus fermentum*).

The three subgenera have comparable susceptibility to antibiotics, characterized by two major features: intrinsic high-level resistance to glycopeptides (except for obligate homofermentative lactobacilli from the subgenus *Thermobacterium* such as *Lactobacillus acidophilus*), and intermediate susceptibility to β-lactams similar to that seen in enterococci, with bactericidal synergy of penicillin G/gentamicin, the first-line treatment of severe infections due to these bacteria.

Erysipelothrix rhusiopathiae, or swine erysipelas, is a pathogenic microorganism responsible for zoonosis that can infect a wide variety of animals and be transmitted to humans through accidental contamination. Human infections are primarily cutaneous and usually benign (Rosenbach's erysipeloid), while septicemic forms, often associated with endocarditis, are rare. The erysipeloid bacillus is also intrinsically resistant to glycopeptides but, in contrast, shows remarkably high-level susceptibility to penicillin G.

METHODS

Until recently there were no official guidelines for antibiotic susceptibility testing in these bacteria. In 2006, the Clinical and Laboratory Standards Institute (CLSI) published guidance M45-A (3) for infrequently isolated or fastidious bacteria, including lactobacilli, *Pediococcus*, *Leuconostoc* and *E. rhusiopathiae*.

The recommended conditions are common to all these bacteria: broth microdilution using cation-adjusted Mueller-Hinton broth supplemented with 2.5-5% (*V/V*) lysed horse blood. The inoculum is prepared by directly suspending colonies and adjusting to the turbidity of a 0.5 McFarland standard. Incubation is at 35°C in ambient air for 20-24 hours. Interpretive criteria are given in Tables 1 and 2.

Table 1. *Lactobacillus*, *Pediococcus* and *Leuconostoc*. Test conditions and interpretive criteria for the microdilution method (adapted from CLSI document M45-A) (3)

Test conditions:

  Medium: Cation-adjusted Mueller-Hinton broth supplemented with 2.5-5% (V/V) lysed horse blood.
  Inoculum: Direct suspension of colonies, turbidity equivalent to a 0.5 McFarland standard.
  Incubation: 35°C; ambient air; 20-24 h.
  Minimal quality control: *Streptococcus pneumoniae* ATCC 49619.

Class	Antibiotic	Interpretive criteria[a] MIC (µg/ml)		
		Susceptible	Intermediate	Resistant
Penicillins	Penicillin G	≤ 8	-	-
	Ampicillin	≤ 8	-	-
Carbapenems	Imipenem	≤ 0.5	-	-
Aminoglycosides	Gentamicin	≤ 4	8	≥ 16
Glycopeptides	Vancomycin	≤ 4	8-16	≥ 32
Macrolides[a]	Erythromycin	≤ 0.5	1-4	≥ 8
Lincosamides[a]	Clindamycin	≤ 0.5	1-2	≥ 4

[a] The M45-A document gives these interpretive criteria only for lactobacilli, but they can be applied to *Pediococcus* and *Leuconostoc*.

Table 2. *Erysipelothrix rhusiopathiae* - Test conditions and interpretive criteria for the broth microdilution method (from CLSI document M45-A) (3)

Test conditions:

  Medium: Cation-adjusted Mueller-Hinton supplemented with 2.5-5% (V/V) lysed horse blood.
  Inoculum: Direct suspension of colonies, turbidity equivalent to a 0.5 McFarland standard.
  Incubation: 35°C; ambient air; 20-24 h.
  Minimal quality control: *Streptococcus pneumoniae* ATCC 49619.

Class	Antibiotic	Interpretive criteria MIC (µg/ml)		
		Susceptible	Intermediate	Resistant
Penicillins	Penicillin G	≤ 8	-	-
	Ampicillin	≤ 8	-	-
Cephalosporins	Cefotaxime	≤ 1	-	-
	Ceftriaxone	≤ 1	-	-
	Cefepime	≤ 1	-	-
Carbapenems	Imipenem	≤ 0.5	-	-
Macrolides	Erythromycin	≤ 0.25	0.5	≥ 1
Lincosamides	Clindamycin	≤ 0.25	0.5	≥ 1
Fluoroquinolones	Ciprofloxacin	≤ 1	-	-
	Levofloxacin	≤ 2	-	-

What can be recommended to laboratories which do not routinely use the broth microdilution method? Document M45-A advises against the disk method because the results cannot be reliably interpreted. Is it possible then to use the E-test®? The antibiotic susceptibility of 104 lactobacillus strains from the *acidophilus* group (obligate homofermenters) was tested by broth microdilution and E-test® (18). For the microdilution method, colonies were suspended in physiological serum (0.85% NaCl) to the turbidity of a 1 McFarland standard, then diluted 1:100 in broth for inoculation (1:500 for inoculation of vancomycin plates). For E-test®, the inoculum consisted of the above suspension with a turbidity equivalent to a 1 McFarland standard. For both methods, plates were incubated for 24 hours at 37°C under an anaerobic atmosphere.

Table 3. Antibiotic susceptibility of lactic acid bacteria

Antibiotic	Genus	MIC$_{50}$ (µg/ml)[a]	Antibiotic	Genus	MIC$_{50}$ (µg/ml)[a]
Vancomycin	*Pediococcus*	>16->256 (2) -1024->1024	Cefuroxime	*Pediococcus*	8-16
	Leuconostoc	>128->256-512-1024		*Leuconostoc*	8
	Lactobacillus	>16->256 (3) ->2048		*Lactobacillus*	32
Teicoplanin	*Pediococcus*	32->256 (2) ->1024-2048	Cefoxitin	*Pediococcus*	-
	Leuconostoc	>128->256-512-1024		*Leuconostoc*	64
	Lactobacillus	>256 (2) -2048		*Lactobacillus*	>128
Daptomycin	*Pediococcus*	0.25-<0.5	Cefixime	*Pediococcus*	>4
	Leuconostoc	<0.5		*Leuconostoc*	-
	Lactobacillus	<0.5-4		*Lactobacillus*	-
Penicillin G	*Pediococcus*	0.25 - 0.5 (2) – 1 - 2	Cefotaxime	*Pediococcus*	4-8-16
	Leuconostoc	0.5 (4)		*Leuconostoc*	8 (3)
	Lactobacillus	0.25 (2) - 0.5 (4) - 2		*Lactobacillus*	2-16
Ampicillin	*Pediococcus*	1-2 (2) - 4	Ceftriaxone	*Pediococcus*	16 (2)
	Leuconostoc	1(2)		*Leuconostoc*	8
	Lactobacillus	0.12 - 0.5 (3) - 1		*Lactobacillus*	16 - > 256
Amoxicillin	*Pediococcus*	1	Ceftazidime	*Pediococcus*	>16
	Leuconostoc	-		*Leuconostoc*	-
	Lactobacillus	1		*Lactobacillus*	-
Oxacillin	*Pediococcus*	2	Cefpirome	*Pediococcus*	8 (2)
	Leuconostoc	-		*Leuconostoc*	-
	Lactobacillus	4		*Lactobacillus*	-
Ticarcillin	*Pediococcus*	16	Imipenem	*Pediococcus*	0.12 (4)
	Leuconostoc	-		*Leuconostoc*	2
	Lactobacillus	-		*Lactobacillus*	0.06 - < 0.12 - 0.5 - 1 - 2
Piperacillin	*Pediococcus*	2	Tobramycin	*Pediococcus*	4 (2)
	Leuconostoc	-		*Leuconostoc*	0.5-1
	Lactobacillus	-		*Lactobacillus*	0.5-8
Piperacillin-tazobactam	*Pediococcus*	-	Gentamicin	*Pediococcus*	1(2) - 2 – 4 (2)
	Leuconostoc	-		*Leuconostoc*	0.25 (2) - < 0.5
	Lactobacillus	0.25 - 1		*Lactobacillus*	< 0.5 – 1 (2) – 8 - 16
Cefalotin	*Pediococcus*	4	Amikacin	*Pediococcus*	4-8-16
	Leuconostoc	4 (2)		*Leuconostoc*	1
	Lactobacillus	4-8-16		*Lactobacillus*	-
Cefaclor	*Pediococcus*	32 (2) - 64	Netilmicin	*Pediococcus*	0.5
	Leuconostoc	16		*Leuconostoc*	0.25
	Lactobacillus	128		*Lactobacillus*	4
Cefazolin	*Pediococcus*	16	Kanamycin	*Pediococcus*	32
	Leuconostoc	-		*Leuconostoc*	4 (2)
	Lactobacillus	-		*Lactobacillus*	4->128
Cefamandole	*Pediococcus*	16	Streptomycin	*Pediococcus*	16-64
	Leuconostoc	16		*Leuconostoc*	2 (2)
	Lactobacillus	8		*Lactobacillus*	4 - 8 - >128

A level of agreement greater than 90% (difference of not more than one dilution between MICs obtained by the two methods) was found for the following antibiotics: ampicillin, streptomycin, gentamicin and vancomycin. The level of agreement was acceptable for erythromycin (80%) and clindamycin (71%) but poor in the case of tetracycline (34%). In general, E-test® gave lower MICs of ampicillin, erythromycin, clindamycin, streptomycin and tetracycline and higher MICs of gentamicin and vancomycin.

However, the test conditions used in this study differed in several respects from the recommendations set forth in document M45-A: not only was

Table 3. Antibiotic susceptibility of lactic acid bacteria (continued)

Antibiotic	Genus	MIC$_{50}$ (µg/ml)[a]	Antibiotic	Genus	MIC$_{50}$ (µg/ml)[a]
Erythromycin	*Pediococcus*	0.03 - 0.06 - 0.12 (3)-0.25	Chloramphenicol	*Pediococcus*	2 (3) - 16
	Leuconostoc	0.03 - 0.06 (2)		*Leuconostoc*	4-8
	Lactobacillus	0.06 (5) - 0.25		*Lactobacillus*	2-4-8
Roxithromycin	*Pediococcus*	< 0.12 - 0.06	Thiamphenicol	*Pediococcus*	8
	Leuconostoc	0.12 (2)		*Leuconostoc*	8
	Lactobacillus	< 0.12 - 0.06		*Lactobacillus*	8
Josamycin	*Pediococcus*	0.25	Fusidic acid	*Pediococcus*	4
	Leuconostoc	0.12		*Leuconostoc*	-
	Lactobacillus	0.12		*Lactobacillus*	64-128
Spiramycin	*Pediococcus*	0.5 (2)	Linezolid	*Pediococcus*	1
	Leuconostoc	0.25		*Leuconostoc*	2
	Lactobacillus	0.25		*Lactobacillus*	1 (2) - 4
Clarithromycin	*Pediococcus*	0.06	Rifampin	*Pediococcus*	0.25 (2) - 0.5 - 2
	Leuconostoc	0.03		*Leuconostoc*	0.5 - 1 - 2
	Lactobacillus	0.015		*Lactobacillus*	0.12 - 0.5 -32
Azithromycin	*Pediococcus*	0.12	Ciprofloxacin	*Pediococcus*	> 4-8-16-32
	Leuconostoc	0,12		*Leuconostoc*	1-2-4
	Lactobacillus	0.06		*Lactobacillus*	0.5 - 1 - 2 - 4 - 8
Lincomycin	*Pediococcus*	0.5	Ofloxacin	*Pediococcus*	> 8-16
	Leuconostoc	-		*Leuconostoc*	-
	Lactobacillus	-		*Lactobacillus*	-
Clindamycin	*Pediococcus*	0.015 (2) - < 0.06 - < 0.25	Levofloxacin	*Pediococcus*	8
	Leuconostoc	0.015 - 0.03		*Leuconostoc*	4
	Lactobacillus	0.03 - 0.06 - 0.25 (2)		*Lactobacillus*	1-4
Telithromycin	*Pediococcus*	0.007	Pefloxacin	*Pediococcus*	-
	Leuconostoc	0.007		*Leuconostoc*	32
	Lactobacillus	0.007		*Lactobacillus*	-
Pristinamycin	*Pediococcus*	0.25	Moxifloxacin	*Pediococcus*	-
	Leuconostoc	-		*Leuconostoc*	0.25
	Lactobacillus	-		*Lactobacillus*	0.25
Quinupristin-dalfopristin	*Pediococcus*	0.5	Trimethoprim	*Pediococcus*	8
	Leuconostoc	2		*Leuconostoc*	4
	Lactobacillus	0.25 (2) - 2		*Lactobacillus*	16
Tetracycline	*Pediococcus*	16 (2) - 32	Sulfonamides	*Pediococcus*	> 512
	Leuconostoc	2-4		*Leuconostoc*	> 512-1024
	Lactobacillus	1 (2) - 16		*Lactobacillus*	> 128->512
Minocycline	*Pediococcus*	2-4-8	Trimethoprim-sulfamethoxazole	*Pediococcus*	2-> 8
	Leuconostoc	1 (2)		*Leuconostoc*	1-2
	Lactobacillus	2		*Lactobacillus*	16-32
Doxycycline	*Pediococcus*	8 (2)	Fosfomycin	*Pediococcus*	-
	Leuconostoc	4		*Leuconostoc*	> 2048
	Lactobacillus	0.25 - 8		*Lactobacillus*	-
			Metronidazole	*Pediococcus*	-
				Leuconostoc	-
				Lactobacillus	> 128

[a] From references 2, 4, 5, 7, 8, 9, 10, 12, 15, 16, 17, 20, 21, 22, 27, and 28.
Numbers in parentheses indicate the number of studies reporting similar values.

the incubation carried out under an anaerobic atmosphere, but another important difference concerned the medium used, which was Lactic acid bacteria Susceptibility test Medium (LSM). This medium was recently developed for antimicrobial susceptibility testing in lactobacilli used in the food industry or as probiotics (11). It was developed because some lactobacillus strains grow poorly or not at all on Mueller-Hinton broth supplemented with lysed blood in an aerobic atmosphere. LSM medium is a mixture of 90% IsoSensiTest broth (IST, Oxoid) and 10% DeMan-Rogosa-Sharpe broth (MRS). It enables good aerobic growth of all strains of lactobacilli, *Pediococcus* and *Leuconostoc*. Since some strains require cysteine, two formulations exist, with or without 0.3 µg/ml L-cysteine hydrochloride.

Can the results obtained by broth microdilution in LSM medium be extrapolated to those obtained in Mueller-Hinton medium supplemented with lysed horse blood? According to the results of Klare et al. (11), the answer is yes. MICs obtained with these two media were very similar; only the MICs of penicillin G were one or two dilutions lower with LSM medium. Furthermore, MICs obtained with LSM medium with or without cysteine showed very good agreement (11).

It may therefore be concluded that the broth microdilution method in Mueller-Hinton medium supplemented with lysed horse blood is the routine reference method for clinical isolates, but that E-test® can be used as an alternative to microdilution and LSM medium as an alternative to supplemented Mueller-Hinton medium.

SUSCEPTIBLE PHENOTYPE

Pediococcus

Almost all the data come from the two medically relevant species, *P. acidilactici* and *P. pentosaceus* (10, 12, 15, 17, 21, 22, 27, 28). Penicillin G, ampicillin, piperacillin and imipenem have moderate *in vitro* activity against *Pediococcus* and are not bactericidal (Table 3) (22). Ticarcillin and all the cephalosporins are basically inactive. However, some agents with low activity, such as ticarcillin or cefotaxime, have been observed to give large inhibition zones (22). This can probably be explained by an imbalance between the diffusion rate of the antibiotic in agar and the slow growth rate of these bacteria. The same is probably true for *Leuconostoc* and lactobacilli. These observations are consistent with the CLSI's recommendation against the use of the disk diffusion method for lactic acid bacteria.

Gentamicin and netilmicin have moderate activity which is nonetheless higher than against streptococci and enterococci. Other aminoglycosides (streptomycin, kanamycin, tobramycin, amikacin) are less active. There are no data on the *in vitro* activity of penicillin/aminoglycoside combinations against *Pediococcus*.

These bacteria display intrinsic high-level resistance to the glycopeptides vancomycin and teicoplanin. The MICs of macrolides and lincosamides are very low, while those of ketolides and especially telithromycin are even lower. Intrinsic resistance to pristinamycin factor A is also observed, but the synergy between the two factors is conserved, hence the susceptibility to pristinamycin and quinupristin-dalfopristin (12, 15, 22).

Rifampin and chloramphenicol are moderately active. While intrinsic resistance to sulfonamides is observed, these bacteria are intermediately susceptible to trimethoprim and trimethoprim-sulfamethoxazole. Tetracyclines are inactive, and this is specific to *Pediococcus* among the lactic acid bacteria. There is also intrinsic resistance to fosfomycin and fusidic acid. The fluoroquinolones ciprofloxacin and levofloxacin have poor activity, while moxifloxacin is somewhat more active (MICs of 0.25-2 µg/ml) (15).

Among the new agents active against Gram-positive species, daptomycin and linezolid show good activity (10, 12, 15, 21). Novobiocin is useful for differentiating between *P. acidilactici* which is susceptible, and *P. pentosaceus* which is resistant (22).

Leuconostoc

The antibiotic susceptibility pattern of *Leuconostoc* is very similar to that of *Pediococcus* with, in particular, intrinsic glycopeptide resistance and moderate activity of penicillin G with absence of a bactericidal effect (2, 7, 9, 15, 21, 27, 28). Synergistic bactericidal activity between penicillin G and streptomycin or gentamicin was observed *in vitro* in six of eight strains studied (2).

Nonetheless several important differences exist:

1. Imipenem has low activity (MIC_{50} 2 µg/ml).

2. As opposed to *Pediococcus*, *Leuconostoc* have higher susceptibility to aminoglycosides and particularly gentamicin: gentamicin $MIC_{50} \leq 0.25$ µg/ml (21). As in the case of *Pediococcus*, gentamicin and netilmicin are the most active aminoglycosides.

3. *Leuconostoc* are susceptible to tetracyclines, with minocycline showing the highest activity.

4. *Leuconostoc* are more susceptible to fluoroquinolones than *Pediococcus* (15).

5. On the other hand they are less susceptible to linezolid (15).

Lactobacilli

The heterofermentative species (*L. brevis, L. casei, L. confusus, L. fermentum, L. paracasei, L. plantarum, L. reuteri* and *L. rhamnosus*), which represent the most common human pathogens, have intrinsic high-level resistance to glycopeptides, whereas the obligate homofermentative species (*L. acidophilus, L. amylovorus, L. crispatus, L. gasseri, L. jensenii* and *L. salivarius*) are susceptible (4, 5, 7, 10, 12, 15, 16, 20, 21, 27, 28).

As far as other antibiotics are concerned, several authors have found differences in susceptibility among different lactobacillus species, notably with respect to β-lactams, fluoroquinolones, tetracyclines, rifampin and daptomycin. However the data tend to be conflicting, obscuring any potential differences that might exist between species. Hence the need to systematically test the antibiotic susceptibility of each strain.

Like *Pediococcus*, the lactobacilli are moderately susceptible to penicillin G, amoxicillin and imipenem, with absence of a bactericidal effect, and not susceptible to cephalosporins.

However, a study by Zarazaga et al. (28) reported higher level resistance for the species *L. plantarum*: the MIC_{50} of penicillin G was 8 µg/ml as compared to 0.5 µg/ml for other species. These authors even found *L. plantarum* isolates with penicillin G MICs > 64 µg/ml, although it is not known if this resistance is intrinsic or acquired. It should be noted that this high-level resistance has not been confirmed in other studies. More recent data suggest that *L. plantarum* as well as *L. reuteri* are intrinsically less susceptible to penicillin G than other lactobacillus species, with MICs as high as 8 or even 16 µg/ml in certain strains (12, 20).

Aminoglycosides and particularly gentamicin have similar activity against lactobacilli and *Pediococcus*, although higher MICs were reported in two studies (MIC_{50}: 16 and 8 µg/ml) (4, 5). In the study reporting the highest MICs, this was probably related to the test conditions: anaerobic atmosphere, high inoculum (suspension equivalent to a 1 McFarland standard) and a rich medium (MRS, suitable for culturing lactic acid bacteria but not for antibiotic susceptibility testing) (4). In the other study, a more reliable medium was used (Mueller-Hinton with 5% sheep blood) but the incubation was carried out in a CO_2-enriched atmosphere (5).

Bactericidal synergy between β-lactams and aminoglycosides has been demonstrated *in vitro* by the checkerboard method and time-kill experiments, and *in vivo* in a rabbit endocarditis model (8).

Macrolides and clindamycin are very active. As in the case of *Pediococcus* and *Leuconostoc*, the ketolides and particularly telithromycin appear to be even more active (28). Quinupristin-dalfopristin is also active (15).

Lactobacilli are also susceptible to tetracyclines and rifampin, although high MICs have been reported for these agents in *L. plantarum* (4) and for rifampin in *L. confusus* (21).

The activity of fluoroquinolones such as ciprofloxacin and levofloxacin is highly variable according to strain or species. This variability might be due to the existence of acquired resistance in certain strains, but this has not been investigated. Moxifloxacin is more active than the older fluoroquinolones (MIC_{50} 0.25 µg/ml) (15).

Lactobacilli are resistant to fosfomycin, fusidic acid, trimethoprim/sulfamethoxazole and metronidazole. However, metronidazole susceptibility has been reported in some lactobacillus isolates.

Lactobacilli are also susceptible to daptomycin (10, 21), although one study reported high MICs of 0.5-8 µg/ml with an MIC_{50} of 4 µg/ml (7). Daptomycin has bactericidal activity and daptomycin/gentamicin exhibit bactericidal synergy (8). Linezolid was found to be active in one study (MIC_{50} 1 µg/ml) although another study reported higher MICs (MIC_{50} 4-8 µg/ml) (7).

Erysipelothrix rhusiopathiae

Penicillin G is very active against *Erysipelothrix rhusiopathiae* (MIC ≤ 0.06 µg/ml) and is also bactericidal (25). This is the drug of first choice for infections caused by this organism, particularly endocarditis. *Erysipelothrix* is also highly susceptible to third generation cephalosporins such as cefotaxime or ceftriaxone, as well as to ciprofloxacin (MIC_{90} 0.06 µg/ml). It is also susceptible to macrolides-lincosamides-streptogramins (MLS), tetracyclines and chloramphenicol. On the other hand, it is intrinsically resistant to aminoglycosides, glycopeptides, sulfonamides and trimethoprim.

RESISTANCE PHENOTYPES

Pediococcus

There are no reports of acquired resistance to penicillin G or imipenem, with a single exception: Yamane and Jones (27) described strains having high MICs of penicillin G (> 16 µg/ml) and imipenem (> 8 µg/ml). These data require confirmation.

A single strain with acquired aminoglycoside resistance has been reported (21). This resistance only concerned streptomycin and the MIC was 2,000 µg/ml.

On the other hand, acquired resistance to macrolides-lincosamides has been described by most authors, albeit at a low frequency. Acquired resistance to quinupristin-dalfopristin has also been observed (15).

Leuconostoc

Three gentamicin-resistant clinical isolates have been reported (MIC 16 µg/ml in two strains, MIC not specified in one case) (9).

Acquired resistance to clindamycin, quinupristin-dalfopristin, cotrimoxazole and fluoroquinolones has also been described (15, 28).

Lactobacillus

An L. rhamnosus isolate with unusually high oxacillin resistance (MIC 32 µg/ml versus 0.58 µg/ml) has been described (4). As noted earlier, high MICs of penicillin G have been noted in some isolates (28), although the existence of acquired resistance to β-lactams in lactobacilli remains to be established.

Strains resistant to streptomycin, macrolides, lincosamides, chloramphenicol, tetracyclines and fluoroquinolones have also been described in different species.

Erysipelothrix rhusiopathiae

Acquired resistance to macrolides, lincosamides, tetracyclines and chloramphenicol has been described (25, 26), but to date there have been no reports of penicillin G resistance.

RESISTANCE MECHANISMS

Lactic acid bacteria

Intrinsic resistance to glycopeptides in *Pediococcus*, *Leuconostoc* and heterofermentative lactobacilli is due to the presence of a late peptidoglycan precursor (UDP-N-acetylmuramyl-pentadepsipeptide) which has only very low affinity for glycopeptides (1). This precursor terminates in D-alanine-D-lactate instead of the usual D-alanine-D-alanine dipeptide, as also seen in acquired glycopeptide resistance in enterococci due to the VanA, VanB and VanD determinants.

Several studies have examined the determinants of resistance to the MLS group, tetracyclines and phenicols in lactobacilli. *erm* genes encoding an rRNA methylase carried on plasmids less than a 20-kb in size have been detected in several MLS-resistant strains (6, 13, 23). These determinants belong to the *erm*(AM) class originally described in *Streptococcus sanguinis* and widely disseminated among streptococci and enterococci. One study detected a determinant with strong homology to *erm*(C) (23). A strain with cross-resistance to macrolides and quinupristin-dalfopristin was found to harbor a 19-kb plasmid encoding an *erm* gene and a *vat*(E) gene coding for a streptogramin A acetyltransferase identical to that in *Enterococcus faecium* (6). Tetracycline resistance is due to the presence of the ribosomal protection determinants *tet*(M) and *tet*(O) (6, 19). A 7-kb plasmid harboring a *cat*(C) gene encoding a Cat-A9 type chloramphenicol acetyltransferase, very similar to that of the staphylococcal plasmid pC194, was found in a chloramphenicol-resistant isolate of *L. reuteri* (14).

A *P. acidilactici* isolate with inducible, non-transferable MLS resistance has been described (22). The determinant, carried on a 46-kb plasmid, is homologous to the *erm*(AM) gene. In another macrolide-resistant strain of *P. acidilactici*, resistance was found to be mediated by a non-conjugative 60-kb plasmid but the gene was not characterized (24). The constant and apparently intrinsic resistance of *Pediococcus* to tetracyclines has yet to be explained; it does not appear to be mediated by any known resistance determinant.

Erysipelothrix rhusiopathiae

For the most part, tetracycline resistance is due to the presence of the *tet*(M) determinant which shows 99% identity to that originally described in *E. faecalis* (26).

ANTIBIOTICS TO BE STUDIED

Standard antibiogram

Lactic acid bacteria

Penicillin G
Ampicillin or amoxicillin

Imipenem
Gentamicin
Erythromycin
Lincomycin or clindamycin
Vancomycin
Novobiocin (for identification of *Pediococcus*)

Erysipelothrix

Penicillin G
Ampicillin or amoxicillin
Cefotaxime
Imipenem
Erythromycin
Lincomycin or clindamycin
Ciprofloxacin
Vancomycin (for identification)

Additional list

Lactic acid bacteria

Pristinamycin
Quinupristin-Dalfopristin
Telithromycin
Chloramphenicol
Tetracycline
Rifampin
Ciprofloxacin
Linezolid
Daptomycin

Erysipelothrix

Pristinamycin
Tetracycline
Chloramphenicol

REFERENCES

(1) **Billot-Klein, D., L. Gutmann, S. Sablé, E. Guittet, and J. van Heijenoort.** 1994. Modification of peptidoglycan precursors is a common feature of the low-level vancomycin-resistant VANB-type *Enterococcus* D366 and of the naturally glycopeptide-resistant species *Lactobacillus casei*, *Pediococcus pentosaceus*, *Leuconostoc mesenteroides*, and *Enterococcus gallinarum*. J. Bacteriol. **176:**2398-2405.

(2) **Buu-Hoï, A., C. Branger, and J.F. Acar.** 1985. Vancomycin-resistant streptococci or *Leuconostoc* sp. Antimicrob. Agents Chemother. **28:**458-460.

(3) **Clinical and Laboratory Standards Institute.** 2006. Methods for antimicrobial dilution and disk susceptibility testing of infrequently isolated or fastidious bacteria. Approved standard M45-A. Clinical and Laboratory Standards Institute, Wayne, PA

(4) **Danielsen, M., and A. Wind.** 2003. Susceptibility of *Lactobacillus* spp. to antimicrobial agents. Int. J. Food Microbiol. **82:**1-11.

(5) **Felten, A., C. Barreau, C. Bizet, P.H. Lagrange, and A. Philippon.** 1999. *Lactobacillus* species identification, H_2O_2 production, and antibiotic resistance and correlation with human clinical status. J. Clin. Microbiol. **37:**729-733.

(6) **Gfeller, K.Y., M. Roth, L. Meile, and M. Teuber.** 2003. Sequence and genetic organization of the 19.3-kb erythromycin- and dalfopristin-resistance plasmid pLME300 from *Lactobacillus fermentum* ROT1. Plasmid **50:**190-201.

(7) **Goldstein, E.J.C., D.M. Citron, C.V. Merriam, Y.A. Warren, K.L. Tyrrell, and H.T. Fernandez.** 2004. In vitro activities of the new semisynthetic glycopeptide telavancin (TD-6424), vancomycin, teicoplanin, daptomycin, linezolid, and four comparator agents against anaerobic gram-positive species and *Corynebacterium* spp. Antimicrob. Agents Chemother. **48:**2149-2152.

(8) **Griffiths, J.K., J.S. Daly, and R.A. Dodge.** 1992. Two cases of endocarditis due to *Lactobacillus* species: Antimicrobial susceptibility, review, and discussion of therapy. Clin. Infect. Dis. **15:** 250-255.

(9) **Handwerger, S., H. Horowitz, K. Coburn, A. Kolokathis, and G.P. Wormser.** 1990. Infection due to *Leuconostoc* species: Six cases and review. Rev. Infect. Dis. **12:**602-610.

(10) **King, A, and I. Phillips.** 2001. The *in vitro* activity of daptomycin against 514 Gram-positive aerobic clinical isolates. J. Antimicrob. Chemother. **48:**219-223.

(11) **Klare, I., C. Konstabel, S. Müller-Bertling, R. Reissbrodt, G. Huys, M. Vancanneyt, J. Swings, H. Goossens, and W. Witte.** 2005. Evaluation of new broth media for microdilution antibiotic susceptibility testing of lactobacilli, pediococci, lactococci, and bifidobacteria. Appl. Environ. Microbiol. **71:**8982-8986.

(12) **Klare, I., C. Konstabel, G. Werner, G. Huys, V. Vankerckhoven, G. Kahlmeter, B. Hildebrandt, S. Müller-Bertling, W. Witte, and H. Goossens.** 2007. Antimicrobial susceptibilities of *Lactobacillus*, *Pediococcus*, and *Lactococcus* human isolates and cultures intended for probiotic or nutritional use. J. Antimicrob. Chemother. **59:**900-912.

(13) **Lin, C.F., and T.C. Chung.** 1999. Cloning of erythromycin-resistance determinants and replication origins from indigenous plasmids of *Lactobacillus reuteri* for potential use in construction of cloning vectors. Plasmid **42:**31-41.

(14) **Lin, C.F., Z.F. Fung, C.L. Wu, and T.C. Chung.** 1996. Molecular characterization of a plasmid-borne (pTC82) chloramphenicol resistance determinant (*cat-TC*) from *Lactobacillus reuteri* G4. Plasmid **36:**116-124.

(15) **Luh, K.-T., P.-R. Hsueh, L.-J. Teng, H.-J. Pan, Y.-C. Chen, J.-J. Lu, J.-J. Wu, and S.-W. Ho.** 2000. Quinupristin-dalfopristin resistance among gram-positive bacteria in Taiwan. Antimicrob. Agents Chemother. **44:**3374-3380.

(16) **Mändar, R., K. Loivukene, P. Hütt, T. Karki, and M. Mikelsaar.** 2001. Antibacterial susceptibility of intestinal lactobacilli of healthy children. Scand. J. Infect. Dis. **33:** 344-349.

(17) **Maugein, J., P. Crouzit, P. Cony Makhoul, and J. Fourche.** 1992. Characterization and antibiotic susceptibility of *Pediococcus acidilactici* strains isolated from neutropenic patients. Eur. J. Clin. Microbiol. Infect. Dis. **11**:383-385.

(18) **Mayrhofer, S., K.J. Domig, C. Mair, U. Zitz, G. Huys, and W. Kneifel.** 2008. Comparison of broth microdilution, E-test, and agar disk diffusion methods for antimicrobial susceptibility testing of *Lactobacillus acidophilus* group members. Appl. Environ. Microbiol. **74**: 3745-3748.

(19) **Robert, M.C., and S.L. Hillier.** 1990. Genetic basis of tetracycline resistance in urogenital bacteria. Antimicrob. Agents Chemother. **34**:261-264.

(20) **Salminen, M.K., H. Rautelin, S. Tynkkynen, T. Poussa, M. Saxelin, V. Valtonen, and A. Jarvinen.** 2006. *Lactobacillus* bacteremia, species identification, and antimicrobial susceptibility of 85 blood isolates. Clin. Infect. Dis. **42**:e35-e44

(21) **Swenson, J.M., R.R. Facklam, and C. Thornsberry.** 1990. Antimicrobial susceptibility of vancomycin-resistant *Leuconostoc*, *Pediococcus*, and *Lactobacillus* species. Antimicrob. Agents Chemother. **34**:543-549.

(22) **Tankovic, J., R. Leclercq, and J. Duval.** 1993. Antimicrobial susceptibility of *Pediococcus* spp. and genetic basis of macrolide resistance in *Pediococcus acidilactici* HM3020. Antimicrob. Agents Chemother. **37**:789-792.

(23) **Tannock, G.W., J.B. Luchansky, L. Miller, H. Connell, S. Thode-Andersen, A.A. Mercer, and T.R. Klaenhammer.** 1994. Molecular characterization of a plasmid-borne (pGT633) erythromycin resistance determinant (*ermGT*) from *Lactobacillus reuteri* 100-63. Plasmid **31**:60-71.

(24) **, S., M. Vescovo, and F. Dellaglio.** 1987. Tracing *Pediococcus acidilactici* in ensiled maize by plasmid-encoded erythromycin resistance. J. Appl. Microbiol. **63**:305-309.

(25) **Venditti, M., V. Gelfusa, A. Tarasi, C. Brandimarte, and P. Serra.** 1990. Antimicrobial susceptibilities of *Erysipelothrix rhusiopathiae*. Antimicrob. Agents Chemother. **34**:2038-2040.

(26) **Yamamoto, K., Y. Sasaki, Y. Ogikubo, N. Noguchi, M. Sasatsu, and T. Takahashi.** 2001. Identification of the tetracycline resistance gene, *tet*(M), in *Erysipelothrix rhusiopathiae*. J. Vet. Med. B. Infect. Dis. Vet. Public Health. **48**:293-301.

(27) **Yamane, N., and R.N. Jones.** 1991. In vitro activity of 43 antimicrobial agents tested against ampicillin-resistant enterococci and gram-positive species resistant to vancomycin. Diagn. Microbiol. Infect. Dis. **14**:337-345.

(28) **Zarazaga, M., Y. Saenz, A. Portillo, C. Tenorio, F. Ruiz-Larrea, R. Del Campo, F. Baquero, and C. Torres.** 1999. In vitro activities of ketolide HMR3647, macrolides, and other antibiotics against *Lactobacillus*, *Leuconostoc*, and *Pediococcus* isolates. Antimicrob. Agents Chemother. **43**:3039-3041.

Chapter 32. *ACINETOBACTER* AND β-LACTAMS

Thierry NAAS and Patrice NORDMANN

INTRODUCTION

Acinetobacter spp. are non-motile Gram-negative coccobacilli. The genus known as *Acinetobacter* has undergone significant taxonomic modification and over thirty genomic species have been identified to date. Its most important representative, *Acinetobacter baumannii*, has emerged as one of the most troublesome pathogens for health care institutions. This organism infects mostly immuno-compromised patients, those who are critically ill with breaches in skin integrity and under mechanical ventilaion. Hospital acquired pneumonia is the most common infection caused by this organism. However, infections involving the central nervous system, skin and soft tissue, and bone are increasingly reported (1, 8, 13, 20, 21, 27).

Antimicrobial resistance among *Acinetobacter* spp. has increased substantially in the past two decades (11, 20-22, 24). The ability of *Acinetobacter* spp. for extensive antimicrobial resistance may be due in part to the organism's relatively impermeable outer membrane and its remarkable ability to accumulate resistance mechanisms, in particular to b-lactams (penicillins, cephalosporins, and carbapenems), tetracyclines, aminoglycosides, and fluoroquinolones (20, 30). A recent comparative genomic study of an epidemic, multidrug-resistant *Acinetobacter* strain identified a large 86-kb genomic "resistance island" containing 45 resistance genes that appeared to have been acquired from *Pseudomonas*, *Salmonella*, or *Escherichia coli* (7).

Outbreaks of *A. baumannii* have been reported worldwide, mainly in intensive care units (ICUs) and involve multidrug-resistant (MDR) isolates for which very few (if any) antibiotic molecules retain significant antibacterial activity. Definitions of MDR *Acinetobacter* vary, referring to a wide array of resistance genotypes and phenotypes (20). Two of the most common definitions of MDR are either resistance to carbapenems or resistance to at least three classes of antimicrobials (20). MDR may be defined (as in our hospital) as resistance to at least two of the following four drug classes: ticarcillin, carbapenems (imipenem or meropenem), fluoroquinolones (ciprofloxacin or levofloxacin), or aminoglycosides (gentamicin or amikacin). Some strains are susceptible only to polymyxins that are not routinely used because of earlier reports about toxicity and pharmacokinetic diffusion limited to blood. Strains resistant to all antimicrobial agents, including polymyxins, may lead to therapeutic dead ends (5, 10, 11, 19).

The resistance mechanisms generally fall into 3 categories: (i) antimicrobial-inactivating enzymes, (ii) reduced access to bacterial targets, or (iii) mutations that alter targets or cellular functions (20, 21, 30). Resistance to β-lactams is related mostly to the production of β-lactamases, whereas alterations of outer-membrane permeability, modification of penicillin-binding proteins, and increased activity of efflux pumps play a secondary role (30).

EPIDEMIOLOGY

The natural reservoir of *A. baumannii* remains to be determined. Nevertheless, it is found in many health care environments and is a very effective human colonizer in the hospital. The combination of its environmental persistence and its wide range of resistances makes it a successful nosocomial pathogen (20). *A. baumannii* is thus emerging as a cause of numerous global outbreaks, displaying ever-increasing rates of resistance (11, 20, 21). There are reports of MDR *A. baumannii* from hospitals in Europe, North America, Argentina, Brazil, China, Taiwan, Hong Kong, Japan, and Korea and from areas as remote as Tahiti or New Caledonia in the South Pacific (14, 16, 20, 21). These MDR strains may be the source of outbreaks throughout cities, countries, and continents (16). The import of MDR strains from areas with high rates of resistance to areas with historically low rates is increasingly documented.

The epidemic MDR *A. baumannii* are usually resistant to all β-lactams, to fluoroquinolones (chromosomal), to aminoglycosides (aminoglycoside inactivating enzymes or 16S rRNA methylases [4, 18, 28]), and remain susceptible only to few antibiotics, such as colistin, tigecycline, and rifampin. However resistance to the latter antibiotics is increasingly reported, leaving almost no therapeutic options (11, 16, 21).

METHODS

The US and European organizations that determine breakpoints, the Clinical and Laboratory Standards Institute [CLSI; (2)] and the European Committee on Antimicrobial Susceptibility Testing [EUCAST; http://www.srga.org/eucastwt/MICTAB/index.html; May 2009]) have set different breakpoints for antibiotics used for therapy of *A. baumannii* infections (Table 1). Up to May 2009, no EUCAST breakpoints existed for penicillins + β-lactamase inhibitor combinations, considering that there was insufficient evidence that *A. baumannii* is a good target for therapy with these drugs and for cephalosporins, rifampin, and tetracyclines. Breakpoints for tigecycline are only available via the British Society for Antimicrobial Chemotherapy (BSAC; http://www.bsac.org.uk/ db/ documents/Version 8 - January 2009.pdf; January 2009) and for rifampin via the Comité de l'Antibiogramme de la Société Française de Microbiologie (SFM; http://www.sfm.asso.fr/publi/general.php?pa=1; January 2009).

CLSI, EUCAST, CA-SFM, and BSAC recommend that MICs of antibiotics *versus Acinetobacter* spp. be determined in broth, using cation-adjusted Mueller-Hinton broth, or on Mueller-Hinton agar. However, there are discrepancies between the results obtained by broth microdilution and disk diffusion (20). Susceptibility by disk diffusion and resistance by broth microdilution has been observed for ampicillin-sulbactam, piperacillin, piperacillin-tazobactam, ticarcillin-clavulanate, ceftazidime, and cefepime. In the absence of human or animal model data, it is impossible to determine which testing method is more clinically relevant. CLSI guidelines for testing piperacillin-tazobactam and ticarcillin-clavulanic acid require fixed concentrations of 4 μg/ml (tazobactam) and 2 μg/ml (clavulanic acid) (2).

Semi-automated methods, such as Vitek 2 (bioMérieux), Microscan (Dade Behring Inc.), and BD Phoenix systems (Becton Dickinson), are commonly used by clinical microbiology laboratories. Unfortunately, there is limited information about the performance of these methods for *A. baumannii*. Nevertheless, the Vitek 2 and BD Phoenix are reliable compared to reference broth microdilution for assessing susceptibility of *A. baumannii* to imipenem and other commonly used antibiotics (20). However, it has been suggested to perform routinely an "all-in-one plate" in which susceptibility to imipenem or meropenem is confirmed by disk diffusion or by E-test® (Fig 1D) and the MIC of colistin is determined on the same plate by E-test® (Fig 1B).

Susceptibility testing of the polymyxins and tigecycline against *A. baumannii* requires special attention since these antibiotics are often used for serious infections due to MDR *A. baumannii* (5, 10, 11, 12).

The CLSI and EUCAST have no established breakpoints for interpretation of susceptibility testing to tigecycline (Table 1). This is partially due to discrepancies in MICs obtained using different methods. Tigecycline susceptibility testing according to several studies seems to be most reliable by microdilution using freshly prepared medium (12-h old) (10). The reliability of disk diffusion or E-test® is still debated (10). While, in some studies, MIC values determined by E-test® were typically fourfold higher than those by broth microdilution, others have found good correlation between E-test® *versus* reference broth microdilution (Fig 1A). The usefulness of automated systems for susceptibility testing of *A. baumannii* and tigecycline has not yet been reported. EUCAST indicates that "there is insufficient evidence that the species in question is a good target for therapy with the drug" (Table 1) (20). Since the mean maximum blood concentration of tigecycline is 0.63 μg/ml after administration of a 100-mg intravenous loading dose followed by 50 mg every 12 h, it would seem prudent not to report bloodstream isolates of *A. baumannii* with tigecycline MICs of 0.5 μg/ml as susceptible (10). The BSAC has established tentative tigecycline breakpoints for *Acinetobacter* spp.: MICs < 1 μg/ml, susceptible; MIC 2 μg/ml, intermediate; and MICs > 2 g/ml, resistant (http://www.bsac.org.uk/ db/ documents/Version 8 - January 2009.pdf). Pending further information, we recommend using these breakpoints for infection sites other than blood.

Testing of *A. baumannii* susceptibility to colistin or polymyxin B should be performed by determination of the MIC, by broth microdilution or E-test® (5, 20) (Fig 1B). Although the agreement between MICs obtained by E-test® and broth microdilution is rather low, within one twofold dilution, clinical categorisationl concordance is 87% to 95%. In an evaluation, there was 100% category agreement between agar dilution and Vitek 2 testing for colistin susceptibility but no colistin-resistant isolates were tested (10, 20). Inherent properties of the polymyxins make disk diffusion testing difficult and not recommended for assessing susceptibility of *A. baumannii* (10, 20).

Rifampin has excellent efficacy in different animal models in combination with other antimicrobials. Its use as monotherapy in animal models,

Table 1. Comparison of EUCAST, CLSI, CA-SFM, and BSAC breakpoints (μg/ml) for various antibiotics versus *Acinetobacter* spp.

Antibiotic	Breakpoints for susceptibility / resistance (μp/ml)			
	EUCAST[a] S≤/>R	CLSI[b] S≤/≥R	CA-SFM[a] S≤/>R	BSAC[a] S≤/>R
Imipenem	2/8	4/16	2/8	2/8
Meropenem	2/8	4/16	2/8	2/8
Doripenem	1/4	-[c]	1/4	1/4
Ciprofloxacin	1/1	1/4	1/2	1/1
Levofloxacin	1/2	2/8	1/2	-
Amikacin	8/16	16/64	8/16	-
Gentamicin	4/4	4/16	4/4	4/4
Tobramycin	4/4	4/16	4/4	-
Netilmicin	4/4	8/32	4/4	-
Ampicillin-sulbactam[d]	IE[e]	8/32	≤ 8	-
Piperacillin-tazobactam[d]	IE	16/128	16/64	16/16
Ticarcillin-clavulanate[d]	IE	16/128	16/64	-
Ceftazidime, cefepime	--[f]	8/32	4/8	-
Ceftriaxone, cefotaxime	--	8/64	-	-
Polymyxin B, colistin	2/2	2/2	2/2	-
Rifampin	--	-	4/16	-
Trimethoprim-sulfamethoxazole[g]	2/4	2/4	2/4	-
Doxycycline, tetracycline	--	4/16	-	-
Minocycline,	IE	4/16	-	-
Tigecycline	IE	-	-	1/2

[a] For EUCAST (http://www.srga.org/eucastwt/MICTAB/index.html; May 2009), SFM (http://www.sfm.asso.fr/publi/general.php?pa=1; January 2009) and BSAC (http://www.bsac.org.uk/_db/_documents/Version_8_-_January_2009.pdf; January 2009) breakpoints, susceptibility is defined by a MIC equal to or lower than the first number and resistance is defined by a MIC greater than the second number.
[b] For CLSI (2) breakpoints, susceptibility is defined by a MIC equal to or lower than the first number and resistance is defined by a MIC equal to or greater than the second number.
[c] "-" No indication
[d] Sulbactam, tazobactam, and clavulanate at fixed concentration of 8, 4, 2 μg/ml, respectively.
[e] IE, There is insufficient evidence that the species in question is a good target for therapy with the drug.
[f] --, Susceptibility testing not recommended as the species is a poor target for therapy with the drug.
[g] Trimethoprim:sulfamethoxazole in the ratio 1:19. Breakpoints are expressed as the trimethoprim concentration.

although effective, is limited by the potential emergence of resistance during treatment (21). The CA-SFM has established rifampin breakpoints for *Acinetobacter* spp. MICs of =<4 μg/ml, susceptible and MICs of >16 g/ml, resistant. Testing of *A. baumannii* susceptibility to rifampin should be performed by determination of the MIC, such as by broth microdilution or E-test® (Fig 1C).

SUSCEPTIBLE PHENOTYPE

Back in the 70s, *Acinetobacter* isolates were reported to be susceptible to all β-lactams except penicillin G (1). This wild-type phenotype may still be observed for *Acinetobacter* species other than *A. baumannii*. The strains termed "susceptible" produce at low level a non-inducible chromosomally encoded AmpC cephalosporinase (20, 21, 22) also known as *Acinetobacter*-derived cephalosporinase (ADCs) (9) (Fig. 2A). This enzyme hydrolyses first and second generation cephalosporins, amoxicillin, and is not inhibited by classical inhibitors such as clavulanic acid. Moxalactam and aztreonam have a reduced activity (MIC from 8 to 32 μg/ml) and mecillinam is inactive. This resistance profile is observed for all *Acinetobacter* with, however, differences in the MICs likely due to differences in AmpC enzymes and their level of expression. In addition *Acinetobacter* is resistant at low level to trimethoprim (MIC of 16-32 μg/ml) and to fosfomycin (Fig. 2B).

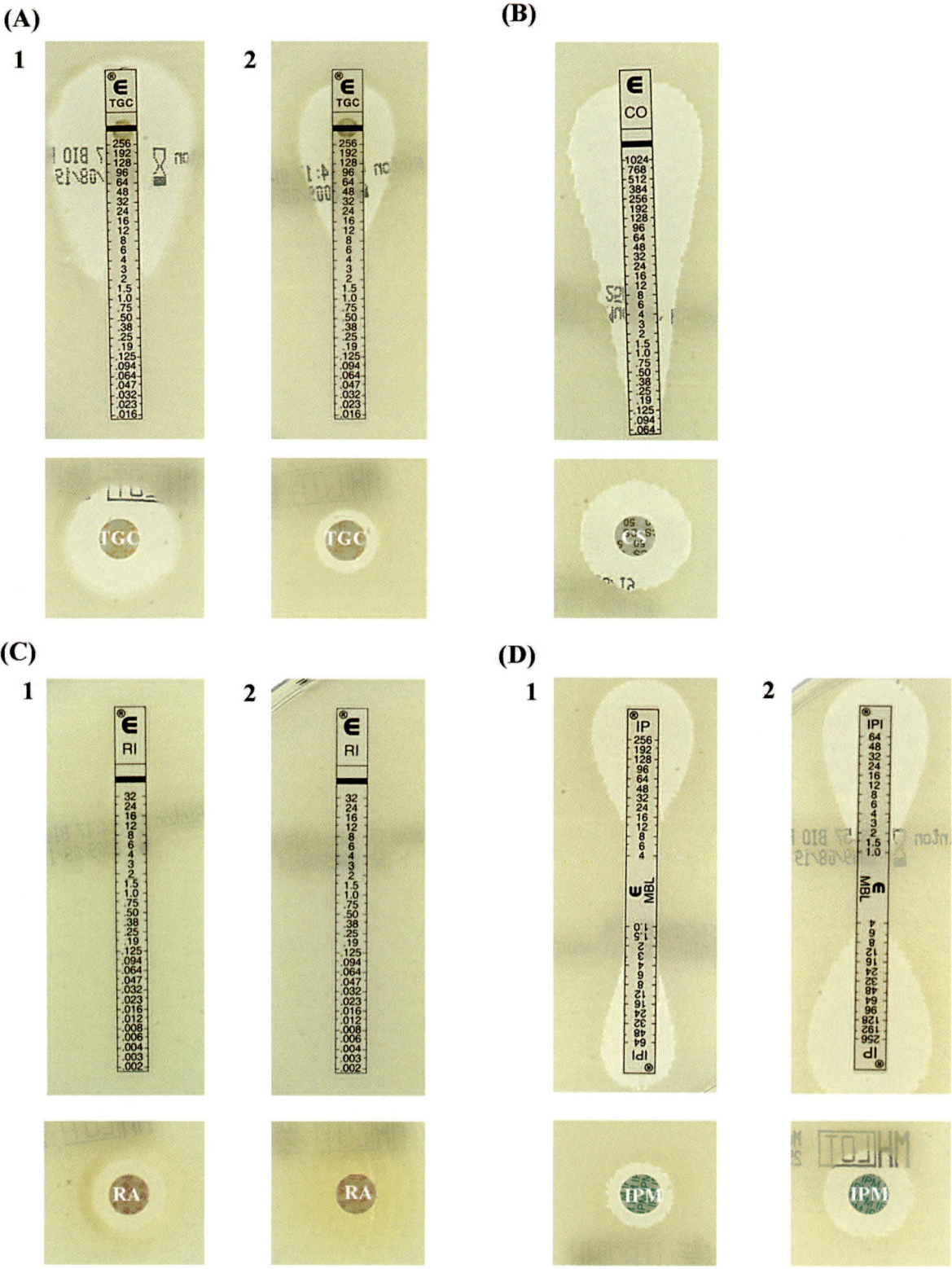

Fig. 1: Disk diffusion and E-test®. **(A)** for tigecycline. (1) *A. baumannii* susceptible; (2) *A. baumannii* over-expressing the AdeABC efflux pump. **(B)** for colistin. (C) for rifampin. (1) *A. baumannii* AYE producing the Arr-2 rifampin ADP ribosylating transferase; (2) *A. baumannii* with an *rpoB* mutation. (D) for imipenem. (1) OXA-23 producer; (2) IMP-4 producer. EDTA inhibition is not always obvious since EDTA may have an intrinsic inhibitory activity against *A. baumannii*, in particular on OXA-23-producers.

Chapter 32. *ACINETOBACTER* AND β-LACTAMS

Table 2. Mechanisms of resistance to β-lactams in *A. baumannii* (from 4, 10, 17, 20, 22, 26, 30, 31)

Antimicrobial class	Mechanism	Resistance[a]
β-lactams		
	ß-Lactamase	
	Natural	AMPCs or ADCs
		OXA-51-like
	Acquired narrow-spectrum	TEM-1, TEM-2
		CARB-5
		SCO-1
		OXA-10
		OXA-20
		OXA-21
	Extended Spectrum β-lactamase	SHV
		VEB
		GES
		PER
		CTX-M
		RTG-4
	Carbapenemase	OXA-23
		OXA-24/40
		OXA-58
		IMP
		VIM
		SIM
	Outer Membrane Protein	CarO (29 kDa)
		47-, 44-, and 37-kDa OMPs
		22- and 33-kDa OMPs
		HMP-AB
		33- to 36-kDa OMPs
		43-kDa OMP
		OmpW
	Efflux	AdeABC
		AdeIJK
	Altered PBP	Altered PBP

[a] ADCs, *Acinetobacter*-derived cephalosporinases; HMP-AB, heat-modifiable protein in *Acinetobacter baumannii*.

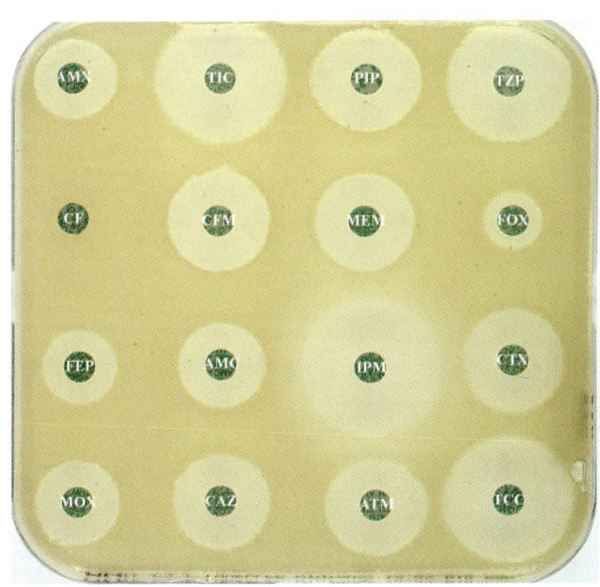

Fig. 2 (A)

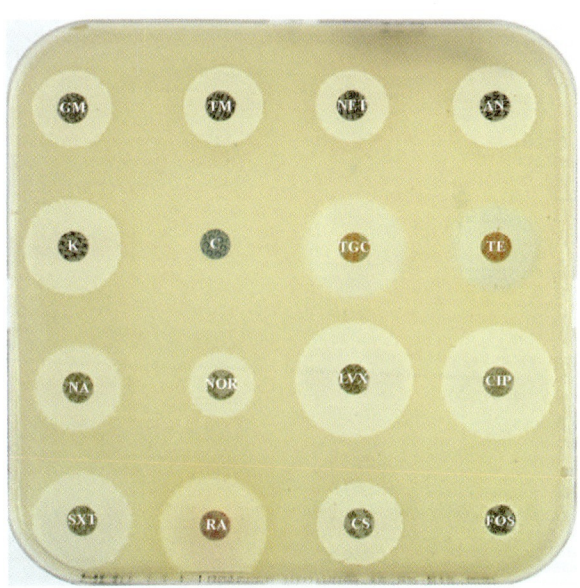

Fig. 2 (B)

Fig. 2: *A. baumannii* susceptible phenotype. (A) β-lactams: AMC, amoxicillin / clavulanic acid; AMX, amoxicillin; ATM, aztreonam; CAZ, ceftazidime, CF, cefalotine; CFM, cefixime; CTX, cefotaxime; FEP, cefepime; FOX, cefoxitin; IPM, imipenem; MEM, meropenem; MOX, moxalactam; PIP, piperacillin; TCC, ticarcillin / clavulanic acid; TIC, ticarcillin; TZP, piperacillin / tazobactam. (B) Non-β-lactams: AN, amikacin; C, chloramphenicol; CIP, ciprofloxacin; CS, colistin; FOS, fosfomycin; GM, gentamicin; KAN, kanamycin; NA, nalidixic acid; NET, netilmicin; NOR, norfloxacin; PEF, pefloxacin; RA, rifampin; SXT, co-trimoxazole; TET, tetracycline; TGC, tigecycline; TM, tobramycin.

Table 3. Main ß-lactam resistance phenotypes and ß-lactamases in *A. baumannii*

ß-lactam	Susceptible	Over-produced AmpC	Narrow-spectrum ß-lactamase	Narrow-spectrum oxacillinas	ESBL	OXA-carbapenemase	Metallo-enzyme
Ticarcillin	S	S/I	R	R	R	R	R
Ticarcillin + Clav acid	S	S/I	I/R	R	I/R	R	R
Piperacillin	S	I/R	I/R	R	R	R	R
Piperacillin + Tazo	S	I/R	I/R	R	I/R	R	R
Ceftazidime	S	R	S	S	R	S	R
Cefepime	S	I/R	S	S	R	S	R
Aztreonam	I/R	R	I/R	I/R	R	I/R	I/R
Imipenem	S	S	S	S	S	I/R	R
Meropenem	S	S	S	S	S	I/R	R

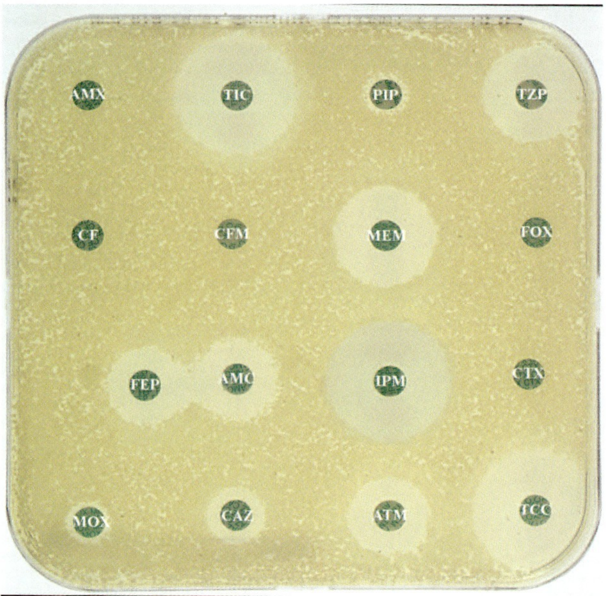

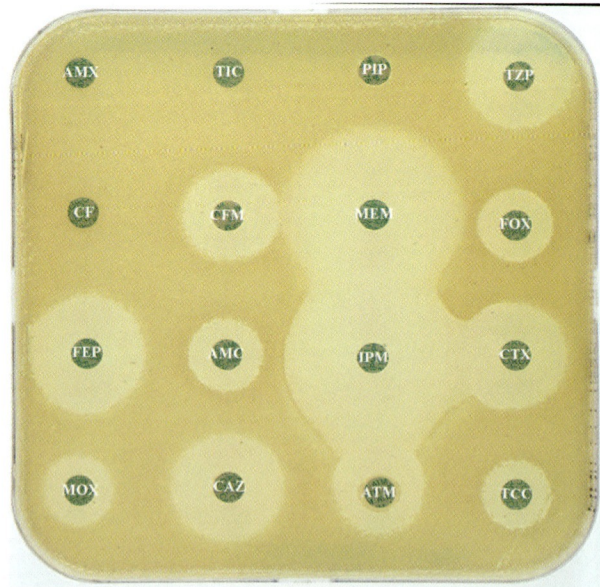

Fig. 3: *A. baumannii* hyperproducing endogenous AmpC cephalosporinase. AMC, amoxicillin / clavulanic acid; AMX, amoxicillin; ATM, aztreonam; CAZ, ceftazidime, CF, cefalotine; CFM, cefixime; CTX, cefotaxime; FEP, cefepime FOX, cefoxitin; IPM, imipenem; MEM, meropenem; MOX, moxalactam, PIP, piperacillin; TCC, ticarcillin / clavulanic acid; TIC, ticarcillin; TZP, piperacillin / tazobactam.

Fig. 4: *A. baumannii* producing acquired penicillinase TEM-1. MC, amoxicillin / clavulanic acid; AMX, amoxicillin; ATM, aztreonam; CAZ, ceftazidime, CF, cefalotine; CFM, cefixime; CTX, cefotaxime; FEP, cefepime FOX, cefoxitin; IPM, imipenem; MEM, meropenem; MOX, moxalactam, PIP, piperacillin; TCC, ticarcillin / clavulanic acid; TIC, ticarcillin; TZP, piperacillin / tazobactam.

RESISTANCE MECHANISMS TO β-LACTAMS

Enzymatic

The most prevalent mechanism of β-lactam resistance in *A. baumannii* is enzymatic degradation by β-lactamases. However, multiple mechanisms often work in concert to produce the same phenotype (20, 22, 30).

Unlike that of AmpC enzymes found in other Gram-negative organisms, inducible AmpC expression does not occur in *A. baumannii* (6, 21). The key determinant regulating overexpression of this enzyme is the presence of an upstream IS*Aba1* copy. The presence of this element correlates with increased expression of the *ampC* gene and resistance to extended-spectrum cephalosporins (Tables 2, 3, Fig. 3). Cefepime and carbapenems appear to be stable to this enzyme.

A few acquired narrow-spectrum β-lactamases are also prevalent in *A. baumannii*, namely clavulanic acid-inhibited penicillinases (TEM-1, TEM-2, and CARB-5) and clavulanic acid-resistant oxacillinases (OXA-20 and OXA-21) (Tables 2, 3, Fig. 4). Their clinical significance is limited given the potency of other resistance determinants. Recently, clavulanic acid-susceptible penicillinase SCO-1 has been identified in *Acinetobacter* spp., including *A. baumannii*, *A. junii*, *A. baylyi*, and *A. johnsonii*. It hydrolyses significantly the penicillins and, at a lower extent, cephalothin, ceftazidime, and cefepime. A combination of narrow-spectrum β-lactamases, such as TEM, with over-production of AmpC may also be observed, leading to isolates being resistant to all β-lactams, except carbapenems (Tables 2, 3, Fig. 5).

Extended-spectrum β-lactamases (ESBLs) from Ambler class A have also been described in *A. baumannii*, but assessment of their true prevalence is hindered by difficulties in laboratory detection, especially in AmpC over-producers. The production of ESBLs in *A. baumannii* may contribute significantly to high-level resistance to the penicillins and extended-spectrum cephalosporins (MICs of ceftazidime, 256 μg/ml and cefepime, 32μg/ml), and to MDR since ESBL genes are often associated with aminoglycoside-resistance genes. *A. baumannii* isolates expressing an ESBL usually remain susceptible to carbapenems (Tables 2, 3, Fig. 6).

The first ESBL identified in *A. baumannii* was PER-1. It is widespread in *P. aeruginosa* and *A. baumannii* isolates, mostly from Turkey and South Korea, and has also been reported in France,

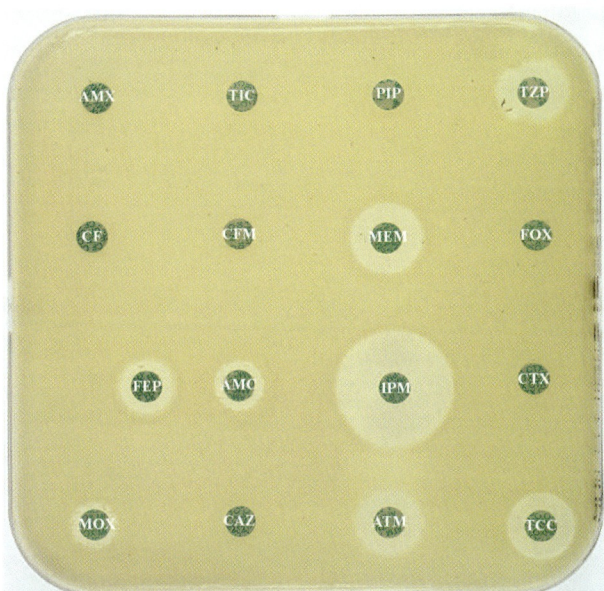

Fig. 5: *A. baumannii* hyperproducing endogenous AmpC cephalosporinase and producing acquired penicillinase TEM-1. AMC, amoxicillin / clavulanic acid; AMX, amoxicillin; ATM, aztreonam; CAZ, ceftazidime, CF, cefalotine; CFM, cefixime; CTX, cefotaxime; FEP, cefepime FOX, cefoxitin; IPM, imipenem; MEM, meropenem; MOX, Moxalactam, PIP, piperacillin; TCC, ticarcillin / clavulanic acid; TIC, ticarcillin; TZP, piperacillin / tazobactam.

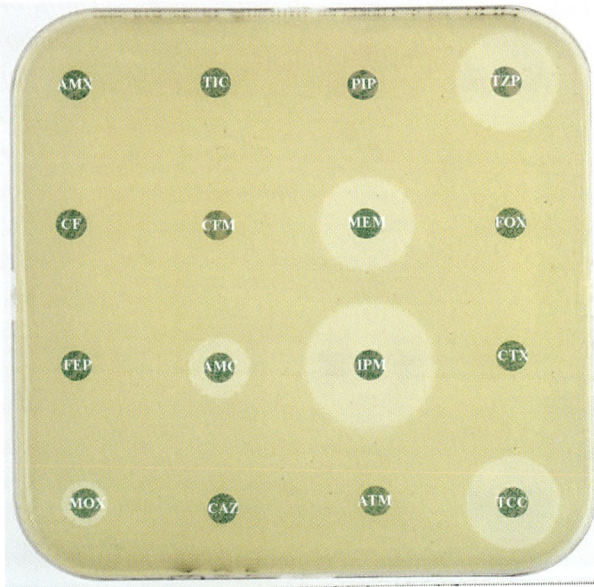

Fig. 6: *A. baumannii* producing extended spectrum β-lactamase VEB-1. AMC, amoxicillin / clavulanic acid; AMX, amoxicillin; ATM, aztreonam; CAZ, ceftazidime, CF, cefalotine; CFM, cefixime; CTX, cefotaxime; FEP, cefepime FOX, cefoxitin; IPM, imipenem; MEM, meropenem; MOX, moxalactam, PIP, piperacillin; TCC, ticarcillin / clavulanic acid; TIC, ticarcillin; TZP, piperacillin / tazobactam.

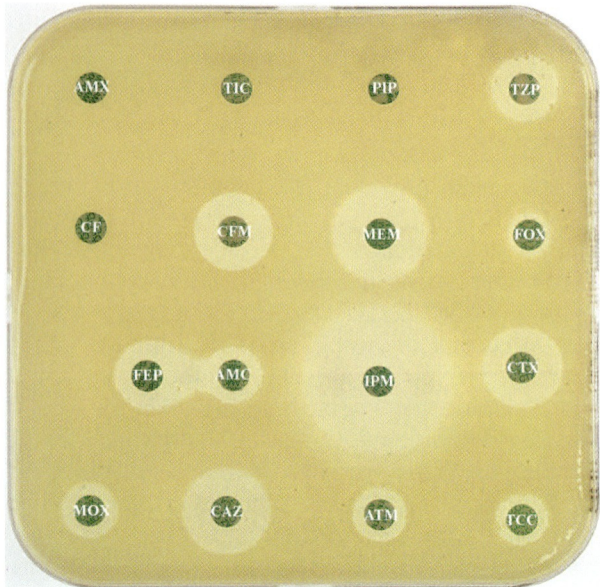

Fig. 7: *A. baumannii* producing extended spectrum carbenicillinase RTG-4. AMC, amoxicillin / clavulanic acid; AMX, amoxicillin; ATM, aztreonam; CAZ, ceftazidime, CF, cefalotine; CFM, cefixime; CTX, cefotaxime; FEP, cefepime FOX, cefoxitin; IPM, imipenem; MEM, meropenem; MOX, moxalactam, PIP, piperacillin; TCC, ticarcillin / clavulanic acid; TIC, ticarcillin; TZP, piperacillin / tazobactam.

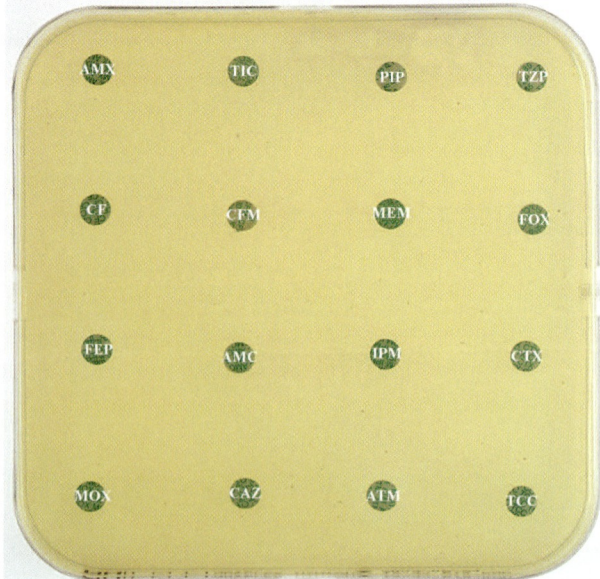

Fig. 8 (B)

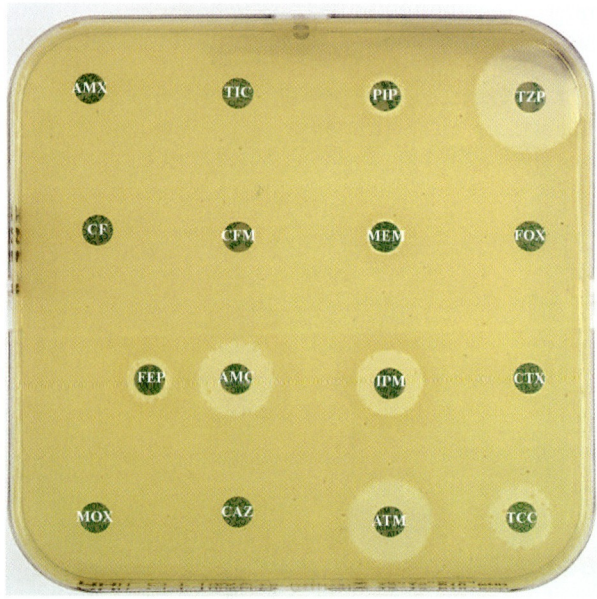

Fig. 8 (C)

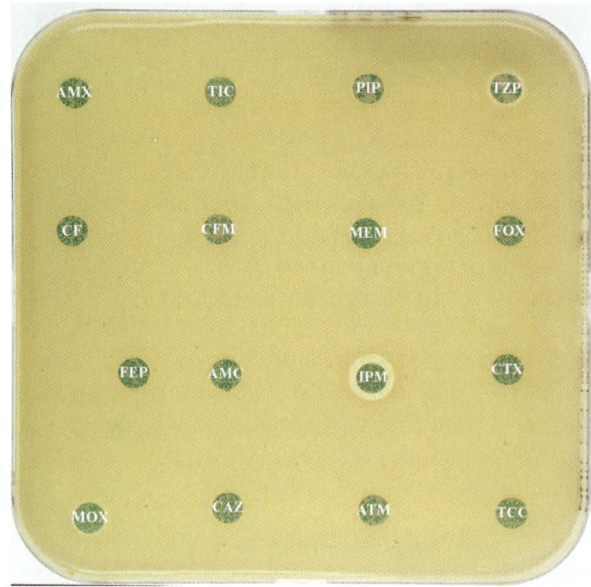

Fig. 8 (A)

Fig. 8: *A. baumannii* producing acquired carbapenemase **(A)** OXA-23; **(B)** OXA-40; and **(C)** IMP-4. AMC, amoxicillin / clavulanic acid; AMX, amoxicillin; ATM, aztreonam; CAZ, ceftazidime, CF, cefalotine; CFM, cefixime; CTX, cefotaxime; FEP, cefepime FOX, cefoxitin; IPM, imipenem; MEM, meropenem; MOX, moxalactam, PIP, piperacillin; TCC, ticarcillin / clavulanic acid; TIC, ticarcillin; TZP, piperacillin / tazobactam.

Hungary, Romania, Russia, China, Belgium, and Bolivia (17, 23). Analysis of MDR *A. baumannii* obtained from soldiers following injury during either Afghanistan or Iraq wars identified PER-1 producers in 3% of the isolates. Analysis of the sequences bracketing a bla_{PER-1} gene in an *A. baumannii* isolate revealed that it was part of transposon Tn*1213* (23). The PER-2 ESBL, which is distantly related to PER-1, has been found so far exclusively in Argentina and Bolivia (17).

The second and most important ESBL in *A. baumannii* is Vietnamese extended-spectrum β-lactamase (VEB-1) (Fig. 6). Initial identification of VEB-1 in *A. baumannii* occurred in France where a single strain was responsible for an hospital and subsequently of nationwide outbreak (16). The bla_{VEB-1} gene was identified in class 1 integrons part of the 96-kb AbaR1 resistance island (7).

Other ESBLs in *A. baumannii* include TEM-92 and -116, SHV-5 and -12, CTX-M-2 and -43, and GES-11 (15, 20). An interspecies transfer of the $bla_{CTX-M-2}$ gene from *P. mirabilis* to *A. baumannii* was hypothesized in the latter case.

Recently, a novel ESBL, RTG-4, was identified, which is the first carbenicillinase to possess ESBL properties (25). This is an atypical ESBL since it hydrolyses significantly cefepime and cefpirome but not ceftazdime nor cefotaxime (Fig. 7).

Resistance to carbapenems is the most serious issue among emerging resistances in *A. baumannii*. *A. baumannii* produces naturally occurring β-lactamases, which are oxacillinases (OXA-51-like variants). These enzymes have low-level carbapenemase activity and, upon overexpression, may be involved in carbapenem resistance in *A. baumannii*. In addition, several acquired β-lactamases have been identified as a source of carbapenem resistance. They belong either to Ambler class D (carbapenem-hydrolysing oxacillinases, CHDLs) or class B (metallo-β-lactamases, MBLs) (22, 24, 31). Thus far, the class A carbapenemases (KPC, GES, SME, NMC, and IMI) have not been described in *A. baumannii* (26).

The carbapenem-hydrolysing oxacillinases have been frequently identified in carbapenem-resistant *A. baumannii* isolates (Tables 2, 3, Fig. 8A, B). They confer low-level resistance to carbapenems (and often not to meropenem) without significant activity against Expanded Spectrum Cephalosporins. The first CHDL, OXA-23 (ARI-1), this is the representative of a first class (OXA-23, OXA-27 and OXA-49). OXA-23-like enzymes are the most widespread CHDLs in *A. baumannii* and have been detected worldwide. The significant contribution of these enzymes to carbapenem-resistance in *A. baumannii* has been emphasized, particularly when they are associated with IS*Aba1* and IS*Aba4* in plasmids (MICs of imipenem and meropenem, 32 µg/ml) (22, 24). The bla_{OXA-23} genes have been identified as part of transposon Tn*2006* and Tn*2007* (22, 24). Interestingly, the reservoir for this gene has been identified as *A. radioresistens* which, with *A. baumannii*, shares the skin of humans eco-system.

A second group of CHDLs, comprising OXA-24/40 (resequencing of its gene showed 100% identity with OXA-40), OXA-25, and OXA-26, has been identified in *A. baumannii*. The corresponding structural genes have been found worldwide either as chromosome- or plasmid-borne. A third group of CHDLs is composed of OXA-58 and its variant OXA-97 that have been identified worldwide (14, 20, 21). $bla_{OXA-58-like}$ genes are part of plasmids and associated with ISs that may play a role in high level expression.

Despite MBLs being less commonly identified in *A. baumannii* than OXA-type carbapenemases, their hydrolytic activity toward carbapenems is significantly more potent (100- to 1,000-fold) (22, 31). These enzymes have the capability of hydrolyzing all β-lactams (including carbapenems), except the monobactams such as aztreonam, which may help in laboratory detection (Tables 2, 3, Fig. 8C). They belong to three groups in *A. baumannii*: the IMP-like, VIM-like, and SIM-1 enzymes. Eight IMP variants belonging to different groups have been identified, namely: IMP-1 in Italy, Japan, and South Korea; IMP-2 in Italy and Japan; IMP-4 in Singapore, Hong Kong, and Australia; IMP-5 in Portugal; IMP-6 in Brazil, IMP-8 in China; IMP-11 and IMP-19 in Japan. VIM enzymes have rarely been identified in *A. baumannii*: VIM-1/VIM-4 in Greece, VIM-2 in South Korea, VIM-6 in India, and VIM-11 in Taiwan. SIM-1 has been reported only in South Korea where this determinant might be widespread.

Analysis of the genetic basis of the MBL structural genes in *A. baumannii* showed that the bla_{IMP}, bla_{VIM}, or bla_{SIM} genes have been embedded in class 1 integrons. Most acquired MBL genes in *A. baumannii* have been found associated with other resistance gene cassettes, in particular those encoding aminoglycoside-modifying enzymes (18, 24). *A. baumannii* strains carrying integrons have been found to be significantly more drug resistant than strains without integrons.

Non enzymatic

β-lactam resistance, including to the carbapenems, has also been ascribed to nonenzymatic mechanisms, including changes in outer membrane proteins, multidrug efflux pumps, and alterations in the affinity or expression of penicillin-binding proteins (30). Relative to other Gram-negative pathogens, very little is known about the outer membrane porins of *A. baumannii*. The loss of a 29-kDa outer-membrane protein, also known as CarO, was shown to be associated with imipenem and meropenem resistance.

Clinical outbreaks of carbapenem-resistant *A. baumannii* due to porin loss, including reduced expression of 47-, 44-, and 37-kDa OMPs and reduced expression of 22- and 33-kDa OMPs in association with OXA-24, have been described. Other OMPs relevant to β-lactam resistance include the heat-modifiable protein HMP-AB, which is homologous to OmpA of *Enterobacteriaceae* and OmpF of *P. aeruginosa*; a 33- to 36-kDa protein; a 43-kDa protein which shows homology with OprD from *P. aeruginosa*; and OmpW, which is homologous to OmpW proteins found in *E. coli* and *P. aeruginosa* (20, 30).

The genome of a MDR *A. baumannii* encodes a wide array of multidrug efflux systems (30). The resistance-nodulation-division (RND) family-type pump AdeABC is the best studied thus far and has a substrate profile that comprises β-lactams (including carbapenems), aminoglycosides, erythromycin, chloramphenicol, tetracycline, fluoroquinolones, and trimethoprim (30). It was also found that overexpression of AdeABC in association with CHDLs may confer high level resistance to carbapenems. Recently, a novel RND pump, AdeIJK, has been identified that contributes to resistance to β-lactams, chloramphenicol, tetracycline, erythromycin, lincosamides, fluoroquinolones, fusidic acid, novobiocin, rifampin, and trimethoprim (3).

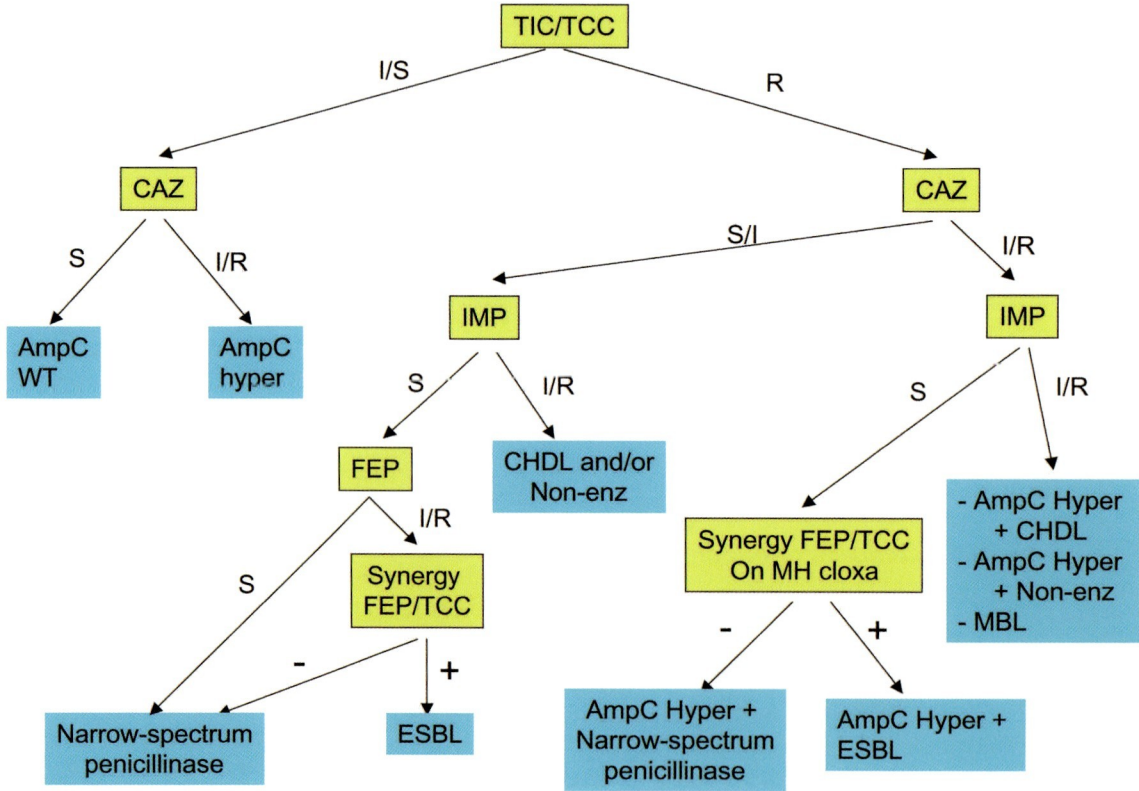

Fig. 9: Diagnostic decision tree for *A. baumannii*. The tested antibiotics are represented yellow. For each antibiotic the results are expressed as S, susceptible; I, Intermediate; R, resistant. CAZ, ceftazidime, FEP, cefepime IMP, imipenem; TCC, ticarcillin / clavulanic acid; TIC, ticarcillin; AmpC hyper, AmpC hyperproduced; CHDL, carbapenem-hydrolyzing oxacillinase; Non-enz, non-enzymatic mechanism; MBL, metallo-β-lactamase; MH-cloxa, Mueller-Hinton containing cloxacillin. + and – close to an arrow indicate the outcome of the synergy test. Blue squares indicate putative resistance mechanisms. This tree is adequate when a single mechanism of resistance is present. The frequent co-existence of several mechanisms makes interpretation difficult and PCR is required. WT, wild type.

Other RND-type pumps have been described in various *Acinetobacter* genomic species. The AdeDE efflux pump has been reported to confer resistance to amikacin, ceftazidime, chloramphenicol, ciprofloxacin, erythromycin, meropenem, rifampin, and tetracycline in *Acinetobacter* genomic DNA group 3 (20, 30).

DETECTION OF RESISTANCE

Surveillance

Surveillance and control of MDR *A. baumannii* outbreaks is based on international guidelines (29) and include usual recommendations for limiting the spread of this pathogen within a hospital (use of standard precautions reinforced by contact precautions, environmental decontamination) but also recommendations for systematic screening in high risk wards (ICU) and appropriate antibiotic use. During the nationwide nosocomial outbreak of VEB-1-producing isolates in France, specific recommendations were dispatched to limit the spread of the strain between hospitals: notification of cases to health authorities and regional infection control teams, limitation of the admissions of infected or colonized patients, and information of other hospitals before transfer (16). Culture of samples from the skin and rectum of patients with recent clinical cultures of *A. baumannii* was thought to have poor sensitivity (25% for any one site) when samples were plated onto Mac-Conkey agar plates containing 8 µg/ml ceftazidime and 2 µg/ml amphotericin. Fig. 9 presents a simplified decision tree for *A. baumannii*. Several phenotypic tests have been proven useful for initial detection of resistance mechanisms but in complex situations molecular tools are required.

Table 4. PCR primers for detection of extended-spectrum resistance genes in *A. baumannii*

β-lactamase	Sequence (5' to 3')	Gene
Cephalosporinase		
AmpC-A1	ACAGAGGAGCTAATCATGCG	
AmpC-A2	GTTCTTTTAAACCATATACC	bla_{AMPC}
ESBL		
VEB-1A	CGACTTCCATTTCCCGATGC	
VEB-1B	GGACTCTGCAACAAATACGC	bla_{VEB}
PER-A	ATGAATGTCATTATAAAAGC	
PER-B	AATTTGGGCTTAGGGCAGAA	bla_{PER}
GES-1A	ATGCGCTTCATTCACGCAC	
GES-1B	CTATTTGTCCGTGCTCAGG	bla_{GES}
TEM-A	GAGTATTCAACATTTCCGTGTC	
TEM-B	TAATCAGTGAGGCACCTATCTC	bla_{TEM}
SWSHV-A	AAGATCCACTATCGCCAGCAG	
SWSHV-B	ATTCAGTTCCGTTTCCCAGCGG	bla_{SHV}
CTXM-A1	SCVATGTGCAGYACCAGTAA	
CTXM-A2	SCVATGTGCAGYACCAGTAA	bla_{CTX-M}
RTG-A	CTCACGCTATCATTAAATGC	
RTG-B	TCAAACGAGGCGTCTGTCTCTG	bla_{RTG-4}
Metallo-β-lactamases		
IMP-2004A	ACAYGGYTTGGTTGTTCTTG	
IMP-2004B	GGTTTAAYAAAACAACCACC	bla_{IMP}
VIM-2004A	GTTTGGTCGCATATCGCAAC	
VIM-2004B	AATGCGCAGCACCAGGATAG	bla_{VIM}
SIM-F	TACAAGGGATTCGGCATCG	
SIM-R	TAATGGCCTGTTCCCATGTG	bla_{SIM}
Carbapenem hydrolyzing oxacillinases		
Oxa-imp1	GCAAATAMAGAATATGTSCC	
Oxa-imp2	CTCMACCCARCCRGTCAACC	$bla_{OXA-23/40-like}$
OXA-58A	CGATCAGAATGTTCAAGCGC	
OXA-58B	ACGATTCTCCCCTCTGCGC	$bla_{OXA-58-like}$
OXA-51A	CGACCGAGTATGTACCTGCTT	
OXA-51B	CTAAGTTAAGGGAGAACGC	$bla_{OXA-51-like}$

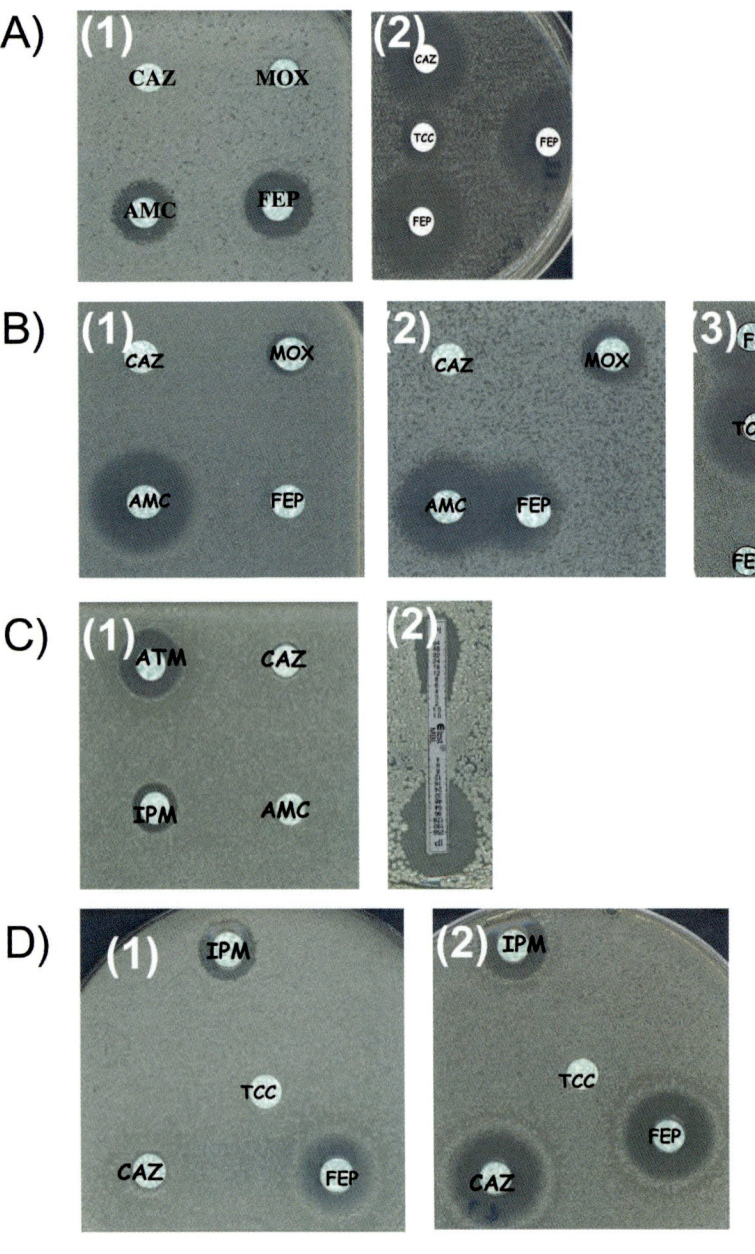

Fig. 10. Phenotypic tests.
(A) *A. baumannii* hyperproducing endogenous cephalosporinase (AmpC). Plates incubated overnight at 37°C and containing (1) Mueller-Hinton and (2) on Mueller-Hinton supplemented with cloxacillin. Susceptibility to 3rd generation cephalosporins is partially restored suggesting that resistance is mostly due to hyperproduced AmpC.
(B) *A. baumannii* producing extended spectrum β-lactamase VEB-1. Plate incubated at (1) 37°C. No synergy is visible due to hyperproduced AmpC. (2) 25°C with the disks of cefepime and clavulanic acid brought closer; synergy indicates the presence of an ESBL; (3) 37°C containing Mueller-Hinton supplemented with cloxacillin; inhibition of the cephalosporinase by cloxacilline reveals synergy. In the absence of clavulanic acid, the inhibition zones around the cefepime disk remain unchanged with or without cloxacillin.
(C) *A. baumannii* producing metallo-enzyme IMP-4. (1) Plate incubated at 37°C containing Mueller-Hinton; (2) E-test® imipenem / imipenem-EDTA. Presence of a metallo-enzyme is indicated by a difference of at least dilutions between the MICs of imipenem and imipenem/EDTA. However, PCR confirmation is required.
(D) *A. baumannii* producing carbapenem-hydrolyzing oxacillinase OXA-23. Plate containing (1) Mueller-Hinton; (2) Mueller-Hinton supplemented with cloxacillin. No synergy is observed since oxacillinases are not inhibited by clavulanic acid nor by EDTA. The inhibition zone of imipenem remains unchanged since cloxacillin does not inhibit oxacillinases. However, partial restoration of susceptibility to 3rd generation cephalosporins is observed, since carbapenem-hydrolyzing oxacillinases do not hydrolyze these molecules. Mechanism identification can only be achieved by PCR.

Phenotypic detection

ESBLs

Detection of ESBLs, based only on susceptibility testing, is not easy due to the variety of β-lactamases, their variable levels of expression, and since they may be associated with overexpression of naturally occurring cephalosporinases (Fig. 10A, B). Several phenotypic tests have been implemented for discrimination between ESBL-producers and those with other mechanisms conferring resistance to extended spectrum cephalosporins. These tests (double-disk synergy, ESBL E-test®, and the combination disk method) are based on clavulanate inhibition and cephalosporin susceptibility testing. They often need slight changes by either reducing the distance between the disks of cephalosporins and clavulanate, the use of cefepime (not hydrolysed by AmpCs) and of cloxacillin-containing plates (200 μg/ml) that inhibits AmpC, or by double inhibition by EDTA and clavulanate (masking metallo-enzymes) (16). Alternatively susceptibility testing performed at room temperature (versus 37°C) has shown to allow better development of synergy images in double-disk synergy tests. Enzymatic tests have also been proposed for identification of ESBL-producers.

Carbapenemases

The most frequently used methods for detection of metallo-β-lactamases (MBLs) are disk approximation methods with imipenem and imipenem plus EDTA (31). Others have used 2-mercaptopropionic acid for this purpose. Screening is performed with imipenem-EDTA synergy tests: (i) the MBL E-test® (AB Biodisk), (ii) the double-disc synergy test (3), and (iii) the combined-disc test (1). E-test® MBL strip has been shown to be reliable in detecting IMP- and VIM-type MBLs in *A. baumannii*. False-positive results were seen for isolates producing OXA-23 likely due to intrinsic activity of EDTA (Fig. 1D, 10C).

Phenotypic tests for detection of serine carbapenemases (OXA type) in *A. baumannii* have not yet been described (24, 26). The detection of a CHDL producer remains based on molecular techniques since the activity of these enzymes is not demonstrated by any of the inhibitors used in clinical microbiology (oxacillin, clavulanic acid, or tazobactam) nor by EDTA (Fig. 10D).

Molecular Detection

PCR-based techniques (end-point or real time) have been developed (Table 4). Several MBLs and ESBL genes can be detected using single- or multiplex-PCR coupled to either pyrosequencing, inverse hybridization, or to fluorescent probes (Taqman). These more specific techniques require knowledge, special equipment, are costly, and detect only known genes, regardless of their expression. For CHDL however, molecular detection is the only way to achieve proper identification (Table 4). Even carbapenem hydrolysis is not easy to detect, since the enzymes hydrolyse only weakly carbapenems, often just above the background level.

Antibiotics to be studied

Minimum

β-lactams should include: ticarcillin, ticarcillin + clavulanate, piperacillin, piperacillin + tazobactam, ceftazidime, and imipenem. Among the aminoglycosides, gentamicin, tobramycin, and amikacin and among the fluoroquinolones, ciprofloxacin or levofloxacin. Rifampin, colistin, co-trimoxazole, tigecycline, and doxycycline.

Enlarged

Several other molecules can be added. Meropenem and doripenem. Cefotaxime (to assess the level of AmpC expression) and cefepime (best substrate to detect synergy indicating the presence of an ESBL). Mecillinam can be used for *Acinetobacter* identification. Kanamycin, netilmicin, and isepamicin to identify the aminoglycoside resistance mechanisms. Sulbactam can be tested only by E-test® in combination with ampicillin.

REFERENCES

Bergogne-Berezin, E., and K. J. Towner. 1996. *Acinetobacter* spp. as nosocomial pathogens: microbiological, clinical, and epidemiological features. Clin. Microbiol. Rev. **9**:148–165.

Clinical and Laboratory Standards Institute. 2007. M7-A7. Dilution antimicrobial susceptibility tests for bacteria that grow aerobically. CLSI, Wayne, PA.

Damier-Piolle, L., S. Magnet, S. Brémont, T. Lambert, and P. Courvalin. 2008. AdeIJK, a resistance-nodulation-cell division pump effluxing multiple antibiotics in *Acinetobacter baumannii*. Antimicrob. Agents Chemother. **52**:557-562.

Doi, Y., and Y. Arakawa. 2007. 16S ribosomal RNA methylation: emerging resistance mechanism against aminoglycosides. Clin. Infect. Dis. **45**:88-94.

Falagas, M. E., and P. I. Rafailidis. 2008. Re-emergence of colistin in today's world of multidrug-resistant organisms: personal perspectives. Expert Opin. Investig. Drugs. **17**:973-981.

Figueiredo, S., L. Poirel, J. Croize, C. Recule, and P. Nordmann. 2009. In vivo selection of reduced susceptibility to carbapenems in *Acinetobacter baumannii* related to ISAba1-mediated overexpression of the natural *bla*(OXA-66) oxacillinase gene. Antimicrob. Agents Chemother. **53**:2657-2659.

Fournier, P. E., D. Vallenet, V. Barbe, S. Audic, H. Ogata, L. Poirel, H. Richet, C. Robert, S. Mangenot, C. Abergel, P. Nordmann, J. Weissenbach, D. Raoult, and J. M. Claverie. 2006. Comparative genomics of multidrug resistance in *Acinetobacter baumannii*. PLoS Genet. **2**(1):e7.

Giamarellou, H., A. Antoniadou, and K. Kanellakopoulou. 2008. *Acinetobacter baumannii*: a universal threat to public health? Int. J. Antimicrob. Agents. **32**:106-119.

Hujer, K. M., N. S. Hamza, A. M. Hujer, F. Perez, M. S. Helfand, C. R. Bethel, J. M. Thomson, V. E. Anderson, M. Barlow, L. B. Rice, F. C. Tenover, and R. A. Bonomo. 2005. Identification of a new allelic variant of the *Acinetobacter baumannii* cephalosporinase ADC-7 beta-lactamase: defining a unique family of class C enzymes. Antimicrob. Agents Chemother. **49**:2941-2948.

Karageorgopoulos, D. E., T. Kelesidis, I. Kelesidis, and M. E. Falagas. 2008. Tigecycline for the treatment of multidrug-resistant (including carbapenem-resistant) *Acinetobacter* infections: a review of the scientific evidence. J. Antimicrob. Chemother. **62**:45-55.

Karageorgopoulos, D. E., and M. E. Falagas. 2008. Current control and treatment of multidrug-resistant *Acinetobacter baumannii* infections. Lancet Infect. Dis. **8**:751-762.

Lee, S. Y., J. W. Lee, D. C. Jeong, S. Y. Chung, D. S. Chung, and J. H. Kang. 2008 Multidrug-resistant *Acinetobacter meningitis* in a 3-year-old boy treated with i.v. colistin. Pediatr. Int. **50**:584-585.

Maragakis, L. L., and T. M. Perl. 2008. *Acinetobacter baumannii*: epidemiology, antimicrobial resistance, and treatment options. Clin. Infect. Dis. **46**:1254-1263.

Marque, S., L. Poirel, C. Heritier, S. Brisse, M. D. Blasco, R. Filip, G. Coman, T. Naas, and P. Nordmann. 2005. Regional occurrence of plasmid-mediated carbapenem-hydrolyzing oxacillinase OXA-58 in *Acinetobacter* spp. in Europe. J. Clin. Microbiol. **43**:4885–4888.

Moubareck, C., S. Brémont, M. C. Conroy, P. Courvalin, and T. Lambert. 2009. GES-11, a novel integron-associated GES variant in *Acinetobacter baumannii*. Antimicrob. Agents Chemother. **53**:3579-3581.

Naas, T., B. Coignard, A. Carbonne, K. Blanckaert, O. Bajolet, C. Bernet, X. Verdeil, P. Astagneau, J. C. Desenclos JC, P. Nordmann and the French Nosocomial Infection Early Warning Investigation and Surveillance Network. 2006 VEB-1 extended-spectrum beta-lactamase-producing *Acinetobacter baumannii*, France. Emerg. Infect. Dis. **12**:1214-1222.

Naas, T., L. Poirel L, and P. Nordmann. 2008. Minor extended-spectrum beta-lactamases. Clin. Microbiol. Infect. Suppl **1**:42-52.

Nemec, A., L. Dolzani, S. Brisse, P. van den Broek, and L. Dijkshoorn. 2004. Diversity of aminoglycoside-resistance genes and their association with class 1 integrons among strains of pan-European *Acinetobacter baumannii* clones. J. Med. Microbiol. **53**:1233–1240.

Paterson, D. L. 2008. Impact of antibiotic resistance in gram-negative bacilli on empirical and definitive antibiotic therapy. Clin. Infect. Dis. **47** Suppl 1:S14-20.

Peleg, A. Y., H. Seifert, and D. L. Paterson. 2008. *Acinetobacter baumannii*: emergence of a successful pathogen. Clin. Microbiol. Rev. **21**:538-582.

Perez, F., A. M. Hujer, K. M. Hujer, B. K. Decker, P. N. Rather, and R. A. Bonomo. 2007. Global challenge of multidrug-resistant *Acinetobacter baumannii*. Antimicrob. Agents Chemother. **51**:3471-3484.

Poirel, L., and P. Nordmann. 2006. Carbapenem resistance in *Acinetobacter baumannii*: mechanisms and epidemiology. Clin. Microbiol. Infect. **12**:826-836.

Poirel, L., T. Naas, and P. Nordmann. 2008. Genetic support of extended-spectrum beta-lactamases. Clin. Microbiol Infect. **Suppl 1**: 75-81.

Poirel, L., J. D. Pitout, and P. Nordmann. 2007. Carbapenemases: molecular diversity and clinical consequences. Future Microbiol. **2**:501-512.

Potron, A., L. Poirel, J. Croizé, V. Chanteperdrix, and P. Nordmann. 2009. Genetic and biochemical characterization of the first extended-spectrum CARB-type beta-lactamase, RTG-4, from *Acinetobacter baumannii*. Antimicrob. Agents Chemother. **53**:3010-3016.

Queenan, A. M., and K. Bush. 2007. Carbapenemases: the versatile beta-lactamases. Clin. Microbiol. Rev. **20**:440-458.

Sebeny, P. J., M. S. Riddle, and K. Petersen. 2008. *Acinetobacter baumannii* skin and soft-tissue infection associated with war trauma. Clin. Infect. Dis. **47**:444-449.

Seward, R. J., T. Lambert, and K. J. Towner. 1998. Molecular epidemiology of aminoglycoside resistance in *Acinetobacter* spp. J. Med. Microbiol. **47**:455-462.

Shlaes, D. M., D. N. Gerding, J. F. J. John, W. A. Craig, D. L. Bornstein, and R. A. Duncan. 1997. Society for Healthcare Epidemiology of America and Infectious Diseases Society of America Joint Committee on the Prevention of Antimicrobial Resistance: guidelines for the prevention of antimicrobial resistance in hospitals. Infect. Control Hosp. Epidemiol. **18**:275-291.

Vila, J., S. Martí, and J. Sánchez-Céspedes. 2007. Porins, efflux pumps and multidrug resistance in *Acinetobacter baumannii*. J. Antimicrob. Chemother. **59**:1210-1215.

Walsh, T. R. 2008 Clinically significant carbapenemases: an update. Curr. Opin. Infect. Dis. **21**:367-371.

Chapter 33. *ACINETOBACTER* AND OTHER ANTIBIOTICS

Thierry LAMBERT

INTRODUCTION

The genus *Acinetobacter* currently comprises 31 species including 19 named species, the remainder being designated as genomic species. Some species are soil organisms and have never been associated with infection, while others may be pathogenic. *Acinetobacter baumannii* is one of the leading causes of nosocomial infections. Antibiotic use has contributed to the selection of resistant strains responsible for epidemic outbreaks in the hospital setting. Some strains of *A. baumannii* are among the most highly resistant Gram-negative bacilli. The other species or genomospecies of the genus *Acinetobacter* isolated from clinical specimens may also be multidrug resistant. Isolates of *Acinetobacter junii*, *Acinetobacter lwoffii*, and *Acinetobacter* genomospecies 13TU show higher antimicrobial susceptibility than *Acinetobacter johnsonii* and *Acinetobacter* genomospecies 3 and 10 (10), themselves more susceptible than *A. baumannii* (1). Multidrug resistance in *A. baumannii* constitutes all the more of a threat because these are the strains responsible for hospital outbreaks (22). Severe *Acinetobacter* infections can ideally be treated by combination therapy with a β-lactam and an aminoglycoside. Imipenem is one of the few β-lactams which is still clinically effective, but reports of imipenem resistance make it necessary to consider treatment options with other antimicrobial agents.

RESISTANCE MECHANISMS

Aminoglycosides

Acinetobacter species are intrinsically susceptible to aminoglycosides, with the exception of proteolytic species like *Acinetobacter haemolyticus* and genomic groups 6, 14, 15, 16, and 17 (14, 15, 26). These organisms naturally harbor a species-specific *aac(6')* gene inherited from a common ancestor (29). These genes are moderately expressed and the level of resistance they confer is detectable by a reduction in the activity of tobramycin compared to gentamicin; the MICs of amikacin are generally unaffected. However, the expression of these genes may be increased by promoters carried by insertion sequences (27, 28). Moreover, *A. baumannii* has the ability to acquire resistance genes. The predominant resistance mechanism is enzymatic inactivation of the antibiotic. Resistance due to methylation of 16S rRNA has been reported but to date this mechanism appears to be rare. On the other hand, resistance due to overexpression of the AdeABC efflux system has frequently been described in clinical isolates.

Enzymatic modification

Aminoglycoside resistance patterns among different bacteria are described in Chapters 16 and 17. Here we will examine the enzymes identified to date and their characteristic distribution in *Acinetobacter* species, which have been found to harbor APH(3')-I, APH(3')-VI, ANT(2"), ANT(3"), AAC(3)-I, AAC(3)-II, AAC(6')-I, and AAC(6')-II (16, 21, 32). AAC(3)-I, which inactivates gentamicin and fortimicin, is found at a high frequency. The same is true for APH(3')-VI which inactivates amikacin, kanamycin and neomycin; interestingly, this enzyme is rarely found in other bacterial genera (12, 13). It is worth mentioning that the strains responsible for hospital outbreaks often harbor several inactivating enzymes (21). The presence of several enzymes results in multiresistance to aminoglycosides which, as a rule, only spares apramycin, since the only enzymes capable of inactivating this aminoglycoside – AAC(1) and AAC(3)-IV - are present at a low frequency.

Ribosome alteration

Resistance due to 16S rRNA methylation, initially described in antibiotic-producing microorganisms, has more recently been found in pathogenic bacteria. This mechanism confers high-level resistance; MICs of 4,6-disubstituted deoxystreptamines (amikacin, gentamicin, netilmicin and tobramycin) are > 512 µg/ml. So far, this mechanism does not appear to be widespread, particularly in *Acinetobacter*, although the fact that the methylase genes are located on transposons, themselves carried by transferable plasmids, poses a significant threat to their dissemination (17).

Efflux

The AdeABC efflux system, a member of the Resistance Nodulation Division (RND) superfamily, has been identified in slightly more than 70% of *A. baumannii* isolates. This efflux pump is expressed under the control of the AdeRS two-component system (19, 20). Certain mutations in the sensor or regulator lead to constitutive expression of the pump, resulting in the extrusion of many antibiotics including aminoglycosides, fluoroquinolones, some β-lactams (such as cefepime), and tetracyclines (20). Thus, aminoglycoside susceptibility is significantly diminished: in strains overexpressing AdeABC, aminoglycoside MICs are 4-32 times higher than in the knock-out strain. The increase in the MIC differs according to the aminoglycoside, ranging from 32-fold for netilmicin and gentamicin, the most affected, to 4-fold for kanamycin, which is much less affected. The reduction in aminoglycoside activity results in low-level resistance: the MIC of gentamicin for a wild-type strain is 0.5-1 μg/ml versus 8 μg/ml (intermediate category) for a variant overexpressing AdeABC. The phenotype associated with AdeABC overexpression is illustrated in Fig. 1. In *Acinetobacter* genomic DNA group 3, inactivation of the AdeABC system resulted in a decrease in the amikacin MIC from 2 to < 0.06 μg/ml (3).

Quinolones

Target modification

Epidemic strains are generally resistant to fluoroquinolones. Resistance is conferred by mutations in the QRDRs of the *gyrA* and *parC* genes encoding DNA gyrase and topoisomerase IV, respectively (33). This results in a $Ser_{80}Leu$ substitution in GyrA and a $Glu_{84}Lys$ substitution in ParC (6, 35, 36). ParC appears to be a secondary target and the GyrA/ParC double mutant confers high-level resistance (33, 36). The MIC of ciprofloxacin in strains harboring both mutations ranges from 32 to 256 μg/ml (34).

Efflux

In *A. baumannii*, overexpression of the AdeABC efflux system leads to a reduction of fluoroquinolone activity (20). Norfloxacin is most sensitive to this type of resistance, with MICs increasing four-fold. The AdeIJK efflux pump also exports fluoroquinolones and its inactivation lowers fluoroquinolone MICs by a factor of two. The AdeDE efflux pump contributes to ciprofloxacin extrusion in *Acinetobacter* genomic DNA group 3 (3). Efflux might constitute a primary mode of adaptation of these bacteria to quinolones, before target modification. Plasmid-mediated fluoroquinolone resistance due to AAC(6')-Ib-cr, Qnr proteins or the QepA pump has not yet been described in *Acinetobacter*, but unfortunately this is probably just a matter of time.

Chloramphenicol

Chloramphenicol resistance is widespread among *Acinetobacter*. It is due to enzymatic inactivation by Cat proteins or an efflux-type mechanism via Cml proteins located on class 1 integrons (23). The latter mechanism also reduces the activity of florphenicol, a fluorinated derivative used in veterinary medicine.

Rifampin

Rifampin has been successfully used to treat *Acinetobacter* infections. MICs in wild-type populations range from 2-4 μg/ml. Resistance is due either to mutations in RNA polymerase selected during treatment, or enzymatic inactivation by an ADP-ribosyltransferase encoded by the *arr2* gene located on a class 1 integron (11).

Tetracyclines

Resistance to tetracyclines and related compounds is due to efflux or ribosomal protection.

Target protection

The *tet*(M) determinant, widely distributed in Gram-positive bacteria, has been described in *A. baumannii* where it confers resistance to tetracyclines and minocycline (25).

Acquired efflux

The *tet*(A), *tet*(B) and *tet*(39) determinants have been detected in *Acinetobacter* (2, 24). The *tet*(A) and *tet*(39) determinants confer resistance to tetracyclines but not to minocycline (MIC < 1 μg/ml), whereas *tet*(B) affects both tetracyclines and minocycline.

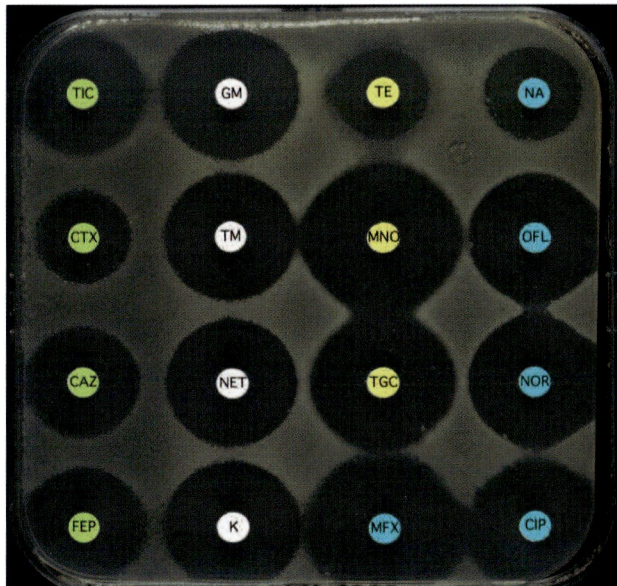 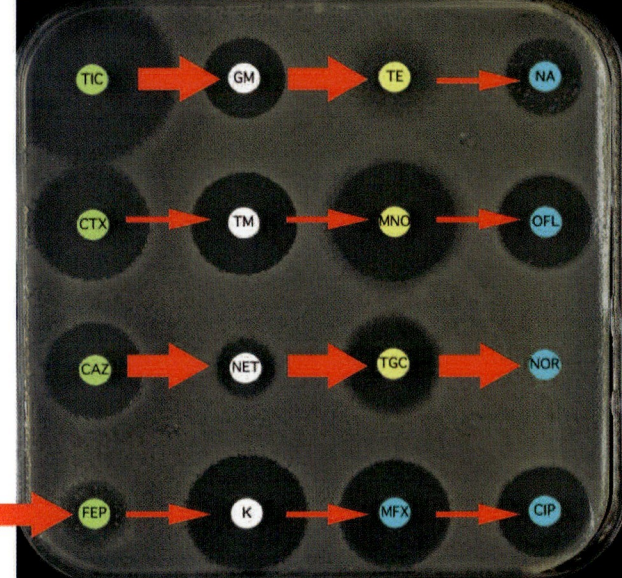

Fig. 1: Left, *A. baumannii* wild type. Right, spontaneous mutant overexpressing the AdeABC pump. Substrate antibiotics are indicated by arrows. CAZ, ceftazidime; CTX, cefotaxime; CIP, ciprofloxacin; FEP, cefepime; G, gentamicin; K, kanamycin; MFX, moxifloxacin; MNO, minocycline; NA, nalidixic acid; NET, netilmicin; NOR, norfloxacin; OFL, ofloxacin; TE, tetracycline; TGC, tigecycline; TIC, ticarcillin; TM, tobramycin.

Table 1. EUCAST and CLSI clinical breakpoints for *Acinetobacter*

Antibiotic	EUCAST S≤/>R	CLSI S≤/≥R
Amikacin	8/16	16/64
Gentamicin	4/4	4/16
Netilmicin	4/4	8/32
Tobramycin	4/4	4/16
Ciprofloxacin	1/1	1/4
Levofloxacin	1/2	2/8
Tetracycline	NA[a]	4/16
Doxycycline	NA	4/16
Minocycline	NA	4/16
Tigecycline	NA	NA
Trimethoprim-sulfamethoxazole	2/4	(2-38)/(4-76)
Colistin	2/2	2/4

[a]NA, not available.

Intrinsic efflux

The AdeABC and AdeIJK efflux pumps export tetracyclines and their role in resistance becomes apparent when they are overexpressed (8). The clinical significance of these efflux pumps concerns tigecycline in particular. Tigecycline is the first glycylcycline, a new class of tetracyclines. The activity of tigecycline is not affected by the Tet proteins involved in acquired efflux, nor by ribosomal protection. Consequently, this drug represents a possible treatment for infections caused by multidrug resistant strains, including strains resistant to carbapenems. Unfortunately, overexpression of the AdeABC system reduces tigecycline activity and this mechanism has been associated with treatment failures due to the selection of constitutive mutants (30). Tigecycline MICs in wild-type strains are < 1 μg/ml but can be as high as 16-32 μg/ml in mutants. Inactivation of the AdeIJK pump lowers the tigecycline MIC twofold. Coordinated hyperproduction of the AdeABC and AdeIJK efflux systems contributes to resistance in a synergistic manner (4). Finally, the AdeFGH efflux pump (unpublished data) also contributes to extrusion of tigecycline. To date, neither EUCAST nor CLSI have defined breakpoints for tigecycline. To assess the activity of this drug, freshly prepared media (within 12 h) should be used in order to avoid underestimating its activity.

Sulfonamides and trimethoprim

Generally, *Acinetobacter* show intrinsic low-level resistance to trimethoprim. The level of resistance varies according to species. The MICs of trimethoprim for *A. baumannii* range from 16-32 µg/ml, but epidemic hospital strains frequently harbor mobile elements – plasmids or transposons – carrying *dfr* genes often contained in integron cassettes (23). The 5' conserved segment of class 1 integrons harbors the *sul*1 gene which confers resistance to sulfonamides.

Polymyxins

The emergence of multidrug resistance and the lack of new antimicrobial agents have revived interest in the polymyxins. Polymyxin B and polymyxin E (colistin) are cationic polypeptides that have long been used in clinical practice. Parental administration of these drugs was abandoned due to reports of nephrotoxicity and neurotoxicity, but more recent studies indicate that they have acceptable toxicity in light of the benefit they procure in the treatment of severe infections caused by multidrug resistant *A. baumannii* or *Pseudomonas aeruginosa* (5, 9).

Colistin is available in two forms, colistin sulfate and colistimethate sodium (also known as colistin methanesulfate, pentasodium colistimethanesulfate or colistin sulfonyl methate) for injection. Colistimethate sodium is less active and less toxic than colistin sulfate. The latter is used for local disinfection and given orally for digestive decontamination. Colistimethate sodium is an inactive prodrug of colistin. In culture media, it is hydrolyzed in an unpredictable manner, releasing intermediates with variable activity. This is why colistin sulfate should be used for *in vitro* tests. The disk diffusion method with 10 µg colistin sulfate disks may give rise to false susceptibility due to poor agar diffusion characteristics; consequently the results should be confirmed with a dilution method. Susceptibility and resistance breakpoints for colistimethate sodium are ≤ 2 µg/ml and > 2 µg/ml (similar for EUCAST and CLSI), respectively. E-test® methodology has proven reliable for MIC determination in several studies (31).

A. baumannii is generally susceptible to polymyxins and colistimethate sodium has been used with success to treat infections caused by multidrug resistant strains. Nevertheless, heteroresistant strains have been identified and colistin-dependent variants have been reported (7, 18). Strains of genomic group 13BG are intrinsically resistant to polymyxins (15). It should be noted that with respect to *Acinetobacter*, there is a divergence between the CLSI and EUCAST breakpoints for certain antibiotics such as aminoglycosides and fluoroquinolones.

Furthermore, EUCAST has not set any breakpoints for tetracyclines, and neither EUCAST nor CLSI has set breakpoints for tigecycline. In this absence, it is possible to use the breakpoints defined for the enterobacteria or to consider the 1/2 breakpoints recommended by the British Society for Antimicrobial Chemotherapy (BSAC).

CONCLUSION

Acinetobacter, and *A. baumannii* in particular, have demonstrated an astonishing ability to acquire and develop resistance to antibiotics. Some *A. baumannii* strains are among the most highly resistant bacteria known. This microorganism has become a formidable nosocomial pathogen. Accordingly, antimicrobial susceptibility testing of clinical isolates must be thorough and carried out with the greatest of care. Furthermore, surveillance of the emergence and dissemination of resistance should not be neglected.

REFERENCES

(1) **Adams-Hauch, J.M., D.L. Paterson, H.E. Sidjabat, A.W. Pasculle, B.A. Potoski, C.A. Muto, L.H. Harrison, and Y. Doi**. 2008. Genetic basis of multidrug resistance in *Acinetobacter baumannii* clinical isolates at a tertiary medical center in Pennsylvania. Antimicrob. Agents Chemother. **52**:3837-3843.

(2) **Agerso, Y., and L. Guardabassi**. 2005. Identification of Tet39, a novel class of tetracycline resistance determinant in *Acinetobacter* spp. of environmental and clinical origin. J. Antimicrob. Chemother. **55**:566-569.

(3) **Chau, S-L., Y-W. Chu, and E.T.S. Houang**. 2004. Novel resistance-nodulation-cell division efflux system AdeDE in *Acinetobacter* genomic DNA group 3. Antimicrob. Agents Chemother. **48**:4054-4055.

(4) **Damier-Piolle, L., S. Magnet, S. Brémont, T. Lambert, and P. Courvalin**. 2008. AdeIJK, a RND pump effluxing multiple antibiotics in *Acinetobacter*

baumannii. Antimicrob. Agents Chemother. **52**:557-562.
(5) **Falagas, M. E., and S.K. Kasiakou.** 2005. Colistin: the revival of polymyxins for the management of multidrug-resistant gram-negative bacterial infections. Clin. Infect. Dis. **40**:1333-1341.
(6) **Hamouda, A., and S.G. Amyes.** 2004. Novel *gyrA* and *parC* point mutations in two strains of *Acinetobacter baumannii* resistant to ciprofloxacin. J. Antimicrob. Chemother. **54**:695-696.
(7) **Hawley, J.S., C.K. Murray, and J.H. Jorgensen.** 2007. Development of colistin-dependent *Acinetobacter baumannii-Acinetobacter calcoaceticus* complex. Antimicrob. Agents Chemother. **51**:4529-4530.
(8) **Higgins, P.G., H. Wisplinghoff, D. Stefanik, and H. Seifert.** 2004. Selection of topoisomerase mutations and overexpression of *adeB* mRNA transcripts during an outbreak of *Acinetobacter baumannii.* J. Antimicrob. Chemother. **54**:821-823.
(9) **Holloway, K.P., N.G. Rouphael, J.B. Wells, M.D. King, and H.M. Blumberg.** 2006. Polymyxin B and doxycycline use in patients with multidrug-resistant *Acinetobacter baumannii* infections in the intensive care unit. Ann. Pharmacother. **40**:1939-1945.
(10) **Horrevorts, A., K. Bergman, L. Kollee, I. Breuker, I. Tjernberg, and L. Dijkshoorn.** 1995. Clinical and epidemiological investigations of *Acinetobacter* genomospecies 3 in a neonatal intensive care unit. J. Clin. Microbiol. **33**:1567-1572.
(11) **Houang, E.T., Y.W. Chu, W.S. Lo, K.Y. Chu, and A.F. Cheng.** 2003. Epidemiology of rifampin ADP-ribosyltransferase (arr-2) and metallo-betalactamase (*bla*IMP-4) gene cassettes in class 1 integrons in *Acinetobacter* strains isolated from blood cultures in 1997 to 2000. Antimicrob. Agents Chemother. **47**:1382-1390.
(12) **Lambert, T., G. Gerbaud, and P. Courvalin.** 1988. Transferable amikacin resistance in *Acinetobacter* spp. due to a new type of 3' aminoglycoside phosphotransferase. Antimicrob. Agents Chemother. **32**:15-19.
(13) **Lambert, T., G. Gerbaud, P. Bouvet, J.F. Vieu, and P. Courvalin.** 1990. Dissemination of the *aphA6* gene in *Acinetobacter* spp. Antimicrob. Agents Chemother. **34**:1244-1248.
(14) **Lambert, T., G. Gerbaud, and P. Courvalin.** 1993. Characterization of *Acinetobacter haemolyticus aac(6')-Ig* gene encoding an aminoglycoside 6'-N-acetyltransferase which modifies amikacin. Antimicrob. Agents Chemother. **37**:2093-2100
(15) **Lambert, T., G. Gerbaud, and P. Courvalin.** 1994. Characterization of the chromosomal *aac(6')-Ij* gene of *Acinetobacter* sp.13 and the *aac(6')-Ih* plasmid gene of *Acinetobacter baumannii.* Antimicrob. Agents Chemother. **38**:1883-1889
(16) **Lambert, T., E. Rudant, P. Bouvet, and P. Courvalin.** 1997. Molecular basis of aminoglycoside resistance in *Acinetobacter* spp. J. Med. Microbiol. **46**:731-735.
(17) **Lee, H., D. Yong. J.H. Yum, K.H. Roh, K. Lee, K. Yamane, Y. Arakawa, and Y. Chong.** 2006. Dissemination of 16S rRNA methylase-mediated highly amikacin-resistant isolates of *Klebsiella pneumoniae* and *Acinetobacter baumannii* in Korea. Diagn. Microbiol. Infect. Dis. **56**:305-312.
(18) **Li, J., C.R. Rayner, R.L. Nation, R.J. Owen, D. Spelman, K. Eng Tan, and L. Liolios.** 2006. Heteroresistance to colistin in multidrug-resistant *Acinetobacter baumannii.* Antimicrob. Agents Chemother. **50**:2946-2950.
(19) **Magnet, S., P. Courvalin, and T. Lambert.** 2001. Resistance-nodulation-cell division-type efflux pump involved in aminoglycoside resistance in *Acinetobacter baumannii* strain BM4454. Antimicrob. Agents Chemother. **45**:3375-3380.
(20) **Marchand, I., L. Damier-Piolle, P. Courvalin, and T. Lambert.** 2004. Expression of the RND-type efflux pump AdeABC in *Acinetobacter baumannii* is regulated by the AdeRS two-component system. Antimicrob. Agents Chemother. **48**:3298-304.
(21) **Nemec, A., L. Dolzani, S. Brisse, P. van den Broek, and L. Dijkshoorn.** 2004. Diversity of aminoglycoside-resistance genes and their association with class1 integrons among strains of pan-European *Acinetobacter baumannii* clones. J. Med. Microbiol. **53**:1233-1240.
(22) **Peleg, A.Y., H. Seifert, and D.L. Paterson.** 2008. *Acinetobacter baumannii*: Emergence of a successful pathogen. Clin. Microbiol. Rev. **21**:538-582.
(23) **Ploy, M-C., F. Denis, P. Courvalin, and T. Lambert.** 2000. Molecular characterization of integrons in *Acinetobacter baumannii* : description of a hybrid class 2 integron. Antimicrob. Agents Chemother. **44**:2684-2688.
(24) **Ribera, A., I. Roca, J. Ruiz, I. Gilbert, and J. Villa.** 2003. Partial characterization of a transposon containing the *tet*(A) determinant in a clinical isolate of *Acinetobacter baumannii.* J. Antimicrob. Chemother. **52**:477-480.
(25) **Ribera, A., J. Ruiz, and J. Villa.** 2003. Presence of the *tet*(M) determinant in a clinical isolate of *Acinetobacter baumannii.* Antimicrob. Agents Chemother. **47**:2310-2312.
(26) **Rudant, E., P. Bourlioux, P. Courvalin, and T. Lambert.** 1994. Characterization of the *aac(6')-Ik* gene of *Acinetobacter* sp. 6. FEMS Microbiol. Lett. **124**:49-54.
(27) **Rudant, E., P. Courvalin, and T. Lambert.** 1997. Loss of intrinsic aminoglycoside resistance in *Acinetobacter haemolyticus* by three types of alterations in the *aac(6')-Ig* gene, including insertion of IS17. Antimicrob. Agents Chemother. **41**:2646-2651.
(28) **Rudant, E., P. Courvalin, and T. Lambert.** 1998. Characterization of IS18, an element capable of activating the silent *aac(6')-Ij* gene of *Acinetobacter* sp. 13 strain BM2716 by transposition. Antimicrob. Agents Chemother. **42**:2759-2761.
(29) **Rudant, E., P. Bouvet, P. Courvalin, and T. Lambert.** 1999. Phylogenetic analysis of proteolytic *Acinetobacter* based on the sequence of genes encoding aminoglycoside 6'-N-acetyltransferases. System. Appl. Microbiol. **22**:59-67
(30) **Ruzin, A., D. Keeney, and P.A. Bradford.** 2007. AdeABC multidrug efflux pump is associated with decreased susceptibility to tigecycline in *Acinetobacter calcoaceticus-Acinetobacter baumannii* complex. J. Antimicrob. Chemother. **59**:1001-1004.
(31) **Sands, M., Y. McCarter, and W. Sanchez.** 2007. Synergy testing of multidrug resistant *Acinetobacter baumannii* against tigecycline and polymyxin using

an E-test methodology. Eur. J. Clin. Microbiol. Infect. Dis. **26**:521-522.

(32) **Seward, R.J., T. Lambert, and K.J. Towner**. 1998. Molecular epidemiology of aminoglycoside resistance in *Acinetobacter* spp. J. Med. Microbiol. **47**:455-462.

(33) **Seward, R.J., and K.J. Towner**. 1998. Molecular epidemiology of quinolone resistance in *Acinetobacter* spp. Clin. Microbiol. Infect. **4**:248-254.

(34) **Vila, J., A. Ribera, F. Marco, J. Ruiz, J. Mensa, J. Chaves, G. Hernandez, and T. Jimenez de Anta**. 2002. Activity of clinofloxacin, compared with six other quinolones, against *Acinetobacter baumannii* clinical isolates. J. Antimicrob. Chemother. **49**:471-477.

(35) **Vila, J., J. Ruiz, P. Goni, A. Marcos, and T. Jimenez de Anta**. 1995. Mutation in the *gyrA* gene of quinolone-resistant clinical isolates of *Acinetobacter baumannii*. Antimicrob. Agents Chemother. **39**:1201-1203.

(36) **Vila, J., J. Ruiz, P. Goni, and T. Jimenez de Anta**. 1997. Quinolone-resistance mutations in the topoisomease IV *parC* gene of *Acinetobacter baumannii*. J. Antimicrob. Chemother. **39**:757-762.

Chapter 34. *HAEMOPHILUS INFLUENZAE*

Olivier GAILLOT

INTRODUCTION

Haemophilus influenzae is a frequent commensal of the upper respiratory tract mucosa whose only natural host is human. It is also a significant pathogen responsible for a variety of invasive and localized infections, due respectively to encapsulated and unencapsulated ("non typeable") strains.

Over the last two decades, the implementation of a worldwide vaccination program with a protein-conjugated polysaccharide b vaccine has dramatically reduced the incidence of the life-threatening *H. influenzae* meningitis, bacteremic pneumonia, and epiglottitis mostly caused by encapsulated serotype b (Hib) strains. Nevertheless, invasive infections which require aggressive antibiotic therapy still occur, especially in children between 4 and 18 months of age and in areas where the vaccine is not used yet (64, 65). Aminopenicillins are standard therapy in the absence of resistance mechanism verified in the laboratory. However, since the emergence and spread of β-lactamase producing strains in the 70s, third-generation cephalosporins such as cefotaxime or ceftriaxone have become the recommended first line treatment for invasive *H. influenzae* infections, with meropenem as an alternative, and possibly fluoroquinolones for adult patients (60). As extended-spectrum β-lactamase (ESBL) have not been described yet in *H. influenzae*, future concerns about the efficacy of third-generation cephalosporins might rather be raised by invasive strains displaying high-level resistance to β-lactams by alteration of their penicillin-binding proteins (PBPs) (28).

Unencapsulated strains are commonly responsible for localized infections of the upper respiratory tract, ear, and eye. In adults, non typeable *H. influenzae* (NTHi) cause community-acquired pneumonia and are predominantly responsible for acute exacerbations of chronic bronchitis (39). Depending on the clinical setting and co-morbidities, recommendations for treatment include amoxicillin, amoxicillin-clavulanate, oral cephalosporins such as cefuroxime axetil and cefpodoxime, third-generation cephalosporins, fluoroquinolones, and macrolides such as azithromycin and clarithromycin, alone or in combination (36). In contrast, the main clinical manifestations of NTHi in children are acute otitis media (AOM), conjunctivitis and acute sinusitis following viral infection. Acute conjunctivitis is usually treated with topical antibiotics, while acute sinusitis and uncomplicated AOM require oral β-lactam treatment. Recent studies (reviewed in 40) showed that the introduction of the conjugate pneumococcal vaccine significantly increased the proportion of aminopenicillin-resistant *H. influenzae* AOM in children failing initial antibiotic therapy. Due to their increasing resistance to antibiotics, and possible persistence in biofilms, some NTHi strains are the leading cause of recurrent and "difficult-to-treat" otitis (38) and require special attention from clinical microbiologists in order to provide therapeutic alternatives to the recommended amoxicillin 80-90 mg/kg/day regimen. As the Hib vaccination has no protective effect on NTHi, an effective vaccine for *H. influenzae* AOM has yet to be developed and would provide considerable health and economic benefits. Interestingly, partial protection (35%) against *H. influenzae* AOM was demonstrated during the evaluation of an 11-valent anti-pneumococcus vaccine in which pneumococcal capsular polysaccharides were conjugated to surface protein D of NTHi used as a carrier (46).

METHODS

The reference method for susceptibility testing of *H. influenzae* is MIC determination by broth or agar dilution (9). Two media, *Haemophilus* test medium (HTM) and Mueller-Hinton supplemented with lysed horse blood and NAD (MH-LHB-NAD) have been specified by the Clinical and Laboratory Standards Institute (CLSI) and the European Committee on Antimicrobial Susceptibility Testing (EUCAST), respectively. Both provide comparable MIC results (30), but the critical breakpoints may differ significantly (Table 1), as EUCAST breakpoints have been determined mainly on the basis of pharmacokinetic and pharmacodynamic (PK/PD) data and CLSI breakpoints generally represent microbiological rather than clinical breakpoints (57).

Table 1. Breakpoints for clinical categorisation of *H. influenzae* as defined in 2009 by the EUCAST and the CLSI

Antimicrobial	MICs interpretative standard (µg/ml)					
	EUCAST			CLSI		
	S[a]	I	R	S	I	R
Ampicillin[b]	≤ 1	-	> 1	≤ 1	2	> 2
Amoxicillin[c]	≤ 1	-	> 1	ND[a]		
Amoxicillin-clavulanate	≤ 1	-	> 1	≤ 4	-	> 4
Piperacillin-tazobactam		Note[d]		≤ 1	-	> 1
Cefaclor	≤ 0.5	-	> 0.5	≤ 8	16	> 16
Cefuroxime axetil	≤ 0.12	0.25-0.5	> 1	≤ 4	8	> 8
Cefpodoxime	≤ 0.25	0.5	> 0.5	≤ 2	-	> 2
Cefixime	≤ 0.12	-	> 0.12	≤ 1	-	> 1
Cefuroxime	≤ 1	2	> 2	≤ 4	8	> 8
Cefotaxime	≤ 0.12	-	> 0.12	≤ 2	-	> 2
Ceftriaxone	≤ 0.12	-	> 0.12	≤ 2	-	> 2
Cefepime	≤ 0.25	-	> 0.25	≤ 2	-	> 2
Ceftazidime, aztreonam		ND		≤ 2	-	> 2
Ertapenem	≤ 0.5	-	> 0.5	≤ 0.5	-	> 0.5
Meropenem	≤ 2	-	> 2	≤ 0.5	-	> 0.5
Meropenem (meningitis)	≤ 0.25[e]	0.5-1	> 1	ND		
Chloramphenicol	≤ 1	2	> 2	≤ 2	4	> 4
Cipro-, moxifloxacin	≤ 0.5	-	> 0.5	≤ 1	-	> 1
Erythromycin	≤ 0.5[f]	1-16	> 16	ND		
Azithromycin		Note[f]		≤ 4	-	> 4
Telithromycin	≤ 0.12	0.25-8	> 8	≤ 4	8	> 8
Tetracycline	≤ 1	2	> 2	≤ 2	4	> 4
Co-trimoxazole[g]	≤ 0.5	1	> 1	≤ 0.5	1-2	> 2
Rifampicin	≤ 0.5	-	> 0.5	≤ 1	2	> 2

[a] S, susceptible I, intermediate; R, resistant; ND, not defined.
[b] Breakpoints relate only to β-lactamase-negative isolates (9, 18).
[c] Result for ampicillin should be used to predict the activity of amoxicillin (9)
[d] Isolates susceptible to amoxicillin-clavulanate are susceptible to piperacillin-tazobactam (18).
[e] Breakpoints based on PK/PD characteristics of meropenem in the CSF. Meropenem is the only carbapenem used in meningitis (18).
[f] As recommended by the EUCAST, erythromycin can be used to determine susceptibility to azithromycin, roxithromycin, clarithromycin (18).
[g] Trimethoprim-sulfamethoxazole in the ratio 1:19. Breakpoints are expressed as the trimethoprim concentration.

E-test® is a gradient diffusion technique providing an alternative to dilution methods for MIC determination in *H. influenzae* when performed on HTM or MH-LHB-NAD agar. However, there is insufficient agreement between E-test® and broth microdilution method for differentiating β-lactamase negative ampicillin-resistant (BLNAR) strains and susceptible isolates (26). Furthermore, in several studies on β-lactamase positive amoxicillin-clavulanate resistant (BLPACR) and BLNAR isolates, MICs of β-lactams, including imipenem and meropenem, were inaccurately higher (up to 6 doubling dilutions) when measured with E-test® as compared to microbroth dilution (3, 6, 57).

Disk diffusion is a cost-effective and convenient alternative and CLSI provides interpretative criteria for 29 antimicrobial agents for *H. influenzae* when tested on HTM agar. However, disk diffusion, including the use of low-strength 2-µg ampicillin disk (63), does not always allow differentiation between ampicillin-resistant (β-lactamase positive or negative) and susceptible isolates. Therefore, production of β-lactamase has to be tested by a chromogenic cephalosporin method, while β-lactamase negative ampicillin-resistance is only accurately detected by microbroth dilution (26).

Semi-automated susceptibility testing methods are not recommended for *H. influenzae* and are not adapted to the detection of BLNAR or low-level resistance to fluoroquinolones.

Eventually, resistance mechanisms can be characterized genetically by amplification and sequencing of resistance genes. Sequences of primers for β-lactam and quinolone resistance are listed in Table 5.

TECHNICAL CONDITIONS

Media

H. influenzae differs from most bacteria by its requirement for growth in both hemin or hematin (X-factor) and NAD (V-factor). Chocolate agar with NAD-containing multivitamin supplement (Choc. A-S) is the medium most commonly used for isolation of *H. influenzae*, but is not suitable for susceptibility testing of all antibiotics. The high cysteine content of the multivitamin supplement markedly increases MICs of imipenem and penicillins (47), and bovine hemoglobin contains large amount of thymidine which inhibits the activity of both sulfonamides and trimethoprim (2). However, Choc. A-S remains an alternative for testing occasional isolates unable to grow on HTM or MH-LHB-NAD agar, although breakpoints are not available for that method.

As mentioned above, CLSI and EUCAST recommend HTM and MH-LHB-NAD, respectively. Both media are adapted to microbroth dilution, or agar dilution and disk diffusion when solidified with agar. HTM is a transparent medium consisting in cation-supplemented Mueller-Hinton broth or agar with addition of 5 mg/ml yeast extract, 15 μg/ml hematin, and 15 μg/ml NAD as growth-promoting additives. MH broth or agar, yeast extract, and hematin are autoclaved together, then cooled and NAD solution is added aseptically after 0.22 μm-pore-size filtration (8). Alternatively, a HTM supplement (Oxoid) containing both hematin and NAD can be added aseptically to autoclaved MH/yeast extract medium. As HTM agar has a rather short shelf-life (4 to 6 weeks at 4°C) due to degradation of hematin and dehydration, it is essential to ensure proper quality control of the freshness of the medium, *e.g.* with *H. influenzae* strain ATCC 10211 which strongly depends on hematin to grow.

MH-LHB-NAD is Mueller-Hinton broth or agar autoclaved, cooled to 50°C, then supplemented with 5% lysed defibrinated horse blood and 20 μg/ml NAD (19) MH-LHB-NAD agar can be kept for at least 6 months at 4°C, longer than HTM agar (30). Thymidine phosphorylase contained specifically in horse erythrocytes inactivates thymidine present in the medium into thymine which does not interfere with sulfonamides and trimethoprim susceptibility testing (22).

Inoculum, inoculation, culture

The inoculum is prepared by suspending isolated colonies from overnight culture on CA-S agar into 0.9% saline. As spontaneous lysis of *H. influenzae* cells occurs rapidly, it is essential that the inoculum is prepared from fresh colonies. The suspension turbidity must be adjusted to that of a 0.5 McFarland standard suspension, corresponding approximately to 10^7 CFU/ml of *H. influenzae*.

For MIC determination by the agar dilution method, 1 μl of suspension (*ca.* 10^4 CFU) is spotted either manually or mechanically with a multipoint inoculator on the agar surface. Plates are dried at room temperature and then incubated at 36° ± 1°C in a humidified 5% CO_2 atmosphere for 24-48 hours. MICs should be read after 20-24 hours of incubation and after 48 hours in the absence of sufficient growth.

For disk diffusion, EUCAST and CLSI recommend that the suspension, as prepared above, is applied on the agar surface by either flooding or swabbing undiluted (8, 15). Swabbing is also recommended for E-test®. Plates must be dried at room temperature before application of the disks or strips and then incubated overnight at 36° ± 1°C in a humidified 5% CO_2 atmosphere. It is noteworthy that the aforementioned inoculum (*ca.* 10^7 CFU/ml) yields a confluent bacterial lawn, as opposed to the semi-confluent growth obtained with lower inocula that are still recommended in 2009 by the Comité de l'Antibiogramme de la Société Française de Microbiologie (CA-SFM) and the British Society for Antimicrobial Chemotherapy (BSAC) working party on susceptibility testing. Indeed, CA-SFM and BSAC recommend that plates are swabbed or flooded with 1:10 and 1:100 dilutions of a suspension adjusted to the 0.5 McFarland standard, respectively (1, 10). As zone diameters depend on the inoculum for many antibiotics, it is crucial that interpretation of the results is only made by comparison with breakpoints corresponding to the chosen inoculum.

For MIC determination by the microbroth dilution method, microtitre plates are inoculated with a final bacterial density of approximately 5 x 10^5 CFU/ml (1:10 dilution in HTM broth of a 10^7 CFU/ml suspension, added v/v to the antibiotic dilutions in each well). Microtitre plates can be incubated in air, but many strains still require 5 % CO_2-enrichment (26).

CONTROL STRAINS

Reference strains available from international collections are used for quality control and in order to ensure the freshness of the media chosen for susceptibility testing. The CLSI recommends *H. influenzae* ATCC 49247, a non β-lactamase ampicillin-resistant (BLNAR) strain also resistant to tetracycline, and ATCC 49766, a wild-type, susceptible strain specified for testing β-lactams (9). *Escherichia coli* ATCC 35218 is also specified as a control when testing amoxicillin-clavulanate (9). Instead of a BLNAR strain, the EUCAST favors *H. influenzae* ATCC 9334 (syn. NCTC 8468, CIP54.94, CCUG23946) which is susceptible to β-lactam antibiotics (20).

The quality of HTM and MH-LHB-NAD media can also be controlled with the fastidious *H. influenzae* ATCC 10211, which is susceptible to ampicillin but strongly depends on hematin/hemin to grow. Ultimately, β-lactamase detection methods may be assessed by using a β-lactamase positive strain, such as *H. influenzae* ATCC 35056.

ANTIBIOTICS TO BE STUDIED

Susceptibility testing of isolates responsible for invasive infections, *i.e.*, meningitis, bacteremia, septicemic pneumonia, epiglottitis, and septic arthritis should include ampicillin with a β-lactamase detection test, a third-generation cephalosporin, a carbapenem (meropenem or possibly doripenem), chloramphenicol, and possibly a fluoroquinolone for adult patients. For CSF isolates, the CLSI recommends that only results of testing with ampicillin, one of the third-generation cephalosporins, meropenem, and chloramphenicol should be reported (9).

As most of the non-invasive infections due to *H. influenzae* are treated empirically, the results of susceptibility tests are often not useful for management of individual patients, except for ampicillin and cotrimoxazole (trimethoprim-sulfamethoxazole). However, management of therapeutic failures and detection of β-lactamase-negative β-lactam resistance or fluoroquinolone resistance may warrant primary testing of amoxicillin-clavulanate, a first generation cephalosporin, oral second- and third-generation cephalosporins, and nalidixic acid. The relevance of testing nalidixic acid is discussed below.

As shown in Table 1, new breakpoints have been provided by both EUCAST and CLSI which allow to interpret the results obtained with oral and parenteral third-generation cephalosporins, carbapenems, macrolides, and telithromycin, in addition to previously available breakpoints for ampicillin, amoxicillin-clavulanate, first- and second generation cephalosporins, cotrimoxazole, tetracycline, rifampicin, and chloramphenicol.

INTRINSIC RESISTANCE

Wild-type strains of *H. influenzae* are susceptible to many antibiotics (Table 2) but are intrinsically resistant to oxacillin, mecillinam and cefsulodin, lipo- and glycopeptides, lincosamides and 16-membered macrolides (spiramycin, josamycin), fusidic acid, linezolid, nitroimidazoles, and bacitracin, which is often used as a selective agent in *H. influenzae*-specific culture media. The intrinsic low-level resistance to the 14- and 15-membered macrolides, ketolides, and streptogramins is discussed below. For wild-type strains, the *in vitro* activity of benzyl penicillin (penicillin G) is similar to that of amoxicillin (MIC_{90} of 0.25 mg/ml). However, due to the prevalence of β-lactamase-producing isolates and to insufficient concentrations achievable therapeutically in the CSF, penicillin G is no longer recommended to treat invasive and respiratory tract infections, and susceptibility breakpoints are not available.

ACQUIRED RESISTANCE

β-Lactams

β-lactams are by far the most prescribed antimicrobials to treat *H. influenzae* infections and although clinical isolates resistant to ampicillin have been reported since 1974 (53), resistance to third-generation cephalosporins remains extremely rare. As the outer membrane of *H. influenzae* offers very little resistance to the penetration into the periplasm of most β-lactams, their intrinsic activity is high and MICs of both susceptible and resistant strains are comparatively lower than those of, *e.g.*, *Enterobacteriaceae* (11). Reduced outer

Table 2. *In vitro* activity of 16 antimicrobial agents against wild-type isolates of *H. influenzae*[a]

Antimicrobial	MICs interpretative standard (μg/ml)		
	50%	90%	Range
Ampicillin	0.125	0.5	0.03-0.5
Amoxicillin	0.25	0.5	0.125-0.5
Cefaclor	2	4	0.5-8
Cefuroxime	0.5	2	0.125-2
Cefpodoxime	0.06	0.12	0.016-0.12
Cefixime	0.03	0.06	0.008-0.06
Cefotaxime	0.016	0.03	0.004-0.06
Ceftriaxone	0.008	0.008	0.004-0.016
Meropenem	0.06	0.06	0.008-0.125
Ciprofloxacin	0.002	0.008	0.002-0.016
Chloramphenicol	0.25	0.5	0.125-1
Erythromycin	2	8	0.06-8
Azithromycin	1	4	0.03-4
Telithromycin	1	4	0.03-8
Tetracycline	0.25	0.5	0.06-0.5
Trimethoprim	0.008	0.25	0.004-0.5

[a] Data from references 26, 28, 29, 31, 32, and 57.

membrane permeability has not been shown to be a resistance mechanism in *H. influenzae* (57) and acquired resistance to ampicillin and other β-lactams is due to either β-lactamase production (BLPAR isolates) or the presence of modified penicillin-binding proteins (PBPs) with lowered affinity for β-lactams (BLNAR isolates). Occasional isolates which express both mechanisms are referred to as β-lactamase-positive amoxicillin-clavulanate-resistant (BLPACR) (16, 37).

β-lactamase production

This is the most common mechanism of resistance in *H. influenzae*. The overall prevalence of β-lactamase-positive isolates is 15-20%, stable or declining in Western Europe, North America, and Japan, while it is higher than 50% in China and Eastern Asia (25, 31, 32, 57, 61, 64). Two enzymes, TEM-1 and ROB-1, account for almost all β-lactamase-mediated resistance in *H. influenzae* and can only be differentiated by their isoelectric point (5.4 and 8.1, respectively) or by PCR-based methods (21, 59) (primers in Table 5). Both are transferable class A β-lactamases that confer resistance to ampicillin and are effectively inhibited by clavulanate. TEM-1 is widely predominant, while ROB-1 is produced by less than 10% of β-lactamase-positive isolates except in Mexico (30%) and the United States (13.2%) (21). Occasional isolates have been reported that express both TEM-1 and ROB-1 (21, 25).

TEM-1 is encoded by a bla_{TEM-1} gene identical to that encountered in *Enterobacteriaceae*. However, as compared to *E. coli*, levels of β-lactam resistance in TEM-1 producing strains are significantly lower in *H. influenzae*. This may be due to the higher intrinsic activity of β-lactams against *H. influenzae* and to lower levels of expression of bla_{TEM-1} in that species.

Sequence analysis suggests that ROB-1 is more closely related to the β-lactamases of Gram-positive bacteria than of Gram-negative bacteria. As ROB-1 is found in other members of the family *Pasteurellaceae* such as *Pasteurella multocida*, *Actinobacillus pleuropneumoniae*, and *Haemophilus parasuis*, the bla_{ROB} gene may have been transferred to *H. influenzae* from these animal pathogens (33, 50).

In clinical isolates, β-lactamase-mediated resistance is usually easily detected, as most positive strains exhibit ampicillin MICs > 4 μg/ml and amoxicillin-clavulanate MICs < 1-2 μg/ml. Occasional TEM-1-producing isolates with ampicillin MICs ≤ 4 μg/ml exist and must be detected by a chromogenic β-lactamase test. If amoxicillin-clavulanate is not tested, or shows increased MIC (BLPACR isolate), a chromogenic detection should also be performed. As β-lactamase production in *H. influenzae* is constitutive, induction, *e.g.* by penicillin, is not necessary for chromogenic detection. Earlier work on ROB-1-producing *H. influenzae* isolates indicated that nitrocefin hydrolysis was weakly positive and could only be detected with a heavy inoculum (48). More recent studies did not confirm such difficulties (21). Few ampicillin-resistant isolates have been reported that were positive for nitrocefin hydrolysis but did not harbor bla_{TEM} or bla_{ROB} genes, which might indicate a previously unrecognized β-lactamase (57). In addition to penicillin G and ampicillin, TEM-1 and ROB-1 inactivate amoxicillin and piperacillin in *H. influenzae* and susceptibility is fully restored by addition of therapeutic doses of clavulanate or tazobactam.

Neither TEM-1 nor ROB-1 affects the susceptibility of *H. influenzae* to second- and third generation cephalosporins. None of the mutations in the bla_{TEM} genes that give rise to extended-spectrum β-lactamases (ESBLs) or inhibitor-resistant β-lactamases (IRTs) in *Enterobacteriaceae* has yet occurred in *H. influenzae*. Several *E. coli* IRT and ESBL genes were cloned into *H. influenzae* strains with limited effects on amoxicillin-clavulanate MICs (≤ 4/2 µg/ml for IRT-expressing strains) or on cefotaxime MICs (≤ 0.5 µg/ml for ESBL-expressing strains) (55). Accordingly, the production of ESBL in clinical *H. influenzae* is unlikely to be detected by a standard double disk diffusion technique. Tristram *et al.* suggested using disks containing a combination of cefpodoxime (10 µg) and clavulanate (1 µg) or cefotaxime (30 µg) and clavulanate (10 µg) in conjunction with a corresponding plain cephalosporin disk. An increase in the zone diameter of ≥ 5 mm for clavulanate-supplemented disk compared with plain disk would be suggestive of an ESBL (56). The potential emergence of *H. influenzae* isolates with high-level cephalosporin resistance resulting from the combination of ESBL with altered PBP3 is a serious concern (5). In 2002, two distinct isolates of *Haemophilus parainfluenzae* were identified in South Africa that expressed the TEM-15 ESBL probably associated with modified PLP, and had cefotaxime MICs of > 16 µg/ml (45, 57).

PBP3 alteration

There are 8 PBPs in *H. influenzae*, referred to as PBPs 1A, 1B, 2, 3A, 3B, 4, 5, and 6 (57). Encoded by the *ftsI* gene, PBP3A and 3B are isoforms that have a transpeptidase activity required for the synthesis of peptidoglycan. Three highly conserved amino acid motifs, Ser327-X-X-Lys, Ser379-Ser-Asn (SSN), and Lys513-Tyr-Gly (KTG) are essential for that function. Resistance to ampicillin in β-lactamase-negative isolates of *H. influenzae* (BLNAR) was reported as early as 1974 (54) and has been related unambiguously to substitutions in PBP3 which result in reduced binding affinity to all β-lactams (review in 57). As opposed to β-lactamase production alone (BLPAR isolates), PBP-mediated resistance (BLNAR and BLPACR isolates) remains infrequent among *H. influenzae* clinical isolates (< 5%) in many countries, but might be underestimated due to inadequate susceptibility testing and to the lack of consensus-defining breakpoints (Table 1). Conversely, 20 to 56% isolates in France, Spain, and the United Kingdom are reported to be BLNAR (13, 23, 24), while in Japan more than 60% of upper respiratory tract and invasive Hib isolates are reported to be BLNAR or BLPACR (28, 29). However, the definition of BLNAR is challenging and does not rely exclusively on raised ampicillin MIC. Thus, all isolates with significant mutations in the *ftsI* gene are designated as genetically BLNAR (gBLNAR), including those with ampicillin MICs lower than the 1.0 µg/ml breakpoint recommended by CLSI and EUCAST (9, 18). Based on the deduced amino acid substitutions in the vicinity of conserved motifs of the PBP3 transpeptidase region, gBLNAR isolates were originally classified in 3 groups (I, II, III) (13, 62). Further subdivisions were later added in attempts to accommodate other mutations (57).

Among the main substitutions listed in Table 3, Arg517 to His and Asp526 to Lys surrounding the KTG motif are present in group I and group II isolates, respectively, and are related to moderate ampicillin resistance (low BLNAR). Isolates possessing a substitution near the KTG motif and Met377 to Ile, Ser385 to Thr, and Leu389 to Phe substitutions near the SSN motif belong to group III, have higher levels of ampicillin resistance, and are designated as BLNAR. Compared to a modal value of 0.12 µg/ml for BLNAS strains, low-BLNAR strains usually have ampicillin MICs of 0.5 to 2.0 µg/ml, and BLNAR strains have ampicillin MICs of 1.0 to 16 µg/ml (Table 3) (27, 62). Decreased susceptibility or sometimes resistance to other β-lactams occurs in both low BLNAR and BLNAR isolates, and strains with ampicillin MIC > 1.0 µg/ml must be considered resistant to amoxicillin-clavulanate, ampicillin-sulbactam, first- and second generation cephalosporins, despite apparent *in vitro* susceptibility of some strains to these antibiotics (9). However, low-BLNAR strains tend to have lower levels of resistance than BLNAR strains, with MIC_{90} of ampicillin of 2.0 µg/ml and 8.0 µg/ml and of cefotaxime of 0.25 µg/ml and 1.0 µg/ml, respectively (57). In BPLACR isolates, the contribution of the β-lactamase to resistance is limited to ampicillin and amoxicillin. BLPACR strains

Table 3. Main a amino acid substitutions in penicillin binding protein 3 associated with β-lactam resistance in *H. influenzae* (from references 13, 24, 27, 57, and 62)

Group[c]	Ampicillin resistance phenotype	PLP3 amino acid substitutions[a,b]							
		Near the SXXK motif	Near the SSN motif				Near the KTG motif		
		Asp-50	Met-377	Ser-385	Leu-389	Gly-490	Ala-502	Arg-517	Asn-526
Wild-type[d]	BLNAS								
Group I	Low BLNAR	Asn	Ileu			Glu	Thr	**His**	
Group II	Low BLNAR	Asn	Ileu			Glu	Val or Thr		**Lys**
Group III	BLNAR	**Asn**	**Ileu**	**Thr**	Phe				**Lys**

[a] Deduced from *fstI* gene sequences.
[b] Bold type, present in all strains; plain text, present in some strains.
[c] BLNAR and low BLNAR strains classification adapted from Ubukata *et al.* (62) and Dabernat *et al.* (13).
[d] *H. influenzae* strain Rd (ATCC 51907).

have higher ampicillin MICs than the BLNAR strains with identical PBP3 amino acid substitutions (2.0 to 64 μg/ml compared to 0.5 to 16 μg/ml) but the MICs of amoxicillin-clavulanate, cefixime, and third-generation cephalosporins are the same (13, 62). In contrast to penicillin-resistant *Streptococcus pneumoniae* isolates, there is great genetic diversity among BLNAR/BLPACR *H. influenzae* isolates and clonal spread is rare (13, 24, 57). Intra- and inter-specific transfer of modified *ftsI* gene in the *Haemophilus* genus has been demonstrated *in vitro* but does not seem to play a major role in the spread of β-lactam resistance among clinical isolates (13). Mutations conferring β-lactam resistance may therefore arise spontaneously to be then selected by antimicrobial therapy.

Third-generation cephalosporin resistance

In accordance with the CLSI breakpoints, resistance to cefixime and cefotaxime (MIC > 2 μg/ml) is extremely rare in *H. influenzae*. Only two isolates have been reported in Spain, with MICs of 4 μg/ml (24). Conversely, if EUCAST breakpoints are considered, resistant isolates (MIC > 0.12 μg/ml) are not unusual, especially in BLNAR group III Hib isolates in Japan (28, 49). Resistance to cefotaxime appears to require at least Met377 to Ile, Ser385 to Thr, and Leu389 to Phe substitutions near the SSN motif of PBP3 and additional mutations in the *ftsI* gene (24, 28, 49). Interestingly, ceftriaxone MICs are usually at least 2 doubling dilutions lower than those of cefotaxime and cefixime (28).

Carbapenem resistance

Resistance to imipenem (MICs of up to 32 μg/ml) has been reported in BLNAR isolates and appears to be related to the accumulation of *ftsI* point mutations, previously described in different BLNAR isolates but not simultaneously (6, 41). Specifically, the conjunction of Asp526 to Lys, Ala502 to Val, Gly490 to Glu and Met377 to Ile substitutions in PBP3 may contribute to high-level imipenem resistance. Surprisingly, the ampicillin susceptibility of imipenem-resistant isolates carrying those 4 mutations is only slightly decreased (MICs of 0.5-0.75 μg/ml) (6).

Other PBPs

In contrast to mutations in *ftsI*, none of the mutations observed so far in the *pbp1A*, *pbp1B*, *pbp2*, *dacB*, and *dacA* genes (encoding PBP1A, PBP1B and PBP2, PBP4, and PBP5, respectively) appear to impact on β-lactam susceptibility of *H. influenzae* (6, 34, 57).

Efflux

An AcrAB-like efflux pump is present in all *H. influenzae* strains that is down-regulated by transcription repressor AcrR. Unusually high ampicillin resistance (MIC of 16 μg/ml) was reported in 2004 in four BLNAR isolates that had both modified PBP3 and overexpression of AcrAB due to the loss of AcrR. In the four isolates, a base pair insertion in the *acrR* gene was found that predicted early termination of the reading frame (34).

Fluoroquinolones

Fluoroquinolones are the most active antibiotics *in vitro* against *H. influenzae* and are also highly effective as treatments for respiratory tract infections in adult patients. Resistant *H. influenzae* isolates have occasionally been reported worldwide and might become a concern in the future (57). In vitro and in vivo, resistance seems to arise only in hypermutable isolates (43). Since hypermutable isolates are frequent in chronic respiratory infections and colonize cystic fibrosis patients, precautions are advised when treating these patients with fluoroquinolones. Recently, clonal expansion of fluoroquinolone-resistant strains among elderly patients has been demonstrated in Japan (66). In *H. influenzae*, quinolone resistance is mainly imparted by mutations in a domain referred to as quinolone-resistance determining region (QRDR) of two genes, *gyrA* and *parC*, respectively encoding the A subunits of DNA gyrase and topoisomerase IV. Mutations in the *gyrB* and *parE* genes, respectively encoding the B subunits of the two enzymes also contribute to lesser extent to the resistance. The most frequent substitutions and their corresponding resistance levels are summarized in Table 4. Mutations in the *gyrA*, *gyrB*, *parC*, and *parE* can be identified by sequencing, using primer listed in Table 5. As in *Neisseria* or other Gram-negative bacteria, low-level fluoroquinolone resistance can be readily detected by testing nalidixic acid (NAL), because single mutations usually confer high-level resistance to this antibiotic (Table 4). In case of resistance to NAL, the EUCAST recommends to "determine the MIC of the fluoroquinolone to be used in therapy". According to the literature, when using disk diffusion an inhibition diameter ≥ 21 mm around a 30-μg NAL disk predicts susceptibility to fluoroquinolones (42). Otherwise, the MICs of fluoroquinolones should be determined. However, a few isolates have been reported which are resistant to fluoroquinolones (*e.g.*, MIC of ciprofloxacin = 32 μg/ml), but not to NAL (MIC = 2 μg/ml) (42). Novel mechanisms could explain this phenotype, such as overexpression of efflux systems or porin defect, but they have not been shown so far to play a role in the quinolone resistance of *H. influenzae*.

Tetracyclines and glycylcyclines

Resistance to tetracyclines was among the first acquired resistances in *H. influenzae*. Its prevalence has been significantly reduced since 1980 as tetracyclines prescription went downward, and is now less than 5% of clinical isolates in European and North American countries. Conversely, resistance rates probably remain higher (≥ 20 % of clinical isolates) in emerging countries like China (51). In *H. influenzae*, resistance is associated with the Tet(B) efflux mechanism which confers high level resistance to tetracycline (128 μg/ml) and lower level resistance to doxycyline and minocyline (MICs, 4-8 μg/ml and 1-2 μg/ml, respectively). The *tet*(B) gene is carried by transposon Tn*10*, usually found on conjugative plasmids. Other resistance genes present in related species of the family *Pasteurellaceae* have been transferred

Table 4. Acquired resistance to quinolones due to substitutions in the quinolone-resistance determining region of DNA gyrase and topoisomerase IV of *H. influenzae* (from ref. 42 and 66)

Substitution(s) in the QRDR of			MIC or MIC range (μg/ml)		
GyrA[a]	ParC	ParE	NAL[b]	LEV	CIP
[Ser84, Asp88][c]	[Gly82, Ser84]	[Asp420]	0.5	0.03	0.008
Asp88Tyr			2-64	0.12	0.12
Asp88Tyr	Gly82Asp		64	2	2
Asp88Asn			16	0.06	0.12
Asp88Asn	Ser84Arg		128	0.5	0.5
Asp88Asn	Gly82Cys, Ser84Arg		128	2	4
Ser84Leu			64	1	1
Ser84Leu	Ser84Ile		128	2-4	2-4
Ser84Leu, Asp88Asn	Ser84Ile		≥ 128	2-16	2-8
Ser84Leu, Asp88Asn	Ser84Ile	Asp420Asn	> 128	16-32	8-16

[a] GyrA, A subunit of DNA gyrase; ParC and ParE, A and B subunits of topoisomerase IV, respectively.
[b] CIP, ciprofloxacin; LEV, levofloxacin; NAL, nalidixic acid.
[c] Corresponding amino acids in strain *H. influenzae* Rd (ATCC 51907).

Table 5. Primers for detection of resistance genes and resistance-related mutations

Gene	Protein	Primer	Amplicon size (positions[a])	Reference
ftsI	PLP3	F: 5'-GAT ACT ACG TCC TTT AAA TTA AG-3' R: 5'-GCA GTA AAT GCC ACA TAC TTA-3'	551 bp (1048-1598)	62
		F: 5'-GTT GCA CAT ATC TCC GAT GAG-3' R: 5'-CAG CTG CTT CAG CAT CTT GC-3'	1029 bp (733-1761)	62
bla$_{TEM}$	TEM-1	F: 5'-TGG GTG CAC GAG TGG GTT AC-3' R: 5'-TTA TCC GCC TCC ATC CAG TC-3'	526 bp (321-846)	27
bla$_{ROB}$	ROB-1	F: 5'-ATC AGC CAC ACA AGC CAC CT-3' R: 5'-GTT TGC GAT TTG GTA TGC GA-3'	692 bp (117-808)	27
Quinolone resistance				
gyrA	GyrA	F: 5'-CCG CCG CGT ACT ATT CTC AAT-3' R: 5'-GTT GCC ATC CCC ACC GCA ATA CCA-3'	400 bp (138-537)	42
parC	ParC	F: 5'-TCT GAA CTT GGC TTA ATT GCC-3' R: 5'-GCC ACG ACC TTG CTC ATA AAT-3'	564 bp (160-723)	42
parE	ParE	F: 5'-TCG TTA GTG GCC CTG CAT TAC-3' R: 5'-GAA CAG GGC ACA GAG TAG GGT-3'	347 bp (1172-1518)	42
gyrB	GyrB	F: 5'-CCT GCT CTT TCT GAA ACT TTA C-3' R: 5'-CCA TCT AAC GCA AGG GTT AAT C-3'	547 bp (1152-1698)	42

[a] Referring to the corresponding coding sequence in *H. influenzae* Rd (ATCC 51907).

in vitro to *H. influenzae* (7) suggesting that ribosomal protection encoded by the *tet*(M) gene or *tet*(K)-mediated efflux might also emerge in *H. influenzae*.

The glycylcycline tigecycline is a derivative of minocycline with higher binding affinity for the ribosomes than earlier tetracyclines. Furthermore, Tet efflux proteins [Tet(A)- to Tet(D) and Tet(K)] do not recognize glycylcyclines and/or are unable to translocate them through the cytoplasmic membrane. Thus tigecycline remains active on *H. influenzae* isolates carrying *tet*(B), *tet*(K), or *tet*(M) genes (44). As tigecycline has been licensed for intra-abdominal and complicated skin and soft tissue infections, neither CLSI nor EUCAST provide *H. influenzae*-related breakpoints, but MIC values (MIC$_{90}$ = 0.25 µg/ml) imply that *H. influenzae* infections might be treated with tigecycline. However, laboratory-derived mutations in *tet*(B) have led to glycylcycline resistance, suggesting that bacterial resistance to tigecycline may develop with clinical use (7).

Sulfonamides and trimethoprim

H. influenzae is intrinsically susceptible to both sulfamethoxazole and trimethoprim, which inhibit the synthesis of tetrahydrofolic acid, thus blocking thymine synthesis, hence preventing DNA replication. Sulfamethoxazole competes with para-aminobenzoic acid as a substrate for dihydropteroate synthetase (DHPS), which is involved in the production of dihydropteroate, a precursor compound of dihydrofolate. Resistance to sulfamethoxazole in *H. influenzae* (MIC = 1,048 µg/ml) is infrequent and is related to mutations in the *folP* gene encoding DHPS or acquisition of supplemental DHPS encoded by plasmid borne *sul* genes (17). Modified or supplemental DHPS have decreased affinity for sulfamethoxazole but retain their affinity for para-aminobenzoic acid.

Trimethoprim is a substrate analog of dihydrofolate and blocks its reduction to tetrahydrofolate by dihydrofolate reductase (DHFR). In *H. influenzae*, resistance to trimethoprim is mostly due to mutations in the sequence and in the promoter region of the *folH* gene encoding the chromosomal DHFR, resulting in the hyperproduction of DHFR with altered affinity to trimethoprim (15). This mechanism is responsible for resistance to co-trimoxazole, which is common among strains of *H. influenzae* worldwide (15 to 50% of clinical isolates) (31, 61).

Other antibiotics

Chloramphenicol

This antibiotic remains a potent alternative therapy for *H. influenzae* meningitis, *e.g.* in developing countries. Resistance occurs in less than 5% of isolates and is usually related to the production of plasmid-mediated chloramphenicol acetyl transferase (CAT). MICs of resistant isolates range from 4 to 16 µg/ml. When present, CAT production is frequently associated with that of β-lactamase.

Macrolides, ketolides and streptogramins

They have limited activity on wild-type strains of *H. influenzae* (*e.g.* MIC of erythromycin, 0.25-4 µg/ml) due to the presence of the AcrAB-like efflux pump and rare isolates that lack this efflux mechanism have lower MICs (erythromycin, 0.06-0.12 µg/ml). In spite of this intrinsic low-level resistance, compounds with specific PK/PD properties like clarithromycin and azithromycin are being used to treat localized NTHi infections such as OMA, although the benefit is not clearly established (14). It was recently shown that azithromycin is active on BLNAR NTHi cells in bacterial biofilms, and might be of interest for treatment of infections involving such biofilms, *e.g.* in recurrent otitis media and early airway infection in cystic fibrosis (52). Less than 1% of *H. influenzae* strains have acquired high-level resistance which is associated with mutations in L4 or L22 ribosomal proteins or in the 23S rRNA domain where those proteins bind. High-level resistance (> 16 µg/ml) is readily detected by disk diffusion or determination of MICs of erythromycin or telithromycin (4) and acquired resistance to azithromycin and clarithromycin can be predicted by testing erythromycin (9).

Rifampin

As oral prophylactic treatment, rifampin is recommended for contacts of a patient with invasive infection and susceptibility should be confirmed by the laboratory. Occasional resistance is due to mutation(s) in the *rpoB* gene encoding the β-subunit of the DNA-dependent RNA polymerase, the target of rifampin. High level resistance (> 32 µg/ml) is frequently related to Asn-516 to Val substitution in the RpoB sequence of clinical isolates as well as *in vitro* generated mutants (12).

Aminoglycosides

Theses drugs are not recommended in the treatment of *H. influenzae* infections, although all strains are susceptible to gentamicin, tobramycin, and amikacin (MICs, 0.25-1 µg/ml). However, resistance to kanamycin due to aminoglycoside 3'-*O*-phosphotranferase [APH(3')-1] is present in more than 95 % of TEM-1 β-lactamase producing isolates.

Fosfomycin

Fosfomycin disodium is not recommended alone in the treatment of *H. influenzae* infections, although it has potent *in vitro* activity (MIC_{90} = 2 µg/ml). Acquired resistance has not been reported so far in *H. influenzae* but could arise as formulations of fosfomycin associated to tobramycin for nebulization have successfully been tested for the treatment of cystic fibrosis and other bronchiectasis-related infections (35).

CONCLUSION

Although systematic anti-Hib vaccination has dramatically reduced the incidence of invasive infections, *H. influenzae* remains one of the leading causes of pneumonia and meningitis in non-vaccinated children and is commonly responsible of numerous respiratory tract infections. Given that most isolates remain susceptible to third-generation cephalosporins and fluoroquinolones, and as it requires specific media and methods, antibiotic susceptibility testing of *H. influenzae* is sometimes overlooked. However, difficult-to-treat respiratory tract *H. influenzae* infections are being reported with increasing frequency, most notably otitis media that are associated to BLNAR or BLPACR isolates. In this setting, the choice of an antibiotic with adequate PK/PD characteristics is essential and clinical laboratories should provide susceptibility testing. Acquired resistance to most antimicrobial agents is readily identified by disk diffusion but accurate susceptibility testing of β-lactams requires to determine MICs with a broth dilution method. When this method is not performed routinely, isolates may be sent to a reference laboratory.

REFERENCES

(1) **Andrews, J. M., for the BSAC Working Party on Susceptibility Testing. 2009.** BSAC standardized disc susceptibility testing method (version 8). J. Antimicrob. Chemother. **64**:454-489.

(2) **Bergeron, M. G., P. Simard, and P. Provencher.** 1987. Influence of growth medium and supplement on growth of *Haemophilus influenzae* and on antibacterial activity of several antibiotics. J. Clin. Microbiol. **7**:650-655.

(3) **Billal, D. S., M. Hotomi, and N. Yamanaka.** 2007. Can the E-test correctly determine the MICs of β-lactam and cephalosporin antibiotics for β-lactamase-negative ampicillin-resistant *Haemophilus influenzae*? Antimicrob. Agents Chemother. **51**:3463-3464.

(4) **Bogdanovich, T., B. Bozdogan, and P. C. Appelbaum**. 2006. Effect of efflux on telithromycin and macrolide susceptibility in *Haemophilus influenzae*. Antimicrob. Agents Chemother. **50**:893-898.

(5) **Bozdogan, B., S. G. Tristram, and P. C. Appelbaum**. 2006. Combination of altered PBPs and expression of cloned extended spectrum β-lactamases confers cefotaxime resistance in *Haemophilus influenzae*. J. Antimicrob. Chemother. **57**:747–749.

(6) **Cerquetti, M., M. Giufrè, R. Cardines, and P. Mastrantonio**. 2007. First characterization of heterogeneous resistance to imipenem in invasive nontypeable *Haemophilus influenzae* isolates. Antimicrob. Agents Chemother. **51**:3155-3161.

(7) **Chopra, I. and M. Roberts**. 2001. Tetracycline antibiotics: mode of action, applications, molecular biology, and epidemiology of bacterial resistance. Microbiol. Mol. Biol. Rev. **65**:232–260.

(8) **Clinical and Laboratory Standards Institute**. 2006. Methods for dilution antimicrobial susceptibility tests for bacteria that grow aerobically, 7th ed. Approved standard. CLSI document M7-A7. Clinical Laboratory Standards Institute, Wayne, PA, USA.

(9) **Clinical and Laboratory Standards Institute**. 2009. Performance Standards for antimicrobial susceptibility testing; nineteenth informational supplement. Standard M100-S19. CLSI. Wayne, PA, USA.

(10) **Comité de l'Antibiogramme de la Société Française de Microbiologie**. 2009. Communiqué 2009, p.5. Comité de l'Antibiogramme de la Société Française de Microbiologie, Paris, France. http://www.sfm.asso.fr/

(11) **Coulton, J. W., P. Mason, and D. Dorrance**. 1983. The permeability barrier of *Haemophilus influenzae* type b against beta-lactam antibiotics. J. Antimicrob. Chemother. **12**:435-449.

(12) **Cruchaga, S., M. Pérez-Vázquez, F. Román, and J. Campos**. 2003. Molecular basis of rifampicin resistance in *Haemophilus influenzae*. J. Antimicrob. Chemother. **52**:1011-1014.

(13) **Dabernat, H., C. Delmas, M. Seguy, R. Pelisser, G. Faucon, S. Bennamani, and C. Pasquier**. 2002. Diversity of β-lactam resistance-conferring amino acid substitutions in penicillin-binding protein 3 of *Haemophilus influenzae*. Antimicrob. Agents Chemother. **46**:2208-2218.

(14) **Dagan, R., and E. Leibovitz**. 2002. Bacterial eradication in the treatment of otitis media. Lancet Infect. Dis. **2**:593-604.

(15) **de Groot, R., M. Sluijter, A. D. de Bruyn, J. Campos, W. H. F. Goessens, A. L. Smith, and P. W. M. Hermans**. 1996. Genetic characterization of trimethoprim resistance in *Haemophilus influenzae*. Antimicrob. Agents Chemother. **40**:2131-2136.

(16) **Doern, G. V., A. B. Brueggemann, G. Pierce, H. P. Holley, Jr., and A. Rauch**. 1997. Antibiotic resistance among clinical isolates of *Haemophilus influenzae* in the United States in 1994 and 1995 and detection of beta-lactamase-positive strains resistant to amoxicillin-clavulanate: results of a national multicenter surveillance study. Antimicrob. Agents Chemother. **41**:292-297.

(17) **Enne, V. I., A. King, D. M. Livermore, and L. M. C. Hall**. 2002. Sulfonamide resistance in *Haemophilus influenzae* mediated by acquisition of *sul*2 or a short insertion in chromosomal *folP*. Antimicrob. Agents Chemother. **46**:1934-1939.

(18) **European Committee on Antimicrobial Susceptibility Testing**. April 2008, accession date. Expert rules in antimicrobial susceptibility testing. http://eucast.www137.server1.mensemedia.net/expert_rules/.

(19) **European Committee on Antimicrobial Susceptibility Testing**. June 2009. EUCAST disk diffusion test methodology http://www.eucast.org/eucast_disk_diffusion_test/disk_diffusion_methodology/.

(20) **European Committee on Antimicrobial Susceptibility Testing**. June 2009. EUCAST recommended strains for internal quality control. http://eucast.www137.server1.mensemedia.net/eucast_disk_diffusion_test/eucast_qc_tables/.

(21) **Farrell, D. J., I. Morrissey, S. Bakker, S. Buckridge, and D. Felmingham**. 2005. Global distribution of TEM-1 and ROB-1 beta-lactamases in *Haemophilus influenzae*. J. Antimicrob. Chemother. **56**:773-776.

(22) **Ferone, R., S. R. M. Bushby, J. J. Burchall, W. D. Moore, and D. Smith**. 1975. Identification of Harper-Cawston factor as thymidine phosphorylase and removal from media of substances interfering with susceptibility testing to sulfonamides and diaminopyrimidines. Antimicrob. Agents Chemother. **7**:91-96.

(23) **Fluit, A. C., A. Florijn, J. Verhoef, and D. Milatovic**. 2005. Susceptibility of European beta-lactamase-positive and -negative *Haemophilus influenzae* isolates from the periods 1997/1998 and 2002/2003. J. Antimicrob. Chemother. **56**:133-138.

(24) **García-Cobos, S., J. Campos, E. Lázaro, F. Román, E. Cercenado, C. García-Rey, M. Pérez-Vázquez, J. Oteo, and F. de Abajo**. 2007. Ampicillin-resistant non-β-lactamase-producing *Haemophilus influenzae* in Spain: recent emergence of clonal isolates with increased resistance to cefotaxime and cefixime. Antimicrob. Agents Chemother. **51**:2564-2573.

(25) **García-Cobos, S., J. Campos, E. Cercenado, F. Román, E. Lázaro, M. Pérez-Vázquez, F. de Abajo, and J. Oteo**. 2008. Antibiotic resistance in *Haemophilus influenzae* decreased, except for beta-lactamase-negative amoxicillin-resistant isolates, in parallel with community antibiotic consumption in Spain from 1997 to 2007. Antimicrob. Agents Chemother. **52**:2760-2766.

(26) **García-Cobos, S., J. Campos, F. Román, C. Carrera, M. Pérez-Vázquez, B. Aracil, and J. Oteo**. 2008. Low beta-lactamase-negative ampicillin-resistant *Haemophilus influenzae* strains are best detected by testing amoxicillin susceptibility by the

broth microdilution method. Antimicrob. Agents Chemother. **52**:2407-2414.

(27) **Hasegawa, K., K. Yamamoto, N. Chiba, R. Kobayashi, K. Nagai, M. R. Jacobs, P. C. Appelbaum, K. Sunakawa, and K. Ubukata.** 2003. Diversity of ampicillin-resistance genes in *Haemophilus influenzae* in Japan and the United States. Microb. Drug Resist. **9**:39-46.

(28) **Hasegawa, K., R. Kobayashi, E. Takada, A. Ono, N. Chiba, M. Morozumi, S. Iwata, K. Sunakawa, and K. Ubukata.** 2006. High prevalence of type β beta-lactamase-non-producing ampicillin-resistant *Haemophilus influenzae* in meningitis: the situation in Japan where Hib vaccine has not been introduced. J. Antimicrob. Chemother. **57**:1077-1082.

(29) **Hotomi, M., K. Fujihara, D. S. Billal, K. Suzuki, T. Nishimura, S. Baba, and N. Yamanaka.** 2007. Genetic characteristics and clonal dissemination of β-lactamase non-producing ampicillin-resistant (BLNAR) *Haemophilus influenzae* isolated from the upper respiratory tract in Japan. Antimicrob. Agents Chemother. **51**:3969-3976.

(30) **Jacobs, M. R., S. Bajaksouzian, A. Windau, P. C. Appelbaum, G. Lin, D. Felmingham, C. Dencer, L. Koeth, M. E. Singer, and C. E. Good.** 2002. Effects of various test media on the activities of 21 antimicrobial agents against *Haemophilus influenzae*. J. Clin. Microbiol. **40**:3269-3276.

(31) **Jacobs, M. R., D. Felmingham, P. C. Appelbaum, and R. N. Gruneberg.** 2003. The Alexander Project 1998-2000: susceptibility of pathogens isolated from community-acquired respiratory tract infection to commonly used antimicrobial agents. J. Antimicrob. Chemother. **52**:229-246.

(32) **Jansen, W. T., A. Verel, M. Beitsma, J. Verhoef, and D. Milatovic.** 2006. Longitudinal European surveillance study of antibiotic resistance of *Haemophilus influenzae*. J. Antimicrob. Chemother. **58**:873-877.

(33) **Juteau, J. M., and R. C. Levesque.** 1990. Sequence analysis and evolutionary perspectives of ROB-1 beta-lactamase. Antimicrob. Agents Chemother. **34**:1364-1369.

(34) **Kaczmarek, F. S., T. D. Gootz, F. Dib-Hajj, W. Shang, S. Hallowell, and M. Cronan.** 2004. Genetic and molecular characterization of β-lactamase negative ampicillin-resistant *Haemophilus influenzae* with unusually high resistance to ampicillin. Antimicrob. Agents Chemother. **48**:1630-1639.

(35) **MacLeod, D. L., L. M. Barker, J. L. Sutherland, S. C. Moss, J. L. Gurgel, T. F. Kenney, J. L. Burns, and W. R. Baker.** 2009. Antibacterial activities of a fosfomycin/tobramycin combination: a novel inhaled antibiotic for bronchiectasis. J. Antimicrob. Chemother. **64**: 829–836.

(36) **Mandell, L. A., R. G. Wunderink, A. Anzueto, J. G. Bartlett, G. D. Campbell, N. C. Dean, S. F. Dowell, T. M. File, Jr, D. M. Musher, M. S. Niederman, A. Torres, and C. G. Whitney.** 2007. Infectious Diseases Society of America/American Thoracic Society consensus guidelines on the management of community-acquired pneumonia in adults. Clin. Infect. Dis. **44**:S27-72.

(37) **Matic, V., B. Bozdogan, M. R. Jacobs, K. Ubukata, and P. C. Appelbaum**. 2003. Contribution of beta-lactamase and PBP amino acid substitutions to amoxicillin/clavulanate resistance in beta-lactamase-positive, amoxicillin/clavulanate-resistant *Haemophilus influenzae*. J. Antimicrob. Chemother. **52**:1018-1021.

(38) **Moriyama, S., M. Hotomi, J. Shimada, D. S. Billal, K. Fujihara, and N. Yamanaka.** 2009. Formation of biofilm by *Haemophilus influenzae* isolated from pediatric intractable otitis media. Auris Nasus Larynx. **36**:525-531.

(39) **Murphy, T. F., A. L. Brauer, A. T. Schiffmacher, and S. Sethi.** 2004. Persistent colonization by *Haemophilus influenzae* in chronic obstructive pulmonary disease. Am. J. Respir. Crit. Care Med. **170**:266-272.

(40) **Murphy, T. F., H. Faden, L. O. Bakaletz, J. M. Kyd, A. Forsgren, J. Campos, M. Virji, S. I. Pelton.** 2009. Nontypeable *Haemophilus influenzae* as a pathogen in children. Pediatr. Infect Dis J. **28**:43-48.

(41) **Osaki, Y., Y. Sanbongi, M. Ishikawa, H. Kataoka, T. Suzuki, K. Maeda, and T. Ida.** 2005. Genetic approach to study the relationship between penicillin-binding protein 3 mutations and *Haemophilus influenzae* beta-lactam resistance by using site-directed mutagenesis and gene recombinants. Antimicrob. Agents Chemother. **49**:2834-2839.

(42) **Pérez-Vázquez, M., F. Román, B. Aracil, R. Cantón, and J. Campos.** 2004. Laboratory detection of *Haemophilus influenzae* with decreased susceptibility to nalidixic acid, ciprofloxacin, levofloxacin, and moxifloxacin due to *gyrA* and *parC* mutations. J. Clin. Microbiol. **42**:1185-1191

(43) **Pérez-Vázquez, M., F. Román, S. García-Cobos, and J. Campos.** 2007. Fluoroquinolone resistance in *Haemophilus influenzae* is associated with hypermutability. Antimicrob. Agents Chemother. **51**:1566-1569.

(44) **Petersen, P. J., N. V. Jacobus, W. J. Weiss, P. E. Sum, and R. T. Testa.** 1999. *In vitro* and *in vivo* antibacterial activities of a novel glycylcycline, the 9-t-butylglycylamido derivative of minocycline (GAR-936). Antimicrob. Agents Chemother. **43**:738-744.

(45) **Pitout, M., K. Macdonald, and H. Musgrave.** Characterisation of extended spectrum β-lactamase (ESBL) activity in *Haemophilus parainfluenzae*. 2002. *In*: Abstracts of the 42nd Interscience Conference on Antimicrobial Agents and Chemotherapy, San Diego, CA. Washington, DC, USA: American Society for Microbiology. Abstract C2-645, p. 96.

(46) **Prymula, R., P. Peeters, V. Chrobok, P. Kriz, E. Novakova, E. Kaliskova, I. Kohl, P. Lommel, J. Poolman, J. P. Prieels, and L. Schuerman.** 2006. Pneumococcal capsular polysaccharides conjugated

to protein D for prevention of acute otitis media caused by both *Streptococcus pneumoniae* and nontypable *Haemophilus influenzae*: a randomised double-blind efficacy study. Lancet **367**:740-748.

(47) **Rhomberg, P. R. and R. N. Jones.** 1994. Evaluations of the E-test for antimicrobial susceptibility testing of *Legionella pneumophila*, including validation of the imipenem and sparfloxacin strips. Diagn. Microbiol. Infect. Dis. **20**:159-162.

(48) **Rubin, L. G., A. A. Medeiros, R. H. Yolken, and E. R. Moxon.** 1981. Ampicillin treatment failure of apparently beta-lactamase-negative *Haemophilus influenzae* type b meningitis due to novel beta-lactamase. Lancet ii:1008-1010.

(49) **Sanbongi, Y., T. Suzuki, Y. Osaki, N. Senju, T. Ida, and K. Ubukata.** 2006. Molecular evolution of beta-lactam-resistant *Haemophilus influenzae*: 9-year surveillance of penicillin-binding protein 3 mutations in isolates from Japan. Antimicrob. Agents Chemother. **50**:2487-2492.

(50) **San Millan, A., J. A. Escudero, A. Catalan, S. Nieto, F. Farelo, M. Gibert, M. A. Moreno, L. Dominguez, and B. Gonzalez-Zorn.** 2007. Beta-lactam resistance in *Haemophilus parasuis* is mediated by plasmid pB1000 bearing bla_{ROB-1}. Antimicrob. Agents Chemother. **51**:2260-2264.

(51) **Shen, X. Z., Q. Lu, L. Deng, S. Yu, H. Zhang, Q. Deng, M. Jiang, Y. Hu, K. H. Yao, and Y. H. Yang.** 2007. Resistance of *Haemophilus influenzae* isolates in children under 5 years old with acute respiratory infections in China between 2000 and 2002. J. Internat. Med. Res. **35**:554-563.

(52) **Starner, T. D., J. D. Shrout, M. R. Parsek, P. C. Appelbaum, and G. Kim.** 2008. Subinhibitory concentrations of azithromycin decrease nontypeable *Haemophilus influenzae* biofilm formation and diminish established biofilms. Antimicrob. Agents Chemother. **52**:137-145.

(53) **Thomas, W. J., J. W. McReynolds, C. R. Mock, and D. W. Bailey.** 1974 Ampicillin-resistant *Haemophilus influenzae* meningitis. Lancet. **1**(7852):313.

(54) **Thornsberry, C., and L. A. Kirven.** 1974. Ampicillin resistance in *Haemophilus influenzae* as determined by a rapid test for beta-lactamase production. Antimicrob. Agents Chemother. **6**:653-654.

(55) **Tristram, S. G.** 2003. Effect of extended spectrum β-lactamases on the susceptibility of *Haemophilus influenzae* to cephalosporins. J. Antimicrob. Chemother. **51**:39-43.

(56) **Tristram S. G., B. Bozdogan B, and P. C. Appelbaum.** 2005. Disk diffusion-based screening tests for extended-spectrum β-lactamases in *Haemophilus influenzae*. J. Antimicrob. Chemother. **55**:570–573.

(57) **Tristram, S. G., M. R. Jacobs, and P. C. Appelbaum.** 2007. Antimicrobial resistance in *Haemophilus influenzae*. Clin. Microbiol. Rev. **20**:368–389.

(58) **Tristram, S. G.** 2008. A comparison of E-test®, M.I.C.Evaluator™ strips and CLSI broth microdilution for determining β-lactam antimicrobial susceptibility in *Haemophilus influenzae*. J. Antimicrob. Chemother. **62**:1464-1466.

(59) **Tristram, S. G.** 2009. Novel *bla* (TEM)-positive ampicillin-susceptible strains of *Haemophilus influenzae*. J. Infect. Chemother. **15**:340-3424.

(60) **Tunkel, A. R., B. J. Hartman, S. L. Kaplan, B. A. Kaufman, K. L. Roos, W. M. Scheld, and R. J. Whitley.** 2004 Practice guidelines for the management of bacterial meningitis. Clin. Infect. Dis. **39**:1267-1284.

(61) **Turnak, M. R., S. I. Bandak, S. K. Bouchillon, B. S. Allen, and D. J. Hoban.** 2001. Antimicrobial susceptibilities of clinical isolates of *Haemophilus influenzae* and *Moraxella catarrhalis* collected during 1999–2000 from 13 countries. Clin. Microbiol. Infect. **7**:671-677.

(62) **Ubukata, K., Y. Shibasaki, K. Yamamoto, N. Chiba, K. Hasegawa, Y. Takeuchi, K. Sunakawa, M. Inoue, and M. Konno.** 2001. Association of amino acid substitutions in penicillin-binding protein 3 with beta-lactam resistance in beta-lactamase-negative ampicillin-resistant *Haemophilus influenzae*. Antimicrob. Agents Chemother. **45**:1693-1699.

(63) **Ubukata, K., N. Chiba, K. Hasegawa, Y. Shibasaki, K. Sunakawa, M. Nonoyama, S. Iwata, and M. Konno.** 2002. Differentiation of beta-lactamase-negative ampicillin-resistant *Haemophilus influenzae* from other *H. influenzae* strains by a disc method. J. Infect. Chemother. **8**:50-58.

(64) **Watt, J. P., L. J. Wolfson, K. L. O'Brien, E. Henkle, M. Deloria-Knoll, N. McCall, E. Lee, O. S. Levine, R. Hajjeh, K. Mulholland, T. Cherian and the Hib and Pneumococcal Global Burden of Disease Study Team.** 2009. Burden of disease caused by *Haemophilus influenzae* type b in children younger than 5 years: global estimates. Lancet. **374**:903-911.

(65) **World Health Organization.** 2005. *Haemophilus influenzae* type B (HiB). WHO fact sheet no. 294. http://www.who.int/mediacentre/factsheets/fs294/en/index.html.

(66) **Yokota S., Y. Ohkoshi, K. Sato, and Fujii N.** 2008. Emergence of fluoroquinolone-resistant *Haemophilus influenzae* strains among elderly patients but not among children. J. Clin. Microbiol. **46**:361-365.

Chapter 35. *NEISSERIA MENINGITIDIS*

Muhamed-Kheir TAHA and Jean-Didier CAVALLO

INTRODUCTION

Neisseria meningitidis, together with *Streptococcus pneumoniae* and *Haemophilus influenzae*, are the main etiological agents of invasive community-acquired infections, including meningococcemia (septicemia) and meningitis (accounting for approximately 30% of acute bacterial meningitis cases), as well as infectious arthritis and pericarditis. Meningococcemia may be complicated by purpura fulminans and fatal septic shock. Antimicrobial therapy with β-lactams is effective at the early phase of bacterial dissemination (sometimes just a few hours), but the inflammatory cascade of septic shock that accompanies the signs of purpura fulminans (disseminated intravascular coagulation) cannot, at present, be countered by any specific treatment. This dual nature of the disease: an easily curable inaugural infectious process followed by an incurable septic complication, requires an emergency diagnostic algorithm and prompt initiation of appropriate antimicrobial therapy (33). Up until to the mid-1980s, acquired resistance rates were low in this species, which characteristically has intrinsic high-level susceptibility to antibiotics (Table 1), with the exception of the sulfonamides (22). Today, the increasing prevalence of strains with reduced penicillin G susceptibility, the emergence of resistance to chloramphenicol - the drug of choice in developing countries - and the reports of resistance to rifampin and ciprofloxacin, recommended for prophylaxis in most countries, highlight the need to systematically perform antibiotic susceptibility testing and to monitor resistance rates to the main therapeutic or prophylactically used antibiotics.

INVASIVE MENINGOCOCCAL INFECTIONS

Invasive meningococcal infections include the bacteremic forms as well as infection of the meninges, joints, pleura or pericardium (26). Other more localized sites are the lungs and genitalia. The human nasopharynx is the specific reservoir of *N. meningitidis* and up to 5-50% of a population may be asymptomatic carriers, depending on climatic conditions and overcrowding. The annual worldwide incidence of invasive infections ranges from 1 to 10 per 100,000 according to the country, with mortality rates exceeding 10% (36). Among the dozen or so serogroups of *N. meningitidis* characterized to date, more than 99% of invasive disease-causing strains isolated worldwide belong to serogroups A, B, C, Y, and W135. However the relative proportion of each serogroup varies considerably on different continents (26). Local outbreaks of serogroup X have recently been reported in Africa (7). Epidemiological surveillance is based on meningococcus genotyping by the Multilocus Sequence Typing (MLST) method, which indexes the variations (polymorphism) of seven meningococcal gene loci in order to determine the genotype of each isolate (sequence type, ST). Phylogenetically related STs are grouped together into clonal complexes (20). Epidemiological surveillance based on antigenic characterization of serogroup (polyosidic capsule antigen), serotype (porin PorB), or sero-subtype (porin PorA) only detects the phenotypic features of a strain. Strains with a same genotype (clonal complex) can express different antigens, illustrating one of the major features of *N. meningitidis*: its diversity and genetic variability through DNA acquisition, transformation and recombination, and more rarely, by mutation (15). Acquisition of rearranged genes by horizontal transfer is responsible for changes in antibiotic susceptibility, particularly to penicillin G (8).

METHODS

The conventional methods for minimal inhibitory concentration (MIC) determination by agar dilution or broth microdilution may be used for *N. meningitidis*. Agar disk diffusion is only suitable for determining susceptibility to certain antibiotics. Automated susceptibility testing systems have not yet been validated for *N. meningitidis*.

Methods for rapid detection of resistance, such as β-lactamase screening with a chromogenic test, can be used to detect the rare β-lactamase-producing strain.

The E-test® which uses antibiotic gradient strips is an acceptable alternative for routine MIC determinations (23, 35).

Although *N. meningitidis* is classified as a group 2 pathogen, there is a real risk of laboratory exposure due to the generation of aerosols when working with the organism. It is therefore necessary to work in a biosafety level 2 laboratory and to take all the necessary precautions to avoid the formation of aerosols. Laboratory personnel should work at microbiological safety stations. Lab coats, gloves and mask should be worn. It is recommended to use biosafety level 3 facilities for high risk procedures (for instance production of high quantities of infectious material). Vaccination with a quadrivalent polysaccharide vaccine directed against serogroups A, C, Y, and W135 is recommended for workers in reference and research laboratories as they have greater risks of exposure. However the risk is only decreased and the vaccination does not provide protection against serogroup B meningococcus (25).

Culture media

N. meningitidis grows within 24 hours on Mueller-Hinton (MH) medium supplemented or not with 5% fresh or heated sheep blood. The Clinical and Laboratory Standards Institute (CLSI) recommends MH broth supplemented with 2.5-5% lysed horse blood for the broth microdilution method and MH agar supplemented with 5% defibrinated sheep blood for agar dilution (12). Specific testing of sulfonamides or trimethoprim/sulfonamide combinations requires MH medium containing 2.5-5% lysed horse blood.

In an attempt to standardize the agar dilution and E-test® method of MIC determination at the European level, the European Monitoring Group on Meningococci (EMGM) recommends the use of MH medium supplemented with 5% defibrinated sheep blood, which gives more reproducible interlaboratory results than MH medium alone and is easier to prepare than MH supplemented with heated blood (35). For routine testing, then, the preferred medium is cation-adjusted MH supplemented with 5% sheep blood for MIC determination on agar medium, agar diffusion with antibiotic disks or strips. This medium is commercially available. For the broth microdilution method, M-H medium should be supplemented with 2-5% lysed horse blood.

Inoculum, inoculation, culture

The inoculum should be prepared from colonies obtained after an 18-24 h culture on PolyVitex® chocolate agar. CLSI recommends direct colony suspension in MH broth or saline to approximately 10^6 CFU/ml, adjusted to a turbidity of a 0.5 McFarland standard. Colonies can also be suspended in phosphate M/15 buffer pH 7.2. For the agar diffusion method or E-test®, the inoculum can be swabbed onto the agar surface. This inoculation method is recommended by the E-test® manufacturer. The overlay method should be avoided for safety reasons.

For MIC determination by agar dilution, the EMGM recommends an inoculum of approximately 10^5 CFU per spot (35). The inoculum can be prepared as a suspension in phosphate buffer equivalent to a 1 McFarland standard (approximately 10^8 CFU/ml), then inoculated manually with a calibrated loop (1 μl) or by applying approximately 1 μl with a multihead inoculator of the Steers type.

For MIC determination by broth microdilution, the inoculum should be adjusted to a final optical density of approximately 5.10^5 CFU/ml.

After inoculation, media are incubated at 35-37°C in a moist 5% CO_2 atmosphere for 18-24 hours. The presence of CO_2 results in an overestimation of macrolide MICs for meningococci, but is necessary because most strains grow poorly in the absence of CO_2.

Control strains

Escherichia coli ATCC®25922, *Staphylococcus aureus* ATCC®25923, *S. aureus* ATCC®29213 and *Streptococcus pneumoniae* ATCC®49619 can be used as internal controls and to validate the MIC series. The CLSI recommends *Escherichia coli* ATCC®25922 incubated in ambient air or 5%CO2 as control for ciprofloxacin, nalidixic acid, minocycline and sulfisoxazole and *Streptococcus pneumoniae* ATCC®49619 incubated in ambient air for azithromycin (11). The MICs of different antibiotics for these strains may be found in the technical documents of the European Committee for Antimicrobial Susceptibility Testing (EUCAST) (//www.escmid.org) or the CLSI. EMGM reference strains may also be used (35).

ANTIBIOTICS TO BE STUDIED

The antibiotics tested in a standard antibiogram should be medically relevant, take into account the guidelines for therapy or prophylaxis, and allow detection of the main types of acquired resistance.

High-dose penicillin G has historically been the treatment of invasive meningococcal infections. Today, ampicillin or amoxicillin and especially the third generation cephalosporins (ceftriaxone, cefotaxime), which diffuse efficiently into cerebrospinal fluid, are the drugs of choice. Meropenem has been proposed as an alternative for treating severe infections. Phenicols (oily chloramphenicol) hold an important place in developing countries. For prophylaxis, rifampin 600 mg per os twice daily for two days in adults, or 10 mg/kg every 12 h in children, is the recommended first-line drug. Ciprofloxacin (500 mg single dose in adults) or ceftriaxone (250 mg IM in adults or 125 mg in infants, single dose) are alternatives (17). Azithromycin 500 mg per os single dose in adults, or minocycline, have also been shown to be effective in this indication. Many other antibiotics are active against N. meningitidis, but their use is limited by either high resistance rates, as with the sulfonamides, or an unsuitable pharmacokinetic profile for the treatment of meningitis.

The minimal antibiogram for N. meningitidis should comprise a penicillin (penicillin G, ampicillin, or amoxicillin), chloramphenicol, rifampin, and ciprofloxacin. So far, there have been no reports of resistance to third generation cephalosporins, but the dissemination of strains with reduced penicillin G susceptibility due to target modification calls for caution and the MICs of these antibiotics for invasive strains should be monitored.

Laboratories employing the agar dilution or broth microdilution method should use antibiotic powders with known potency, stored at –20°C in the presence of a dessicant (unless otherwise indicated by the supplier). Stock solutions should be prepared immediately after dissolution, then sterilized by passage through a 0.22 μm membrane filter. Table 2 shows the range of dilutions to be prepared for different antibiotics.

RESISTANCE

N. meningitidis is intrinsically susceptible to many antibiotic classes and MIC_{50} and MIC_{90} values (antibiotic concentrations respectively inhibiting 50% and 90% of a sample of strains) are very low (Table 1). It is intrinsically resistant to trimethoprim, glycopeptides, lincosamides, and polymyxins. Over time it has acquired many resistance mechanisms. Vancomycin is used in selective media.

β-lactams

Strains susceptible to penicillin G are inhibited in vitro by 0.03 μg/ml penicillin G. While many strains with reduced penicillin susceptibility and a few isolated β-lactamase producing strains have been described, so far there have been no reports of resistance to third generation cephalosporins (ceftriaxone, cefotaxime), which have very low MICs, even against strains with reduced susceptibility to penicillin G (Table 3).

β-lactamase production by N. meningitidis was first described in 1983 (14) in a only a very small number of strains isolated in Canada, Spain, and South Africa. Penicillin G MICs were always 2 μg/ml and in some cases exceeded 256 μg/ml (21). These plasmid-borne TEM-1 type enzymes (14) had previously been described in Neisseria gonorrhoeae. They are transferable in vitro from gonococci to meningococci (19). This penicillinase strongly inactivates penicillins, whose activity can be partially restored by clavulanic acid. However, it does not hydrolyze second or third generation cephalosporins which remain active. β-lactamase production can be easily detected with the aid of a chromogenic cephalosporin disk.

Since 1985, the number of clinical isolates with reduced penicillin G susceptibility (MICs 0.125-1 μg/ml) has been increasing. This reduced susceptibility is due to alterations in the penA gene, modifying the affinity as well as the enzymatic activity of the penicillin binding protein PBP2, which alters the peptidoglycan structure (3). Alterations of penA in N. meningitidis result from interspecies recombination of homologous sequences from commensal Neisseria (8). Neisseria are spontaneously transformable, which enables horizontal DNA transfer leading to mosaicism of the penA gene. Reduced penicillin G susceptibility in meningococci is transferable through transformation and horizontal DNA transfer and can occur during pharyngeal carriage between commensal Neisseria species (like N. cinerea, N. flavescens and N. lactamica) and N. meningitidis (8, 31). This target modification mechanism results in cross-resistance to all β-lactams displaying affinity for PBP2 but with different levels of expression. In terms of MICs values, penicillins are more affected than third generation cephalosporins

Table 1. Minimal inhibitory concentrations (μg/ml) 50% (MIC_{50}) and 90% (MIC_{90}) for wild strains of *N. meningitidis* (adapted from reference 21)

Antibiotic	MIC_{50}	MIC_{90}
Penicillin G	0.06	0.12
Ampicillin	0.06	0.25
Amoxicillin	0.125	0.25
Cefotaxime	0.003	0.007
Ceftriaxone	≤ 0.0015	≤ 0.0015
Meropenem	0.007	0.015
Chloramphenicol	0.5	1
Rifampin	0.03	0.125
Nalidixic acid	1	1
Ciprofloxacin	0.003	0.003
Levofloxacin	0.007	0.007
Azithromycin		
with CO_2	0.25	0.5
without CO_2	0.06	0.12
Tetracycline	0.25	1
Minocycline	0.12	0.25
Sulfisoxazole	8	> 64
Trimethoprim-sulfamethoxazole	0.5	2

Table 2. Solvents and diluents for preparation of stock solutions of antibiotics for *N. meningitidis*

Antibiotic	Range of concentrations (μg/ml)	Solvent	Diluent
Penicillin G	0.003 – 4	Phosphate buffer, 0.1mol/l, pH 6.0	
Ampicillin, Amoxicillin	0.015 – 4	Phosphate buffer, 0.1mol/l, pH 6.0	
Cephalosporins	0.003 – 4	Phosphate buffer, 0.1mol/l, pH 6.0	
Chloramphenicol	0.125 - 32	Distilled water	
Rifampin	0.125-128	Methanol	Distilled water
Ciprofloxacin	0.007 - 4	Water + NaOH 1M until dissolution	Distilled water
Tetracycline	0.125 – 32	Distilled water	
Minocycline			
Macrolides	0.03 - 32	95% Ethanol	Distilled water
Sulfonamides	0.03 - 256	Water + NaOH 1M until dissolution	Distilled water

whose MICs remain very low (Table 3). Periodically isolated in Spain and the United States since the late 1980s, these strains have spread rapidly to Europe and North and South America.

While reduced penicillin G susceptibility is somewhat more frequent among serogroups W135 and C, the emergence of such strains does not appear to be due to expansion of a particular clone, but more likely to independent recombination events promoted selected by antibiotic pressure (31).

Although treatment failures have been described for strains with the highest MICs (34), the severe infections caused by these strains generally resolve favorably with high doses of penicillin G or amoxicillin, which allow bactericidal concentrations to be reached in cerebrospinal fluid. Right now the biggest fear is the emergence of

Table 3. MICs (µg/ml) of three β-lactams for *N. meningitidis* according to susceptibility to penicillin G (4).

β-lactam[a]	MIC (µg/ml) according to susceptibility to penicillin G		
	MIC_{50}	MIC_{90}	Range
Penicillin G			
Pen[S]	0.04	0.09	0.006 - 0.09
Pen[I]	0.25	0.75	0.125 - 1
Amoxicillin			
Pen[S]	0.06	0.19	0.016 - 0.38
Pen[I]	0.38	1	0.03 - 1.5
Cefotaxime			
Pen[S]	0.006	0.0012	0.002 - 0.023
Pen[I]	0.008	0.023	0.002 - 0.25

[a] Pen[s], susceptible to penicillin G (MIC E-test® < 0.125 µg/ml); Pen[IR], MIC of penicillin G ≥ 0.125 µg/ml.

strains with a penicillin G MIC above the critical therapeutic threshold of 1 µg/ml or, even worse, resistant to third generation cephalosporins. Emergence of such strains might make it necessary to resort to the less commonly used antibiotics such as chloramphenicol, or to seek alternative treatments (6).

The classical agar disk diffusion method is not suitable for detection of strains with reduced β-lactam susceptibility (Fig. 1 and 2). This is because there is an overlap between inhibition zone diameters for susceptible and intermediate strains, making it impossible to determine critical diameters for amoxicillin disks (25 µg), ampicillin (10 µg) or penicillin G (10 IU) (21). Other detection methods using disks with a low β-lactam content, such as 2 IU penicillin G or 1 or 5 µg oxacillin, have been proposed (9, 21), but these methods produce many false positives and their value is controversial (5). Screening methods are considerably less useful when reduced susceptibility strains are common, in which case it is better to determine β-lactam MICs directly by agar dilution which, together with broth microdilution, remains the reference method.

For routine testing, the E-test® is a good alternative and shows 95-100% agreement (± 1 log2) with MICs of penicillin G and third generation cephalosporins determined by agar dilution (35). It thus enables reliable identification of strains with reduced penicillin G susceptibility.

Molecular methods for characterizing strains with reduced penicillin G susceptibility are currently being developed. Studies of *penA* gene polymorphism by restriction profiling and sequencing have identified a single (or highly conserved) *penA* allele in susceptible strains. On the other hand, many mosaic alleles of *penA* are present in strains with reduced susceptibility. Five amino acids are always modified in strains with reduced penicillin G susceptibility, located in the C-terminal extremity of PBP2 in the vicinity of the active site. Analysis of altered *penA* alleles in a large series of strains isolated in 22 countries over a 60-year period revealed a correlation between the critical value of 0.125 µg/ml and alteration of PBP2. These findings clearly highlight the importance of studying *penA* polymorphism, both to identify reduced penicillin G susceptibility strains, and as a novel tool for molecular typing (31). Rapid, culture-free PCR methods are also under development for detection of reduced penicillin G susceptibility strains (2, 29).

Phenicols

MICs of chloramphenicol for susceptible strains range from 1-4 µg/ml for concentrations of 6-23 µg/ml in CSF. The first reports of high-level resistance (MICs 16-64 µg/ml) date back to 1987 in a small number of *N. meningitidis* serogroup B strains isolated in Vietman, France and Australia (18, 27). This resistance is easy to detect by agar disk diffusion (27) or E-test® which shows good agreement with the reference method (23). Resistance is mediated by a chloramphenicol acetyltransferase encoded by the *catP* gene carried on a mobile genetic element (18). These strains can be identified by molecular detection of the *catP* gene. Dissemination of this type of resistance could pose major problems in developing countries where oily chloramphenicol is widely used as a single intramuscular dose to treat meningococcal meningitis. Nevertheless, no such strains were detected among isolates from an epidemic outbreak in Africa (32).

ANTIBIOTIC PROPHYLAXIS

Currently, rifampin is the recommended first-line prophylactic agent. Several other antibiotics have been proposed as alternatives for the prophylaxis of invasive infections. A recent meta-analysis confirmed the efficacy of rifampin, ciprofloxacin and ceftriaxone in this indication (17).

Rifampin

The MICs for all rifampin-susceptible strains are comprised between 0.007 and 0.25 µg/ml. After an oral dose of 600 mg rifampin, peak concentrations reach 0.25 µg/ml in saliva and 4-5 µg/ml in serum. Acquired resistance to rifampin is still rare. It is due to mutations in the *rpoB* gene, combined or not with decreased permeability, and confers high-level resistance with MICs ranging from 25 to > 256 µg/ml (1). Resistance is easily detectable by agar diffusion or E-test®, although MICs determined by the latter method showed only 82% (± 1 log2) agreement with the agar diffusion method in a European multicenter study (35). Chemoprophylaxis with rifampin cannot be used to prevent secondary infections caused by these resistant strains (37).

Macrolides

Macrolides such as azithromycin (MIC_{50} and MIC_{90} = 0.5 µg/ml) have been proposed for the prophylaxis of invasive meningococcal infections. The mechanisms underlying acquired resistance to macrolides include efflux systems (*mef* genes) or production of methylases (*erm* genes); one or both of these mechanisms may be present (13).

Quinolones

Ciprofloxacin given as a single 500 mg oral dose has been proposed as prophylaxis (17). MICs for susceptible strains range from 0.007 to 0.03 µg/ml. Resistant strains (MIC > 0.12 µg/ml) have been reported very infrequently in Argentina, Australia, France, India, Israel, Spain and the United States; resistance is due to point mutations in the *gyrA* gene (10, 28, 30). These strains are heterogeneous and have not spread through clonal propagation. This low-level fluoroquinolone resistance can be easily detected by agar diffusion with a 30 µg nalidixic acid disk: an inhibition zone diameter ≤ 25 mm is correlated with reduced fluoroquinolone susceptibility (11).

Sulfonamides

Sulfonamides were widely used as prophylaxis until the early 1980s and MICs of these agents were < 1 µg/ml. Since that time, resistance due to mutations in the chromosomal dihydropteorate synthase gene *folP* has become extremely frequent (16). Sulfonamide susceptibility testing has there-

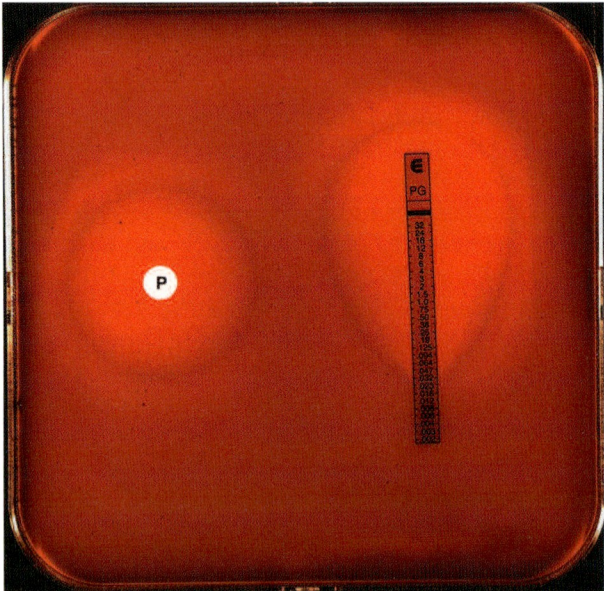

Fig. 1. Penicillin G susceptible *N. meningitidis*. Left, P, penicillin G; inhibition diameter: 34 mm; Right, E-test®; MIC: 0.032 µg/ml.

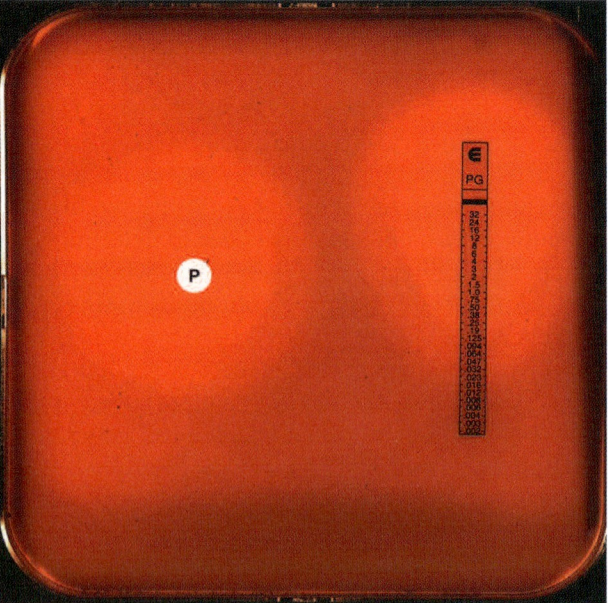

Fig. 2. Lack of correlation between MICs and diameters for β-lactams. *N. meningitidis* with reduced susceptibility to penicillin G. Left, P, penicillin G; inhibition diameter: 34 mm, false susceptibility; Right, E-test®; MIC: 0.190 µg/ml.

Table 4. Breakpoints for *N. meningitidis* as defined by the European Committee for Antimicrobial Susceptibility Testing (EUCAST) and the Clinical and Laboratory Standards Institute (CLSI)

Antibiotic (disk content)[a]	MICs interpretative standard (µg/ml)					
	EUCAST			CLSI		
	S	I	R	S	I	R
Penicillin G	≤ 0.06	0.12-0.25	> 0.25	≤ 0.06	0.12-0,25	≥ 0.5
Ampicillin	≤ 0.12	0.25-1	> 1	≤ 0.12	0,25-0.5	≥ 1
Amoxicillin	≤ 0.12	0.25-1	> 1	-	-	-
Ceftriaxone / Cefotaxime	≤ 0.12	-	> 0.12	≤ 0.12	-	-
(30 µg)[a]	-	-	≥ 34 mm	-	-	-
Meropenem	≤ 0.25	-	> 0.12	≤ 0.25	-	-
(10 µg)[a]				≥ 30 mm		
Chloramphenicol	≤ 2	4	> 4	≤ 2	4	≥ 8
(30 µg)[a]				≥ 26 mm	20-25	≤ 19 mm
Nalidixic acid	-	-	-	≤ 4	-	≥ 8
(30 µg)[a]				≥ 26 mm		≤ 25 mm
Ciprofloxacin	≤ 0.03	0.06	> 0.06	≤ 0.03	0.06	≥ 0.12
(30 µg)[a]	-	-	-	≥ 35 mm	33-34 mm	≤ 32 mm
Levofloxacin	-	-	-	≤ 0.06	0.12-0.5	≥ 1
Tetracycline	≤ 1	2	> 2	-	-	-
(30 µg)[a]						
Minocycline	≤ 1	2	> 2	≤ 2	-	-
(30 µg)[a]	-	-	-	≥ 26 mm		
Rifampin	≤ 0.25	-	> 0.25	≤ 0.5	1	≥ 2
(5 µg)[a]	-	-	-	≥ 25 mm	20-24 mm	≤19 mm
Azithromycin	-	-	-	≤ 2	-	-
(15 µg)[a]	-	-	-	≥ 20 mm	-	-
Sulfisoxazole	-	-	-	≤ 2	4	≥ 8
Trimethoprim-sulfamethoxazole	-	-	-	≤ 0.12/2.4	4	≥ 8

[a] Disk content and inhibition zone diameter as defined by CLSI.

fore lost much of its interest. Moreover, it requires special conditions for MIC determination by agar dilution, including the use of M-H medium supplemented with 5% lysed horse blood, i.e., with a high thymidine phosphorylase content, to avoid false resistance.

Tetracyclines

Tetracyclines such as minocycline have also been proposed as prophylaxis. Tetracycline MICs for susceptible strains range from 0.25 to 1 µg/ml. High-level resistance (MIC > 8 µg/ml) is still uncommon and is usually related to plasmid-encoded *tet*(M) genes (24).

CONCLUSION

At the dawn of the twenty-first century, *N. meningitidis* is still globally susceptible to antibiotics, with the exception of sulfonamides, and the current guidelines for treatment and prophylaxis remain valid. Nevertheless, this species has demonstrated its ability to acquire resistance to different classes of antibiotics. The rising incidence of strains with reduced penicillin G susceptibility, which might evolve in parallel to that of multiresistant pneumococci, under the same selective pressures, calls for sustained vigilance. Likewise, the emergence of rifampin- and ciprofloxacin-resistant strains poses a problem for prophylaxis. Antibiotic susceptibility testing of meningococci should be systematically performed in order to ensure optimum treatment of individual patients and enable surveillance of emerging resistances. Indeed, surveillance is an essential tool to rapidly adapt, if the need exists, the treatment and prophylaxis strategies for invasive meningococcal infections. Breakpoints and critical diameters allowing clinical categorization of laboratory strains are determined by national and international working groups on the basis of pharmacokinetic and pharmacodynamic (PK/PD) data, MIC distribution according to species, and clinical efficacy. For *N. meningitidis*, the most recent values proposed by the European Committee for Antimicrobial Susceptibility Testing and the Clinical and Laboratory Standards Institute (11) are summarized in Table 4.

Molecular detection of antibiotic resistance in *N. meningitidis* is a tool of the future. Even if treatment is initiated before cultures are performed, the development of molecular methods will make it possible to detect resistance to the main antibiotics used for the treatment and prophylaxis of meningococcal infections.

REFERENCES

(1) **Abadi, F.J.R., P.E. Carter, P. Cash, and T.H. Pennington.** 1996. Rifampin resistance in *Neisseria meningitidis* due to alterations in membrane permeability. Antimicrob. Agents Chemother. **40**:646-651.

(2) **Antignac, A., J.M. Alonso, and M.K. Taha.** 2001. Nonculture prediction of *Neisseria meningitidis* susceptibility to penicillin. Antimicrob. Agents Chemother. **45**:3625-3628.

(3) **Antignac, A., I.G. Boneca, J.C. Rousselle, A. Namane, J.P. Carlier, J.A. Vazquez, A. Fox, J.M. Alonso, and M.K. Taha.** 2003. Correlation between alterations of the penicillin-binding protein 2 and modifications of the peptidoglycan structure in *Neisseria meningitidis* with reduced susceptibility to penicillin G. J. Biol. Chem. **278**:31529-31535.

(4) **Antignac, A., M. Ducos-Galand, A. Guiyoule, R. Pires, J.M. Alonso, and M.K. Taha.** 2003. *Neisseria meningitidis* strains isolated from invasive infections in France (1999-2002): phenotypes and antibiotic susceptibility patterns. Clin. Infect. Dis. **37**: 912-920.

(5) **Block, C., Y. Davidson, and N. Keller.** 1998. Unreliability of disc diffusion test for screening for reduced penicillin susceptibility in *Neisseria meningitidis*. J. Clin. Microbiol. **36**:3103-3104.

(6) **Blondeau, J.M., and Y. Yaschuk.** 1995. In vitro activities of ciprofloxacin, cefotaxime, ceftriaxone, chloramphenicol, and rifampin against fully susceptible and moderately penicillin-resistant *Neisseria meningitidis*. Antimicrob. Agents Chemother. **39**:2577-2579.

(7) **Boisier, P., P. Nicolas, S. Djibo, M.K. Taha, I. Jeanne, H.B. Mainassara, B. Tenebray, K.K. Kairo, D. Giorgini, and S. Chanteau.** 2007. Meningococcal meningitis: unprecedented incidence of serogroup X-related cases in 2006 in Niger. Clin. Infect. Dis. **44**:657-663.

(8) **Bowler, L.D., Q.Y. Zhang, J.Y. Riou, and B.G. Spratt.** 1994. Interspecies recombination between the *penA* genes of *Neisseria meningitidis* and commensal *Neisseria* species during the emergence of penicillin resistance in *N. meningitidis*: natural events and laboratory simulation. J. Bacteriol. **176**:333-337.

(9) **Campos, J., M.C. Fuste, G. Trujillo, J. Saez-Nieto, J. Vazquez, J.G. Loren, M. Vinas, and B.G. Spratt.** 1992. Genetic diversity of penicillin-resistant *Neisseria meningitidis*. J. Infect. Dis. **166**:173-177.

(10) **Centers for Disease Control and Prevention (CDC).** Emergence of fluoroquinolone- ,resistant *Neisseria meningitidis*--Minnesota and North Dakota, 2007-2008. MMWR Morb. Mortal. Wkly. Rep. 2008. **57**:173-175.

(11) **Clinical and Laboratory Standards Institute.** 2009. Performance standards for Antimicrobial susceptibility testing; Nineteenth informational supplement. Clinical and Laboratory Standards Institute. Wayne, PA.

(12) **Clinical and Laboratory Standards Institute.** 2009. Methods for Dilution Antimicrobial Susceptibility Tests for Bacteria That Grow Aerobically. Approved Standard. 8th ed. M07-A8. Clinical and Laboratory Standards Institute. Wayne, PA.

(13) **Cousin, S., Jr., W.L. Whittington, and M.C. Roberts.** 2003. Acquired macrolide resistance genes in pathogenic *Neisseria* spp. isolated between 1940 and 1987. Antimicrob. Agents Chemother. **47**:3877-3880.

(14) **Dillon, J.R., M. Pauze, and K.H. Yeung.** 1983. Spread of penicillinase-producing and transfer plasmids from the gonococcus to *Neisseria meningitidis*. Lancet **1**:779-781.

(15) **Feil, E.J., M.C. Maiden, M. Achtman, and B.G. Spratt.** 1999. The relative contributions of recombination and mutation to the divergence of clones of *Neisseria meningitidis*. Mol. Biol. Evol. **16**:1496-1502.

(16) **Fiebelkorn, K.R., S.A. Crawford, and J.H. Jorgensen.** 2005. Mutations in *folP* associated with elevated sulfonamide MICs for *Neisseria meningitidis* clinical isolates from five continents. Antimicrob. Agents Chemother. **49**:536-540.

(17) **Fraser, A., A. Gafter-Gvili, M. Paul, and L. Leibovici.** 2006. Antibiotics for preventing meningococcal infections. Cochrane Database Syst. Rev.:CD004785.

(18) **Galimand, M., G. Gerbaud, M. Guibourdenche, J.Y. Riou, and P. Courvalin.** 1998. High-level chloramphenicol resistance in *Neisseria meningitidis*. N. Engl. J. Med. **339**:868-874.

(19) **Ikeda, F., A. Tsuji, Y. Kaneko, M. Nishida, and S. Goto.** 1986. Conjugal transfer of beta-lactamase-producing plasmids of *Neisseria gonorrhoeae* to *Neisseria meningitidis*. Microbiol. Immunol. **30**:737-742.

(20) **Maiden, M.C., J.A. Bygraves, E. Feil, G. Morelli, J.E. Russell, R. Urwin, Q. Zhang, J. Zhou, K. Zurth, D.A. Caugant, I.M. Feavers, M. Achtman, and B.G. Spratt.** 1998. Multilocus sequence typing: a portable approach to the identification of clones within populations of pathogenic microorganisms. Proc. Natl. Acad. Sci. USA **95**:3140-3145.

(21) **Nicolas, P., J.D. Cavallo, R. Fabre, and G. Martet.** 1998. Standardization of the *Neisseria meningitidis* antibiogram. Detection of strains relatively resistant to penicillin. Bull. World Health Organ. **76**:393-400.

(22) **Oppenheim, B.A.** 1997. Antibiotic resistance in *Neisseria meningitidis*. Clin. Infect. Dis. **24 Suppl 1**:S98-101.

(23) **Pascual, A., P. Joyanes, L. Martinez-Martinez, A.I. Suarez, and E.J. Perea.** 1996. Comparison of broth

microdilution and E-test for susceptibility testing of *Neisseria meningitidis*. J. Clin. Microbiol. **34**:588-591.

(24) **Roberts, M.C., and J.S. Knapp.** 1988. Host range of the conjugative 25.2-megadalton tetracycline resistance plasmid from *Neisseria gonorrhoeae* and related species. Antimicrob. Agents Chemother. **32**:488-491.

(25) **Rosenstein, N.E., M. Fischer, and J.W. Tappero.** 2001. Meningococcal vaccines. Infect. Dis. Clin. North Am. **15**:155-169.

(26) **Rosenstein, N.E., B.A. Perkins, D.S. Stephens, T. Popovic, and J.M. Hughes.** 2001. Meningococcal disease. N. Engl. J. Med. **344**:1378-1388.

(27) **Shultz, T.R., J.W. Tapsall, P.A. White, C.S. Ryan, D. Lyras, J.I. Rood, E. Binotto, and C.J. Richardson.** 2003. Chloramphenicol-resistant *Neisseria meningitidis* containing *catP* isolated in Australia. J. Antimicrob. Chemother. **52**:856-859.

(28) **Skoczynska, A., J.M. Alonso, and M.K. Taha.** 2008. Ciprofloxacin resistance in *Neisseria meningitidis*, France. Emerg. Infect. Dis. **14**:1322-1323.

(29) **Stefanelli, P., A. Carattoli, A. Neri, C. Fazio, and P. Mastrantonio.** 2003. Prediction of decreased susceptibility to penicillin of *Neisseria meningitidis* strains by real-time PCR. J. Clin. Microbiol. **41**:4666-4670.

(30) **Strahilevitz, J., A. Adler, G. Smollan, V. Temper, N. Keller, and C. Block.** 2008. Serogroup A *Neisseria meningitidis* with reduced susceptibility to ciprofloxacin. Emerg. Infect. Dis. **14**:1667-1669.

(31) **Taha, M.K., J.A. Vazquez, E. Hong, D.E. Bennett, S. Bertrand, S. Bukovski, M.T. Cafferkey, F. Carion, J.J. Christensen, M. Diggle, G. Edwards, R. Enriquez, C. Fazio, M. Frosch, S. Heuberger, S. Hoffmann, K.A. Jolley, M. Kadlubowski, A. Kechrid, K. Kesanopoulos, P. Kriz, L. Lambertsen, I. Levenet, M. Musilek, M. Paragi, A. Saguer, A. Skoczynska, P. Stefanelli, S. Thulin, G. Tzanakaki, M. Unemo, U. Vogel, and M.L. Zarantonelli.** 2007. Target gene sequencing to characterize the penicillin G susceptibility of *Neisseria meningitidis*. Antimicrob. Agents Chemother. **51**:2784-2792.

(32) **Tondella, M.L., N.E. Rosenstein, L.W. Mayer, F.C. Tenover, S.A. Stocker, M.W. Reeves, and T. Popovic.** 2001. Lack of evidence for chloramphenicol resistance in *Neisseria meningitidis*, Africa. Emerg. Infect. Dis. **7**:163-164.

(33) **Tunkel, A.R., B.J. Hartman, S.L. Kaplan, B.A. Kaufman, K.L. Roos, W.M. Scheld, and R.J. Whitley.** 2004. Practice guidelines for the management of bacterial meningitis. Clin. Infect. Dis. **39**:1267-1284.

(34) **Turner, P.C., K.W. Southern, N.J. Spencer, and H. Pullen.** 1990. Treatment failure in meningococcal meningitis. Lancet **335**:732-733.

(35) **Vazquez, J.A., L. Arreaza, C. Block, I. Ehrhard, S.J. Gray, S. Heuberger, S. Hoffmann, P. Kriz, P. Nicolas, P. Olcen, A. Skoczynska, L. Spanjaard, P. Stefanelli, M. K. Taha, and G. Tzanakaki.** 2003. Interlaboratory comparison of agar dilution and E-test methods for determining the MICs of antibiotics used in management of *Neisseria meningitidis* infections. Antimicrob. Agents Chemother. **47**:3430-3434.

(36) **WHO.** 1998. Control of epidemic meningococcal disease. WHO Practical Guidelines. 2nd edition. WHO Geneva.

(37) **Yagupsky, P., S. Ashkenazi, and C. Block.** 1993. Rifampicin-resistant meningococci causing invasive disease and failure of chemoprophylaxis. Lancet **341**:1152-1153.

Chapter 36. *NEISSERIA GONORRHOEAE*

Jean-Didier CAVALLO

INTRODUCTION

Neisseria gonorrhoeae, also known as "gonococcus", is a strictly human pathogen responsible for sexually transmitted infections. The incidence of gonococcal infections started to decrease considerably in the early 1980s as prevention programs were established and reinforced in response to the AIDS epidemic. Yet since the late 1990s these measures have slackened somewhat, with an attendant stabilization, or even an increase, in gonococcal infection rates in certain countries (12). Gonococcal infections are initially localized to the genitals, presenting mainly as acute urethritis in men or cervicitis in women. Other mucosal sites of infection such as the pharynx and anorectum are also on the rise and may accompany the genital forms. If left untreated or treated inappropriately, locoregional complications such as epididymitis, salpingitis, infection of the ovaries or fallopian tubes or pelvic inflammatory disease may result, as well as disseminated infection and secondary localizations, usually joint involvement. Gonococcal infections that are neglected may result in functional sequelae of chronic inflammation, such as urethral stricture in men or tubal scarring, a common cause of infertility, in women. *N. gonorrhoeae* is intrinsically susceptible to many antibiotics (Table 1). According to the treatment guidelines issued by the World Health Organization (WHO) and the Centers for Disease Control and Prevention (CDC) (4), uncomplicated local infections are usually treated with single-dose antibiotic regimens whereas longer treatment regimens are used in complicated infections (4, 21). Over the past thirty years there has been a significant increase in acquired plasmid or chromosome-mediated resistance to all the antibiotic classes normally active against *N. gonorrhoeae*. This rising prevalence of acquired resistance is a major concern which justifies systematic antibiotic susceptibility testing of all *N. gonorrhoeae* isolates. This is all the more important since clinical outcomes on treatment are generally well correlated to the level of susceptibility *in vitro*.

METHODS

Antibiotic susceptibility testing in *N. gonorrhoeae* requires a clear definition of the culture media, inoculum, the method itself and the reference strains. MIC determination by agar dilution is the reference method for *N. gonorrhoeae* (6). The results obtained by agar diffusion with antibiotic disks are far too random for the majority of antibiotics used to treat gonococcal infections (15). The E-test® based on strips with a predefined antibiotic gradient is an acceptable alternative for routine laboratory MIC determinations since it shows good concordance with the agar dilution method (2, 15, 31). Rapid screening methods to infer underlying resistance mechanisms, such as the use of a chromogenic substrate to test for the presence of β-lactamases or a nalidixic acid disk to detect low-level quinolone resistance, illustrate the concept of interpretative reading of the antibiogram in this species.

TECHNICAL CONDITIONS

Media

The medium recommended for antibiotic susceptibility testing must be both readily available and allow a 24-hour culture of the very fastidious

Table 1. Minimal inhibitory concentrations (μg/ml) 50% (MIC_{50}) and 90% (MIC_{90}) for wild strains of *N. gonorrhoeae*

Antibiotic	MIC_{50}	MIC_{90}
Penicillin G	0.06	0.125
Amoxicillin/Ampicillin	0.06	0.125
Cefixime	0.008	0.03
Ceftriaxone	0.002	0.008
Spectinomycin	16	32
Nalidixic acid	1	2
Ciprofloxacin	0.002	0.008
Tetracycline	0.125	0.25
Chloramphenicol	0.005	1
Erythromycin	0.25	1
Azithromycin	0.06	0.125

N. gonorrhoeae. Supplemented media which best meet these requirements include chocolate agar with multivitamin supplement such as PolyviteX® (bioMérieux) or IsoVitaleX® (Becton-Dickinson) (30), or GC agar supplemented with cysteine-free 1% multivitamin supplement, recommended by the Clinical and Laboratory Standards Institute (CLSI) (6). The high cysteine content in multivitamin supplements can strongly influence the results for carbapenems and β-lactamase inhibitors. Susceptibility tests on these antibiotics, which are of little use in common practice, require media supplemented with cysteine-free IsoVitaleX®. The presence of cysteine has little effect for other antibiotics and the use of a cysteine-free growth supplement is not required for testing these antibiotics by disk-diffusion or agar broth dilution (1).

Inoculum, inoculation, culture

The inoculum is prepared from an 18-24 hours culture on chocolate agar supplemented with 1% PolyviteX® by using a No. 1 MacFarland standard suspension of approximately 10^8 CFU/ml in 0.9% phosphate buffer pH 7.2.

For MIC determination by the agar dilution method, the agar is inoculated either manually with a calibrated loop (1 µl) or mechanically with a Steers multipoint inoculator. Each head of the inoculator applies 1 µl of suspension (approximately 10^5 bacteria per spot) on the agar. Plates are dried at room temperature, then incubated at 36°+/- 1°C in a humidified 5% CO_2 atmosphere for 20-48 hours. MICs should be read if possible after 20-24 hours of incubation, and after 48 hours in the absence of sufficient growth. Studies have shown that there are no significant differences in the MICs determined with inocula of 10^3, 10^4 or 10^5 bacteria per spot, with the exception of an increase in the MICs of penicillin G for penicillinase-producing strains at the highest inocula (30). There may however be a difference of approximately one dilution, higher for MICs read after 48 hours than for those read after 24 hours (30).

For the agar diffusion method (antibiotic disks or antibiotic gradient strips), the bacterial suspension as prepared above is diluted 1:100 or adjusted to equal a MacFarland 0.5 turbidity standard (approximately 10^6 bacteria per ml). The inoculum is applied on the agar surface by swabbing as recommended by the manufacturer of the E-test®. The surface is dried for about fifteen minutes at room temperature before application of the disks or strips. Plates are incubated at 36° +/- 1°C in a humidified 5% CO_2 atmosphere for 20-24 hours.

CONTROL STRAINS

N. gonorrhoeae ATCC 49226, which is susceptible to all antibiotics active against *N. gonorrhoeae*, is used as internal control. WHO reference strains A to E which have different resistance phenotypes can also be used as quality controls in multicenter studies for penicillin G, tetracycline, and spectinomycin. Strain A is resistant to spectinomycin. Strain B is susceptible to all antibiotics active against *N. gonorrhoeae*. Strain C is streptomycin-resistant and has low-level chromosome-mediated resistance (intermediate) to penicillin G and tetracycline. Strain D is resistant to streptomycin and highly resistant (chromosomal) to penicillin G and tetracycline, and has low-level resistance to chloramphenicol. Strain E produces a plasmid-encoded TEM-type penicillinase resulting in high-level penicillin resistance, low-level tetracycline resistance and resistance to streptomycin. The emergence of new resistance mechanisms has driven the search for new reference strains expressing these mechanisms (15). Thus, the CDC proposes a quality control panel of strains harboring different resistance mechanisms. These include a spectinomycin-resistant strain, a strain harboring a conjugative plasmid encoding a penicillinase and a TetM protein conferring cycline resistance, a strain with reduced susceptibility (MIC = 0.125-0.5 µg/ml), a ciprofloxacin-resistant strain (MIC ≥ 1 µg/ml), a strain with an azithromycin MIC ≥ 1 µg/ml and a strain with reduced cefixime susceptibility (MIC = 0.25-0.5 µg/ml).

ANTIBIOTICS TO BE STUDIED

The antibiotics to be tested in a standard susceptibility test must have a practical clinical use, be consistent with treatment guidelines, and allow screening of the main acquired resistance mechanisms. The antibiotics recommended for single-dose treatment of uncomplicated urogenital infections as well as rectal and pharyngeal infections include principally the third generation injectable (ceftriaxone, cefotaxime, ceftizoxime) and oral (cefixime) cephalosporins (4). Fluoroquinolone resistance has become increasingly widespread and as of 2007 these drugs are no longer recommended (5). Spectinomycin is also recommended in urogenital and rectal infections but not for pharyngitis (4, 5). Another factor to be taken into account is the national or European marketing authorization status of the antibiotics being tested.

While many antibiotics are active against *N. gonorrhoeae*, today their use is limited by either a high level of acquired resistance, a pharmacokinetic profile which does not permit a single dose regimen, or an unfavorable benefit/risk ratio. The penicillins, tetracyclines, chloramphenicol and macrolides fall into this category. Taking all these considerations into account, the following antibiotics can be proposed for standard susceptibility testing in *N. gonorrhoeae* for purposes of guiding treatment or for epidemiological surveillance (those suggested by CLSI are marked by an asterisk): penicillin G* (or ampicillin or amoxicillin), ceftriaxone* or cefotaxim*, cefixime* or cefpodoxime*, spectinomycin*, tetracyclines*, chloramphenicol, azithromycin, and a fluoroquinolone (ciprofloxacin*, ofloxacin*, or levofloxacin). For fluoroquinolones, low-level resistance can be detected with a nalidixic acid disk. β-lactamases can be easily detected with a chromogenic test.

Laboratories which determine MICs by the agar dilution method should use an antibiotic powder with defined potency, stored at –20°C in the presence of a dessicant (unless otherwise indicated by the manufacturer). Stock solutions are prepared immediately before use after dissolution and sterilization through a 0.22 μm membrane filter. Table 2 shows the range of dilutions to be prepared for different antibiotics, as well as the solvents and diluents to be used.

INTRINSIC RESISTANCE

N. gonorrhoeae is intrinsically resistant to trimethoprim, lincosamides, polymyxins, and glycopeptides. These intrinsic resistances can be used to prepare antibiotic supplements for selective media. Such media are routinely used when the isolate is taken from an open site which may be contaminated by commensal flora. However, the existence of a small percentage of mutant vancomycin-susceptible strains (MIC ≤ 1 μg/ml) requires the use of a nonselective medium in addition to the selective media.

ACQUIRED RESISTANCE

Acquired resistance has been described for every class of antibiotic used in the treatment of gonococcal infections, and bears witness to the extreme adaptability of this species. Acquired resistance is due to an accumulation of chromosomal mutations or gene transfer. The latter results from the acquisition of mobile genetic elements or of genetic material by transformation on contact with other strains of *N. gonorrhoeae* or with commensal bacteria.

β-lactams

Strains susceptible to penicillin G are inhibited *in vitro* by 0.03 μg/ml penicillin G. Over the past thirty years, two main types of β-lactam resistance mechanisms have emerged, each of which has a different impact on the MICs (Table 3).

The acquisition of a plasmid-encoded penicillinase (penicillinase-producing *Neisseria gonorrhoeae* or PPNG) was described as early as 1976 (24). These penicillinases are TEM-1-type enzymes encoded by several types of plasmids with a variable geographical distribution (10, 26). All penicillins are inactivated by this enzyme, which was found in over 12% of isolates from western Europe in 2004 and only 1% of isolates

Table 2. Solvents and diluents for preparation of stock solutions of antibiotics for *N. gonorrhoeae*

Antibiotic	Range of concentrations (μg/ml)	Solvent	Diluent
Penicillin G	0.007 - 4	Phosphate buffer, 0.1 mol/l, pH 6.0	
Amoxicillin	0.015 - 4	Phosphate buffer, 0.1 mol/l, pH 6.0	
Cephalosporins	0.0015 - 1	Phosphate buffer, 0.1 mol/l, pH 6.0	
Fluoroquinolones	0.015 - 16	Distilled water	
Spectinomycin	8 - 256	Distilled water	
Tetracycline	0.125 - 32	Distilled water	
Chloramphenicol	0.125 - 32	Distilled water	
Erythromycin	0.015 - 8	95% Ethanol	Distilled water
Azithromycin	0.015 - 8	95% Ethanol	Distilled water

Table 3. Minimal inhibitory concentrations (µg/ml) of four β-lactams according to the mechanism of resistance (adapted from 7 and 25)

Antibiotic	Mechanism of resistance	MIC$_{50}$	MIC$_{90}$
Penicillin G	No mechanism	0.03	0.25
	Chromosomal	2	8
	PPNG[a]	32	> 64
Amoxicillin + clavulanic acid	No mechanism	0.06	0.25
	Chromosomal	2	4
	PPNG[a]	4	16
Cefixime	No mechanism	0.008	0.03
	Chromosomal	0.03	0.125
	PPNG[a]	0.008	0.03
Ceftriaxone	No mechanism	0.008	0.03
	Chromosomal	0.03	0.125
	PPNG[a]	0.008	0.03

[a] PPNG, penicillinase producing *N. gonorrhoeae*.

Table 4. Chromosomal non enzymatic resistance to β-lactams in *N. gonorrhoeae* (adapted from 27)

Mechanism of resistance	MIC (µg/ml)		
	Penicillin G	Tetracycline	Erythromycin
No mechanism	0.02	0.15	0.3
penA	0.12	0.15	0.3
penA + *mtr*	0.12	0.15	4
penA + *mtr* + *penB*	1	1	4
penA + *mtr* + *penB* + *penC*	2	2	4
penA + *mtr* + *penB* + *penC* + *ponA1*	4	2	4

from the United States in 2003 (19, 33); MICs of penicillin G are generally high (from 1 to > 64 µg/ml) with partial restoration by clavulanic acid, although not enough for amoxicillin-clavulanic acid to have a therapeutic effect (Table 3). Second and third generation cephalosporins remain active.

Chromosomal β-lactam resistance emerged in the early 1970s and involves a number of mechanisms, often found in combination (Table 4). The level of penicillin resistance is lower than that seen with PPNG (MIC of penicillin G = 0.125-8 µg/ml) but cross-resistance occurs with all β-lactams and in some cases with other antibiotic classes (Table 4). Approximately 9% of *N. gonorrhoeae* strains isolated in western Europe in 2004 and 4% of strains isolated in the United States in 2003 had chromosome-mediated resistance with penicillin G MICs ≥ 2 µg/ml in the absence of β-lactamases and tetracycline MICs of 2-8 µg/ml (19, 33). MICs vary according to the β-lactam and the mechanism of resistance. Third generation cephalosporins like cefixime, cefotaxime, and especially ceftriaxone are the least affected, retaining low MIC values which are usually compatible with therapeutic use (Table 3). This resistance may be related to an alteration of one or both essential PBPs of *N. gonorrhoeae*: PBP-2 (*penA* gene) and PBP-1 (*penC* and *ponA* genes), to a modification of the major porin PI (*penB* gene), or to overexpression of the MtrCDE efflux system (*mtr* genes). Mutations in PBP genes only modify β-lactam activity (27) while mutations affecting the major porin PI result in cross-resistance to other hydrophilic antibiotics such as tetracyclines and a slight decrease in quinolone susceptibility (14, 27). MtrCDE efflux system overexpression mainly affects the most hydrophobic antibiotics such as macrolides, to a greater extent than β-lactams, quinolones or tetracyclines (27, 32). The synergistic action of these different mechanisms on resistance to β-lactams has been clearly established (14, 32).

Penicillinases can be screened with a chromogenic test as soon as the strain is isolated. A positive result indicates penicillin resistance. Penicillin activity is partially restored when a β-lactamase inhibitor is added. The failure rate of intramuscular penicillin G (5 MU) + probenecid (1 g) is about 2% for strains having an MIC of penicillin ≤ 0.06 µg/ml, 4% for MICs between 0.125 and 0.5 µg/ml and 14% for MICs > 0.5 µg/ml (11). Reduced penicillin susceptibility can be detected on a routine basis by determining the MIC of penicillin G. Strains with high penicillin G MICs due to a chromosomal mechanism (MIC 1-8 µg/ml) may have significantly higher MICs of cephalosporins such as cefixime or, to a lesser extent, ceftriaxone. Treatment failure has been described for oral cephalosporins such as cefixime with this type of strain (MIC of cefixime = 0.125-0.5 µg/ml or higher) (9). The recent description of strains with MICs of ceftriaxone ≥ 0.5 µg/ml calls for increased vigilance (16). The increase in resistance rates to third generation cephalosporins is more pronounced for oral cephalosporins and is mainly due to altered affinity of PBP-2 resulting from mosaic alleles of the *penA* gene which integrated fragments of *penA* genes from *Neisseria cinerea* and *Neisseria perflava*, more or less associated with polymorphisms of the *mtrR*, *porB1b* and *ponA* genes (18, 23). With this in mind, MICs should be routinely determined for therapeutically used cephalosporins when the strain harbors high-level chromosomal resistance to penicillin G.

Fluoroquinolones

N. gonorrhoeae is normally susceptible to quinolones. Due to the recent and significant emergence of fluoroquinolone resistance, these drugs are no longer used in probabilistic treatment (5). Cross-resistance occurs with all quinolones, to a variable extent according to the drug (8, 29). Resistance is mainly due to single or multiple mutations in DNA gyrase (*gyrA* gene) or the topoisomerase IV subunit C (*parC* gene) (Table 5). Overexpression of the MtrCDE efflux system plays only a secondary role in quinolone resistance. A recent literature review reports success rates with single dose ciprofloxacin in uncomplicated urogenital infections ranging from 90-100% for MICs ≤ 0.06 µg/ml to approximately 80% for MICs of 0.125-0.5 µg/ml and 30% for MICs > 0.5 µg/ml. This acquired fluoroquinolone resistance, when it is low level, can be easily detected with a nalidixic acid disk (30 µg) because a single mutation suffices to confer high-level resistance to this antibiotic (Table 5). According to the Comité de l'Antibiogramme de la Société Française de Microbiologie, an inhibition diameter ≥ 25 mm around the nalidixic acid disk (30 µg) predicts susceptibility to fluoroquinolones. Otherwise, the MICs of fluoroquinolones should be determined. Fluoroquinolone disks readily detect high-level fluoroquinolone resistance which, currently, is by far the most prevalent.

Spectinomycin

Resistance of *N. gonorrhoeae* to this aminoglycoside, used exclusively to treat gonococcal infections, was first described in 1973 but generally has remained rare. MICs of spectinomycin for susceptible strains range from 1-32 µg/ml. Resistance results from mutations in the 30S ribosomal subunit. Treatment failure has been described for strains with MICs > 64 µg/ml and inhibition zone diameters ≤ 15 mm around a 100 µg spectinomycin disk (20).

Tetracyclines

All the tetracyclines have comparable activity against *N. gonorrhoeae* and antibiogram results for tetracycline predict those for minocycline and doxycycline. Tetracycline-susceptible strains have MICs comprised between 0.03 and 0.5 µg/ml. Failure of tetracycline therapy has been reported in 20% of strains with tetracycline MICs of 1-2 µg/ml and is more frequent for MICs above 2 µg/ml (11, 17). Resistance is chromosome or plasmid-mediated and has been found respectively in 39% and 12% of strains isolated in western Europe in 2004 and 14% and 4% of strains isolated in the United States in 2003 (19, 33). Chromosome-mediated resistance (MIC of tetracycline = 2-8 µg/ml) generally confers cross-resistance to β-lac-

Table 5. Minimal inhibitory concentrations of quinolones according the main mechanisms of resistance (adapted from 8)

Resistance mechanism	MICs (µg/ml)		
	Nalidixic acid	Ofloxacin	Ciprofloxacin
Wild type	0.5 - 4	0.008 - 0.06	0.004 - 0.03
gyrA	128 - 256	0.25 - 1	0.06 - 0.5
gyrA + parC	128 - 256	0.5 - 8	0.25 - 8

tams since common mechanisms are involved, including alteration of the major porin PI associated with the MtrCDE efflux system (32). Plasmid-mediated resistance, first described in 1985, is high-level (MIC = 16-64 µg/ml) and related to acquisition of the tet(M) gene originally described in streptococci and carried on a transposon located in N. gonorrhoeae on large conjugative plasmids (13). The TetM protein encoded by the tet(M) gene protects the ribosomal target from the action of tetracyclines. High-level tetracycline resistance and plasmid-encoded resistance in particular can be detected by using a tetracycline disk (30 IU). TetM-producing strains all show an inhibition zone diameter < 19 mm.

Other antibiotics

Single-dose thiamphenicol (2.5 g) was long used with success in the treatment of gonococcal infections. However, there is a strong correlation between chromosomal β-lactam resistance and reduced phenicol susceptibility. Treatment failure has been described mainly for strains with MICs of chloramphenicol ≥ 1 µg/ml (3). While high-level resistance is rare, as many as 20% of strains have reduced chloramphenicol susceptibility.

Macrolides are rarely used to treat gonococcal infections because they are only moderately active against N. gonorrhoeae. Moreover, they cannot be given by a single dose regimen, except for azithromycin 2 g which is effective but causes frequent gastrointestinal side effects at this high dose. Erythromycin only works against strains with low MICs (≤ 0.125 µg/ml). Failure rates of a five-day course of erythromycin 2 g daily were 12%, 30%, 70% and 80% for MICs of 0.25, 0.5, 1 and 2 µg/ml, respectively (11). Low-level acquired resistance is due mainly to overexpression of the MtrCDE or MacAB efflux systems with MICs of erythromycin and azithromycin of 2-4 and 0.25-0.5 µg/ml, respectively (28, 34). Higher-level resistance is due to the production of methylases encoded by the erm genes or ribosomal mutations (22); these enzymes methylate the 23S rRNA and reduce the affinity of macrolides, lincosamides and streptogramin B for the ribosome.

Table 6. Breakpoints for N. gonorrhoeae as defined by the European Committee for Antimicrobial Susceptibility Testing (EUCAST), the Clinical and Laboratory Standards Institute (CLSI) and completed by the Centers for Disease Control (CDC)

Antibiotic (disk content)	MICs interpretative standard (µg/ml)					
	EUCAST			CLSI		
	S[a]	I	R	S	I	R
Penicillin G [b] (10 units)	≤ 0.06	0.12-1	> 1	≤ 0.06 ≥ 47 mm	0.12-0.5 27-46 mm	≥ 1 ≤26 mm
Cefixime [b] (5 µg)	≤ 0.12	-	> 0.12	≤ 0.25 ≥ 31 mm	- -	- -
Ceftriaxone [b] (30 µg)	≤ 0.12	-	≤ 0.12	≤ 0.25 ≥ 35 mm	- -	- -
Cefotaxime [b] (30 µg)	≤ 0.12	-	> 0.12	≤ 0.5 ≥ 31 mm	- -	- -
Ciprofloxacin [b] (5 µg)	≤ 0.03 -	0.06 -	> 0.06 -	≤ 0.06 ≥ 41 mm	0.12-0.5 28-40 mm	≥ 1 ≤ 27 mm
Ofloxacin [b] (5 µg)	≤ 0.12 -	0.12 -	> 0.25 -	≤ 0.25 ≥ 31 mm	0.5-1 25-30 mm	≥ 2 ≤ 25 mm
Levofloxacin [c]	-	-	-	-	-	≥ 1
Spectinomycin [b] (100 µg)	≤ 64 -	- -	> 64 -	≤ 32 ≥ 18 mm	64 15-17mm	≥ 128 ≤ 14 mm
Tetracycline (30 µg)	≤0.5 -	0.5 -	>1 -	≤ 0.25 ≥ 38 mm	0.5-1 31-37 mm	≥ 2 ≤ 30 mm
Azithromycin [c] (15 µg)	≤ 0.25 -	0.5 -	> 0.5 -	- -	- -	≥ 1[c] ≤ 30 mm

[a] I, intermediate; R, resistant; S, susceptible.

[b] Disk contents and zone inhibition diameters as defined by CLSI.

[c] Breakpoints and diameters as defined by the CDC.

CONCLUSION

The rising rate and spread of acquired resistance in *N. gonorrhoeae* make it essential to perform antibiotic susceptibility testing on a routine basis and not only in the case of treatment failure. Breakpoints and critical diameters allowing clinical categorization of laboratory isolates have been determined by national and international scientific committees based on pharmacokinetic and pharmacodynamic (PK/PD) data, MIC distribution by species, and *in vivo* efficacy data. For *N. gonorrhoeae*, the most recent values proposed by the European Committee for Antimicrobial Susceptibility Testing (EUCAST) (http://www.srga.org/eucastwt:MICTAB/) and the CLSI (6) completed by the CDC are summarized in Table 6. This antibiogram not only documents the choice of treatment at the individual level but also enables epidemiological surveillance of antibiotic resistance in multicenter studies or national or international surveillance programs. Continuing surveillance of the emergence and spread of antibiotic resistance makes it possible to modify and adapt treatment guidelines for gonococci both nationally and internationally. For instance, the recent spread of fluoroquinolone resistance worldwide and the emergence of multi-resistant strains with reduced susceptibility to third generation cephalosporins, particularly oral ones, are factors to be taken into account when adapting treatment guidelines. MIC determination by the agar dilution method is the reference method for evaluating antibiotic susceptibility of *N. gonorrhoeae*. In everyday practice, penicillinase producing strains can be detected by a rapid chromogenic test and strains resistant to the main therapeutically used antibiotics can be detected by agar diffusion method with antibiotic disks or by MIC determination using antibiotic gradient strips.

REFERENCES

(1) **Barry, A.L., and P.C. Fuchs**. 1991. Comparison of agar media used for determining antimicrobial susceptibility of *Neisseria gonorrhoeae*. J. Antimicrob. Chemother. **28**:149-151.

(2) **Biedenbach, D.J., and R.N. Jones**. 1996. Comparative assessment of E-test for testing susceptibilities of *Neisseria gonorrhoeae* to penicillin, tetracycline, ceftriaxone, cefotaxime and ciprofloxacin: investigation using 510(k) review criteria recommended by the Food and Drug Administration. J. Clin. Microbiol. **34**:3214-3217.

(3) **Bogaerts, J., W. Martinez Tello, L. Verbist, P. Piot, and J. Vandepitte**. 1987. Norfloxacin versus thiamphenicol for treatment of uncomplicated gonorrhea in Rwanda. Antimicrob. Agents Chemother. **31**:434-437.

(4) **Centers for Disease Control and Prevention**. 2006. Sexually transmitted diseases treatment guidelines, 2006. M.M.W.R. Recomm. Rep. **55** (RR-11):1-78.

(5) **Centers for Disease Control and Prevention**. 2007. Update to CDC's Sexually transmitted diseases treatment guidelines, 2006: Fluoroquinolones no longer recommended for treatment of gonococcal infections M.M.W.R. **56**:332-336.

(6) **Clinical and Laboratory Standards Institute.** Performance Standards for antimicrobial susceptibility testing; nineteenth informational supplement. Standard M100-S19. CLSI. Wayne, PA, USA, 2009.

(7) **Cohen, M., M.H. Cooney, E. Blackman, and P.F. Sparling**. 1983. In vitro antimicrobial susceptibility of penicillinase-producing and intrinsically resistant *Neisseria gonorrhoeae* strains. Antimicrob. Agents Chemother. **24**:597-599.

(8) **Deguchi, T., M. Yasuda, M. Nakano, S. Ozeki, T. Ezaki, I. Saito, and Y. Kawada**. 1996. Quinolone-resistant *Neisseria gonorrhoeae*: correlation of alterations in the GyrA subunit of DNA gyrase and the ParC subunit of topoisomerase IV with antimicrobial susceptibility profiles. Antimicrob. Agents Chemother. **40**:1020-1023.

(9) **Deguchi, T., M. Yasuda, S. Yokoi, K. Ishida, M. Ito, S. Ishihara, K. Minamidate, Y. Harada, K. Tei, K. Kojima, M. Tamaki, and S. Maeda**. 2003. Treatment of uncomplicated gonococcal urethritis by double-dosing of 200 mg cefixime at a 6-h interval. J. Infect. Chemother. **9**:35-39.

(10) **Dillon, J.A.R., and K. Yeung**. 1989. β-lactamase plasmids and chromosomally mediated antibiotic resistance in pathogenic *Neisseria* species. Clin. Microbiol. Rev. **2** (suppl.):S125-S133.

(11) **Fekete, T**. 1993. Antimicrobial susceptibility testing of *Neisseria gonorrhoeae* and implications for epidemiology and therapy. Clin. Microbiol. Rev. **6**:22-33.

(12) **Fenton, K.A., and C.M. Lowndes**. 2004. European surveillance of STIs network. Recent trends in the epidemiology of sexually transmitted infections in the European Union. Sex Trans. Infect. **80**:255-263.

(13) **Gascoyne, D.M., J. Heritage, P.M. Hawkey, A. Turner, and B. van Klingeren**. 1991. Molecular evolution of tetracycline-resistance plasmids carrying *tet*(M) found in *Neisseria gonorrhoeae* from different countries. J. Antimicrob. Chemother. **28**:173-183.

(14) **Gill, M.J., S. Simjee, K. Al-Hattaw, B.D. Robertson, C.S.F. Easmon, and C.A. Ison**. 1998. Gonococcal resistance to β-lactams and tetracycline involves mutation in loop3 of the porin-encoded at the *penB* locus. Antimicrob. Agents Chemother. **42**:2799-2803.

(15) **Ison, C.A., I.C.M. Martin, C.M. Lowndes, and K.A. Fenton on behalf of the European Surveillance of Sexually Transmitted Infections (ESSTI) network**. 2006. Comparability of laboratory diagnosis and antimicrobial susceptibility testing of *Neisseria gonorrhoeae* from reference laboratories in Western Europe. J. Antimicrob. Chemother. **58**:580-586.

(16) **Ito, M., M. Yasuda, S. Yokoi, S. Ito, Y. Takahashi, S. Ishihara, S. Maeda, and T. Deguchi**. 2004. Remarkable increase in central Japan in 2001-2002 of *Neisseria gonorrhoeae* isolates with decreased sus-

ceptibility to penicillin, tetracycline, oral cephalosporins, and fluoroquinolones. Antimicrob. Agents Chemother. **48**: 3185-3187.

(17) **Karney, W.W., A.H. Pedersen, M. Nelson, H. Adams, R.T. Pfeifer, and K.K. Holmes**.1977. Spectinomycin versus tetracycline for the treatment of gonorrhea. N. Engl. J. Med. **296**:889-894.

(18) **Lindberg, R., H. Fredlund, R. Nicholas, and M. Unemo**. 2007. *Neisseria gonorrhoeae* isolates with reduced susceptibility to cefixime and ceftriaxone: association with genetic polymorphisms in *penA*, *mtrR*, *porB1b*, and *PonA*. Antimicrob. Agents Chemother. **51**:2117-2122.

(19) **Martin, IM.C., S. Hoffmann, and C.A. Ison on behalf of the European Surveillance of Sexually Transmitted Infections (ESSTI) network**. 2006. European Surveillance of Sexually Transmitted Infections (ESSTI): the first combined antimicrobial susceptibility data for *Neisseria gonorrhoeae* in Western Europe. J. Antimicrob. Chemother. **58**:587-593.

(20) **Mc Chesney, D.G., J.W. Boslego, and W.N. Khan**. 1988. Spectinomycin disk zone diameter as a predictor of outcome in clinical treatment of gonorrhoea. Antimicrob. Agents Chemother. **32**:775-776.

(21) **Moran, J.S., and W.C. Levin**. 1995. Drugs of choice for the treatment of uncomplicated gonococcal infections. Clin. Infect. Dis. **20** (suppl I):S47-65.

(22) **Ng, L.K., I. Martin, G. Liu, and L. Bryden**. 2002. Mutation in 23S rRNA associated with macrolide resistance in *Neisseria gonorrhoeae*. Antimicrob. Agents Chemother. **46**:3020-3025.

(23) **Ochiai, S., S. Sekiguchi, A. Hayashi, M. Shimadzu, H. Ishiko, R.Matsushima-Nishiwaki, O. Kozawa, and Y. Deguchi**. 2007. Decreased affinity of mosaic-structure recombinant penicillin-binding protein 2 for oral cephalosporins in *Neisseria gonorrhoeae*. J. Antimicrob. Chemother. **60**:54-60.

(24) **Philips, I**. 1976. Beta-lactamase producing, penicillin-resistant gonococcus. Lancet. **2**: 656-657.

(25) **Rice, R., and J.S. Knapp**. 1994. Antimicrobial susceptibilities of *Neisseria gonorrhoeae* strains representing five distinct resistance phenotypes. Antimicrob. Agents Chemother. **38**:155-158.

(26) **Roberts, M.C**. 1989. Plasmids of *Neisseria gonorrhoeae* and other *Neisseria* species. Clin. Microbiol. Rev. **2** (suppl):S18-S23.

(27) **Ropp, P.A., M. Hu, M. Olesky, and R.A. Nicholas**. 2002. Mutations in *ponA*, the gene encoding penicillin-binding protein 1, and a novel locus *penC* are required for high-level chromosomally mediated penicillin resistance in *Neisseria gonorrhoeae*. Antimicrob. Agents Chemother. **46**:769-777.

(28) **Rouquette-Louglglin, C.E., J.T. Balthazar, and W.M. Shafer**. 2005. Characterization of the MacA-MacB efflux system in *Neisseria gonorrhoeae*. J. Antimicrob. Chemother. **56**: 856-860.

(29) **Tanaka, M., H. Nakayama, M. Haraoka, T. Saika, I. Kobayashi, and S. Naito**. 2000. Susceptibilities of *Neisseria gonorrhoeae* isolates containing amino acid substitutions in GyrA, with or without substitutions in ParC, to newer fluoroquinolones and other antibiotics. Antimicrob. Agents Chemother. **44**:192-195.

(30) **Thabaut, A., J.L. Durosoir, et P. Saliou**. 1981. La sensibilité de *Neisseria gonorrhoeae* aux antibiotiques : considérations méthodologiques. Bull. O.M.S. **59**:561-566.

(31) **Van Dyck, E., H. Smet, and P. Piot**. 1994. Comparison of the E-test with agar dilution for antimicrobial susceptibility testing of *Neisseria gonorrhoeae*. J. Clin. Microbiol. **32**:1586-1588.

(32) **Veal, W.L., R.A. Nicholas, and W.M. Shafer**. 2002. Overexpression of the MtrC-MtrD-MtrE efflux pump due to an *mtrR* mutation is required for chromosomally mediated penicillin resistance in *Neisseria gonorrhoeae*. J. Bacteriol. **184**:5619-5624.

(33) **Wang, S.A., A.B. Harvey, S.M. Conner, A.A. Zaidi, J.S. Knapp, W.L.H. Whittington, C. del Rio, F.N. Judson, and K.K. Holmes**. 2007. Antimicrobial resistance of *Neisseria gonorrhoeae* in the United States, 1988 to 2003: the spread of fluoroquinolone resistance. Ann. Intern. Med. **147**:81-88.

(34) **Zarantonelli, L., G. Borthagaray, E.H. Lee, and W. Shafer**. 1999. Decreased azithromycin susceptibility of *Neisseria gonorrhoeae* due to *mtr* mutations. Antimicrob. Agents Chemother. **43**:2468-2472.

Chapter 37. HELICOBACTER PYLORI

Francis MEGRAUD

INTRODUCTION

Helicobacter pylori was cultured for the first time in 1982 in Australia (15). This bacterium is found only in the human stomach and was rapidly shown to be a major pathogen. Infection with *H. pylori* can be acquired early in life and causes a gastritis that can last a lifetime unless treated. This infection can cause gastric and duodenal ulcers (17), and lymphoma of the gastric mucosa associated lymphoid tissue (MALT). It is a risk factor for gastric adenocarcinoma (9) and can contribute to the gastric side effects of nonsteroidal anti-inflammatory drugs and aspirin consumption, as well as some of the non-ulcer dyspepsias. In addition, it has a role in extra-digestive conditions such as idiopathic thrombocytopenic purpura, certain iron deficiency anemias and possibly even some cardiovascular diseases.

Because of the serious consequences for human health, *H. pylori* eradication is necessary in many indications and the possibility of thereby preventing gastric cancer is an issue under discussion (14). Antibiotic treatment first used only single antibiotics but was not effective. The necessity to use a combination of two antibiotics became rapidly evident in order to 1) increase effectiveness since diffusion of antibiotics at the gastric mucosal site of infection is limited and 2) avoid selection of resistant bacteria. In addition, since the antibiotics have optimal activity at neutral pH, it was necessary to add an anti-secretory agent. The group of pharmaceutical agents called proton pump inhibitors (PPI) was selected for their maximum activity.

The antibiotic - PPI combination proposed by all of the consensus conferences held in the world was clarithromycin (500 mg x 2), amoxicillin (1 g x 2) and PPI in double dose given for at least seven days. Clarithromycin was shown to be the macrolide of choice because of its low MIC and good diffusion at the gastric mucosa level. The major problem of this treatment is the selection of bacteria resistant to clarithromycin. Epidemiological studies have shown that in several countries, 15% to 20% or more of bacteria are resistant to this antibiotic. One alternative is replacing it by the fluoroquinolone levofloxacin but there is a significant risk of resistance arising with this antibiotic. Metronidazole is also used successfully despite frequent resistance *in vitro*. Tetracycline and rifabutin have a small risk for resistance as well as the problem of being sometimes contraindicated in children. Susceptibility studies of *H. pylori* to antibiotics are now even more necessary than ever.

METHODS

Agar dilution

This is considered to be the reference method to assess the reliability of other methods and was selected by the National Committee for Clinical Laboratory Standards (NCCLS) as the method of choice to study clarithromycin susceptibility (22). In Europe, a task force of the European *H. pylori* Study Group has published recommendations that are similar to NCCLS recommendations (6) (Table 1).

The proposed critical concentrations for clarithromycin are: susceptible < 0.25 µl/ml, intermediate 0.25-0.5 µg/ml, and resistant ≥ 1 µl/ml. These concentrations have shown excellent predictive value for therapeutic failure when the combination PPI - clarithromycin - amoxicillin is used. Even though the same standardization work has not been done for the other antibiotics (amoxicillin, tetracycline, rifabutin, and levofloxacin), the agar dilution method can still be used.

Minimal inhibitory concentrations (MIC) greater than 0.5 µg/ml for amoxicillin are unusual. MICs from 0.25 to 0.5 µg/ml are considered as decreased susceptibility but the clinical impact has not been evaluated.

The critical concentrations used for other antibiotics are as follows: tetracycline, 2 µg/ml; rifabutin, 1 µg/ml; ciprofloxacin (representative for fluoroquinolones), 1 µg/ml.

Metronidazole is a special case because most studies have shown lack of reproducibility of the results, for an unknown reason, in both inter-laboratory and even intra-laboratory comparisons (5).

Table 1. Recommendations for *H. pylori* susceptibility testing by agar dilution

Method	USA – CLSI	European *H. pylori* Study Group
Medium	Mueller-Hinton agar sheep blood (5% v/v) over 2 weeks old	Mueller Hinton agar + horse blood (10% v/v)
Inoculum	$1 \times 10^7 - 1 \times 10^8$ CFU/ml (McFarland opacity standard 2, prepared from a 3-day culture on solid medium)	0.5 to 1×10^9 CFU/ml (McFarland opacity standard 4, prepared from a 2-day culture on solid medium)
Incubation	35°C; microaerobic atmosphere	37°C; microaerobic atmosphere
Reading	3 days	3 days
H. pylori for quality control	ATCC 43504	CCUG 38770, CCUG 38771, CCUG 38772
Quality control cut-off standards	Amoxicillin, ciprofloxacin, clarithromycin, metronidazole, tetracycline	Amoxicillin, clarithromycin, metronidazole

The intracellular redox potential is important for reduction of metronidazole into its active metabolite. Not monitoring and controlling this parameter could be responsible for variations in the results. Preincubation of the media in anaerobic conditions has been shown to increase the activity of metronidazole (3). The absence of laboratory and clinical correlation is also a problem because even the strains with higher MICs can sometimes be eradicated. This is perhaps due to the variable redox potential within the stomach. The critical value generally used to define resistance is >8 µg/ml. Because of this lack of correlation and despite the use of the best method to determine susceptibility of *H. pylori*, the European Consensus (Maastricht-3 2005) has recommended not to routinely test this antibiotic (14).

Broth dilution

This method has the advantage to be easily automated. It is, however not commonly used for *H. pylori* since it is difficult to grow these bacteria in liquid medium. Supplemented media such as Brucella and Mueller-Hinton broth have given satisfactory results. Excellent correlation has been found with the E-test® except for metronidazole.

Point Limit

This is the ultimate simplified version of agar dilution. It consists of the inoculation in one stroke of a medium containing a critical concentration of antibiotic (e.g. 1 µg/ml of clarithromycin). Two separate media with concentrations of 0.25 and 1 µg/ml can be used to classify the strain in one of the three clinical categories. This method is easy to perform and theoretically excellent but the media must be prepared in the laboratory. It has been used for comparisons with diffusion by E-test® or disks in order to test metronidazole. A correlation of 94% was found but reproducibility has not been studied. One variation of this method is to use an agar plate divided into four sectors. One sector is without antibiotic and serves as a control, while the three others have the critical concentrations of clarithromycin, amoxicillin, and metronidazole, respectively.

Diffusion

For routine use this method is the simplest and most economical to study susceptibility to several antibiotics. However as a rule, it is not recommended for fastidious slowly growing bacteria. It has been validated in France for the detection of *H. pylori* resistance to macrolides. Because of the significant difference in the MIC against susceptible and resistant strains, a clear separation is possible by disk diffusion. The critical diameter which corresponds to a MIC ≥ 1 µg/ml is 22 mm for clarithromycin and 17 mm for erythromycin. Erythromycin is the antibiotic recommended for the study of macrolides (8). However, discordant results were found for metronidazole. As was already mentioned, it might be due to a lack of standardization of parameters that are not usually taken into account. For example, the redox potential is affected by the delay between preparation of media and performance of the test. This method has not been validated for the other antibiotics but in general a good correlation with other methods has been found.

E-test®

This method has the advantage to be quantitative and to provide the MIC directly. It is adapted to slow-growing bacteria such as *H. pylori*. Good correlation has been found with agar diffusion except for metronidazole. Resistance to metronidazole is overestimated by 10 to 20% by the E-test®, possibly because of the difference of redox potential. In fact, media used to determine the MIC by agar dilution are generally prepared at the time of use and have a greater chance to have a redox potential lower than media for E-test® which are prepared usually long in advance. The European multicenter study reported differences of more than two dilutions between E-test® and agar dilution for metronidazole with five of the 10 strains of *H. pylori* in four laboratories using the same technique (5). The difference resulted in changes in clinical category for two of the strains. Moreover, the two methods showed lack of reproducibility. The existence of mixtures of strains that can occur in 10 to 15% of cases in developed countries might also contribute to the variability of the results.

SUSCEPTIBLE PHENOTYPE

Wild strains of *H. pylori* are intrinsically resistant to certain antibiotics and antifungal agents. Some of these are used in the isolation media, including glycopeptides, cefsulodin, lincosamides, streptogramins, polymyxins, nalidixic acid, trimethoprim, sulfonamides, nystatin, amphotericin B, and cycloheximide. They are naturally susceptible to β-lactams (except cefsulodin), fosfomycin, macrolides, aminosides, tetracyclines, chloramphenicol, rifamycins, fluoroquinolones, nitroimidazoles, nitrofuranes, and bismuth salts.

The MICs of clarithromycin, amoxicillin, and metronidazole that were reported in the European multicentric study are presented in Fig. 1 to 3. MIC_{50} and MIC_{90} of amoxicillin and clarithromycin for susceptible strains are 0.03 and 0.125 µg/ml, respectively (18). They are 0.5 and 1 µl/ml for tetracycline, 0.008 and 0.008 µg/ml for rifabutin, and 0.06 µg/ml and 0.125 µl/ml for ciprofloxacin. When the MICs are determined at an acid rather than at neutral pH, they increase in significant amounts except for metronidazole (Table 2).

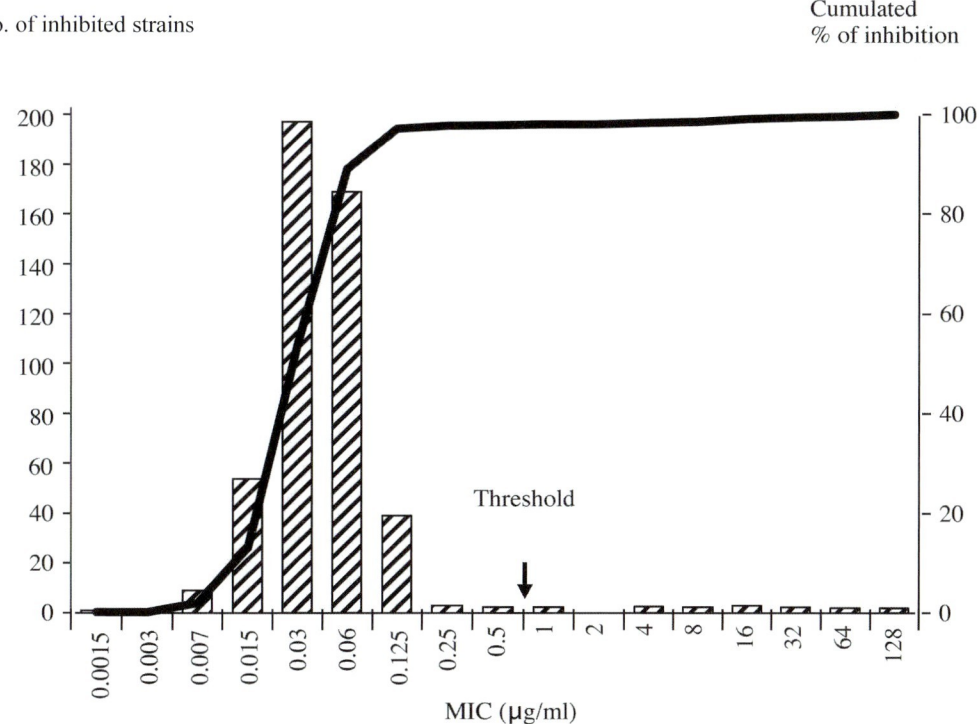

Fig. 1. MICs of clarithromycin against *H. pylori*. MACH2 study by agar dilution (18). Susceptible strains MIC_{50} = 0.03 µg/ml; MIC_{90} = 0.125 µg/ml.

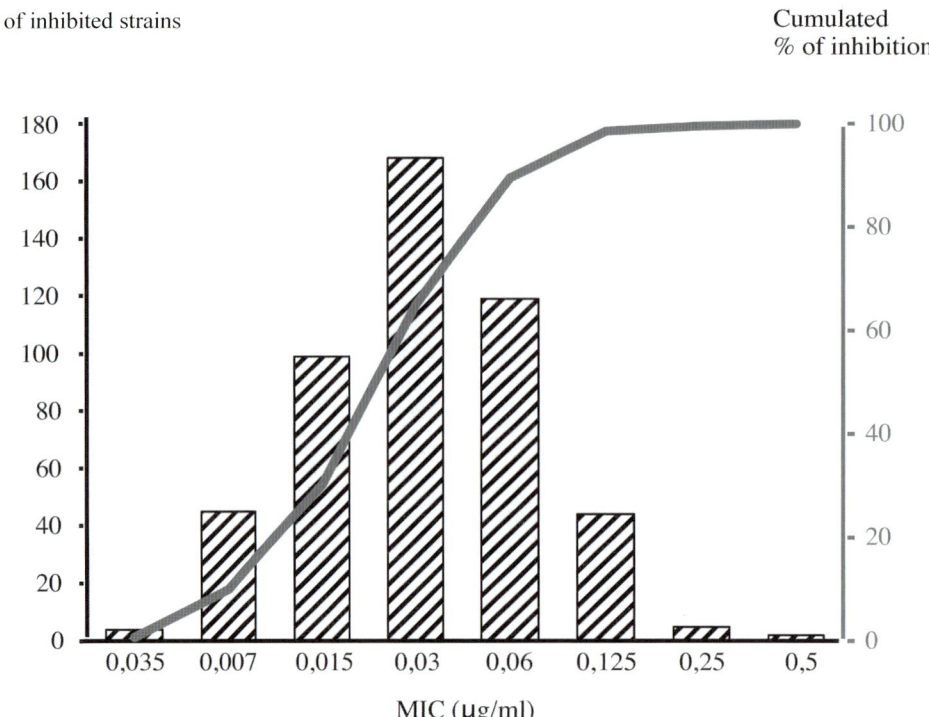

Fig. 2. MICs of amoxicillin against *H. pylori*. MACH2 study by agar dilution (18). Susceptible strains $MIC_{50} = 0.03$ μg/ml; $MIC_{90} = 0.125$ μg/ml.

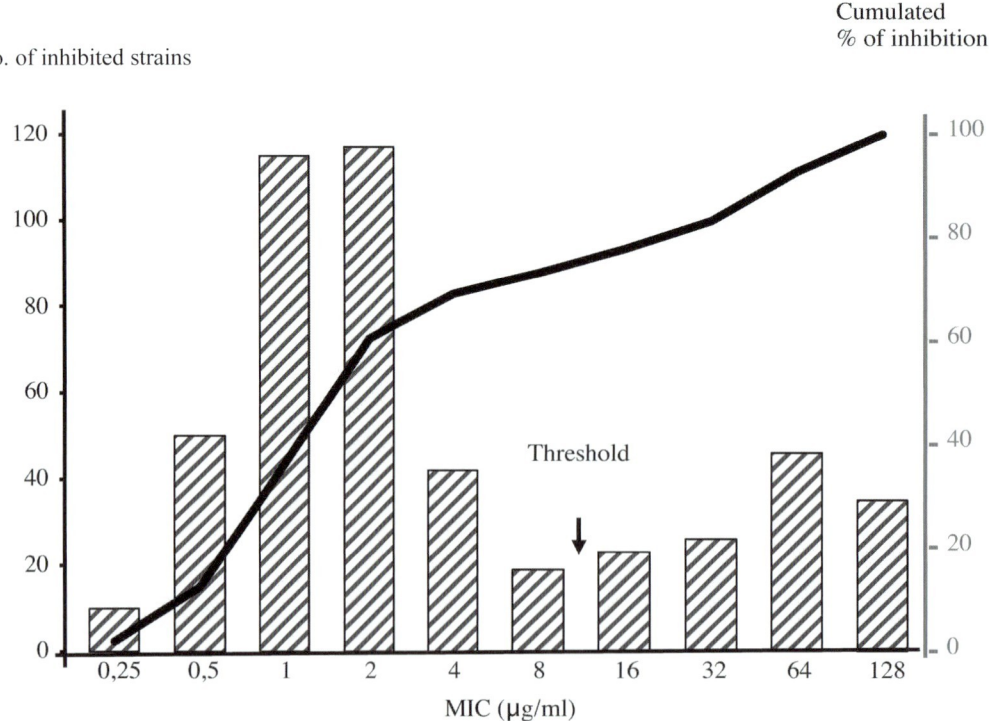

Fig. 3. MICs of metronidazole against *H. pylori*. MACH2 study by agar dilution (9). Susceptible strains $MIC_{50} = 2$ μg/ml; $MIC_{90} = 4$ μg/ml.

Table 2. MIC$_{90}$ of various antibiotics on wild-type strains of *H. pylori* at various pH

Antibiotic	MIC$_{90}$ (µg/ml)		
	pH 7.5	pH 6.0	pH 5.5
Penicillin G	3	5	0.5
Ampicillin	6	25	0.5
Cephalexin	2	16	32
Erythromycin	6	2	8
Clarithromycin	3	6	0.25
Ciprofloxacin	12	5	2
Tetracycline	12	25	0.5
Nitrofurantoin	1	2	2
Metronidazole	2	2	2
Bismuth subcitrate	16	8	–

Minimal bactericidal concentrations (MBC) are rarely studied. They have a one-dilution difference with the MIC for most of the antibiotics. However, when *H. pylori* is cultivated in chemostat, i.e. under conditions which mimic growth conditions *in vivo* where the generation time is very long compared to growth conditions *in vitro*, a weak bactericidal activity is observed. Only amoxicillin and bismuth salts are still bactericidal. These conditions probably better reflect the situation in the infected patient. The study of MBCs for adherent strains compared to those for strains in suspension also showed that amoxicillin was less effective on adherent strains (19).

RESISTANCE MECHANISMS

H. pylori has the distinctive characteristic found in a small number of bacterial species, notably *Mycobacterium tuberculosis*, of acquiring resistance essentially by mutation (Table 3). This is true for all the antibiotics used in therapy. It is, however, unusual for amoxicillin and tetracycline. There are sporadic chromosomal mutations and it is theoretically possible that resistance is transmitted horizontally by transformation. However, this implies that two strains are present simultaneously in the stomach. Our current understanding is that this seems to be a rare event. On the other hand it is possible, and even relatively frequent, that the same strain contains a double population of susceptible and resistant bacteria. Vertical transmission of resistance causes a progressive increase in resistance rates because of the selection pressure exerted. Resistance by efflux does not appear to play a major role in *H. pylori* except perhaps for metronidazole and tetracycline.

Macrolides

The target of macrolides is the peptidyl transferase loop of the domain V of 23S ribosomal RNA. Their binding at this site blocks the elongation of the peptide chain. Clarithromycin, and erythromycin from which it was derived, and its metabolite 14OH clarithromycin are all macrolides that bind with high affinity to the ribosome. Macrolide resistance of the MLS$_B$ type, which involves methylation of an adenine residue, is not observed in *H. pylori*. Another mechanism was described in *Escherichia coli* in 1992 and then was reported in other bacteria including *M. tuberculosis*, *M. intracellulare*, *Mycoplasma pneumoniae*, and in *H. pylori* in 1996: transitions adenine → guanine at positions 2142 (A$_{2142}$G) and 2143 (A$_{2143}$G) as well as transversion adenine → cytosine at position 2142 (A$_{2142}$C) (Fig. 4). These mutations result in decreased binding of erythromycin to the ribosomes of *H. pylori* (23, 30) and are probably due to a conformational change of the attachment site.

Other mutations A$_{2143}$C, A$_{2142}$T, A$_{2143}$T were induced *in vitro* by site-directed mutagenesis. Unlike the previous examples, the mutated bacte-

Table 3. Antibiotic resistance genes in *H. pylori*

Antibiotic	Gene
Macrolides	*rrl*
Metronidazole	*rdxA, frxA*
Quinolones	*gyrA*
Rifamycins	*rpoB*
Amoxicillin	*plp1*
Tetracycline	*rrn 16S*

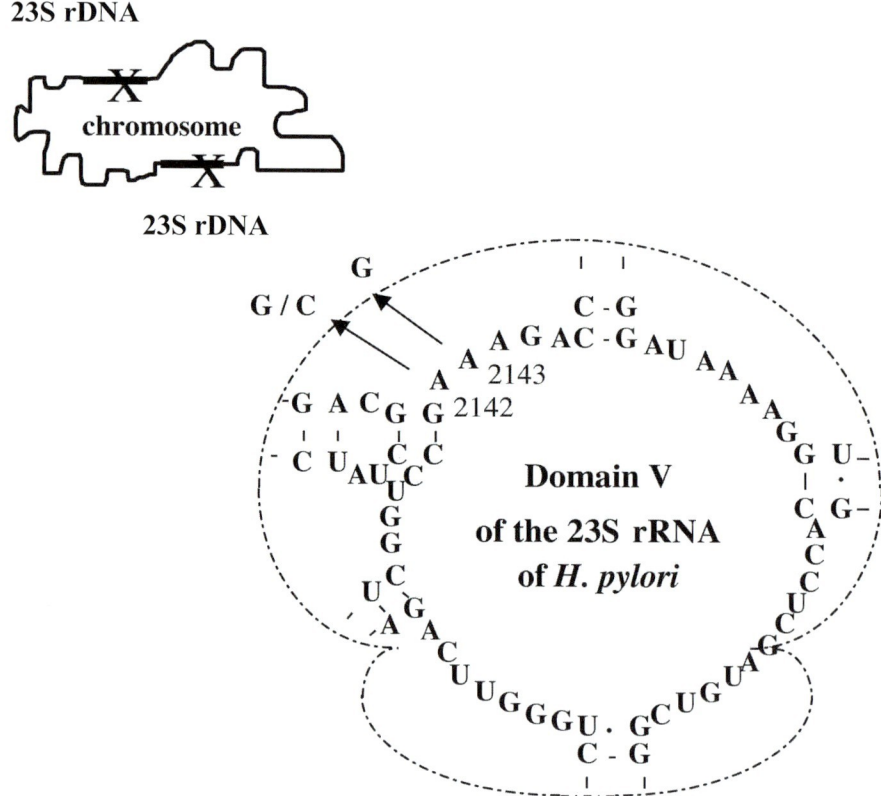

Fig. 4. Mutations in domain V of 23S rRNA of *H. pylori* leading to clarithromycin resistance.

ria had a low growth rate. Mutant $A_{2143}T$ had an intermediate MIC of 0.5 µg/ml and was isolated in an Italian study. The mutation could induce changes in free energy and conformation sufficient to have an impact on the vital properties of the bacteria. It is likely that other mutations were not found because they are lethal. Other mutations have been described but never confirmed: simultaneous mutations $A_{2115}G$ and $G_{2141}A$, as well as the mutations $T_{2717}C$, $T_{2182}C$, and more recently $C_{2147}G$ and $C_{2694}A$. The consequences of these mutations on the MICs have also been studied. In most of the studies mutation $A_{2142}G$ was more frequent in strains having a MIC > 64 µg/ml (65%) than those having a MIC < 64 µg/ml (30%). A greater variety of mutations was seen in strains isolated in cases of treatment failure compared to those cultured before treatment.

These mutations confer cross-resistance to all macrolides. However, clarithromycin seems to be the least affected. In rare cases, for mutation $A_{2143}G$, the MIC can remain even lower than the breakpoint for clarithromycin while the strain is clearly resistant to erythromycin.

H. pylori has two rRNA operons (*rrn*) but when a mutation occurs, it is usually found on both copies. Heterozygoty was only seen four times. Mutations arise spontaneously and then are selected by exposure to antibiotics. There are many examples in which a small proportion of resistant bacteria are found within a larger population of susceptible bacteria, even if the patient has not received macrolides before. This is more easily detected using genotypic methods of detection of resistance. *In vitro* frequency of mutations leading to macrolide resistance is from 3.2×10^{-7} to 6×10^{-8}. This rate can be higher *in vivo* since it can increase under conditions of oxidative stress. In fact, it has been shown *in vitro* that peroxynitrite that is generated *in vivo* in the context of inflammatory reactions is a significant cause of mutations. The hypothesis that *H. pylori* is a naturally hypermutating bacteria has been put forth. No association has been shown with *H. pylori* pathogenicity factors such as the *cag* pathogenicity island and VacA cytotoxin. The stability of mutants $A_{2142}G$ and $A_{2143}G$ has been studied because resistance usually carries a biological cost. In two studies where strains were sub-cultured from 10 to 50 times *in vitro* or obtained from a patient several months after, with confirmation of strain's identity by molecular typing, resistance was still present indicating stability of the mutations. In contrast, authors in another study concluded that reversion to the wild phenotype was possible.

Amoxicillin

Amoxicillin is the β-lactam used to treat *H. pylori* infections. As for all β-lactams, its mechanism of action is the inhibition of peptidoglycan synthesis. In 1996, the Hardenberg strain of *H. pylori* with stable resistance to amoxicillin (MIC = 8 µg/ml) was described in The Netherlands in a patient who had received several treatment courses of amoxicillin for a respiratory infection. This resistance could be transferred by transformation with a frequency of 10^{-5}. The transformants remained stable even after freezing and subculture. Their MIC was 400 times higher than the MIC of susceptible strains and similar to that of the resistant donor strain. These results were not due to production of a β-lactamase since there was no β-lactamase activity nor any corresponding gene in the genome of *H. pylori*. Mutations of the penicillin binding protein PBP-1A partially explain this resistance. Replacing the PBP-1A gene of a wild strain by that of the Hardenberg strain resulted in a 100-fold increase of amoxicillin MIC. Several amino acid substitutions were found by sequence determination but only $Ser_{414}Arg$ was involved in resistance. It is interesting to note that growing an *H. pylori* strain susceptible to amoxicillin, in the presence of progressively increasing concentrations of the antibiotic results in the increase of the MIC from 0.03 - 0.06 µg/ml to 4 - 8 µg/ml, which represents a 100-fold increase. The resistance was stable and no β-lactamase activity was detected. However a decrease in affinity of PBP-1A for β-lactams was observed.

A similar study showed that the MIC increased from 0.02 to 15 µg/ml after 35 passages. The resistant strain had PBP-1A mutations that involved four amino acids. However, transformation of a susceptible strain by the mutated PBP-1 gene resulted in moderately resistant strains. This suggests that another mechanism might be involved. In a study of two strains isolated from the same patient that were identical with the exception of susceptibility to amoxicillin (MIC = 0.06 µg/ml and 2 µg/ml), two mutations at the third motif of PBP-1A were shown to be involved in resistance. Another study showed that PBP-2 and PBP-3 were involved.

A recent alarming event is the isolation of a strain resistant to high levels of amoxicillin (256 µg/ml) in Taiwan in 2009. A TEM-1 β-lactamase was detected in this strain (29). The existence of such a strain raises concerns of its spread in a bacterial species where amoxicillin resistance is rare.

In addition, another type of resistance was described in 17 strains of *H. pylori* that were isolated in Sardinia and in the USA with MIC > 256 µg/ml. However, this resistant phenotype was unstable and lost after freezing of the strains at -80°C but could be restored by culture on an amoxicillin gradient. The isolated strains grown that way had MICs ranging from 0.5 to 32 µl/ml and MBCs of 32 to 1024 µg/ml with a MBC/MIC ratio greater than 32 for all the strains indicating tolerance to amoxicillin. The proposed mechanism was the absence of a fourth PBP, called PBP-D. Four of these strains have been studied further. Transformants had a MIC of 8 µg/ml, which is less than the MIC of the clinical isolates. It has been suggested that this resistance is due to a mosaicism of the C-terminal end of PBP-1A that seems to always be transferred as a unit. The concomitant presence of resistance to multiple antibiotics including fluoroquinolone, chloramphenicol, metronidazole, rifampicin, and tetracycline might be caused by a decrease in membrane permeability and not by active efflux. In summary, even if the mechanism of resistance to amoxicillin is not completely understood, it is now clear that it involves primarily the PBPs.

Tetracyclines

Tetracycline binds to the 30S subunit of the ribosome where it blocks the binding of aminoacyl-tRNA resulting in the synthesis of a truncated peptide. The first strain resistant to tetracycline (MIC >256 µg/ml) was described in Australia in 1996 in a patient whose *H. pylori* eradication by triple therapy had failed. Since then, other studies have reported the existence of strains resistant to tetracyclines but always in small numbers.

No efflux has been found in these strains and two research groups have found modifications of the triplet $AGA_{926-928}TTC$ (position 965-967 according to the numbering system of *E. coli*) of 16S rRNA that is located in the h1 loop where tetracycline binds to the ribosome. This change would result in a lack of binding of tetracycline. This modification of the triplet involves the two 16S *rrn* operons and affects minocycline and doxycycline.

Mutations at the same site involving one or two bases have also been described. These result in a lower level of resistance to tetracycline (4 µg/ml) and a lower growth rate. The need for three mutations to be present might explain why resistance to tetracycline is rare. Resistant strains that do not have a mutation at this triplet have also been described. As in the cells with mutations, these strains show decreased accumulation of tetracycline that can be prevented by an efflux pump inhibitor.

Rifamycins

Rifamycins, especially rifabutin that is used to treat *H. pylori*, inhibit the ß subunit of RNA polymerase coded for by the *rpoB* gene. The first study of the genetic basis of resistance was carried out in 1999 on mutants obtained in the laboratory. It showed changes in codons 524, 525, and 585 of *rpoB*, which are at the same positions as those already implicated in *M. tuberculosis* and *E. coli* studies confirmed transformation that these mutations were indeed the cause of the resistance. Another mutation $V_{149}F$ acquired while the patient was being treated has been described. These mutations affect all the members of the rifamycin group.

Quinolones

Quinolones inhibit the A subunit of DNA gyrase. This enzyme is a tetramer composed of two A subunits encoded by the *gyrA* gene and two B subunits by the *gyrB* gene. Similarly to *M. tuberculosis*, *H. pylori* does not have a type IV topoisomerase.

H. pylori has intrinsic resistance to nalidixic acid whose mechanism has not been studied. Resistance to fluoroquinolones, especially ciprofloxacin, was associated in 1995 to mutations at the Quinolone Resistance Determining Region (QRDR) of *gyrA* which is located mainly at positions 87 and 91. A single mutation can lead to high level resistance (27). However, there are resistant strains that do not have these mutations and whose mechanism requires further study. Susceptible strains can be transformed into resistant strains with amplified DNA fragments from the mutated genes.

New fluoroquinolones, such as sitafloxacin, garenoxacin, and finafloxacin, can avoid the effect of these mutations. Finafloxacin has the characteristic of having increased activity when the pH decreases.

5-Nitroimidazoles

Metronidazole must be reduced within the bacterial cell in order to be active. It alters cellular structures, and cause lethal mutations. Whether metronidazole can be reduced depends on the redox potential of the intracellular environment. Any redox system having a potential less than that of metronidazole (- 415 mV) can reduce metronidazole. Such systems are present in anaerobic bacteria but not in aerobic bacteria. *H. pylori* is a microaerobic bacterium that can nonetheless reduce metronidazole. Hoffman's group has contributed important work to our understanding of resistance to 5-nitroimidazoles. They showed that mutations in the gene of a nitroreductase that is insensitive to oxygen (*rdxA*) were responsible for resistance (7). Another study established that resistance to 5-nitroimidazoles in *H. pylori* ATCC 43504 was due to an insertion sequence (mini-IS*605*) and deletions in the same gene.

Other electron donor candidates have been suggested in previous studies using biochemical and genetic approaches. These include ferredoxin, ferredoxin-like proteins, flavodoxin, flavin oxydoreductase (*frxA*), 2 oxoglutarate oxydoreductase, and pyruvate ferredoxin oxydoreductase. Inactivation of genes involved in some of these systems causes resistance to metronidazole. These data imply that many bacterial enzymes can reduce metronidazole. In other words, the maintenance of an appropriate redox potential depends on multiple enzymatic systems. It has since been shown that point mutations in the *frxA* gene are involved in resistance to metronidazole, either in association with mutations in *rdxA*, or alone. The *frxA* gene of a susceptible *H. pylori* was successfully expressed in an intrinsically resistant *E. coli* that became susceptible while expression of nonfunctional *frxA* could restore the resistant phenotype (21). Variations in the upstream sequences of genes *rdxA* and *frxA* can also be associated with resistance.

Inactivation of a TolC type efflux mechanism increases susceptibility to metronidazole suggesting that it could also be involved. It is of interest to note that aspirin can also increase susceptibility of *H. pylori* to metronidazole by modifying the expression of certain outer membrane proteins.

RESISTANCE FREQUENCY

Many studies have been performed to determine the prevalence of *H. pylori* resistance to antibiotics. However, many of these studies had limitations, particularly concerning the number of strains and how representative they were. Most of these studies were conducted in specialized centers where there were more difficult cases and which were not representative of the general population. In addition, some of these studies originate from a single center with low numbers of patients leading to larger confidence intervals for the prevalence rate. Few of these studies included sufficient numbers of patients who were representative of their region. There was one study of this type where there was random sampling of a Swedish population of 3,000 adults who were contacted by mail. The response rate was 74%. One third of the responders selected randomly accepted an endoscopy and the *H. pylori* strains were then tested for antibiotic susceptibility (26). Another alternative is to analyze the data from clinical trials that were conducted to evaluate new drugs or new therapeutic drug combinations. Since resistance prevalence is by nature an evolving phenomenon, only the most recent data are presented in Table 5.

Clarithromycin

A European multicenter study was conducted in 1998. Bacteriologists from 22 centers in 17 countries were involved and used the E-test®. A total of 1279 strains were studied with an average of 64 strains per center with a range from 21 to 115. The overall primary resistance rate to clarithromycin was 9.9% [CI 95% 0-10.8]. The rate was higher in Central and Eastern Europe (9.3%), [CI 95% 0-22] and the greatest in Southern Europe [CI 95%, 2.1-34.8] (6).

The study was repeated in 2008 and 2009. Preliminary results on almost 2000 strains indicated a resistance rate close to 20%, which represents a doubling in the last decade. Results of individual studies are presented in Table 5 and confirm the difference between Northern Europe with limited resistance and Southern Europe where resistance is higher.

A European multicenter study was carried out in 16 pediatric centers of 14 countries from 1999 until 2002. It showed overall clarithromycin resistance to be 24% in children (11). Individual studies concur with data showing greater prevalence in children (Table 6).

Outside of Europe the prevalence of resistance to clarithromycin seems lower. A systematic review of studies conducted before 2000 estimated it to be less than 4% in Canada. It reached 10 to 15% in the USA based on tests done during clinical trials, regardless of the state, except Alaska. A prospective study from 1998 to 2002 (HARP project) in 11 centers in the USA confirmed these results. The resistance to clarithromycin was 12.9%. Concerning the Far East, prevalence was greater in Japan (22%) than in Hong Kong (7.8%) or Taiwan (6.7-9.5%). Very high rates of resistance were reported in Alaska (31%) and in Turkey (48%).

The main risk factor for *H. pylori* resistance to clarithromycin is the patient's consumption of macrolides. If the resistance is higher in children, it is because of increased prescription of these antibiotics, especially in children for respiratory infections in recent years. One study done on a Japanese family showed that although the strains found in the children were identical to those of their parents by molecular typing they became resistant to clarithromycin after treatment with this antibiotic. In Estonia, resistance of *H. pylori* to clarithromycin appeared in 1998 after the introduction of this drug in 1997. In Japan the consumption of clarithromycin was multiplied by four between 1993 and 2000 and led to a four-fold increase of resistance of *H. pylori* to this antibiotic. However, this was not the case in the Netherlands: even though prescriptions of clarithromycin tripled between 1993 and 1997, no increase of resistance of *H. pylori* was observed. This might be explained by the prudent use of antibiotics in this country. The Dutch have the lowest rate of consumption of antibiotics of all the countries of the European Union. When prevalence of resistance to clarithromycin, as reported in the European multicenter study of 1998, is compared to the consumption of macrolides in the same countries at the same time, then a perfect correlation is found.

Even though there is *in vitro* cross-resistance between the various macrolides, it is not obvious that they have the same potential for selection of resistant strains *in vivo* because of their different abilities to diffuse in the gastric mucosa. Based on *in vitro* data, one can predict that when clarithromycin is present at subinhibitory concentrations, it can select resistant mutants. Perhaps other macrolides cannot reach these subinhibitory concentrations since they have little impact on the selection of resistant strains.

Table 4. MICs for *H. pylori* strains that are resistant to antibiotics

Antibiotic	MIC (µg/ml)
Clarithromycin	1 - 256
Amoxicillin	1 - 8
Metronidazole	16 - 256
Tetracycline	4 - 64
Rifabutin	2 - 64
Ciprofloxacin	2 - 32

Table 5. Primary resistance of *H. pylori* in adults worldwide[a]

Country	Years	Study	Method	No. strains	Clari[R] (%)	Metro[R] (%)	Tetra[R] (%)	Amoxi[R] (%)	FQ[R] (%)	Authors
Europe										
Germany	01-05	MultiC	E-test®	126	9.5	42	ND	0	9.6	Glocker et al.
Belgium	02	MonoC	DD	164	3	31	0	0	ND	Aguemon et al.
Belgium	03-04	MultiC	E-test®	488	ND	ND	ND	ND	16.8	Bogaerts et al.
Bulgaria	05-07	MultiC	AD	613	17.8	25	4.4	ND	7.7	Boyanova et al.
Croatia	01	MonoC	E-test®	196	8	33	ND	0	ND	Bago et al.
Croatia	02-05	MonoC	AD	592	8.2	32.9	ND	ND	ND	Filipec Kanizay et al.
Finland	00-02	MultiC	E-test®	292	2	38	ND	ND	ND	Kovisto et al.
France	04-05	MonoC	AD	128	ND	ND	ND	ND	17.2	Cattoir et al.
Hungary	04-06	MonoC	FISH	238	17.3	ND	ND	ND	ND	Buzas et al.
Italy	04-06	MultiC	E-test®	255	16.9	29.4	ND	ND	19.1	Zullo et al.
Italy	98-02	MonoC	AD	406	23.4	36.7	ND	0.2	ND	Toracchio et al.
Italy	04-05	MonoC	RT-PCR	178	21.3	ND	ND	ND	3	De Francesco et al.
Italy	07	MultiC		109	18	27	0	ND	ND	Romano et al.
Italy	04-05	MultiC	RT-PCR	232	26.7	ND	ND	ND	ND	De Francesco et al.
Netherlands	97-02	MonoC	DD	1,125	1	14.4	ND	ND	ND	Janssen et al.
Poland	01-04	MultiC	E-test®	130	15	42	0	0	ND	Dzierzanowska-Fangrat et al.
UK (Wales)	00-03	MonoC	E-test®	363	7	24	0	0	ND	Elviss et al.
UK (Wales)	00-05	MonoC	E-test®	664	8.4	36.3	<0.5	0	ND	Chisholm et al.
UK (England)	00-05	MonoC	E-test®	646	12.7	28.6	<0.5	0	ND	Chisholm et al.
Sweden	98-01	MultiC	AD	333	1.5	16.2	0.3	0	ND	Storskrubb et al.
North America										
USA (Alaska)	99-03	MultiC	AD	352	31	44	0	2	ND	Bruce et al.
USA	00-01	MultiC	AD	106	12.2	33.9	ND	ND	ND	Laine et al.
USA	98-02	MultiC	AD	347	12.9	25.1	0	0.9	ND	Duck et al.
Middle East										
Iran	01-02	BiC	DD	120	16.7	57.5	0	1.6	ND	Mohammadi et al.
Israel	00-01	MonoC	E-test®	110	8.2	38.2	0	0.9	ND	Samra et al.
Turkey		MonoC	RT-PCR	110	48.2	ND	ND	ND	ND	Onder et al.
Far East										
Korea	01-05	MonoC	E-test®	144	16.7	34.7	ND	11.8	ND	Bang et al.
Hong Kong	03-04	MonoC	E-test®	102	7.8	39.2	ND	0	ND	Gu et al.
Hong Kong	04-05	MonoC	AD	191	ND	ND	ND	ND	11.5	Lee et al.
Japan	01-04	MonoC	E-test®	507	22.7	ND	ND	ND	15	Miyachi et al.
Japan	02-05	MultiC	AD	3,707	ND	2.7	ND	0.08	ND	Kobayashi et al.
Singapore	02	MonoC	AD	120	9.5	31.7	ND	1	ND	Lui et al.
Taiwan	98-07	MonoC	AD	210	9.5	27.6	0.5	ND	5.7	Hung et al.
Taiwan	01-04	MonoC	E-test®	134	6.7	25.4	ND	ND	ND	Poon et al.
Taiwan	04-05	MonoC	E-test®	133	13.5	51.9	0	0.7	ND	Hu et al.
Africa										
Kenya	03-04	MonoC		114	6.4	100	1.9	4.6	ND	Lwai-Lume et al.

[a] Data from studies including more than 100 strains conducted completely or partially since 2000. AD, agar dilution; Amoxi, amoxicillin; BD, broth dilution; BiC, two centers; C, centre; Clari, clarithromycin; DD., disk-diffusion ; FQ, fluoroquinolone; Metro, metronidazole; MonoC, one centre; MultiC, multicentre; ND, not done; R, resistant; Tetra, tetracycline.

Table 6. Primary resistance of *H. pylori* in children in Europe[a]

Country	Years	Study	Method	No. strains	Clari[R] (%)	Metro[R] (%)	Amoxi[R] (%)	FQ (%)	Reference
Bulgaria	00-01	MonoC	AD	115	12.4	15.8	0	ND	Boyanova et al.
France	94-05	MultiC	E-test®	377	22.8	36.7	0	ND	Kalach et al.
Iran	03-05	MonoC		100	16	95	ND	7	Rafeery et al.
Poland	01-04	MultiC	E-test®	139	28	40	0	ND	Dzierzanowska-Fangrat et al.
Portugal	99-03	MonoC	E-test®	109	39.4	16.5	0	4.5	Lopes et al

[a] Data from studies including more than 100 strains conducted completely or partially since 2000. AD, agar dilution; Amoxi, amoxicillin; centre; Clari, clarithromycin; FQ, fluoroquinolone; Metro, metronidazole; MonoC, one centre; MultiC, multicentre; ND, not done; R, resistant.

When treatment with clarithromycin fails, resistant mutants are selected in two thirds of the cases. This is not the case with azithromycin: in a French study the secondary resistance rate was only 23% after triple therapy that included this antibiotic despite a high failure rate of 62%. The impact of erythromycin on selection of resistant strains may be more important. For example, in Iran the prevalence of resistance to clarithromycin was already 17% before the drug was introduced into the country whereas erythromycin was mainly used. A similar situation existed in France in 1993. The prevalence of resistance to clarithromycin was already 8% before the drug was on the market. This was likely the result of significant utilization of other macrolides such as erythromycin and josamycin during the preceding decade.

Few studies report differences in the prevalence of resistance to clarithromycin according to patient type. Strains isolated in a French prospective study from ulcer patients were less often resistant than those isolated from patients with non-ulcer dyspepsia or other diseases: OR = 0.08 [CI 95% 0.011–0.66] versus 1, respectively. The same result was found in a study analyzing causes of treatment failure in clinical trials conducted in France. In the subgroup in which susceptibility had been tested, 5.6% of the strains isolated from ulcer patients were resistant versus 16.5% of those from patients with non-ulcer dyspepsia (p =0.0005) (2). A similar observation was made in Germany. One explanation might be that ulcer patients are infected by *cag* positive strains whereas only half of those with non-ulcer dyspepsia carry these strains (1). These strains are easier to eradicate, perhaps because of their shorter generation time or because they are in closer contact with gastric cells and are therefore more accessible to the antibiotics. Another possibility might be simply that patients with non-ulcer dyspepsia have taken more antibiotics than the others, as was shown in Croatia.

Prevalence of secondary resistance to clarithromycin, i.e. after failure of a treatment regimen including this antibiotic, is extremely high at approximately 60%. Another possible cause of resistance that must be considered is the frequency of mutations.

Mutation $A_{2143}G$ is most often found and mutation $A_{2142}C$ is rarely found (Table 7).

Amoxicillin

In most of the studies, resistance to amoxicillin is either none or less than 1% and is not yet a prob-

Table 7. Mutations associated with clarithromycin resistance

Country	No. strains	$A_{2143}G$ No. (%)	$A_{2142}G$ No. (%)	$A_{2142}C$ No. (%)	Double mutation (%)	Not detected (%)	Authors
Germany (adults)	16	9 (52.7)	3 (16)			4 (11)	Wolle et al.
Brazil	19	14 (73.6)[a]	3 (18.7)			2 (10.5)	Prazeres-Magalhaes et al.
Spain (children)	28	23 (82.1)	2 (7.1)			3 (10.7)	Alarcon et al.
France	50	45 (90)	5 (10)				Raymond et al.
Hong Kong	23	22 (95.6)	1 (4.3)				Ling et al.
Italy	62	35 (56.4)	14 (22.6)	8 (12.9)	5 (8.12)		De Francesco et al.
Iran	20	15 (75)	1 (5)	3 (15)		1 (5)	Mohammadi et al.
Japan	9	2 (22.2)	6 (66.6)			1 (11.1)	Umegaki et al.
Poland	79	50 (62.5)	19 (24)	6 (7.5)	2 (2.5)	2 (2.5)	Dzierzanowska-Fangrat et al.
Taiwan	12	10 (83.3)	1 (8.3)			1 (8.3)	Yang et al.
Total	318	225 (71)	55 (17)	17 (5)	7 (2)	14 (4)	

[a] Two strains also had an $A_{2142}G$ mutation.

lem. No resistant strains are found in France, only strains with decreased susceptibility (0.25-0.5 µg/ml). When very high resistance rates are reported, the results must be considered cautiously until the strains are studied in detail.

Tetracyclines

This resistance has been reported in the past in Spain (0.7%), Great Britain (0.5%), Hong Kong (0.5%), and now the U.K. (<0.5%), Sweden (0.3%), Taiwan (0.5%), Kenya (1.9%), and at a higher rate in Korea (5.3%) and Bulgaria (4.4%) (Table 5). As is true for other antibiotics, this resistance increases with the use of tetracyclines.

Rifamycins

Prevalence of resistance to rifamycins has rarely been studied but it is probably extremely low because these drugs are not used except in patients with mycobacterial infections. Three studies carried out in Germany, Italy, and Japan have not found a single resistant strain. Treatment of tuberculosis with rifampin has been shown to be a risk factor for resistance.

Fluoroquinolones

Prevalence of resistance to fluoroquinolones was only later studied. It was 3-4% in France in the decade from 1990 to 2000. Cross-resistance has been demonstrated in the Netherlands where 4.7% of the strains are resistant to trovafloxacin despite the fact that this drug had not been marketed. Prevalence depends on the selection pressure. In Portugal where fluoroquinolones were used more than in any other European country, prevalence of resistance was 20.9% in 1999. In Portuguese children for whom fluoroquinolones are not prescribed, this resistance was 4.5%. This suggests transmission of resistant strains from the parents. Use of fluoroquinolones for eradication of H. pylori led to an increase in resistance rates which are currently 13% in Europe.

Metronidazole

As mentioned above, results concerning resistance to metronidazole are poorly reproducible and the value of detection on an individual basis is limited. For this reason, the Maastricht-3 Consensus Conference recommended that testing not be done routinely any more. Nonetheless, the low, intermediate, or high trends observed at the population level seem valid.

In the 1998 European multicenter study, overall prevalence of resistance to metronidazole was 33.1% [CI 95% 7.5 - 58.9] with no significant difference between the North (33% [CI 95% 7.1 - 69.2]) and the South (40.8% [CI 95% 27.3 - 54.3]) but with a significantly lower prevalence in Central Europe and Eastern Europe (29.2% [CI 95% 17.9 - 41.95]) (p < 0.01) (6). Overall resistance rose to a small degree with respect to the results of a similar study conducted in Europe in 1991 but not conducted at the same medical centers (27.5% [CI 95% 23.4 - 32]). In the 2008 - 2009 European multicenter study overall resistance was approximately 32%.

The prevalence seen in the individual European studies (Table 5) varies between 14% and 38% and in the USA between 25% and 44%. In the European multicenter pediatric study the prevalence was found to be 25%.

As is true for other antibiotics, prevalence depends upon the selection pressure. It is very high (50 - 80%) in developing countries where metronidazole is often used for certain parasitic diseases and very low in countries where it is rarely used such as Japan (2.7%). Strains isolated from women in industrialized countries are in general more resistant than those isolated from men because of gynecological treatments. Use of metronidazole in treatment of dental infections may also contribute to selection.

The prevalence of secondary resistance is approximately 65% to 75%.

Double Resistance

Since clarithromycin and metronidazole are among the most used antibiotics, it was of interest to see if double resistance occurred randomly. The results showed that twice as many were found as would have been predicted. The proportion of strains is, however, still below 10% in most centers in Europe and Asia, but it is seen much more in developing countries like Mexico (18%). The situation is different after failure of a therapy combining both antibiotics where up to 50% of strains may have this dual resistance. Strains with resistance to 3, 4, or even 5 antibiotics are encountered in 15% of cases in Germany in patients who have been treated multiple times without success (31).

CLINICAL IMPACT OF RESISTANCE

Treatments to eradicate *H. pylori* are complex. They always include two antibiotics and a PPI and may also use bismuth salts. The currently recommended treatments are presented in Table 8.

The clinical impact of antibiotic resistance is significant if it leads to therapeutic failure. Until 1998 few therapeutic trials included the study of antibiotic resistance. A systematic review was published in 1999. We conducted a systematic review of trials published from 1999 to 2003. They dealt mainly with clarithromycin resistance but also looked at metronidazole in the context of triple therapy (16). Few studies have been published since then. Some authors have used 3 antibiotics with a PPI, but antibiotic susceptibility was not tested.

Clarithromycin

Twenty studies involving 1,975 patients during the period 1999-2003 were reported in which the reference triple therapy was administered and where susceptibility to clarithromycin was determined. These studies represent only a small proportion of all those carried out and sometimes the results are not presented so as to be usable.

A major difference in eradication rate was observed. The rate was 87.8% when the strain was susceptible and only 18.3% when it was resistant. The pooled Mantel-Haenzel OR was highly significant (24.5 [CI 95% 17.2-35]), ($p < 0.001$) (Fig. 5). This lower treatment efficacy of 70% is higher than the 53% reported in 1999 and this was found for many more patients. The percentage reduction in the eradication rate reported in the meta-analysis of Fischbach *et al.* published in 2007 was 66.2% [58.2-74.2] on the basis of 24 studies representing 64 treatment arms and 2,556 patients (4). Resistance to clarithromycin appears to be the main cause of the reference treatment's failure. High success rates with susceptible strains were found regardless of which PPI was used, the dose of the various drugs or treatment duration.

Fewer studies have addressed resistance to clarithromycin in the context of combination therapy with PPI - clarithromycin - metronidazole. The number of cases where the strain was resistant to clarithromycin and susceptible to metronidazole was low (22 cases). There was, however, a trend to

Table 8. Combination therapy used to treat *H. pylori* infection with a 7-day course

1- Double dose of proton pump inhibitor (omeprazole, lansoprazole, pantoprazole, rabeprazole, esomeprazole)
    + clarithromycin (2 x 500 mg)
    + amoxicillin (2 x 1 g)
(most commonly used first line treatment)

2- Double dose of proton pump inhibitor (omeprazole, lansoprazole, pantoprazole, rabeprazole, esomeprazole)
    + clarithromycin (2 x 500 mg)
    + metronidazole (2 x 500 mg)

3- Double dose of proton pump inhibitor (omeprazole, lansoprazole, pantoprazole, rabeprazole, esomeprazole)
    + amoxicillin (2 x 1 g)
    + metronidazole (2 x 500 mg)
(Used primarily as a second line treatment for 14 days after failure of other therapies)

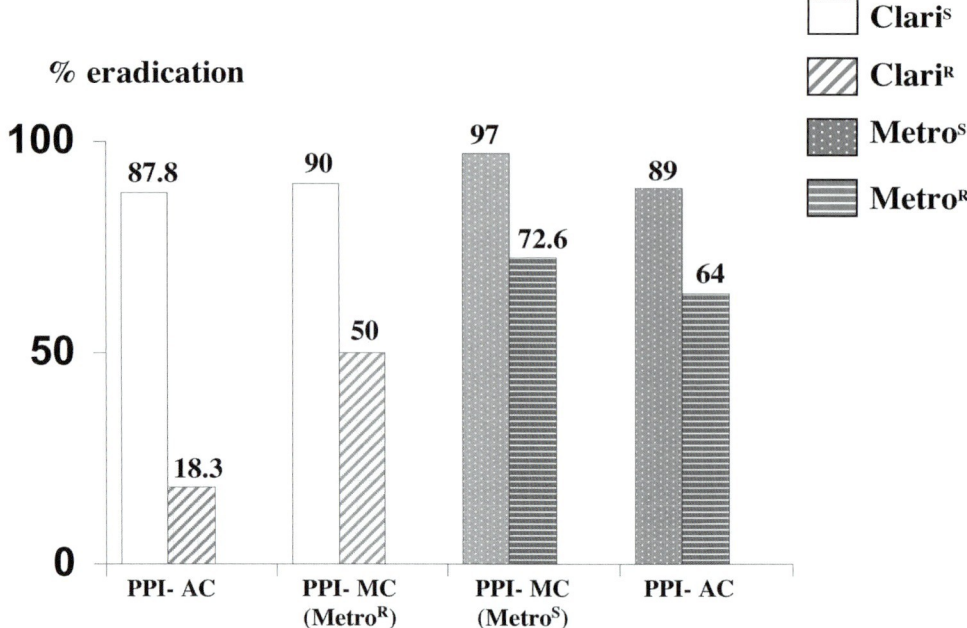

Fig. 5. *H. pylori* eradication using clarithromycin and metronidazole based triple therapies (studies carried out from 1999 to 2003). PPI-AC, proton pump inhibutor – amoxicillin – clarithromycin; PPI-MC, proton pump inhibitor – metronidazole – clarithromycin.

better efficacy of this treatment for these strains with a 50% success rate reported. Eradication was achieved in 97% of cases when strains were susceptible to both antibiotics in our study (16). Fischbach *et al.* analyzed 34 studies representing 99 treatment arms and 3,128 patients. They reported a reduction in the eradication rate of 35.4% [25.4-45.4] (4).

In three studies a compound called ranitidine bismuth citrate, which combines an anti-H_2 agent and bismuth salts, was used in place of a PPI with clarithromycin and metronidazole. Only three strains were resistant to clarithromycin and susceptible to metronidazole. Since all three were eradicated, this suggests a possible synergy. Eradication was achieved for 97.2% of susceptible strains.

Metronidazole

In the context of triple therapy combining PPI, clarithromycin and metronidazole for strains susceptible to clarithromycin, the success rate was 97% for strains susceptible to metronidazole and 72.6% for resistant strains. The existence of resistance to metronidazole is thus associated with a decrease in the success rate of only 25% (16) and only 18% in the study of Fischbach *et al.* (4). The use of ranitidine bismuth citrate instead of a PPI seems to give comparable results for eradication, whether the strain is susceptible or resistant (98%). When metronidazole was used with a PPI and amoxicillin, which is the second-line treatment recommended in France, the success rate for susceptible strains was 89% but 64% for resistant strains, a difference of 25% (16); it was 30% in the study of Fischbach *et al.* (4). The same survey reported a decrease in efficacy of 26% [14.2-37.8] for triple therapy with bismuth (bismuth + metronidazole + tetracycline) (14 studies) and only 14% [5.4-22.6] in the quadruple therapy with bismuth (16 studies). A heterogeneity of the results was observed in the case of strains resistant to metronidazole.

Clarithromycin and metronidazole

Few patients carrying strains with this double resistance have been treated. Treatment by clarithromycin-metronidazole-PPI in 14 patients never led to eradication of *H. pylori*. Only two out of five were successful when ranitidine bismuth citrate was used in place of a PPI.

Fluoroquinolones

Few studies have evaluated the clinical impact of fluoroquinolone resistance on the eradication rates. PPI - amoxicillin - levofloxacin triple therapy for 10 days resulted in an eradication rate of 75% for 33 strains susceptible to levofloxacin and only 33% for resistant strains. The use of gatifloxacin instead of levofloxacin for 7 days led to an eradication rate of 100% for susceptible strains and 33% for resistant strains.

Other antibiotics

Resistance to other antibiotics used for eradication of *H. pylori* such as tetracycline and rifabutin may have an impact on the treatment success but most clinical trials either showed no resistant strains or did not include the study of antibiotic susceptibility. Resistance to amoxicillin is often investigated but the low number of reported cases does not allow any conclusions to be drawn.

ANTIBIOTICS TO TEST

The minimum susceptibility test should include clarithromycin and either levofloxacin or ciprofloxacin. Of the two antibiotics of the recommended first line treatment protocol, clarithromycin is the only one for which the result has a very higher predictive value. In recent years the importance of fluoroquinolones such as levofloxacin or moxifloxacin as alternatives to clarithromycin has emerged. Resistance to these drugs is best assessed by testing levofloxacin or ciprofloxacin, the latter not being used in therapy.

Clinical trials comparing empirical treatment with regimens based on antibiotic susceptibility studies have shown the benefits of the second approach.

In addition to clarithromycin and levofloxacin, susceptibility testing can include antibiotics that might be used for eradication of *H. pylori*, namely amoxicillin, tetracycline, and rifabutin. Including metronidazole in routine testing is of limited value because of lack of reproducibility of the results. It is no longer recommended since the Maastricht Consensus Conference.

RESISTANCE DETECTION

Phenotypic

Clarithromycin

An Erythromycin disk-diffusion is the most attractive method for routine testing because of its optimal cost-effectiveness (8). It is recommended by the « Comité de l'Antibiogramme de la Société Française de Microbiologie ». The reference method using agar dilution or E-test® may also be used for MIC determination.

Amoxicillin

The E-test® is the method of choice since it allows determination of the MIC which can vary from 0.015 to 0.5 µg/ml for susceptible strains.

Table 9. Genotypic detection of macrolide resistance in *H. pylori*

Amplification of 23S rRNA gene	Hybridization without amplification
Sequencing, pyrosequencing	FISH (Fluorescence in situ Hybridization)
RFLP (Restriction Fragment Length Polymorphism)	
OLA (Oligonucleotide Ligation Assay)	
DEIA (DNA Enzyme Immunoassay)	
INNO-LiPA (Line Probe Assay)	
Quadruplex real-time PCR	
PCR-based denaturing HPLC	
Allele-specific primer PCR	
Dual priming Oligonucleotide multiplex PCR	
PHFA (Preferential Homoduplex Formation Assay)	
3' mismatched PCR and 3' mismatched reverse PCR	
Real Time PCR (FRET-MCA)	
Oligonucleotide microarray	
Microelectronic chip array	
Electrocatalytic detection	

Tetracycline, rifabutin, and levofloxacin

Diffusion can be used for its convenience and low cost because it allows detection of resistant strains that have a significant decrease in inhibition diameter. If the diameter is less than 20 mm, an E-test® can be performed to determine the MIC.

Metronidazole

Diffusion methods such as E-test® and agar disk diffusion are not recommended. Of the remaining but not yet recommended methods, the best choice would be agar dilution or its simplified version the limit point test with a concentration of 8 µg/ml.

Genotypic

As previously mentioned, *H. pylori* resistance most often results from a limited number of point mutations which are easily detected by molecular testing.

Clarithromycin

Many genotypic techniques have been developed to detect resistance because of its clinical importance and the small number of mutations involved (Table 9). The main methods are PCR-RFLP, real-time PCR followed by melting curve analysis of the amplicons, the FISH technique, and multiplex PCR followed by strip hybridization.

- PCR-RFLP - This method has been used since 1996. It is based on the fact that mutations generate restriction sites in the amplicon obtained with specific primers complementary to 23S rDNA (30). These sites are recognized by enzymes *Bsa*I for mutation $A_{2142}G$ and *Bsb*I for $A_{2143}G$. Therefore, two bands are present in the gel if either of these mutations is present. In case of an incomplete digestion, a mixture is observed. More recently, *Bce*AI has been proposed to detect $A_{2142}C$ (20). PCR-RFLP is simple but has the same pitfalls as standard PCR including response time and need to handle the amplicon products. It can be used directly on stool specimens.

- Real-time PCR - This method was developed to make PCR quantitative but also allows for detection of mutations by means of melting curve analysis of the amplicons. It was first used in 1999 with the fluorophore SYBR Green I which is specific for double stranded DNA to detect the presence of *H. pylori* and the second fluorophore, Cy5, on a probe specific for *H. pylori* to detect the mutations associated with clarithromycin resistance; first on cultured strains and then directly on biop-

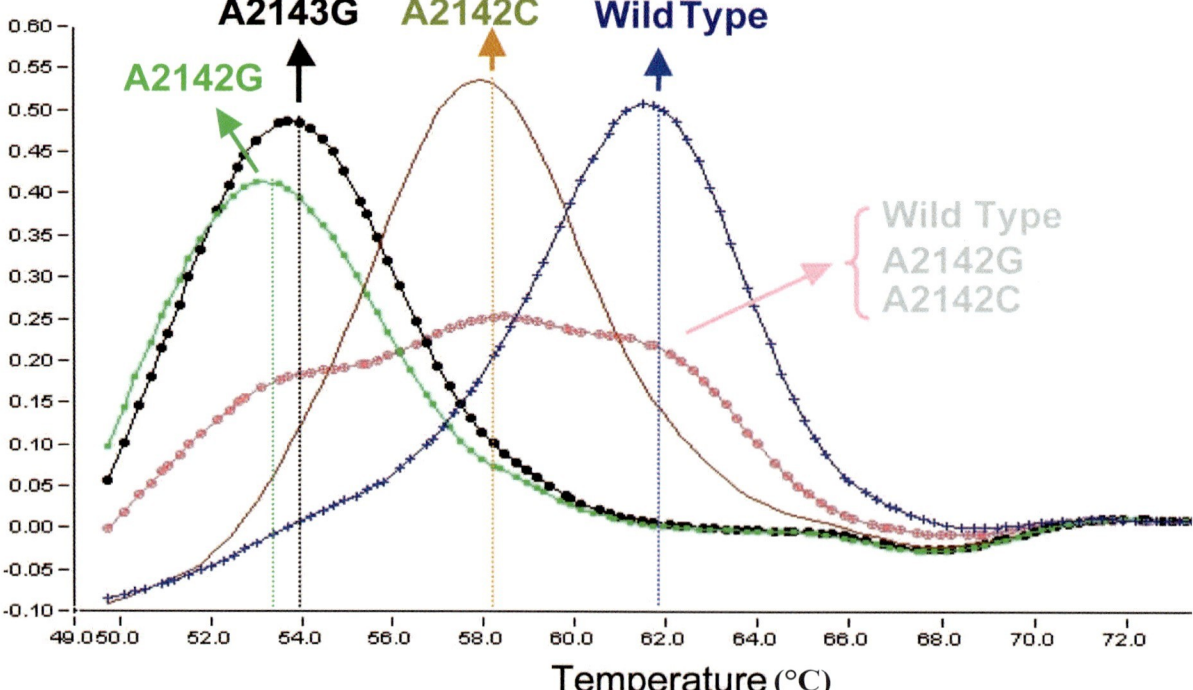

Fig. 6. Detection of clarithromycin resistance in *H. pylori* by real-time PCR using a biprobe according to the FRET-MCA principle. Melting curve of the amplicons allowing to detect the mutations.

sies. FRET (Fluorescence Resonance Energy Transfer) was then used with a dual probe comprised of a detection probe marked in 5' with the LC-Red 640 dye, which hybridizes at the mutation site and a second attachment probe marked in 3' by fluorescein that hybridizes 3 to 5 bases upstream from the previous one. When the attachment probe receives an excitation, an energy transfer occurs to the detection probe because of its proximity and a light signal is emitted. This allows to follow the synthesis of the amplicon in real time on an apparatus such as the LightCycler™. This first step therefore enables detection of *H. pylori* directly on a gastric biopsy. After amplification, a melting curve of the amplicons is performed and the melting points obtained differ for the wild strain and the mutants (Fig. 6) (24). This is a significant improvement for diagnosis because the result can be obtained in two hours and the contaminations are limited because the reaction occurs in the same tube that is never open.

A limitation of this method for *H. pylori* is the fact that there are few 23S rRNA sequences of closely related species available in databases. In our experience, *Helicobacter heilmannii* can also give a positive result.

A variant of this method developed by Lascols *et al.* (12) is to perform the procedure in two steps using different probes for detection of the bacteria and of resistance.

Molecular methods, such as PCR-RFLP and especially real-time PCR, have allowed direct detection of *H. pylori* and a search for clarithromycin resistance mutations in stool specimens.

The first work was published in 2004 by Schabereiter-Gurtner *et al.* using real-time PCR targeting the 23S rRNA gene and a melting curve for amplicons. Susceptibility and specificity of 98% were obtained for detection of *H. pylori* and only one out of 9 cases of resistance was not detected (25). This test has since been marketed (ClariRes® assay, Ingenetix, Vienna, Austria). A Japanese team used nested PCR to amplify the gene for 23S rRNA of *H. pylori* in the feces, and this was then followed by amplicon restriction or by sequencing. A key issue with stool specimens is DNA extraction because of the presence of Taq polymerase inhibitors.

• DNA test strip - A new molecular test has been recently developed which allows detection of *H. pylori* and of the mutations associated with clarithromycin and fluoroquinolone resistance. The protocol (Genotype HelicoDR®, Hain Life Sciences, Nehren, Germany) includes 2 steps: first DNA amplification using multiplex PCR and second hybridization with biotin-labeled specific oligonucleotides immobilized on a strip visualized by a streptavidin/alkaline phosphatase-mediated staining reaction.

This test can be used on *H. pylori* strains or directly on biopsy specimens. Susceptibility and specificity are 96% and 100% for clarithromycin and 89% and 98.5% for fluoroquinolones, respectively.

• Fluorescence *In Situ* Hybridization (FISH) - The FISH method offers the possibility of detecting clarithromycin resistance without performing PCR. In practice, two probes are used. The first one targets 16S rRNA and is labeled with fluorochrome Cy3 (red) that allows detection of *H. pylori*. The second targets the mutated 23S rRNA and is labeled with fluorescein (green). Both probes are used simultaneously. Therefore, susceptible *H. pylori* appear red and resistant strains yellow because of superimposition of green and red as seen by microscopic observation (28). This method has yielded good results, although sometimes the slides are difficult to interpret. It can be used in pathology laboratories on fixed specimens who are embedded in paraffin.

Molecular methods detect more often mutations associated with clarithromycin resistance than phenotypic methods detect resistant strains. In fact, there are generally mixtures of wild and mutant phenotypes in various proportions. No correlation studies of these discordant results in relation to the eradication of *H. pylori* using standard triple agent therapy have yet been done that would allow to conclude which of these methods is the most reliable.

Fluoroquinolones

FRET-MCA was also used to detect resistance of *H. pylori* to fluoroquinolones. However, not all mutations that can be present and detected lead to resistance. Nonetheless, with two biprobes it is possible to detect important mutations at triplets *aa87* and *aa91*. The technique called allele-specific PCR was also used. The hybridization strip (GenoType HelicoDR®) described above has the advantage of detecting mutations associated with resistance to fluoroquinolones with good susceptibility and specificity.

Tetracyclines

A PCR-RFLP was developed with primers amplifying a portion of 16S rDNA and the amplicon is then subjected to restriction enzyme *Hinf1*.

Strains with the triple mutation associated with a high level of resistance exhibit three bands, whereas there are only two bands in susceptible strains or in strains with low level resistance.

In 2005, two real-time PCR using the LightCycler™ to detect these mutations were published simultaneously. However, in one of these studies the mutations were identified in only 10 out of 18 strains that had decreased susceptibility.

Metronidazole

The excessive number of mutations in the *rdxA* gene, some of which are not associated with resistance, did not allow the development of molecular methods to detect resistance. A novel approach is detection of the RdxA protein by immunoblotting using an anti-RdxA rabbit serum (13). It is thus possible to visualize an immunoreactive band of 24 kDa corresponding to RdxA in susceptible strains which does not appear in resistant strains. However, there could be 10% false positives. This promising technique needs to be confirmed by determination of its predictive value for successful treatment regimens that include metronidazole.

Other antibiotics

No molecular method has yet been proposed to detect strains resistant to rifabutin probably because of the rarity of resistance. A deeper understanding of *rpoB* gene mutations may allow development of a molecular test in the future.

CONCLUSION

Although the study of susceptibility of *H. pylori* to antibiotics is difficult, as is the case for many slow-growing bacteria, it is nonetheless essential for patient care. Clarithromycin is the best antibiotic when the strain is susceptible but, since the rate of resistance can be high, this calls into question its use without prior study of susceptibility. The development of molecular methods, including real-time PCR, is an answer to this challenge, especially since it can be carried out on stool specimens which makes it a non-invasive test. Additional molecular methods will have to be developed for other antibiotics to which *H. pylori* can become resistant.

REFERENCES

(1) **Broutet, N., A. Marais, H. Lamouliatte, A. de Mascarel, R. Samoyeau, R. Salamon, and F. Mégraud**. 2001. *cagA* status and eradication treatment outcome of anti-*Helicobacter pylori* triple therapies in non-ulcer dyspeptic patients. J. Clin. Microbiol. **39**:1319-1322.

(2) **Broutet, N., S. Tchamgoué, E. Pereira, H. Lamouliatte, R. Salamon, and F. Mégraud**. 2003. Risk factors for failure of *Helicobacter pylori* therapy - results of an individual data analysis of 2751 patients. Aliment. Pharmacol. & Ther. **17**:99-109.

(3) **Cederbrant, G., G. Kahlmeter, and A. Ljungh**. 1992. Proposed mechanism for metronidazole resistance in *Helicobacter pylori*. J. Antimicrob. Chemother. **29**:115-120.

(4) **Fischbach, L., and E. L. Evans**. 2007. Meta-analysis: the effect of antibiotic resistance status on the efficacy of triple and quadruple first-line therapies for *Helicobacter pylori*. Aliment Pharmacol. Ther. **26**:343-57.

(5) **Glupczynski, Y., N. Broutet, A. Cantagrel, L. P. Andersen, T. Alarcon, M. Lopez-Brea, and F. Mégraud**. 2002. Comparison of the E-test® and agar dilution method for antimicrobial susceptibility testing of *Helicobacter pylori*. Eur. J. Clin. Microbiol. Infect. Dis. **21**:549-552.

(6) **Glupczynski, Y., F. Mégraud, M. Lopez-Brea, and L. Andersen**. 2001. European multicentre survey of *in vitro* antimicrobial resistance in *Helicobacter pylori*. Eur. J. Clin. Microbiol. Infect. Dis. **20**:820-823.

(7) **Goodwin, A., D. Kersulyte, G. Sisson, S. J. O. Veldhuyzen van Zanten, D. E. Berg, and P. S. Hoffman**. 1998. Metronidazole resistance in *Helicobacter pylori* is due to null mutations in a gene (*rdxA*) that encodes an oxygen-insensitive NADPH nitroreductase. Mol. Microbiol. **28**:383-393.

(8) **Grignon, B., J. Tankovic, F. Mégraud, Y. Glupczynski, M. O. Husson, M. C. Conroy, L. P. Emond, J. Loulergue, J. Raymond, and J. L. Fauchère**. 2002. Validation of diffusion methods for macrolide susceptibility testing of *Helicobacter pylori*. Microbial. Drug. Resistance. **8**:61-66.

(9) **International Agency for Research on Cancer**. 1994. IARC monographs on the evaluation of carcinogenic risks to humans, Vol. 61, Schistosomes, liver flukes and *Helicobacter pylori*. Lyon; 1994.

(10) **Kobayashi, I., T. Saika, H. Muraoka, K. Murakami, and T. Fujioka**. 2006. *Helicobacter pylori* isolated from patients who later failed *H. pylori* eradication triple therapy readily develop resistance to clarithromycin. J. Med. Microbiol. **55**:737-740.

(11) **Koletzko, S., F. Richy, F., P. Bontems, J. Crone, N. Kalach, M.L. Monteiro, F. Gottrand, D. Celinska-Cedro, E. Roma-Giannikou, G. Orderda, S. Kolacek, P. Urruzuno, M. J. Martínez-Gómez, T. Casswall, M. Ashorn, H. Bodanszky, and F. Mégraud**. 2006. Prospective multicentre study on antibiotic resistance of *Helicobacter pylori* strains obtained from children living in Europe. Gut **55**:1711-1716.

(12) **Lascols, C., D. Lamarque, J. M. Costa, C. Copie-Bergman, J. M. Le Glaunec, L. Deforges, C. J. Soussy, J. C. Petit, J. C. Delchier, and J. Tankovic**. 2003. Fast and accurate quantitative detection of *Helicobacter pylori* and identification of clarithromycin resistance mutations in *H. pylori* isolates

from gastric biopsy specimens by real-time PCR. J. Clin. Microbiol. **41**:4573-4577.

(13) **Latham, S. R., A. Labigne, and P. J. Jenks.** 2002. Production of the RdxA protein in metronidazole-susceptible and -resistant isolates of *Helicobacter pylori* cultured from treated mice. J. Antimicrob. Chemother. **49**:675-678.

(14) **Malfertheiner, P., F. Mégraud, C. O'Morain, F. Bazzoli, E. El-Omar, D. Graham, R. Hunt, T. Rokkas, N. Vakil, and E. J. Kuipers.** 2007. Current concepts in the management of *Helicobacter pylori* infection. The Maastricht-III Consensus Report. Gut **56**:772-781

(15) **Marshall, B. J., and J. R. Warren.** 1983. Unidentified curved bacilli on gastric epithelium in active chronic gastritis. Lancet **i**, 1273-1275.

(16) **Mégraud, F.** 2004. *Helicobacter pylori* antibiotic resistance. Prevalence, importance, and advances in testing. Gut **53**:1374-1384.

(17) **Mégraud, F., and H. Lamouliatte.** 1992. *Helicobacter pylori* and duodenal ulcer. Evidence suggesting causation. Dig. Dis. Sci. **37**:769-772.

(18) **Mégraud, F., N. Lehn, T. Lind, E. Bayerdorffer, C. O'Morain, R. Spiller, P. Unge, S. V. Van Zanten, M. Wrangstadh, and C. F. Burman.** 1999. Antimicrobial susceptibility testing of *Helicobacter pylori* in a large multicenter trial: the MACH 2 study. J. Antimicrob. Chemother. **43**:2747-2752.

(19) **Mégraud, F., P. Trimoulet, H. Lamouliatte, and L. Boyanova.** 1991. Bactericidal effect of amoxicillin on *Helicobacter pylori* in an *in vitro* model using epithelial cells. J. Antimicrob. Chemother. **35**:869-872.

(20) **Ménard, A., A. Santos, F. Mégraud, and M. Oleastro.** 2002. PCR-restriction fragment length polymorphism can also detect point mutation $A_{2142}C$ in the 23S rRNA gene, associated with *Helicobacter pylori* resistance to clarithromycin. Antimicrob. Agents Chemother. **46**: 1156-1157.

(21) **Mendz, G. L., and F. Mégraud.** 2002. Is the molecular basis of metronidazole resistance in microaerophilic organisms understood? Trends Microbiol. **10**:370-375.

(22) **National Committee for Clinical Laboratory Standards.** 1999. Performance Standards for Antimicrobial Susceptibility testing. VIth informational supplement M100 S9. 19,1. National Committee for Clinical Laboratory Standards, Villanova, PA.

(23) **Occhialini, A., M. Urdaci, F. Doucet-Populaire, C.M. Bébéar, H. Lamouliatte, and F. Mégraud.** 1997. Macrolide resistance in *Helicobacter pylori*: rapid detection of point mutations and assays of macrolide binding to ribosomes. Antimicrob. Agents Chemother. **41**: 2724-2728.

(24) **Oleastro, M., A. Ménard, A. Santos, H. Lamouliatte, L. Monteiro, C. Barthélémy, and F. Mégraud.** 2003. Real-time PCR assay for rapid and accurate detection of point mutations conferring resistance to clarithromycin in *Helicobacter pylori*. J. Clin. Microbiol. **41**:397-402.

(25) **Schabereiter-Gurtner, C., A. M. Hirschl, B. Dragosics, P. Hufnagl, S. Puz, Z. Kovach, M. Rotter, and A. Makristathis.** 2004. Novel real-time PCR assay for detection of *Helicobacter pylori* infection and simultaneous clarithromycin susceptibility testing of stool and biopsy specimens. J. Clin. Microbiol. **42**:4512-4518.

(26) **Storskrubb, T., P. Aro, J. Ronkainen, K. Wreiber, H. Nyhlin, E. Bolling-Sternevaid, N. J. Talley, L. Engstrand, and L. Agréus.** 2006. Antimicrobial susceptibility of *Helicobacter pylori* strains in a random adult Swedish population. Helicobacter **11**:224-30.

(27) **Tankovic, J., C. Lascols, Q. Sculo, J. C. Petit, and C. J. Soussy.** 2003. Single and double mutations in *gyrA* but not in *gyrB* are associated with low- and high-level fluoroquinolone resistance in *Helicobacter pylori*. Antimicrob. Agents Chemother. **47**:3942-3944.

(28) **Trebesius, K., K. Panthel, S. Strobel, K. Vogt, G. Faller, T. Kirchner, M. Kist, J. Heeseman, and R. Haas.** 2000. Rapid and specific detection of *Helicobacter pylori* macrolide resistance in gastric tissue by fluorescent *in situ* hybridisation. Gut **46**:608-614.

(29) **Tseng, Y. S., D.C. Wu, C. Y. Chang, C.H. Kuo, Y. C. Yang, C. M. Jan, Y. C. Su, F. C. Kuo, and L. L. Chang.** 2009. Amoxicillin resistance with beta-lactamase production in *Helicobacter pylori*. Eur. J. Clin. Invest. **39**:807-812.

(30) **Versalovic, J., D. Shortridge, K. Kliber, V. Griffy, J. Beyer, R. K. Flamm, S. K. Tanaka, D. Y. Graham, and M. F. Go.** 1996. Mutations in 23S rRNA are associated with clarithromycin resistance in *Helicobacter pylori*. Antimicrob. Agents Chemother. **40**:477-480.

(31) **Wueppenhorst, N., H. P. Stueger, M. Kist, and E. Glocker.** 2009. Identification and molecular characterization of triple and quadruple-resistant *Helicobacter pylori* clinical isolates in Germany. J Antimicrob Chemother. **63**:648-653.

Chapter 38. *CAMPYLOBACTER*

Patrick F. McDERMOTT

INTRODUCTION

Campylobacter is a Gram-negative, spiral, flagellated microaerophilic bacterium that causes diseases of the gastrointestinal tract. The role of this genus in infectious disease was not established until the 1970s, when improvements in culture methods permitted systematic study of *Campylobacter* in diarrheal disease (109). Today, it is recognized as one of the leading bacterial causes of foodborne gastroenteritis worldwide, causing 31% of laboratory-confirmed cases in the U.S.A in 2008 (15). Thermophilic *Campylobacter jejuni* and *C. coli* are the most commonly isolated species in human infections, accounting for about 90% and 9% of cases, respectively (13). *C. concisus* and *C. upsaliensis* have also been linked to diarrheal disease.

Campylobacteriosis is usually a self-limiting diarrheal disease. In immunocompromised hosts, especially those with humoral deficiency, severe, prolonged, or relapsing disease occurs, with extraintestinal infections such as bacteremia, osteomyelitis, and arthritis (63). In these cases, antimicrobial therapy may be necessary. There is no consensus on the optimal antibiotic regimen in *Campylobacter*. Most treatment recommendations are based on *in vitro* susceptibility data, anecdotal evidence, and case reports. Treatment with erythromycin may be effective early in the course of infection (132) and is currently considered the drug of choice for treating culture-confirmed cases (4). Treatment with a fluoroquinolone is often given empirically and is the treatment of choice for traveler's diarrhea (45). In some regions, tetracycline or doxycycline has been used for intestinal illness. In bacteraemic infections, aminoglycosides in conjunction with other parenteral drugs have been used successfully (89). Gentamicin, meropenem, clindamycin, telithromycin, and azithromycin all show potent *in vitro* activity and may prove valuable alternative treatments. Use of third-generation cephalosporins to treat bacteremia due to species other than *C. fetus* is not recommended (93).

Campylobacter gastroenteritis is difficult to distinguish clinically from gastroenteritis caused by other pathogens such as *Salmonella* and *Shigella*. It typically presents as diarrhea (with or without blood) with severe abdominal pain and fever. Headache, myalgia, and nausea are also common symptoms. Depending on host factors, inoculum size, and strain virulence, symptoms follow one to seven days after ingesting the organism. Symptoms usually resolve within three to seven days, and primary treatment consists of fluid and electrolyte replacement. Extra-intestinal infections are rare and include bacteremia, peritonitis, cholecystitis, pancreatitis, and hepatitis (110). *Campylobacter* is also important as the most common antecedent microbial infection of Guillain–Barré syndrome (82), preceeding 20 to 50% of Guillain–Barré cases (55). Other sequelae include irritable bowel syndrome and reactive arthritis.

Campylobacter are enteric commensals in several animal hosts, which include various avian and mammalian species. Most *Campylobacter* infections are sporadic, resulting mostly from the consumption of contaminated meats. Among food animals, *C. jejuni* is most often isolated from chickens and cattle while *C. coli* is more common in pigs and turkeys. Case control studies point to mishandled or undercooked foods of animal origin, mainly poultry, as the most important sources of infection (19, 28, 70, 115). Therefore, interventions have taken an ecological approach, focused on reducing the prevalence of *Campylobacter*-positive poultry flocks destined for human consumption, the freezing of meats derived from colonized birds, (133), and the use of carcass decontamination agents in order to reduce bacterial loads (102). Other sources include untreated surface waters, contact with companion and farm animals, and non-pasteurized milk. Large outbreaks are uncommon and have been linked to ingestion of milk and water (29) presumably contaminated from animal sources. Because food animals are considered the most important reservoirs of infection for humans, interventions to limit or reduce resistance in *Campylobacter* spp. have focused largely on the use of antimicrobial agents in food animals, although the human use of antibiotics can be considered to play a significant role.

METHODS

Agar diffusion

For years, a variety of laboratory methods have been used to measure the *in vitro* susceptibility of *Campylobacter* to antimicrobial agents. Disk diffusion is an attractive method because of its flexibility, convenience, and low cost. However, attempts to standardize disk diffusion in a multi-laboratory validation protocol showed a lack of intra- and inter-laboratory reproducibility, which was greater for certain antimicrobial agents (McDermott, unpublished observation). This problem is exacerbated by variations in zone sizes according to medium manufacturer. These confounding elements have prevented the establishment of quality control (QC) ranges for testing *Campylobacter* by disk diffusion to date. Without such controls in place, disk diffusion should not be relied on for susceptibility testing of *Campylobacter* (127).

A variation on disk diffusion is the use of specific disks to screen clinical strains for resistance. This approach uses the lack of a zone of inhibition as an indicator of resistance, making it cost-effective and suitable to clinical situations. This method works very well to predict resistant to ciprofloxacin and erythromycin (17, 80) using 5 µg and 15 µg disk potencies, respectively; but has not been validated with other disks. Another widely used method is the E-test® (34, 90). This technique is convenient and has the advantage of providing MIC values over a wide range (15 $\log_2$ dilutions). Using incubation at 36°C, it has been observed that, for many agents, the E-test® endpoints fall one or more dilutions above or below those observed using agar dilution (34, 125). The two methods compare favorably for some drugs, with a reported overall agreement between E-test® and agar dilution ranging from 62% (34) to 83% (51). For ciprofloxacin, the E-test® compares favorably with the reference method for predicting resistance (34).

Broth microdilution

Following the standardization of agar dilution (77) a broth microdilution susceptibility testing method for *Campylobacter* was developed that established QC ranges for fourteen antimicrobial agents (79). The method requires testing in Mueller-Hinton broth supplemented with 2-5 % lysed horse blood and incubation in a humid atmosphere of 10% CO_2 and 5% O_2. QC ranges are established for testing at both 36-37°C for 48 h or 42°C for 24 h, the latter applying only to thermophilic species (77). It is important that testing be done using a well controlled gas mixture (plastic bags are not acceptable) and constant temperature, since not all isolates will grow at incubation temperatures of 35°C or 43°C, and not all commercially available gas-generating systems produce consistent results (79). In the U.S. National Antimicrobial Resistance Monitoring System, this method has been in place since 2005 for monitoring susceptibility trends in *Campylobacter*.

Clinical breakpoints

Currently, there are no validated breakpoints for any antimicrobial agent for *Campylobacter*. Establishing interpretive criteria for laboratory tests requires data on population MIC distributions, information on the pharmacokinetic/pharmacodynamic properties at the site of infection, and most importantly clinical outcome studies from drug efficacy trials. Because controlled clinical studies are few, breakpoints used at different institutions often vary considerably, thereby complicating the comparison of resistance rates. Standards setting organizations and best practices organizations must rely mainly on population MIC distributions (epidemiological cut-off values) in order to guide therapy and report resistance trends.

The Clinical and Laboratory Standards Institute (CLSI, June, 2006) used population MIC distributions to set tentative *Campylobacter* MIC breakpoints for resistance to ciprofloxacin (MIC ≥ 4 µg/ml), erythromycin (MIC ≥ 32 µg/ml), doxycycline (MIC ≥ 8 µg/ml), and tetracycline (MIC ≥ 16 µg/ml) (17). The CLSI approach set cut-off values based chiefly on the MIC distributions of resistant populations with a view toward guiding therapy. These values are highly correlated with the presence of know resistance determinants.

The European Committee on Antimicrobial Susceptibility Testing (EUCAST) sets cut-off values based on the MIC distributions of susceptible populations, with a view toward harmonized surveillance reporting of non-wild type organisms (57). This approach identifies strains results in the grouping of intermediate and resistant populations. Both approaches identify strains with acquired resistance determinants and permit a direct comparison of testing results such that local interpretive criteria can be applied. Both methodologies, however, should be considered with caution as guidelines to anti-infective therapy until supporting clinical outcome data are available.

Clinical significance of resistance

There is conflicting evidence on whether antimicrobial resistance *per se* presents a greater burden of illness in patients with *Campylobacter* infections. Smith *et al.* (112) compared cases of campylobacteriosis from 1992-1998 and calculated that, among subjects treated with a quinolone, the median duration of diarrhea was seven days if the causative strain was susceptible *vs.* 10 days if it was resistant. Similarly, in a Danish study of macrolide and quinolone resistant *C. jejuni* and *C. coli* infections, Engberg *et al.* (24) showed a longer duration of illness for patients with a quinolone-resistant *C. jejuni* infection (median 13.2 days) compared to patients infected with a susceptible strain (median 10.3, p = 0.001). Based on the analysis of 3471 patients with *Campylobacter* infections, a quinolone-resistant strain was associated with a 6-fold increased risk of an adverse event within 30 days of infection compared with infections cause by susceptible strains (50). Infection with erythromycin-resistant strains was associated with a > 5-fold risk of an adverse event within 90 days of the date of illness (50). Comparing infections caused by quinolone-resistant and -susceptible strains, a Centers for Disease Control (CDC) study estimated a two-day increase in duration of diarrhea caused by resistant strains (9 *vs.* 7 days) (84). This difference was greater among subjects who did not take antidiarrheal medications or antimicrobial agents (12 vs. 6 days).

A study of domestically acquired campylobacteriosis cases in England and Wales compared infection by ciprofloxacin-resistant and -susceptible strains. This analysis found no differences between persons infected with ciprofloxacin-resistant and pansusceptible strains with regard to average length of illness or hospitalization (12). Subsequently, Wassenarr *et al.* (130) undertook a re-analysis of the reported data on risks attributed to ciprofloxacin-resistant *Campylobacter* infections and concluded that there are no significant differences in duration of disease between susceptible and resistant infections. Moreover, a recent Finnish study examining the impact of fluoroquinolone resistance on disease outcome in 192 cases concluded that ciprofloxacin-susceptible *Campylobacter* isolates tended to result more frequently in bloody diarrhea and hospitalization when compared with infections caused by resistant strains (27).

MECHANISMS OF RESISTANCE

The known genetic elements underlying *Campylobacter* resistance include the common chromosomal and plasmid-borne mechanisms present in other bacteria, namely, target modification, structural gene mutation, enzymatic inactivation, and energy-dependent drug efflux. An overview of resistance for the major antimicrobial drug classes is presented below.

Macrolides

Erythromycin has long been considered as a primary treatment for laboratory-confirmed cases of *Campylobacter* infections. Macrolides are bacteriostatic agents that function by binding to the 50S subunit of the bacterial ribosome and obstructing peptide chain elongation (131). Resistance is stably low in *C. jejuni* from the U.S. (14), Canada (43), Japan (52), Denmark (111), and other countries. Higher rates have been reported in parts of Europe (101) and Thailand (107). Resistance to macrolides (and other antimicrobials) is typically higher in *C. coli*, where resistance to erythromycin resistance ranges from 4-6% in the U.S. (13) to 29.4% in Germany (71) and up to 50% among pediatric isolates in Singapore (40). Among strains isolated from animals, resistance is generally higher in isolates from swine and poultry production environments, (1) where macrolides are used routinely.

As in other bacteria, macrolide resistance in *C. jejuni* and *C. coli* is due to target mutations and efflux. The only example of an extrachromosomal macrolide resistance determinant in *Campylobacter* is a plasmid-encoded rRNA methylase (*erm*), which has been found only in *C. rectus* to date (104). There is no evidence that *Campylobacter* produce drug modifying enzymes.

Target-site mutations occur in two positions of domain V (peptidyl transferase region) of the 23S rRNA. *Campylobacter* contains three copies of the rRNA gene. At least two copies must be mutated to cause resistance (36, 62), but it is usually mutated in all three copies (36) that can confer high MICs (> 128 µg/ml). *In vitro* transformation experiments demonstrated that these mutations are readily transferred and stably incorporated into the chromosomes of susceptible *C. jejuni* and *C. coli* (36, 58).

Ribosomal gene mutations are present only in isolates with erythromycin MICs ≥ 32 µg/ml, (62,96) supporting the use of 32 µg/ml as a breakpoint denoting acquired erythromycin resistance.

Nucleotide changes at positions A2074 and A2075 are most common, corresponding in *E. coli* to positions 2058 and 2059 (23). An $A_{2075}G$ transition is the most frequent mutation observed in clinical strains, although A-T and A-C mutations also occur (36, 85, 86, 124). Mutation in ribosomal proteins L4 and L22 have also been reported to contribute to macrolide resistance in *Campylobacter* (10).

Ribosomal mutations in *Campylobacter* can confer cross-resistance to tylosin, azithromycin, clarithromycin, and clindamycin to varying degrees. Erythromycin MICs are identical to those of clarithromycin, therefore, erythromycin can be used as a surrogate for this compound. Ribosomal mutations imparting erythromycin resistance also impact susceptibility to tylosin and azithromycin, but the MICs of those latter drugs are not equivalent to those of erythromycin (11, 62). Cross-resistance between erythromycin and clindamycin also has been observed (26).

The role of efflux in both baseline erythromycin susceptibility levels and in elevated MICs conferring clinical resistance has been described in several studies. Multidrug efflux in *C. jejuni* was first described by Charvalos *et al*. (16) using mutants selected *in vitro* with pefloxacin and cefotaxime. The MDR phenotype includes macrolides along with ß-lactams, quinolones, chloramphenicol, and tetracycline but the underlying genetic mechanisms were not characterized.

Sequence analysis implies the presence of at least ten efflux systems in *Campylobacter* (35). Studies by Lin *et al*. (69) and Pumbwe *et al*. (99) identified an efflux system encoded by the *cmeABC* locus. CmeB extrudes a variety of structurally unrelated antimicrobials, including macrolides, and appears to be nearly ubiquitous in the genus (18, 31) Activity of CmeB is down-regulated by CmeR (68), a repressor protein of the TetR family of regulatory proteins (105). Inhibition of *cme* expression yielded a 4- to 16-fold reduction in erythromycin MICs in wild-type susceptible strains (69, 100) and also reduced the selection of erythromycin-resistant mutants *in vitro* (11). Overexpression of *cmeB* also confers resistance to ampicillin, chloramphenicol, and tetracycline. Mameli *et al*. have described a second macrolide efflux pump (74) whose inactivation increased erythromycin susceptibility to wild-type levels in intermediately-susceptible strains, and to a lesser degree in resistant strains, and it rendered a wild-type isolate hyper-susceptible (73).

Fluoroquinolones

As in other genera, resistance to quinolones in *Campylobacter* occurs by target mutation (*gyrA*), energy-dependent efflux (*cmeABC*), and decreased cell permeability (*porA*). A hyper-mutable state (mediated by the *mfd* locus) (48) also influences the emergence of fluoroquinolone resistance in *Campylobacter*, as occurs in other bacteria. Plasmid-mediated target protection or drug modification mechanisms of quinolone resistance have been described in various enteric organisms that are mediated by the *qnr* genes and variant *aac* genes, respectively. Homologues of the plasmid-borne genes have not yet been detected in quinolone-resistant *Campylobacter*.

In regard to antibiotic resistance in *Campylobacter*, increasing resistance to fluoroquinolones has caused the greatest concern. Fluoroquinolone-resistant *Campylobacter* has emerged in many geographic regions over the past two decades (8, 14, 22, 23, 46, 53, 71, 76). The foodborne zoonotic nature of most infections has focused on the antimicrobial selection pressures in animal production environments as the primary means of limiting the development of resistance. Fluoroquinolone resistance develops rapidly in treated broilers (72, 78, 126), appearing within 24h in animals treated with enrofloxacin (78). It is commonly present in retail poultry products and animals at slaughter (25), highlighting the need for interventions in food production and processing settings.

Ciprofloxacin resistance in *Campylobacter* results from mutation in *gyrA* along with efflux mediated by the CmeABC pump (35, 72). Unlike other enterics such as *E. coli* and *Salmonella*, acquired fluoroquinolone resistance in *Campylobacter* does not require multiple stepwise mutations in *gyrA*. A single point mutation in *gyrA* confers high level ciprofloxacin MICs (≥ 32 µg/ml), occurring spontaneously at rates ranging from 10^{-3} to 10^{-9} (49, 136). The most common substitution is $Thr_{86}Ile$ (3, 7, 47, 83, 128). Mutations at Asp90 and Ala70 (72, 128) impart intermediate levels of resistance (MICs 1-4 µg/ml). The small proportion of isolates exhibiting resistance to nalidixic acid but not to ciprofloxacin, show a Thr_{86} substitution by Ala rather than by Ile in *gyrA* (56). No changes in GyrB have been associated with resistance, and *C. jejuni* lacks the *parC-parE* genes encoding topoisomerase IV (95). The requirement of only a single base change for high-level ciprofloxacin MICs is an important feature of *Campylobacter*. Recent work by Han *et al.* (48) showed that this process in *C. jejuni* is potentiated by induction of the *mfd* locus in an adaptive response to ciprofloxacin exposure. Mdf expression increased the fluoroquinolone resistance mutation rate by about 10-fold (48). The sufficiency of a single mutation and the hyper-mutable state of *C. jejuni* under selection pressure, help explain the rapid evolution of ciprofloxacin resistance in *Campylobacter* from treated animals and humans (134), as well as the widespread occurrence of resistant strains in retail raw meats (26) and human clinical isolates (14).

Similar to what is observed in resistance to macrolides, the CmeB multidrug efflux pump contributes to baseline susceptibility and acquired fluoroquinolone resistance in *Campylobacter* (35, 69, 72, 99, 136). In susceptible strains, deletion of *cme* decreased ciprofloxacin MICs by 8-fold (69). In resistant strains containing *gyrA* mutations, *cme* inactivation reduced ciprofloxacin MICs near to that of wild-type isolates (72). In addition, overexpression of *cmeABC* impaired ciprofloxacin intracellular accumulation and increased MICs in strains carrying *gyrA* mutations. These findings show that *cmeB* functions cooperatively in isolates with target-site mutations to acquire and maintain fluoroquinolone resistance.

Aminoglycosides

Aminoglycosides, particularly in combination with other antibiotics, are effective in treating severe cases of campylobacteriosis, particularly bacteremia in compromised patients where fluoroquinolones and macrolides may not succeed (122). Case reports show that oral kanamycin plus intravenous antibiotics proved effective in clearing intestinal infections from which recurrent bacteremia can be seeded in immune deficient patients (89). Resistance to aminoglycosides is not common in *Campylobacter*, accounting for < 1% of clinical isolates in the U.S., for example (14).

The genetic determinants that cause aminoglycoside resistance are well characterized in several bacteria. Resistance is mediated mainly by three types of transferases that inactivate aminoglycosides by chemical modification. These enzymes are classified according to the type of reaction they mediate (108): aminoglycoside phosphotransferase (APH), aminoglycoside nulceotidyltransferase/adenylyltransferase (AAD/ANT), and aminoglycoside acetyltransferases (AAC). While all three mechanisms have been detected in *Campylobacter*, aminoglycoside resistance is due mainly to the APH(3') class of phosphorylases, belonging to subclasses I, III, IV, and VII, which impart resistance to at least kanamycin and neomycin (39, 64, 118-121).

Sequence analysis of the type I enzymes point to an origin in *E. coli* (91) while the type III enzymes appear to have been acquired from *Enterococcus* (64), perhaps via a *Helicobacter* intermediate (39, 92). An APH(3')-IV enzyme has been identified in an isolate of *C. coli* (103). The APH(3')-VII phosphotransferase class, first described by Tenover *et al.*, was associated with very high kanamycin MICs (5,000 µg/mL) but did not confer gentamicin resistance (121). The G+C content of the coding sequence suggested evolution of this allele within the genus.

Adenylyltransferases (nucleotidyltransferases) are also associated with aminoglycoside resistance in *Campylobacter* and may be present in strains also carrying APH genes (91, 97). Enzymes belonging to ANT(3')-Ia and ANT(6')-Ia subclasses encode streptomycin and/or spectinomycin resistance (97, 108). O'Halloran *et al.* described a collection of *Campylobacter* strains in which 16.4% were found to carry an *ant(3')-Ia* gene cassette within a class I integron (88). Class I integrons very often serve as vehicles for these genes in *Salmonella* and *E. coli*. The sequences of the *ant(3')-Ia* cassettes are identical to those found in a *Salmonella* serovar Hadar integron and an *E. coli* plasmid (88). The *Campylobacter ant(6)-Ia* gene, conferring streptomycin resistance, is closely related to that found in *Staphylococcus* (97, 108). An integron in *Campylobacter* carrying and AAC(3')-IV has been described in a poultry isolate, encoding resistance to tobramycin and gentamicin (66). Resistance to the aminoglycoside streptothricin has been linked to the *sat4* gene product in animal and clinical isolates from Europe (54).

β-lactams

The susceptibility of *Campylobacter* to β-lactams varies due to the combination of various resistance mechanisms. While methods for *in vitro* susceptibility to β-lactams [except meropenem (77)] have not been standardized for *Campylobacter*, *C. jejuni* and *C. coli* appear to be intrinsically resistant to the penicillins and many cephalosporins (44, 61) including cefoperazone, which is used in some *Campylobacter* selective media. Intrinsic β-lactam resistance is due in part to the presence of low-affinity penicillin-binding proteins and size and charge exclusion by cell wall porins (94). Along with both poor target affinity and low uptake, β-lactamases are common. Several studies report that more than 80% of *C. jejuni* and *C. coli* produce beta-lactamases (44, 60, 116, 135). The role of these enzymes in conferring clinical resistance is not clear. In *C. jejuni*, carriage of β-lactamases renders cells less susceptible to ampicillin, amoxicillin, and ticarcillin (60). The most active β-lactams include amoxicillin/clavulanate, cefpirome, meropenem, ertapenem, and cefotaxime (44, 60, 116). Based on the genome sequence of *C. jejuni* 11168, Alfredson and Korolik cloned a β-lactamase, bla_{OXA-61}, from a clinical strain of *C. jejuni*. Recombinant plasmids encoding this enzyme conferred a ≥ 32-fold rise in the MICs of ampicillin, piperacillin, and carbenicillin but did not affect susceptibility to cefotaxime or imipenem in a susceptible recipient *C. jejuni* (2). Griggs et al. detected OXA-61 in 91% of ampicillin-resistant poultry isolates (44) and showed evidence of a second β-lactamase, CjBla2, that was not fully characterized. These findings support the potential therapeutic value of the penem class of drugs for treating severe *Campylobacter* infections (9, 81).

Tetracyclines

Tetracycline is considered a second-line treatment for *Campylobacter*. It is used more often in developing regions due to its low cost and low toxicity. Tetracycline resistance has increased in many countries, making this class of antimicrobials less useful for therapy. In Canada, tetracycline resistance increased from 7% - 9% in 1980 - 1981 (32) to 43% - 68% in 1998 – 2001, (33) with more recent resistant strains also showing even higher MIC values (41). A German study showed tetracycline resistance increasing from 16.2% to 38.5% between 1991 and 2002 (71). In Denmark, tetracycline resistance rose from approximately 8% to 16% between 1997 and 2007 (20). In the U.S. tetracycline resistance has been stably high at 38% - 48% of isolates during the same time period (14). In Norway, doxycycline resistance declined in domestically acquired cases from 9.5% in 2003 to 0% in 2006 (87). In The Netherlands, tetracycline resistance increased from 3% in 1992 to 24% in 1997 (20). In some countries, the proportion of resistant isolates is much higher (67, 106).

In general, tetracycline resistance is caused by efflux, drug modification, target (ribosome) protection, and target (16S rDNA) mutation. In *Campylobacter*, tetracycline resistance is chiefly the result of ribosomal protection mediated by the *tet*(O) gene (75) in conjunction with the multidrug pump encoded by *cmeABC* (42, 69, 99). Tet(O) confers resistance by allosterically displacing tetracycline from its primary binding site on the ribosome (114, 123). The *tet*(O) gene is widespread in *Campylobacter* worldwide and is also present in various Gram-positive species from which it is though to originate (113). Alleles of *tet*(O) in *C. jejuni* usually impart MIC levels of tetracycline ranging from 32 to 128 μg/ml, but mutations in *tet*(O) can lead to MICs as high as 512 μg/ml (41).

The *tet*(O) gene is usually carried by transmissible plasmids in *C. jejuni* (30) but may be located on the chromosome (41, 65, 98) Evidence suggests that it may be localized to the chromosome more often in *C. coli* (21, 21, 98). Horizontal spread of tetracycline resistance plasmids has been demonstrated *in vitro* (117) and in the gut of chickens (5) where *Campylobacter* is a common constituent. The sequence of two large self-transmissible tetracycline resistance plasmids, one from *C. jejuni* and one from *C. coli*, isolated on separate continents about 20 years apart was determined by Batchelor et al. (6). These plasmids showed 94.3% DNA sequence identity and are widespread in plasmid-containing tetracycline-resistant *Campylobacter*.

The function of the CmeABC multidrug efflux pump in tetracycline resistance is analogous to its role in macrolide and fluoroquinolone resistance. Inactivation of *cmeABC* increases tetracycline susceptibility in *tet*(O)-positive and -negative strains (42, 69, 99).

Other Resistances

Most *Campylobacter* are resistant to β-lactams with over 80% of *C. jejuni* producing β-lactamases (116). *C. jejuni* are resistant to cefamandole, cefoxitin, and cefoperazone. Most isolates are also resistant to cephalothin and cefazolin, and resistance is variable for cefotaxime, moxalactam, piperacillin, and ticarcillin (60). The most active β-lactams include ampicillin, amoxicillin, cefotaxime, ceftazidime, and cefpirome (116). The penems (meropenem, imipenem) show good *in vitro* activity (26, 59, 116) and have been recommended as a treatment option (9, 81).

Campylobacter are generally resistant to trimethoprim and sulfonamides, through mechanisms common to other bacteria. Trimethoprim resistance in *C. jejuni* is due to the chromosomal presence of acquired dihydrofolate reductase gene cassettes (*dfr1*, *dfr9*) (38). Sulfonamide resistance, as in other bacteria, results from mutations in dihydropteroate synthase (37). Chloramphenicol resistance is rare in *Campylobacter* and results from acetylation encoded by *cat* genes (129).

CONCLUSION

As one of the most common causes of diarrheal disease worldwide, *Campylobacter* will continue to pose a major public health and medical challenge. While most cases of campylobacteriosis resolve without antimicrobial intervention, the availability of effective drugs is necessary. Antimicrobial resistance in *Campylobacter* has reached high levels for tetracycline and ciprofloxacin, making empirical therapy problematic. Resistance in *C. jejuni*, which causes 90-99% of infections, remains low for erythromycin, chloramphenicol, gentamicin, amoxicillin/clavulanate, and meropenem in many regions where data are available. Resistance in *C. coli* is generally more common for most antimicrobial drugs. Limiting the development of resistance in *Campylobacter*, as with all zoonotic foodborne pathogens, is complicated by the need for antimicrobial agents in food animal production. It also highlights the need for public health monitoring of resistance in different environments, which is ongoing in several countries (15, 20, 25, 76, 87).

REFERENCES

(1) **Aarestrup, F. M., E. M. Nielsen, M. Madsen, and J. Engberg**. 1997. Antimicrobial susceptibility patterns of thermophilic *Campylobacter* spp. from humans, pigs, cattle, and broilers in Denmark. Antimicrob. Agents Chemother. **41**:2244-2250.

(2) **Alfredson, D. A., and V. Korolik**. 2005. Isolation and expression of a novel molecular class D beta-lactamase, OXA-61, from *Campylobacter jejuni*. Antimicrob. Agents Chemother. **49**:2515-2518.

(3) **Alonso, R., E. Mateo, C. Girbau, E. Churruca, I. Martinez, and A. Fernandez-Astorga**. 2004. PCR-restriction fragment length polymorphism assay for detection of *gyrA* mutations associated with fluoroquinolone resistance in *Campylobacter coli*. Antimicrob. Agents Chemother. **48**:4886-4888.

(4) **Anonymous**. 2003. The Sanford Guide to Antimicrobial Therapy. Antimicrobial Therapy, Inc., Hyde Park, VT.

(5) **Avrain, L., C. Vernozy-Rozand, and I. Kempf**. 2004. Evidence for natural horizontal transfer of *tet*(O) gene between *Campylobacter jejuni* strains in chickens. J Appl Microbiol **97**:134-140.

(6) **Batchelor, R. A., B. M. Pearson, L. M. Friis, P. Guerry, and J. M. Wells**. 2004. Nucleotide sequences and comparison of two large conjugative plasmids from different *Campylobacter* species. Microbiology **150**:3507-3517.

(7) **Beckmann, L., M. Muller, P. Luber, C. Schrader, E. Bartelt, and G. Klein**. 2004. Analysis of *gyrA* mutations in quinolone-resistant and -susceptible *Campylobacter jejuni* isolates from retail poultry and human clinical isolates by non-radioactive single-strand conformation polymorphism analysis and DNA sequencing. J. Appl. Microbiol. **96**:1040-1047.

(8) **Boonmar, S., Y. Morita, M. Fujita, L. Sangsuk, K. Suthivarakom, P. Padungtod, S. Maruyama, H. Kabeya, M. Kato, K. Kozawa, S. Yamamoto, and H. Kimura**. 2007. Serotypes, antimicrobial susceptibility, and *gyrA* gene mutation of *Campylobacter jejuni* isolates from humans and chickens in Thailand. Microbiol. Immunol. **51**:531-537.

(9) **Burch, K. L., K. Saeed, A. D. Sails, and P. A. Wright**. 1999. Successful treatment by meropenem of *Campylobacter jejuni* meningitis in a chronic alcoholic following neurosurgery. J. Infect. **39**:241-243.

(10) **Cagliero, C., C. Mouline, A. Cloeckaert, and S. Payot**. 2006. Synergy between efflux pump CmeABC and modifications in ribosomal proteins L4 and L22 in conferring macrolide resistance in *Campylobacter jejuni* and *Campylobacter coli*. Antimicrob. Agents Chemother. **50**:3893-3896.

(11) **Cagliero, C., C. Mouline, S. Payot, and A. Cloeckaert**. 2005. Involvement of the CmeABC efflux pump in the macrolide resistance of *Campylobacter coli*. J. Antimicrob. Chemother. **56**:948-950.

(12) **Campylobacter Sentinel Surveillance Scheme Collaborators**. 2002. Ciprofloxacin resistance in *Campylobacter jejuni*: case-case analysis as a tool for elucidating risks at home and abroad. J. Antimicrob. Chemother. **50**:561-568.

(13) **CDC**. 2006. 2003 National Antimicrobial Resistance Monitoring System (NARMS) For Enteric Bacteria. [Online.] (http://www.cdc.gov/ncidod/dbmd/narms/).

(14) **CDC**. 2009. National Antimicrobial Resistance Monitoring System (NARMS): Human Isolates Final Report, 2006. Atlanta, Ba: U.S. Department of Health and HHuman Services, CDC. [Online.] (http://www.cdc.gov/narms).

(15) **CDC**. 2009. Preliminary FoodNet Data on the incidence of infection with pathogens transmitted commonly through food—10 States, 2008. MMWR Morb Mortal Wkly Rep **58**:333-337.

(16) **Charvalos, E., Y. Tselentis, M. M. Hamzehpour, T. Kohler, and J. C. Pechere**. 1995. Evidence for an efflux pump in multidrug-resistant *Campylobacter jejuni*. Antimicrob. Agents Chemother. **39**:2019-2022.

(17) **CLSI**. 2008. Clinical and Laboratory Standards Institute (CLSI). Methods for Antimicrobial Dilution and Disk Susceptibility Testing of Infrequently-Isolated or Fastidious Bacteria; Approved Guideline. CLSI document M45-A (ISBN 1-56238-607-7). Clinical and Laboratory Standards Institute, 940 West Valley Road, Suite 1400, Wayne, Pennsylvania 19087-1898 USA, 2005.

(18) **Corcoran, D., T. Quinn, L. Cotter, F. O'Halloran, and S. Fanning**. 2005. Characterization of a *cmeABC* operon in a quinolone- resistant *Campylobacter coli* isolate of Irish origin. Microb. Drug Resist. **11**:303-308.

(19) **Danis, K., M. Di Renzi, W. O'Neill, B. Smyth, P. McKeown, B. Foley, V. Tohani, and M. Devine**. 2009. Risk factors for sporadic *Campylobacter* infec-

tion: an all-Ireland case-control study. Euro Surveill. 14.(7).
(20) **DANMAP.** 2008. DANMAP 2007 - pp. 40-41. *In*. V. F. Jensen, Use of antimicrobial agents and occurrence of antimicrobial resistance in bacteria from food animals, foods and humans in Denmark. ISSN 1600-2032,
(21) **Dasti, J. I., U. Gross, S. Pohl, R. Lugert, M. Weig, and R. Schmidt-Ott**. 2007. Role of the plasmid-encoded *tet*(O) gene in tetracycline-resistant clinical isolates of *Campylobacter jejuni* and *Campylobacter coli*. J. Med. Microbiol. **56**:833-837.
(22) **Endtz, H. P., G. J. Ruijs, B. van Klingeren, W. H. Jansen, T. van der Reyden, and R. P. Mouton**. 1991. Quinolone resistance in *Campylobacter* isolated from man and poultry following the introduction of fluoroquinolones in veterinary medicine. J. Antimicrob. Chemother. **27**:199-208.
(23) **Engberg, J., F. M. Aarestrup, D. E. Taylor, P. Gerner-Smidt, and I. Nachamkin**. 2001. Quinolone and macrolide resistance in *Campylobacter jejuni* and *C. coli*: resistance mechanisms and trends in human isolates. Emerg. Infect. Dis. **7**:24-34.
(24) **Engberg, J., J. Neimann, E. M. Nielsen, F. M. Aerestrup, and V. Fussing**. 2004. Quinolone-resistant *Campylobacter* infections: risk factors and clinical consequences. Emerg. Infect. Dis. **10**:1056-1063.
(25) **FDA**. 2009. National Antimicrobial resistance Monitoring System - Enteric Bacteria (NARMS): 2005 Executive report. Rockville, MD: U.S. Department of Health and Human Services, Food and Drug Administration. NARMS. [Online.] http://www.fda.gov/AnimalVeterinary/SafetyHealth/AntimicrobialResistance/NationalAntimicrobialResistanceMonitoringSystem/ucm093532.htm.
(26) **FDA**. 2009. National Antimicrobial Resistance Monitoring System for Enteric Bacteria (NARMS): NARMS Retail Meat Annual Report, 2007. Rockville, MD : U.S. Department of Health and Human Services, FDA, [Online] http://www.fda.gov/AnimalVeterinary/SafetyHealth/AntimicrobialResistanceMonitoringSystem/ucm16466
(27) **Feodoroff, F. B., A. R. Lauhio, S. J. Sarna, M. L. Hanninen, and H. I. Rautelin**. 2009. Severe diarrhoea caused by highly ciprofloxacin-susceptible *Campylobacter* isolates. Clin. Microbiol. Infect. **15**:188-192.
(28) **Friedman, C. R., R. M. Hoekstra, M. Samuel, R. Marcus, J. Bender, B. Shiferaw, S. Reddy, S. D. Ahuja, D. L. Helfrick, F. Hardnett, M. Carter, B. Anderson, and R. V. Tauxe**. 2004. Risk factors for sporadic *Campylobacter* infection in the United States: A case-control study in FoodNet sites. Clin. Infect. Dis. **38** Suppl 3:S285-S296.
(29) **Friedman, C. R., J. Neimann, H. C. Wegener, and R. V. Tauxe**. 2000. Epidemiology of *Campylobacter jejuni* infections in the United States and other industrialized nations, pp. 121-138. *In* I. Nachamkin, and M. J. Blaser (ed.), *Campylobacter* (2nd edition). American Society for Microbiology, Washington, DC.
(30) **Friis, L. M., C. Pin, D. E. Taylor, B. M. Pearson, and J. M. Wells**. 2007. A role for the *tet*(O) plasmid in maintaining *Campylobacter* plasticity. Plasmid **57**:18-28.
(31) **Frye, J. G., T. Jesse, F. Long, G. Rondeau, S. Porwollik, M. McClelland, C. R. Jackson, M. Englen, and P. J. Fedorka-Cray**. 2006. DNA microarray detection of antimicrobial resistance genes in diverse bacteria. Int. J. Antimicrob. Agents **27**:138-151.
(32) **Gaudreau, C., and H. Gilbert**. 1998. Antimicrobial resistance of clinical strains of *Campylobacter jejuni* subsp. *jejuni* isolated from 1985 to 1997 in Quebec, Canada. Antimicrob. Agents Chemother. **42**:2106-2108.
(33) **Gaudreau, C., and H. Gilbert**. 2003. Antimicrobial resistance of *Campylobacter jejuni* subsp. *jejuni* strains isolated from humans in 1998 to 2001 in Montreal, Canada. Antimicrob. Agents Chemother. **47**:2027-2029.
(34) **Ge, B., S. Bodeis, R. D. Walker, D. G. White, S. Zhao, P. F. McDermott, and J. Meng**. 2002. Comparison of the E-test and agar dilution for *in vitro* antimicrobial susceptibility testing of *Campylobacter*. J. Antimicrob. Chemother. **50**:487-494.
(35) **Ge, B., P. F. McDermott, D. G. White, and J. Meng**. 2005. Role of efflux pumps and topoisomerase mutations in fluoroquinolone resistance in *Campylobacter jejuni* and *Campylobacter coli*. Antimicrob. Agents Chemother. **49**:3347-3354.
(36) **Gibreel, A., V. N. Kos, M. Keelan, C. A. Trieber, S. Levesque, S. Michaud, and D. E. Taylor**. 2005. Macrolide resistance in *Campylobacter jejuni* and *Campylobacter coli*: molecular mechanism and stability of the resistance phenotype. Antimicrob. Agents Chemother. **49**:2753-2759.
(37) **Gibreel, A., and O. Skold**. 1999. Sulfonamide resistance in clinical isolates of *Campylobacter jejuni*: mutational changes in the chromosomal dihydropteroate synthase. Antimicrob. Agents Chemother. **43**:2156-2160.
(38) **Gibreel, A., and O. Skold**. 2000. An integron cassette carrying *dfr1* with 90-bp repeat sequences located on the chromosome of trimethoprim-resistant isolates of *Campylobacter jejuni*. Microb. Drug Resist. **6**:91-98.
(39) **Gibreel, A., O. Skold, and D. E. Taylor**. 2004. Characterization of plasmid-mediated *aphA-3* kanamycin resistance in *Campylobacter jejuni*. Microb. Drug Resist. **10**:98-105.
(40) **Gibreel, A. and D. E. Taylor**. 2006. Macrolide resistance in *Campylobacter jejuni* and *Campylobacter coli*. J. Antimicrob. Chemother. **58**:243-255.
(41) **Gibreel, A., D. M. Tracz, L. Nonaka, T. M. Ngo, S. R. Connell, and D. E. Taylor**. 2004. Incidence of antibiotic resistance in *Campylobacter jejuni* isolated in Alberta, Canada, from 1999 to 2002, with special reference to *tet*(O)-mediated tetracycline resistance. Antimicrob. Agents Chemother. **48**:3442-3450.
(42) **Gibreel, A., N. M. Wetsch, and D. E. Taylor**. 2007. Contribution of the CmeABC efflux pump to macrolide and tetracycline resistance in *Campylobacter jejuni*. Antimicrob. Agents Chemother. **51**:3212-3216.
(43) **Government of Canada**. 2009. Canadian Integrated Program for Antimicrobial Resistance Surveillance (CIPARS) 2006, *In* . Public Health Agency of Canada, Guelph, ON.

(44) **Griggs, D. J., L. Peake, M. M. Johnson, S. Ghori, A. Mott, and L. J. Piddock**. 2009. β-lactamase-mediated β-lactam resistance in *Campylobacter* species: prevalence of Cj0299 (*bla* OXA-61) and evidence for a novel β-lactamase in *C. jejuni*. Antimicrob. Agents Chemother. **53**:3357-3364.

(45) **Guerrant, R. L., T. Van Gilder, T. S. Steiner, N. M. Thielman, L. Slutsker, R. V. Tauxe, T. Hennessy, P. M. Griffin, H. DuPont, R. B. Sack, P. Tarr, M. Neill, I. Nachamkin, L. B. Reller, M. T. Osterholm, M. L. Bennish, and L. K. Pickering**. 2001. Practice guidelines for the management of infectious diarrhea. Clin. Infect. Dis. **32**:331-351.

(46) **Gupta, A., J. M. Nelson, T. J. Barrett, R. V. Tauxe, S. P. Rossiter, C. R. Friedman, K. W. Joyce, K. E. Smith, T. F. Jones, M. A. Hawkins, B. Shiferaw, J. L. Beebe, D. J. Vugia, T. Rabatsky-Ehr, J. A. Benson, T. P. Root, and F. J. Angulo**. 2004. Antimicrobial resistance among *Campylobacter* strains, United States, 1997-2001. Emerg. Infect. Dis. **10**:1102-1109.

(47) **Hakanen, A. J., M. Lehtopolku, A. Siitonen, P. Huovinen, and P. Kotilainen**. 2003. Multidrug resistance in *Campylobacter jejuni* strains collected from Finnish patients during 1995-2000. J. Antimicrob. Chemother. **52**:1035-1039.

(48) **Han, J., O. Sahin, Y. W. Barton, and Q. Zhang**. 2008. Key role of Mfd in the development of fluoroquinolone resistance in *Campylobacter jejuni*. PLoS Pathog. **4**:e1000083.

(49) **Hanninen, M. L., and M. Hannula**. 2007. Spontaneous mutation frequency and emergence of ciprofloxacin resistance in *Campylobacter jejuni* and *Campylobacter coli*. J. Antimicrob. Chemother. **60**:1251-1257.

(50) **Helms, M., J. Simonsen, K. E. Olsen, and K. Molbak**. 2005. Adverse health events associated with antimicrobial drug resistance in *Campylobacter* species: a registry-based cohort study. J. Infect. Dis. **191**:1050-1055.

(51) **Huang, M. B., C. N. Baker, S. Banerjee, and F. C. Tenover**. 1992. Accuracy of the E-test for determining antimicrobial susceptibilities of staphylococci, enterococci, *Campylobacter jejuni*, and gram-negative bacteria resistant to antimicrobial agents. J. Clin. Microbiol. **30**:3243-3248.

(52) **Igimi, S., Y. Okade, A. Ishiwa, M. Yamasaki, N. Morisaki, Y. Kubo, H. Asakura, and S. Yamamoto**. 2008. Antimicrobial resistance of *Campylobacter*: prevalence and trends in Japan. Food Addit. Contam. **25**:1080-1083.

(53) **Isenbarger, D. W., C. W. Hoge, A. Srijan, C. Pitarangsi, N. Vithayasai, L. Bodhidatta, K. W. Hickey, and P. D. Cam**. 2002. Comparative antibiotic resistance of diarrheal pathogens from Vietnam and Thailand, 1996-1999. Emerg. Infect. Dis. **8**:175-180.

(54) **Jacob, J., S. Evers, K. Bischoff, C. Carlier, and P. Courvalin**. 1994. Characterization of the *sat4* gene encoding a streptothricin acetyltransferase in *Campylobacter coli* BE/G4. FEMS Microbiol. Lett. **120**:13-17.

(55) **Jacobs, B. C., A. van Belkum, and H. P. Endtz**. 2008. Guillain-Barre syndrome and *Campylobacter* infection, pp. 245-261. *In* I. Nachamkin, C. M. Szymanski, and M. J. Blaser (ed.), *Campylobacter* (2nd edition). American Society for Microbiology, Washington, DC.

(56) **Jesse, T. W., M. D. Englen, L. G. Pittenger-Alley, and P. J. Fedorka-Cray**. 2006. Two distinct mutations in *gyrA* lead to ciprofloxacin and nalidixic acid resistance in *Campylobacter coli* and *Campylobacter jejuni* isolated from chickens and beef cattle. J. Appl. Microbiol. **100**:682-688.

(57) **Kahlmeter, G., and D. F. J. Brown**. 2004. Harmonization of antimicrobial breakpoints in Europe - can it be achieved? Clin. Microbiol. Newslett. **26**:187-192.

(58) **Kim, J. S., D. K. Carver, and S. Kathariou**. 2006. Natural transformation-mediated transfer of erythromycin resistance in *Campylobacter coli* strains from turkeys and swine. Appl. Environ. Microbiol. **72**:1316-1321.

(59) **Kwon, S. Y., D. H. Cho, S. Y. Lee, K. Lee, and Y. Chong**. 1994. Antimicrobial susceptibility of *Campylobacter fetus* subsp. *fetus* isolated from blood and synovial fluid. Yonsei Med. J. **35**:314-319.

(60) **Lachance, N., C. Gaudreau, F. Lamothe, and L. A. Lariviere**. 1991. Role of the β-lactamase of *Campylobacter jejuni* in resistance to β-lactam agents. Antimicrob. Agents Chemother. **35**:813-818.

(61) **Lachance, N., C. Gaudreau, F. Lamothe, and F. Turgeon**. 1993. Susceptibilities of β-lactamase-positive and -negative strains of *Campylobacter coli* to β-lactam agents. Antimicrob. Agents Chemother. **37**:1174-1176.

(62) **Ladely, S. R., R. J. Meinersmann, M. D. Englen, P. J. Fedorka-Cray, and M. A. Harrison**. 2009. 23S rRNA gene mutations contributing to macrolide resistance in *Campylobacter jejuni* and *Campylobacter coli*. Foodborne Pathog. Dis. **6**:91-98.

(63) **Ladron, D. G., J. Gonzalez, and P. Pena**. 1994. Bacteraemia caused by *Campylobacter* spp. J. Clin. Pathol. **47**:174-175.

(64) **Lambert, T., G. Gerbaud, P. Trieu-Cuot, and P. Courvalin**. 1985. Structural relationship between the genes encoding 3'-aminoglycoside phosphotransferases in *Campylobacter* and in gram-positive cocci. Ann. Inst. Pasteur Microbiol. **136B**:135-150.

(65) **Lee, C. Y., C. L. Tai, S. C. Lin, and Y. T. Chen**. 1994. Occurrence of plasmids and tetracycline resistance among *Campylobacter jejuni* and *Campylobacter coli* isolated from whole market chickens and clinical samples. Int. J. Food Microbiol. **24**:161-170.

(66) **Lee, M. D., S. Sanchez, M. Zimmer, U. Idris, M. E. Berrang, and P. F. McDermott**. 2002. Class 1 integron-associated tobramycin-gentamicin resistance in *Campylobacter jejuni* isolated from the broiler chicken house environment. Antimicrob. Agents Chemother. **46**:3660-3664.

(67) **Li, C. C., C. H. Chiu, J. L. Wu, Y. C. Huang, and T. Y. Lin**. 1998. Antimicrobial susceptibilities of *Campylobacter jejuni* and *coli* by using E-test in Taiwan. Scand. J. Infect. Dis. **30**:39-42.

(68) **Lin, J., M. Akiba, O. Sahin, and Q. Zhang**. 2005. CmeR functions as a transcriptional repressor for the multidrug efflux pump CmeABC in *Campylobacter jejuni*. Antimicrob. Agents Chemother. **49**:1067-1075.

(69) **Lin, J., L. O. Michel, and Q. Zhang**. 2002. CmeABC functions as a multidrug efflux system in

Campylobacter jejuni. Antimicrob. Agents Chemother. **46**:2124-2131.

(70) **Lindmark, H., S. Boqvist, M. Ljungstrom, P. Agren, B. Bjorkholm, and L. Engstrand.** 2009. Risk factors for campylobacteriosis: an epidemiological surveillance study of patients and retail poultry. J. Clin. Microbiol. **47**:2616-2619.

(71) **Luber, P., J. Wagner, H. Hahn, and E. Bartelt.** 2003. Antimicrobial resistance in *Campylobacter jejuni* and *Campylobacter coli* strains isolated in 1991 and 2001-2002 from poultry and humans in Berlin, Germany. Antimicrob. Agents Chemother. **47**:3825-3830.

(72) **Luo, N., O. Sahin, J. Lin, L. O. Michel, and Q. Zhang.** 2003. In vivo selection of *Campylobacter* isolates with high levels of fluoroquinolone resistance associated with *gyrA* mutations and the function of the CmeABC efflux pump. Antimicrob. Agents Chemother. **47**:390-394.

(73) **Mamelli, L., J. P. Amoros, J. M. Pages, and J. M. Bolla.** 2003. A phenylalanine-arginine beta-naphthylamide sensitive multidrug efflux pump involved in intrinsic and acquired resistance of *Campylobacter* to macrolides. Int. J. Antimicrob. Agents **22**:237-241.

(74) **Mamelli, L., V. Prouzet-Mauleon, J. M. Pages, F. Megraud, and J. M. Bolla.** 2005. Molecular basis of macrolide resistance in *Campylobacter*: role of efflux pumps and target mutations. J. Antimicrob. Chemother. **56**:491-497.

(75) **Manavathu, E. K., K. Hiratsuka, and D. E. Taylor.** 1988. Nucleotide sequence analysis and expression of a tetracycline-resistance gene from *Campylobacter jejuni*. Gene **62**:17-26.

(76) **MARAN.** 2007. pp. 54-57. *In* D. J. Mevius, and I. B. Wit (ed.), Monitoring of antimicrobial resistance and antibiotic usage in animals in The Netherland in 2006/2007.

(77) **McDermott, P. F., S. M. Bodeis, F. M. Aarestrup, S. Brown, M. Traczewski, P. Fedorka-Cray, M. Wallace, I. A. Critchley, C. Thornsberry, S. Graff, R. Flamm, J. Beyer, D. Shortridge, L. J. Piddock, V. Ricci, M. M. Johnson, R. N. Jones, B. Reller, S. Mirrett, J. Aldrobi, R. Rennie, C. Brosnikoff, L. Turnbull, G. Stein, S. Schooley, R. A. Hanson, and R. D. Walker.** 2004. Development of a standardized susceptibility test for *Campylobacter* with quality-control ranges for ciprofloxacin, doxycycline, erythromycin, gentamicin, and meropenem. Microb. Drug Resist. **10**:124-131.

(78) **McDermott, P. F., S. M. Bodeis, L. L. English, D. G. White, R. D. Walker, S. Zhao, S. Simjee, and D. D. Wagner.** 2002. Ciprofloxacin resistance in *Campylobacter jejuni* evolves rapidly in chickens treated with fluoroquinolones. J. Infect. Dis. **185**:837-840.

(79) **McDermott, P. F., S. M. Bodeis-Jones, T. R. Fritsche, R. N. Jones, and R. D. Walker.** 2005. Broth microdilution susceptibility testing of *Campylobacter jejuni* and the determination of quality control ranges for fourteen antimicrobial agents. J. Clin. Microbiol. **43**:6136-6138.

(80) **McDermott, P. F., S. M. Bodeis-Jones, and I. Nachamkin.** 2003. The use of disk diffusion to screen for antimicrobial resistance in *Campylobacter*. Abstracts of the 12th International Workshop on *Campylobacter, Helicobacter* and Related Organisms. Aarhus, Denmark.

(81) **Monselise, A., D. Blickstein, I. Ostfeld, R. Segal, and M. Weinberger.** 2004. A case of cellulitis complicating *Campylobacter jejuni* subspecies jejuni bacteremia and review of the literature. Eur. J. Clin. Microbiol. Infect. Dis. **23**:718-721.

(82) **Nachamkin, I., B. M. Allos, and T. Ho.** 1998. *Campylobacter* species and Guillain-Barre syndrome. Clin. Microbiol. Rev. **11**:555-567.

(83) **Nachamkin, I., H. Ung, and M. Li.** 2002. Increasing fluoroquinolone resistance in *Campylobacter jejuni*, Pennsylvania, USA,1982-2001. Emerg. Infect. Dis. **8**:1501-1503.

(84) **Nelson, J. M., K. E. Smith, D. J. Vugia, T. Rabatsky-Ehr, S. D. Segler, H. D. Kassenborg, S. M. Zansky, K. Joyce, N. Marano, R. M. Hoekstra, and F. J. Angulo.** 2004. Prolonged diarrhea due to ciprofloxacin-resistant *Campylobacter* infection. J. Infect. Dis. **190**:1150-1157.

(85) **Niwa, H., T. Chuma, K. Okamoto, and K. Itoh.** 2001. Rapid detection of mutations associated with resistance to erythromycin in *Campylobacter jejuni/coli* by PCR and line probe assay. Int. J. Antimicrob. Agents **18**:359-364.

(86) **Niwa, H., T. Chuma, K. Okamoto, and K. Itoh.** 2003. Simultaneous detection of mutations associated with resistance to macrolides and quinolones in *Campylobacter jejuni* and *C. coli* using a PCR-line probe assay. Int. J. Antimicrob. Agents **22**:374-379.

(87) **NORM.** 2008. pp. 41-44. *In.* J. Mikalsen, and G. S. Simonsen (ed.), Usage of antimicrobial agents and occurrence of antimicrobial resistance in Norway. ISSN 1502-2307,

(88) **O'Halloran, F., B. Lucey, B. Cryan, T. Buckley, and S. Fanning.** 2004. Molecular characterization of class 1 integrons from Irish thermophilic *Campylobacter* spp. J. Antimicrob. Chemother. **53**:952-957.

(89) **Okada, H., T. Kitazawa, S. Harada, S. Itoyama, S. Hatakeyama, Y. Ota, and K. Koike.** 2008. Combined treatment with oral kanamycin and parenteral antibiotics for a case of persistent bacteremia and intestinal carriage with *Campylobacter coli*. Intern. Med. **47**:1363-1366.

(90) **Oncul, O., P. Zarakolu, O. Oncul, and D. Gur.** 2003. Antimicrobial susceptibility testing of *Campylobacter jejuni*: a comparison between E-test and agar dilution method. Diagn. Microbiol. Infect. Dis. **45**:69-71.

(91) **Ouellette, M., G. Gerbaud, T. Lambert, and P. Courvalin.** 1987. Acquisition by a *Campylobacter*-like strain of *aphA-1*, a kanamycin resistance determinant from members of the family *Enterobacteriaceae*. Antimicrob. Agents Chemother. **31**:1021-1026.

(92) **Oyarzabal, O. A., R. Rad, and S. Backert.** 2007. Conjugative transfer of chromosomally encoded antibiotic resistance from *Helicobacter pylori* to *Campylobacter jejuni*. J. Clin. Microbiol. **45**:402-408.

(93) **Pacanowski, J., V. Lalande, K. Lacombe, C. Boudraa, P. Lesprit, P. Legrand, D. Trystram, N. Kassis, G. Arlet, J. L. Mainardi, F. Doucet-Populaire, P. M. Girard, and J. L. Meynard.** 2008. *Campylobacter* bacteremia: clinical features and fac-

tors associated with fatal outcome. Clin. Infect. Dis. **47**:790-796.

(94) **Page, W. J., G. Huyer, M. Huyer, and E. A. Worobec**. 1989. Characterization of the porins of *Campylobacter jejuni* and *Campylobacter coli* and implications for antibiotic susceptibility. Antimicrob. Agents Chemother. **33**:297-303.

(95) **Parkhill, J., B. W. Wren, K. Mungall, J. M. Ketley, C. Churcher, D. Basham, T. Chillingworth, R. M. Davies, T. Feltwell, S. Holroyd, K. Jagels, A. V. Karlyshev, S. Moule, M. J. Pallen, C. W. Penn, M. A. Quail, M. A. Rajandream, K. M. Rutherford, A. H. van Vliet, S. Whitehead, and B. G. Barrell**. 2000. The genome sequence of the food-borne pathogen *Campylobacter jejuni* reveals hypervariable sequences. Nature **403**:665-668.

(96) **Payot, S., L. Avrain, C. Magras, K. Praud, A. Cloeckaert, and E. Chaslus-Dancla**. 2004. Relative contribution of target gene mutation and efflux to fluoroquinolone and erythromycin resistance in French poultry and pig isolates of *Campylobacter coli*. Int. J. Antimicrob. Agents **23**:468-472.

(97) **Pinto-Alphandary, H., C. Mabilat, and P. Courvalin**. 1990. Emergence of aminoglycoside resistance genes *aadA* and *aadE* in the genus *Campylobacter*. Antimicrob. Agents Chemother. **34**:1294-1296.

(98) **Pratt, A. and V. Korolik**. 2005. Tetracycline resistance of Australian *Campylobacter jejuni* and *Campylobacter coli* isolates. J. Antimicrob. Chemother. **55**:452-460.

(99) **Pumbwe, L. and L. J. Piddock**. 2002. Identification and molecular characterisation of CmeB, a *Campylobacter jejuni* multidrug efflux pump. FEMS Microbiol. Lett. **206**:185-189.

(100) **Pumbwe, L., L. P. Randall, M. J. Woodward, and L. J. Piddock**. 2004. Expression of the efflux pump genes *cmeB*, *cmeF* and the porin gene *porA* in multiple-antibiotic-resistant *Campylobacter jejuni*. J. Antimicrob. Chemother. **54**:341-347.

(101) **Rao, D., J. R. Rao, E. Crothers, R. McMullan, D. McDowell, A. McMahon, P. J. Rooney, B. C. Millar, and J. E. Moore**. 2005. Increased erythromycin resistance in clinical *Campylobacter* in Northern Ireland—an update. J. Antimicrob. Chemother. **56**:435-437.

(102) **Riedel, C. T., L. Brondsted, H. Rosenquist, S. N. Haxgart, and B. B. Christensen**. 2009. Chemical decontamination of *Campylobacter jejuni* on chicken skin and meat. J. Food Prot. **72**:1173-1180.

(103) **Rivera, M. J., J. Castillo, C. Martin, M. Navarro, and R. Gomez-Lus**. 1986. Aminoglycoside-phosphotransferases APH(3')-IV and APH(3'') synthesized by a strain of *Campylobacter coli*. J Antimicrob Chemother. **18**:153-158.

(104) **Roe, D. E., A. Weinberg, and M. C. Roberts**. 1995. Mobile rRNA methylase genes in *Campylobacter* (*Wolinella*) *rectus*. J. Antimicrob. Chemother. **36**:738-740.

(105) **Routh, M. D., C. C. Su, Q. Zhang, and E. W. Yu**. 2009. Structures of AcrR and CmeR: insight into the mechanisms of transcriptional repression and multidrug recognition within the TetR family of regulators. Biochim. Biophys. Acta **1794**:844-851.

(106) **Schwartz, D., H. Goossens, J. Levy, J. P. Butzler, and J. Goldhar**. 1993. Plasmid profiles and antimicrobial susceptibility of *Campylobacter jejuni* isolated from Israeli children with diarrhea. Zentralbl. Bakteriol. **279**:368-376.

(107) **Serichantalergs, O., A. Dalsgaard, L. Bodhidatta, S. Krasaesub, C. Pitarangsi, A. Srijan, and C. J. Mason**. 2007. Emerging fluoroquinolone and macrolide resistance of *Campylobacter jejuni* and *Campylobacter coli* isolates and their serotypes in Thai children from 1991 to 2000. Epidemiol. Infect. **135**:1299-1306.

(108) **Shaw, K. J., P. N. Rather, R. S. Hare, and G. H. Miller**. 1993. Molecular genetics of aminoglycoside resistance genes and familial relationships of the aminoglycoside-modifying enzymes. Microbiol. Rev. **57**:138-163.

(109) **Skirrow, M. B.** 1977. *Campylobacter* enteritis: a «new» disease. Br. Med. J. **2**:9-11.

(110) **Skirrow, M. B., and M. J. Blaser**. 2002. *Campylobacter jejuni*, pp. 719-739. *In* M. J. Blaser, P. D. Smith, J. I. Ravdin, H. B. Greenberg, and R. L. Guerrant (ed.), Infections of the gastrointestinal tract. Lippincott Williams and Wilkins, Baltimore, MD.

(111) **Skjot-Rasmussen, L., S. Ethelberg, H. D. Emborg, Y. Agerso, L. S. Larsen, S. Nordentoft, S. S. Olsen, T. Ejlertsen, H. Holt, E. M. Nielsen, and A. M. Hammerum**. 2009. Trends in occurrence of antimicrobial resistance in *Campylobacter jejuni* isolates from broiler chickens, broiler chicken meat, and human domestically acquired cases and travel associated cases in Denmark. Int. J. Food Microbiol. **131**:277-279.

(112) **Smith, K. E., J. M. Besser, C. W. Hedberg, F. T. Leano, J. B. Bender, J. H. Wicklund, B. P. Johnson, K. A. Moore, and M. T. Osterholm**. 1999. Quinolone-resistant *Campylobacter jejuni* infections in Minnesota, 1992-1998. Investigation Team. N. Engl. J. Med. **340**:1525-1532.

(113) **Sougakoff, W. B., B. Papadopoulou, P. Nordmann, and P. Courvalin**. 1987. Nucleotide sequence and distribution of gene *tetO* encoding tetracycline resistance in *Campylobacter coli*. FEMS Microbiol. Lett. **44**:153-159.

(114) **Spahn, C. M., G. Blaha, R. K. Agrawal, P. Penczek, R. A. Grassucci, C. A. Trieber, S. R. Connell, D. E. Taylor, K. H. Nierhaus, and J. Frank**. 2001. Localization of the ribosomal protection protein Tet(O) on the ribosome and the mechanism of tetracycline resistance. Mol. Cell **7**:1037-1045.

(115) **Studahl, A. and Y. Andersson**. 2000. Risk factors for indigenous campylobacter infection: a Swedish case-control study. Epidemiol. Infect. **125**:269-275.

(116) **Tajada, P., J. L. Gomez-Graces, J. I. Alos, D. Balas, and R. Cogollos**. 1996. Antimicrobial susceptibilities of *Campylobacter jejuni* and *Campylobacter coli* to 12 β-lactam agents and combinations with β-lactamase inhibitors. Antimicrob. Agents Chemother. **40**:1924-1925.

(117) **Taylor, D. E., S. A. DeGrandis, M. A. Karmali, and P. C. Fleming**. 1980. Transmissible tetracycline resistance in *Campylobacter jejuni*. Lancet **2**:797.

(118) **Taylor, D. E., W. Yan, L. K. Ng, E. K. Manavathu, and P. Courvalin**. 1988. Genetic characterization of kanamycin resistance in *Campylobacter coli*. Ann. Inst. Pasteur Microbiol. **139**:665-676.

(119) **Tenover, F. C., and P. M. Elvrum**. 1988. Detection of two different kanamycin resistance genes in naturally occurring isolates of *Campylobacter jejuni* and *Campylobacter coli*. Antimicrob. Agents Chemother. **32**:1170-1173.

(120) **Tenover, F. C., C. L. Fennell, L. Lee, and D. J. LeBlanc**. 1992. Characterization of two plasmids from *Campylobacter jejuni* isolates that carry the *aphA-7* kanamycin resistance determinant. Antimicrob. Agents Chemother. **36**:712-716.

(121) **Tenover, F. C., T. Gilbert, and P. O'Hara**. 1989. Nucleotide sequence of a novel kanamycin resistance gene, *aphA-7*, from *Campylobacter jejuni* and comparison to other kanamycin phosphotransferase genes. Plasmid **22**:52-58.

(122) **Tokuda, K., J. Nishi, H. Miyanohara, J. Sarantuya, M. Iwashita, A. Kamenosono, K. Hizukuri, N. Wakimoto, and M. Yoshinaga**. 2004. Relapsing cellulitis associated with *Campylobacter coli* bacteremia in an agammaglobulinemic patient. Pediatr. Infect. Dis. J. **23**:577-579.

(123) **Trieber, C. A., N. Burkhardt, K. H. Nierhaus, and D. E. Taylor**. 1998. Ribosomal protection from tetracycline mediated by Tet(O): Tet(O) interaction with ribosomes is GTP-dependent. Biol. Chem. **379**:847-855.

(124) **Vacher, S., A. Menard, E. Bernard, A. Santos, and F. Megraud**. 2005. Detection of mutations associated with macrolide resistance in thermophilic *Campylobacter* spp. by real-time PCR. Microb. Drug Resist. **11**:40-47.

(125) **Valdivieso-Garcia, A., R. Imgrund, A. Deckert, B. Varughese, K. Harris, N. Bunimov, R. Reid-Smith, and S. McEwen**. 2003. Cost analysis and antimicrobial susceptibility testing comparing the E-test and the agar dilution method in *Campylobacter* spp. Diagn. Microbiol. Infect. Dis. **65**:168-174.

(126) **van Boven, M., K. T. Veldman, M. C. de Jong, and D. J. Mevius**. 2003. Rapid selection of quinolone resistance in *Campylobacter jejuni* but not in *Escherichia coli* in individually housed broilers. J. Antimicrob. Chemother. **52**:719-723.

(127) **van der Beek, M. T., E. C. Claas, D. J. Mevius, W. van Pelt, J. A. Wagenaar, and E. J. Kuijper**. 2009. Inaccuracy of routine susceptibility tests for detection of erythromycin resistance of *Campylobacter jejuni* and *Campylobacter coli*. Clin. Microbiol. Infect. (in press).

(128) **Wang, Y., W. M. Huang, and D. E. Taylor**. 1993. Cloning and nucleotide sequence of the *Campylobacter jejuni gyrA* gene and characterization of quinolone resistance mutations. Antimicrob. Agents Chemother. **37**:457-463.

(129) **Wang, Y., and D. E. Taylor**. 1990. Chloramphenicol resistance in *Campylobacter coli*: nucleotide sequence, expression, and cloning vector construction. Gene **94**:23-28.

(130) **Wassenaar, T. M., M. Kist, and A. de Jong**. 2007. Re-analysis of the risks attributed to ciprofloxacin-resistant *Campylobacter jejuni* infections. Int. J. Antimicrob. Agents **30**:195-201.

(131) **Weisblum, B**. 1995. Erythromycin resistance by ribosome modification. Antimicrob. Agents Chemother. **39**:577-585.

(132) **Williams, M. D., J. B. Schorling, L. J. Barrett, S. M. Dudley, I. Orgel, W. C. Koch, D. S. Shields, S. M. Thorson, J. A. Lohr, and R. L. Guerrant**. 1989. Early treatment of *Campylobacter jejuni* enteritis. Antimicrob. Agents Chemother. **33**:248-250.

(133) **Wingstrand, A., J. Neimann, J. Engberg, E. M. Nielsen, P. Gerner-Smidt, H. C. Wegener, and K. Molbak**. 2006. Fresh chicken as main risk factor for campylobacteriosis, Denmark. Emerg. Infect. Dis. **12**:280-285.

(134) **Wretlind, B., A. Stromberg, L. Ostlund, E. Sjogren, and B. Kaijser**. 1992. Rapid emergence of quinolone resistance in *Campylobacter jejuni* in patients treated with norfloxacin. Scand. J. Infect. Dis. **24**:685-686.

(135) **Wright, E. P. and M. A. Knowles**. 1980. Beta-lactamase production by *Campylobacter jejuni*. J. Clin. Pathol. **33**:904-905.

(136) **Yan, M., O. Sahin, J. Lin, and Q. Zhang**. 2006. Role of the CmeABC efflux pump in the emergence of fluoroquinolone-resistant *Campylobacter* under selection pressure. J. Antimicrob. Chemother. **58**:1154-1159.

Chapter 39. *MORAXELLA (BRANHAMELLA) CATARRHALIS*

Hubert CHARDON

INTRODUCTION

Moraxella catarrhalis has always been a topic for lively discussions: controversy over its nomenclature (*Branhamella* or *Moraxella*) and over its family (*Branhamaceae* or *Moraxellaceae*), doubts on its pathogenicity, on the genetic determinants of its β−lactamase, on any real impact of this enzyme on susceptibility to aminopenicillins and cephalosporins, on explanations for the rapid increase in percentage of strains producing β-lactamase, and on the mechanism of acquiring this resistance. Its classification in the genus *Neisseria*, as *Neisseria catarrhalis*, based on similarity to other *Neisseria* of the oro-pharynx, and its lack of its identification by microbiologist for a long time are partly responsible for the ignorance regarding this species.

METHODS

For determination of MICs, CLSI recommends broth microdilution in the guideline M45 (16). Cation-adjusted Mueller-Hinton broth (unsupplemented) should be directly inoculated with a colony suspension equivalent to a 0.5 McFarland standard and incubated at 35°C in ambient air for 20-24 h. Breakpoints for amoxicillin-clavulanic acid, some cephalosporins, macrolides, tetracyclines, trimethoprim-sulfamethoxazole, chloramphenicol, rifampin, and fluoroquinolones are available (Table 1). EUCAST also recommends broth microdilution but provides different breakpoints (Table 1).

So far, CLSI and EUCAST have not provided any recommendation for testing *M. catarrhalis* by disk diffusion. However, both committees

Table 1. MIC breakpoints for some antimicrobials and *M. catarrhalis* according to CLSI (16) and EUCAST (http://www.eucast.org/clinical_breakpoints/)

Antibiotic	CLSI breakpoints (µg/ml)		EUCAST breakpoints (µg/ml)	
	S (≤)	R (≥)	S (≤)	R (>)
β-lactams				
Amoxicillin-clavulanic acid	4/2	8/4	1[a]	1[a]
Cefaclor	8	32	0.5	0.5
Cefuroxime	4	16	0.12 (oral)	2 (oral)
			1 (intravenous)	2 (intravenous)
Cefixime	NA[b]	NA	0.5	1
Cefotaxime/ceftriaxone	2	NA	1	2
Macrolides				
Erythromycin	0.5	8	0.25	0.5
Azithromycin	2	8	0.5	0.5
Clarithromycin	2	8	0.25	0.5
Tetracyclines				
Tetracycline	2	8	1[c]	2[c]
Quinolones				
Levofloxacin	2	NA	1	1
Ciprofloxacin	1	NA	0.5	0.5

[a] The concentration of clavulanate is fixed at 2 µg/ml; same breakpoints for ampicillin, amoxicillin, and ampicillin-sulbactam (sulbactam concentration fixed at 2 µg/ml).
[b] NA, not available.
[c] Same breakpoints for doxycycline and minocycline.

recommend β-lactamase testing as a routine test since there is overlap in MICs of ampicillin or amoxicillin for β-lactamase positive and negative isolates. Only chromogenic cephalosporin methods (Nitrocefin®) should be used. However, since > 90% of *M. catarrhalis* strains produce a β-lactamase, EUCAST (http://www.eucast.org/expert_rules/) discourages testing of penicillinase production. These isolates should be reported as resistant to benzylpenicillin, ampicillin, and amoxicillin. Recently, Bell *et al.* (2) developed a disk-diffusion test for *M. catarrhalis* that is performed on Mueller-Hinton agar and incubated for 20 to 24 h in 5% CO_2.

SUSCEPTIBLE PHENOTYPE AND INTRINSIC RESISTANCE

Moraxella spp. are naturally susceptible to antibiotics of the following classes: penicillins, aminoglycosides, chloramphenicol, tetracyclines, macrolides, rifamycins, quinolones, and sulfonamides. They are naturally resistant to vancomycin, teicoplanin, and trimethoprim. Their natural resistance is used for the purposes of identification and for designing selective media.

ACQUIRED RESISTANCE

β-lactams

Non β-lactamase producers

Populations of strains of *M. catarrhalis* that are β-lactamase non-producers are not homogenous in terms of susceptibility to ampicillin: some are more susceptible than others. Based on distribution of MICs among 40 β-lactamase non-producing strains (11), two populations could be distinguished:
- one with a mode ≤ 0.01 µg/ml
- one with a mode of 0.12 µg/ml
- MICs for all the strains were ≤ 0.5 µg/ml. A similar distribution had been previously described (31).

The characteristics of these two populations are not yet clearly defined. As in the case of *Neisseria gonorrhoeae*, one can suspect occurrence of mutations which could reduce the affinity of PBPs for the penicillins or could modify the outer membrane resulting in reduced permeability and cross-resistance to other antibiotics (25). In fact, MICs for the least susceptible population do not reach the critical concentration that would justify classification of such β-lactamase non-producing strains as resistant to aminopenicillins. So far, there has been no report of treatment failure with aminopenicillins of infection with such strains.

β-lactamase producers

Study of β-lactamases was carried out by several authors (7, 14, 31, 40, 44). However, a comprehensive review proves difficult. For example, values for isoelectric points vary for the same enzyme depending on the authors who have not consistently referred to the enzyme(s) described in the previous studies. The discrepancies are likely due to the low level of β-lactamase production and studies based on non-purified enzymes, purification being rendered difficult due to the strong membrane association of the enzyme. Indeed, during isoelectric point determination, one often observes several major or minor bands for the same enzyme activity. An excellent review was provided by Wallace *et al.* (44) who compared two strains of *B. catarrhalis* from Belgium, previously called Ravasio and 1908 (20) and two strains described by Nash *et al.* (29). Presence of two β-lactamases was confirmed in both and they were renamed:
- Ravasio renamed BRO-1 pI = 5.3 – 5.5, 6.1-6.4 – 6.65
- 1908 renamed BRO-2 pI = 5.3 – 5.5 – 6.1 – 6.55 – 7.7

In fact, only the bands corresponding to a pI greater than 6.1 are discriminatory.

In the same study, the authors report that the two enzymes are also present in *Moraxella nonliquefaciens* and *M. lacunata*, which explains their new nomenclature: BR for *Branhamella* and O for *Moraxella*. Noticeably, BRO-1 and BRO-2 had also appeared in *M. non liquefaciens* and *M. lacunata* in 1978 (44). β-lactamases present in other species, *M. urethralis*, *M. osloensis*, and *M. phenylpyruvica* are different.

In 1991, a new enzyme, called BRO-3, was described by Christensen *et al.* (15). Some authors (39) considered that BRO-3, an enzyme linked to the cytoplasmic membrane, could only be a precursor of BRO-1 and BRO-2, and hence BRO-3 has not been included in subsequent classifications. Enzymes of the BRO-1 type are the most commonly encountered in *B. catarrhalis*: in 90% of the cases in the United States (29) and 87% in France (31), as reported in earlier investigations, and also in the more recent ones (94% in an European investigation in 2002) (35). Both enzymes have a similar substrate utilization profile

(44). Penicillins, aminopenicillins, methicillin, and cefaclor are hydrolysed by both. Nitrocefin® proves to be an excellent substrate, explaining its efficiency in detection of β-lactamase production. BRO-1 and BRO-2 are both strongly inhibited by β-lactamase inhibitors: clavulanic acid (I_{50}: 0.005μg/ml) and sulbactam (I_{50}: 0.025μg/ml) (44). BRO-1 appears to be produced in large amounts as judged by the nanomoles of Nitrocefin® hydrolysed per minute per mg protein: 149 ± 57 for BRO-1 versus 66 ± 43 for BRO-2, which likely explains the differences in their activity.

Inhibition zone diameters for ampicillin are on the average smaller for cultures producing BRO-1 (17mm) than for those producing BRO-2 (28mm). However, this is not useful in distinguishing between the types of the enzyme due to a significant overlap of the diameters and hence genotypic methods are required.

MICs of penicillin G tend to be higher against BRO-1 producing isolates than the BRO-2 producers (32, 35). MIC_{50} of β-lactamase non-producer strains of M. catarrhalis, are ≤ 0.03μg/ml. These values reach 4μg/ml for BRO-1 producing isolates and 1μg/ml for those producing BRO-2. However, these phenotypes are not discriminatory enough to differentiate between the two enzymes because the MIC values overlap, ranging from 0.06 to 32μg/ml for BRO-1 producers and from 0.06 to 1 μg/ml for BRO-2. Once again, genotypic methods seem to be required.

The nature of the β-lactamases is better defined by analysis of their genetic determinants. The corresponding bro gene is located in the chromosome and is easily transferable by conjugation to M. nonliquefaciens and M. lacunata (44). The percentage of GC in the bro gene is 31%, which is very different from that of rest of the genome of M. catarrhalis which is 41%, suggesting that it has been acquired from an unrelated species. BRO proteins carry a lipoprotein characteristic motif, LTGC. Lipoproteinic β-lactamases are strongly membrane-bound. These are rare in Gram-negative bacilli (Pseudomonas pseudomallei and Capnocytophage species) but seen more frequently in Gram-positive bacteria (Bacillus cereus, Bacillus licheniformis, Staphylococcus aureus) (4). The lipoproteinic nature of the β-lactamase suggests that it has originated in a Gram-positive bacterium (4). The sequences of BRO-1 and BRO-2 (314 amino acids) are largely identical (5, 35) except at position 294. At this position, there is a substitution of aspartic acid (BRO-1) by glycine (BRO-2). Another difference in the two genes was revealed by sequence analysis of promoter regions. There appear to be deletions in the BRO-2 promoter sequence, which likely explains its lower level of production.

Aminoglycosides

A rare, plasmid-borne resistance associated with β-lactams was reported in M. catarrhalis (34). This had been attributed to the synthesis of an aminoglycoside 3'-O-phosphotranferase [APH(3')] which inactivates kanamycin, neomycin, and to a lesser extent, amikacin. However, a multi-centric French study conducted in 2001-2002 (9) did not report any resistance to aminoglycosides.

Tetracyclines

Resistance to tetracyclines though rare, is constitutive, non-transferable, and most often encoded by the tet(B) gene (33), which is most probably located in the chromosome. Minocycline is effective, although resistance to this antibiotic was reported from USA (6), England (2%) (38), and France (9, 12). In another study, a tet (K) gene was identified in a single strain (13).

Macrolides

Isolates resistant to erythromycin have been described very rarely (6). Nevertheless, in Sweden, two strains with a MIC of erythromycin of 8 μg/ml and three strains with a MIC greater than 8 μg/ml have been reported (25). More recently, a strain with a MIC of clarithromycin of 32 μg/ml was reported (37). In French multicentric studies, no resistant strains have been detected (9, 12, 13). Depending on whether resistance was independent or associated with co-resistance to other antibiotics, a modification of the 50S subunit of the ribosome or a reduction in permeability, respectively, have been suspected to be involved. The activity of five macrolides has been studied on strains susceptible to erythromycin (Table 2) (10). Spiramycin appears less active. Resistance to pristinamycin and to telithromycin (8) has not been reported.

Rifampin, quinolones, colistin, and sulfonamides

Resistance to rifampin is rare. Of note, a strain (MIC = 64 μg/ml) has been isolated in France in a multicentric study in 1994-1995 (12). A strain with reduced susceptibility to pefloxacin, a fluoroquinolone, (MIC = 2μg/ml) has been detected in France (11). Rarely, strains resistant to ciprofloxacin and levofloxacin have also been reported (17, 18). Strains capable of growth on selective media containing 7.5 µg/ml of colistin have also been described.

Although *M. catarrhalis* is intrinsically resistant to trimethoprim, combination of trimethoprim-sulfamethaxole is synergistic against *M. catarrhalis*, as this species is susceptible to sulfonamides. Strains resistant to sulfonamides have been rarely reported (9, 41). Media used to study this antibiotic have to be depleted in thymidine, otherwise the medium is inhibitory and leads to a false resistance. A rare resistance to trimethoprim-sulfamethaxole combination was reported in Spain (34). It is plasmid-borne, transferable, and associated with other resistances. The mechanisms of resistance to these antibiotics, although well studied in other bacterial genera, have not been investigated in *M. catarrhalis*.

RESISTANCE PHENOTYPES

The MICs of antimicrobials against 185 isolates (2001-2002) are shown in Table 2 (9).

Table 2. Activity of macrolides (µg/ml) against 200 strains of *M. catarrhalis* (10).

Macrolide	MIC_{50}	MIC_{90}	MIC range
Erythromycin	0.25	0.5	0.125 - 1
Josamycin	0.5	1	0.25 - 1
Midecamycin	2	2	0.5 - 4
Spiramycin	4	8	1 - 16
Roxithromycin	0.5	0.5	0.125 - 1

β-lactams

β-lactamase non-producers

β-lactamase non-producing strains having an MIC of ampicillin > 4 µg/ml have been reported. In a study published in 1986 using disk diffusion, Luman *et al.* (28) observed that 60 β-lactamase non-producers displayed diameters of 40.6 ± 4.3 mm (range 33 to 50 mm) around a disk of ampicillin; a single strain had a diameter ≤ 26 mm. There was no information about the MIC of ampicillin for this strain, which also had a reduced diameter around a disk of penicillin G. MICs of amoxicillin ≤ 0.5 µg/ml for 41 strains were reported in a French survey (11). The MIC of ampicillin needs to be constantly determined by a reference method on the rare β-lactamase non-producer strains of *M. catarrhalis* that display a reduced diameter around the disk of ampicillin or against strains that may be responsible for clinical failures.

β-lactamase producers

In a study using disk diffusion, as recommended by NCCLS, Luman *et al.* (28) reported that 52.6% of the β-lactamase producing strains had inhibition zone diameters of ≥ 18 mm, which would classify them as susceptible. Moreover, inter-laboratory reproducibility is also barely satisfactory, probably related to the size of the inoculum. Jones *et al.* (23) reported inhibition zone diameters for ampicillin (disk containing 10 µg) obtained by 534 laboratories in the USA on the same β-lactamase producing strain. The range of inhibition zone diameters was as follows: ten measured 6-10 mm, ten 11-13 mm, seventy-six 14-19 mm, one hundred and nine 20-21 mm, two hundred seventy-two 22-28 mm, and fifty-seven ≥ 29mm. In view of the lack of efficiency of disk diffusion for testing ampicillin susceptibility, this technique has a little interest for detection of β-lactamase production.

Screening for β-lactamase production is thus mandatory in routine. It is detectable by various methods: the microbiological method (Gots test) is not used in practice as the results can be obtained only after 24 h. In practice, iodometric tests, acidimetric methods, and chromogenic techniques (Padac® and Nitrofecin®) are used. The choice of the method is important. Philippon *et al.* (31) found 100% efficiency for iodometric and chromogenic tests (Nitrocefin®); in contrast, the acidimetric method proved to be inefficient yielding 4.1% false negatives and 15.4% false positives. Jones *et al.* (23) reported results from 487 tests carried out in different laboratories on the same β-lactamase producing strain: acidimetric method, 78% of positives over 182 tests, iodometric test, 64% positives over 11 tests, Nitrocefin®, 96% positives over 262 tests, Padac®, 69% positives on 32 tests

Evidently, Nitrocefin® is the method of choice based on the excellent affinity of the β-lactamases from *M. catarrhalis* for this substrate and especially in view of low level enzyme production in this species.

Table 3. Activity of eleven antibiotics (μg/ml) against 185 strains of *M. catarrhalis* (9)

Antibiotic	0.02	0.03	0.06	0.13	0.25	0.5	1	2	4	8	16	32	64	128	256	MIC_{50}	MIC_{90}
Amoxicillin	13	2	2	1	3	47	9	57	36	11	1					2	4
Amoxicillin-clavulanic acid	74	8	28	49	23	1										0.06	0.25
Cefalotin			1		1	3	8	8	17	130	16	1				8	8
Cefotaxim	4	19	43	6	26	68	19									0.25	1
Gentamicin				6	69	107										0.5	0.5
Tetracycline				2	2	180					1					0.5	0.5
Erythromycin			3	3	61	102	15									0.5	0.5
Co-trimoxazole									20	95	48	20	1	0	1	8	32
Nalidixic acid						1	22	110	52							2	4
Pefloxacin	1	0	160	4	24		1									0.125	0.25
Ciprofloxacin	43	138	4													0.06	0.06

MIC DETERMINATION

Ampicillin resistance has not been clearly defined for *M. catarrhalis*. Should all strains producing a β-lactamase be considered as resistant, in particular those that produce a low level of the enzyme and have a MIC < 2 μg/ml? Or should ampicillin susceptibility be assessed in terms of critical concentrations? Moreover, the reported MIC values are highly variable for various reasons: inoculum size effect of β-lactamase producing strains, difficulty in accurately estimating the inoculum size (due to clumping of the bacteria) and use of liquid or solid medium. Thus, Doern *et al*. (19) found that the MICs of ampicillin for 58 β-lactamase producers ranged from 0.03 to 4 μg/ml (MIC_{90} = 2 μg/ml), overlapping those for non-producers, the MICs for the latter being in the range of 0.004 to 0.125 μg/ml (MIC_{90} = 0.06).

The effect of the inoculum size is important since the MICs increase from 0.5 to 64 μg/ml while the inoculum size increases from 10^4 to 10^6 CFU/ml. By using a heavy inoculum (11), which could be considered clinically relevant, there is good discrimination between producers and non-producers of β-lactamase (Fig. 1). All producing strains had a MIC ≥ 2 μg/ml and a MIC_{90} of 128 μg/ml, while non-producers had MICs ≤ 0.5 μg/ml.

In view of the uncertainties in the determination of ampicillin MIC, it is rather difficult to use this value for classifying strains as resistant or susceptible. Several failures have been reported while using this antibiotic for treating *M. catarrhalis* β-lactamase producers (30, 36, 42, 43). Hence, it is recommended that strains be considered as resistant to amoxicillin and ampicillin if they are β-lactamase producers, even if these are classified as susceptible by MIC determination.

The efficacy of β-lactamase inhibitors available in therapy is remarkable (Table 4). MIC_{90} drop from 128 μg/ml to 0.12 μg/ml for ampicillin in the presence of 1 μg/ml of sulbactam and to 0.25 μg/ml for amoxicillin in the presence of same concentration of clavulanic acid (14).

The problems encountered for determination of MICs of ampicillin and amoxicillin are also common to cephalosporins, with a similar discordance between authors. Thus, 58 β-lactamase producing strains were shown to have MIC of cefalotin ranging from 1 to 8 μg/ml (MIC_{90} = 8 μg/ml) according to Doern *et al*. (19) while the corresponding values ranged from 4 to 32 μg/ml (MIC_{90} = 32) for other authors (14).

First generation cephalosporins are inactive. V_{max} values for hydrolysis of cefaclor could vary

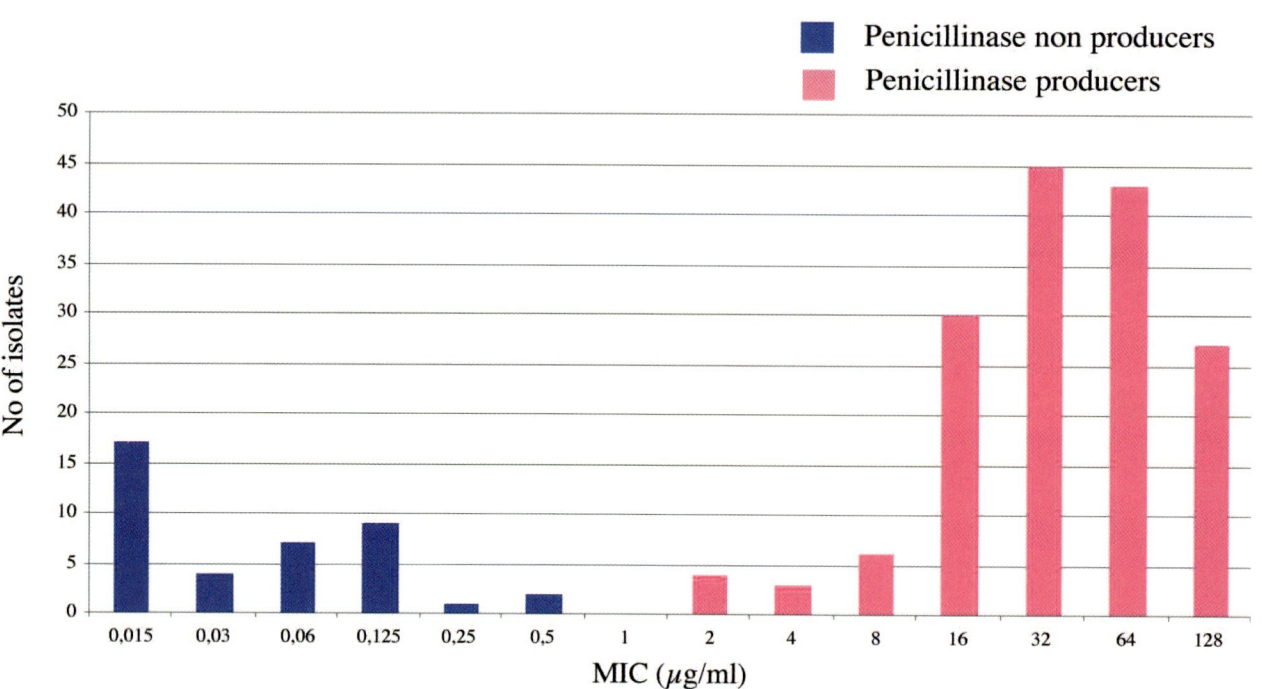

Fig. 1. MIC of amoxicillin as a function of β-lactamase production (11)

Table 4. MIC (µg/ml) of β-lactams against 43 strains of *M. catarrhalis*, including 35 penicillinase producers (14).

Antibiotic	β-lactamase	MIC$_{50}$	MIC$_{90}$	Extreme values
Penicillin G	−	0.008	0.12	0.008-0.12
	+	64	128	4-256
Ampicillin	−	0.008	0.06	0.004-0.06
	+	64	128	2-128
Ampicillin + sulbactam	+	0.06	0.12	0.001-0.12
Amoxicillin	−	0.008	0.06	0.008-0.06
	+	64	128	4-256
Amoxicillin + clavulanic acid	+	0.12	0.25	0.002-0.25
Cefalotin	−	0.5	2	0.5-2
	+	16	32	4-32
Cefoxitin	−	0.25	0.5	0.03-0.5
	+	0.25	0.5	0.03-1
Cefotaxime	−	0.016	0.5	0.016-0.5
	+	1	1	0.06-1
Ceftazidime	−	0.12	0.25	0.004-0.25
	+	0.03	0.12	0.004-0.25
Ceftriaxone	−	0.25	0.25	0.004-0.25
	+	1	2	0.016-4
Imipenem	−	0.008	0.03	0.008-0.03
	+	0.03	0.12	0.008-0.12
Aztreonam	−	0.5	2	0.25-2
	+	2	2	0.25-4

from 108 to 240 nmol min^{-1} mg protein^{-1} compared to a value of 100 for penicillin G (44). MIC$_{90}$ of cefalotin for β-lactamase non-producers or producers are 2 µg/ml and 32 µg/ml, respectively (Table 4) (14). Treatment failures have been reported during use of this antibiotic against β-lactamase producing strains (42).

Second and third generation cephalosporins are bacteriostatic (Table 4). Cefuroxime is bacteriostatic with a MIC$_{90}$ of 2 µg/ml for β-lactamase producers (27) which is four times higher than that (0.5 µg/ml) for non-producers. This probably reflects low level hydrolysis of the molecule. Cefoxitin and moxalactam, known for their resistance to hydrolysis by β-lactamases, are effective. Moxalactam has very low MICs (MIC$_{90}$ = 0.016 µg/ml for producing strains). The MIC$_{90}$ of cefoxitin is identical (0.5 µg/ml) regardless of whether the strain is non-producer or producer of β-lactamase, and independent of the presence of clavulanic acid. Nevertheless, cephalosporins of the second and third generation are mildly hydrolysed by the β-lactamase of *M. catarrhalis*. Thus, the MIC$_{90}$ of cefotaxime is 0.06 µg/ml for β-lactamase negative strains and 1 µg/ml for β-lactamase positive isolates (Table 4).

In order to accurately estimate the efficiency of cephalosporins, kinetic studies of this bactericidal agent had been initiated on β-lactamase producers (3). It appears that certain cephalosporins, such as cefaclor and cefuroxime, are not bactericidal; while cefixime, and above all the combination amoxicillin-clavulanic acid, are bactericidal. It should be noted that cefuroxime is definitely bactericidal on β-lactamase non-producers.

Serious infections by strains of *M. catarrhalis* are rare but have been reported: endocarditis, meningitis, and infections in immunosuppressed patients, in particular, septicaemia. In case of severe infections with β-lactamase producing strains of *M. catarrhalis*, for which a bactericidal antibiotic therapy needs to be used, the use of third generation cephalosporins or the combination amoxicillin-clavulanic acid is advisable.

PREVALENCE OF RESISTANCE

β-µµlactamase producers

Strains isolated up to 1976 were non β-lactamase producers (31, 44). The first resistant strains were simultaneously reported in 1977 in France (7), Sweden, England, and Belgium. In a retrospective study on a collection of strains acquired between 1952 and 1980 in the U.S., Wallace *et al.* (44) reported two strains isolated in 1976 which were β-lactamase producers. After 1977, antibiotic resistance was reported to rise spectacularly across the globe: in Japan, China, Australia, and Finland. Moreover, there was an extraordinary increase in the percentage of β-lactamase producers: less than 10% before 1980 and more than 80% currently. The percentage of β-lactamase producing strains in France, as compiled from several multicentric surveys, is as follows: 82.7% in 1987 (13), 90% in 1994-1995 (12), and 95% in 2001-2002 (9). A study conducted between November 2002 and April 2003 in 20 countries in Europe, Asia, and Africa reported 94% of strains to be β-lactamase producers among the 1,047 strains collected (80% to 100% depending on the country) (1). In the U.S., a multicentric study including children and adults (26) conducted between September 2001 and April 2002 showed that the percentage of β-lactamase producers reached 95% regardless of age.

Tetracyclines

The MICs against strains resistant to tetracyclines are moderately high (16 µg/ml) (Table 3). These strains are rare in France: 0.6% in 1987 (13), 0.3% in 1994-1995 (12) and 0.3% in 2001-2002 (9); In an European study, MIC$_{90}$ was found to be ≤ 0.5 µg/ml in all countries (22). These results were confirmed by a global multicentric study conducted in 1999-2002 (Table 5) (8). MIC$_{90}$ was ≤ 0.5 µg/ml but strains with MIC ≥ 32 µg/ml have been isolated in each study period. For the period 1999-2000, the percentage of tetracycline resistant strains was 1.6% (21). However, a focused study in Saudi Arabia reported 14.5% of strains to be resistant (24).

Other antibiotics

In a global study (PROTEKT) from 1999-2000, one notes the absence of acquired resistance against other antibiotic classes: erythromycin, telithromycin, chloramphenicol, and levofloxacin (Table 5) (8). In another study, 100% of the strains were found to be susceptible to clarithromycin and azythromycin (21). These results have been confirmed in a recent European study which reported MICs$_{90}$ (µg/ml) as follows: erythromycin, 0.25; azithromycin, 0.06; levofloxacin, 0.06; moxifloxacin, 0.06; cotrimoxazole, 0.25 in four countries, but 0.5 in France and 1 in Spain (22). Clarithromycin resistance in one strain (MIC: 32 µg/ml) should be confirmed as the MIC of ery-

Table 5. MIC (μg/ml) of antibiotics against M. catarrhalis (8)

Time period	Tetracycline	Chloramphenicol	Erythromycin	Telithromycin	Co-trimoxazole	Levofloxacin
2000 (1158 isolates)						
MIC_{50}	0.25	0.5	0.25	0.06	0.25	0.03
MIC_{90}	0.5	0.5	0.25	0.12	0.5	0.03
MIC range	≤ 0.12 - ≥ 32	≤ 0.12 - 1	0.25 - 1	0.004 - 0.5	0.03 - 4	0.015 - 1
2001 (1156 isolates)						
MIC_{50}	0.25	0.5	0.25	0.06	0.12	0.03
MIC_{90}	0.25	0.5	0.25	0.12	0.25	0.03
MIC range	≤ 0.12 - ≥ 32	≤ 0.12 - 1	0.25 - 1	0.004 - 0.5	0.03 - 4	0.015 - 1
2002 (1170 isolates)						
MIC_{50}	0.25	0.5	0.25	0.06	0.12	0.03
MIC_{90}	0.5	0.5	0.25	0.12	0.5	0.06
MIC range	≤ 0.12 - ≥ 32	≤ 0.12 - 4	0.25 - 1	0.004 - 1	0.03 - 4	0.008 - 2

thromycin for the same strain was ≤ 0.5 μg/ml (37). In France, multicentric studies in 1987 (13) and 2002 (9) showed that 100% of the strains were susceptible to the amoxicillin-clavulanic acid combination, as well as to gentamicin, pefloxacin, ciprofloxacin, erythromycin, and pristinamycin. The level of susceptibilty to erythromycin (MIC_{50}, 0.25 μg/ml) was identical in both studies.

Fluoroquinolones are effective against all isolates (Table 5) (8, 9, 22). Rare strains which were resistant and for which antibiotic treatment failed, have also been described (17, 18); one strain had a MIC of ciprofloxacin equal to 4 μg/ml (17) and another was resistant to levofloxacin (18). It should be noted that in these cases, patients had received several fluoroquinolone treatments in the months preceding isolation of these strains.

Resistance to co-trimoxazole is very rare (Tables 3 and 5). A strain recovered in a French multicentric study from 2002 was resistant to this antibiotic. In a global study from 1999-2000, 97.8% of the strains were found to be susceptible (21).

ANTIBIOTICS TO BE STUDIED

The percentage of resistance to various antibiotic classes in this organism is so remarkably stable that some believe that antibiogram is unnecessary. A minimal testing would consist in detection of β-lactamase production using Nitrocefin®, as only this acquired resistance is frequent in *M. catarrhalis*. Presence of β-lactamase should be interpreted as resistance to amoxicillin, ampicillin, ticarcillin, and ureidopenicillins. For the first generation cephalosporins, presence of a β-lactamase, should be considered to cause "intermediate" resistance, due to lack of consensus in the literature regarding this antibiotic. As previously mentioned, EUCAST considers that *M. catharralis* isolates may be reported as resistant to benzylpenicillin, ampicillin, and amoxicillin, without any β-lactamase screening since the vast majority of *M. catarrhalis* strains produce a β-lactamase.

A more comprehensive antibiogram would include gentamicin, tetracycline, erythromycin, co-trimoxazole, nalidixic acid, and ciprofloxacin. A comprehensive monitoring should ensure absence of acquired resistance to amoxicillin-clavulanic acid combination, second generation cephalosporins, cefotaxamin, chloramphenicol, and telithromycin.

GENOTYPIC DETECTION OF RESISTANCE

These methods are not used routinely. Epidemiological studies of β-lactamases, BRO-1 and BRO-2 (5) suggested the use of primers (5'CTTG-GCGATGTCTACACC-3' and 5'AAGTTTG-GCATTGACACG) for amplification of the structural gene and part of the promoter region.

CONCLUSION

M. catarrhalis is an organism that displays weak virulence but may, in rare cases, cause severe infections. Therapeutic failures against this species arising from acquired resistance to antibiotics are infrequent. Nevertheless, previous treatment failures with aminopenicillins and first generation cephalosporins during infections with β-lactamase producing strains and recent failures against strains resistant to fluoroquinolones signal a need for vigilance.

REFERENCES

(1) **Beekmann, S. E., K. P. Heilmann, S. S. Richter, J. Garcia-de-Lomas, G. V. Doern, and the GRASP Group**. 2005. Antimicrobial resistance in *Streptococcus pneumoniae*, *Haemophilus influenzae*, *Moraxella catarrhalis* and group A beta-haemolytic streptococci in 2002-2003. Results of the multinational GRASP Surveillance Program. Int. J. Antimicrob. Agents **25**:148-156.

(2) **Bell, J. M., J. D. Turnidge, and R. N. Jones**. 2009. Development of a disk diffusion method for testing *Moraxella catarrhalis* susceptibility using clinical and laboratory standards institute methods: a SENTRY antimicrobial surveillance program report. J. Clin. Microbiol. **47**:2187-2193.

(3) **Bingen, E., F. Bourgeois, H. Chardon, C. Doit, and N. Lambert-Zechovsky**. 1992. Killing kinetics of five orally administered antibiotics at clinically achievable concentrations against *Moraxella catarrhalis*. Eur. J. Clin. Microbiol. Infect. Dis. **11**: 923-926.

(4) **Bootsma, H. J., P. C. Aerts, G. Posthuma, T. Harmsen, J. Verhoef, H. Van Dijk, and F. R. Mooi**. 1999. *Moraxella (Branhamella) catarrhalis* BRO β-lactamase : a lipoprotein of Gram-positive origin ? J. Bacteriol. **181**:5090-5093.

(5) **Bootsma, H. J., H. Van Dijk, J. Verhoef, A. Fleer, and F. R. Mooi**. 1996. Molecular characterization of the BRO beta-lactamase of *Moraxella (Branhamella) catarrhalis*. Antimicrob. Agents Chemother. **40**:966-972.

(6) **Brown, B. A., R. J. Wallace, C. W. Flanagan, R. W. Wilson, J. I. Luman, and S. D. Reddite**. 1989. Tetracycline and erythromycin resistance among clinical isolates of *Moraxella catarrhalis*. Antimicrob. Agents Chemother. **33**:1631-1633.

(7) **Buu Hoi-Dang Van, A., C. Brive le Bouguenec, M. Barthélemy, and R. Labia**. 1978. Novel β-lactamase from *Branhamella catarrhalis*. Ann. Microbiol. **129**:397-406.

(8) **Canton, R**. 2004. Resistance trends in *Moraxella catarrhalis* (PROTEKT Years 1-3 1999-2002). J. Chemother. **16 (Supp. 6)**: 63-70.

(9) **Chardon, H., T. Bensaid, O. Bellon, E. Lagier et réseau COLBVH**. 2002. Sensibilité de *Branhamella catarrhalis* aux antibiotiques : activité de la gatifloxacine. Enquête multicentrique du réseau COLBVH. Réunion Interdisciplinaire de Chimiothérapie Anti-Infectieuse (RICAI), Paris. Poster : 130/P1.

(10) **Chardon, H., O. Bellon, F. Bourgeois et E. Lagier**. 1989. Activité comparée de 5 macrolides sur 190 souches de *Branhamella catarrhalis*. Path. Biol. **37**:382-385.

(11) **Chardon, H., O. Bellon et E. Lagier**. 1989. Activité in vitro du céfixime (Oroken®) sur 200 souches de *Branhamella catarrhalis*. Comparaison au céfotaxime. Presse Méd. **18**:1556-1559.

(12) **Chardon, H., O. Bellon, L. Talon, C. May, E. Lagier et COLBVH**. 1997. Activité in vitro de la pristinamycine (Pyostacine®), de l'association quinupristine / dalfopristine (Synercid®) et du RPR106972 sur 200 souches de *Branhamella catarrhalis*. Réunion Interdisciplinaire de Chimiothérapie Anti-Infectieuse (RICAI), Paris. Abstract 63 / P6.

(13) **Chardon, H., E. Lagier, M. Thibault, P. Geslin, A. Boisivon, J. C. Ghnassia, P. Allouch, A. Sedallian, A. Marmonier, J. Tous, J. Y. Leberre , J. P. Darchis, P. Ross, Y. Boucaud Maître, A. Dublanchet, D. Fèvre, M. C. Letouzey et M. Melon**. 1988. Enquête multicentrique sur les isolements de *Branhamella catarrhalis* dans les centres hospitaliers généraux. Réunion Interdisciplinaire de Chimiothérapie Anti-Infectieuse (RICAI), Paris. Abstract : 72/P6.

(14) **Chardon, H., C. Meiffre, E. Lagier, A. Kazmierczak et R. Labia**. 1989. Activité in vitro des β-lactamines sur *Branhamella catarrhalis*. Méd. Mal. Infect. H.S. mai , 86-94.

(15) **Christensen, J. J., J. Keiding, H. Schumacher, and B. Bruun**. 1991. Recognition of new *Branhamella catarrhalis* β-lactamase BRO-3. J. Antimicrob. Chemother. **5**:774-775.

(16) **Clinical and Laboratory Standards Institute**. 2006. Methods for antimicrobial dilution and disk susceptibility testing of infrequently isolated or fastidious bacteria. Approved standard M45-A. Wayne, PA: Clinical and Laboratory Standards Institute.

(17) **Cunliffe, N. A., F. X. S. Emmanuel, and C. J. Thomson**. 1995. Lower respiratory tract infection due to ciprofloxacin resistant *Moraxella catarrhalis*. J. Antimicrob. Chemother. **36**:273-274.

(18) **DiPersio, J. R., R. N. Jones, T. Barret, G. V. Doern, and M. A. Pfaller**. 1998. Fluoroquinolone-resistant *Moraxella catarrhalis* in a patient with pneumonia: report from SENTRY Antimicrobial Surveillance Programm (1998). Diagn. Microbiol. Infect. Dis. **32**:131-135.

(19) **Doern, G. V., and T. A. Tubert**. 1988. In vitro activities of 39 antimicrobial agents for *Branhamella catarrhalis* and comparison of results with different quantitative susceptibility test methods. Antimicrob. Agents Chemother. **32**:259-261.

(20) **Farmer, T., and C. Reeading**. 1982. β-lactamases of *Branhamella catarrhali*s and their inhibition by clavulanic acid. Antimicrob. Agents Chemother. **21**:506-508.

(21) **Hoban, D., and D. Felmingham**. 2002. The PROTEKT surveillance study: antimicrobial susceptibility of *Haemophilus influenzae* and *Moraxella catarrhalis* from community-acquired respiratory tract infections. J. Antimicrob. Chemother. **50 (suppl. S1)**:49-59.

(22) **Jones, M. E., R. S. Blosser-Middleton, I. A. Critchley, J. A. Karlowsky, C. Thornsberry, and D. J. Sahm**. 2003. In vitro susceptibility of *Streptococcus pneumoniae*, *Haemophilus influenzae* and *Moraxella catarrhalis*: a European multicenter study during 2000-2001. Clin. Microbiol. Infect. **9**:590-599.

(23) **Jones, R. N., and H. M. Sommers**. 1986. Identification and antimicrobial susceptibility testing of *Branhamella catarrhalis* in United States laboratories, 1983-1985. Drugs **31 (Suppl. 3)**:34-37

(24) **Kadry, A. A., S. I. Fouda, N. A. Elkhizzi, and A. M. Shibl**. 2003. Correlation between susceptibility and BRO type enzyme of *Moraxella catarrhalis* strains. Int. J. Antimicrobial. Agents. **22**:532-536.

(25) **Kallings, I**. 1986. Sensitivity of *Branhamella catarrhalis* to oral antibiotics. Drugs **31, S 3**:17-22.

(26) **Karlowsky, J., C. Thornsberry, I. A. Critchley, M. E. Jones, A. T. Evangelista, G. J. Noel, and D. J. Sahm**. 2003. Susceptibilities to levofloxacin in *Streptococcus pneumoniae, Haemophilus influenzae*, and *Moraxella catarrhalis* clinical isolates from Children: results from 2000-2001 and 2001-2002 TRUST Studies in the United States. Antimicrob. Agents Chemother. **47**:1790-1797.

(27) **Laurans, G., and J. Orfila**. 1991. *Moraxella (Branhamella) catarrhalis* dans les infections respiratoires : activité du céfuroxime. Med. Mal. Infect. **21 (H. S.)**:34-40.

(28) **Luman, L., R. W. Wilson, R. J. Wallace, and D. R. Nash**. 1986. Disk diffusion susceptibility of *Branhamella catarrhalis* and relationship of β-lactam zone size to β-lactamase production. Antimicrob. Agents Chemother. **30**:774-776.

(29) **Nash, D. R., R. J. Wallace, V. A. Steingrube, and P. A. Shurin**. 1986. Isoelectric focusing of β-lactamases from sputum and middle ear isolates of *Branhamella catarrhalis* recovered in the United States. Drugs **31 (Suppl.3)**:48-54.

(30) **Ninane, G., J. Joly, and M. Kraytman**. 1978. Bronchopulmonary infection due to *Branhamella catarrhalis*: 11 cases assessed by transtracheal puncture. Br. Med. J. **1**:276-278.

(31) **Philippon, A., J. Y. Riou, M. Guibourdenche, and F. Sotolongo**. 1986. Detection, distribution, inhibition of *Branhamella catarrhalis* β-lactamases. Drugs. **31**:S64-S69.

(32) **Richter S. S., P. L. Winokur, A. B. Brueggemann, H. K. Huynh, P. R. Rhomberg, E. M. Wingert, and G. V. Doern**. 2000. Molecular characterization of the β-lactamases from clinical isolates of *Moraxella (Branhamella) catarrhalis* obtained from 24 U. S. medical centers during 1994-1995 and 1997-1998. Antimicrob. Agents Chemother. **44**:444-446.

(33) **Roberts, M. C., B. A. Brown, V. A. Steingrube, and R. J. Wallace**. 1990. Genetic basis of tetracycline resistance in *Moraxella (Branhamella) catarrhalis*. Antimicrob. Agents Chemother. **34**:1816-1818.

(34) **Robledano, L., M. J. Rivera, I. Otal, and R. Gomez-Lus**. 1987. Enzymatic modification of aminoglycoside antibiotics by *Branhamella catarrhalis* carrying an R factor. Drugs Exp. Clin. Res. **13**:137-143.

(35) **Schmitz, F. J., A. Beeck, M. Perdikouli, M. Boos, S. Mayer, S. Scheuring, K. Köhrer, J. Verhoef, and A. C. Fluit**. 2002. Production of BRO β-lactamases and resistance to complement in European *Moraxella catarrhalis* isolates. J. Clin. Microbiol. **40**:1546-1548.

(36) **Slevin, N. J., J. Aitken, and P. E. Thornley**. 1984. Clinical and microbiological features of *Branhamella catarrhalis* bronchopulmonary infections. Lancet **i**:782-783.

(37) **Soriano, F., J. J. Granizo, P. Coronel, M. Gimeno, E. Rodenas, M. Gracia, C. Garcia, R. Fernandez-Roblas, J. Esteban, and I. Gadea**. Antimicrobial susceptibility of *Haemophilus influenzae, Haemophilus parainfluenzae* and *Moraxella catarrhalis* isolated from adult patients with respiratory tract infections in four Southern European countries. The ARISE project. Int. J. Antimicrob. Agents. **23**:296-299.

(38) **Spencer, R. C., and P. F. Wheat**. 1990. In vitro activity of roxithromycin against *Branhamella catarrhalis*. J. Antimicrob. Chemother. **26**:153-154.

(39) **Steingrube, V. A., R. J. Wallace, and D. Beaulieu**. 1993. A membrane-bound precursor β-lactamase in strains of *Moraxella catarrhalis* and *Moraxella nonliquefaciens* that produce periplasmic BRO-1 and BRO-2 β-lactamases. J. Antimicrob. Chemother. **31**:237-244.

(40) **Stobberingh, E. E., B. I. Davies, and C. P. A. Van Boven**. 1984. *Branhamella catarrhalis*: antibiotic sensitivities and β-lactamases. J. Antimicrob. Chemother. **13**:55-64.

(41) **Sweeney, K. G., A. Verghese, and C. A. Needham**. 1985. In vitro susceptibilities of isolates from patients with *Branhamella catarrhalis* pneumonia compared with those of colonizing strains. Antimicrob. Agents Chemother. **27**:499-502.

(42) **Van Hare, G. F., P. A. Shurin, C. D. Marchant, N. A. Cartelli, C. E. Johnson, D. Fulton, S. Cartlin, and C. H. Kim**. 1987. Acute otitis media caused by *Branhamella catarrhalis*: biology and therapy. Rev. Infect. Dis. **9**:16-27.

(43) **Wald, E. R., D. D. Rohn, D. M. Chiponis, M. M. Blattner, K. S. Reisiger, and F. P. Wucher**. 1983. Quantitative cultures of middle-ear fluid in acute otitis media. J. Pediatr. **102**:259-261.

(44) **Wallace, R. J., V. A. Steingrube, D. R. Nash, D. G. Hollis, C. Flanagan, B. A. Brown, A. Labidi, and R. E. Weaver**. 1989. BRO β-lactamase of *Branhamella catarrhalis* and *Moraxella* subgenus *Moraxella* including evidence for chromosomal β-lactamase transfer by conjugation in *B. catarrhalis, M. nonliquefaciens*, and *M. lacunata*. Antimicrob. Agents Chemother. **33**:1845-1854.

Chapter 40. *PASTEURELLA*

Pierre-Yves DONNIO

INTRODUCTION

The choice of antibiotic therapy for treatment of human or animal pasteurelloses is rather broad as the causative bacteria are naturally susceptible to several classes of antibiotics and acquired resistance is seldom seen (3). All β-lactams, except a few first-generation cephalosporins, are effective against pasteurellae, including chloramphenicol, tetracyclines, quinolones, sulfonamides, trimethoprim, and co-trimoxazole (3, 4). In contrast, these bacteria display variable susceptibility to aminoglycosides: while 80% of the strains are susceptible to gentamicin, most are intermediate or resistance to amikacin (MIC range of 8 – 64 µg/ml, MIC_{90} = 32 µg/ml) (unpublished data). Further, these have an intermediate susceptibility to macrolides and are resistant to lincosamides (4).

ACQUIRED RESISTANCE

Among the species and subspecies of the *Pasteurella multocida* "complex" that cause, zoonosis (*P. multocida* subsp. *multocida*, *P. multocida* subsp. *septica*, *P. multocida* subsp. *gallicida*, *P. canis*, and *P. stomatis*) acquired resistance is rare and may be seen against β-lactams, tetracyclines, and quinolones.

Resistance to β-lactams by β-lactamase production

Resistance due to production of the ROB-1 type of β-lactamase has been reported in 12% of the strains of *P. multicoda* of bovine origin in France (6, 9) but is rare in strains isolated from human infections (10, 12). Like that from *Haemophilus influenzae*, the enzyme inactivates aminopenicillins, carboxypenicillins, ureidopenicillins, and first-generation cephalosporins and is inhibited by clavulanic acid.

Recently, two human isolates that produced TEM-1 β-lactamases have been described (8, 11). Both ROB-1 and TEM-1 enzymes have substrate profiles that are too similar to allowphenotypic differentiation.

Resistance to tetracyclines

Resistance to tetracyclines is mostly due to the *tet*(H) gene, putatively encoding an efflux protein (5). The *tet*(H) gene, which is apparently indigenous to *Pasteurella* spp., was detected on plasmids and also in the chromosome, as part of complete or truncated transposons (5, 6). Other resistance genes that have been reported in *Pasteurella* spp. are responsible for efflux [*tet*(B), *tet*(D), *tet*(G), and *tet*(L)] or ribosomal protection [*tet*(M)] (13).

Resistance to quinolones

Resistance to quinolones is linked to mutations in the structural genes for type II topoisomerases, *gyrA* and *parC*, comprising the *q*uinolone *r*esistance *d*etermining *r*egion (QRDR). In clinical isolates, the level of resistance to nalidixic acid may sometimes be high, but stays low for fluoroquinolones. In the long term, accumulation of mutations may lead to high level fluoroquinolone resistance (1).

METHODS

For determination of MICs, both the Clinical and Laboratory Standards Institute (CLSI) and the European Committee on Antimicrobial Susceptibility Testing (EUCAST) recommend the broth microdilution technique (http://www.eucast.org/, 2). Cation-adjusted Mueller-Hinton broth supplemented with 2.5-5% lysed horse blood should be inoculated with a direct colony suspension equivalent to a 0.5 McFarland standard and incubated at 35°C in ambient air for 18-24 h. For disk diffusion, CLSI and EUCAST recommend Mueller-Hinton agar with 5% sheep blood and Mueller-Hinton supplemented with lysed horse blood and NAD, respectively. Agar plates are inoculated with a direct colony suspension equivalent to a 0.5 McFarland standard and incubated at 35°C in ambient air for 18-24 h. CLSI breakpoints for penicillins, cephalosporins, quinolones, tetracyclines, macrolides, trimethoprim-sulfamethoxazole, and chloramphenicol are available. However, for most antimicrobials, only breakpoints for the "susceptible" category are provided since resistant isolates are rare or absent. EUCAST does not provide specific breakpoints for *Pasteurella spp*. However, non-species related breakpoints determined mainly on the basis of PK/PD data may be used.

E-test® may be used as a routine method for determination of MICs for various bacterial species. However, correlation with the reference MIC method has been poorly studied for *Pasteurella spp*. The manufacturer recommends Mueller-Hinton agar with 5% sheep blood swabbed with a colony suspension equivalent to a 1 McFarland standard and incubated at 35°C with 5% CO_2 for 48 h.

CONTROL STRAINS

The CLSI recommends *Streptococcus pneumoniae* ATCC 49619, *Escherichia coli* ATCC 35218 when testing b-lactam/b-lactamase inhibitor combinations, and *Staphylococcus aureus* ATCC 25923 for disk diffusion (amoxicillin-clavulanic acid and doxycycline) (2).

ANTIBIOTICS TO BE STUDIED

The minimal panel of antibiotics to be tested should include those molecules that are most suitable for treatment or prevention of pasteurellosis:
- an aminopenicillin (ampicillin or amoxicillin), amoxicillin-clavulanic acid,
- a third-generation injectable cephalosporin (cefotaxime or ceftriaxone),
- a tetracycline (the response is valid for the entire class),
- nalidixic acid and a fluoroquinolone (ciprofloxacin or ofloxacin). A reduced susceptibility to nalidixic acid necessitates determination of fluoroquinolones MIC (1).

Other therapeutically useful molecules that could be tested are trimethoprim-sulfamethoxazole and third-generation oral cephalosporins (cefixime, cefpodoxime). However, it is not advisable to study aminoglycosides for which the disk diffusion method usually gives false susceptibility results. The same is true for the macrolides for which the report is usually intermediate.

β-LACTAMASE SCREENING

The synergy between aminopenicillin and the β-lactamase inhibitor could be discrete, especially for strains that produce ROB-1 (9). Monitoring for a β-lactamase should hence be routinely carried out by the chromogenic method (Nitrocefin®).

REFERENCES

(1) **Cardenas, M., J. Barbe, M. Llagostera, E. Miro, F. Navarro, B. Mirelis, G. Prats, and I. Badiola.** 2001. Quinolone resistance-determining regions of *gyrA* and *parC* in *Pasteurella multocida* strains with different levels of nalidixic acid resistance. Antimicrob. Agents Chemother. **45**:990-991.

(2) **Clinical and Laboratory Standards Institute.** 2006. Methods for antimicrobial dilution and disk susceptibility testing of infrequently isolated or fastidious bacteria. Approved standard M45-A. Wayne, PA: Clinical and Laboratory Standards Institute.

(3) **Goldstein, E. J., D. M. Citron, M. Hudspeth, S. Hunt Gerardo, and C. V. Merriam.** 1997. In vitro activity of Bay 12-8039, a new 8-methoxyquinolone, compared to the activities of 11 other oral antimicrobial agents against 390 aerobic and anaerobic bacteria isolated from human and animal bite wound skin and soft tissue infections in humans. Antimicrob. Agents Chemother. **41**:1552–1557.

(4) **Goldstein, E. J., D. M. Citron, and G. A. Richwald.** 1988. Lack of in vitro efficacy of oral forms of certain cephalosporins, erythromycin, and oxacillin against *Pasteurella multocida*. Antimicrob. Agents Chemother. **32**:213-215.

(5) **Hansen, L. M., P. C. Blanchard, and D. C. Hirsh.** 1996. Distribution of *tet*(H) among *Pasteurella* isolates from the United States and Canada. Antimicrob. Agents Chemother. **40**:1558-1560

(6) **Joly, B., J.L. Martel, R. Michel, A. Reynaud, et R. Cluzel.** 1986. Sensibilité aux antibiotiques et production de β-lactamases chez les souches de *Pasteurella* d'origine bovine isolées en France. Méd. Mal. Inf. **16**:S52-S56.

(7) **Kehrenberg C., C. Werckenthin, and S. Schwarz.** 1998. Tn*5706*, a transposon-like element from *Pasteurella multocida* mediating tetracycline resistance. Antimicrob. Agents Chemother. **42**:2116-2118.

(8) **Lion C., A. Lozniewski, V. Rosner, and M. Weber.** 1999. Lung abscess due to β-lactamase producing *Pasteurella multocida*. Clin. Infect. Dis. **29**:1345-1346.

(9) **Livrelli, V. O., A. Darfeuille-Michaud, C. D. Rich, B. H. Joly, and J. L. Martel.** 1988. Genetic determinant of the ROB-1 β-lactamase in bovine and porcine *Pasteurella* strains. Antimicrob. Agents Chemother. **32**:1282-1284.

(10) **Mesnard, R., P.-Y. Donnio, F. Denis, A. Philippon, et J.-L. Avril.** 1989. Une deuxième souche de *Pasteurella multocida* d'origine humaine productrice d'une β-lactamase. Méd. Mal. Inf. **19**:422-423.

(11) **Naas T., F. Benaoudia, L. Lebrun, and P. Nordmann.** 2001. Molecular identification of TEM-1 β-lactamase in a *Pasteurella multocida* isolate of human origin. Eur. J. Clin. Microbiol. Infect. Dis. **20**:210-213.

(12) **Rosenau, A., F. Laporte-Tron, M. Boulot-Tolle, A. Philippon, T. N'Guyen-Phuong, F. Escande, E. N. Moyen, et J. L. Fauchère.** 1988. Infection pulmonaire humaine par une souche de *Pasteurella multocida* productrice de β-lactamase. Méd. Mal. Inf. **10**:440-444.

(13) **Roberts, M. C.** 2005. Update on acquired tetracycline resistance genes. FEMS Microbiol. Lett. **245**:195-203.

Chapter 41. *LEGIONELLA*

Sophie JARRAUD and Jerome ETIENNE

INTRODUCTION

Legionella are facultative intracellular bacteria that multiply in the environment in protozoans, especially amoebas, and in man in various types of cells such as alveolar macrophages, monocytes or pulmonary epithelial cells. Although about twenty species have been isolated at least once in human medicine (*L. longbeachae, L. micdadei, L. jordanis, L. bozemanii*, etc.), *L. pneumophila* is responsible for more than 95% of all legionellosis and serogroup 1 of this species (Lp1) is associated with more than 80% of cases. Despite this diversity, the antibiotic susceptibility and clinical manifestations of the various species appear to be similar to those of *L. pneumophila*, the most extensively studied species. Data on the potential efficacy and utility of anti-*Legionella* antibiotics are based on four methods: (i) *in vitro* study of extracellular activity, (ii) *in vitro* study of intracellular activity, (iii) activity in animal models, and (iv) clinical studies. *Legionella* are characterized by marked susceptibility to the antibiotics commonly used for the treatment of legionellosis, making systematic antibiotic susceptibility testing of these strains clinically irrelevant. Tests of extracellular activity of antibiotics by determination of minimum inhibitory concentrations (MICs) can be used, but standardization of MIC determination against *Legionella* is difficult, especially regarding the choice of medium, inoculum, and incubation times, because of particular culture conditions.

METHODS

In vitro susceptibility

Extracellular activity

The extracellular activity of antibiotics on *Legionella* can be studied by conventional methods for determination of MICs on agar medium or by E-test® (11, 23, 31). However, no standardized method is available for the study of *Legionella* and published studies vary considerably in terms of culture medium, inoculum, incubation temperature and atmosphere, and incubation time. BCYE (Buffered Charcoal-Yeast Extract) is the medium of choice for isolation of *Legionella* and initial susceptibility studies were performed on this medium due to the optimal growth. Various studies have shown that the choice of the culture medium is essential, as culture media can inhibit the activity of many antibiotics (28, 29). This inhibition can be due to the presence of charcoal in the BCYE medium but also to the acidity of the media, their iron content, or factors generated during autoclaving (6). The binding of antibiotics to charcoal has been well documented. Quinolones, erythromycin, and rifampin are rapidly and almost completely bound to charcoal, and the free fraction represents less than 8% of the total antibiotic concentration (33). Some authors have proposed the calculation of a corrected geometric MIC derived from the MIC determined on BCYE and corrected according to the free fraction of each antibiotic. In these studies, correction of MICs leads to a greater than tenfold reduction of the original value. These corrected MICs become comparable to those obtained on media not containing charcoal (33). Several charcoal-free media have been proposed: BYE (Buffered Yeast Extract) (23), BSYE (Buffered Starch Yeast Extract) (22, 28) or YEB (Yeast Extract Broth) (30). Several investigators have recommended the BSYE medium rather than BCYE. However, growth of *Legionella* spp. on BSYE is weaker than that of *L. pneumophila* and therefore not reproducible (28) and requires an inoculum of 10^6 CFU/spot. BYE is the most widely used medium and the MICs obtained are globally 4 to 6 dilutions lower than those obtained with the BCYE medium (12). Studies by Rhomberg *et al.* suggest that charcoal has little or no effect on the results by E-test® (31). However, these findings have not been confirmed by other authors (23).

The inoculum effect on the MIC values is generally negligible. The inoculum is prepared from a 48-h culture on BCYE medium. For dilution in agar medium, the turbidity of the bacterial suspension obtained in sterile water is adjusted to 1 unit of McFarland's range, which corresponds to about 10^8 CFU/ml. Petri dishes are inoculated to obtain a final concentration of 10^5 CFU. For the E-test®, the same suspension is spread onto a 140 mm Petri dish of BYE and an antibiotic strip is applied to each plate. Due to the large inhibition zones, it is not recommended to use several strips on the same Petri dish. In view of the long generation time, Legionella cultures should be examined after aerobic incubation at 35°C (without CO_2) for a minimum of 48 h. Cultures can be examined at 72 h, as the incubation time does not alter the activity of the antibiotics (23, 29, 34). Using the macrodilution technique, the MIC for each drug could be determined also in 96-well microtitres plates using liquid BYE-α medium (22, 32). MICs correspond to the lowest antibiotic concentrations with no visible growth after 48h incubation of the plates at 37°C.

According to the conventional method, three reference strains, L. pneumophila serogroup 1 (ATCC 33152), Staphylococcus aureus ATCC 29213 and Escherichia coli ATCC 25922, are studied in parallel on BYE and Mueller-Hinton media to assess a possible interference with the specific culture medium and to control antibiotic concentrations. The inoculum of S. aureus and E. coli reference strains is that recommended for the MIC technique chosen.

Intracellular activity

Studies of the extracellular activity of antibiotics are technically easy but do not take into account the intracellular penetration of the antibiotic. Many antibiotics, including β-lactams, have a very good activity against extracellular Legionella (29, 35). However, as β-lactams do not penetrate the cells, they are inactive on intracellular Legionella. Conversely, some antibiotics such as the tetracyclines appear to be less active on extracellular Legionella than on intracellular Legionella. This is also the case for azithromycin which has MICs equivalent to those of erythromycin (Table 1) but which is more active than erythromycin on intracellular Legionella.

The intracellular activity of antibiotics can be studied after growth of L. pneumophila on various types of cell cultures such as alveolar guinea-pig macrophages, human monocyte-macrophage cell lines (HL-60 and HeLa cell line) (17, 36, 37), human monocyte cell line THP-1 (21), alveolar epithelial cells A 549 (21), murine macrophage cell line J774.1 (17). The intracellular activity of antibiotics and the intracellular growth of L. pneumophila vary as a function of the various cell types used (21). The capacity of antibiotics to inhibit the intracellular growth of bacteria is determined by quantification of bacterial concentrations over time. The concept of minimal extracellular concentration inhibiting intracellular multiplication of L. pneumophila (MIEC) has been defined to evaluate the intracellular activity of antimicrobial agents. The MIECs of β-lactams and aminoglycosides are clearly higher than conventional MICs, while MIECs and MICs are similar for macrolides, quinolones, rifampin, and minocycline (17, 38).

The results obtained by studying the intracellular activity are globally well correlated with those of studies in animal models. This technique is long, expensive, requires cell culture skills and therefore cannot be easily applied in routine practice. Colorimetric quantification systems have been developed for the analysis of larger numbers of samples (17) and real-time PCR quantification systems have been developed to allow more rapid results (32).

Table 1. MICs (μg/ml) of various antibiotics for L. pneumophila

Antibiotic	MIC_{90}	Range	Reference
Macrolides			
Erythromycin	0.06 - 1.0	≤ 0.015 - 1.0	6, 7, 13, 15, 22, 23, 28, 30, 33, 34
Spiramycin	1 - 5	1 - 5	6, 14
Clarithromycin	≤ 0.004 - 0.12	≤ 0.004 - 0.12	7, 28, 30, 34
Azithromycin	0.06 - 2.77	0.03 - 4.0	7, 13, 15, 19, 22, 28
Roxithromycin	0.12 - 0.25	0.03 - 0.5	7, 34
Quinolones			
Ofloxacin	0.015 - 0.25	0.015 - 0.25	7, 15
Pefloxacin	0.5	0.25 - 0.5	18
Ciprofloxacin	0.015 - 0.38	0.008 - 0.38	7, 15, 19, 22, 23, 28, 30, 33
Levofloxacin	0.015 - 0.125	0.015 - 0.125	7, 15, 19, 28, 34
Moxifloxacin	0.016 - 0.06	0.016 - 0.06	7, 33, 34
Lomefloxacin	0.06	0.06 - 0.12	18
Rifampin	0.0028 - 0.008	< 0.002 - 0.003	7, 15, 22, 23, 30, 33, 34
Quinupristin/dalfopristin	0.008 - 1	0.008 - 2	5

Animal models

The activity of antibiotics can also be studied experimentally in guinea-pigs or rats by inhalation of infected aerosols or by direct intratracheal inoculation. Several studies have also used intraperitoneal infection in guinea-pigs (11).

USUAL SUSCEPTIBILITY

All published studies confirm the excellent *in vitro* activity of the main antibiotics used to treat Legionellosis: macrolides, fluoroquinolones, and rifampin (7, 11).

Macrolides and streptogramins

Erythromycin is active against extracellular *Legionella* with MICs ranging from 0.06 µg/ml to 1 µg/ml depending on the culture conditions. The MICs of erythromycin are equivalent to those of josamycin and azithromycin (0.06 to 2.7 µg/ml) but erythromycin is less active than clarithromycin ($\leq$ 0.004 to 0.12 µg/ml) and more active than spiramycin (1 to 5 µg/ml) (Table 1). Evaluation of the activity of macrolides on cell culture showed that the most active inhibitors of intracellular multiplication of *L. pneumophila* are, in decreasing order of activity: azithromycin, erythromycin, roxithromycin, and clarithromycin (36). Azithromycin exerts a bactericidal effect in guinea-pig alveolar macrophages unlike erythromycin (bacteriostatic) and has a higher post-antibiotic effect. In experimental models, azithromycin appears to be more active than erythromycin or clarithromycin (12). Although it has a poor *in vitro* activity, spiramycin is as active as erythromycin in guinea-pig experimental models of legionellosis (8). The MBC/MIC ratio is 8 for erythromycin and azithromycin.

The dalfopristin-quinupristin combination is more active (MICs 0.008 to 1 µg/ml) (10) or just as active (MICs of 0.06 to 2 µg/ml) (5) *in vitro* on extracellular *L. pneumophila* as erythromycin. While this antibiotic combination penetrates easily into murine macrophages with a concentration 30- to 50-fold higher than the extracellular concentration (5), it appears to be only partially active against intracellular *L. pneumophila* and is less effective than azithromycin and erythromycin (13, 34). No experience is available in animal models due to the toxicity of the combination for guinea-pigs and no clinical studies have been reported.

Ketolides are active on extracellular and intracellular *Legionella* (34) and are effective in guinea-pig models of pneumonia.

Quinolones

All fluoroquinolones have an excellent extracellular activity against *Legionella* with low MICs, often less than 0.01 µg/ml (Table 1). Levofloxacin, moxifloxacin, ciprofloxacin, lomefloxacin, and ofloxacin have similar MICs between 0.06 and 0.38 µg/ml, while pefloxacin is the least active molecule (MICs of 0.25 to 0.5 µg/ml). In HL-60 cells, Stout *et al.* reported the superior intracellular activity and post-antibiotic effect of levofloxacin compared to ciprofloxacin and ofloxacin (in decreasing order of activity) (37). Other studies have reported similar activities for these fluoroquinolones on guinea-pig alveolar macrophages (15). Studies on cell cultures and animal models show that fluoroquinolones are more active than erythromycin (1, 11, 36). Quinolones enter and are readily concentrated in the intracellular compartment. Their advantages include an intracellular bactericidal activity and a prolonged post-antibiotic effect. MBC/MIC ratios are identical (value of 4) for all fluoroquinolones (levofloxacin, moxifloxacin, ciprofloxacin, ofloxacin) (15). The post-antibiotic effect of fluoroquinolones and rifampin is greater than that of erythromycin and azithromycin (15).

Rifampin

Rifampin is very active on extracellular (very low MICs ranging from 0.0028 to 0.008 µg/ml) and intracellular *Legionella* and is effective in guinea-pig experimental models (3, 30, 34). In vitro, rifampin-resistant strains of *L. pneumophila* have been selected and become predominant in culture medium containing rifampin only (4). The MBC/MIC ratio is 4 for rifampin (15).

β-lactams and β-lactamase inhibitors

β-lactams (amoxicillin and cephalosporins) and especially imipenem are active *in vitro* on extracellular *Legionella* but are inactive against intracellular bacteria and ineffective in animal models. Various studies have demonstrated the intracellular activity of clavulanic acid alone in a MRC5 cell model, while amoxicillin was not active in the same culture system (35). Other authors reported the inefficacy of clavulanic acid and amoxicillin on Mono-Mac 6 cells, but at lower antibiotic concentrations (19). The *in vivo* activity of clavulanic acid, with or without amoxicillin, was demonstrated in studies of rat respiratory tract infections, while amoxicillin alone was ineffective.

Aminoglycosides

Aminoglycosides (gentamicin and amikacin) are active against extracellular *Legionella* with MICs between 0.5 and 1 µg/ml (14, 29) and gentamicin has demonstrated an intracellular activity in several studies, but this antibiotic has little or no efficacy in guinea-pig experimental models. These discordant results are probably due to inhibition of intracellular bacterial growth that is too slow to be effective in human or animal infections (11).

Other molecules

Cotrimoxazole possesses an intracellular activity against *Legionella* and is effective in the treatment of experimental legionellosis in guinea-pigs. Few clinical data are available, but successes and failures of treatment have both been reported (11).

Tetracyclines are inactive *in vitro* against extracellular *Legionella* probably because of inactivation of these antibiotics by agar culture media. MICs are between 16 and 32 µg/ml for tetracycline and between 1 and 8 µg/ml for doxycycline and minocycline (14). The intracellular activity and that in animal models varies according to the study, but tetracyclines are always less active than macrolides, quinolones, and rifampin (11).

Antibiotic combinations

Barker and Farrel showed *in vitro* that the combination of rifampin and a bactericidal concentration of erythromycin was synergistic (4). Similar results were also observed for combinations of ciprofloxacin and erythromycin or rifampin. Clarithromycin and azithromycin are more active in combination with a fluoroquinolone than with erythromycin. In intracellular models using human monocytes, the addition of rifampin or erythromycin (at a concentration tenfold higher than their MICs) did not affect the antibacterial activity of levofloxacin (2). The value of fluoroquinolone plus macrolide combinations compared to fluoroquinolone monotherapy has not been demonstrated clinically (11). Similarly, no convincing data have demonstrated the benefit of adding rifampin to fluoroquinolones or macrolides compared to monotherapy without rifampin (3, 16).

INCIDENCE OF RESISTANCE

Intrinsic resistance

In vitro, most antibiotics are active against *Legionella* except vancomycin, lincosamides, colistin, and sulfonamides. Noninducible β-lactamases have been detected in almost all *Legionella* species (except in *L. micdadei*, *L. feelei* and *L. maceachernii*) which hydrolyze penicillins (penicillin G and ampicillin) and most cephalosporins. Cefoxitin and cefuroxime are not hydrolyzed and imipenem is very active *in vitro*. β-lactamase inhibitors (such as clavulanic acid) partially prevent hydrolysis of penicillins and cephalosporin (24).

Selection of resistance

Antibiotic-resistant strains have not yet been isolated in clinical practice. However, several early studies demonstrated the ease with which erythromycin-, ciprofloxacin-, and rifampin-resistant mutants can be selected *in vitro* (9, 25, 26). In the presence of rifampin or ciprofloxacin, the frequency of mutation of *Legionella* was estimated to be between 10^8 to 10^7 (25). In vitro selection of *L. pneumophila* mutants against which the MICs of fluoroquinolones are eightfold higher is obtained in less than thirty subcultures on media containing a sub-inhibitory concentration of antibiotic. These mutants are stable and cross-resistant to the various quinolones (ciprofloxacin, levofloxacin, moxifloxacin, trovafloxacin, and clinafloxacin) (20). For some mutants, the decreased susceptibility to fluoroquinolones is associated with a mutation of codon 83 of *gyrA*. As not all of the mutants observed present this mutation, other targets and resistance mechanisms are probably involved, such as topoisomerase IV and efflux pumps. More recently, mutations that affected also topoisomerase II – encoding genes *parC* and *gyrB* have been described (Almahmoud et al, 2009). Rifampin resistance in four species, *L. bozemanii*, *L. longbeachae*, *L. micdadei* and *L. pneumophila*, is associated with *rpoB* mutations (27).

Unlike in vitro tests, treatments of experimental pneumonia in guinea-pigs have not demonstrated any selection of resistance of *L. pneumophila* to rifampin.

RELEVANCE OF ANTIBIOTIC SUSCEPTIBILITY TESTING

As *Legionella* are intracellular organisms, *in vitro* studies of the extracellular antibiotic susceptibility of these bacteria cannot be directly correlated with the clinical activity of these molecules. *In vitro* extracellular susceptibility studies must be considered to be screening tests to determine whether an antibacterial agent is inactive without being predictive of its intracellular efficacy and its *in vivo* efficacy. Systematic antibiotic susceptibility testing of *Legionella* strains is therefore not recommended. Some authors suggest that treatment failures are unlikely to be related to the emergence of resistance following the use of antimicrobial agents. As legionellosis is not transmitted from human to human, but is related to exposure to contaminated water aerosols, there is a low potential for exposure of *Legionella* to antibiotics before infection. The absence of antibiotic resistance in clinical strains is probably due to the absence of selection pressure in the *Legionella* natural environment. Nevertheless, at the individual level, *Legionella* could acquire resistance during treatment. An antibiotic susceptibility study of *Legionella* isolated from patients in treatment failure can be recommended together with more global surveillance of antibiotic resistance by specialized microbiology laboratories. Depending on the treatment prescribed, the *in vitro* activity of erythromycin, azithromycin, ciprofloxacin, levofloxacin, moxifloxacin, or rifampin could be studied by E-test® as described above.

REFERENCES

(1) **Baltch, A. L., L. H. Bopp, R. P. Smith, P. B. Michelsen, and W. J. Ritz.** 2005. Antibacterial activities of gemifloxacin, levofloxacin, gatifloxacin, moxifloxacin and erythromycin against intracellular *Legionella pneumophila* and *Legionella micdadei* in human monocytes. J Antimicrob Chemother **56**:104-9.

(2) **Baltch, A. L., R. P. Smith, M. A. Franke, and P. B. Michelsen.** 1998. Antibacterial effects of levofloxacin, erythromycin, and rifampin in a human monocyte system against *Legionella pneumophila*. Antimicrob Agents Chemother **42**:3153-6.

(3) **Baltch, A. L., R. P. Smith, and W. Ritz.** 1995. Inhibitory and bactericidal activities of levofloxacin, ofloxacin, erythromycin, and rifampin used singly and in combination against *Legionella pneumophila*. Antimicrob Agents Chemother **39**:1661-6.

(4) **Barker, J. E., and I. D. Farrell.** 1990. The effects of single and combined antibiotics on the growth of *Legionella pneumophila* using time-kill studies. J Antimicrob Chemother **26**:45-53.

(5) **Bebear, C., and D. H. Bouanchaud.** 1997. A review of the in-vitro activity of quinupristin/dalfopristin against intracellular pathogens and Mycoplasmas. J Antimicrob Chemother 39 Suppl **A**:59-62.

(6) **Bornstein, N., C. Roudier, and J. Fleurette.** 1985. Determination of the activity on *Legionella* of eight macrolides and related agents by comparative testing on three media. J Antimicrob Chemother **15**:17-22.

(7) **Dedicoat, M., and P. Venkatesan.** 1999. The treatment of Legionnaires' disease. J Antimicrob Chemother **43**:747-52.

(8) **Dournon, E., and P. Rajagopalan.** 1988. Comparison of spiramycin and erythromycin in the treatment of experimental guinea pig legionellosis. J Antimicrob Chemother 22 Suppl **B**:69-72.

(9) **Dowling, J. N., D. A. McDevitt, and A. W. Pasculle.** 1985. Isolation and preliminary characterization of erythromycin-resistant variants of *Legionella micdadei* and *Legionella pneumophila*. Antimicrob Agents Chemother **27**:272-4.

(10) **Dubois, J., and J. R. Joly.** 1992. In-vitro activity of RP 59500, a new synergic antibacterial agent, against *Legionella* spp. J Antimicrob Chemother 30 Suppl **A**:77-81.

(11) **Edelstein, P. H.** 1995. Antimicrobial chemotherapy for legionnaires' disease: a review. Clin Infect Dis 21 Suppl 3:S265-76.

(12) **Edelstein, P. H.** 1995. Review of azithromycin activity against *Legionella* spp. Pathol Biol (Paris) **43**:569-72.

(13) **Edelstein, P. H., and M. A. Edelstein.** 2000. In vitro activity of quinupristin/dalfopristin (Synercid, RP 59500) against *Legionella* spp. Diagn Microbiol Infect Dis **36**:49-52.

(14) **Edelstein, P. H., and R. D. Meyer.** 1980. Susceptibility of *Legionella pneumophila* to twenty antimicrobial agents. Antimicrob Agents Chemother **18**:403-8.

(15) **Gomez-Lus, R., F. Adrian, R. del Campo, P. Gomez-Lus, S. Sanchez, C. Garcia, and M. C. Rubio.** 2001. Comparative in vitro bacteriostatic and bactericidal activity of trovafloxacin, levofloxacin and moxifloxacin against clinical and environmental isolates of *Legionella* spp. Int J Antimicrob Agents **18**:49-54.

(16) **Grau, S., J. M. Antonio, E. Ribes, M. Salvado, J. M. Garces, and J. Garau.** 2006. Impact of rifampicin addition to clarithromycin in *Legionella pneumophila* pneumonia. Int J Antimicrob Agents **28**:249-52.

(17) **Higa, F., N. Kusano, M. Tateyama, T. Shinzato, N. Arakaki, K. Kawakami, and A. Saito.** 1998. Simplified quantitative assay system for measuring activities of drugs against intracellular *Legionella pneumophila*. J Clin Microbiol **36**:1392-8.

(18) **Hoogkamp-Korstanje, J. A.** 1997. In-vitro activities of ciprofloxacin, levofloxacin, lomefloxacin, ofloxacin, pefloxacin, sparfloxacin and trovafloxacin against gram-positive and gram-negative pathogens from respiratory tract infections. J Antimicrob Chemother **40**:427-31.

(19) **Jonas, D., I. Engels, F. D. Daschner, and U. Frank.** 2000. The effect of azithromycin on intracellular *Legionella pneumophila* in the Mono Mac 6 cell line at serum concentrations attainable in vivo. J Antimicrob Chemother **46**:385-90.

(20) **Jonas, D., I. Engels, D. Hartung, J. Beyersmann, U. Frank, and F. D. Daschner.** 2003. Development and mechanism of fluoroquinolone resistance in *Legionella pneumophila*. J Antimicrob Chemother **51**:275-80.

(21) **Kunishima, H., H. Takemura, H. Yamamoto, K. Kanemitsu, and J. Shimada.** 2000. Evaluation of

the activity of antimicrobial agents against *Legionella pneumophila* multiplying in a human monocytic cell line, THP-1, and an alveolar epithelial cell line, A549. J Infect Chemother **6**:206-10.

(22) **Liebers, D. M., A. L. Baltch, R. P. Smith, M. C. Hammer, and J. V. Conroy.** 1989. Susceptibility of *Legionella pneumophila* to eight antimicrobial agents including four macrolides under different assay conditions. J Antimicrob Chemother **23**:37-41.

(23) **Marques, T., and J. Piedade.** 1997. Susceptibility testing by E-test and agar dilution of 30 strains of *Legionella* spp. isolated in Portugal. Clin Microbiol Infect **3**:365-368.

(24) **Marre, R., A. A. Medeiros, and A. W. Pasculle.** 1982. Characterization of the beta-lactamases of six species of *Legionella*. J Bacteriol **151**:216-21.

(25) **Moffie, B. G., and R. P. Mouton.** 1988. Sensitivity and resistance of *Legionella pneumophila* to some antibiotics and combinations of antibiotics. J Antimicrob Chemother **22**:457-62.

(26) **Nielsen, K., J. M. Bangsborg, and N. Hoiby.** 2000. Susceptibility of *Legionella* species to five antibiotics and development of resistance by exposure to erythromycin, ciprofloxacin, and rifampicin. Diagn Microbiol Infect Dis **36**:43-8.

(27) **Nielsen, K., P. Hindersson, N. Hoiby, and J. M. Bangsborg.** 2000. Sequencing of the rpoB gene in *Legionella pneumophila* and characterization of mutations associated with rifampin resistance in the Legionellaceae. Antimicrob Agents Chemother **44**:2679-83.

(28) **Pendland, S. L., S. J. Martin, C. Chen, P. C. Schreckenberger, and L. H. Danziger.** 1997. Comparison of charcoal- and starch-based media for testing susceptibilities of *Legionella* species to macrolides, azalides, and fluoroquinolones. J Clin Microbiol **35**:3004-6.

(29) **Pohlod, D. J., L. D. Saravolatz, E. L. Quinn, and M. M. Somerville.** 1981. The effect of inoculum, culture medium and antimicrobial combinations on the in-vitro susceptibilities of *Legionella pneumophila*. J Antimicrob Chemother **7**:335-41.

(30) **Reda, C., T. Quaresima, and M. C. Pastoris.** 1994. In-vitro activity of six intracellular antibiotics against *Legionella pneumophila* strains of human and environmental origin. J Antimicrob Chemother **33**:757-64.

(31) **Rhomberg, P. R., M. J. Bale, and R. N. Jones.** 1994. Application of the Etest to antimicrobial susceptibility testing of *Legionella* spp. Diagn Microbiol Infect Dis **19**:175-8.

(32) **Roch, N., and M. Maurin.** 2005. Antibiotic susceptibilities of *Legionella pneumophila* strain Paris in THP-1 cells as determined by real-time PCR assay. J Antimicrob Chemother **55**:866-71.

(33) **Ruckdeschel, G., and A. Dalhoff.** 1999. The in-vitro activity of moxifloxacin against *Legionella* species and the effects of medium on susceptibility test results. J Antimicrob Chemother 43 Suppl B:25-9.

(34) **Schulin, T., C. B. Wennersten, M. J. Ferraro, R. C. Moellering, Jr., and G. M. Eliopoulos.** 1998. Susceptibilities of *Legionella* spp. to newer antimicrobials in vitro. Antimicrob Agents Chemother **42**:1520-3.

(35) **Stokes, D. H., B. Slocombe, and R. Sutherland.** 1989. Bactericidal effects of amoxycillin/clavulanic acid against *Legionella pneumophila*. J Antimicrob Chemother **23**:43-51.

(36) **Stout, J. E., B. Arnold, and V. L. Yu.** 1998. Activity of azithromycin, clarithromycin, roxithromycin, dirithromycin, quinupristin/dalfopristin and erythromycin against *Legionella* species by intracellular susceptibility testing in HL-60 cells. J Antimicrob Chemother **41**:289-91.

(37) **Stout, J. E., B. Arnold, and V. L. Yu.** 1998. Comparative activity of ciprofloxacin, ofloxacin, levofloxacin, and erythromycin against *Legionella* species by broth microdilution and intracellular susceptibility testing in HL-60 cells. Diagn Microbiol Infect Dis **30**:37-43.

(38) **Takemura, H., H. Yamamoto, H. Kunishima, H. Ikejima, T. Hara, K. Kanemitsu, S. Terakubo, Y. Shoji, M. Kaku, and J. Shimada.** 2000. Evaluation of a human monocytic cell line THP-1 model for assay of the intracellular activities of antimicrobial agents against *Legionella pneumophila*. J Antimicrob Chemother **46**:589-94.

Chapter 42. *AEROMONAS, VIBRIO AND PLESIOMONAS*

Thierry FOSSE

INTRODUCTION

The family *Vibrionaceae* comprises the genera *Vibrio* and *Plesiomonas*. The genus *Aeromonas* was recently removed from the *Vibrionaceae* to form the family *Aeromonadaceae*. These three genera comprise water-borne human pathogens responsible for gastroenteritis and other types of infection. The clinical picture depends on the species and mode of contamination (Table 1) and the frequency varies according to season and sanitation conditions. The pathogenic species possess potent virulence factors including enterotoxins, cytoxins and hemolysins.

Vibrio cholerae O1 and more recently O139 have historically been associated with cholera pandemics. Over the past several years, multidrug resistant *V. cholerae* non-O1, non-O139 strains have been isolated. Other species appear to be increasingly prevalent but only a few are human pathogens.

The genus *Aeromonas* is expanding rapidly and now counts seventeen species or hybridization groups (32). The main species or phenospecies identified in the laboratory are *Aeromonas hydrophila, A. salmonicida, A. caviae (A. punctata), A. veronii* subsp. *sobria, A. jandaei, A. schubertii,* and *A. trota*. These species are isolated at different frequencies according to whether they are environmental or pathogenic strains. All species are intrinsically resistant to β-lactams but resistance phenotypes vary widely due to the intrinsic production of one to three β-lactamases, a phenomenon unique in the bacterial world.

The genus *Plesiomonas* comprises a single species, *P. shigelloides*, which causes gastroenteritis. The antimicrobial susceptibility of this species is much less well known.

Aeromonas, and particularly the genus *Vibrio*, are capable of acquiring antibiotic resistance genes and contributing to their spread from the environment to animals and humans (18, 40, 52). Environmental factors promote the horizontal transfer of resistance genes, in particular by activation of the SOS system (6). The numerous contacts with environmental microbes as well as the biodiversity of the *Vibrionaceae* (5, 57, 65) play an important role in the evolution and emergence of pathogenic species.

Table 1. Principal species, sources of contamination, and infections observed in the group *Vibrio, Aeromonas,* and *Plesiomonas*

Species	Source of contamination	Type of infection
Vibrio cholerae O1, O139		Diarrhea, epidemic or not
Vibrio cholerae Non-O1 non-O139		Sporadic diarrhea, skin wound
V. parahaemolyticus	Salt or brackish water, drinking water, seafood	Diarrhea, skin wound
V. alginolyticus		ENT infection, skin wound
V. vulnificus		Skin wound
Vibrio fluvialis, V. mimicus, V. metschnikovii, V. hollisae[a]		Diarrhea
A caviae, A. hydrophila, A. veronii sobria	Ubiquitous, fresh water, water systems, drinking water, seafood	Diarrhea, skin wound, bacteremia, respiratory tract or ocular infections
Plesiomonas shigeloides	Fresh or brackish water	Diarrhea, bacteremia in immunocompromised patients

[a] *Grimontia hollisae.*

METHODS

Identification

Identification is an important step in classifying medically relevant strains to the species level and interpreting antibiotic susceptibility tests (15, 32, 65). Errors of identification are common, especially for the genus *Aeromonas*. Resistance to the vibriostatic agent 0/129 (2,4-diamino-6,7-diisopropylopteridine) was described in *V. cholerae* in 1986 and may lead to bacterial misidentification (25). Commercially available galleries must be completed by individual tests (1) and where necessary by *gyrB* gene sequencing (67).

Susceptibility testing

Dilution and diffusion methods can be modified to take into account the culture requirements of these bacteria. Most species can be cultured at an incubation temperature of 35°C ± 2°C but grow better at 28-30°C. Salt-supplemented (NaCl 3%) Mueller-Hinton medium for halophilic vibrios (*V. alginolyticus*, *V. parahaemolyticus*) is not mandatory but may be useful if growth is difficult. A larger inoculum (MacFarland 2 suspension) makes it easier to detect low-level β-lactamase expression in *Aeromonas*, particularly for imipenem (carbapenemase) and in some cases cephalothin (cephalosporinase). For the same reasons, the interpretation of rapid automated β-lactam susceptibility tests in liquid medium should be adapted to the resistance phenotypes most likely to be found for the species (19, 59).

The CLSI has produced recommendations for the antimicrobial susceptibility testing of *V. cholerae* in the document M11-S19 (2009) and of *Aeromonas hydrophila* complex and *Plesiomonas shigelloides* in the document M45-A (2006). The guidelines include the antibiotics to be tested and interpretive criteria for reporting results. Testing conditions are the same as for enterobacteria, with some modifications: for *Vibrio* spp. (other than *V. cholerae*), inoculum should be prepared in 0.85% NaCl which allows most isolates of *Vibrio* spp. to grow without adding NaCl to the MH medium, and for disk diffusion and *V. cholerae*, incubation time is 16-18 h.

EUCAST (http://www.eucast.org/clinical_breakpoints/) does not provide specific breakpoints for the *Vibrionaceae* and *Aeromonadaceae* and therefore non species related breakpoints should be used.

β-LACTAMS

Resistance to β-lactams can be readily interpreted for the genera *Vibrio* and *Plesiomonas* with the frequent presence of a penicillinase phenotype (Fig. 1 to 3) and no inducibility. Interpretation is more difficult for *Aeromonas* because two or three β-lactamases are often present (Fig. 4 to 8). Nonetheless, each of these β-lactamases, when sufficiently expressed, can be identified on the basis of its substrate profile.

Vibrio cholerae

Clinical isolates of *V. cholerae* show intrinsic *in vitro* susceptibility to penicillins and cephalosporins (Fig. 1). A *V. cholerae* isolate with acquired resistance to ampicillin due to a plasmid TEM-1-type β-lactamase was described in 1977 (14, 29). However, with the identification of a SAR-1 β-lactamase in 1986 (Table 4) in a strain of *V. cholerae El Tor* (54), it is likely that the penicillinase profile of multiresistant strains was already, at this time, due to the dissemination of a plasmid carbenicillinase (11, 47).

Starting in the 1990s, ampicillin resistance began to be observed at a high prevalence in *V. cholerae* non-O1, non-O139 strains. The ampicillin resistance gene was carried by a class I integron (66). Altogether, four new carbenicillinases were described: CARB-2 (PSE-1), CARB-6, CARB-7, and CARB-9 (Table 4) (11, 13, 42, 50, 54). CARB-2 has also been detected in strains of *V. cholerae* O1.

This major group of carbenicillinases is characterized by an RSG amino acid triad in positions 234-236 instead of the K-T/S-G motif present in other class A β-lactamases (36). The bla_{CARB} genes are encoded by a cassette located in the VCR region of the superintegron on the second *V. cholerae* chromosome (57) but in different positions (42). The oldest bla_{CARB} genes (bla_{CARB-7} and bla_{CARB-9}) probably evolved from a unique ancestral cassette in *V. cholerae* located in a superintegron. These cassettes later migrated to class 1 integrons by *in vivo* capture (50).

Other *Vibrio*

Resistance to ampicillin and carbenicillin is very common among other vibrio species that cause human disease (15, 34). Most of these strains have a similar β-lactam resistance profile, probably due to the production of related β-lactamases. Class A β-lactamases sharing 50% homology with

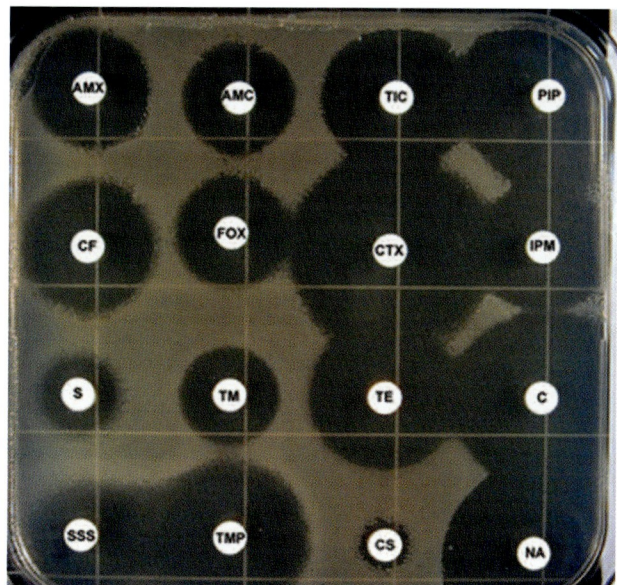

Fig. 1. *V. cholerae* V101 wild-type phenotype, β-lactam-susceptible and colistin-resistant

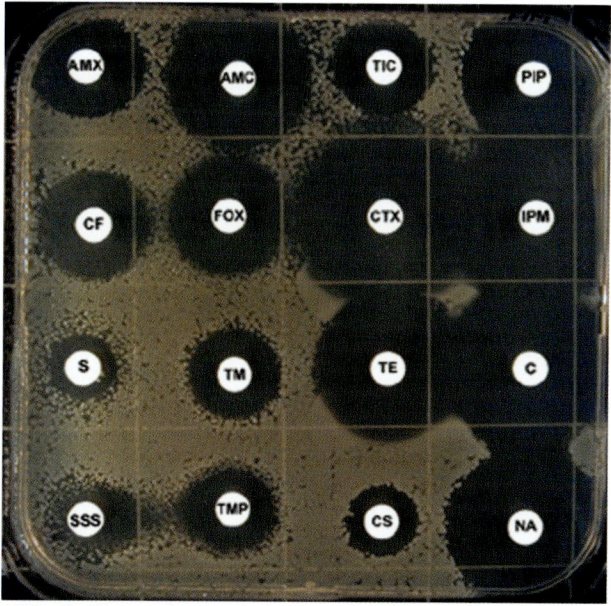

Fig. 2. *V. parahaemolyticus* penicillinase phenotype

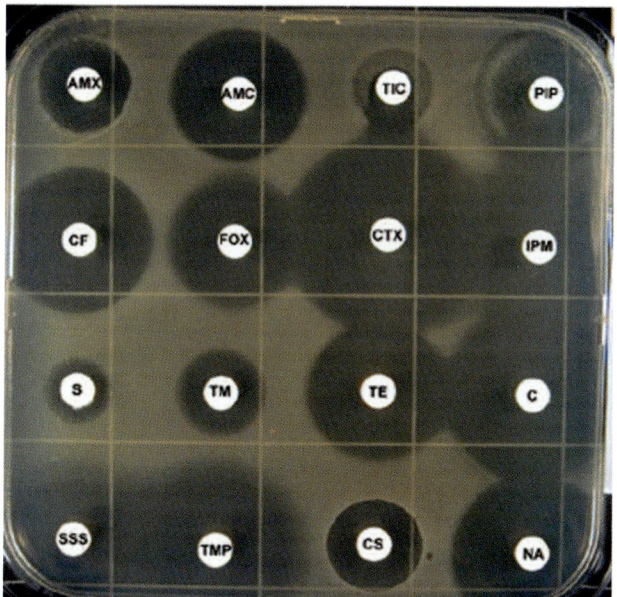

Fig. 3. *P. shigelloides* penicillinase phenotype

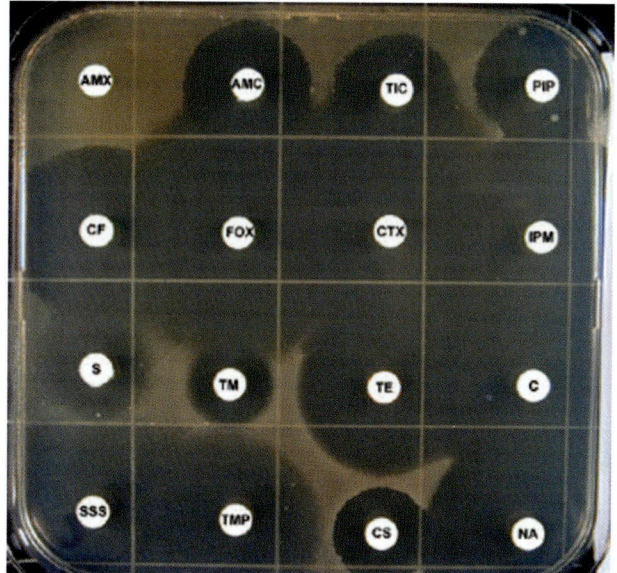

Fig. 4. *A. schubertii* penicillinase phenotype

AMC, amoxicillin + clavulanic acid; AMX, amoxicillin; C, chloramphenicol; CF, cephalothin; CS, colistin; CTX, cefotaxime; FOX, cefoxitin; I, imipenem; NA, nalidixic acid; PIP, piperacillin; S, streptomycin; SSS, sulfonamides; TE, tetracycline; TIC, ticarcillin; TM, tobramycin; TMP, trimethoprim.

the carbenicillinases described in *V. cholerae* (Table 3) were studied in two environmental species, *V. harveyi* (64), and *V. fischeri* (70). Genomic sequencing of a *V. parahaemolyticus* strain (37) revealed a class A β-lactamase gene with 80% homology to that of *V. harveyi*, and 54% to that of *V. fischeri* and *V. cholerae* carbenicillinases (Table 3). Among the sequenced genomes, several other species from the genus *Vibrio* also harbored a class A β-lactamase, probably of the carbenicillinase type with a conserved RSG motif (Genbank references, *V. alginolyticus* EAS75483, *V. splendidus* EAP95935, *V. campbellii* EDP59525, *V. angustum* EAS64703 and *V. shilonii* EDL55389). Additional data are needed to understand the genetic determinism of the penicillinase phenotype in clinically relevant *Vibrio*: species-specific β-lactamase or transferable carbenicillin-hydrolyzing β-lactamase with transfer possible between *V. cholerae* O1 and non-O1 and *V. fluvialis*, *V. parahaemolyticus*, and

Table 2. Carbenicillinases of *Vibrio*, *Aeromonas*, and *Plesiomonas*

Gene	Species	Location	pI	Reference
bla_{SAR-1}	*V. cholerae*	Plasmid	4.9	44
bla_{CARB-2}	*V. cholerae*	Plasmid, class 1 integron	5.7	12
bla_{CARB-6}	*V. cholerae* non-O1 non-O139	Chromosome	5.35	10
bla_{CARB-7}	*V. cholerae* non-O1 non-O139	VCR Superintegron	5.4	36
bla_{CARB-9}	*V. cholerae* non-O1 non-O139	VCR Superintegron	5.2	42
bla_{AER-1}	*A. hydrophila*	Transposon ($\Omega 7711$)	5.9	27
bla_{CARB-x}	*P. shigelloides*	Chromosome	5.2	4

V. vulnificus (40, 57). Plasmid-encoded CTX-M-2 and PER-2 extended spectrum β-lactamases were detected in *V. cholerae* isolates from an epidemic in Argentina (49, 61).

Plesiomonas shigelloides

P. shigelloides is intrinsically resistant to amoxicillin, ticarcillin, and piperacillin (4, 12, 63) but susceptible to amoxicillin/clavulanic acid (Table 3; Fig. 3) and to cephalosporins. A large inoculum effect is observed with an increase in the MICs of cefoperazone and ceftazidime (63, 71) which does not appear to be related to β-lactamase induction.

This penicillinase phenotype is due to the production of a β-lactamase, probably chromosomally encoded, with an acidic pI and substrate selectivity for ticarcillin (carbenicillinase type) or oxacillin (4). Further studies are needed to determine the type of β-lactamase(s) (carbenicillinase or oxacillinase) produced in *Plesiomonas*.

Aeromonas spp.

Intrinsic resistance

Five basic phenotypes according to the type of β-lactamase produced in relation to the species or species group can be described (Tables 3 and 4). They are based on the possible production by the species of one to three class B, C and D β-lactamases (8, 19, 21). These phenotypes have been validated by PCR amplification of the corresponding genes (Table 4). Expression may be very low, particularly in some environmental strains. The genes encoding the three β-lactamases are very far apart on the chromosome of the two species whose genomes have been sequenced: *A. salmonicida* (55) and *A. hydrophilia* (60). However, the three β-lactamases are inducible and their production is governed by a coordinated regulation of the "quorum sensing" type (3, 45), and is therefore strictly dependent on culture conditions.

Penicillinase phenotype

This is due to the class D β-lactamase, or oxacillinase, (pI > 8.5) produced by all species except *A. trota* (Table 4). It is usually highly expressed and confers resistance to ticarcillin (MIC > 256 μg/ml). It is weakly inhibited by clavulanic acid and tazobactam. OXA-12 was the first oxacillinase studied and is representative of the genus *Aeromonas* (53). This phenotype is rarely observed in clinical isolates. *A. schubertii* appears to be the only species (19, 48) to produce a single oxacillinase-type β-lactamase (Fig. 4) with less than 75% homology to the other class D β-lactamases studied in *Aeromonas* (21).

Cephalosporinase phenotype

This phenotype is due to the production of a cephalosporinase (class C, pI 7 ± 0.5) which confers resistance to cephalothin (MIC > 256 μg/ml). *A. trota* is apparently the only species to produce a single β-lactamase of the cephalosporinase type (24). This species is amoxicillin-susceptible or intermediate (9) (Fig. 5) and susceptible to ticarcillin, which is a better marker.

Penicillinase - cephalosporinase phenotype

This common phenotype is found in the phenospecies *A. caviae* (*A. caviae* or *A. punctata*, *A. eucronophila*, *A. media*). It is characterized by resistance to amoxicillin, ticarcillin, cephalothin and sometimes cefoxitin. Antagonism is often observed between a disk containing a strong inducer (cefoxitin or imipenem) and one containing a good β-lactam substrate (cefuroxime or cefotaxime). Strains which have become resistant to cefotaxime after therapeutic use of this antibiotic have been observed; this phenomenon is due to hyperproduction of a chromosomal cephalosporinase resulting from a regulatory mutation.

Chapter 42. *AEROMONAS, VIBRIO* AND *PLESIOMONAS*

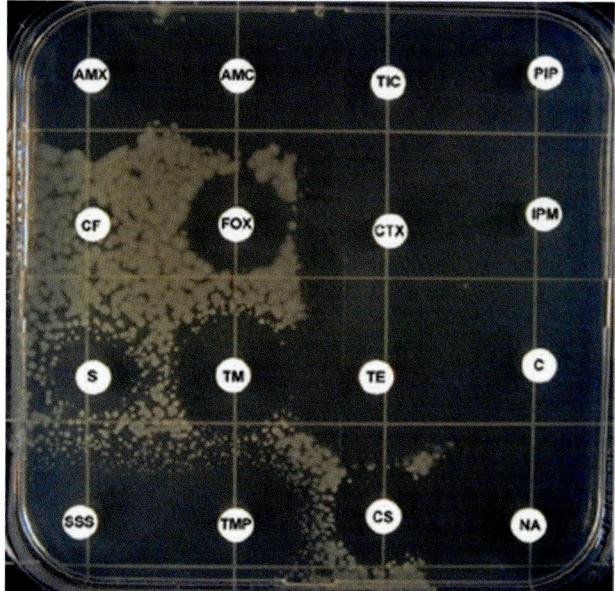

Fig. 5. *A. tructi* cephalosporinase phenotype

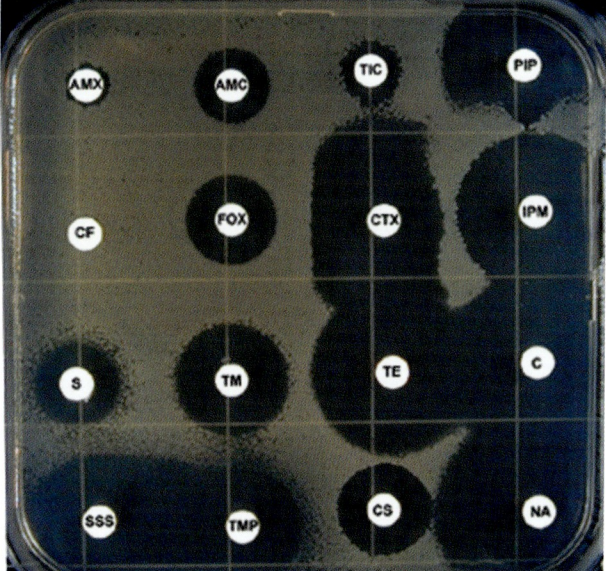

Fig. 6. *A. caviae* penicillinase + cephalosporinase phenotype.

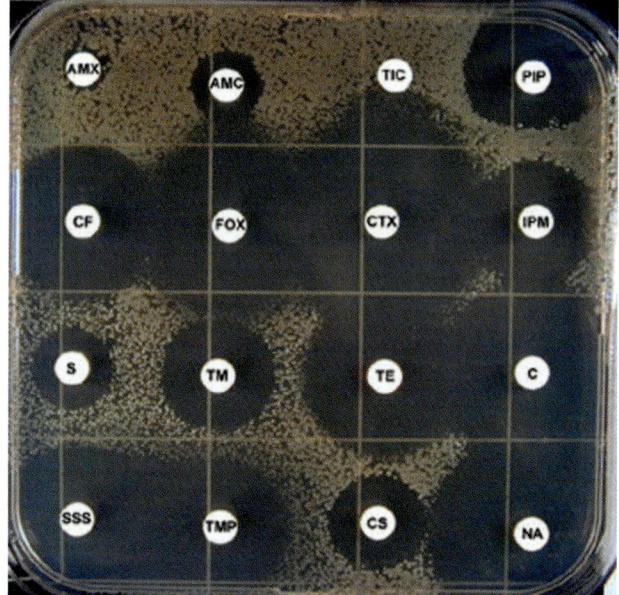

Fig. 7. *A. veronii* penicillinase + carbapenemase phenotype

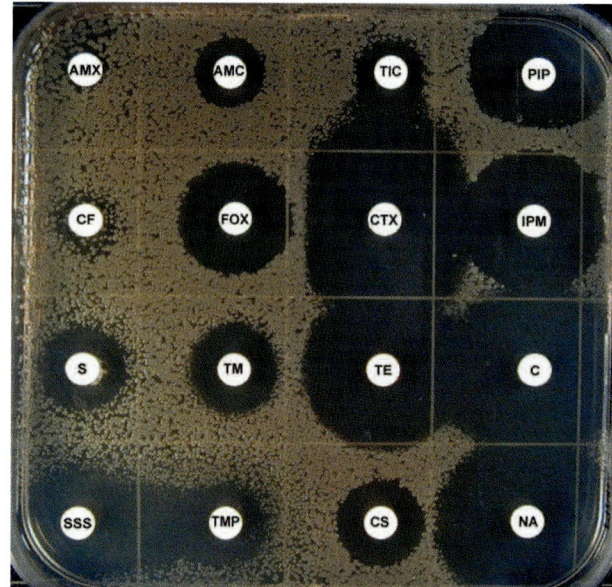

Fig. 8. *A. hydrophila* penicillinase + cephalosporinase + carbapenemase phenotype

AMC, amoxicillin + clavulanic acid; AMX, amoxicillin; C, chloramphenicol; CF, cephalothin; CS, colistin; CTX, cefotaxime; FOX, cefoxitin; I, imipenem; NA, nalidixic acid; PIP, piperacillin; S, streptomycin; SSS, sulfonamides; TE, tetracycline; TIC, ticarcillin; TM, tobramycin; TMP, trimethoprim.

Penicillinase - carbapenemase phenotype

This is another common phenotype found in the phenospecies *A. veronii* (*A. veronii sobria*, *A. veronii veronii*, *A. ichtiosmia*, *A. sobria*), characterized by amoxicillin and ticarcillin resistance, imipenem-intermediate, and cephalothin susceptibility. These strains produce an oxacillinase which confers the penicillinase profile and a very narrow spectrum carbapenemase which mainly hydrolyzes imipenem. This carbapenemase is a class B, group B2 enzyme (22). The first two enzymes described in this group were CphA (39, 56) and ImiS (68). This β-lactamase has a pI of about 8 and confers fairly low-level resistance (19, 28). A larger inoculum and a breakpoint adapted for imipenem (MIC

513

> 1 μg/ml) allow categorization of the majority of strains. The very narrow specificity profile is due in part to the binding of a single zinc ion to the active site for the enzyme to conserve its activity, as opposed to subgroups B1 and B2 which bind two zinc ions (23). This is illustrated by the double mutant N116H/N220G which allows a second zinc ion to bind, thus broadening the substrate profile (7).

Penicillinase - cephalosporinase - carbapenemase phenotype

This phenotype is found in the phenospecies *A. hydrophila* (*A. hydrophila, A. bestiarum, A. popoffii, A. salmonicida, A. allosaccharophila*). Strains are resistant to amoxicillin, ticarcillin, and cephalothin. As for *A. caviae*, antagonism which reveals the induction of cephalosporinase can be observed but is usually less pronounced. Reduced imipenem susceptibility is more difficult to observe than for *A. veronii*; it may be necessary to use a larger inoculum and to incubate the antibiogram at 22°C for an additional 24-48 h in order to see growth of colonies in the inhibition zone.

Acquired resistance

An acquired class A β-lactamase can be suspected if the antibiogram shows a high-level penicillinase phenotype (piperacillin + tazobactam resistance) or an extended spectrum β-lactamase phenotype (synergy between cefotaxime or ceftazidime and clavulanic acid). The carbenicillin-hydrolyzing β-lactamase AER-1 was described in an *A. hydrophila* strain in 1985 (30, 58). The gene is carried by a transposon but has not been found in other *Aeromonas* strains nor in another bacterial species. The most closely related β-lactamase (61% homology) is the class A enzyme found on the Rms149 plasmid in *P. aeruginosa* (27). The bla_{AER-1} gene may have been acquired by horizontal transfer of an integron cassette (58). TEM-1 β-lactamases are very uncommon (2/417 strains in our collection). A TEM-24 extended spectrum β-lactamase was found in *A. caviae* (38) and *A. hydrophila* through acquisition of an *E. aerogenes* plasmid (20). In parallel to the outbreak of *V. cholerae* harboring a CTX-M-2 type β-lactamase, this enzyme was found in *Aeromonas* spp. in Argentina (49). A PER-1-like extended spectrum β-lactamase was detected in an *A. caviae* strain isolated during an epidemic (43) and in an environmental strain of *A. media* (51).

Acquired class B β-lactamases conferring extended spectrum resistance including to

Table 3. Main resistance phenotypes of *Vibrio*, *Aeromonas* and *Plesiomonas*

Species or phenospecies	β-lactamase class	Amoxicillin	Ticarcillin	Amoxicillin + clavulanic acid	Cephalothin	Imipenem	Colistin	O/129
Vibrio spp.	A	S/R[a]	S/R	S	S	S	R	S/R
Plesiomonas spp.	A ou D	R	R	S	S	S	S	R
A. schubertii	D	R	R	S	S	S	S	R
A. trota	C	S/I	S	S	R	S	S	R
A. caviae	C+D	R	R	I/R	R	S	S	R
A. veronii	B+D	R	R	I/R	S	I	S	R
A. jandaei	B+D	R	R	I/R	S	I	R[b]	R
A. hydrophila	B+C+D	R	R	I/R	R	S/I	S/R[b]	R

[a] I, intermediate; R, resistant; S, susceptible.
[b] Better expression of resistance in liquid medium, MIC > 2 μg/ml.

Table 4. β-lactamases and resistance phenotypes in *Aeromonas*

Species or phenospecies	β-lactamase[a]			Phenotype[b]			
	B	C	D	Amoxicillin	Ticarcillin	Cephalothin	Imipenem[c]
A. schubertii			+	R	R	S	S
A. trota		+		S/I	S	R	S
A. caviae		+	+	R	R	R	S
A. eucronophila		+	+	R	R	R	S
A. veronii sobria	+		+	R	R	S	I
A. veronii veronii	+		+	R	R	S	I
A. allosaccharophila	+	+	+	R	R	R	S/I
A. hydrophila	+	+	+	R	R	R	S/I
A. bestiarum	+	+	+	R	R	R	S/I
A. salmonicida	+	+	+	R	R	R	S/I

[a] Class B, primers MEI1 and MEI2; Class C, primers AERCP1 and AERCP2; Class D, primers AERD1 and AERD2.
[b] I, intermediate; R, resistant; S, susceptible.
[c] Phenotype: imipenem (S < 1 µg/ml; I or R ≥ 1 µg/ml).

imipenem have been described in *A. hydrophila* (VIM-4) (35) and *A. caviae* (IMP-19) (44). Unusual resistance to imipenem or to third generation cephalosporins should suggest the acquisition of a transferable extended spectrum β-lactamase (class A or B) or a mutation in the AheABC efflux system (31).

OTHER ANTIBIOTICS

Polymyxins

Intrinsic colistin resistance is frequently observed in a number of *Vibrio* (Table 2) and *Aeromonas* species (15, 17). However, in the *Aeromonas* species concerned (*A. jandaei* and *A. hydrophila*), broth medium must be used in order for resistance to be expressed (MIC > 2 µg/ml) (17).

Sulfonamides

Halophilic *Vibrio* are frequently resistant to sulfonamides.

Acquired resistance to other antibiotics

Vibrio, *Aeromonas* and *Plesiomonas* are usually intrinsically susceptible to aminoglycosides, tetracyclines, chloramphenicol, sulfonamides (except halophilic *Vibrio*), trimethoprim, nitrofurans, nalidixic acid, and fluoroquinolones. Multidrug resistance acquired through transferable genetic elements like conjugative transposons or plasmids has become very common in the family *Vibrionaceae*, but also in other Gram-negative bacilli (2, 5, 33, 47, 66). Transposable resistance to trimethoprim and the vibriostatic agent 0/129 was described in *V. cholerae* in 1986 (25). The streptomycin-sulfonamides-trimethoprim-chloramphenicol resistance phenotype is due to the dissemination of the conjugative transposon SXT (69) among strains of *V. cholerae* O139 and more recently in non-O1 and non-O139 strains (66). An SXT variant has been found in *V. fluvialis* (2). Analysis of SXT shows similarity with a multiresistance region of *Salmonella enterica* serovar Typhimurium DT104 (33).

Tetracycline resistance determinants are located in a class 1 integron (*tetA* and *aadA1* cassettes) but also in the conjugative transposon SXT in strains of *V. cholerae* El Tor O1 isolated after 1997 (33). Transferable plasmid-mediated florfenicol resistance has been described in *A. salmonicida* (41) and *A. bestiarum* (Genbank EF495198).

The transferable plasmid pRAS1 conferring resistance to tetracyclines, trimethoprim, and sulfonamides has been described in *A. salmonicida*; the genes are located in a class 1 integron (62).

The prevalence of fluoroquinolone resistance is high among environmental strains of *Aeromonas* spp. (10, 26) and in *V. parahaemolyticus* (46). As in other Gram-negative bacilli, resistance is due to mutations in GyrA (primary target) and ParC (secondary target) or to the presence of *qnr* genes in plasmid cassettes (10) or superintegrons (16).

CONCLUSION

Knowledge of resistance phenotypes among *Aeromonas* has taxonomic as well as therapeutic implications. Fluoroquinolones are still the most active drugs. However, a third generation cephalosporin like ceftriaxone can be used for severe infections caused by cephalothin -susceptible *A. veronii*, or a carbapenem like imipenem for *A. caviae* infections. A wide diversity of resistance genes and transferable genetic elements are found in *Vibrionaceae* and *Aeromonadaceae*. These bacteria can serve as vectors for the transfer of genes between the environment, animals and humans. Constant surveillance of resistance in this group of bacteria should be continued, especially now that multiresistant strains have been isolated from patients, limiting treatment options (20, 35, 49).

REFERENCES

(1) **Abbott, S.L., W.K.W. Cheung, and J.M. Janda.** 2003. The genus *Aeromonas*: biochemical characteristics, atypical reactions, and phenotypic identification schemes. J. Clin. Microbiol. **41**:2348-2357.

(2) **Ahmed, A.M, S. Shinoda, and T. Shimamoto.** 2005. A variant type of *Vibrio cholerae* SXT element in a multidrug-resistant strain of *Vibrio fluvialis*. FEMS Microbiol. Lett. **242**:241-247.

(3) **Alksne, L.E., and BA. Rasmussen.** 1997. Expression of AsbA1, OXA-12, and AsbM1 -lactamases in *Aeromonas jandaei* AER14 is regulated by a two-component regulon. J. Bacteriol. **179**:2006-2013.

(4) **Avison, M.B., P.M. Bennett, and T.R. Walsh.** 2000. β-lactamase expression in *Plesiomonas shigelloides*. J. Antimicrob. Chemother. **45**:877–880.

(5) **Beaber, J.W., V. Burrus, B. Hochhut, and M.K. Waldor.** 2002. Comparison of SXT and R391, two conjugative integrating elements: definition of a genetic backbone for the mobilization of resistance determinants. Cell. Mol. Life Sci. **59**:2065-2070.

(6) **Beaber J.W., B. Hochhut, and M.K. Waldor.** 2004. SOS response promotes horizontal dissemination of antibiotic resistance genes. Nature **427**:72–74.

(7) **Bebrone, C., C. Anne, K. De Vriendt, B. Devreese, G.M. Rossolini, J. Van Beeumen, J.M. Frere, and M. Galleni.** 2005. Dramatic broadening of the substrate profile of the *Aeromonas hydrophila* CphA metallo-β-lactamase by site-directed mutagenesis. J. Biol. Chem. **280**:28195-28202.

(8) **Bush, K., G.A. Jacoby, and A.A. Medeiros.** 1995. A functional classification scheme for -lactamases and its correlation with molecular structure. Antimicrob. Agents Chemother. **39**:1211-1233.

(9) **Carnahan, A.M., T. Chakraborty, G.R. Fanning, D. Verma, A. Ali, J.M. Janda, and S.W. Joseph.** 1991. *Aeromonas trota* sp. nov., an ampicillin-susceptible species isolated from clinical specimens. J. Clin. Microbiol. **29**:1206-1210.

(10) **Cattoir, V., L. Poirel, C. Aubert, C.J. Soussy, and P. Nordmann.** 2008. Unexpected occurrence of plasmid-mediated quinolone resistance determinants in environmental *Aeromonas spp*. Emerg. Infect. Dis. **14**:231-237

(11) **Choury, D., G. Aubert, M. Szajnert, K. Azibi, M. Delpech, and G. Paul.** 1999. Characterization and nucleotide sequence of CARB-6, a new carbenicillin-hydrolyzing β-lactamase from *Vibrio cholerae*. Antimicrob. Agents Chemother. **43**:297-301.

(12) **Clark, R.B., P.D. Lister, L. Arneson-Rotert, and J.M. Janda.** 1990. *In vitro* susceptibilities of *Plesiomonas shigelloides* to 24 antibiotics and antibiotic–β-lactamase-inhibitor combinations. Antimicrob. Agents Chemother. **34**:159–160.

(13) **Dalsgaard, A., A. Forslund, O. Serichantalergs, and D. Sandvang.** 2000. Distribution and content of class 1 integrons in different *Vibrio cholerae* O-serotype strains isolated in Thailand. Antimicrob. Agents Chemother. **44**:1315-1321.

(14) **Dupont, M.J., M. Jouvenot, G. Couetdic, and Y. Michel-Briand.** 1985. Development of plasmid-mediated resistance in *Vibrio cholerae* during treatment with trimethoprim-sulfamethoxazole. Antimicrob. Agents Chemother. **27**:280-281.

(15) **Farmer, J.J. III, J.M. Janda, and K. Birkhead.** 2003. *Vibrio*, p. 706-718, *In* P.R. Murray, E.J. Baron, M.A. Pfaller, J.H. Jorgensen, and R.H. Yolken (ed.), Manual of clinical microbiology, 8th ed. American Society for Microbiology, Washington, D.C.

(16) **Fonseca E.L., Dos Santos Freitas F., Vieira V.V., and A.C. Vicente .** 2008. New *qnr* gene cassettes associated with superintegron repeats in *Vibrio cholerae* O1. Emerg. Infect. Dis. **14**:1129-1131.

(17) **Fosse, T., C. Giraud-Morin, and I. Madinier.** 2003. Induced colistin resistance as an identifying marker for *Aeromonas* phenospecies groups. Lett. Appl. Microbiol. **36**:25-29.

(18) **Fosse, T., C. Giraud-Morin, I. Madinier, and R. Labia.** 2003. Sequence analysis and biochemical characterisation of chromosomal CAV-1 (*Aeromonas caviae*), the parental cephalosporinase of plasmid-mediated AmpC 'FOX' cluster. FEMS Microbiol. Lett. **16**:93-98.

(19) **Fosse, T, C . Giraud-Morin, and I. Madinier.** 2003. Phenotypes de resistance aux ☐lactamines dans le genre *Aeromonas*. Path. Biol. **51**:290-296.

(20) **Fosse, T., C. Giraud-Morin, I. Madinier, F. Mantoux, J.P. Lacour, and J.P. Ortonne.** 2004. *Aeromonas hydrophila* with plasmid-borne class A extended-spectrum β-lactamase TEM-24 and three chromosomal class B, C, and D β-lactamases, isolated from a patient with necrotizing fasciitis. Antimicrob. Agents Chemother. **48**:2342-2343.

(21) **Fosse, T.** 2005. Distribution and phylogeny of class B, C and D β-lactamases in the genus *Aeromonas*. 6th international β-lactamase meeting, LEONESSA (abstract 21)

(22) **Garau, G., I. Garcia-Saez, C. Bebrone, C. Anne, P. Mercuri, M. Galleni, J.M. Frere, and O. Dideberg.** 2004. Update of the standard numbering scheme for class B β-lactamases. Antimicrob. Agents Chemother. **48**:2347-2349.

(23) **Garau, G., C. Bebrone, C. Anne, M. Galleni, J.M. Frere, and O. Dideberg.** 2005. A metallo-β-lactamase enzyme in action: crystal structures of the

monozinc carbapenemase CphA and its complex with biapenem. J. Mol. Biol. **345**:785-795.

(24) **Giraud-Morin, C., F. De Luca, G.M. Rossolini, J.D. Docquier, and T. Fosse.** 2007. Genetic and biochemical characterization of TRU-1, the endogenous Class C β-Lactamase from *Aeromonas trota*. Abstr. 48th Intersci. Conf. Antimicrob. Agents Chemother., abstr. C1-592.

(25) **Goldstein, F., G. Gerbaud, and P. Courvalin.** 1986. Transposable resistance to trimethoprim and 0/129 in *Vibrio cholerae*. J. Antimicrob. Chemother. **17**:559-569.

(26) **Goñi-Urriza, M., C. Arpin, M. Capdepuy, V. Dubois, P. Caumette, and C. Quentin.** 2003. Type II Topoisomerase Quinolone Resistance-Determining Regions of *Aeromonas caviae*, *A. hydrophila*, and *A. sobria* complexes and mutations associated with quinolone resistance. Antimicrob. Agents Chemother. **46**:350-359.

(27) **Haines, S.A, K. Jones, M., Cheung, and C.M. Thomas.** 2005. The IncP-6 plasmid Rms149 consists of a small mobilizable backbone with multiple large insertions. J. Bacteriol. **187**:4728-4738.

(28) **Hayes, M.V., C.J. Thomson, and S.G.B. Amyes.** 1996. The "hidden" carbapenemase of *Aeromonas hydrophila*. J. Antimicrob. Chemother. **37**:33-44.

(29) **Hedges, R.W., J.L. Vialard, N.J. Pearson, and F. O'Grady.** 1977. R plasmids from Asian strains of *Vibrio cholerae*. Antimicrob. Agents Chemother. **11**:585-588

(30) **Hedges, R.W., A.A. Medeiros, M. Cohenford, and G.A. Jacoby.** 1985. Genetic and biochemical properties of AER-1, a novel carbenicillin-hydrolyzing β-lactamase from *Aeromonas hydrophila*. Antimicrob. Agents Chemother. **27**:479-484.

(31) **Hernould, M., S. Gagne, M. Fournier, C. Quentin, and C. Arpin.** 2008. Role of the AheABC efflux pump in *Aeromonas hydrophila* intrinsic multidrug resistance. Antimicrob. Agents Chemother. **52**:1559-1563.

(32) **Janda, J.M., and S.L. Abbott.** 1998. Evolving concepts regarding the genus *Aeromonas*: an expanding panorama of species, disease presentations, and unanswered questions. Clin. Infect. Dis. **27**:332-344.

(33) **Iwanaga, M., C. Toma, T. Miyazato, S. Insisiengmay, N. Nakasone, and M. Ehara.** 2004. Antibiotic resistance conferred by a class I integron and SXT constin in *Vibrio cholerae* O1 strains isolated in Laos. Antimicrob. Agents Chemother. **48**:2364-2369.

(34) **Joseph, S.W., R.M. DeBell, and W.P. Brown.** 1978. In vitro response to chloramphenicol, tetracycline, ampicillin, gentamicin, and beta-lactamase production by halophilic vibrios from human and environmental sources. Antimicrob. Agents Chemother. **13**:244-248.

(35) **Libisch B., C.G. Giske, B. Kovács, T.G. Tóth, and M. Füzi.** 2008. Identification of the first VIM metallo-beta-lactamase-producing multiresistant *Aeromonas hydrophila* strain. J. Clin. Microbiol. **46**:1878-1880.

(36) **Lim, D., F. Sanschagrin, L. Passmore, L. De Castro, R.C. Levesque, and N.C. Strynadka.** 2001. Insights into the molecular basis for the carbenicillinase activity of PSE-4 beta-lactamase from crystallographic and kinetic studies. Biochemistry **40**:395-402.

(37) **Makino, K., K. Oshima, K. Kurokawa, K. Yokoyama, T. Uda, K. Tagomori, Y. Iijima, M. Najima, M. Nakano, A. Yamashita, Y. Kubota, S. Kimura, T. Yasunaga, T. Honda, H. Shinagawa, M. Hattori, and T. Iida.** 2003. Genome sequence of *Vibrio parahaemolyticus*: a pathogenic mechanism distinct from that of *V. cholerae*. Lancet **361**:743-749.

(38) **Marchandin, H., S. Godreuil, H. Darbas, H. Jean-Pierre, E. Jumas-Bilak, C. Chanal, and R. Bonnet.** 2003. Extended-spectrum β-lactamase TEM-24 in an *Aeromonas* clinical strain: Acquisition from the prevalent *Enterobacter aerogenes* clone in France. Antimicrob. Agents Chemother. **47**:3994-3995

(39) **Massidda, O., G.M. Rossolini, and G. Satta.** 1991. The *Aeromonas hydrophila cphA* gene: molecular heterogeneity among class B metallo-β-lactamases. J. Bacteriol. **173**:4611-4617.

(40) **Mazel, D., B. Dychinco, V. Webb, and J. Davies.** 1998. A distinctive class of integron in the *Vibrio cholerae* genome. Science **280**:605-608.

(41) **McIntosh, D., M. Cunningham, B. Ji, F.A. Fekete, E.M. Parry, S.E. Clark, Z.B. Zalinger, I.C. Gilg, G.R. Danner, K.A. Johnson, M. Beattie, and R. Ritchie.** 2008. Transferable, multiple antibiotic and mercury resistance in Atlantic Canadian isolates of *Aeromonas salmonicida* subsp. *salmonicida* is associated with carriage of an IncA/C plasmid similar to the *Salmonella enterica* plasmid pSN254. J. Antimicrob. Chemother. **61**:1221-1228.

(42) **Melano, R., A. Petroni, A. Garutti, H.A. Saka, L. Mange, F. Pasterán, M. Rapoport, A. Rossi, and M. Galas.** 2002. New carbenicillin-hydrolyzing beta-lactamase (CARB-7) from *Vibrio cholerae* non-O1, non-O139 strains encoded by the VCR region of the *V. cholerae* genome. Antimicrob. Agents Chemother. **46**:2162-2168.

(43) **Neuwirth, C., R. Heller, E. Siebor, E. Parisi, L. Clerget, C. Bochaton, I. Grawey, M. Martinot, G. Laplatte, and D.A. Debriel.** 2004. Outbreak of *Aeromonas caviae* Producing a PER-1-Like Beta-Lactamase. Abstr. 46th Intersci. Conf. Antimicrob. Agents Chemother., abstr. C1-300.

(44) **Neuwirth, C., E. Siebor, F. Robin, and R. Bonnet.** 2007. First occurrence of an IMP metallo-β-lactamase in *Aeromonas caviae*: IMP-19 in an isolate from France. Antimicrob. Agents Chemother. **51**:4486-4488.

(45) **Niumsup, P., A.M. Simm, K. Nurmahomed, T.R. Walsh, P.M. Bennett, and M.B. Avison.** 2003. Genetic linkage of the penicillinase gene, *amp*, and *blrAB*, encoding the regulator of β-lactamase expression in *Aeromonas* spp. J Antimicrob. Chemother. **51**: 1351-1358.

(46) **Okuda, J., E. Hayakawa, M. Nishibuchi, and T. Nishino.** 1999. Sequence analysis of the *gyrA* and *parC* homologues of a wild-type strain of *Vibrio parahaemolyticus* and its fluoroquinolone-resistant mutants. Antimicrob. Agents Chemother. **43**:1156-1162.

(47) **Ouellette, M., G. Gerbaud, and P. Courvalin.** 1988. Genetic, biochemical and molecular characterization of strains of *Vibrio cholerae* multiresistant to antibiotics. Ann. Microbiol. (Inst. Pasteur) **139**:105-113.

(48) **Overman, T.L., and J.M. Janda.** 1999. Antimicrobial susceptibility patterns of *Aeromonas jandaei*, *A. schubertii*, *A. trota*, and *A. veronii* biotype *veronii*. J. Clin. Microbiol. **37** : 706–708

(49) **Petroni, A., A. Corso, R. Melano, M.L. Cacace, A.M. Bru, A. Rossi, and M. Galas.** 2002. Plasmidic extended-spectrum beta-lactamases in *Vibrio cholerae* O1 El Tor isolates in Argentina. Antimicrob. Agents Chemother. **46**:1462-1468.

(50) **Petroni, A., R.G. Melano, H.A. Saka, A. Garutti, L. Mange, F. Pasteran, M. Rapoport, M. Miranda, D. Faccone, A. Rossi, P.S. Hoffman, and M.F. Galas.** 2004. CARB-9, a carbenicillinase encoded in the VCR region of *Vibrio cholerae* Non-O1, Non-O139 belongs to a family of cassette-encoded β-lactamases. Antimicrob. Agents Chemother. **48**: 4042-4046.

(51) **Picao, R.C., L. Poirel, A. Demarta, O. Petrini, A.R. Corvaglia, and P. Nordmann.** 2008. Expanded-spectrum beta-lactamase PER-1 in an environmental *Aeromonas media* isolate from Switzerland. Antimicrob. Agents Chemother. **52**:3461-3462.

(52) **Poirel, L., A. Liard, J.M. Rodriguez-Martinez, and P. Nordmann.** 2005. *Vibrionaceae* as a possible source of *qnr*-like quinolone resistance determinants. J. Antimicrob. Chemother. **56**:1118-1121.

(53) **Rasmussen, B.A., D. Keeney, Y. Yang, and K. Bush.** 1994. Cloning and expression of a cloxacillin-hydrolyzing enzyme and a cephalosporinase from *Aeromonas sobria* AER 14M in *Escherichia coli*: requirement for an *E. coli* chromosomal mutation for efficient expression of the class D enzyme. Antimicrob. Agents Chemother. **38**:2078-2085.

(54) **Reid, A.J., and S.G.B. Amyes.** 1986. Plasmid penicillin resistance in *Vibrio cholerae*: identification of new β-lactamase SAR-1. Antimicrob. Agents Chemother. **30**:245-247.

(55) **Reith, M.E., R.K. Singh, B. Curtis, J.M. Boyd, A. Bouevitch, J. Kimball, J. Munholland, C. Murphy, D. Sarty, J. Williams, J.H. Nash, S.C. Johnson, and L.L. Brown.** 2008. The genome of *Aeromonas salmonicida subsp. salmonicida* A449: insights into the evolution of a fish pathogen. BMC Genomics. **9**:427.

(56) **Rossolini, G.M., A. Zanchi, A. Chiesurin, G. Amicosante, G. Satta, and P. Guglielmetti.** 1995. Distribution of *cphA* or related carbapenemase-encoding genes and production of carbapenemase activity in members of the genus *Aeromonas*. Antimicrob. Agents Chemother. **39**:346-349.

(57) **Rowe-Magnus, D.A., A.M. Guerout, L. Biskri, P. Bouige, and D. Mazel.** 2003. Comparative analysis of superintegrons: engineering extensive genetic diversity in the *Vibrionaceae*. Genome Res. **13**:428-442.

(58) **Sanschagrin, F., N. Bejaoui, and R.C. Levesque.** 1998. Structure of CARB-4 and AER-1 carbenicillin-hydrolyzing β-lactamases. Antimicrob. Agents Chemother. **42**:1966-1972.

(59) **Schadow, K.H., D.K. Giger, and C.C. Sanders.** 1993. Failure of the Vitek AutoMicrobic system to detect beta-lactam resistance in *Aeromonas* species. Am. J. Clin. Pathol. **100**:308-310.

(60) **Seshadri, R., S.W. Joseph, A.K. Chopra, J. Sha, J. Shaw, J. Graf, D. Haft, M. Wu, Q. Ren, M.J. Rosovitz, R. Madupu, L. Tallon, M. Kim, S. Jin, H. Vuong, O.C. Stine, A. Ali, A.J. Horneman, and J.F. Heidelberg.** 2006. Genome sequence of *Aeromonas hydrophila* ATCC 7966T: Jack of all trades. J. Bacteriol. **188**:8272-8282.

(61) **Soler Bistue, A.J., F.A. Martin, A. Petroni, D. Faccone, M. Galas, M.E. Tolmasky, and A. Zorreguieta.** 2006. *Vibrio cholerae* InV117, a class 1 integron harboring *aac(6')-Ib* and $bla_{CTX-M-2}$, is linked to transposition genes. Antimicrob. Agents Chemother. **50**:1903-1907.

(62) **Sorum, H., T.M. L'Abee-Lund, A. Solberg, and A. Wold.** 2003. Integron-containing IncU R plasmids pRAS1 and pAr-32 from the fish pathogen *Aeromonas salmonicida*. Antimicrob. Agents Chemother. **47**:1285-1290.

(63) **Stock, I., and B. Wiedemann.** 2001. Natural antimicrobial susceptibilities of *Plesiomonas shigelloides* strains. J. Antimicrob. Chemother. **48**:803-811.

(64) **Teo, J.W., A. Suwanto, and C.L. Poh.** 2000. Novel β-lactamase genes from two environmental isolates of *Vibrio harveyi*. Antimicrob. Agents Chemother. **44**:1309-1314.

(65) **Thompson, F.L., T. Iida, and J. Swings.** 2004. Biodiversity of Vibrios. Microbiol. Mol. Biol. Rev. **68**:403-431

(66) **Thungapathra, M., K.K. Amita Sinha, S.R. Chaudhuri, P. Garg, T. Ramamurthy, G.B. Nair, and A. Ghosh.** 2002. Occurrence of antibiotic resistance gene cassettes *aac(6')-Ib*, *dfrA5*, *dfrA12*, and *ereA2* in class I integrons in non-O1, non-O139 *Vibrio cholerae* strains in India. Antimicrob. Agents Chemother. **46**:2948-2955.

(67) **Yáñez, M.A., V. Catalán, D. Apráiz, M.J. Figueras, and A.J. Martínez-Murcia.** 2003. Phylogenic analysis of members of the genus *Aeromonas* based on *gyrB* gene sequences. Int. J. Syst. Evol. Microbiol. **53**:875-883

(68) **Walsh, T.R., W.A. Neville, M.H. Haran, D. Tolson, D.J. Payne, J.H. Bateson, A.P. Macgowan, and P.M. Bennett.** 1998. Nucleotide and amino acid sequences of the metallo-beta-lactamase, ImiS, from *Aeromonas veronii bv. sobria*. Antimicrob. Agents Chemother. **42**:436-439

(69) **Waldor, M.K., H. Tschäpe, and J.J. Mekalanos.** 1996. A new type of conjugative transposon encodes resistance to sulfamethoxazole, trimethoprim, and streptomycin in *Vibrio cholerae* O139. J. Bacteriol. **178**:4157-4165

(70) **Weng, S.F., Y.F. Chao, and J.W. Lin.** 2004. Identification and characteristic analysis of the *ampC* gene encoding beta-lactamase from *Vibrio fischeri*. Biochem. Biophys. Res. Commun. **314**:838-843.

(71) **Wiegand, I., and S. Burak.** 2004. Effect of inoculum density on susceptibility of *Plesiomonas shigelloides* to cephalosporins. J. Antimicrob. Chemother. **54**: 418-423.

Chapter 43. *MYCOPLASMA, UREAPLASMA*

Cécile M. BEBEAR

INTRODUCTION

Four species of mycoplasmas, bacteria which belong to the class *Mollicutes*, are pathogenic in humans. *Mycoplasma pneumoniae* causes atypical pneumonia but also benign respiratory disorders such as tracheobronchitis. This species has been incriminated in the onset and exacerbation of asthma in children and adults (39). Genital species include *Mycoplasma genitalium*, *Mycoplasma hominis* and *Ureaplasma urealyticum*. The latter has recently been separated into two new species: *U. parvum* (formerly *U. urealyticum* biovar 1) and *U. urealyticum* (*U. urealyticum* biovar 2) which, in this chapter, will be grouped together under the term *Ureaplasma* spp. They are part of the commensal genital flora but can also be etiological agents of infections (9). With the development of molecular diagnostic methods, a large body of new data has accrued concerning the pathogenic potential of *M. genitalium* (19). Mycoplasmas can also cause infections in immunocompromised patients, typically at extra-pulmonary or extra-genital sites (9).

The tetracyclines, macrolides, and related antibiotics, and fluoroquinolones constitute the main classes of antibiotics active against these bacteria, although *M. hominis* and *Ureaplasma* spp. are intrinsically resistant to certain macrolides. Acquired resistance leading to treatment failure has been reported in clinical isolates of *M. hominis* and *Ureaplasma* spp. This resistance is primarily to tetracyclines and is mediated by the presence of the *tet*(M) determinant. Acquired resistance to macrolides and fluoroquinolones in these two species is much less common and has been described mainly in immunocompromised patients. In this case, resistance is due to mutations in the targets of these antibiotics. For *M. pneumoniae*, only macrolide resistance has been described *in vivo* in a growing number of clinical isolates, whereas fluoroquinolone and tetracycline-resistant mutants have been selected *in vitro*. Resistance is starting to emerge in *M. genitalium* as well, with the isolation of macrolide-resistant strains and resultant reports of treatment failures. This chapter will review the methods used for antibiotic susceptibility testing of mycoplasmas, the intrinsic and acquired resistance mechanisms in the different pathogenic species, and the antibiotics to be studied (list of drugs and indications for antibiotic susceptibility testing).

METHODS

The nutritional requirements and culture conditions of mycoplasmas, bacteria which can multiply both intracellularly and extracellularly, are very different from the standard conditions recommended for conventional bacteria. The mycoplasmas require complex culture media and their growth rates differ according to species. While there has been no true standardization of antibiotic susceptibility testing methods, guidelines have been proposed (36) and a subcommittee of the Clinical and Laboratory Standards Institute (CLSI) has been created with the aim of drawing up standardized protocols for *in vitro* antibiotic susceptibility testing in *M. pneumoniae*, *M. hominis* and *Ureaplasma* spp. Broth and agar dilution methods have been adapted for use with mycoplasmas. These methods share several common features. There is no single medium that can be used for all species. Thus, SP4 or Hayflick's modified media are recommended for species from the genus *Mycoplasma* while Shepard's or 10B media are recommended for *Ureaplasma* spp. (36). The recommended pH of the medium is 7.0-7.5 for *Mycoplasma* spp. while an acidic pH of 6.0-6.5 is necessary for growth of *Ureaplasma* spp. It should be noted that this acidic pH may affect the activity of macrolides *in vitro*. Incubation is carried out at a temperature of 35-37°C in a 5% CO_2 atmosphere for agar media. Incubation times vary according to species (24-48 hours for *Ureaplasma* spp., 48-72 hours for *M. hominis* and 5-7 days for *M. pneumoniae* and *M. genitalium*). An inoculum of 10^4-10^5 color changing units or colony forming units per milliliter is recommended (36). When available, a control strain with known MICs of the drugs being tested can be included. The choice of the method is influenced, in particular, by the number of strains tested and the species.

Broth dilution

Broth dilution methods, particularly in microtiter plates, are widely used for mycoplasmas. The MIC is defined as the lowest antibiotic concentration inhibiting the color change of the pH indicator in the broth medium when the antibiotic-free growth control has changed color. The change in the color of the indicator (usually phenol red) is related to acidification due to glucose fermentation for *M. pneumoniae* and *M. genitalium*, to alkalinization due to arginine hydrolysis for *M. hominis* and to urea degradation for *Ureaplasma* spp.

Broth dilution is the most widely used method and is less labor-intensive than agar dilution. It is particularly useful when testing a small number of strains or for time-kill studies. However, it has the drawback that the MIC value for some antibiotics may change over time. Also, the inoculum may comprise a mixture of both susceptible and resistant bacterial populations.

Test kits have been commercialized for *Ureaplasma* spp. and *M. hominis*. They take the form of microtiter plates containing antibiotic powders at one or two breakpoint concentrations (36). Some kits combine detection, counting and antibiotic susceptibility testing and are used directly on the specimen. Overall, they give results comparable to those obtained by broth dilution methods. However, they cannot always detect tetracycline resistance because of a poorly standardized small inoculum taken directly from the specimen. These kits can also be used after primary culture of the specimen.

Agar dilution

Agar dilution is considered the reference method (36). The MIC is defined as the lowest antibiotic concentration inhibiting the formation of colonies when the growth control has formed colonies. Agar media are especially suited to species which form colonies easily visible with a binocular magnifier, that is, practically all species of the genus *Mycoplasma*. From a practical standpoint, this method is more labor-intensive but it has the advantage of giving a stable MIC value, detecting possible mixtures of populations and allowing a large number of strains to be tested simultaneously. Moreover, the preliminary results of the CLSI subcommittee indicate that this method has superior inter-laboratory reproducibility than the broth dilution method.

Agar gradient diffusion (E-test®)

The disk diffusion technique cannot be used for mycoplasmas due to the long growth times of these microorganisms. However, the agar gradient diffusion technique, or E-test®, has recently been adapted for use in *M. hominis* and *Ureaplasma* spp. (36). The results agree within two dilutions with the values obtained by broth or agar dilution methods. The results are not always easy to read, but this method is useful for occasional testing, mainly of *M. hominis* isolates.

Bactericidal testing

The bactericidal activity of antibiotics against mycoplasmas can be measured directly after susceptibility testing with the broth dilution method, by subculturing the broth from microtiter wells that do not show any visible growth (36). After passage through a 0.22 µm pore-size filter to retain mycoplasmas and eliminate any antibiotic remaining in the medium, the culture is placed in antibiotic-free broth medium or subcultured onto agar to allow growth of remaining viable organisms. The Minimum Bactericidal Concentration (MBC) is then defined as the lowest antibiotic concentration inhibiting a color change of the pH indicator in broth medium or colony formation on agar. The MBC can also be determined by time-kill studies adapted to mycoplasmas (37), in which case the MBC is defined as the amount of antibiotic required to produce 99% killing of the original inoculum.

Molecular tests

Molecular biology techniques including real-time quantitative PCR have been adapted for antimicrobial susceptibility testing in *M. genitalium*, an extremely fastidious species which is very difficult to isolate by culture (18). A real-time PCR method with melt-curve analysis was recently developed to detect mutations in the 23S rRNA gene which confer macrolide resistance in *M. pneumoniae* (40). The advantage of this method is that it can be used directly on respiratory specimens, thus allowing rapid screening for resistance and avoiding the need for lengthy isolation of the fastidious *M. pneumoniae* by culture.

Interpretation of results

Since no recommended breakpoints are available, it is preferable to simply report MICs. Some laboratories have adopted the breakpoints used for interpretation of MICs for conventional bacteria. MICs < 1 µg/ml are often considered to predict an efficient treatment outcome (36). MBCs are rarely determined.

INTRINSIC RESISTANCE

Two types of intrinsic resistance are found in mycoplasmas, the first common to all species in the class *Mollicutes*, and the other specific to certain species. These properties have been used to isolate mycoplasmas from specimens contaminated by other bacteria, or else to separate mycoplasma species within a same specimen.

Related to class

Since they lack a cell wall, all microorganisms in the class *Mollicutes* are resistant to cell wall synthesis inhibitors such as β-lactams, glycopeptides, and fosfomycin. They are also resistant to polymyxins, sulfonamides, trimethoprim, nalidixic acid, and rifampin (2, 4). Rifampin resistance has been studied in the plant mycoplasma *Spiroplasma citri* and was found to be due to a natural mutation in the *rpoB* gene of the RNA polymerase β subunit which prevents the antibiotic from binding to its target. *M. pneumoniae*, *M. hominis* and *Ureaplasma* spp. are resistant to linezolid (Table 1).

Related to species

This type of intrinsic resistance concerns mainly the macrolide-lincosamide-streptogramin group and the ketolides (MLSK antibiotics) (2, 4). Among the human mycoplasmas, *M. pneumoniae* and *M. genitalium* are intrinsically susceptible to MLSK, with the exception of lincomycin which has modest activity against these two species (Table 1). *Ureaplasma* spp. are susceptible to macrolides, ketolides, and streptogramins but resistant to lincosamides. Conversely, *M. hominis* is resistant to macrolides with a 14 or 15-membered ring but susceptible to certain 16-membered ring macrolides (josamycin and midecamycin) and to lincosamides, but not to spiramycin, another 16-membered ring macrolide. *M. fermentans*, a human commensal species, has a similar profile. Among the ketolides, *M. hominis* is resistant to telithromycin but susceptible to cethromycin (Table 1).

The genetic basis underlying intrinsic resistance to erythromycin has been studied by comparing the molecular target of macrolides (domains V and II of 23S rRNA) in *M. hominis* and *M. fermentans* with that of *M. pneumoniae*, an erythromycin-susceptible species (28). Resistance is due to a G (*M. pneumoniae*) to A (*M. hominis* and *M. fermentans*) transition at position 2057 in the peptidyltransferase loop of the domain V region of 23S rRNA (*Escherichia coli* numbering). This transition has been found in two ribosomal operons of reference strains *M. hominis* PG21 and *M. fermentans* PG18 and is associated with macrolide resistance in other bacteria. An additional $C_{2610}U$ transition may be responsible for the higher MICs of macrolides, lincosamides, and telithromycin for *M. hominis* as compared to *M. fermentans*. High-level erythromycin resistance is related to an absence of intracellular erythromycin accumulation and binding to the ribosome (28).

ACTIVE ANTIBIOTICS

Antibiotics with potential activity against mycoplasmas and used in clinical practice include the tetracyclines, MLSK antibiotics, and fluoroquinolones (2, 4). These drugs achieve high intracellular concentrations in mammalian cells and are thereby able to reach the intracellular mycoplasmas. Only the fluoroquinolones and ketolides have a potential bactericidal action. All three classes have the advantage of being active against other bacteria which may be associated with mycoplasmas in respiratory and genital tract infections. Other antibiotics such as aminoglycosides and chloramphenicol may also show activity against mycoplasmas but are only rarely used.

Tetracyclines

Tetracyclines are the first-line treatment of mycoplasmal urogenital infections such as urethritis and pelvic inflammatory disease (4). They are also indicated in the treatment of infections due to *M. pneumoniae* in adults (39). They cannot be used in children under 8 years or during pregnancy. However, there have been several reports that doxycycline has been effective in the treatment of central nervous system infections in neonates (34).

A recent study compared the efficacy of doxycycline versus azithromycin in men and women with a urogenital infection caused by *M. genitalium* (16). Whereas all patients treated with a five-day course of azithromycin were *M. genitalium* negative at the follow-up visit, the majority of doxycycline-treated patients still harbored the mycoplasma. These results suggest that tetracyclines are not always efficient against *M. genitalium* infections *in vivo* and highlight the need for randomized clinical trials.

The glycylcyclines were designed to circumvent tetracycline resistance due to efflux pumps or ribosomal protection (11). Tigecycline shows comparable activity to tetracyclines against *M. pneumoniae* and *M. hominis* but is less active against wild-type strains of *Ureaplasma* spp. (Table 1). In mycoplasma strains with acquired tetracycline resistance, tigecycline retains its activity against *M. hominis* but not against *Ureaplasma* spp. (4).

Macrolides-lincosamides-streptogramins, and ketolides

MLSK are the antibiotics of choice for the treatment of *M. pneumoniae* respiratory tract infections affecting mainly children (39) or when tetracyclines or fluoroquinolones are contraindicated. They are also the drugs of choice for mycoplasmal infections in neonates. Azithromycin and ketolides (telithromycin and cethromycin) have better activity *in vitro* against *M. pneumoniae* while lincosamides, particularly lincomycin, have modest activity (Table 1). Erythromycin was recently shown to have bactericidal activity *in vitro* against *M. genitalium* (3).

Table 1. MIC (µg/ml) of antibiotics for *M. pneumoniae, M. genitalium, M. hominis,* and *Ureaplasma* spp.[a] (adapted from 2, 4).

Antibiotic	*M. pneumoniae*	*M. genitalium*	*M. hominis*	*Ureaplasma* spp.
Tetracycline	0.63 - 0.25	0.06 - 0.5	0.2 - 2	0.05 - 2
Doxycycline	0.02 - 0.5	≤ 0.01 - 0.3	0.03 - 2	0.02 - 1
Minocycline	0.06 - 0.5	≤ 0.01 - 0.2	0.03 - 1	0.06 - 1
Tigecycline	0.06 - 0.25	ND[b]	0.125 - 0.5	1 - 16
Erythromycin	≤ 0.004 - 0.06	≤ 0.01	32 - >1000	0.02 - 4
Roxithromycin	≤ 0.01 - 0.03	≤ 0.01	>16 - > 64	0.06 - 4
Clarithromycin	≤ 0.004 - 0.125	≤ 0.01 - 0.06	16 - > 256	≤ 0.004 - 2
Azithromycin	≤ 0.004 - 0.01	≤ 0.01 - 0.03	4 - > 64	0.5 - 4
Josamycin	≤ 0.01 - 0.02	0.01 - 0.02	0.05 - 2	0.03 - 4
Spiramycin	≤ 0.01 - 0.25	0.12 - 1	32 - > 64	4 - 32
Midecamycin	≤ 0.015	ND	0.25	ND
Clindamycin	≤ 0.008 - 2	0.2 - 1	≤ 0.008 - 2	0.2 - 64
Lincomycin	4 - 8	1 - 8	0.2 - 4	8 - 256
Pristinamycin	0.02 - 0.05	ND	0.1 - 0.5	0.1 - 1
Quinupristin/Dalfopristin	0.008 - 0.12	0.05	0.03 - 2	0.03 - 0.5
Telithromycin	0.0002 - 0.06	≤ 0.015	2 - 32	≤ 0.015 - 0.25
Cethromycin	≤ 0.001 - 0.016	ND	≤ 0.008 - 0.031	≤ 0.008 - 0.031
Pefloxacin	2	ND	1 - 4	1 - 8
Norfloxacin	ND	ND	4 - 16	4 - 16
Ciprofloxacin	0.5 - 2	2	0.5 - 4	0.1 - 4
Ofloxacin	0.05 - 2	1 - 2	0.5 - 4	0.2 - 4
Sparfloxacin	≤ 0.008 - 0.5	0.05 - 0.1	≤ 0.008 - 0.1	0.003 - 1
Levofloxacin	0.5 - 1	0.5 - 1	≤ 0.008 - 0.5	0.12 - 2
Gatifloxacin	0.06 - 1	0.12	0.06 - 0.25	0.25 - 2
Moxifloxacin	0.06 - 0.3	0.03	0.06	0.12 - 0.5
Gemifloxacin	≤ 0.008 - 0.12	0.05	0.0025 - 0.01	≤ 0.008 - 0.25
Garenoxacin	0.015 - 0.12	0.06 - 0.12	0.008 - 0.25	0.06 - 0.25
Chloramphenicol	2 - 10	0.5 - 25	4 - 25	0.4 - 8
Gentamicin	4	ND	2 - 16	0.1 - 13
Linezolid	64 - 256	ND	2 - 8	> 64

[a] Strains without acquired resistance.
[b] ND, not determined.

Fluoroquinolones

The newest fluoroquinolones have the highest activity (Table 1) and are an interesting alternative in the treatment of mycoplasmal respiratory and genital tract infections, particularly in the treatment of disseminated infections in immunocompromised patients because of their bactericidal activity *in vitro* (4).

Susceptible phenotype

Table 1 shows the MICs of different antibiotics for mycoplasmas pathogenic to humans (2, 4). There is a large body of data for *M. pneumoniae*, *M. hominis* and *Ureaplasma* spp. For *M. genitalium*, the results obtained with the very small number of available strains indicate that *M. genitalium* and *M. pneumoniae* have similar susceptibility profiles. For *M. pneumoniae*, recent *in vitro* susceptibility tests carried out in Europe and North America gave comparable results with no major changes from the older studies (39).

ACQUIRED RESISTANCE

Among the various mechanisms of acquired resistance, the only ones described *in vivo* for mycoplasmas are target modification and protection. An active efflux mechanism has also been demonstrated *in vitro* (4). Resistance is mediated either by chromosomal mutations or acquisition of a transposon.

Mycoplasmas are characterized by high mutation rates. Sequencing studies of several mycoplasma genomes have revealed that only a small amount of genetic information is dedicated to DNA repair (9). These high mutation rates have been linked to antibiotic resistance in mycoplasmas, as shown in other bacteria. Resistance through mutation concerns all classes of antibiotics used to treat mycoplasma infections.

Acquisition of plasmids harboring exogenous genes has been described in mollicutes but not in human mycoplasmal pathogens. However, transposons carrying antibiotic resistance genes have been found in the latter, the main example being the *tet*(M) determinant conferring tetracycline resistance.

Until recently, few studies on *in vitro* or *in vivo* resistance of mycoplasmas to antibiotics were available. Research has since intensified and is now focusing not only on *M. hominis* and *Ureaplasma* spp., two species long known to be tetracycline-resistant, but also on *M. pneumoniae* and *M. genitalium*, two species with high antibiotic susceptibility in which macrolide resistance is now becoming a problem (5, 10, 20).

Tetracyclines

Mechanisms

Acquired resistance to tetracyclines has long been known in *Ureaplasma* spp. and *M. hominis* and is due to the presence of the *tet*(M) determinant (4). In mycoplasmas this determinant is located on the conjugative transposon Tn*916*. This transposon, present in *M. hominis* and *Ureaplasma* spp., is the only naturally acquired antibiotic resistance determinant in human mycoplasmas. It codes for the Tet(M) protein which protects the ribosome from the action of tetracyclines. The Tet(M) protein is homologous to elongation factors EF-Tu and EF-G and upon binding to the ribosome induces a conformational change which is thought to prevent tetracycline binding without altering protein synthesis (11).

M. hominis and *M. pneumoniae* strains with reduced tetracycline susceptibility (MIC ≤ 2 µg/ml) have been obtained *in vitro* in the presence of increasing tetracycline concentrations (14). Reduced susceptibility to tetracyclines is related to mutations of the tetracycline binding pocket of 16S rRNA.

Phenotypes and prevalence

High-level tetracycline resistance (MIC ≥ 8 µg/ml) is associated with the presence of the *tet*(M) determinant which confers cross-resistance to all tetracyclines (Table 2). Such strains are easily detected in susceptibility tests with categorization of strains as intermediate or resistant to tetracycline, doxycycline, and minocycline. Genotypic detection can be performed by PCR amplification of the *tet*(M) gene (12).

The prevalence of acquired tetracycline resistance among the genital mycoplasma *M. hominis* and *Ureaplasma* spp. varies according to the country and the antibiotic exposure of the population. Resistance was estimated to be present in about 10% of patients consulting for a sexually transmitted infection in the United Kingdom (4) and 3% in France in 1992 (1). A more recent study carried out in France between 1999 and 2002 showed a significant increase in resistance rates for *M. hominis*, with 19% of isolates showing reduced tetracycline susceptibility (13). On the other hand,

Table 2. MIC (µg/ml) of macrolides and tetracyclines for clinical isolates of *Mycoplasma* and *Ureaplasma* (adapted from 2, 5)

Species	No. of resistant isolates	TET[a]	DOX	MIN	ERY	JOS	AZM	CLI	Q-D	TEL
M. pneumoniae										
macrolide S[b]	—	—	—	—	0.015–256	0.03–0.12	0.002–>64	1–2	0.25–1	0.002–>64
macrolide R[c]	30	—	—	—	8–>256	0.25–256	0.03–>64	4–256	0.25–1	2–>64
M. hominis										
macrolide S	—	0.25	0.06	0.06	512	0.25	32	0.25	0.25	32
macrolide R[c]	2	32–>64	8–32	2–32	512	512	512	16–64	0.5	256
tetracycline S	—									
tetracycline R[d]	Nmr[f]									
Ureaplasma spp.										
macrolide R[e]	1	—	—	—	0.12–1	0.03–0.12	>100	>100	—	—
			0.25	0.12	>100	88	>100	>100		
tetracycline S	—	1	—	—	—	—	—	—	—	—
tetracycline R[d]	Nmr	>32	>32	8–32						
M. genitalium										
macrolide S	—	0.25–0.5	0.25	—	≤0.015	—	≤0.015	—	—	—
macrolide R[e]	12	0.25–4	0.25–1	—	≥16	—	≥8	—	—	—

[a] AZM, azithromycin; CLI, clindamycin; DOX, doxycycline; ERY, erythromycin; JOS, josamycin; MIN, minocycline; Q-D, quinupristin-dalfopristin; TEL, telithromycin; TET, tetracycline.
[b] R, resistant; S, susceptible.
[c] Mutations in 23S rRNA.
[d] *tet*(M) gene.
[e] Unknown mechanism.
[f] Nmr, numerous.

---

no such increase was found in *Ureaplasma* spp. for which the percentage of tetracycline-resistant isolates was 2% over the same period. In contrast to our findings, a recent American study reported that the *tet*(M) gene was present in 45 of 100 *Ureaplasma* spp. clinical isolates obtained in different regions between 2000 and 2004 (38).

There has been a considerable number of treatment failures of tetracyclines in *M. genitalium* urethritis although the cause for this remains obscure (19).

Macrolides-lincosamides-streptogramins, and ketolides

Mechanisms

Macrolide resistance in mycoplasmas, which have a small number of ribosomal operons, is conferred by mutations in the ribosomal target (23S rRNA or riboproteins L4 and L22). It has been described mainly in *M. pneumoniae* but resistant strains of *M. hominis*, *Ureaplasma* spp. (2, 4) and, more recently, *M. genitalium* (10, 20), have been reported.

Most resistant strains of *M. pneumoniae* harbor a $A_{2058}G$ mutation in the peptidyltransferase loop of 23S rRNA (5) (Fig. 1). The other *in vivo* mutations at positions 2059 and 2611 (23, 26) have been identified as macrolide resistance hot spots in other bacteria. No mutations in domain II or in the ribosomal proteins L4 or L22 genes have been described *in vivo*. Resistant strains do not show cross-resistance to other classes of antibiotics.

Resistant mutants of *M. pneumoniae* have been obtained by selection *in vitro* on erythromycin (22, 26). Resistance is due to mutations at positions 2058 and 2059 which were previously described *in vivo*. A recent, very exhaustive *in vitro* study describes the selection of mutants resistant to different macrolides, streptogramins and a ketolide, testing a total of eight antibiotics (29). The selected mutations were in domain V of 23S rRNA at positions 2611 and 2062 and in the genes encoding ribosomal proteins L4 and L22; these were point mutations, insertions or deletions. No mutations were detected in domain II of 23S rRNA. The different antibiotics did not select mutants in the same manner. A mutation appeared after the first passages in erythromycin or azithromycin but these drugs remained active after 50 passages. Conversely, josamycin and clindamycin selected mutants after more than 20 passages but ultimately lost all activity against these mutants. With

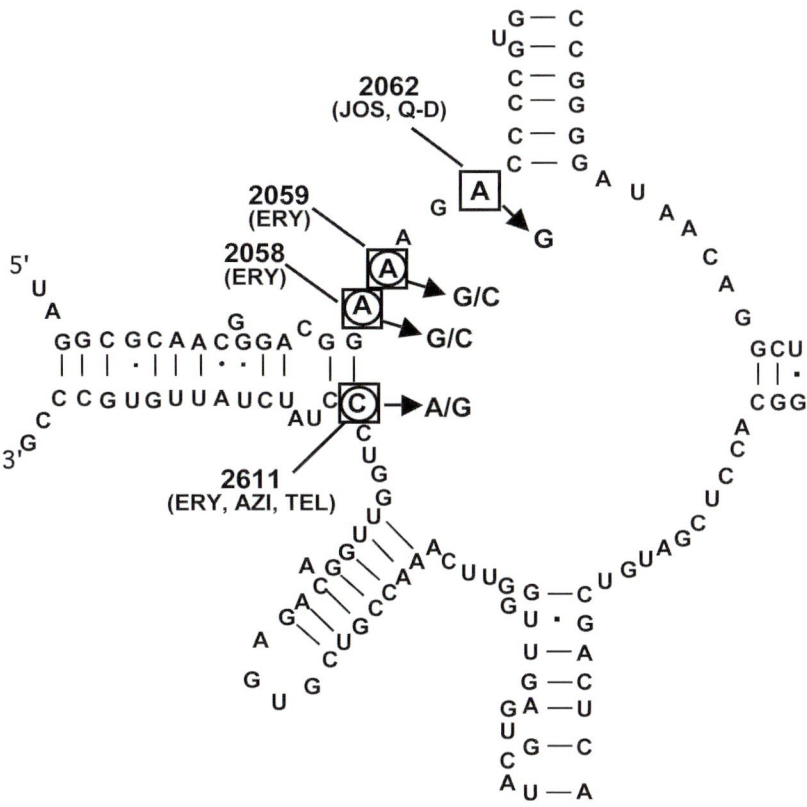

Fig. 1. Secondary structure of the peptidyltransferase loop of domain V of 23S rRNA of *M. pneumoniae* (*E. coli* numbering). Squared nucleotides indicate positions mutated *in vitro*. Antibiotics in parentheses (AZM, azithromycin, ERY, erythromycin, JOS, josamycin, Q-D, quinupristin-dalfopristin and TEL, telithromycin) indicate the selective agent. Circled nucleotides indicate positions mutated *in vivo*. Adapted from (5).

telithromycin, 32 passages and three mutational events were required to categorize the mutant as resistant.

Among urogenital mycoplasmas, a clinical isolate of *Ureaplasma* spp. resistant to 14 and 16-member macrolides was isolated from a patient with urethritis treated with erythromycin (4) (Table 2). Antibiotic binding to the ribosome was decreased but the molecular mechanism was not identified. Two *M. hominis* clinical isolates resistant to 16-member macrolides and lincosamides were obtained from respiratory specimens in a patient with chronic obstructive pulmonary disease with multiple antibiotic exposure (28). These strains were resistant to fluoroquinolones through target modification and to tetracyclines through acquisition of the *tet*(M) gene. Macrolide resistance was related to the presence of two transitions, $A_{2059}G$ and $C_{2611}U$, in domain V of one of the two ribosomal operons for one strain, while the other strain harbored a single mutation at position 2059 of the same operon. These clinical descriptions have been confirmed by *in vitro* selection of resistant mutants of *M. hominis* and *Ureaplasma* spp. in which mutations were found in the 23S rRNA and ribosomal proteins L4 and L22 (30, 31).

Twelve macrolide resistant clinical isolates of *M. genitalium* were recently described in Australian and Scandinavian patients with urethritis treated with azithromycin (Table 2) (10, 20). All isolates harbored a $A_{2058}G$ or $A_{2059}G$ mutation. In the majority of cases these macrolide resistant mutants were selected during azithromycin therapy (20).

Phenotypes and prevalence

The resistant *M. pneumoniae* clinical isolates that were studied had an MLS_B phenotype and were resistant to macrolides, lincosamides, streptogramin B and ketolides, with different increases in the MICs according to the mutation (5). For example, for 16-membered macrolides there was a larger increase in the MICs for the mutation at position 2059 than at position 2058 whereas the reverse was true for ketolides. The mutation at position 2611 was associated with the lowest levels of resistance. Quinupristin-dalfopristin retained activity against the mutants (Table 2).

Molecular detection of resistance by PCR-RFLP (23) or real-time PCR (40) on PCR-positive respiratory specimens has been developed for the mutations at positions 2058 and 2059 in *M. pneumoniae*.

Prior to the year 2000, very few clinical isolates of *M. pneumoniae* were resistant to macrolides (5). In contrast, since 2000 several Japanese studies (23, 25) have reported a significant increase in macrolide resistance rates in *M. pneumoniae*, affecting up to 30% (37/121) of strains in 2006 according to Morozumi et al. (24). In a recent *M. pneumoniae* epidemic in the United States (40), three of eleven isolates were resistant to macrolides. In France, only two macrolide-resistant clinical isolates were described within a series of 155 strains isolated between 1994 and 2006 (27). More recently, however, macrolide resistance in *M. pneumoniae* has been on the rise in France, with a 10% rate (5/51) of resistant genotypes reported between 2005 and 2007 (Bébéar et al., unpublished data). The isolation of macrolide-resistant *M. pneumoniae* may lead to treatment failure which, for the patients concerned, translates into more febrile days and more frequent changes of the initially prescribed macrolide (35).

The prevalence of acquired macrolide resistance in clinical isolates of *M. hominis* and *Ureaplasma* spp. is unknown but probably very low. In contrast, macrolide resistance rates appear to be increasing in M. *genitalium*; this has resulted in failure of azithromycin treatment (10, 20) and justifies epidemiological surveillance using molecular technologies that can detect mutations in the 23S rRNA directly on the specimen without requiring a culture step.

Fluoroquinolones

Mechanisms

Mutations in the target genes *gyrA* and *gyrB* of DNA gyrase and *parC* and *parE* of topoisomerase IV are the main mechanisms conferring fluoroquinolone resistance in mycoplasmas (4).

Resistance *in vivo* has been described only in genital mycoplasmas. Mutations in the Quinolone Resistance Determining Regions (QRDR) of the two targets (*gyrA*, *parC* and *parE* genes) have been detected in clinical isolates of *M. hominis* (7, 8) and *Ureaplasma* spp. (7). Treatment failure has been described in patients with nongonococcal urethritis in whom *M. genitalium* was isolated following treatment with levofloxacin. Mutations in the *gyrA* and *parC* genes of *M. genitalium* have been detected by molecular methods (15).

Similar results have been obtained by *in vitro* selection of resistant mutants of *M. hominis* and *M. pneumoniae* on different fluoroquinolones, including the most recent ones (levofloxacin, trovafloxacin, gatifloxacin, moxifloxacin, and gemifloxacin) (6, 17, 21). Regardless of which drug was used for selection, fluoroquinolone resistance hot spots in the QRDRs of other bacteria were found to be mutated in the resistant strains. Mutation rates however were lower for the newer fluoroquinolones than for the older ones like ofloxacin or ciprofloxacin. Moreover, in *M. pneumoniae* as in *M. hominis*, the primary target depends on the fluoroquinolone used for selection. For example, in *M. hominis* the primary target of ciprofloxacin is topoisomerase IV while the primary target of sparfloxacin is DNA gyrase (6).

An active efflux system of the ATP binding cassette (ABC) transporter type has been described in *M. hominis* strains selected on ethidium bromide displaying a multiresistant phenotype with increased MICs of ciprofloxacin and ethidium bromide (32). Two genes, *md1* and *md2*, encoding putative ABC transporters are constitutively expressed in the reference strain *M. hominis* PG21 and overexpressed in the resistant strains (33).

Phenotypes

Resistant clinical isolates of *M. hominis* and *Ureaplasma* spp. show cross-resistance to fluoroquinolones (Table 3). The level of resistance depends on the number and positions of the mutations. High-level resistance is associated with target modification on DNA gyrase and topoisomerase IV. It is the newest molecules, moxifloxacin and gatifloxacin, which remain most effective against these mutants, although they lose their bactericidal activity *in vitro* (3).

Here again, the prevalence of fluoroquinolone resistance is unknown but probably very low, estimated at less than 1% for *Ureaplasma* spp. (7). The clinical isolates described so far were from patients treated with fluoroquinolones and most of whom were immunocompromised.

It should be noted that fluoroquinolone-resistant strains of *M. hominis* and *M. fermentans*

Table 3. MIC (µg/ml) of fluoroquinolones against clinical isolates of urogenital *Mycoplasma* (adapted from 2)

Species	No. of resistant isolates	OFX[a]	CIP	LVX	GAT	MXF
M. hominis						
Fluoroquinolone S[b]	–	0.5	1	0.25	0.12	0.06
Fluoroquinolone R (2 to 3 mutations)	6	8 – 16	16 – 32	2 – 32	1 – 4	0.5 – 4
Ureaplasma spp.						
Fluoroquinolone S	–	1	1	0.5	1	0.25
Fluoroquinolone R						
1 mutation	5	> 4	4 – 16	0.5 – 2	2	0.5 – 1
2 mutations	7	> 4	8 – 64	2 – 16	2 – 8	1 – 4

[a] CIP, ciprofloxacin; GAT, gatifloxacin; LVX, levofloxacin; OFX, ofloxacin; MXF, moxifloxacin.
[b] R, resistant; S, susceptible.

have been isolated from cell cultures infected with these mycoplasmas after treatment with these antibiotics (4).

ANTIBIOTICS TO BE STUDIED

First-line and alternativs

The number and classes of antibiotics to be studied depends on the mycoplasma species, the patient's pathology, age and concomitant diseases, as well as the consensus guidelines. Not all antibiotics active against mycoplasma can be used for all clinical syndromes.

Three main classes should be tested: tetracyclines, macrolides group and fluoroquinolones. Among the tetracyclines, tetracycline, doxycycline, and minocycline are recommended. In the macrolides group, a 14-membered (erythromycin) or 15-membered (azithromycin) macrolide, a 16-membered macrolide (josamycin, in countries using this antibiotic), a lincosamide (clindamycin) and a streptogramin (pristinamycin, in countries using this antibiotic) should be used. Where necessary a ketolide (telithromycin) can be added. Fluoroquinolones should include ofloxacin or ciprofloxacin and, depending on the indication, a fluoroquinolone with higher intrinsic activity such as levofloxacin or moxifloxacin.

There are few alternative treatments. Chloramphenicol has been used to treat neonatal meningitis since it diffuses well into cerebrospinal fluid. In this case it is not necessary to test the susceptibility of the strain, since acquired resistance to chloramphenicol has never been described *in vivo*. However, since chloramphenicol has been associated with a risk of gray baby syndrome, ciprofloxacin can be used as an alternative treatment.

Indications of antibiotic susceptibility testing

Should antibiotic susceptibility testing of mycoplasmas be a routine practice? What is important to consider is the relative prevalence of resistance and its possible impact on therapy. The action to take differs according to the species and depends on whether individual or collective surveillance is the goal.

Today, only the genital mycoplasmas (*Ureaplasma* spp. and *M. hominis*) should be routinely tested for resistance when these bacteria are incriminated in infection. Resistance is especially worrisome when these bacteria are isolated from extra-genital sites in immunocompromised patients with multiple drug exposure.

Resistance is still rare in *M. pneumoniae* and *M. genitalium* and the time needed to detect it due to the lengthy isolation of these fastidious bacteria by culture, if they are even cultivable, is such that there is no immediate impact on treatment. Susceptibility testing may therefore be useful in immunocompromised patients, for epidemiological studies or in new drug development. However, recent data from Japan as well as the United States and France point toward a rising prevalence of macrolide resistance in *M. pneumoniae*, which makes epidemiological surveillance a necessity in Europe, the United States and Asia. The development of real-time PCR for rapid detection of mutations in the 23S rRNA conferring macrolide resistance, directly from respiratory specimens, appears very promising and should allow treatment to be adjusted rapidly in case a resistant genotype is detected.

REFERENCES

(1) **Bébéar, C., B. de Barbeyrac, A. Dewilde, D. Edert, C. Janvresse, M.P. Layani, A. Le Faou, J.C. Lefèvre, I. Mendel, H. Renaudin, M.J. Sanson le Pors, D. Thouvenot, and Groupe MST.** 1993. Etude multicentrique de la sensibilité in vitro des mycoplasmes génitaux aux antibiotiques. Pathol. Biol. **41:**289-293.

(2) **Bébéar, C.M., B. de Barbeyrac, S. Pereyre, and C. Bébéar.** 2007. Mycoplasmes et chlamydiae: sensibilité et résistance aux antibiotiques. Revue Française des Laboratoires **392:**77-85.

(3) **Bébéar, C.M., B. de Barbeyrac, S. Pereyre, H. Renaudin, M. Clerc, and C. Bébéar.** 2008. Activity of moxifloxacin against the urogenital mycoplasmas *Ureaplasma* spp., *Mycoplasma hominis* and *Mycoplasma genitalium* and *Chlamydia trachomatis*. Clin. Microbiol. Infect. **14:**801-805.

(4) **Bébéar, C.M., and I. Kempf.** 2005. Antimicrobial therapy and antimicrobial resistance, p. 535-568. *In* A. Blanchard and G.F. Browning (ed.), Mycoplasmas: pathogenesis, molecular biology, and emerging strategies for control. Horizon Bioscience, Wymondham.

(5) **Bébéar, C.M., and S. Pereyre.** 2005. Mechanisms of drug resistance in *Mycoplasma pneumoniae*. Current Drug Targets - Infectious Disorders **5:**263-271.

(6) **Bébéar, C.M., H. Renaudin, A. Charron, J.M. Bové, C. Bébéar, and J. Renaudin.** 1998. Alterations in topoisomerase IV and DNA gyrase in quinolone-resistant mutants of *Mycoplasma hominis* obtained in vitro. Antimicrob. Agents Chemother. **42:**2304-2311.

(7) **Bébéar, C.M., H. Renaudin, A. Charron, M. Clerc, S. Pereyre, and C. Bébéar.** 2003. DNA gyrase and topoisomerase IV mutations in clinical isolates of *Ureaplasma* spp. and *Mycoplasma hominis* resistant to fluoroquinolones. Antimicrob. Agents Chemother. **47:**3323-3325.

(8) **Bébéar, C.M., J. Renaudin, A. Charron, H. Renaudin, B. de Barbeyrac, T. Schaeverbeke, and C. Bébéar.** 1999. Mutations in the *gyrA*, *parC*, and *parE* genes associated with fluoroquinolone resistance in clinical isolates of *Mycoplasma hominis*. Antimicrob. Agents Chemother. **43:**954-956.

(9) **Blanchard, A., and C.M. Bébéar.** 2002. Mycoplasmas of humans, p. 45-71. *In* S. Razin and R. Herrmann (ed.), Molecular biology and pathogenicity of mycoplasmas. Kluwer Academic/Plenum Publishers, London.

(10) **Bradshaw, C.S., J.S. Jensen, S.N. Tabrizi, T.R. Read, S.M. Garland, C.A. Hopkins, L.M. Moss, and C.K. Fairley.** 2006. Azithromycin failure in *Mycoplasma genitalium* urethritis. Emerg. Infect. Dis. **12:**1149-1152.

(11) **Chopra, I., and M. Roberts.** 2001. Tetracycline antibiotics: mode of action, applications, molecular biology, and epidemiology of bacterial resistance. Microbiol. Mol. Biol. Rev. **65:**232-260.

(12) **de Barbeyrac, B., M. Dupon, P. Rodriguez, H. Renaudin, and C. Bébéar.** 1996. A Tn*1545*-like transposon carries the *tet*(M) gene in tetracycline resistant strains of *Bacteroides ureolyticus* as well as *Ureaplasma urealyticum* but not *Neisseria gonorrhoeae*. J. Antimicrob. Chemother. **37:**223-232.

(13) **Dégrange, S., H. Renaudin, A. Charron, C. Bébéar, and C.M. Bébéar.** 2008. Tetracycline resistance in *Ureaplasma* spp. and *Mycoplasma hominis*: prevalence in Bordeaux, France, from 1999 to 2002 and description of two *tet*(M)-positive isolates of *M. hominis* susceptible to tetracyclines. Antimicrob. Agents Chemother. **52:**742-744.

(14) **Dégrange, S., H. Renaudin, A. Charron, S. Pereyre, C. Bébéar, and C.M. Bébéar.** 2008. Reduced susceptibility to tetracyclines is associated *in vitro* with the presence of 16S rRNA mutations in *Mycoplasma hominis* and *Mycoplasma pneumoniae*. J. Antimicrob. Chemother. **61:**1390-1392.

(15) **Deguchi, T., S. Maeda, M. Tamaki, T. Yoshida, H. Ishiko, M. Ito, S. Yokoi, Y. Takahashi, and S. Ishihara.** 2001. Analysis of the *gyrA* and *parC* genes of *Mycoplasma genitalium* detected in first-pass urine of men with non-gonococcal urethritis before and after fluoroquinolone treatment. J. Antimicrob. Chemother. **48:**742-744.

(16) **Falk, L., H. Fredlund, and J.S. Jensen.** 2003. Tetracycline treatment does not eradicate *Mycoplasma genitalium*. Sex. Transm. Infect. **79:**318-319.

(17) **Gruson, D., S. Pereyre, A. Charron, H. Renaudin, C. Bébéar, and C.M. Bébéar.** 2005. In vitro development of resistance to six and four fluoroquinolones in *Mycoplasma pneumoniae* and in *Mycoplasma hominis*. Antimicrob. Agents Chemother. **49:**1190-1193.

(18) **Hamasuna, R., Y. Osada, and J.S. Jensen.** 2005. Antibiotic susceptibility testing of *Mycoplasma genitalium* by TaqMan 5' nuclease real-time PCR. Antimicrob. Agents Chemother. **49:**4993-4998.

(19) **Jensen, J.S.** 2004. *Mycoplasma genitalium*: the aetiological agent of urethritis and other sexually transmitted diseases. J. Eur. Acad. Dermatol. Venereol. **18:**1-11.

(20) **Jensen, J.S., C.S. Bradshaw, S.N. Tabrizi, C.K. Fairley, and R. Hamasuna.** 2008. Azithromycin treatment failure in *Mycoplasma genitalium*-positive patients with nongonococcal urethritis is associated with induced macrolide resistance. Clin. Infect. Dis. **47:**1546-1553.

(21) **Kenny, G.E., P.A. Young, F.D. Cartwright, K.E. Sjostrom, and W.M. Huang.** 1999. Sparfloxacin selects gyrase mutations in first-step *Mycoplasma hominis* mutants, whereas ofloxacin selects topoisomerase IV mutations. Antimicrob. Agents Chemother. **43:**2493-2496.

(22) **Lucier, T.S., K. Heitzman, S.K. Liu, and P.C. Hu.** 1995. Transition mutations in the 23S rRNA of erythromycin-resistant isolates of *Mycoplasma pneumoniae*. Antimicrob. Agents Chemother. **39:**2770-2773.

(23) **Matsuoka, M., M. Narita, N. Okazaki, H. Ohya, T. Yamazaki, K. Ouchi, I. Suzuki, T. Andoh, T. Kenri, Y. Sasaki, A. Horino, M. Shintani, Y. Arakawa, and T. Sasaki.** 2004. Characterization and molecular analysis of macrolide-resistant *Mycoplasma pneumoniae* clinical isolates obtained in Japan. Antimicrob. Agents Chemother. **48:**4624-4630.

(24) **Morozumi, M., S. Iwata, K. Hasegawa, N. Chiba, R. Takayanagi, K. Matsubara, E. Nakayama, K. Sunakawa, and K. Ubukata.** 2008. Increased macrolide resistance of *Mycoplasma pneumoniae* in

pediatric patients with community-acquired pneumonia. Antimicrob. Agents Chemother. **52**:348-350.

(25) **Morozumi, T., K. Hasegawa, R. Kobayashi, N. Inoue, S. Iwata, H. Kuroki, N. Kawamura, E. Nakayama, T. Tajima, K. Shimizu, and K. Ubukata.** 2005. Emergence of macrolide-resistant *Mycoplasma pneumoniae* with a 23S rRNA gene mutation. Antimicrob. Agents Chemother. **49**:2302-2306.

(26) **Okazaki, N., M. Narita, S. Yamada, K. Izumikawa, M. Umetsu, T. Kenri, Y. Sasaki, Y. Arakawa, and T. Sasaki.** 2001. Characteristics of macrolide-resistant *Mycoplasma pneumoniae* strains isolated from patients and induced with erythromycin in vitro. Microbiol. Immunol. **45**:617-620.

(27) **Pereyre, S., A. Charron, H. Renaudin, C. Bébéar, and C.M. Bébéar.** 2007. First report of macrolide-resistant strains and description of a novel nucleotide sequence variation in the P1 adhesin gene in *Mycoplasma pneumoniae* clinical strains isolated in France over 12 years. J. Clin. Microbiol. **45**:3534-3539.

(28) **Pereyre, S., P. Gonzalez, B. de Barbeyrac, A. Darnige, H. Renaudin, A. Charron, S. Raherison, C. Bébéar, and C.M. Bébéar.** 2002. Mutations in 23S rRNA account for intrinsic resistance to macrolides in *Mycoplasma hominis* and *Mycoplasma fermentans* and for acquired resistance to macrolides in *M. hominis*. Antimicrob. Agents Chemother. **46**:3142-3150.

(29) **Pereyre, S., C. Guyot, H. Renaudin, A. Charron, C. Bébéar, and C.M. Bébéar.** 2004. In vitro selection of resistance to macrolides and related antibiotics in *Mycoplasma pneumoniae*. Antimicrob. Agents Chemother. **48**:460-465.

(30) **Pereyre, S., M. Métifiot, C. Cazanave, H. Renaudin, A. Charron, C. Bébéar, and C.M. Bébéar.** 2007. Characterisation of *in vitro*-selected mutants of *Ureaplasma parvum* resistant to macrolides and related antibiotics. Int. J. Antimicrob. Agents **29**:207-211.

(31) **Pereyre, S., H. Renaudin, A. Charron, C. Bébéar, and C.M. Bébéar.** 2006. Emergence of a 23S rRNA mutation in *Mycoplasma hominis* associated with a loss of the intrinsic resistance to erythromycin and azithromycin. J. Antimicrob. Chemother. **57**:753-756.

(32) **Raherison, S., P. Gonzalez, H. Renaudin, A. Charron, C. Bébéar, and C.M. Bébéar.** 2002. Evidence of an active efflux in resistance to ciprofloxacin and ethidium bromide by *Mycoplasma hominis*. Antimicrob. Agents Chemother. **46**:672-679.

(33) **Raherison, S., P. Gonzalez, H. Renaudin, A. Charron, C. Bébéar, and C.M. Bébéar.** 2005. Increased expression of two multidrug transporter-like genes is associated with ethidium bromide and ciprofloxacin resistance in *Mycoplasma hominis*. Antimicrob. Agents Chemother. **49**:421-424.

(34) **Sarlangue, J., and C. Bébéar.** 1999. Infections néonatales à mycoplasmes. Médecine Thérapeutique Pédiatrie **2**:105-109.

(35) **Suzuki, S., T. Yamazaki, M. Narita, N. Okazaki, I. Suzuki, T. Andoh, M. Matsuoka, T. Kenri, Y. Arakawa, and T. Sasaki.** 2006. Clinical evaluation of macrolide-resistant *Mycoplasma pneumoniae*. Antimicrob. Agents Chemother. **50**:709-712.

(36) **Waites, K.B., C.M. Bébéar, J.A. Roberston, D.F. Talkington, and G.E. Kenny** (ed.). 2001. Cumitech 34, Laboratory diagnosis of mycoplasmal infections. American Society for Microbiology, Washington D.C.

(37) **Waites, K.B., D.M. Crabb, X. Bing, and L.B. Duffy.** 2003. In vitro susceptibilities to and bactericidal activities of garenoxacin (BMS-284756) and other antimicrobial agents against human mycoplasmas and ureaplasmas. Antimicrob. Agents Chemother. **47**:161-165.

(38) **Waites, K.B., B. Katz, and R.L. Schelonka.** 2005. Mycoplasmas and ureaplasmas as neonatal pathogens. Clin. Microbiol. Rev. **18**:757-789.

(39) **Waites, K.B., and D. Talkington.** 2004. *Mycoplasma pneumoniae* and its role as a human pathogen. Clin. Microbiol. Rev. **17**:697-728.

(40) **Wolff, B.J., W.L. Thacker, S.B. Schwartz, and J.M. Winchell.** 2008. Detection of macrolide resistance in *Mycoplasma pneumoniae* by real-time PCR and high-resolution melt analysis. Antimicrob. Agents Chemother. **52**:3542-3549.

Chapter 44. *CHLAMYDIA*

Bertille de BARBEYRAC

INTRODUCTION

Chlamydia are obligate intracellular bacteria capable of developing in different cell lines. They have a unique life cycle wherein they adopt different forms:
- the elementary body (EB), which is infectious and can survive in the extracellular milieu but cannot replicate,
- the reticulate body (RB), which is the intracellular replicative form,
- the intermediate body (IB), which represents the transition between RB and EB.

In broad outline, the EB attaches to and enters the cell, then differentiates to the RB which replicates inside a membrane-bound compartment called an inclusion. RBs then convert back to IBs and then to EBs which are released from the inclusion. A fourth form, called the aberrant body, has been observed in certain conditions; it corresponds to a viable but non-culturable alternative form which appears to be responsible for persistent infection.

This mode of development explains:
- why so few antibiotics are effective, since the drug must penetrate the host cell membrane as well as that of the inclusion and the bacterial wall;
- why antibiotic susceptibility testing is difficult and not routinely performed.

In addition, as cell culture is not a good diagnostic tool, few strains are available, which is a limiting factor for antibiotic susceptibility testing. This is especially true for *C. pneumoniae*, whose culture is problematic and done in only a few specialized laboratories, and for *C. psittaci* which, due to its contagiousness, requires a level P3 facility. With respect to *C. trachomatis*, cell cultures were used for many years but have since been replaced by newly available and more practical molecular methods with greater sensitivity.

METHODS

Principle

Antibiotic susceptibility testing of chlamydiae comprises a step of culturing the bacteria on a species-appropriate cell line in the presence of increasing antibiotic concentrations (25). Usually, cells seeded with an inoculum of 10^3-10^5 IFU (Inclusion Forming Units) per coverslip are centrifuged at 2,500-3,000 x g for 1 h at 37°C and incubated in a 5% CO_2 atmosphere at 37°C, for 2 to 3 h according to whether the species is *C. trachomatis* or *C. pneumoniae*, respectively. Elementary bodies unattached to cells are then eliminated and medium containing antibiotic and supplemented with glucose and cycloheximide is added. After a 40-60 h incubation, growth inhibition can be determined by immunofluorescence staining of the inclusions or by molecular methods.

Determination of growth inhibition

Immunofluorescence staining of inclusions

The infected cell monolayers are stained with a fluorescent fluorescein-labeled monoclonal antibody with variable specificity for a species or genus.

Microscopic examination

Coverslips are examined on a fluorescence microscope to visualize inclusions, which appear fluorescent green against a background of cells counterstained in red (Fig. 1). The level of susceptibility of a strain is evaluated by determining the minimum inhibitory concentration (MIC) and the minimum bactericidal concentration (MBC). The MIC is the lowest antibiotic concentration which inhibits the formation of any typical inclusions. The MBC is the lowest antibiotic concentration inhibiting the production of infectious bodies that can reinfect other cells (5). After one round of infection in the presence of antibiotic to determine the MIC, the cells are detached and reinoculated on new cells in the absence of antibiotic. The MBC is generally determined after one or two passages in antibiotic-free cell culture.

Ultimately, this method is subjective because it is difficult to differentiate an inclusion from residual inoculum under the microscope. In fact, at concentrations close to the MIC, there is a significant reduction in the size and fluorescence of the inclusions, making MIC determination tricky (Fig. 1D).

This explains the large variations that were found in the MICs of five antibiotics determined against five *C. trachomatis* strains in a multicenter study carried out by six laboratories, despite the fact that all the laboratories used the same protocol. The MICs of some antibiotics like azithromycin or ofloxacin differed by more than six-fold (22). It was recently suggested that the MIC be defined as the antibiotic concentration corresponding to the dilution following that at which 90% or more of the inclusions have altered size and morphology (29).

Flow cytometry

To remedy this problem, we have developed a more objective fluorescence reading method based on flow cytometry (7). Cells infected and incubated in the presence of antibiotic are resuspended, permeabilized, and immunolabeled with the same antibodies as above. In this method, labeled infected cells appear as a fluorescence peak on the histograms. Antibiotic activity is evaluated by calculating the IC_{50}, *i.e.,* the antibiotic concentration which produces a 50% decrease in fluorescence intensity, relative to a control of infected cells cultured without antibiotic representing 100%. The IC_{50} values are extrapolated from plots of the percentage of remaining fluorescence versus antibiotic concentration. These values have the advantage of being reproducible and independent of the concentration range tested.

Fig. 2 illustrates the results obtained with ofloxacin and grepafloxacin against a clinical isolate. The activity curves of the two drugs are clearly separated and IC_{50} values extrapolated from the curves (IC_{50} grepafloxacin = 0.004 µg/ml and IC_{50} ofloxacin = 0.25 µg/ml) indicate that grepafloxacin has higher activity (23). MICs differ from IC_{50} values because the MIC represents total inhibition defined as absence of inclusions, whereas IC_{50} represents 50% inhibition of the inoculum. Flow cytometry will detect antibiotic resistance in a strain only if a large fraction of the bacterial population expresses this resistance. Flow cytometry is useful for comparing *in vitro* activity of different antibiotics, but is limited by the availability and cost of the equipment.

Molecular methods

These methods consist in measuring bacterial growth inhibition by quantification of either DNA or transcripts by real time PCR.

Real time PCR quantification of DNA has recently been used for other intracellular bacteria such as *Tropheryma whipplei* and *Coxiella burnetii*. We have evaluated this method on *C. trachomatis*. Real time PCR is based on the use of a fluorescent tracer and a fluorescence detection system. Amplification of the PCR products generates an exponential function which depends on the number of cycles performed and on fluorescence intensity. Each sample is defined by the threshold cycle which corresponds to the number of cycles for which the fluorescence signal is significantly higher than background. The lower the number of cycles, the more targets there are in the sample. The MIC is defined as the lowest antibiotic concentration for which the threshold cycle determined by real time PCR is greater than or equal to that obtained with the bacterial inoculum (Fig. 3). In the example in Fig. 3, the MIC is equal to 0.5 µg/ml.

A RT-PCR method for testing antibiotic susceptibility has previously been described for *C. trachomatis* (4) and *C. pneumoniae* (11).

By using cDNA quantification, theoretically, the antibiotic concentration for which no RNA is transcripted, corresponds to a bactericidal concentration since the RNA transcripts measure the expression of viable bacteria. In our experience, at 40h post infection, the cDNA quantification never showed a complete absence of transcription whatever the gene target studied and whatever the antibiotics tested for both reference strains D and L2. For all antibiotic tested, *C. trachomatis* still transcribes groEL gene even at concentrations well above MIC (personnal data).

Antibiotics inhibit the multiplication of bacteria but not exert a lethal effect on the organism. A potential problem with bacteriostatic antibiotics in the therapy of chlamydia infections is the induction of latent or persistent forms of chlamydiae which result in apparent eradication but which may allow subclinical progressions of persistent infections. In C. trachomatis infection treated with bacteriostatic antibiotics, the clearance of bacteria depends on not only the activity of antibiotic but also the capacity of host to eliminate the remaining bacteria.

Limitations

Antibiotic susceptibility testing in cell culture has not been standardized. A recent review examining the influence of different parameters (29) found that:

- Cell type has little influence on MIC values. However, these authors recommend using McCoy cells to study antibiotic activity in *C. trachomatis* and Hep-2 cells for *C. pneumo-*

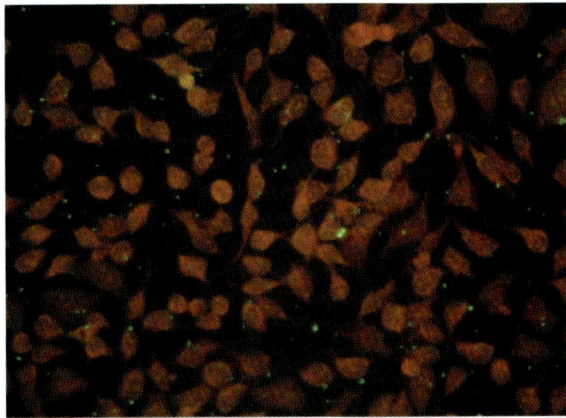

A : Cell culture infected after 2h incubation without antibiotics: inoculum control

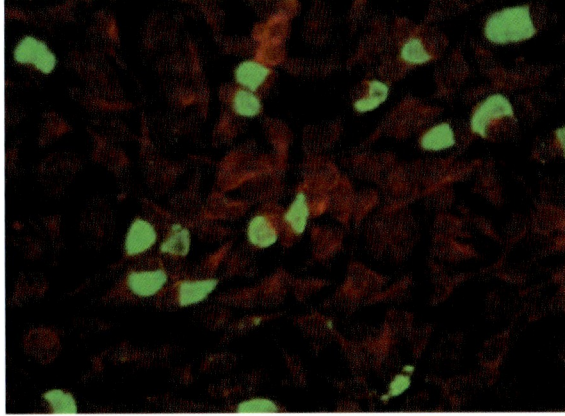

B : Cell culture infected after 40h incubation without antibiotic : positive control.

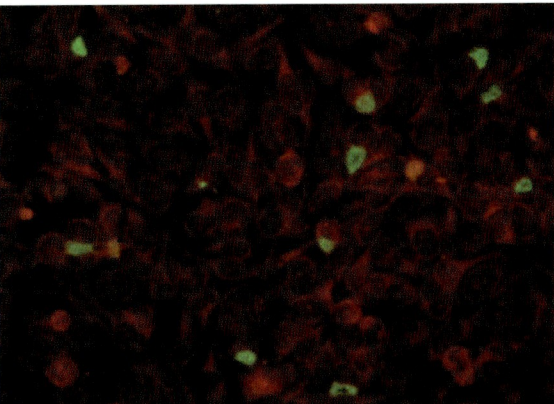

C : Cell culture infected after 40h incubation with 0.25 mg/L of ofloxacin.

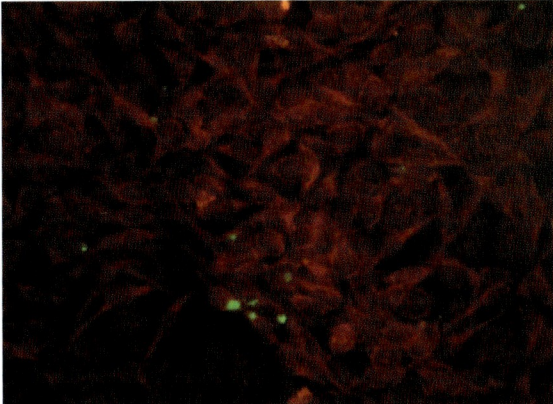

D : Cell culture infected after 40h incubation with 0.5mg/L of ofloxacin corresponding to the MIC.

Fig. 1. MIC determination by fluorescence microscopy reading. MIC was defined as the lowest antibiotic concentration for which there is no typical inclusion.

niae. In fact, the MIC of azithromycin against the reference strain *C. trachomatis* serovar D increased from 0.008 µg/ml in monkey BGMK cells to 1 µg/ml in HL cells.

- Inoculum size has no effect on MIC values between 300 and 300,000 IFU per well. On the other hand, MBCs after three passages are far higher than MICs for an inoculum > 5,000 IFU/well, suggesting that the survival rate is about 1 bacterium per 5,000 infected cells. In fact, for all chlamydia strains, so-called "heterotypic" survivors persist at concentrations above the MIC. After subculturing, these heterotypic survivors have the same MICs as the parent strains and do not represent resistant mutants. Survivors have been described in strains isolated post therapy from patients with either recurrent or persistent infection defined as three or more infectious episodes with the same serovar, or single-incident infections (29). This therefore appears to be a common phenomenon with chlamydiae.

- The time between infection and addition of antibiotic is crucial. MICs are identical during the first 8 h post-infection and then increase dramatically, reflecting the lower efficacy of the antibiotic after 8 h of *C. trachomatis* proliferation.

It is likely that the culture systems used *in vitro* poorly reflect the natural conditions of infection. First, epithelia *in vivo* are differentiated and polarized and secondly, *C. pneumoniae* in particular can multiply in monocytes. Studies of the effect of culture conditions on the pathogenicity and azithromycin-susceptibility of *C. trachomatis* show that on polarized cells, the cultured bacteria

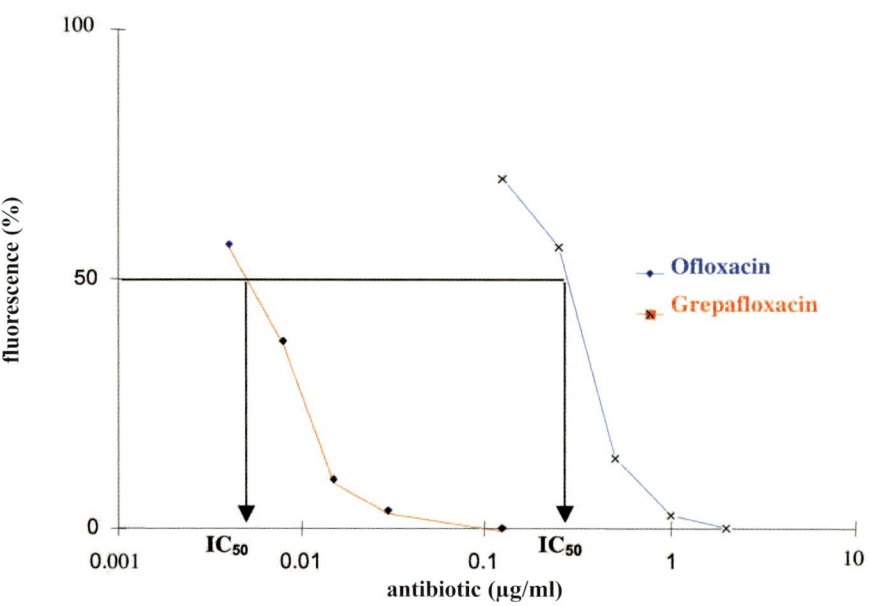

Fig. 2. Ofloxacin and grepafloxacin activity on *C. trachomatis* studied by using flow cytometry.

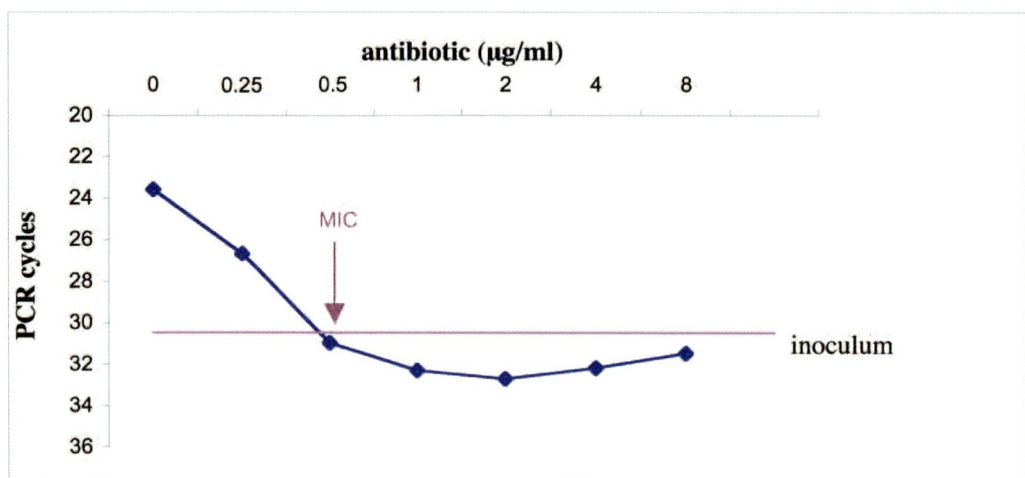

Fig. 3. MIC determination of ofloxacine on *C. trachomatis* by using real time PCR. The antibiotic concentration for which the concentration of *C. trachomatis* was near or equal to that of the inoculum control at T0 corresponds to MICs

are more infectious and MBCs are lower (0.125 versus 0.5 µg/ml on non-polarized cells) (31). Based on *in vitro* studies and *ex vivo* infection of monocytes in the presence of antibiotics, it appears that *C. pneumoniae* within monocytes is refractory to antibiotics (10).

INTRINSIC SUSCEPTIBILITY

Table 1 presents the MICs of the main active drugs. Rifampin has the highest *in vitro* activity and the lowest MICs. Tetracyclines, particularly doxycycline and minocycline, have good *in vitro* activity. Among macrolides and related compounds, those with 14-member rings (erythromycin and roxithromycin) have good activity and among these, roxithromycin has the lowest MICs. Among macrolides with 16-member rings, josamycin is more active than spiramycin and the 15-member ring azithromycin has activity comparable to roxithromycin. Telithromycin has twice the activity of roxithromycin, azithromycin and erythromycin but is less active than clarithromycin (19).

Table 1. MIC range values (µg/ml) of antibiotics against *C. trachomatis* and *C. pneumoniae*.

Antibiotic	*C. trachomatis*	*C. pneumoniae*
Rifampin	0.005 - 0.2	0.00125 - 0.0025
Minocycline	0.001 - 0.2	0.015 - 0.03
Doxycycline	0.01 - 0.2	0.03 - 0.5
Erythromycin	0.1 - 1	0.063 - 0.25
Roxithromycin	0.125 - 0.25	0.06 - 0.2
Azithromycin	0.03 - 1	0.125 - 0.5
Josamycin	0.01 - 1	0.25
Clarithromycin	ND[a]	0.016 - 0.063
Telithromycin	ND	0.031 - 0.25
Ofloxacin	0.5 - 4	0.5 - 2
Levofloxacin	0.5 - 2	0.5 - 1
Moxifloxacin	0.03 - 0.06	0.125 - 1
Gatifloxacin	0.25	0.125 - 0.25
Gemifloxacin	0.015 - 0.03	0.015 - 0.03

[a] ND, not determined.

Chlamydia are resistant to first-generation quinolones and different fluoroquinolones have different activities: norfloxacin and enoxacin are inactive, pefloxacin has intermediate activity while ofloxacin, ciprofloxacin, levofloxacin, gatifloxacin, moxifloxacin, and gemifloxacin are active. Gemifloxacin is the most active of the fluoroquinolones.

INTRINSIC RESISTANCE

Other antibiotic classes have little or no activity. MICs of gentamicin and spectinomycin, which have antigonococcal activity, are > 256 µg/ml and 32-256 µg/ml, respectively. Metronidazole (MIC > 256 µg/ml), colistin (MIC > 500 µg/ml) and vancomycin (MIC > 256 µg/ml) are ineffective. Gentamicin and vancomycin are also used as selective agents in culture media.

The β-lactams deserve special attention due to their paradoxical activity. Susceptibility of chlamydiae to penicillin G is similar to that of peptidoglycan-containing bacteria, such that amoxicillin has been proposed for the treatment of chlamydial infections when the recommended drugs are contraindicated. The growth of reversible, aberrant forms is observed *in vitro* in the presence of penicillin G. The activity of an antibiotic, whose mechanism of action is to block peptidoglycan synthesis in a bacterium that does not possess peptidoglycan, raises many questions. Our current state of knowledge can be summarized as follows (21): (i) only minute quantities of muramic acid, an essential peptidoglycan constituent, have been detected in EBs; (ii) three penicillin-binding proteins (PBPs) are present in the EB and RB forms of the bacteria and are thought to be the presumed target of penicillin G in Chlamydia; (iii) in the presence of penicillin G, synthesis of the major 40 kDa outer membrane protein is not affected while that of the 60 kDa protein is inhibited; (iv) the latter protein is synthesized at a late stage of RB differentiation back to EBs.

Knowledge of the genomic sequence of *C. trachomatis* and *C. pneumoniae* has shed light on the matter. It appears that these species possess all the genes involved in peptidoglycan synthesis and that these genes are grouped as in *Escherichia coli* (3). These genes account for 1.8% of the genome, a proportion which precludes the possibility that they are cryptic. It might be speculated that in chlamydiae, peptidoglycan is synthesized by RBs, that it plays an essential role in division and that, during back-differentiation of RBs to EBs, amidases (whose genes have been identified in the chlamydial genome) are activated to degrade it. This transient peptidoglycan synthesis would explain the action of the penicillins, although this hypothesis remains to be demonstrated. From a therapeutic standpoint, it is highly inadvisable to use penicillins since this may induce persistent infection without eradicating the bacteria.

RESISTANCE MECHANISMS

Data on acquired antibiotic resistance in chlamydiae are scarce due to the small number of strains isolated in culture. However, evidence pointing towards acquired resistance does exist, including the occurrence of treatment failure and the repeated isolation of the same *C. trachomatis* serovar despite appropriate antibiotic therapy (2). While in sexually transmitted infections treatment failure is hard to distinguish from reinfection, bacterial persistence post-treatment has also been described for *C. pneumoniae*. Some publications have reported the isolation of strains with increased MICs. Lastly, it has also been possible to select resistant mutants *in vitro*.

Resistance *in vivo*

There are few reports of resistance among clinical isolates. In 1990 Jones et al. (12) described five patients infected with tetracycline- and erythromycin-resistant but ofloxacin-susceptible strains. Resistance was only demonstrated with a high inoculum and less than 1% of the bacterial population had high-level resistance. Furthermore, these resistant phenotypes were not viable or else lost their resistance after passage on antibiotic-free medium. Treatment failure was suspected in four of these patients. Such heterogeneous resistance has also been described by Lefevre et al. (15) in a *C. trachomatis* endocervical isolate, in which high-level tetracycline resistance (MIC > 64 µg/ml) was only detected in a small fraction of the bacterial population, the remainder being inhibited at antibiotic concentrations ≤ 0.125 µg/ml. In contrast to the American strains, the French strain remained susceptible to the antibiotics tested: azithromycin, erythromycin, ofloxacin, and pristinamycin. In 2000, Somani et al. (27) described three isolates resistant to ofloxacin, doxycycline, and azithromycin in three patients, two of whom had failed treatment. Finally, this same phenomenon of heterotypic survival was recently described in 44 strains with respect to doxycycline, azithromycin, and ofloxacin, although the molecular mechanism remains obscure (29).

C. suis respiratory and conjunctival isolates from swine which are highly resistant to tetracyclines (MIC 5-10 µg/ml) and/or sulfadiazine (growth in the presence of 20 µg/ml) have been described (16). The mechanism of tetracycline resistance was recently elucidated by the identification of a *tet(C)* resistance gene (9). The presence of genomic islands carrying the *tet(C)* gene is the first demonstration of horizontal acquisition of genetic information in this family of bacteria.

A recent report describes six *C. trachomatis* clinical isolates from four patients showing cross-resistance to erythromycin, azithromycin, and josamycin (18). These strains harbored mutations in genes encoding the 23S rRNA and protein L22. On the other hand, no mutations were found in three *C. pneumoniae* clinical strains isolated after treatment with azithromycin and which showed a four-fold increase in the MIC (24). No highly resistant mutants have been obtained by *in vitro* selection.

Resistance *in vitro*

Although there are few published data on acquisition of resistance during therapy, the *in vitro* selection of resistant strains in the presence of antibiotics has been described, particularly with rifampin, sulfonamides, trimethoprim, and fluoroquinolones. Mutations in the *rpoB* gene have been identified in *C. trachomatis* variants with high-level rifampin resistance (8). As with other bacterial species, there is a correlation between the level of resistance and the position of the mutation, particularly $His_{526}Tyr$ (*E. coli* numbering). Suchland et al. (28) recently reported the selection of *C. trachomatis* mutants with high-level rifampin resistance (MIC > 512 µg/ml) which remained susceptible to rifalazil (MIC 0.064 µg/ml), a new ansamycin. For *C. pneumoniae*, selection of mutants is more difficult. Kutlin et al. (13) describe the selection of *C. pneumoniae* TW-183 mutants with low-level resistance to rifampin (MIC 0.25 µg/ml) and rifalazil (MIC 0.016 µg/ml) after twelve passages whereas no mutants could be selected with strain CWL-029. Rifalazil therefore appears to be of major potential for the treatment of chlamydial infections due to its potent activity (MIC 0.00025 µg/ml), its pharmacokinetic properties (high intracellular concentrations, long half-life) and its low propensity to select resistant mutants.

Sulfonamides are effective against *C. trachomatis* (MICs of sulfamethoxazole range from 0.5-4 µg/ml) but not *C. pneumoniae*. *C. trachomatis* normally synthesizes the purine and pyrimidine bases required for DNA synthesis from ribonucleotide precursors supplied by the host cell. Sulfonamides are active against *C. trachomatis* because they block the biosynthesis of dTTP. By successive passage of reference strain L2 on increasing concentrations of trimethoprim and sulphisoxazole, Wang et al. (30) successfully selected mutants with high-level resistance to these antibiotics that were incapable of *de novo* dTTP synthesis. Resistance is thought to be due to the ability of the mutants to use the host cell thymidine and thymidine kinase activity to effectively bypass the action of the sulfonamide.

With respect to fluoroquinolones, *in vitro* selection studies with *C. trachomatis* and *C. pneumoniae* have led to the isolation of highly resistant *C. trachomatis* mutants after four passages on ofloxacin or sparfloxacin (6). These mutants carried a single point mutation resulting in a $Ser_{83}Ile$ substitution in the Quinolone Resistance Determining Region (QRDR) sequence of the *gyrA* gene for the DNA gyrase subunit. This mutation, previously described in other bacterial genera, is responsible for fluoroquinolone resistance. These data suggest that these two quinolones mainly target the DNA gyrase in this species. These strains were cross-resistant to the five fluoroquinolones studied whereas there was no increase in MICs of other antibiotic classes (doxycycline, erythromycin). The G→T mutation creates a cleavage site for endonuclease *Tsp*5091 which can be detected on the restriction profile of the *gyrA* gene QRDR amplification product. Using this simple PCR-RFLP method for rapid identification of this mutation, it is possible to analyze clinical isolates. However the method can only detect this point mutation.

Selection of mutants is much more problematic in the case of *C. pneumoniae*. Morrissey et al. (20) were unable to select mutants of respiratory strain IOL 207 after thirty passages on moxifloxacin or ofloxacin and resistant mutants could not be kept viable on sparfloxacin. More recently, Rupp et al. (26) selected a viable variant of the *C. pneumoniae* vascular isolate CV-6 with an MIC of 6.4 µg/ml, which is 256 times higher than that of the parent strain. A single point mutation $Ser_{83}Asn$ was identified.

Persistence of infection

Persistent infection is a phenomenon described *in vitro* for *C. pneumoniae* and *C. trachomatis*. It is reversible when the inducing factor is removed. Persistent infection is defined as the inability to produce infectious EBs, altered gene expression, and the production of morphologically aberrant bodies (1). Geiffers et al. (11) showed that all antibiotics active against chlamydiae are capable of inducing the phenomenon of persistence. The heterotypical resistance observed in clinical isolates may result from the formation of these persistent forms. The aberrant body, whose altered membrane probably affects permeability, is a stress response as demonstrated by the large amounts of stress proteins produced.

In vitro, persistence is detected by the presence of inclusions in infected cells from the infected cell monolayer that was in contact with antibiotic concentrations above the MIC. Persistence is comparable to bacteriostasis although the mechanism appears to differ. Yet, unlike extracellular bacteria, persistent intracellular bacteria are protected from the immune system in their cellular niche and may be responsible for failure of therapy. It might be speculated that when antibiotic concentrations are close to the MIC, the bacterium enters this state of persistence and is reactivated when the antibiotic is withdrawn.

To study antibiotic activity on persistent forms of *C. pneumoniae in vitro*, a continuous infection Hep2 cell model was developed. The authors showed that a thirty day course of azithromycin, clarithromycin, or levofloxacin at concentrations comparable to those achieved in the pulmonary parenchyma reduced the bacterial inoculum but did not eradicate it (14). These data suggest that the usual dosage and duration of therapy used to treat *C. pneumoniae* pulmonary infections are not sufficient. The inconclusive data from clinical trials in atherosclerosis also raise questions about the effective dosages and treatment durations needed to reach persistent forms and their cycle of reactivation.

CONCLUSION

Antibiotic susceptibility testing of *C. trachomatis* requires a good mastery of cell culture techniques. The absence of standardization does not make it easy to compare data from the few studies that have been performed, generally on only a small number of strains. The use of flow cytometry allows a comparison of calculated IC_{50} values which are more accurate and objective. Molecular methods have an important contribution to make. Potentially active antibiotics, in decreasing order of *in vitro* activity, include rifampin with the lowest MICs, tetracyclines, macrolides, and the newer fluoroquinolones. Failure of therapy due to acquired resistance is rare. The possibility of selecting resistant mutants *in vitro* merits special attention and calls for epidemiological surveillance of strains. Such surveillance is not justified at the individual level. On the other hand, the persistence of infection following therapy, particularly in the case of sexually transmitted infections, highlights the need for post-therapeutic monitoring by direct testing of the bacterium (17); the modalities of these controls have yet to be established. The major problem is the ability of chlamydiae to enter into a persistent state which is refractory to antibiotics.

REFERENCES

(1) **Beatty, W.L., R.P. Morrison, and G.I. Byrne.** 1994. Persistent chlamydiae: from cell culture to a paradigm for chlamydial pathogenesis. Microbiol. Rev. **58:** 686-699.

(2) **Bébéar, C., B. de Barbeyrac, S. Pereyre, and C. Bébéar.** 2004. Résistance aux antibiotiques chez les mycoplasmes et les chlamydiae. Antibiotiques **6:** 263-272.

(3) **Chopra, I., C. Storey, T.J. Falla, and J.H. Pearce.** 1998. Antibiotics, peptidoglycan synthesis and genomics: the chlamydial anomaly revisited. Microbiology **144:** 2673-2678.

(4) **Cross, N.A., D.J. Kellock, G.R. Kinghorn, M. Taraktchoglou, E. Bataki, K.M. Oxley, P.M. Hawkey, and A. Eley.** 1999. Antimicrobial susceptibility testing of *Chlamydia trachomatis* using a reverse transcriptase PCR-based method. Antimicrob. Agents Chemother. **43:** 2311-2313.

(5) **de Barbeyrac, B., S. Dessus-Babus, F. Poutiers, C.M. Bébéar, A. Allery, and C. Bébéar.** 1999. *Chlamydia trachomatis*: sensibilité et résistance aux antibiotiques. Méd. Mal. Inf. **29:** 60-67.

(6) **Dessus-Babus, S., C.M. Bébéar, A. Charron, C. Bébéar, and B. de Barbeyrac.** 1998. Sequencing of gyrase and topoisomerase IV quinolone-resistance-determining regions of *Chlamydia trachomatis* and characterization of quinolone-resistant mutants obtained *in vitro*. Antimicrob. Agents Chemother. **42:** 2474-2481.

(7) **Dessus-Babus, S., F. Belloc, C.M. Bébéar, F. Poutiers, F. Lacombe, C. Bébéar, and B. de Barbeyrac.** 1998. Antibiotic susceptibility testing for *Chlamydia trachomatis* using flow cytometry. Cytometry **31:** 37-44.

(8) **Dreses Werringloer, U., I. Padubrin, L. Kohler, and A.P. Hudson.** 2003. Detection of nucleotide variability in *rpo*B in both rifampin-sensitive and rifampin-resistant strains of *Chlamydia trachomatis*. Antimicrob. Agents Chemother. **47:** 2316-2318.

(9) **Dugan, J., D.D. Rockey, L. Jones, and A.A. Andersen.** 2004. Tetracycline resistance in *Chlamydia suis* mediated by genomic islands inserted into the chlamydial *inv*-like gene. Antimicrob. Agents Chemother. **48:** 3989-3995.

(10) **Gieffers, J., J. Fullgraf, J. Jahn, M. Klinger, K. Dalhoff, H. A. Katus, W. Solbach, and M. Maass.** 2001. *Chlamydia pneumoniae* infection in circulating human monocytes is refractory to antibiotic treatment. Circulation **103:** 351-356.

(11) **Gieffers, J., J. Rupp, A. Gebert, W. Solbach, and M. Klinger.** 2004. First-choice antibiotics at subinhibitory concentrations induce persistence of *Chlamydia pneumoniae*. Antimicrob. Agents Chemother. **48:** 1402-1405.

(12) **Jones, R. B., B. Van der Pol, D.H. Martin, and M.K. Shepard.** 1990. Partial characterization of *Chlamydia trachomatis* isolates resistant to multiple antibiotics. J. Infect. Dis. **162:** 1309-1315.

(13) **Kutlin, A., S. Kohlhoff, P. Roblin, M.R. Hammerschlag, and P. Riska.** 2005. Emergence of resistance to rifampin and rifalazil in *Chlamydophila pneumoniae* and *Chlamydia trachomatis*. Antimicrob. Agents Chemother. **49:** 903-907.

(14) **Kutlin, A., P.M. Roblin, and M.R. Hammerschlag.** 2002. Effect of prolonged treatment with azithromycin, clarithromycin, or levofloxacin on *Chlamydia pneumoniae* in a continuous-infection model. Antimicrob. Agents Chemother. **46:** 409-412.

(15) **Lefèvre, J.C., J.P. Lepargneur, D. Guion, and S. Bei.** 1997. Tetracycline-resistant *Chlamydia trachomatis* in Toulouse, France. Path. Biol. **45:** 376-378.

(16) **Lenart, J., A.A. Andersen, and D.D. Rockey.** 2001. Growth and development of tetracycline-resistant *Chlamydia suis*. Antimicrob. Agents Chemother. **45:** 2198-2203.

(17) **Mardh, P.A., and K. Persson.** 2002. Is there a need for rescreening of patients treated for genital chlamydial infections? Int. J. Std Aids **13:** 363-367.

(18) **Misyurina, O.Y., E.V. Chipitsyna, Y.P. Finashutina, V.N. Lazarev, T.A. Akopian, A.M. Savicheva, and V.M. Govorun.** 2004. Mutations in a 23S rRNA gene of *Chlamydia trachomatis* associated with resistance to macrolides. Antimicrob. Agents Chemother. **48:** 1347-1349.

(19) **Miyashita, N., H. Fukano, Y. Niki, and T. Matsushima.** 2001. *In vitro* activity of telithromycin, a new ketolide, against *Chlamydia pneumoniae*. J. Antimicrob. Chemother. **48:** 403-405.

(20) **Morrissey, I., H. Salman, S. Bakker, D. Farrell, C.M. Bebear, and G. Ridgway.** 2002. Serial passage of *Chlamydia* spp. in sub-inhibitory fluoroquinolone concentrations. J. Antimicrob. Chemother. **49:** 757-761.

(21) **Moulder, J. W.** 1993. Why is *Chlamydia* sensitive to penicillin in the absence of peptidoglycan? Infect. Agents Dis. **2:** 87-99.

(22) **Peeling R.W., Bowie W.R., Dillon J.R., Johnson R., Jones R.B., Van del Pol B., Low D.T., Martin D.H., Newhall J., Orfila J., Rice R., Schachter J., and M.J.** 1994. Standardisation of antimicrobial susceptibility testing for *Chlamydia trachomatis*, pp. 346-349. *In* G. I. B. J. Orfila, M.A. Chernesky, J.T. Grayston, R.B. Jones, G.L. Saikku, J. Schachter, W.E. Stamm, R.S. Stephens (ed.), Chlamydial Infections. Societa Editrice Esculapio, Italy.

(23) **Poutiers, F., S. Dessus-Babus, F. Leblanc, C. Bébéar, and B. de Barbeyrac.** 1999. In vitro activity of grepafloxacin against *Chlamydia trachomatis*. Drugs **58:** 404-405.

(24) **Riska, P.F., A. Kutlin, P. Ajiboye, A. Cua, P.M. Roblin, and M.R. Hammerschlag.** 2004. Genetic and culture-based approaches for detecting macrolide resistance in *Chlamydia pneumoniae*. Antimicrob. Agents Chemother. **48:** 3586-3590.

(25) **Rodriguez, P., B. de Barbeyrac, H. Renaudin, and C. Bébéar.** 1995. Antibiogramme des Chlamydia et des mycoplasmes. Rev. Française des Lab. **277**: 75-80.

(26) **Rupp, J., A. Gebert, W. Solbach, and M. Maass.** 2005. Serine-to-asparagine substitution in the *gyrA* gene leads to quinolone resistance in moxifloxacin-exposed *Chlamydia pneumoniae*. Antimicrob. Agents Chemother. **49**: 406-407.

(27) **Somani, J., V.B. Bhullar, K.A. Workowski, C.E. Farshy, and C.M. Black.** 2000. Multiple drug-resistant *Chlamydia trachomatis* associated with clinical treatment failure. J. Infect. Dis. **181**: 1421-1427.

(28) **Suchland, R.J., A. Bourillon, E. Denamur, W.E. Stamm, and D.M. Rothstein.** 2005. Rifampin-resistant RNA polymerase mutants of *Chlamydia trachomatis* remain susceptible to the ansamycin rifalazil. Antimicrob. Agents Chemother. **49**: 1120-1126.

(29) **Suchland, R.J., W.M. Geisler, and W.E. Stamm.** 2003. Methodologies and cell lines used for antimicrobial susceptibility testing of *Chlamydia* spp. Antimicrob. Agents Chemother. **47**: 636-642.

(30) **Wang, L.L., E. Henson, and G. McClarty.** 1994. Characterization of trimethoprim- and sulphisoxazole-resistant *Chlamydia trachomatis*. Mol. Microbiol. **14**: 271-281.

(31) **Wyrick, P.B., C.H. Davis, J.E. Raulston, S.T. Knight, and J. Choong.** 1994. Effect of clinically relevant culture conditions on antimicrobial susceptibility of *Chlamydia trachomatis*. Clin. Infect. Dis. **19**: 931-936.

Chapter 45. HACEK AND DYSGONIC FERMENTERS

Michel VERGNAUD

INTRODUCTION

"Difficult to cultivate" Gram-negative bacilli can be divided into two groups:
- The HACEK organisms (*Haemophilus aphrophilus/paraphrophilus*, *Actinobacillus/ Haemophilus actinomycetemcomitans*, *Cardiobacterium hominis*, *Eikenella corrodens*, *Kingella kingae*) are part of the commensal oropharyngeal flora. They are causative agents of subacute endocarditis but are also responsible for septicemia, suppurations, and periodontitis. The species *H. aphrophilus/paraphrophilus*, *A. actinomycetemcomitans* and *H. segnis* have been classified into the newly created genus *Aggregatibacter*. This new nomenclature will be used in the text (33).
- The Centers for Disease Control (CDC) "dysgonic fermenters" comprise *Capnocytophaga* [part of the oropharyngeal flora of humans (DF1) or animals (DF2)] and *Dysgonomonas* (DF3) present in the digestive tract. Species present in both human (DF1 and DF3) and animal (DF2) hosts are known to cause bacteremia or septicemia.
- The DF1 group includes three main species: *Capnocytophaga ochracea*, *C. sputigena* and *C. gingivalis*; DF2 comprises *C. canimorsus*, and *C. cynodegmi*. The genus *Dysgonomonas* comprises three species: *D. gadei*, *D. capnocytophagoides*, and *D. mossii*.

Antimicrobial susceptibility testing in this disparate group is complex, heterogeneous and poorly documented. Since there are no standardized test methods, extreme caution should be exercised when interpreting and reporting results, which should be based on an analysis of the literature (24).

For these reasons, antibiotic susceptibility testing should be limited to cases of severe infection, in particular when reference treatments fail or when intolerance necessitates a switch to an alternative treatment.

The interpretive criteria defined by the working groups for other bacteria cannot be applied due to the particular testing conditions required for these fastidious organisms. Nevertheless, some authors use the specific data validated for other closely related genera or species: *Haemophilus influenzae* for *A. aphrophilus* or *A. actinomycetemcomitans*, anaerobic Gram-negative bacilli for metronidazole, etc. (24).

The Clinical and Laboratory Standards Institute (CLSI) has recently published provisional guidance for the HACEK group (*Aggregatibacter aphrophilus*, *A. segnis*, *A. actinomycetemcomitans*, *Cardiobacterium* spp., *Eikenella corrodens* and *Kingella* spp.) (8).

These guidelines recommend systematic screening for β-lactamase production with the chromogenic cephalosporin test (Nitrocefin®) and suggest that antibiotic susceptibility in these species should only be tested when it can truly be helpful (blood cultures, specimens from deep sites, prosthetic materials), particularly in immunocompromised patients. It is recommended that test results not be interpreted if there is insufficient growth of the culture.

METHODS

Susceptibility testing methods for these bacteria have not been standardized since each organism has its own special requirements relative to normally cultured species and also relative to each other. It is generally agreed that the media should be supplemented with blood or blood components, the atmosphere enriched in CO_2 or even anaerobic (which affects the activity of certain antibiotics) and the incubation times should be long (48 h). There is no consensus as to any one method and no reference method exists, since each parameter can affect the results (preparation and size of inoculum, inoculation medium and presence of supplements, atmosphere and incubation time, etc.). Moreover, the relative scarcity of isolates and their fastidious nature means that only a small number of strains have been studied. The E-test® has been a major advance for some genera, although there are still few published data. The methods described below have not, in most cases, been the object of a consensus or validation, but were used in the publications cited.

A. aphrophilus

Disks

The method has been validated using Haemophilus test medium or Columbia chocolate agar medium (for strains which do not grow on HTM) by applying the conditions and interpretive criteria used for *H. influenzae* (23).
- Inoculum: 10^6 CFU/ml suspension of colonies from a 24-48 h culture on chocolate-Polyvitex® agar plates;
- Inoculation: swab or overlay;
- Incubation: 48 h at 35-37°C.

E-test®

The method has been validated for this species (26, 37).
- Medium: Mueller-Hinton agar supplemented with hemoglobin and Isovitalex® or HTM medium;
- Inoculum: suspension adjusted to match the turbidity of a No. 1 McFarland standard;
- Incubation: 35-37°C, aerobic 5% CO_2 atmosphere for 24-72 h.

Agar or broth dilution (3, 25, 35, 47)

- Solid media: trypticase-soy agar supplemented with 5% sheep blood or Fildes extract, chocolate agar, HTM agar. Liquid media: Mueller-Hinton broth supplemented with NAD and hemin or lysed blood (5%), or HTM broth (culture sometimes difficult);
- Inoculum: 10^3-10^5 CFU per spot or suspension of 10^5 CFU/ml or equivalent to a 0.5 McFarland standard in liquid medium;
- Incubation: 35-37°C, aerobic atmosphere (enriched with 5% CO_2 for agar dilution) for 48 h.

A. actinomycetemcomitans

Disks

Not recommended.

E-test®

Brucella agar supplemented with 5% blood or HTM (25, 33).

Agar or broth dilution (17, 35, 38, 46)

- Solid media: Mueller-Hinton agar, trypticase soy agar, Wilkins-Chalgren agar supplemented with 5-10% blood or HTM agar. Liquid media: Mueller-Hinton, thioglycollate or trypticase-soy broth supplemented with yeast extract and hemin or lysed horse blood;
- Inoculum: 10^3-10^5 CFU per spot or suspension of 10^5 CFU/ml or equivalent to a 0.5 McFarland standard in liquid medium;
- Incubation: 35-37°C, aerobic atmosphere (enriched with 5% CO_2 for agar dilution) for 24-48 h.

C. hominis

Disks

- Medium: chocolate agar or supplemented with erythrocyte lysate;
- Inoculum: 10^6 CFU/ml suspension of colonies from a 24-48 h culture on chocolate-Polyvitex® agar;
- Inoculation: swab or overlay;
- Incubation 35-37°C, 5% CO_2 atmosphere for 48 h.

E-test®

Mueller-Hinton or Brucella agar supplemented with 5% blood (26).

Broth dilution (28, 49)

- Medium: Mueller-Hinton, trypticase-soy or Schaedler broth supplemented with erythrocyte lysate, yeast extract and Isovitalex® or lysed horse blood (5%);
- Inoculum: 10^5-10^6 CFU/ml suspension or equivalent to a 0.5 McFarland standard in liquid medium;
- Incubation: 35-37°C, aerobic or 5% CO_2 atmosphere for 24-48 h.

E. corrodens

Disks

- Medium: Mueller-Hinton agar supplemented with 5% sheep blood (11);
- Inoculum: 10^6 CFU/ml suspension of colonies from a 24-48 h culture on chocolate-Polyvitex® agar;
- Inoculation: swab or overlay;
- Incubation: 48 h at 35-37°C.

E-test®

Validated for this species on Mueller-Hinton agar supplemented with hemoglobin and Isovitalex® or HTM or Brucella agar supplemented with 5% blood (26).

Agar or broth dilution (1, 12, 27)

- Solid media: Wilkins-Chalgren or Mueller-Hinton agar supplemented with 5% sheep blood. Liquid media: Mueller-Hinton broth supplemented with 5% lysed horse blood, blood components (Fildes extract), or HTM broth;
- Inoculum: 10^5-10^6 CFU per spot or a suspension of 10^5-10^6 CFU/ml or equivalent to a 0.5 McFarland standard in liquid medium;
- Incubation: 35-37°C, aerobic or 5% CO_2 atmosphere for 24-48 h.

K. kingae

Disks (7, 20, 50)

- Medium: Mueller-Hinton agar supplemented with 5% horse or sheep blood or chocolate agar;
- Inoculum: Mac Farland 0.5 suspension.
- Incubation: 35-37°C, 5% CO_2 atmosphere for 24-48 h.

E-test®

On Brucella or Mueller-Hinton agar supplemented with 5% blood (26).

Agar or broth dilution (19, 20, 40)

- Solid medium: Mueller-Hinton agar supplemented with 5% horse blood;
- Liquid medium: Mueller-Hinton broth supplemented with 5% lysed horse blood;
- Inoculum: 10^5-10^6 CFU per spot or a suspension of 10^5-10^6 CFU/ml or equivalent to a 0.5 McFarland standard in liquid medium;
- Incubation: 37°C, aerobic or 5% CO_2 atmosphere for 24 h.

Capnocytophaga DF1 and DF2

Disks

Method validated against the agar dilution (6, 32).
- Medium: Mueller-Hinton agar supplemented with 5% fresh blood or chocolate agar and vitamin K1;
- Incubation: 37°C, 5% CO_2 atmosphere for 48 h.

E-test®

Excellent correlation with the reference methods.
- Medium: Brucella agar supplemented with 5% blood or chocolate agar;
- Inoculum: prepared from a suspension adjusted to the turbidity of a 1 McFarland standard;
- Incubation: 35-37°C, aerobic or 5% CO_2 atmosphere for 24-48 h.

Agar or broth dilution (2, 9, 16, 21, 42, 45, 48)

- Solid media: Brucella chocolate agar, Wilkins-Chalgren agar supplemented with 10% blood or Columbia agar supplemented with hemoglobin and Polyvitex®.
- Liquid media: trypticase-soy broth containing dextrose, Mueller-Hinton or Schaedler broth;
- Inoculum: 10^3-10^5 CFU per spot or 10^7 CFU/ml in liquid medium;
- Incubation: 37°C, 5-10% CO_2 or anaerobic atmosphere for 48-72 h.

Dysgonomonas spp.

Disks

Mueller-Hinton agar supplemented according to the conditions and interpretive criteria used for *H. influenzae*: incubation at 35-37°C in a 5% CO_2 atmosphere for 18 h (5).

E-test® (15, 18)

- Medium: Mueller-Hinton agar or anaerobic medium supplemented with 5% sheep blood;
- Incubation: 35-37°C, aerobic or 5% CO_2 atmosphere for 24-48 h.

Agar dilution

- HTM or Mueller-Hinton broth medium containing 5% Fildes extract.

SUSCEPTIBLE PHENOTYPE

Considering the diversity of test methods, the data on some antibiotics are not always concordant and may be based on a only small number of isolates. The MICs presented in the tables have been compiled from the literature. The variations in these values stem from differences in methodology.

A. aphrophilus

β-lactams and particularly injectable and oral (cefixime) third generation cephalosporins are active. *A. aphrophilus* is susceptible to fluoroquinolones, cotrimoxazole, chloramphenicol, tetracyclines, and rifampin, whereas macrolides and aminoglycosides usually have weak activity (Table 1) (5, 21, 23, 24, 32, 34, 42). Clindamycin, vancomycin, and metronidazole are inactive. The bactericidal activity of some reputedly active antibiotics (β-lactam + aminoglycoside combination, fluoroquinolones) is low.

A. actinomycetemcomitans

Apart from the injectable and oral (cefixime) cephalosporins which have very low MICs, β-lactams are basically inactive. Most other antibiotics, except for lincomycin, clindamycin and vancomycin, are active. Macrolides and aminoglycosides have more variable activity and the activity of metronidazole is controversial (Table 2) (18, 26, 35, 36, 37, 38, 46). Finally, there are large differences in the activity of different antibiotics according to the source of the isolate and its serotype; this is particularly true for β-lactams.

C. hominis

This species is highly susceptible to β-lactams and to all antibiotics tested except vancomycin. Macrolide activity is variable and often low. Lincosamides, in contrast to streptogramins, are inactive (Table 3) (26, 28, 49).

Table 2. MIC (µg/ml) of antibiotics against *A. actinomycetemcomitans*

Antibiotic	Range	MIC$_{90}$
Penicillin G	0.5 - 8	8
Oxacillin	16 - > 128	128
Ampicillin - amoxicillin	0.25 - 4	1
Cephalothin	0,5 - 4	2
Cefoxitin	0.25 - 4	2
Cefotaxime	0.03 - 0.06	0.03
Imipenem	0.25 - 1	0.5
Gentamicin	1 - 8	8
Chloramphenicol	0.4 - 0.8	0.8
Tetracyclines	0.5 - 2	2
Erythromycin	1 - 8	8
Azithromycin	0.5 - 4	2
Lincomycin	16 - 128	128
Clindamycin	2 - 16	16
Ciprofloxacin	< 0,03 - 0,12	< 0.06
Sulfamides	0.8 - 50	ND[a]
Cotrimoxazole	0.03 - 0.25	0.12
Colistin	0.1 - 2	ND
Rifampicin	0.15 - 2	1
Vancomycin	16 - 128	64
Metronidazole	4 - > 256	32

[a] ND, not determined.

Table 1. MIC (µg/ml) of antibiotics against *A. aphrophilus*

Antibiotic	Range	MIC$_{90}$
Penicillin G	0.012 - 0.5	0.5
Ampicillin-amoxicillin	0.25 - 0.5	0.25
Oxacillin	1 - > 8	> 8
Cephalosporins 1st gen.	1 - 4	2
Cephalosporins 2nd gen.	0.25 - 1	0.5
Cephalosporins 3rd gen.	0.06 - 0.25	0.125
Gentamicin	1 - 8	4
Chloramphenicol	0.5 - 5	5
Tétracyclines	0.03 - 1	1
Erythromycin	0.5 - 5	5
Azithromycin	0.5 - 4	4
Clindamycin	1 - 32	>16
Trovafloxacin	< 0.03 - 0.25	0.25
Cotrimoxazole	0.25 -1	ND[a]
Rifampin	0.25 - 2	1
Vancomycin	> 16	> 16
Metronidazol	12 - > 256	> 256

[a] ND, not determined.

Table 3. MIC (µg/ml) of antibiotics against *C. hominis*

Antibiotic	Range	MIC$_{90}$
Penicillin G	0.006 - 0.064	0.012
Oxacillin	0.5 - 4	ND[a]
Ampicillin	< 0.016 - 0.047	< 0.016
Cephalothin	0.001 - 0.25	0.125
Cefoxitin	< 0.016 - 0.023	< 0.016
Cefotaxime	0.047 - 0.125	0.064
Imipenem	< 0.016 - 0.023	0.016
Aminoglycosides	0.2 - 0.8	0.8
Chloramphenicol	< 0.4 - 1.6	ND
Tetracyclines	0.1 - 0.4	ND
Ciprofloxacin	0.004 - 0.5	0.008
Levofloxacin	0.012 - 1	0.016
Cotrimoxazole	0.5 - 1.5	1
Rifampin	0.047 - 0.125	0.064
Vancomycin	1 - 32	8

[a] ND, not determined.

E. corrodens

β-lactams are usually active, although oxacillin and first generation cephalosporins have higher MIC values (2, 13, 14, 15, 26). *E. corrodens* is susceptible to most other antibiotics with the exception of aminoglycosides and macrolides, which have variable, often low, activity. Lincosamides as well as metronidazole and vancomycin are inactive (Table 4).

K. kingae

This species is highly susceptible to the majority of antibiotics with the exception of vancomycin, trimethoprim, and lincomycin (Table 5) (10, 19, 20, 26, 40, 50).

Capnocytophaga DF1

This species is susceptible to β-lactams other than first generation cephalosporins which are inactive. Most other antibiotics are active although resistance to aminoglycosides, glycopeptides, colimycin and trimethoprim has been reported. Data on metronidazole susceptibility are conflicting, probably due to differences in methodology (Table 6) (2, 6, 16, 21, 42, 45).

Table 4. MIC (µg/ml) of antibiotics against *E. corrodens*

Antibiotic	Range	MIC_{90}
Penicillin G	0.16 - 4	2
Oxacillin	2 - >16	> 16
Ampicillin	0.25 - 4	1
Amoxicillin	0.125 - 0.5	0.5
Amoxicillin+clavulanic acid	0.06 - 0.5	0.5
Piperacillin	0.06 - 0.25	0.12
Cephalothin	4 - 16	16
Cefoxitin	0.2 - 1.5	0.5
Cefotaxime	0.016 - 0.06	0.03
Imipenem	0.12 - 0.5	0.5
Gentamicin	0.4 - 4	4
Tetracyclines	0.25 - 2	1
Chloramphenicol	2 - 8	2
Erythromycin	2 - 8	8
Azithromycin	2 - 4	4
Lincomycin	128 - 256	256
Clindamycin	4 - 128	64
Linezolid	4 - 16	16
Ciprofloxacin	0.06 - 0.125	0.03
Levofloxacin	0.06 - 0.25	0.125
Cotrimoxazole	0.06 - 0.5	0.25
Metronidazole	8 - 64	64
Rifampin	0.5 - 2	1
Vancomycin	4 - 64	16

Table 5. MIC (µg/ml) of antibiotics against *K. kingae*.

Antibiotic	Range	MIC_{90} (MIC_{50})
Penicillin G	0.004 - 0.03	0.015
Oxacillin	0.25 - 1	0.5
Ampicillin	< 0.016 - 0.06	0.008
Piperacillin	< 0.016	(< 0.016)
Cephalothin	0.125 - 0.25	0.25
Cefoxitin	0.008 - 0.06	0.03
Cefotaxime	0.008 - 0.015	0.015
Imipenem	0.023 - 0.094	(0.047)
Aminoglycosides	0.03 - 0.5	0.5
Tetracyclines	0.5	0.5
Chloramphenicol	0.25 - 2	1
Erythromycin	0.06 - 2	0.5
Lincomycin	32 à 64	(32)
Ciprofloxacin	< 0.002 - 0.008	0.004
Trimethoprim	16 - > 32	> 32
Cotrimoxazole	0.032 - 0.5	(0.064)
Rifampin	0.064 - 0.5	(0.125)
Vancomycin	32	32

Table 6. MIC (µg/ml) of antibiotics against *Capnocytophaga* DF1

Antibiotic	Range	MIC_{90} (MIC_{50})
Penicillin G	0.016 - 2	1
Ampicillin or amoxicillin	0.03 - 1	(0.5)
Piperacillin	0.03 - 0.25	(0.06)
Cephalothin	2 - 64	32
Cefoxitin	0.03 - 1	(0.06)
Cefotaxime	< 0.03	(< 0.03)
Imipenem	< 0.03 - 0.5	(< 0.03)
Aztreonam	< 0.03 - 0.5	(< 0.12)
Aminoglycosides	128	128
Tetracyclines	0.125 - 2	1
Chloramphenicol	0.2 - 2	0.39
Erythromycin	0.2 - 1	0.5
Clindamycin	0.03 - 0.06	0.03
Ciprofloxacin	< 0.06 - 0.5	0.06
Trimethoprim	32 - >128	> 128
Metronidazole	2 - 64	64
Vancomycin	1 - 128	64

Capnocytophaga DF2

C. canimorsus is susceptible to many antibiotics but resistant to aminoglycosides, even though MICs determined in liquid medium may appear low. This species is also resistant to fosfomycin, colimycin, and trimethoprim (Table 7) (6, 32, 48).

Dysgonomonas spp.

Antibiotic susceptibility has only been evaluated in *D. capnocytophagoides*. These bacteria are consistently resistant to all β-lactams, apart from combinations containing a β-lactamase inhibitor and imipenem. Aminoglycosides, fluoroquinolones, and glycopeptides are inactive. Erythromycin, clindamycin, tetracycline, chloramphenicol, cotrimoxazole, and rifampin are usually active (Table 8) (5, 15, 18).

RESISTANCE MECHANISMS

Since so few strains have been studied, resistance mechanisms have been incompletely or sketchily described.

A. aphrophilus

No β-lactamases have been detected in this species, although several strains with high MICs of penicillin G, amoxicillin and even second and third generation cephalosporins have been described. In the absence of inhibition by clavulanic acid and in the presence of a negative chromogenic cephalosporin (Nitrocefin®) test, mechanisms involving alterations of penicillin binding proteins or cell wall permeability have been invoked, but this has not been investigated (34). The presence of the *tet*(K) determinant conferring tetracycline resistance through an efflux mechanism was demonstrated in a systematic study of oropharyngeal organisms resistant to these antibiotics (44). Macrolide resistance has also been described in some strains but the mechanisms have not been elucidated.

A. actinomycetemcomitans

No β-lactamase producing strains have been described. The low susceptibility of some strains to β-lactams is thought to be related to modification of penicillin-binding proteins. The *tet*(B) determinant has been detected in a high percentage of periodontal strains associated with the presence of conjugative plasmids, and confers resistance through an efflux mechanism. The *erm* (B, C, F, Q) genes coding for a ribosomal methylase have been identified in periodontal isolates and could have been transferred to *H. influenzae* and *Enterococcus faecalis*, conferring high-level erythromycin resistance.

Table 7. MIC (µg/ml) of antibiotics against *Capnocytophaga* DF2

Antibiotic	Mean MIC
Penicillin G	0.04
Ampicillin/amoxicillin	0.03
Piperacillin	1
Cephalothin	0.5
Cefamandole	0.03
Cefotaxime	0.23
Imipenem	0.13
Aztreonam	12.6
Chloramphenicol	0.39
Erythromycin	0.48
Clindamycin	0.05
Ciprofloxacin	0.37
Cotrimoxazole	8.2
Rifampin	0.006
Vancomycin	0.29

Table 8. MIC (µg/ml) of antibiotics against *Dysgonomonas* sp.

Antibiotic	Mean MIC
Penicillin G	> 32
Amoxicillin	6
Amoxicillin+clavulanic acid	1
Cephalothin	256
Cefoxitin	32
Cefotaxime	256
Aztreonam	256
Imipenem	0.5
Aminoglycosides	256
Tetracycline	0.2
Chloramphenicol	4
Erythromycin	0.25
Clindamycin	0.25
Ciprofloxacin	32
Cotrimoxazole	0.125
Rifampicin	2
Vancomycin	48
Metronidazole	1.5

C. hominis

Two β-lactamase producing strains have been described but the enzymes have not been characterized (29, 30). The enzyme was detected by a chromogenic cephalosporin test and could be inhibited by clavulanic acid. These β-lactamases appear to be most active on penicillins but might also affect third generation cephalosporins, possibly resulting in clinical failure. Some strains are resistant to aminoglycosides, sulfonamides and cotrimoxazole.

E. corrodens

Penicillinase-producing strains are found with variable frequency (≤ 5%). Resistance is either plasmid-mediated encoding a TEM enzyme similar to a resistance plasmid described in *Neisseria sicca* (44), or chromosomally encoded and inhibited by clavulanic acid, classified as Bush group 2a (27). Some β-lactamase producers are also resistant to streptomycin and sulfonamides. A tetracycline-resistant strain was found to harbor a plasmidic *tet*(M) determinant conferring resistance by a ribosomal protection mechanism. The *mef* gene has been successfully transferred *in vitro* from a *Streptococcus pneumoniae* strain but has never been found in clinical isolates.

K. kingae

Several β-lactamase producing strains have been described but the enzyme has not been characterized. Strains resistant to cotrimoxazole, ciprofloxacin and erythromycin have also been reported. Thirty to fifty percent of strains are resistant to clindamycin.

Capnocytophaga DF1

β-lactamase producing strains were first described in 1986 and 1987 (2, 45), but interest in this mechanism of resistance really began to intensify with widespread reports of strains resistant to third generation cephalosporins, isolated from bacteremia patients with hematologic diseases.

Two β-lactamases have been described:
- An enzyme similar to CfxA found in *Prevotella* and *Bacteroides*, with a pI 5.6, encoded on a plasmid or chromosome, inhibited by clavulanic acid and belonging to Bush group 2e. This enzyme is active on most β-lactams except imipenem and perhaps cefoxitin and aztreonam (22).
- A plasmid-encoded extended spectrum TEM-17 penicillinase, pI 5.5, derived from TEM-1a by an amino acid substitution $Glu_{104}Lys$ (43).

Strains resistant to erythromycin, clindamycin, ciprofloxacin, chloramphenicol and tetracycline [*tet*(Q) determinant conferring ribosomal protection] have also been reported.

Dysgonomonas

Erythromycin, clindamycin, tetracycline, chloramphenicol, and cotrimoxazole resistance has been described, but not rifampin. With respect to imipenem the data are discordant, possibly suggesting acquired resistance, or else a methodological problem. β-lactamase production detected by a chromogenic cephalosporin test or suggested by the activity of drug combinations including a penicillinase inhibitor has not been further investigated (15,31).

RESISTANCE PHENOTYPES

A. aphrophilus

One strain with abnormal susceptibility to β-lactams has been described, for which the MIC of third generation cephalosporins was > 8 μg/ml. In a second strain the MIC of penicillin was high but that of amoxicillin was 0.25 μg/ml. Modification of the β-lactam target was suggested but no further studies were performed.

A. actinomycetemcomitans

In erythromycin-resistant strains the MIC values range from 32-256 μg/ml. In strains harboring a *tet* gene, the MICs of tetracycline range from 4-8 μg/ml.

C. hominis

In β-lactamase producers, the MICs of penicillins are high (penicillin G, amoxicillin > 256 μg/ml) but these values decrease in the presence of clavulanic acid (MIC of amoxicillin + clavulanic acid: 4 μg/ml). In one strain the MIC of cefotaxime was high (1 μg/ml).

E. corrodens

β-lactamase production results in high MICs of penicillins (penicillin G ≥ 64 μg/ml, amoxicillin ≥ 64 μg/ml) which decrease in the presence of clavulanic acid (MIC of amoxicillin + clavulanic acid: 0.5 μg/ml). Cephalosporins are unaffected (MIC of cephalothin: 8 μg/ml and cefotaxime: 0.03 μg/ml). These strains are found at a low frequency of about 2%.

K. kingae

β-lactamase producing *Kingella* are very rare, and no such strains were found in a series of 145 isolates studied by Yagupsky *et al.* (50). They are resistant to penicillin G and amoxicillin but susceptible to amoxicillin + clavulanic acid and to second generation cephalosporins. The three β-lactamase producing strains isolated in Iceland were also resistant to cotrimoxazole (5).

Capnocytophaga DF1

β-lactamase producing strains of *Capnocytophaga* DF1 are resistant to many β-lactams, although aztreonam, imipenem, and cefoxitin remain active. In all these cases, combination of a β-lactam with a β-lactamase inhibitor resulted in excellent synergy (Table 9). The frequency of these strains differs according to the population being studied and can reach 50% or more in immunocompromised patients on antibiotic therapy.

ANTIBIOTICS TO BE STUDIED

Acquired resistance is uncommon and mainly concerns the β-lactams. Since resistance may be difficult to detect by susceptibility testing, it is necessary to systematically screen for β-lactamase production with the chromogenic cephalosporin test (Nitrocefin®). The lists presented below include antibiotics that should be tested.

Table 9. MIC (μg/ml) of β-lactams against β-lactamase producing *Capnocyto phaga* DF1 [from (21)]

Antibiotic	MIC_{90}
Penicillin G	> 128
Amoxicillin	> 128
Amoxicillin+clavulanic acid	2
Ticarcillin	> 128
Ticarcillin+clavulanic acid	2
Piperacillin	64
Piperacillin+tazobactam	2
Cephalothin	> 128
Cefoxitin	4
Cefotaxime	16
Cefotaxime+clavulanic acid	0.06
Ceftazidime	64
Ceftazidime+clavulanic acid	1 - 4
Imipenem	0.5
Aztreonam	0.5

Practically, only those for which National Committees have provided breakpoints can be tested, which limits considerably the choice.

HACEK group

The antibiotics used in the treatment of endocarditis should be tested.

Minimum antibiogram

Penicillin G, ampicillin or amoxicillin, amoxicillin + clavulanic acid, third generation cephalosporin (cefotaxime or ceftriaxone) and fluoroquinolone (ciprofloxacin or levofloxacin).

Standard antibiogram

In addition: other third generation cephalosporins (ceftazidime, cefixime), imipenem, erythromycin, clindamycin, chloramphenicol, tetracycline and co-trimoxazole.

Aminoglycosides should be tested in the case of serious infections (endocarditis). Extreme caution should always be used when interpreting the results.

Capnocytophaga and *Dysgonomonas*

Minimum antibiogram

Penicillin G, ampicillin or amoxicillin, amoxicillin + clavulanic acid, third generation cephalosporins (cefotaxime, ceftazidime), aztreonam, imipenem, erythromycin, clindamycin, and ciprofloxacin.

Standard antibiogram

Add to the previous antibiotics: ticarcillin, piperacillin, ticarcillin + clavulanic acid and piperacillin + tazobactam combinations, cefoxitin, cotrimoxazole, chloramphenicol, tetracycline, and rifampin.

Alternatives and additional tests

- Detection of β-lactamases with a chromogenic cephalosporin test (Nitrocefin®) is essential since β-lactamase producing strains exist.
- β-lactam/β-lactamase inhibitor synergy should be sought by a method used to detect extended spectrum β-lactamases in enterobacteria. For instance, the double disk synergy test allows to observe a champagne cork or more often a funnel-shaped zone in case of positivity.

Table 10. CLSI critical concentrations for HACEK[a]

Antibiotic		MIC (µg/ml)[a]		
Class	Molecule	Susceptible	Intermediate	Resistant
β-lactams	Penicillin	≤ 1	2	≥ 4
	Ampicillin	≤ 1	2	≥ 4
	Ampicillin + sulbactam	≤ 2/1	-	≥ 4/2
	Amoxicillin + clavulanic acid	≤ 4/2	-	≥ 8/4
	Ceftriaxone	≤ 2	-	-
	Cefotaxime	≤ 2	-	-
Carbapenems	Imipenem (*Haemophilus* spp.) [b]	≤ 4	8	≥ 16
	Meropenem (*Haemophilus* spp.) [b]	≤ 4	8	≥ 16
	Imipenem (other species)	≤ 0.5	1	≥ 2
	Meropenem (other species)	≤ 0.5	1	≥ 2
Macrolides	Azithromycin	≤ 4	-	-
	Clarithromycin	≤ 8	16	≥ 32
Quinolones	Ciprofloxacin	≤ 1	2	≥ 4
	Levofloxacin	≤ 2	4	≥ 8
Tetracyclines	Tetracycline	≤ 2	4	≥ 8
Phenicols	Chloramphenicol	≤ 4	8	≥ 16
Ansamycins	Rifampin	≤ 1	2	≥ 4
Folate inhibitors	Trimethoprim-sulfamethoxazole	≤ 0.5/9.5	1-2/19-38	≥ 4/76

[a] Determined by dilution in liquid medium.
[b] *Haemophilus* spp. correspond to the new species *Aggregatibacter* (*A. aphrophilus*, *A. aphrophilus* requiring V factor [*H. paraphrophilus*], *A. segnis*, and *A. actinomycetemcomitans*).

INTERPRETIVE CRITERIA

The CLSI critical concentrations for HACEK group bacteria are given in Table 10.

Interpretive criteria are based on the MIC distribution for β-lactams (mainly penicillin G) or adapted from those for *Haemophilus influenzae*.

REFERENCES

(1) **Alcala, L., F. Garcia-Garrote, E. Cercenado, T. Pelaez, G. Ramos, and E. Bouza**. 1998. Comparison of broth microdilution method using *Haemophilus* test medium and agar dilution method for susceptibility testing of *Eikenella corrodens*. J. Clin. Microbiol. **36**:2386-2388.

(2) **Arlet, G., M. J. Sanson-Le Pors, I. M. Casin, M. Ortenberg, and Y. Perol**. 1987. In vitro susceptibility of 96 *Capnocytophaga* strains, including a β-lactamase producer, to new β-lactam antibiotics and six quinolones. Antimicrob. Agents Chemother. **31**:1283-1284.

(3) **Bieger, R. C., N. S. Brewer, and J. A. Washington 2nd**. 1978.. *Haemophilus aphrophilus* : a microbiologic and clinical review and report of 42 cases. Medicine. **57**:345-355.

(4) **Birgisson, H., O. Steingrimsson, and T. Gudnason,**. 1997. *Kingella kingae* infections in paediatric patients: 5 cases of septic arthritis, osteomyelitis and bacteraemia. Scandinavian Journal of Infectious Diseases **29**, 495–498.

(5) **Blum, R. N., C. D. Berry, M. G. Phillips, D. L. Hamilos, and E. W. Koneman**. 1992. Clinical illnesses associated with isolation of dysgonic fermenter 3 from stool samples. J. Clin. Microbiol. **30**:396-400.

(6) **Bremmelgaard, A., C. Pers, J. E. Kristiansen, B. Korner, O. Heltberg, and W. Frederiksen**. 1989. Susceptibility testing of Danish isolates of *Capnocytophaga* and CDC group DF-2 bacteria. APMIS. **97**:43-48.

(7) **Claesson, B., E. Falsen, and B. Kjellman**. 1985. *Kingella kingae* infections : a review and a presentation of data from 10 swedish cases. Scand. J. Infect. Dis. **17**: 233-243.

(8) **Clinical and Laboratory Standards Institute**. 2006. Methods for antimicrobial dilution and disk susceptibility testing of infrequently isolated or fastidious bacteria. Approved standard M45-A. Wayne, PA: Clinical and Laboratory Standards Institute.

(9) **Forleiza, S. W., M. G. Newman, A. L. Horikoshi, and U. Blachman**. 1981. Antimicrobial susceptibility of *Capnocytophaga*. Antimicrob. Agents Chemother. **19**:144-146.

(10) **Foweraker, J. E., P. M. Hawkey, J. Heritage, and H. W. Van Landuyt**. 1990. Novel beta-lactamase from *Capnocytophaga* spp. Antimicrob. Agents Chemother. **34**:1501-1504.

(11) **Goldstein, E. J., E. O. Agyare, and R. Silletti**. 1981. Comparative growth of *Eikenella corrodens* on 15 media in three atmospheres of incubation. J. Clin. Microbiol. **13**:951-953.

(12) **Goldstein, E. J., C. E. Cherubin, and M. Shulman**. 1983. Comparison of microtiter broth dilution and agar dilution methods for susceptibility testing of

(12) *Eikenella corrodens*. Antimicrob. Agents Chemother. **23**:42-45.

(13) **Goldstein, E. J., and D. M. Citron**. 1984. Susceptibility of *Eikenella corrodens* to penicillin, apalcillin, and twelve new cephalosporins. Antimicrob. Agents Chemother. **26**:947-948.

(14) **Goldstein, E. J., D. M. Citron, C. V. Merriam, Y. A. Warren, K. L. Tyrrell, and H. Fernandez**. 2002. In vitro activities of a new des-fluoroquinolone, BMS 284756, and seven other antimicrobial agents against 151 isolates of *Eikenella corrodens*. Antimicrob. Agents Chemother. **46**:1141-1143.

(15) **Grob, R., R. Zbinden, C. Ruef, M. Hackenthal, I. Diesterweg, M. Altwegg, and A. von Graevenitz**. 1999. Septicemia caused by dysgonic fermenter 3 in a severely immunocompromised patient and isolation of the same microorganism from a stool specimen. J. Clin. Microbiol. **3**:1617-1618.

(16) **Hawkey, P. M., S. D. Smith, J. Haynes, H. Malnick, and S. W. Forlenza**. 1987. In vitro susceptibility of *Capnocytophaga species* to antimicrobial agents. Antimicrob. Agents Chemother. **31**:331-332.

(17) **Hoffler, U., W. Niederau, and G. Pulverer**. 1980. Susceptibility of *Bacterium actinomycetem comitans* to 45 antibiotics. Antimicrob. Agents Chemother. **17**:943-946.

(18) **Hofstad, T., I. Olsen, E. R. Eribe, E. Falsen, M. D. Collins, and P. A. Lawson**. 2000. *Dysgonomonas* gen. nov. to accommodate *Dysgonomonas gadei* sp. nov., an organism isolated from a human gall bladder, and *Dysgonomonas capnocytophagoides* (formerly CDC group DF-3). Int. J. Syst. Evol. Microbiol. **50**:2189-2195.

(19) **Jeff L., M.B. Marques, E. S. Brookings, and K. B. Waites**. 1997. Detection of *Kingella kingae* bacteremia and identification of the organism in the clinical laboratory: Experience from two cases. Clin. Microbiol. Newsl. **19**:73-76

(20) **Jensen, K. T., H. Schonheyder, and V. F. Thomsen**. 1994. In-vitro activity of β-lactam and other antimicrobial agents against *Kingella kingae*. J. Antimicrob. Chemother. **33**:635-640.

(21) **Jolivet-Gougeon, A., A. Buffet, C. Dupuy, J. L. Sixou, M. Bonnaure-Mallet, S. David, and M. Cormier**. 2000. In vitro susceptibilities of *Capnocytophaga* isolates to beta-lactam antibiotics and beta-lactamase inhibitors. Antimicrob. Agents Chemother. **44**:3186-3188.

(22) **Jolivet-Gougeon, A., Z Tamanai-Shacoori, L. Desbordes, N. Burggraeve, M. Cormier, and Bonnaure-Mallet**. 2004. Genetic analysis of an ambler class A extended-spectrum beta-lactamase from *Capnocytophaga ochracea*. J. Clin. Microbiol. **42**:888-890.

(23) **Jorgensen, J. H., A. W. Howell, and L. A. Maher**. 1990. Antimicrobial susceptibility testing of less commonly isolated *Haemophilus species* using *Haemophilus* test medium. J. Clin. Microbiol. **28**:985-988.

(24) **Jorgensen, J. H**. 2004. Need for susceptibility testing guidelines for fastidious or less-frequently isolated bacteria. J. Clin. Microbiol. **42**:493-498

(25) **King, E. O., and H.W. Tatum**. 1962. *Actinobacillus actinomycetemcomitans* and *Haemophilus aphrophilus*. J. Infect. Dis. **111**:85-94.

(26) **Kugler, K. C., D. J. Biedenbach, and R. N. Jones**. 1999. Determination of the antimicrobial activity of 29 clinically important compounds tested against fastidious HACEK group organisms. Diagn. Microbiol. Infect. Dis. **34**:73-76.

(27) **Lacroix, J. M., and C. Walker**. 1991. Characterization of a β-lactamase found in *Eikenella corrodens*. Antimicrob. Agents Chemother. **35**:886-891.

(28) **Lane, T., R. R. MacGregor, D. Wright, and J. Hollander**. 1983. *Cardiobacterium hominis:* an elusive cause of endocarditis. J. Infect. **6**:75-80.

(29) **Le Quellec, A., D. Bessis, C. Perez, and A. J. Ciurana**. 1994. Endocarditis due to beta-lactamase-producing *Cardiobacterium hominis*. Clin. Infect. Dis. **19**:994-995.

(30) **Lu, P. L., P. R. Hsueh, C. C. Hung, L. J. Teng, T. N. Jang, and K. T. Luh**. 2000. Infective endocarditis complicated with progressive heart failure due to beta-lactamase-producing *Cardiobacterium hominis*. J. Clin. Microbiol. **38**:2015-2017.

(31) **Matsumoto T., Y. Kawakami, K. Oana, T. Honda, K. Yamauchi, Y. Okimura, M. Shiohara, and E. Kasuga**. 2006. First isolation of *Dysgonomonas mossii* from intestinal juice of a patient with pancreatic cancer. Arch. Med. Res. **37**:914–916

(32) **Ndon, J. A**. 1992. *Capnocytophaga canimorsus* septicemia caused by a dog bite in a hairy cell leukemia patient. J. Clin. Microbiol. **30**:211-213.

(33) **Nørskov-Lauritsen N. and M. Kilian**. 2006. Reclassification of *Actinobacillus actinomycetemcomitans*, *Haemophilus aphrophilus*, *Haemophilus paraphrophilus* and *Haemophilus segnis* as *Aggregatibacter actinomycetemcomitans* gen. nov., comb. nov., *Aggregatibacter aphrophilus* comb. nov. and *Aggregatibacter segnis* comb. nov., and emended description of *Aggregatibacter aphrophilus* to include V factor-dependent and V factor-independent isolates. Int. J. Syst. Evol. Microbiol. **56**, 2135-2146

(34) **O'Driscoll J. C., G. S. Keene, M. J. Weinbren, A. P. Johnson, M. F. Palepou, R. C. George**. 1995. *Haemophilus aphrophilus* discitis and vertebral osteomyelitis. Scand. J. Infect. Dis. **27**:291-293

(35) **Page, M. I., and E. O. King**. 1966. Infection due to *Actinobacillus actinomycetemcomitans* and *Haemophilus aphrophilus*. N. Engl. J. Med. **275**:181-188.

(36) **Paju, S., P. Carlson, H. Jousimies-Somer, and S. Asikainen**. 2000. Heterogeneity of *Actinobacillus actinomycetemcomitans* strains in various human infections and relationships between serotype, genotype, and antimicrobial susceptibility. J. Clin. Microbiol. **38**:79-84.

(37) **Paju, S., P. Carlson, and H. Jousimies-Somer**. 2003. Asikainen S. *Actinobacillus actinomycetemcomitans* and *Haemophilus aphrophilus* in systemic and nonoral infections in Finland. APMIS. **111**:653-657.

(38) **Pajukanta, R., S. Asikainen, M. Saarela, S. Alaluusua, and H. Jousimies-Somer**. 1992. In vitro activity of azithromycin compared with that of erythromycin against *Actinobacillus actinomycetemcomitans*. Antimicrob. Agents Chemother. **36**:1241-1243.

(39) **Pang, Y., T. Bosch, and M. C. Roberts**. 1994. Single polymerase chain reaction for the detection of tetra-

cycline resistant determinants Tet K and Tet L. Mol. Cell. Probes **8:**417–422.

(40) **Prère, M F., M. Seguy, Y. Vezard, and M. B. Lareng**. 1986. Sensibilité aux antibiotiques de *Kingella kingae*. Pathol. Biol. **34**:604-607.

(41) **Roe, D. E., A. Weinberg, and M.C. Roberts**. 1996. Mobile rRNA methylase genes coding for erythromycin resistance in *Actinobacillus actinomycetemcomitans*. J. Antimicrob. Chemother. **37**:457-464.

(42) **Roscoe, D. L., S. J. Zemcov, D. Thornber, R. Wise, and A. M. Clarke**. 1992. Antimicrobial susceptibilities and beta-lactamase characterization of *Capnocytophaga species*. Antimicrob. Agents Chemother. **36**:2197-2200.

(43) **Rosenau, A., B. Cattier, N. Gousset, P. Harriau, A. Philippon, and R. Quentin.** 2000. *Capnocytophaga ochracea*: characterization of a plasmid-encoded extended-spectrum TEM-17 beta-lactamase in the phylum *Flavobacter-bacteroides*. Antimicrob. Agents Chemother. **44**:760-762.

(44) **Rotger, R., E. Garcia-Valdes, and E. P. Trallero**. 1986. Characterization of a β-lactamase specifying plasmid isolated from *Eikenella corrodens* and its relationship to a commensal *Neisseria* plasmid. Antimicrob. Agents Chemother. **30**:508-509.

(45) **Rummens, J. L., B. Gordts, and H. W. Van Landuyt**. 1986. In vitro susceptibility of *Capnocytophaga species* to 29 antimicrobial agents. Antimicrob. Agents Chemother. **30**:739-742.

(46) **Slots, J., R. T. Evans, P. M. Lobbins, and R. J. Genco**. 1980. In vitro antimicrobial susceptibility of *Actinobacillus actinomycetemcomitans*. Antimicrob. Agents Chemother. **18**:9-12.

(47) **Sutter, V. L, and S. M. Finegold**. 1970. *Haemophilus aphrophilus* infections : clinical and bacteriological studies. Ann. N. Y. Acad. Sci. **174**:468-487.

(48) **Verghese, A., F. Hamati, S. Berk, B. Franzus, and J. K. Smith**. 1988. Susceptibility of dysgonic fermenter 2 to antimicrobial agents in vitro. Antimicrob. Agents Chemother. **32**:78-80.

(49) **Wormser, G. P., and E. J. Bottone.** 1983. *Cardiobacterium hominis:* review of microbiologic and clinical features. Rev. Infect. Dis. **5**:680-691.

(50) **Yagupsky, P., O. Katz, and N. Peled.** 2001. Antibiotic susceptibility of *Kingella kingae* isolates from respiratory carriers and patients with invasive infections. J. Antimicrob. Chemother. **47**:191-193.

Chapter 46. METHODS FOR ANTIMICROBIAL SUSCEPTIBILITY TESTING OF ANAEROBIC BACTERIA

Luc DUBREUIL

"Anaerobes may be a colossal hoax perpetrated by a cabal of investigators who claim special powers to culture these malodorous creatures."
                                                Anonymous

INTRODUCTION

The isolation and identification of strict anaerobes from pathological specimens is labor-intensive and time-consuming. The delay in obtaining definitive results is very long, which is why antimicrobial susceptibility testing of anaerobic bacteria has remained a subject of controversy in which progress has come only slowly. Apart from the agar dilution method, no consensus has emerged as to which methods should be used. Whether confronted with strict anaerobic or mixed infections, initially the therapy must be empirical, based on the usual flora of such infections and on knowledge of antimicrobial susceptibility patterns.

IS ANTIMICROBIAL SUSCEPTIBILITY TESTING OF ANAEROBES NECESSARY?

Many arguments have been advanced both for and against antimicrobial susceptibility testing in strict anaerobes (Table 1), since treatment has usually been initiated long before the definitive bacteriology report becomes available. However, changing resistance patterns and the emergence of new types of resistance, such as imidazole and carbapenem resistance in *B. fragilis*, have led to changes in susceptibility patterns. The species most highly resistant to antimicrobial agents include the *Bacteroides fragilis* group, *Clostridium* RIC group (*C. ramosum, C. innocuum, C. clostridioforme*), *Fusobacterium varium*, and *Bilophila wadsworthia*. When a dozen or so species are isolated from the same specimen (appendectomy, for example), it is not necessary to test all the strains (3), since in such cases the aim of antibiotic therapy is to reduce the initial bacterial load and/or abolish the bacterial synergies which govern these types of infections. Finally, there is no need for susceptibility testing of strains which are not clinically relevant or which are part of the normal flora in proximity to the infection site. Antimicrobial susceptibility testing should be limited to clinically relevant species (Table 2).

Special attention should be paid to strains isolated from specimens obtained in good conditions (bone or joint biopsy; biopsy of muscle or other sterile sites). Furthermore, distinguishing between *B. fragilis* isolates for which the MIC of cefoxitin or cefotetan ranges from 16-64 µg/ml is less important than detecting a strain for which the imipenem MIC is 64 µg/ml, when generally it is 0.25 µg/ml.

Table 1. Arguments for antimicrobial susceptibility testing of strict anaerobes

For	Against
- Why study only aerobes and facultative aero-anaerobes; is there less mortality and morbidity in anaerobic infections?	Anaerobes are not always the greatest cause of concern for the clinician.
- Failure of empirical therapy increases hospitalization times and costs.	Empirical treatment is generally satisfactory.
- Development of antibiotic resistance.	Susceptibility of strains is well established.
- There are variations in the susceptibility of bacterial species according to the ecosystem.	
- Susceptibility testing establishes a susceptibility profile for the species which is useful for future patients.	Response time: results only become available after the patient has already left the hospital!
- Essential if patients respond poorly to treatment or in case of clinical failure.	Difficulty and cost of testing.

Table 2. Anaerobes for which antibiotic susceptibility should be tested

Bacteroides fragilis group	*Clostridium perfringens*
Prevotella and *Porphyromonas*	*Clostridium ramosum*
	Clostridium butyricum
	Clostridium clostridioforme
	Clostridium innocuum
Other *Bacteroides*	
Fusobacterium spp.	*Fusobacterium varium*
Fusobacterium necrophorum	
Fusobacterium mortiferum	*Bilophila wadsworthia*

If the infection proves refractory, or if prolonged therapy is required, then the bacteriological findings become essential. Susceptibility testing is therefore carried out when the response to empirical therapy is insufficient, when patients require prolonged therapy, or when there are no clinical data available in the literature to guide the empirical choice (13).

Antimicrobial susceptibility testing is recommended in the following situations:
- when an anaerobe is isolated in pure culture or from a blood culture;
- in severe infections such as osteomyelitis, brain abscess, endocarditis, infections on prosthetic materials or vascular grafts, or in persisting or recurring bacteremia;
- in case of failure of empirical therapy, the CLSI working group on anaerobic bacteria has clearly indicated the value of susceptibility testing (33):
- to determine the activity of new antimicrobial agents;
- to establish susceptibility patterns of different species or species groups in a region or even a hospital;
- to monitor resistance patterns;
- to aid clinicians in treating the patients described above.

METHODS

In any susceptibility test method, it is essential to clearly define and standardize the test conditions, including culture media, addition or not of blood and other supplements, inoculum preparation (size, source, physiological condition), incubation time, and anaerobic atmosphere. As far as anaerobes are concerned, two factors are important but have not yet been satisfactorily resolved: anaerobiosis and the effect of pH on anaerobiosis.

General points about anaerobic techniques
Media

All culture media, whether solid or liquid, must be prereduced before use by incubation in a boiling water bath for 20 min. Agar should be dried rapidly (20 min at 42°C) and all media should be stored in an anaerobic atmosphere (chamber or jar). As soon as the medium is inoculated it must be placed in conditions of anaerobiosis without delay. Since no single medium supports the growth of all anaerobes, different agar media have been developed: Wilkins Chalgren, brain-heart infusion, Schaedler, Brucella, FAA (Fastidious Anaerobes Agar), TGY (trypticase, glucose, yeast extract), and Columbia. Solid or liquid media are supplemented with 5% horse or sheep blood, hemin, vitamin K1, and sodium bicarbonate (concentrations are indicated in the "inoculum" section). Imipenem is inactivated in thioglycollate broth. The CLSI currently recommends Brucella medium because it supports growth of the largest number of anaerobes. Not all commercially available Brucella media have the same composition; only those media whose composition is identical to the formula shown in the appendix permit adequate growth of anaerobic bacteria.

Anaerobiosis

To minimize oxygen exposure, culture media should preferably be placed in an anaerobic atmosphere as rapidly as possible. Anaerobic chambers are the ideal system. When these are unavailable, it is possible to use jars containing gas generator envelopes which create an anaerobic environment in under 2 h. Anaerobic jars equipped with a gas inlet and outlet valve or else an Anoxomat anaerobic generator (TTO, NL) are preferable. Connected to an anaerobic jar with an inlet/outlet valve, the Anoxomat system insufflates the gas mixture and provides an airtight seal between the jar and the lid at each use. With these atmosphere replacement systems, bacterial growth in anaerobic jars is quite similar to that achieved in an anaerobic chamber and has proved superior to that obtained with gas generator envelopes. Incorrect anaerobiosis produces false resistance data for imidazoles.

Effect of pH on anaerobiosis

Carbon dioxide concentrations in the different anaerobic systems are highly variable. When testing macrolides, large decreases in activity may be observed due to a change in the pH of the medium resulting from increased carbon dioxide levels. A

1% increase in carbon dioxide concentrations led to a pH decrease of 0.05 units (18). The fall in pH at the agar surface has also been attributed to bacterial growth.

Although these variations occur less frequently in anaerobic chambers as compared to jars, rigorous quality control is essential when testing macrolides. In our experience, the modal MICs of erythromycin and roxithromycin were respectively 2 and 4 µg/ml for *C. perfringens* ATCC13124, 16 and 32 µg/ml for *B. thetaiotaomicron* ATCC29741, and 1 µg/ml with both drugs for *B. fragilis* ATCC 25285. In Wilkins Chalgren medium (pH 7.3), the MICs of erythromycin and azithromycin for *B. fragilis* ATCC 25285 determined in an anaerobic jar using the Gas Pak® system were 1 and 2 µg/ml, respectively; the medium had a pH of 6.8. With the Oxyrase® system which traps oxygen without supplying carbon dioxide, the MICs were 0.06 µg/ml and the initial pH of the medium did not change (28). Although this system gets around the problems with pH changes resulting from the presence of carbon dioxide, it has not yet been validated. Moreover, it should not be forgotten that the pH within an intra-abdominal abscess is in the range of 5.5 to 6.8.

Variations in pH have little effect on metronidazole or piperacillin + tazobactam but greatly influence the results for imipenem, clindamycin and, to a lesser extent, cefoxitin (35).

Inoculum

Since bacteria of different sizes and shapes can generate errors when determining the density of an inoculum by turbidimetry, the only method that can be used with anaerobes is to consider that a McFarland 0.5 standard is equivalent to approximately 1.5×10^8 CFU/ml.

A sterile loop is used to pick up at least five colonies from a Columbia blood agar plate (supplemented with 5 µg/ml hemin and 1 µg/ml vitamin K1) which are inoculated in Brucella or Schaedler broth supplemented with 5 µg/ml hemin, 1 µg/ml sodium bicarbonate, and 1 µg/ml vitamin K1. The broth is incubated for 6-24 h until the turbidity matches a McFarland 0.5 standard. This is possible for *Bacteroides fragilis* group strains and *Clostridium perfringens*. If the turbidity obtained 24 h after inoculation is too high, the culture may be diluted in anaerobic broth to a McFarland 0.5 standard. For slow growing strains, colonies picked from Petri dishes may be directly suspended in anaerobic broth until reaching the desired turbidity. Colonies less than 72 h old should not be removed from the anaerobic atmosphere for more than 30 min. Suspensions are prepared in Brucella or Schaedler broth (prereduced by placing in a boiling water bath for 20 min, then cooled to room temperature before use). These two media remain sufficiently clear after prereduction.

The different bacterial suspensions obtained in this way (approximately 10^8 CFU/ml) are then:

- loaded in a multipoint inoculator which delivers 1-5 µl per spot, for a final inoculum of 10^5 to 5×10^5 CFU per spot.
- again diluted 100-fold in anaerobic broth so as to obtain, for microdilution techniques, a final inoculum of 10^5 CFU per 100 µl well.

Breakpoints

Any strain for which the MIC is higher than the upper breakpoint is categorized as resistant. On the other hand, the fact that anaerobic or mixed infections require high doses of antibiotics means that strains categorized as intermediate are considered accessible to treatment. CLSI (7) and EUCAST breakpoints (tentative values) are given in Table 3. EUCAST breakpoints are lower than those of the CLSI. In particular, the following differences may be noted:

- For the amoxicillin + clavulanic acid combination, the latter is used in a 2/1 ratio by the CLSI and at a fixed concentration of 2 µg/ml in Europe.
- There is no CLSI breakpoint for amoxicillin because intravenous amoxicillin is not available in the US.
- An important difference is that CLSI breakpoints do not enable the detection of strains with reduced metronidazole susceptibility (MIC of 8 and 16 µg/ml) responsible for clinical failures (11, 23, 30).

Agar dilution

Petri dishes containing increasing antibiotic concentrations should be prepared immediately before use (7, 26). They may be prepared the day before use (with the exception of imipenem and certain β-lactamase inhibitor combinations) provided that they are either stored in an anaerobic chamber or else kept overnight at 4°C, brought to room temperature, dried if necessary and placed in anaerobiosis for 3 h prior to use.

In Brucella blood agar

This is considered the reference method of MIC determination for anaerobic bacteria (7). Brucella agar is supplemented with 5 µg/ml hemin, 1 µg/ml

Table 3. CLSI breakpoints (µg/ml) (7) and EUCAST tentative breakpoints for anaerobic bacteria.

Antibiotic	CLSI[a]		EUCAST[b] tentative breakpoints			
			Gram-negative		Gram-positive	
	c	C	c	C	c	C
Amoxicillin	ND[c]	ND	0,5	2	4	8
Amoxicillin + clavulanic acid	≤ 4/2	≥ 16/8	4/2	8/2	4/2	8/2
Ampicillin	≤ 2	≥ 8[c]	0,5	2	4	8
Ampicillin + sulbactam	≤ 8/4	≥ 32/16	ND	ND	ND	ND
Cefotaxime	≤ 16	≥ 64	IE	IE	IE	IE
Cefotetan	≤ 16	≥ 64	IE	IE	IE	IE
Cefoxitin	≤ 16	≥ 64	ND	ND	ND	ND
Chloramphenicol	≤ 8	≥ 32	8	16	8	16
Clindamycin	≤ 2	≥ 8	4	4	4	4
Doripenem	ND	ND	1	1	1	1
Ertapenem	≤ 4	≥ 16	1	1	1	1
Imipenem	≤ 4	≥ 16	2	8	2	8
Meropenem	≤ 4	≥ 16	2	8	2	8
Metronidazole	≤ 8	≥ 32	4	4	4	4
Moxifloxacin	≤ 2	≥ 8	IE	IE	IE	IE
Penicillin G	≤ 2	≥ 8[c]	0.25	0.5	0.25	0.5
Piperacillin	≤ 2	≥ 128	16	16	8	16
Piperacillin + tazobactam	≤ 32/4	≥ 128/4	16/4	16/4	8/4	16/4
Ticarcillin	≤ 32	≥ 128	16	16	8	16
Ticarcillin + clavulanic acid	≤ 32/2	≥ 128/2	8/2	16/2	8/2	16/2
Vancomycin	ND	ND	-	-	4	8

[a] CLSI: MIC ≤ c, susceptible strain; MIC ≥ C, resistant strain; c < MIC < C, intermediate strain.
[b] EUCAST: MIC ≤ c, susceptible strain; MIC > C, resistant strain; c < MIC ≤ C, intermediate strain.
[c] ND, not determined.
[d] IE, there is insufficient evidence that the species in question is a good target for therapy with the drug.
According to EUCAST with tigecycline: for anaerobic bacteria there is clinical evidence of activity in mixed intra-abdominal infections, but no correlation between MIC values, Pk/Pd data and clinical outcome. Therefore no breakpoint for susceptibility testing is given.

vitamin K and 5% lysed sheep blood (may be obtained by successive freezing/thawing).

In addition to antibiotic-containing plates, two antibiotic-free plates are inoculated at the beginning and end of the test. At the beginning of the test, one plate is incubated aerobically to check that the strain is pure; the other is incubated anaerobically to check strain viability. The two plates inoculated at the end of the test serve to detect any contamination (aerobes or anaerobes) occurring during the test. After the plates are inoculated with a multipoint inoculator, the inoculum should be allowed to diffuse into the agar for 5-10 min. All these steps should be carried out rapidly in an aerobic atmosphere, and the plates should then be incubated anaerobically at 35-37°C **for 48 h**. It is important to keep in mind that **introduction of the multipoint inoculator or any other electrical device into the anaerobic chamber is prohibited due to the risk of explosion in the presence of hydrogen**. When using anaerobic jars, it is recommended that an antibiotic-free control plate is placed in each jar, even if an anaerobiosis indicator is added. This is done to ensure that each inoculated strain grows. Technical details may be found in CLSI standard M11A7 (7).

Advantages:
- Excellent intra- and inter-laboratory reproducibility.
- Can be carried out simultaneously on a large number of strains and with several antibiotics.
- Bacteria collected *in vivo* are more similar to those cultivated in agar medium than to those cultivated in broth medium (20).

Drawbacks:
- Too labor-intensive, complex and costly for routine use. A multipoint inoculator and at least eight plates per antibiotic are required.
- In the previous NCCLS standards, Wilkins Chalgren medium was recommended, but this medium does not support the growth of certain anaerobes like pigmented *Porphyromonas* and *Prevotella* or *Fusobacterium* spp. Gram-positive cocci grow more or less efficiently on this medium. Addition of 5% defibrinated or lysed blood or appropriate supplements can partially remedy this problem. In the latest CLSI guidance, Brucella blood agar has supplanted Wilkins Chalgren medium.

Broth dilution

Macrodilution

This method is quite long and can only be used on a small number of antibiotics and strains. It is suitable for certain *Clostridium* strains which colonize solid media in the manner of *Proteus* strains. Survivor counts give an indication of the bactericidal potency of the antibiotic.

Microdilution

Several broth media have been used, including Brucella, Wilkins West, Wilkins Chalgren, brain-heart infusion, and Schaedler (24). As there is no single broth medium that supports the growth of all anaerobic bacteria, one must first make sure that the strain under study grows in the chosen medium. It is possible to supplement the media, for example with blood, in order to improve growth. This method has been validated for the *Bacteroides fragilis* group.

Preparation of plates

Either a microtiter plate well filler or a multichannel pipette is needed. In either case, frequent quality controls must be performed to check the volume delivered to the wells. Volumes smaller than 100 μl should be avoided so as to minimize the inoculum effect, which is very large in small volumes, and to reduce any evaporation occurring after long incubation times. In the older anaerobic chambers, traces of oxygen are converted into water which in turn is trapped by a dessicant. To avoid concentrating the antibiotic in the well through evaporation, plates are placed in plastic bags before being put in the incubator. A perforated film protects against evaporation while allowing gas exchange, which can occur provided that no more than four plates are stacked on top of each other. Higher stacks lead to uneven heating within the incubator. Prereduction of medium is not necessary since the volumes used are so small, as long as the plates are placed in anaerobiosis immediately after inoculation. Plates are incubated for **48 h at 35°C**.

The problem of storage arises when antibiotic plates are prepared in advance (36). Plates should be stored at –60°C. Plates containing imipenem or clavulanic acid should be stored at –70°C. At these temperatures, and depending on the antibiotic, they may be kept for 4-6 months. Thawed plates should be discarded, as successive freezing and thawing causes degradation of the antibiotic (beware of automatic defrosting freezers).

Advantages:
- The results show good correlation with the reference method, although MICs are generally one dilution lower than those determined by agar dilution.
- Partial automation is possible.
- It is possible to test a small number of strains every day, as well as *Clostridium* strains which colonize agar media.

Drawbacks:
- Plate preparation times and storage.
- Many quality controls are required when preparing and using microtiter plates and the duration must be established.
- Reading difficulties: for some species like *Fusobacterium* spp., there is no clear transition from growth to no-growth but rather a trailing effect. This usually corresponds to lysed forms which hinder the reading of MIC endpoints. This problem can be resolved by adding a few drops of 1% Andrade indicator (0.5% acid fuchsin) or triphenyltetrazolium chloride (blue in color) which, in the presence of bacterial growth, is converted to formazan (red).
- The method cannot be used to test β-lactam activity in strains that produce β-lactamases (R.J. Zabranski, personal communication).

Commercial plates

Commercial microtiter plates have made the microdilution method more accessible, provided that wells are filled with 100 µl of broth for a final inoculum of 10^5 CFU/100 µl well. Plates are read after 48 h incubation in an anaerobic atmosphere.

Antibiotics are incorporated into the plates which are stored in frozen or lyophilized form. Different systems include MicroScan® (containing West Wilkins broth), MSI/MicroMedia® (containing Wilkins Chalgren broth), Sceptor® (Becton Dickinson), ANA MIC 20® (Innovative Diagnostics Systems) which must be stored at –20°C, and ANA MIC 70® which must be stored at –70°C because it contains imipenem which is less stable than other antibiotics. These systems are not available in all countries.

Advantages and drawbacks:

These methods generally show good correlation with MIC determination by the agar dilution method: 91% agreement for MicroMedia® (Micro Media Systems) except for clindamycin (56%); 83% for MicroScan®; 92% for Sceptor Anaerobic Panel® (Becton Dickinson). Using three clinical categories to classify strains, the MHK-Anaerob-Biotest® (Biotest Serum Institute), Dynatech MIC® (Dynatech), Sceptor Anaerobic MIC®, and ATB ANA® (bioMérieux) systems respectively showed 97, 93, 97, and 96% essential agreement (excluding false susceptible and false resistance results) (14).

Agar diffusion

Diffusion methods have been criticized because they cannot be used on all species or all antibiotics. Their reproducibility is low and the results may correlate poorly with dilution methods. Standardization is difficult, essentially due to the highly varied growth rates and critical times that characterize the anaerobes, even within a same species. For instance, the inhibition zone diameters measured in nine consecutive tests of metronidazole against a *B. fragilis* isolate showed a difference of 16 mm (4). On the other hand, the diffusion method can be used to test imipenem, tetracycline, and clindamycin against the *B. fragilis* group since susceptible and resistant populations are clearly distinct. Agar diffusion techniques cannot be analyzed if growth is insufficient or in the presence of a film or haze at the agar surface, double inhibition zones, large inhibition zones, excessively small inhibition zones, or in the absence of an antibiotic diffusion gradient in anaerobiosis due to antibiotic degradation and resultant absence of critical diameters. Very major discrepancies are common, occurring at a frequency of about 13%.

The first diffusion technique, described by Horn et al. (16), allowed susceptibility testing of rapidly growing species like *B. fragilis* and *C. perfringens*. In this diffusion method, Mueller-Hinton medium, which is poorly suited to the growth of anaerobes, is replaced by Wilkins Chalgren agar (34). Interpretive criteria for inhibition zone diameters differ from those of aerobes. Few of the antibiotics usable in anaerobic infections have been studied. Only strains able to grow on unsupplemented Wilkins Chalgren medium can be tested, which excludes *Porphyromonas*, *Prevotella*, some *Fusobacterium*, and *Peptostreptococcus*.

To our knowledge, no critical diameters have been published for interpretation of diffusion antibiograms for all the antibiotics active against anaerobic bacteria.

In Wilkins Chalgren agar

Without being more enthusiastic than the cause deserves, a very large inhibition zone allows the conclusion that the strain is susceptible, while conversely, the presence of colonies in contact with the disk provides confirmation of resistance. It is often by comparing inhibition zone diameters with those of a wild type strain that one can suspect a resistance mechanism at work. If the difference is large, MIC determination is the only way to categorize the strain for the clinician.

In 1990, A. Dublanchet (8) described the detection of reduced susceptibility strains by a diffusion method using Rosco® tablets. Metronidazole-susceptible strains of *B. fragilis* (MIC 0.5-1 µg/ml, inhibition zone diameters 43 mm, Fig. 1) could be distinguished from reduced susceptibility strains (MIC 2-4 µg/ml, inhibition zone diameters 21 mm, Fig. 2), while resistant strains (MIC 64 µg/ml, Fig. 3) grew in contact with the tablet. In case of reduced susceptibility, an incubation period of four or more days was necessary to be able to observe delayed growth of colonies in the inhibition zone.

In Brucella blood agar

We have performed a preliminary study on approximately 100 strains in order to define critical diameters in Brucella medium. Correlation coefficients between inhibition zone diameters and MIC values were usually low, ranging from 0.4 to 0.94.

Table 4. Detection of strains resistant or with reduced susceptibility to metronidazole by diffusion in Brucella blood agar (personal data)

Antibiotic	Detection system	Species	Strains tested	Positive detection
Amoxicillin	25 µg disk	Peptostreptococcus	1	1
Amoxicillin+ clav. acid	20/10 µg disk	B. fragilis	10	7
Amoxicillin+ clav. acid	Rosco® tablet	B. fragilis	10	8 (+ 1 strain I)
Ticarcillin	75 µg disk	B. fragilis	22	21
Ticarcillin + clav. acid	75/10 µg disk	B. fragilis	3	3
Imipenem	10 µg disk	B. fragilis	3	3
Clindamycin	2 I.U. disk	Anaerobes	33	28
Metronidazole	4 µg disk	B. fragilis	1	1
Metronidazole	10 µg disk	B. fragilis	1	1
Metronidazole	Rosco® tablet	B. fragilis	1	1
Metronidazole RS[a]	4 µg disk	B. fragilis	9	6
Metronidazole RS[a]	10 µg disk	B. fragilis	9	5
Metronidazole RS[a]	Rosco® tablet	B. fragilis	9	6

RS = strain with reduced susceptibility

Although the diffusion method cannot be recommended for routine testing, it is preferable to no testing at all. The main advantage lies in the detection of resistant strains (Table 4). We were able to detect resistance of a *Peptostreptococcus* isolate to amoxicillin, resistance of *Bacteroides fragilis* group strains to ticarcillin, ticarcillin + clavulanic acid, and metronidazole, as well as high-level clindamycin resistance (MIC > 128 μg/ml) in the series of anaerobes tested (28/33 strains). Imipenem resistance in *B. fragilis* was demonstrated in 3/3 cases.

Reduced metronidazole susceptibility was detected in *B. fragilis* strains 5 or 6 out of 9 times with the conventional disks versus 6 out of 9 times with Rosco® tablets.

The detection of amoxicillin + clavulanic acid resistance in imipenem-susceptible strains of *B. fragilis* is difficult by any method which does not determine the MIC. We purposely included ten such strains in our study. Resistance was detected in 8 out of 10 strains with conventional disks or Rosco® tablets.

Summary

In practice, the diffusion method readily detects resistance to imipenem, clindamycin, and metronidazole in *B. fragilis*, and to amoxicillin in penicillinase-producing *Clostridium* and *Fusobacterium*. The only difficulty lies in the detection of the rare *B. fragilis* strains resistant to β-lactam + β-lactamase inhibitor combinations among imipenem-susceptible *B. fragilis*. The diffusion method can detect *B. fragilis* strains with reduced metronidazole susceptibility, provided that plates are read a second time after 4-5 days of incubation (see Gram-negative anaerobes).

Molecular detection of resistance genes such as *nim* and *cfiA* does not resolve the problem in so far as the expression of these genes depends on promoters which themselves are regulated.

Alternative methods

The complexity of agar dilution and the limitations of the diffusion method have made it necessary to turn to alternative methods. Broth disk elution is no longer recommended, and the spiral inoculation technique is not very widespread. These two techniques will be reviewed briefly before moving on to the most widely used routine methods: ATB ANA® and E-test®.

Broth disk elution (not recommended)

This method, used by some US laboratories for routine testing, consists in dropping antibiotic disks commercialized for the diffusion method into an anaerobic broth medium. The number of disks to be added to the tubes per antibiotic (24) is calculated so as to obtain a final concentration as close as possible to the two breakpoints in a final volume of 5 ml. The medium is inoculated with 100 μl of a 24-48 h

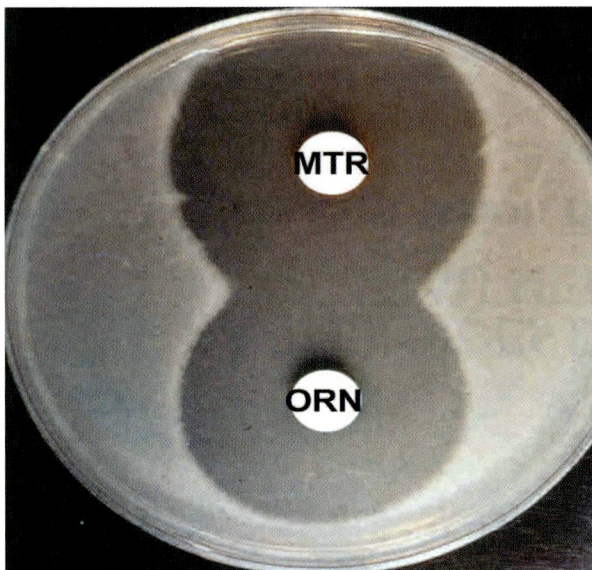

Fig.1. Strain susceptible to metronidazole (Rosco® tablets; MTR, metronidazole; ORN, ornidazole) (with permission of A. Dublanchet).

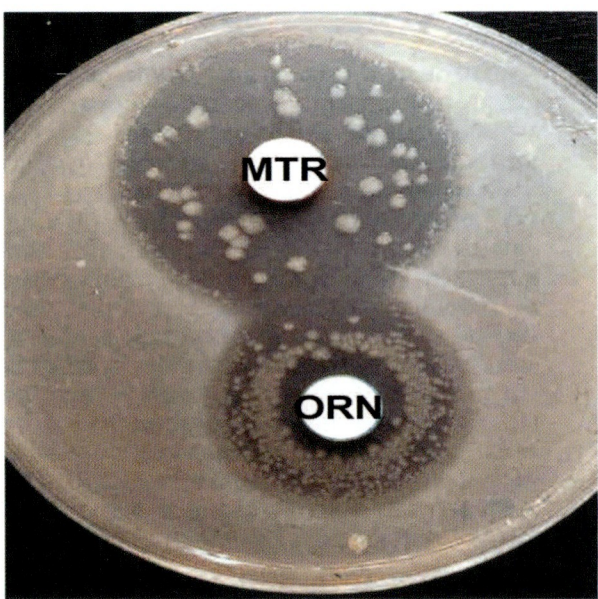

Fig.2. Strain with reduced susceptibility to metronidazole (Rosco® tablets; MTR, metronidazole; ORN, ornidazole) (with permission of A. Dublanchet).

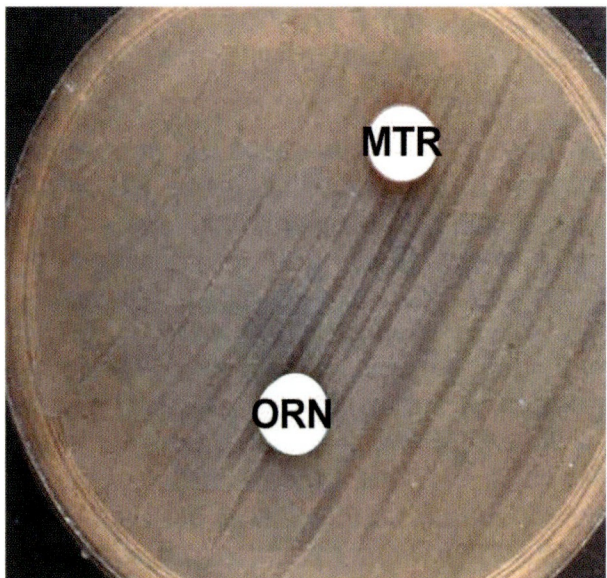

Fig.3. Strain resistant to metronidazole (Rosco® tablets; MTR, metrnidazole; ORN, ornidazole) (with permission of A. Dublanchet).

Spiral® (SGE: Spiral Gradient Endpoint) System

To avoid the labor-intensive preparation of Petri dishes containing the different dilutions of antibiotics needed for the reference method, the spiral system uses a stylus that deposits, on a rotating Petri dish, a fixed amount of antibiotic at the agar surface, forming concentric lines that create a concentration gradient of drug from the center (highest concentration) outwards. After the antibiotic diffuses in the agar for 3-4 hours, the plates are inoculated by streaking each strain in radial lines from the center to the edge of the plate, either using a swab or a Spiral® plater (Steers inoculator producing star-shaped streaks and thus better standardization). In this manner it is possible to simultaneously inoculate 17 strains on a 150 mm plate containing a concentration gradient corresponding to 8 dilutions. After a 48 h incubation, a caliper or Spiral® graduated plate is used to measure, for each streak, the distance between the center of the plate and the first visible growth. The MIC, which is proportional to the radial location of the transition from growth to no-growth, is computed by dedicated software. MICs measured with this technique showed 90% concordance with the reference method (± 1 dilution) (15).

Advantages:
- Technique similar to reference method but requires only one plate per antibiotic.
- Short preparation time (only one antibiotic concentration is needed, as the system automatically creates the concentration gradient).

culture and incubated for 24-48 hours, after which an absence of turbidity indicates that the strain is susceptible, while growth indicates resistance. Some concentrations can only be reached if a large number of disks is used, resulting in a "disk soup" which makes it difficult to read the results. The same happens when particles detach from the disk.

- Easy to read: the growth to no-growth transition can be accurately measured.
- Precise MIC determinations: (e.g.: 2.8 µg/ml)

Drawbacks:
- The system is expensive.
- The method has been evaluated by only a few investigators.
- Need to allow the antibiotic to diffuse for 4 h before inoculation.
- Petri dishes have to be prepared daily.

ATB ANA® system (bioMérieux)

The ATB® system can be used to test the following antibiotics: amoxicillin, amoxicillin + clavulanic acid, ticarcillin, ticarcillin + clavulanic acid, piperacillin, piperacillin + tazobactam, cefoxitin, cefotetan, imipenem, chloramphenicol, clindamycin, rifampin, levofloxacin, moxifloxacin, metronidazole, and vancomycin.

Colonies of the strain to be tested are introduced into the suspension medium to a turbidity matching a McFarland 3 standard (9×10^8 CFU/ml). Two hundred microliters of this suspension are introduced into the ATB S® medium tube; and 135 µl are then transferred into each well of the device. After 48 h incubation, growth is read either visually or with an ATB® automatic reader. When expressed as S, I and R clinical categories and in comparison to the agar dilution method, the results showed 94% agreement, with 4.8% minor errors, 0.4% major errors and 0.6% very major errors (9). The device therefore meets the generally accepted criteria (false susceptibility < 1%, false resistance < 4%, major and very major errors < 7%, complete category agreement > 90%).

Advantages:
- Easy and rapid.
- Low cost.
- Results correlate well with the reference method (14, 22, 31).

Drawbacks:
- Wilkins Chalgren broth is used, which did not support the growth of 40 out of 200 strains studied (20%), resulting in negative growth controls and an absence of results. This is the main fault of this method (9).
- Since the starting inoculum must have the turbidity of a McFarland 3 standard, for some strains of *Peptostreptococcus* spp. which produce little turbidity in broth medium, two plates of Columbia blood agar must be used so as to be able to harvest a sufficient number of bacteria to prepare the inoculum.
- Ten microliters of the above suspension are inoculated for rapidly growing strains (*B. fragilis, C. perfringens*) and 200 µl for slow growing strains. What volume should be used with intermediate growth strains?
- Absence of choice of antibiotics.
- There have not been many independent evaluations of the system.
- Reading difficulties with strains that produce abundant black pigment.

Epsilometer (E-test®)

An E-test® strip (AB Biodisk) is placed on Wilkins Chalgren or Brucella agar previously inoculated with the strain under study (McFarland 1 standard). One side of the strip contains an antibiotic which, when the strip comes in contact with the agar, is released into the agar in a concentration gradient. After incubation an inhibition ellipse forms. The MIC is read directly on a graduated scale on the other side of the strip at the point where the ellipse intersects the strip. E-test® results have been compared with MICs determined by the reference method. The results depended on the antibiotics and media used, the size of the inoculum and above all, the incubation times. Some resistances, particularly to clindamycin, were only detected if the incubation time was extended to 48 h. For *Clostridia*, up to 37% of strains tested falsely susceptible after 24 h of incubation; all these discrepancies disappeared after 48 h of incubation. 85-91% of E-test® results were within ± 1 dilution of those obtained by the reference method, and 92-98% were within ± 2 dilutions; the rate of major errors (false resistance) plus very major errors (false susceptibility) was < 4%.

The E-test® can sometimes give lower values (by approximately 1 dilution), depending on the antibiotic. For this reason, when the point of intersection of the inhibition ellipse falls between two graduations we suggest rounding up to the higher value.

Advantages:
- Simple method of MIC determination.
- Low rate of major errors (false susceptibility or false resistance).
- Available for the newest antibiotics.

Drawbacks:
- The MIC of only one antibiotic can be determined per strip. Testing more than one antibiotic, even if the strips are placed head to tail, consumes a large amount of agar.
- High cost which limits the number of antibiotics to test.

- Some β-lactam + β-lactamase inhibitor combinations have not been widely studied.

Laboratory practice

No method is satisfactory. One can choose between two alternatives: either the ATB ANA® system, or diffusion coupled with E-test®.

While the ATB ANA® device is satisfactory from a methodological standpoint, it does not support growth of about 20% of species. In case of metronidazole resistance, use E-test® to check for contamination arising from handling or incorrect anaerobiosis.

When using the diffusion method and by taking the proper precautions, it is possible to categorize strains as susceptible or resistant. The intermediate zone is unusable, and in this case an E-test® should be performed. The diffusion method is capable of detecting resistance to clindamycin, imipenem, and metronidazole.

Testing for β-lactamase production

Detection

The principal β-lactamase-producing species are shown in Table 5. The chromogenic cephalosporin test is a simple detection method in *B. fragilis*. If the test is negative after 15 min, it is recommended to incubate the disk for 1 h at 37°C (1). However, β-lactam resistance is not always due to β-lactamase production (27), particularly in *Bilophila wadsworthia* (2) and some strains of *B. distasonis* (21). Furthermore, this test does not detect imipenem resistance in *B. fragilis* or *B. distasonis*. Testing for β-lactamase production in the *B. fragilis* group is therefore of little interest (12). On the other hand, β-lactamase testing should be done in *Prevotella, Porphyromonas, Fusobacterium,* and the few penicillin-resistant strains of *Clostridium* (17). *Prevotella* strains are highly penicillin susceptible, but when a β-lactamase is detected by the chromogenic cephalosporin test, the MICs of amoxicillin became higher (0.5 to 128 μg/ml) than those of non-β-lactamase producing strains (Table 6). In this case it is easier to perform an E-test® and check that the amoxicillin MIC is < 0.5 μg/ml rather than carry out a chromogenic cephalosporin test, which may be difficult to interpret.

Frequency

β-lactamase production has been detected in 95-100% of species of the *fragilis* group. In France, 56% of *Prevotella* strains produce β-lacta-

Table 5. Anaerobic species in which β-lactamase production has been demonstrated

Bacteroides spp.
    B. capillosus
    B. coagulans
    B. splanchnicus
	Prevotella spp.
	    P. bivia
	    P. melaninogenica
	    P. buccae
	    P. disiens
	    P. oralis
	    P. ruminicola
	    P. oris

Bacteroides fragilis group
    B. fragilis
    B. thetaiotaomicron
    B. distasonis
    B. uniformis
    B. vulgatus
    B. ovatus
    and other members of this group
	Other Gram-negative bacilli
	Megamonas hypermegas
	Mitsuokella multiacida
	Porphyromonas asaccharolytica
	Porphyromonas uenonis
	Bilophila wadsworthia
	Alistipes finegoldii

Fusobacterium spp.
    F. nucleatum
    F. mortiferum
    F. varium
	Clostridium spp.
	    C. butyricum
	    C. clostridioforme
	    C. ramosum
	    C. bolteae

Gram-positive anaerobes *Acidaminococcus fermentans*	*C. innocuum*

Table 6. MICs of antibiotics according to β-lactamase production in *Prevotella* spp. after (10).

Antibiotic	MIC (µg/ml)			
	Non β-lactamase producing		Producing β-lactamase	
	MIC_{50}	MIC_{90}	MIC_{50}	MIC_{90}
Penicillin G	0.03	0.06	0.5	16
Amoxicillin	0.12	0.25	8	> 64
Amoxicillin + clavulanic acid	0.06	0.06	0.06	2
Cephalothin	0.25	1	16	> 64
Cefuroxime	0.12	1	8	> 64
Cefixime	0.25	1	16	> 64
Cefpodoxime	0.12	0.5	4	> 64
Ceftriaxone	0.12	0.5	4	> 64

mases that hydrolyze amoxicillin, cephalothin, and cefuroxime (10). β-lactamase production has been described in 85% of *P. bivia* strains whereas less than 5% of *Fusobacterium* strains produce a β-lactamase. The β-lactamases produced by *Prevotella* are sensitive to inhibitors such as clavulanic acid, tazobactam, and sulbactam (1, 19).

In the presence of a *Bacteroides fragilis* group strain and for any strain of *Prevotella*, *Fusobacterium,* or *Clostridium*, the technical data sheet should be consulted for interpretive reading of the antibiogram.

Quality control strains

The MICs of antibiotics for the four main strains are given in the technical data sheet.

Antibiotics to be studied

Most authors who follow CLSI guidance (25) consider it unnecessary to test the susceptibility of strict anaerobes to the following drugs, since these agents are active against virtually all strains: amoxicillin/ticarcillin + clavulanic acid combinations (except *Bilophila wadsworthia*), imipenem, meropenem, and metronidazole (except non-spore-forming Gram-positive bacilli and some *Peptostreptococcus* strains). Although resistance to these agents is very rare, it important that it be detected, which is why we have included these drugs in the list of antibiotics to be studied according to species groups (see technical data sheet).

Interpretive reading

See the technical data sheet.

In vitro-in vivo correlation

Many parameters play a role in the healing of anaerobic or mixed infections, including bacterial synergies, inoculum effect (5), time to treatment initiation, antibiotic concentration at the infection site, condition of the patient, to name a few. When surgical procedures such as abscess drainage, tissue debridement, or exeresis are combined with antibiotic or even hyperbaric oxygen therapy, it is difficult to discern the precise role of antibiotics in the cure of the infection. For instance, following surgery, some patients respond favorably with no antibiotics or with an inappropriate antibiotic, while on the other hand, if surgery is not performed, cure may not be achieved even with appropriate antibiotic therapy. The correlation between *in vitro* susceptibility tests and clinical response is therefore difficult to establish (32). However, many studies have shown that antibiotics which show activity against anaerobes have a higher success rate that agents inactive against these organisms; the same is true when considering mortality rates in anaerobic septicemias (13). Clinical failures have been described in metronidazole-treated patients harboring resistant strains (6, 29) but also in the presence of reduced imidazole susceptibility strains (11, 23, 30).

Antibiotic susceptibility testing of anaerobes, while desirable, does not *a priori* affect the likelihood of cure. Some agents like metronidazole, penicillin + β-lactamase inhibitor combinations, chloramphenicol, or imipenem allow clinicians to efficiently treat the majority of anaerobic infections without knowing the susceptibility of the causal strains. In case of treatment failure or in the specific clinical situations mentioned above, knowledge of antibiotic susceptibility is necessary so that treatment can be adjusted accordingly. Rare cases of resistance (to metronidazole or imipenem) can be detected by agar diffusion for some rapidly growing species (*B. fragilis* group, *C. perfringens*) and antibiotic susceptibility of other anaerobes can be tested by E-test® or ATB ANA®. Last but not least, empirical therapy should be based on the epidemiological data collected in a hospital.

CONCLUSION

Bacteroides of the *fragilis* group are among the most highly antibiotic resistant species of bacteria. These organisms are often found in association with other anaerobes, raising the problem of antibiotic efficacy against the largest number of anaerobes.

No antibiotic is 100% effective. If one accepts 95% efficacy, anaerobic bacteria will be inhibited by carbapenems, chloramphenicol, and penicillin + β-lactamase inhibitor combinations. While imidazoles are often combined with another antimicrobial agent, insufficiently active against Gram-negative anaerobes, a third generation cephalosporin + imidazole combination, though useful, does not necessarily cover all the anaerobes, particularly Gram-positive organisms.

Carbapenems in severe infections and penicillin + β-lactamase inhibitor combinations provide almost full coverage of the strict anaerobes, but other agents still have a place: spiramycin (available in some countries) + metronidazole in odontology, cefoxitin as prophylaxis in abdominal surgery. Gram-positive anaerobes have remained highly susceptible to penicillin G and amoxicillin. Imidazoles are almost always active against Gram-negative bacteria and *Clostridium*. Finally, thiamphenicol, whose susceptibility can be tested with a chloramphenicol disk, should be part of the therapeutic arsenal in brain infections; in some cases it is the only drug active against multiresistant *B. fragilis*. Moxifloxacin and linezolid are alternatives when other treatment options fail. All these considerations argue for susceptibility testing of anaerobic bacteria. Diffusion coupled with E-test® or the bioMérieux ATB ANA® system are useful substitutes for the dilution reference method. The availability of ready-to-use plates should, in the future, allow easier determination of MICs so as to better guide clinicians in their choice of antibiotics for mixed infections.

REFERENCES

(1) **Appelbaum, P.C., A. Philippon, R. Jacobs, S.K. Spangler, and L. Gutmann**. 1990. Characterization of β-lactamases from non *B. fragilis* group *Bacteroides* spp belonging to seven species and their role in β-lactam resistance. Antimicrob. Agents Chemother. **34**:2169-2176.

(2) **Baron, E.J., J.P. Summanen, J. Downes, M.C. Roberts, H.M. Wexler, and S.M. Finegold**. 1989. *Bilophila wadsworthia*, gen. nov. and sp. nov., a unique gram-negative anaerobic rod recovered from appendicitis specimens and human faeces. J. Gen. Microbiol. **135**:3405-3411.

(3) **Baron, E.J., R. Bennion, J. Thompson, C. Strong, P. Summanen, M. Mc Teague, and S.M. Finegold**. 1992. A microbiological comparison between acute and complicated appendicitis. Clin. Infect. Dis. **14**:227-231.

(4) **Barry, A.L, P.C. Fuchs, E.H. Gerlach, S.D. Allen, J.F. Acar, K.E. Aldridge, A-M. Bourgault, H. Grimm, G.S. Hall, W. Heizmann, R.N. Jones, J.W. Swenson, C. Thornsberry, H. Wexler, and J. Wüst**. 1990. Multilaboratory evaluation of an agar diffusion disk susceptibility test for rapidly growing anaerobic bacteria. Rev. Infect. Dis. **12** (Suppl. 2):S210-S217.

(5) **Brook, I.** 1991. In vitro susceptibility vs in vivo efficacy of various antimicrobial agents against the *B. fragilis* group. Rev. Infect. Dis. **13**:1170-1180.

(6) **Chauldhry, R., P. Mathur, B. Dhawan, and L. Kumar.** 2001. Emergence of metronidazole-resistant *B. fragilis*, India. Emerg. Infect. Dis. **7**:485-486.

(7) **Clinical and Laboratory Standards Institute**. 2007. Methods for antimicrobial susceptibility testing of anaerobic bacteria; approved standard -7th Edition. M11-A7, 27, No. 2, 1-4 , CLSI Wayne, PA, USA.

(8) **Dublanchet, A.** 1990. *Bacteroides* de sensibilité réduite au métronidazole. Une expression phénotypique inhabituelle. Med. Mal. Infect. **20** (Hors série):113-116.

(9) **Dubreuil, L., E. Singer, and I. Houcke.** 1999. Susceptibility testing of anaerobic bacteria: evaluation of the redesigned (version 96) bioMérieux ATB ANA device. J. Clin. Microbiol. **37**:1824-1828.

(10) **Dubreuil, L, J. Behra-Miellet, C. Vouillot, S. Bland, A. Sedallian, and F. Mory.** 2003. β-lactamase production in *Prevotella* and in vitro susceptibilities to selected beta-lactam antibiotics. Int. J. Antimicrob. Agents. **21**:267-273.

(11) **Elsaghier, A.A., J.S. Brazier, and E.A. James.** 2003. Bacteraemia due to *Bacteroides fragilis* with reduced susceptibility to metronidazole. J. Antimicrob. Chemother. **51**:1436-1437.

(12) **Finegold, S.M., and the National Committee for Clinical Laboratory Standards working group on anerobic susceptibility testing**. 1988. Susceptibility testing of anaerobic bacteria. J. Clin. Microbiol. **26**:1253-1256.

(13) **Finegold, S.M.** 1990. Anaerobes: problems and controversies in bacteriology, infections and susceptibility testing. Rev. Infect. Dis. **12** (Suppl. 2):S223-S230.

(14) **Heizmann, W., H. Werner, and B. Herb.** 1988. Comparison of four commercial microdilution systems for susceptibility testing of anaerobic bacteria. Eur. J. Clin. Microbiol. Infect. Dis. **7**:758-763.

(15) **Hill, G.B.** 1991. Spiral gradient endpoint method compared to standard agar dilution for susceptibility testing of anaerobic gram-negative bacilli. J. Clin. Microbiol. **29**:975-979.

(16) **Horn, R., A.M. Bourgault, and F. Lamothe.** 1987. Disk diffusion susceptibility testing of the *B. fragilis* group. Antimicrob. Agents Chemother. **31**:1596-1599.

(17) **Jacobs, M.R., S.K. Spangler, and P.C. Appelbaum.** 1990. Susceptibility of B. non-fragilis and fusobacteria to amoxicillin, amoxicillin/clavulanate, ticarcillin, ticarcillin/clavulanate, cefoxitin, imipenem and metronidazole. Eur. J. Clin. Microbiol. Infect. Dis. **9**:417-421.

(18) **Jansen, J.E., and A. Bremmelgaard.** 1986. Effect of culture medium and carbon dioxide concentration on growth of anaerobic bacteria and medium pH. Acta Path. Microbiol. Immun. Scand. Sect B. **94**:319-323.

(19) **Lacroix, J.M., F. Lamothe, and F. Malouin.** 1984. Role of *B. bivius* β-lactamase in β-lactam susceptibility. Antimicrob. Agents Chemother. **26**:694 - 698.

(20) **Lorian, V.** 1989. In vitro simulation of in vivo conditions: physical state of the culture media. J. Clin. Microbiol. **27**:2403-2406.

(21) **Malouin, F., and F. Lamothe.** 1987. The role of β-lactamase and the permeability barrier on the activity of cephalosporins against members of the *B. fragilis* group. Can. J. Microbiol. **33**:262-266.

(22) **Monteil, H., D. Rasoamananjara, and M.T. Vetter.** 1986. Evaluation de la sensibilité aux antibiotiques de *Bacteroides* et *Fusobacterium* à l'aide de la galerie ATB ANA. Path. Biol. **34**:648-652.

(23) **Mory F., J.P. Carlier, M. Thouvenin, H. Schuchmacher, and A. Losniewski.** 2004. Bacteremia caused by *Prevotella spp.* with reduced susceptibility to metronidazole. Int. J. Antimicrob. Agents 24 (Suppl 2):S152.

(24) **National Committee for Clinical Laboratory Standards.** 1985. Alternative methods for antimicrobial testing of anaerobic bacteria; Approved standard. NCCLS publication M-17P. National Committee for Clinical Laboratory Standards, Villanova, Pa.

(25) **National Committee for Clinical Laboratory Standards.** 1990. Methods for antimicrobial testing of anaerobic bacteria-second edition; Approved standard, NCCLS publication M11-A2. National Committee for Clinical Laboratory Standards, Villanova, Pa.

(26) **National Committee for Clinical Laboratory Standards.** 2003 Methods for antimicrobial testing of anaerobic bacteria, approved standard 6th edition. NCCLS document M11A6,NCCLS Wayne, PA.

(27) **Nord, C.E.** 1986. Mechanisms of β-lactams in anaerobic bacteria. Rev. Infect. Dis. **8** (Suppl.5):S543-548.

(28) **Retsema, J.A., L.A. Brennam, and A. E. Girard.** 1991. Effects of environmental factors on the in vitro potency of azithromycin. Eur. J. Clin. Microbiol. Infect. Dis. **10**:834-842.

(29) **Rotimi, V.O., M. Khoursheed, J.S. Brazier, W.Y. Jamal, and F.B. Khodakhast.** 1999. *Bacteroides* species highly resistant to metronidazole: an emerging clinical problem. Clin. Microbiol. Infect. **5**:166-169.

(30) **Sandoe, J.A.T., J.K. Struthers, and J.S. Brazier.** 2001. Subdural empyema caused by *Prevotella loescheii* with reduced susceptibilty to metronidazole. J. Antimicrob. Chemother. **47**: 66-367.

(31) **Sedallian, A., M. Derriennic, and L. Dubreuil.** 1988. Anaérobies stricts, p. 119-129. In P. Courvalin, J.P. Flandrois, F. Goldstein, A. Philippon, C. Quentin, and J. Sirot. (ed.), L'antibiogramme automatisé. MPC Vigot, Paris.

(32) **Snydman, D.R., G.J. Cuchural, J.R.L. McDermott, and M. Gill.** 1992. Correlation of in vitro testing methods with clinical outcomes in patients with *B. fragilis* group infections treated with cefoxitin: a retrospective analysis. Antimicrob. Agents Chemother. **36**:540-544.

(33) **Thornsberry, C.** 1990. Antimicrobial susceptibility testing of anaerobic bacteria: review and update on the role of the National Committee for Clinical Laboratory Standards. Rev. Infect. Dis. **12** (Suppl. 2):S218-S222.

(34) **Wilkins, T.D., and S. Chalgren.** 1976. Medium for use in antibiotic susceptibility testing of anaerobic bacteria. Antimicrob. Agents Chemother. **10**:926-928.

(35) **Wistanley, T.G., M.H. Wilcox, and R.C. Spencer.** 1992. Effect of pH on antibiotics used to treat anaerobic infection. J. Antimicrob. Chemother. **29**:594-595.

(36) **Zabransky, R.J., and K.J. Hauser.** 1977. Stability of antibiotics in Wilkins Chalgren anaerobic susceptibility testing medium after prolonged storage. Antimicrob. Agents Chemother. **12**:440-441.

Chapter 47. GRAM-POSITIVE ANAEROBES

Jean-Louis PONS and Frédéric BARBUT

INTRODUCTION

This chapter will examine the antimicrobial susceptibility patterns of the main groups of Gram-positive anaerobic bacteria:
- cocci (*Peptostreptococcus* and related genera),
- spore-forming bacilli (*Clostridium*),
- non-spore-forming bacilli (*Propionibacterium*, *Actinomyces*, *Bifidobacterium*, *Eubacterium*).

Available data on the latest antimicrobial agents including the new carbapenems, oxazolidinones and glycylcyclines will also be analyzed. Interpretative criteria for susceptibility data are based on guidance from the Clinical and Laboratory Standards Institute (CLSI, M11-A7, vol. 2) (11) and the European Committee on Antimicrobial Susceptibility Testing (EUCAST) (17).

GRAM-POSITIVE COCCI

Analysis of antimicrobial susceptibility in anaerobic Gram-positive cocci has been hindered by taxonomic revisions which have generated a proliferation of different synonyms. Presently, several newly defined genera have been separated from *Peptococcus niger* and *Peptostreptococcus anaerobius*; these include *Micromonas* (*M. micros*), *Anaerococcus* (*A. prevotii*), *Peptoniphilus* (*P. asaccharolyticus*), and *Finegoldia* (*F. magna*). The susceptibility patterns of different species are shown in Table 1.

Penicillins

Although a French study reported that "*Peptostreptococcus*" strains were always susceptible to amoxicillin (34), a multicenter study on a large series of isolates collected in Europe and North American revealed the existence of resistant strains, particularly of *P. anaerobius* (26%) (MIC$_{90}$ = 16 µg/ml) and more rarely *M. micros* (2%) (MIC$_{90}$ = 0.5 µg/ml) (28). Amoxicillin resistance appears to be due to a modification of penicillin-binding-proteins (PBPs), since there is no indisputable evidence for β-lactamase production.

Imipenem

High imipenem MICs (0.5 - 2 µg/ml) have been reported in some strains of *P. anaerobius* (7).

Macrolides

Macrolide resistance in the genus *Peptostreptococcus* is usually mediated by the *ermTR* gene, the most common resistance determinant in *Streptococcus pyogenes* (41). Clindamycin resistance rates have been estimated at approximately 28% (34) although resistance is highly species-dependent: a study of North American and European isolates which took the new taxons into account reported clindamycin resistance rates of 13.3% for *F. magna*, 0.7% for *M. micros*, and 1.1% for *P. anaerobius* (28).

Metronidazole

Susceptibility testing of metronidazole requires conditions of optimal anaerobiosis and the identification of an authentic *Peptostreptococcus* (and not *Streptococcus*) strain. Metronidazole resistance has been detected in strains of *F. magna* and *P. anaerobius* (28). A *nimB* gene (encoding a nitroimidazole reductase which reduces nitroimidazole to aminoimidazole, which is less toxic to DNA than the reduced intermediates produced by pyruvate:ferredoxin oxidoreductase in susceptible strains) has been detected in two strains of *F. magna* displaying high-level metronidazole resistance (MIC > 128 µg/ml). However, the *nimB* gene has also been demonstrated in susceptible strains and its expression depends on the presence of insertion sequences carrying strong or weak promoters (51).

SPORE-FORMING GRAM-POSITIVE BACILLI: GENUS *CLOSTRIDIUM*

Bacteria from the genus *Clostridium* display broad intrinsic susceptibility, particularly to β-lactams and macrolides. However, resistance phenotypes differ according to species, justifying the identification of clinical isolates to the species level.

Table 1. Activity (µg/ml) of amoxicillin or ampicillin (+/- clavulanic acid), erythromycin, clindamycin, and metronidazole against Gram-positive cocci

Species	Antibiotic	MIC	MIC$_{50}$	MIC$_{90}$	Reference
P. anaerobius	Amoxicillin	0.06 - 32	0.25	16	28
	Amoxicillin-clavulanate	0.094 - 48	0.25	12	9
	Erythromycin	0.023 - 16	0.04	4	9
	Clindamycin	< 0.016 - 32	< 0.06	0.25	28
		0.016 - 1	0.094	0.38	9
	Metronidazole	0.06 - 2	0.5	1	28
		0.023 - 0.75	0.19	0.39	9
F. magna	Amoxicillin	0.06 - 1	0.25	0.5	28
	Amoxicillin-clavulanate	0.016 - 1	0.064	0.25	9
	Erythromycin	0.064 - > 256	4	256	9
	Clindamycin	< 0.016 - 256	0.5	32	28
		0.023 - 256	1	4	9
	Metronidazole	0.06 - > 64	0.5	1	28
		0.032 - 1	0.125	0.38	9
M. micros	Amoxicillin	0.03 - >128	< 0.125	0.5	28
	Clindamycin	< 0.016 - 8	0.125	0.5	28
		0.125 - 1	0.25	0.25	12
	Metronidazole	0.06 - >64	0.25	0.5	28
		≤ 0.125 - 1	0.25	0.5	12
P. asaccharolyticus	Ampicillin	< 0.03 - 1	≤ 0.03	0.25	10
	Clindamycin	< 0.03 - 128	0.25	64	10
		0.06 - > 32	0.125	>32	12
	Metronidazole	0.125 - 2	0.5	1	10
		< 0.125 - 1	1	1	12

Breakpoints : amoxicillin /ampicillin 0.5-2 µg/ml (CLSI, 2007) or 4-16 µg/ml (EUCAST, 2006); clindamycin 2-8 µg/ml (CLSI, 2007) or 4-8 µg/ml (EUCAST, 2006); metronidazole 8-32 µg/ml (CLSI, 2007) or 4-8 µg/ml (EUCAST, 2006).

Clostridia other than C. difficile

The main resistances observed in the genus *Clostridium* are to cefoxitin (20%), cefotetan (32%) and clindamycin (32%) (34). Susceptibility patterns of *C. perfringens* and *C. innocuum* are shown in Table 2.

C. perfringens. This species is particularly susceptible to β-lactams (penicillins, cephalosporins, carbapenems) and also to clindamycin, although resistance to the latter agent may be observed (6, 10, 12, 34). Macrolide MLS$_B$ resistance is inducible and its expression requires a prolonged incubation of 48 hours.

C. innocuum. This species has intrinsic low-level resistance to vancomycin (35). The MICs of vancomycin range from 8-16 µg/ml (MIC$_{90}$ 16 µg/ml) while teicoplanin remains active (MIC 0.25-1 µg/ml, MIC$_{90}$ 0.5 µg/ml). This intrinsic resistance may not be detected by diffusion methods. Resistance is due to the synthesis of UDP-MurNac-pentapeptide [D-serine] peptidoglycan precursors (13).

Among the β-lactams, cefoxitin resistance is almost always observed (MIC$_{90}$ 128 µg/ml), and some strains are imipenem-intermediate.

Other clostridia

- Some species such as *C. tertium* may have low susceptibility to penicillins (MIC of penicillin G = 0.75 – 1 µg/ml) and cephalosporins (MIC of cefoxitin = 0.38 – 1 µg/ml) (50).
- β-lactamase production (diffusible, therefore detected by a chromogenic cephalosporin) has been reported in three species:
- *C. butyricum* (enzyme sensitive to β-lactamase inhibitors) (32);
- *C. clostridioforme* (enzyme resistant to β-lactamase inhibitors) (4); however, in penicillin G-resistant strains of this species, resistance is believed to due mainly to modification of PBPs (3);
- *C. ramosum* (enzyme resistant to β-lactamase inhibitors).

Table 2. Activity (µg/ml) of β-lactams and clindamycin against *C. perfringens*, *C. difficile*, and *C. innocuum*

Species	Antibiotic	MIC	MIC$_{50}$	MIC$_{90}$	Reference
C. perfringens	Ampicillin	< 0.03 - 0.06	< 0.03	0.06	10
	Cefoxitin	0.5 - 2	1	1	10
	Imipenem	0.06 - 0.25	0.125	0.25	21
		0.03 - 1	0.125	0.25	12
	Clindamycin	< 0.03 - 128	0.5	2	10
		0.06 - > 32	0.5	2	12
C. difficile	Ampicillin	2 - 4	2	4	10
	Cefoxitin	128 - >128	128	> 128	10
		32 - 128	64	128	34
	Cefotaxime	32 - 128	64	64	34
	Imipenem	2 - >16	4	16	21
		1 - 8	4	4	34
	Clindamycin	2 - >128	4	> 128	10
		0.12 - >128	4	> 128	34
		0.016 - > 256	3	256	6
C. innocuum	Ampicillin	0.06 - 0.25	0.25	0.25	10
	Cefoxitin	8 - 128	64	128	10
	Imipenem	1 - 2	2	2	21
	Clindamycin	0.125 - 128	0.5	128	10

Breakpoints : ampicillin 0.5-2 µg/ml (CLSI, 2007) or 4-16 µg/ml (EUCAST, 2006); cefoxitin 16-64 µg/ml (CLSI, 2007); cefotaxime 16-64 µg/ml (CLSI, 2007); imipenem 4-16 µg/ml (CLSI, 2007) or 2-16 µg/ml (EUCAST, 2006); clindamycin 2-8 µg/ml (CLSI, 2007) or 4-8 µg/ml (EUCAST, 2006).

Among the quinolones, the MICs of garenoxacin are 2-4 times lower than those of moxifloxacin (Table 3). The species *C. clostridioforme* and *C. symbiosum* are normally resistant to moxifloxacin (23).

C. difficile

With respect to β-lactams, *C. difficile* is characterized by (Table 2):
- Intrinsic resistance to cefoxitin (MIC 32-128 µg/ml) which can be used for selective media (cefoxitin-lysozyme medium, cycloserine-cefoxitin-fructose-agar medium). Cross-resistance to cefotetan is rare (3% of strains) (34).
- Over 90% of strains are resistant to cefotaxime (34).
- Low susceptibility to imipenem, as also seen with *C. innocuum*. MICs range from 1 to > 16 µg/ml (21, 34), so a large proportion of strains is categorized as intermediate or resistant.

Clindamycin resistance has been detected in over 50% of *C. difficile* isolates (5, 6, 34). Resistance rates for chloramphenicol and tetracycline are approximately 15 and > 20%, respectively (5).

Metronidazole resistance has been reported in some studies, although this has never been correlated with clinical failure. Resistance is not due to the presence of *nim* genes (40). Detection of resistance requires conditions of optimal anaerobiosis (low partial pressure of oxygen can interfere with intracellular penetration of metronidazole) and incubation times of up to 3 or even 4 days (inducible and possibly heterogeneous resistance) (40). While equine isolates have been categorized as intermediate or resistant (MICs ranging from ≤ 0.125 to 32 µg/ml) (26), human isolates show variable susceptibility according to geographic origin: no resistance detected in France (34), Germany (1) or Europe (7) but resistance rate reported as 6% in Spain (MIC = 8 – 16 µg/ml) (39).

Vancomycin susceptibility appears to be a constant characteristic (MICs < 4 µg/ml) (6, 12, 24) although 3% of isolates collected in Spain between 1993 and 2000 were reported as vancomycin-intermediate (39).

Characterization of moxifloxacin-resistant strains of *C. difficile* has revealed the presence of mutations in the *gyrA* or *gyrB* genes (2, 14, 49). The mutant GyrA protein harbors mainly a Thr$_{82}$Ile mutation (position known to be a resis-

Table 3. Activity (µg/ml) of quinolones against Gram-positive anaerobes

Species	Antibiotic	MIC	MIC$_{50}$	MIC$_{90}$	Reference
Clostridium spp.	Ciprofloxacin	0.25 - 256	2	16	15
	Levofloxacin	0.25 - 8	1	4	15
	Gatifloxacin	0.25 - 8	0.5	2	15
	Garenoxacin	0.06 - 2	0.5	1	25
	Moxifloxacin	0.125 - 8	1	2	25
C. perfringens	Garenoxacin	0.03 - 0,5	0.25	0.25	25
	Moxifloxacin	0.125 - 2	0.25	0.5	25
C. difficile	Levofloxacin	2 - 64	4	32	24
	Gatifloxacin	0.5 - 64	1	16	24
	Moxifloxacin	0.5 - 32	1	16	24
Gram-positive cocci	Ciprofloxacin	< 0.125 - 8	1	2	15
	Levofloxacin	0.25 - 8	2	4	15
	Gatifloxacin	< 0.06 - 4	0.25	1	15
P. asaccharolyticus	Garenoxacin	0.03 - 0.125	0.125	0.125	25
	Moxifloxacin	< 0.015 - 1	0.25	0.25	25
Gram-positive bacilli (other than Propionibacterium)	Ciprofloxacin	0.5 - 64	8	32	15
	Levofloxacin	< 0.125 - 8	1	2	15
	Gatifloxacin	0.125 - 16	0.5	1	15
Propionibacterium spp.	Ciprofloxacin	0.5			15
	Levofloxacin	0.125 - 0.5			15
	Gatifloxacin	0.125			15
	Garenoxacin	0.06 - 0.5	0.25	0.5	25
	Moxifloxacin	0.125 - 0.25	0.125	0.25	25
Actinomyces spp.	Garenoxacin	0.06 - 1	1		25
	Moxifloxacin	0.125 - 2	0.5		25

Breakpoint : moxifloxacin 2-8 µg/ml (CLSI, 2007).

tance determinant in different species) while the GyrB mutation is Asp$_{426}$Asn (position involved in resistance in *E. coli*). DNA gyrase therefore appears to be the primary target of quinolones in *C. difficile*. Efflux has not been shown to be a mechanism of reduced quinolone susceptibility. The frequency of moxifloxacin-intermediate or resistant strains of *C. difficile* varies in different studies, ranging from 7% in France (14) to 26% in Germany (2).

Genetic determinants of resistance in clostridia

Macrolides

In *C. perfringens*, MLS$_B$ resistance is associated with *erm*(B) or more frequently *erm*(Q) genes (8) which methylate an adenine of the ribosomal RNA. In *C. difficile*, resistance is encoded by the *erm*(B) resistance determinant located on the non-conjugative but mobilizable transposon Tn*5398* (18).

Chloramphenicol

The *cat* resistance genes encoding a chloramphenicol acetyltransferase have been characterized in *C. perfringens* (*catP*) and *C. difficile* (*catD*) (31). They are located on mobilizable non-conjugative transposons (Tn*4451* and Tn*4452* in *C. perfringens*, Tn*4453* in *C. difficile*) which share a close structural and functional relationship (31). In *C. perfringens*, Tn*4451* also confers resistance to tetracycline.

Tetracyclines

In *C. perfringens* the *tet*(P) determinant, located on a conjugative plasmid, consists of two genes, *tetA*(P) and *tetB*(P) (27):
- *tetA*(P) encodes a transmembrane protein which actively exports tetracycline outside the cell;
- *tetB*(P) directs the synthesis of a protein with significant homology to Tet(M), which confers

tetracycline resistance through ribosomal protection.

However, other genetic organizations have been described, involving in particular the *tet*(M) gene which is also found on conjugative transposons of *C. difficile* (Tn*5397*) and *Enterococcus faecalis* (Tn*916*) (42, 48).

NON-SPORE-FORMING GRAM-POSITIVE BACILLI

An analysis of this very heterogeneous group of anaerobic bacteria on the basis of morphological features distinguishes:
- diphtheromorphic bacilli, which sometimes form pseudo-branches, such as the genera *Propionibacterium*, *Actinomyces*, *Bifidobacterium*;
- regular, more or less elongated bacilli: *Eubacterium* and related genera.

This distinction usually corresponds to the practical orientation of the bacteriological identification, even though it only partially agrees with the phylogenetic classification. The antibiotic susceptibilities of these different genera, which generally do not take into account the recent taxonomic changes (genera *Eggerthella*, *Slackia*, *Collinsella*, etc.), are shown in Table 4.

Propionibacterium

Intrinsic metronidazole resistance

Intrinsic metronidazole resistance in *Propionibacterium* is due to an absence of pyruvate:ferredoxin oxidoreductase activity, thus preventing the reduction of metronidazole to a form which is toxic to DNA (37). The *nimA* gene encoding a nitroreductase which produces nontoxic aminoimidazole intermediates has been detected in some strains (30).

β-lactams

It is generally established that bacteria from the genus *Propionibacterium* are highly susceptible to penicillins (38). Susceptibility to cefotaxime is also common and bactericidal synergy is observed when combined with vancomycin (33).

Macrolides

Clindamycin resistance has been detected in 15-20% of *P. acnes* isolates in Europe (38), although no resistant strains were found in a study of central nervous system isolates (33).

Erythromycin resistant strains of *Propionibacterium* spp. can be divided into four phenotypic classes (43): class I, constitutive MLS resistance; class II, inducible MLS resistance; class III low-level erythromycin resistance (susceptible to 16-carbon macrolides); class IV, high-level resistance to 14, 15 and 16 carbon macrolides, low-level lincosamide resistance.

Strains from groups I, III and IV respectively harbor the point mutations $A_{2058}G$, $G_{2057}A$ and $A_{2059}G$ in 23S rRNA. Group II strains possess the *ermX* gene (located on the non-conjugative transposon Tn*5432*) which methylates the 23S rRNA (43).

Tetracyclines

The susceptibility of *P. acnes* to tetracyclines explains the widespread use of these agents in the treatment of acne vulgaris. In a study of isolates from Europe, North America, Japan and Australia, the rate of resistance (due to a $G_{1058}C$ mutation in the 16S rRNA) was 52% (44) as compared to 2.6% in European strains isolated in 2005 (38).

Fluoroquinolones

The activity of the fluoroquinolones against *P. acnes* is noteworthy because these agents diffuse efficiently, enabling the treatment of bone and joint infections. In one study, isolates were found to be intermediate to ofloxacin (MIC 0.25-2 µg/ml, 62.5% susceptible strains) but all susceptible to ciprofloxacin (MIC 0.25-1 µg/ml) (33). Moxifloxacin has excellent activity (MIC 0.125-0.25 µg/ml, MIC_{90} 0.25 µg/ml) (25).

Actinomyces

β-lactams

Bacteria from the genus *Actinomyces* are usually susceptible to penicillins and imipenem (20). Cephamycin susceptibility is variable, with MICs ranging from ≤ 0.008 to 32 µg/ml for cefoxitin and 0.015 to > 128 µg/ml for cefotetan. Resistance to third generation cephalosporins has been described in some isolates (54).

Metronidazole

Actinomyces are considered resistant to metronidazole, although a few susceptible strains have been reported (21, 54). As in *Propionibacterium*, resistance is due to an absence of pyruvate:ferredoxin oxidoreductase activity, as demonstrated in *A. israelii* (37).

Table 4. Activity (µg/ml) of β-lactams, erythromycin, clindamycin, tetracycline, and metronidazole against non-spore-forming Gram-positive bacilli

Species	Antibiotic	MIC	MIC$_{50}$	MIC$_{90}$	Reference
Propionibacterium spp.	Ampicillin	< 0.03 - 0.25	0.125	0.25	10
	Erythromycin	< 0.064 - > 128	0.25	0.50	38
	Clindamycin	< 0.03 - 0.5	< 0.03	< 0.03	10
		< 0.064 - 64	< 0.064	0.25	38
	Tetracycline	< 0.064 - 32	0.5	1	38
	Metronidazole	64 - >128	> 128	> 128	10
Actinomyces spp.	Ampicillin	< 0.03 - 0.5	0.06	0.25	10
	Cefoxitin	< 0.008 - 32	0.25	16	54
	Ceftriaxone	< 0.008 - >128	0.12	4	54
	Clindamycin	< 0.03 - 0.5	0.06	0.25	10
	Metronidazole	< 0.03 - >128	32	> 128	10
Bifidobacterium spp.	Ampicillin	< 0.03 - 1	0.125	0.5	10
	Cefoxitin	0.25 - 64	4	16	36
	Clindamycin	< 0.03 - 0.25	< 0.03	< 0.03	10
	Metronidazole	4 - >128	8	16	10
Eubacterium spp.	Ampicillin	< 0.03 - 1	0.125	0.25	10
	Clindamycin	< 0.03	≤ 0.03	0.5	10
	Metronidazole	< 0.03 - >128	0.25	4	10

Breakpoints : ampicillin 0.5-2 µg/ml (CLSI, 2007) or 4-16 µg/ml (EUCAST, 2006); clindamycin 2-8 µg/ml (CLSI, 2007) or 4-8 µg/ml (EUCAST, 2006); metronidazole 8-32 µg/ml (CLSI, 2007) or 4-8 µg/ml (EUCAST, 2006).

Fluoroquinolones

Ciprofloxacin resistance is common in *Actinomyces* spp., particularly in *A. israelii* (MIC 0.19- > 32 µg/ml, MIC$_{90}$ > 32 µg/ml) (45). Moxifloxacin appears to be more active, although strains with intermediate susceptibility have been described (MIC 0.125-4 µg/ml) (23, 25).

Bifidobacterium

The few available data for *Bifidobacterium* indicate susceptibility to penicillins and cefoxitin but a 26% resistance rate for cefotetan (36). Susceptibility to clindamycin is constant. Metronidazole resistance has been detected in many strains (10, 36).

Eubacterium

β-lactams are the most active agents although a cefotaxime-resistant strain has been described (34). On the other hand, metronidazole susceptibility is variable (MIC 0.125-16 µg/ml; MIC$_{50}$ 0.5 µg/ml; MIC$_{90}$ 1 µg/ml) (16).

Mobiluncus

These motile, curved rods stain Gram-negative or Gram-variable but have a Gram-positive cell wall. Most studies of antimicrobial susceptibility concern strains of *Mobiluncus* spp. which are always reported to be resistant to metronidazole. However, resistance is species-dependent: it has been detected in all *M. curtisii* but only half of *M. mulieris* isolates. *Mobiluncus* spp. are also intrinsically susceptible to ampicillin, cefotaxime, and erythromycin (47).

NEW ANTIBIOTICS

Carbapenems

Carbapenems generally possess significant activity against Gram-positive anaerobes, apart from the genus *Clostridium* where their efficacy is inconstant (Table 5).

In comparative studies, imipenem and ertapenem exhibited similar activity. *Peptostreptococcus*, *Actinomyces*, and *Propionibacterium* are highly susceptible to ertapenem. Among *Clostridium*, *C. difficile*, and *C. innocuum* are the least susceptible species (52).

Faropenem has a similar spectrum of activity (53). *C. difficile* may be cross-resistant to imipenem, ertapenem, and faropenem whereas this resistance is dissociated in *C. innocuum* (faropenem MIC: 8 µg/ml; imipenem MIC: 1-2 µg/ml) as well as in two *P. anaerobius* isolates (faropenem MIC: 8-16 µg/ml; imipenem MIC: 1-2 µg/ml) (53).

Table 5. Activity (μg/ml) of carbapenems against Gram-positive anaerobes

Species	Antibiotic	MIC	MIC$_{50}$	MIC$_{90}$	Reference
C. perfringens	Imipenem	0.06 - 0.50	0.12	0.25	53
	Faropenem	0.12 - 1	0.5	0.5	53
	Doripenem	0.06 - 0.125	0.06	0.125	46
C. difficile	Imipenem	1 - 8	4	4	34
		4 - 8	4	8	19
	Ertapenem	4 - 8	4	8	19
	Faropenem	0.5 - 32	8	16	53
	Doripenem	1 - 2	-	-	46
		0.5 - 4	1	2	24
Peptostreptococcus spp.	Imipenem	< 0.03 - 8	< 0.03	0.25	7
		< 0.015 - 0.5	0.03	0.06	19
	Ertapenem	< 0.015 - 1	0.06	0.125	19
P. asaccharolyticus	Imipenem	0.12 - 0.12	0.12	0.12	53
	Faropenem	0.12 - 2	0.12	1	53
Gram-positive cocci	Doripenem	0.06 - 2	0.06	0.5	46
Actinomyces spp.	Imipenem	< 0.015 - 0.5	0.06	0.5	19
	Ertapenem	0.06 - 2	0.125	1	19
Non-spore-forming Gram-positive bacilli	Imipenem	< 0.03 - 1	0.06	0.5	7
	Faropenem	0.12 - 2	0.12	0.5	53

Breakpoint : imipenem 4-16 μg/ml (CLSI, 2007) or 2-16 μg/ml (EUCAST, 2006)

Table 6. Activity (μg/ml) of linezolid against Gram-positive anaerobes

Species	MIC	MIC$_{50}$	MIC$_{90}$	Reference
Clostridium spp.	0.5 - 4	1	4	21
	0.5 - 2	1	1	7
C. perfringens	1 - 2	2	2	21
	2 - 4	2	4	46
C. difficile	1 - 16	2	8	21
	1 - 2	-	-	46
Peptostreptococcus spp.	0.5 - 2	0.5	2	21
	0.25 - 2	0.5	2	7
Gram-positive cocci	1.25 - 4	1	2	46
Non-spore-forming Gram-positive bacilli	0.25 - 4	1	2	7
Propionibacterium spp.	0.25 - 1	0.5	1	21
	0.25 - 0.5	0.5	0.5	7
	0.5 - 1	0.5	0.5	46
Actinomyces spp.	0.25 - 1	0.5	1	21
Eubacterium spp.	0.25 - 8	2	4	21

Doripenem is active against Gram-positive anaerobes, particularly C. difficile (MIC 1-2 μg/ml), C. perfringens (0.06-125 μg/ml), F. magna (0.06-125 μg/ml), Gram-positive cocci (0.05-2 μg/ml), and P. acnes (0.06 μg/ml) (46).

Oxazolidinones

Linezolid has been evaluated in several studies (7, 20, 21, 25, 46). With reference to EUCAST breakpoints of ≤2 and >4 μg/m, Peptostreptococcus and Propionibacterium are always susceptible whereas a few resistant strains of Eubacterium have been reported (Table 6). Among Clostridium, some C. difficile strains may be resistant (with possible associated-resistance between linezolid, clindamycin and moxifloxacin) (1).

Glycylcyclines

Tigecycline is very active against Gram-positive cocci (MIC ≤ 0.015-0.25 μg/ml) and Clostridium, particularly C. difficile (MIC ≤ 0.06 μg/ml) (22). Bacteria from the genus Actinomyces, including doxycycline-resistant strains, are susceptible to tigecycline (MIC ≤ 1 µg/ml) (22).

CONCLUSION

In conclusion, the importance of antimicrobial susceptibility surveillance in Gram-positive anaerobes should be emphasized, taking taxonomic revisions into account. Overall, these microorganisms continue to show susceptibility to penicillins. On the other hand, clindamycin activity varies considerably between species and in different isolates of a same species. Among the quinolones, moxifloxacin is of potential interest although resistant strains have already been described.

The molecular mechanisms underlying antibiotic resistance and their genetic determinants have not been widely studied, with the exception of agents like chloramphenicol or tetracyclines which have fallen out of use today. Consequently, it is virtually impossible to reason in terms of resistance phenotypes. This should serve as an impetus for further research into this underexplored aspect of the antibiogram.

REFERENCES

(1) **Ackermann, G., A. Degner, S.H. Cohen, J. Silva Jr, and A.C. Rodloff**. 2003. Prevalence and association of macrolide-lincosamide-streptogramin B (MLS$_B$) resistance with resistance to moxifloxacin in *Clostridium difficile*. J. Antimicrob. Chemother. **51**:599-603.

(2) **Ackermann, G., Y.J. Tang, R. Kueper, P. Heisig, A.C. Rodloff, J. Silva Jr, and S.H. Cohen**. 2001. Resistance to moxifloxacin in toxigenic *Clostridium difficile* isolates is associated with mutations in *gyrA*. Antimicrob. Agents Chemother. **45**:2348-2253.

(3) **Alexander, C.J., D.M. Citron, J.S. Brazier, and E.J.C. Goldstein**. 1995. Identification and antimicrobial resistance patterns of clinical isolates of *Clostridium clostridioforme*, *Clostridium innocuum*, and *Clostridium ramosum* compared with those of clinical isolates of *Clostridium perfringens*. J. Clin. Microbiol. **33**:3209-3215.

(4) **Appelbaum, P.C., S.K. Spangler, G.A. Pankuch, A. Philippon, M.R. Jacobs, R. Shiman, E.J.C. Goldstein, and D.M. Citron**. 1994. Characterization of a beta-lactamase from *Clostridium clostridioforme*. J. Antimicrob. Chemother. **33**:33-40.

(5) **Barbut, F., D. Decre, B. Burghoffer, D. Lesage, F. Delisle, V. Lalande, M. Delmee, V. Avesani, N. Sano, C. Coudert, and J.C. Petit**. 1999. Antimicrobial susceptibilities and serogroups of clinical strains of *Clostridium difficile* isolated in France in 1991 and 1997. Antimicrob. Agents Chemother. **43**:2607-2611.

(6) **Barbut F., P. Mastrantonio, M. Delmée, J. Brazier, E. Kuijper, and I. Poxton, for the European study group on *Clostridium difficile* (ESGCD)**. 2007. Prospective study of *Clostridium difficile*-associated infections in Europe with phenotypic and genotypic characterisation of the isolates. Clin. Microbiol. Infect. **13**:1048-1057.

(7) **Behra-Miellet, J., L. Calvet, and L. Dubreuil**. 2003. Activity of linezolid against anaerobic bacteria. Int. J. Antimicrob. Agents. **22**:28-34.

(8) **Berryman, D.I., M. Lyristis, and J.I. Rood**. 1994. Cloning and sequence analysis of *ermQ*, the predominant macrolide-lincosamide-streptogramin B resistance gene in *Clostridium perfringens*. Antimicrob. Agents Chemother. **38**:1041-1046.

(9) **Brazier, J.S., V. Hall, T.E. Morris, M. Gal, and B.I. Duerden**. 2003. Antibiotic susceptibilities of Gram-positive anaerobic cocci: results of a sentinel study in England and Wales. J. Antimicriobial. Chemother. **52**:224-228.

(10) **Citron, D.M., C.V. Merriam, K.L. Tyrrell, Y.A. Warren, H. Fernandez, and E.J.C. Goldstein**. 2003. In vitro activities of ramoplanin, teicoplanin, vancomycin, linezolid, bacitracin, and four other antimicrobials against intestinal anaerobic bacteria. Antimicrob. Agents Chemother. **47**:2334-2338.

(11) **Clinical and Laboratory Standards Institute (CLSI)**. Methods for antimicrobial susceptibility testing of anaerobic bacteria; approved standards-seventh edition. CLSI document M11-A7, Wayne (PA), 2007.

(12) **Credito K.L., and P.C. Appelbaum**. Activity of OPT80, a novel macrocycle, compared with those of eight other agents against selected anaerobic species. 2004. Antimicrob. Agents Chemother. **48**:4430-4434.

(13) **David, V., B. Bozdogan, J.L. Mainardi, R. Legrand, L. Gutmann, and R. Leclercq**. 2004. Mechanism of intrinsic resistance to vancomycin in *Clostridium innocuum* NCIB 10674. J. Bacteriol. **186**:3415-3422.

(14) **Dridi, L., J. Tankovic, B. Burghoffer, F. Barbut, and J.C. Petit**. 2002. *gyrA* and *gyrB* mutations are implicated in cross-resistance to ciprofloxacin and moxifloxacin in *Clostridium difficile*. Antimicrob. Agents Chemother. **46**:3418-3421.

(15) **Dubreuil, L., J. Behra-Miellet, C. Neut, and L. Calvet**. 2003. In vitro activity of gatifloxacin, a new fluoroquinolone, against 204 anaerobes compared to seven other compounds. Clin. Microbiol. Infect. **9**:1133-1138.

(16) **Dubreuil L., I. Houcke, Y. Mouton, and J.F. Rossignol**. 1996. In vitro evaluation of activities of nitazoxanide and tizoxanide against anaerobes and aerobic organisms. Antimicrob. Agents Chemother. **40**:2266-2270.

(17) **European Committee on Antimicrobial Susceptibility Testing. (EUCAST)**. http://www.srga.org/eucastwt/MICTAB/index.html.

(18) **Farrow, K.A., D. Lyras, and J.I. Rood**. 2001. Genomic analysis of the erythromycin resistance element Tn*5398* from *Clostridium difficile*. Microbiology **147**:2717-2728.

(19) **Goldstein, E.J.C., D.M. Citron, C.V. Merriam, Y.A. Warren, K.L. Tyrrell, and H.T. Fernandez**. 2002. Comparative in vitro activities of ertapenem (MK-0826) against 469 less frequently identified

anaerobes isolated from human infections. Antimicrob. Agents Chemother. **46**:1136-1140.

(20) **Goldstein, E.J.C., D.M. Citron, C.V. Merriam, Y.A. Warren, K.L. Tyrrell, and H.T. Fernandez.** 2003. In vitro activities of daptomycin, vancomycin, quinupristin-dalfopristin, linezolid, and five other antimicrobials against gram-positive anaerobic and 31 *Corynebacterium* clinical isolates. Antimicrob. Agents Chemother. **47**:337-341.

(21) **Goldstein, E.J.C., D.M. Citron, C.V. Merriam, Y.A. Warren, K.L. Tyrrell, and H.T. Fernandez.** 2003. In vitro activities of dalbavancin and nine comparator agents against anaerobic gram-positive species and corynebacteria. Antimicrob. Agents Chemother. **47**:1968-1971.

(22) **Goldstein, E.J.C., D.M. Citron, C.V. Merriam, Y.A. Warren, K.L. Tyrrell, and H.T. Fernandez.** 2006. Comparative in vitro susceptibilities of 396 unusual anaerobic strains to tigecycline and eight other antimicrobial agents. Antimicrob. Agents Chemother. **50**:3507-3513.

(23) **Goldstein, E.J.C., D.M. Citron, Y.A. Warren, K.L. Tyrrell, C.V. Merriam, and H.T. Fernandez.** 2006. In vitro activity of moxifloxacin against 923 clinical anaerobes isolated from human intra-abdominal infections. Antimicrob. Agents Chemother. **50**:148-155.

(24) **Hecht D.W., M.A. Galang, S.P. Sambol, J.R. Osmolski, S. Johnson, and D.L. Gerding.** 2007. In vitro activities of 15 antimicrobial agents against 110 toxigenic *Clostridium difficile* clinical isolates collected from 1983 to 2004. Antimicrob. Agents Chemother. **51**:2716-2719.

(25) **Hecht, D.W., and J.R. Osmolski.** 2003. Activities of garenoxacin (BMS-284756) and other agents against anaerobic clinical isolates. Antimicrob. Agents Chemother. **47**:910-916.

(26) **Jang, S.S., L.M. Hansen, J.E. Breher, D.A. Riley, K.G. Magdesian, J.E. Madigan, Y.J. Tang, J. Silva Jr, and D.C. Hirsh.** 1997. Antimicrobial susceptibilities of equine isolates of *Clostridium difficile* and molecular characterization of metronidazole-resistant strains. Clin. Infect. Dis. **25**:S266-S267.

(27) **Johanesen, P.A., D. Lyras, T.L. Bannam, and J.I. Rood.** 2001. Transcriptional analysis of the *tet*(P) operon from *Clostridium perfringens*. J. Bacteriol. **183**:7110-7119.

(28) **Koeth, L.M., C.E. Good, P.C. Appelbaum, E.J.C. Goldstein, A.C. Rodloff, M. Claros, and L.J. Dubreuil.** 2004. Surveillance of susceptibility patterns in 1297 European and US anaerobic and capnophilic isolates to co-amoxiclav and five other antimicrobial agents. J. Antimicrob. Chemother. **53**:1039-1044.

(29) **Liebetrau, A., A.C. Rodloff, J. Behra-Miellet, and L. Dubreuil.** 2003. In vitro activities of a new desfluoro(6) quinolone, garenoxacin, against clinical anaerobic bacteria. Antimicrob. Agents Chemother. **47**:3667-3671.

(30) **Lubbe, M.M., K. Stanley, and L.J. Chalkley.** 1999. Prevalence of *nim* genes in anaerobic/facultative anaerobic bacteria isolated in South Africa. FEMS Microbiol. Lett. **172**:79-83.

(31) **Lyras, D., C. Storie, A.S. Huggins, P.K. Crellin, T.L. Bannam, and J.I. Rood.** 1998. Chloramphenicol resistance in *Clostridium difficile* is encoded on Tn*4453* transposons that are closely related to Tn*4451* from *Clostridium perfringens*. Antimicrob. Agents Chemother. **42**:1563-1567.

(32) **Magot, M.** 1981. Some properties of the *Clostridium butyricum* group beta-lactamase. J. Gen. Microbiol. **127**:113-119.

(33) **Mory, F., S. Fougnot, C. Rabaud, H. Schuhmacher, and A. Lozniewski.** 2005. In vitro activities of cefotaxime, vancomycin, quinupristin/dalfopristin, linezolid and other antibiotics alone and in combination against *Propionibacterium acnes* isolates from central nervous system infections. J. Antimicrob. Chemother. **55**:265-268.

(34) **Mory, F., A. Lozniewski, S. Bland, A. Sedallian, G. Grollier, F. Girard-Pipau, M.F. Paris, and L. Dubreuil.** 1998. Survey of anaerobic susceptibility patterns: a French multicentre study. Int. J. Antimicrob. Agents **10**:229-236.

(35) **Mory, F., A. Lozniewski, V. David, J.P. Carlier, L. Dubreuil, and R. Leclercq.** 1998. Low-level vancomycin resistance in *Clostridium innocuum*. J. Clin. Microbiol. **36**:1767-1768.

(36) **Moubareck, C., F. Gavini, L. Vaugien, M.J. Butel, and F. Doucet-Populaire.** 2005. Antimicrobial susceptibility of bifidobacteria. J. Antimicrob. Chemother. **55**:38-44.

(37) **Narikawa, S.** 1986. Distribution of metronidazole susceptibility factors in obligate anaerobes. J. Antimicrob. Chemother. **18**:565-574.

(38) **Oprica C., C.E. Nord.** 2005. European surveillance study on the antibiotic susceptibility of *Propionibacterium acnes*. Clin. Microbiol. Infect. **11**:204-213.

(39) **Pelaez, T., L. Alcala, R. Alonso, M. Rodriguez-Creixems, J.M. Garcia-Lechuz, and E. Bouza.** 2002. Reassessment of *Clostridium difficile* susceptibility to metronidazole and vancomycin. Antimicrob. Agents Chemother. **46**:1647-1650.

(40) **Peláez T, E. Cercenado, L. Alcalá, M. Marín, A. Martín-López, J. Martínez-Alarcón, P. Catalán, M. Sánchez-Somolinos, and E. Bouza.** 2008. Metronidazole resistance in *Clostridium difficile* is heterogeneous. J. Clin. Microbiol. **46**:3026-3032.

(41) **Reig, M., J. Galan, F. Baquero, and J.C. Perez-Diaz.** 2001. Macrolide resistance in *Peptostreptococcus* spp. mediated by *ermTR*: possible source of macrolide-lincosamide-streptogramin B resistance in *Streptococcus pyogenes*. Antimicrob. Agents Chemother. **45**:630-632.

(42) **Roberts, A.P., P.A. Johanesen, D. Lyras, P. Mullany, and J.I. Rood.** 2001. Comparison of Tn*5397* from *Clostridium difficile*, Tn*916* from *Enterococcus faecalis* and the CW459*tet*(M) element from *Clostridium perfringens* shows that they have similar conjugation regions but different insertion and excision modules. Microbiology **147**:1243-1251.

(43) **Ross, J.I., E.A. Eady, E. Carnegie, and J.H. Cove.** 2002. Detection of transposon Tn*5432*-mediated macrolide-lincosamide-streptogramin B (MLS$_B$) resistance in cutaneous propionibacteria from six European cities. J. Antimicrob. Chemother. **49**:165-168.

(44) **Ross, J.I., A.M. Snelling, E.A. Eady, J.H. Cove, W.J. Cunliffe, J.J. Leyden, P. Collignon, B. Dreno, A. Reynaud, J. Fluhr, and S. Oshima.** 2001.

Phenotypic and genotypic characterization of antibiotic-resistant *Propionibacterium acnes* isolated from acne patients attending dermatology clinics in Europe, the U.S.A., Japan and Australia. Br. J. Dermatol. **144**:339-346.

(45) **Smith, A.J., V. Hall, B. Thakker, and C.G. Gemmell.** 2005. Antimicrobial susceptibility testing of *Actinomyces* species with 12 antimicrobial agents. J. Antimicrob. Chemother. **56**:407-409.

(46) **Snydman D.R., N.V. Jacobus, and L.A. McDermott.** 2008. In vitro activities of doripenem, a new broad-spectrum carbapenem, against recently collected clinical anaerobic isolates, with emphasis on the *Bacteroides fragilis* group. Antimicrob. Agents Chemother. **52**:4492-4496.

(47) **Spiegel, C.A.** 1987. Susceptibility of *Mobiluncus* species to 23 antimicrobial agents and 15 other compounds. Antimicrob. Agents Chemother. **31**:249-252.

(48) **Spigaglia P., F. Barbanti, and P. Mastrantonio.** 2006. New variants of the *tet*(M) gene in *Clostridium difficile* clinical isolates harbouring Tn*916*-like elements. J. Antimicrob. Chemother. **57**:1205-1209.

(49) **Spigaglia P, F. Barbanti, P. Mastrantonio, J.S. Brazier, F. Barbut F, M. Delmée, E. Kuijper, and I.R. Poxton, for the European study group on *Clostridium difficile* (ESGCD).** 2008. Fluoroquinolone resistance in *Clostridium difficile* isolates from a prospective study of *C. difficile* infections in Europe. J Med Microbiol. **57**: 784-789.

(50) **Steyaert, S., R. Peleman, M. Vaneechoutte, T. De Baere, G. Claeys, and G. Verschraegen.** 1999. Septicemia in neutropenic patients infected with *Clostridium tertium* resistant to cefepime and other expanded-spectrum cephalosporins. J. Clin. Microbiol. **37**:3778-3779.

(51) **Theron, M.M., M.N. Janse Van Rensburg, and L.J. Chalkley.** 2004. Nitroimidazole resistance genes (*nimB*) in anaerobic Gram-positive cocci (previously *Peptostreptococcus* spp.). J. Antimicrob. Chemother. **54**:240-242.

(52) **Wexler, H.M.** 2004. In vitro activity of ertapenem: review of recent studies. J. Antimicrob. Chemother. **53**: 11-21.

(53) **Wexler, H.M., D. Molitoris, S. St John, A. Vu, E.K. Read, and S.M. Finegold.** 2002. In vitro activities of faropenem against 579 strains of anaerobic bacteria. Antimicrob. Agents Chemother. **46**:3669-3675.

(54) **Wootton, M., K.E. Bowker, H.A. Holt, and A.P. MacGowan.** 2002. BAL 9141, a new broad-spectrum pyrrolidinone cephalosporin: activity against clinically significant anaerobes in comparison with 10 other antimicrobials. J. Antimicrob. Chemother. **49**:535-539.

Chapter 48. GRAM-NEGATIVE ANAEROBES

Luc DUBREUIL

INTRODUCTION

Considering the diversity of the Gram-negative anaerobes (Table 1), this chapter will successively address the main groups of species according to antimicrobial susceptibility patterns. Likewise, it is not possible to exhaustively describe the many resistance mechanisms found in *B. fragilis*. Methodology is discussed in Chapter 46 "Methods for antimicrobiol susceptibility testing of anaerobic bacteria".

INTRINSIC RESISTANCE IN GRAM-NEGATIVE BACILLI

Anaerobic Gram-negative bacilli are resistant to aminoglycosides, glycopeptides (except *Porphyromonas*), fosfomycin (except *Fusobacterium*), trimethoprim, fusidic acid, older quinolones like nalidixic acid, and, for most species, ofloxacin and ciprofloxacin. Selective medium for the *Bacteroides fragilis* group contains a combination of vancomycin 7.5 µg/ml and kanamycin 75 µg/ml. *Bacteroides* Bile Esculine medium (BBE), widely used in the US, contains gentamicin 40 µg/ml. These intrinsic resistances are a valuable aid in the presumptive identification of Gram-negative anaerobes (Table 2).

Several points should nonetheless be emphasized. Gentamicin MICs exceed 32 µg/ml for the majority of anaerobes with the exception of *Bacteroides ureolyticus* (MIC 2-8 µg/ml). The MIC_{50} and MIC_{90} of amikacin range from 8-32 µg/ml for *B. ureolyticus*. With regard to aztreonam, MICs are generally above 128 µg/ml although

Table 1. Main anaerobic species isolated in humans

Gram-negative bacilli:

Bacteroides fragilis group: *B. caccae, B. distasonis, B. dorei, B. eggerthii, B. finegoldii, B. fragilis, B. goldsteinii, B. helcogenes, B. intestinalis, B. johnsonii, B. massiliensis, B. merdae, B. nordii, B. ovatus, B. plebeius, B. salyersae, B. stercoris, B. thetaiotaomicron, B. uniformis, B. vulgatus*.

Prevotella: *P. corporis, P. denticola, P. intermedia, P. loescheii, P. melaninogenica, P. nigrescens, P. pallens, P. tannaerae,* (**pigmented**), *P. amnii, P. baroniae, P. bergensis, P. bivia, P. buccae, P. buccalis, P. copri, P. disiens P. heparinolytica, P. maculosa, P. marshii, P. multisaccharivorax, P. nanceiensis, P. oralis, P. oris, P. oulora, P. pleuritidis, P. salivae, P. shahii, P. stercorea, P. timonensis, P. veroralis, P. zoogleoformans* (**non pigmented**).

Porphyromonas: *P. assacharolytica, P. appendicitis, P. cangingivalis, P. canoris, P. cansulci, P. catoniae, P. circumdentaria, P. crevioricanis, P. endodontalis, P. gingivalis, P. gingivicanis, P. gulae, P. salivosa, P. somaerae, P. unenonis*

Other Bacteroides: *B. capillosus, B. coagulans, B. galacturonicus, B. pectinophilus, B. tectus*; **agar-corroding Bacteroides**: *B. ureolyticus*;

Former Bacteroides newly reclassified into different genera: *Alistipes finegoldii, A. onderdonkii, A. putredinis A. shahii. Anaerorhabdus furcosus, Dialister pneumosintes, Dialister invisus, Megamonas hypermegas, Mitsuokella multiacida, Mitsuokella dentalis, Tanerella forsythia, Tisierella praeacuta, O. splanchnicus*

Fusobacterium and related organisms: *F. gonidiaformans, F. mortiferum, F. necrogenes, F. necrophorum, F. nucleatum* (three sub-species: *F. nucleatum, F. polymorphum, F. vincentii*), *F. periodonticum, F. pseudonecrophorum, F. rusii, F. sulci, F. ulcerans, F. varium. Filifactor alocis, Faecalibacter prausnitzii, Subdoligranulum variabile*

Other bacilli: *Anaerobiospirillum succiniciproducens, Bilophila wadsworthia, Butyrivibrio crossotus, B. fibrosolvens, Campylobacter concisus, Centipeda periodontii, Desulfomonas pigra, Desulfovibrio piger, D. farfieldensis, D. desulfiricans, D.vulgaris, Leptotrichia amnionii, L. buccalis, L. goodfellowii, L. hofstadii, L. shahii, L. trevisani, L. wadei, Selenomonas artemidis, S. dianae, S. flueggei, S. infelix, S. noxia, S. sputigena, Sneathia sanguinegens*.

Other Gram-negative bacilli: *Leptotrichia buccalis.*

values ranging from 0.25-4 µg/ml have been reported for *B. fragilis*, *Prevotella* and *Fusobacterium* isolates. *B. ureolyticus* is susceptible to aztreonam (modal MIC 0.5 µg/ml).

Bacteroides fragilis group

Wild-type phenotype

Virtually all strains (> 97%) produce a chromosomal β-lactamase encoded by the *cepA* gene (35). This is an extended spectrum β-lactamase which hydrolyzes first, second, third, and fourth generation cephalosporins but is less active on penicillins. Cefamycins (cefoxitin and cefotetan) and latamoxef are not substrates. The enzyme has an isoelectric point of 4.7-4.8 and is strongly inhibited by clavulanic acid, sulbactam, tazobactam, and cloxacillin. In practice, the *Bacteroides fragilis* group is resistant to aminopenicillins, first generation cephalosporins, cefamandole, cefuroxime, cefixime, cefpodoxime, and cefepime. Due to low-level expression of this β-lactamase, some strains may appear falsely susceptible on the antibiogram, in which case they should be reported as resistant. Third generation cephalosporins exhibit low and variable activity (Table 3). Cefotaxime and ceftizoxime are more active than ceftazidime, which basically has no activity. None of these drugs should be considered active. We use the following rule for the *Bacteroides fragilis* group: any S result for third generation cephalosporins should be interpreted as I.

The *Bacteroides fragilis* group is susceptible to ticarcillin and piperacillin, to the combinations amoxicillin + clavulanic acid, ticarcillin + clavulanic acid and piperacillin + tazobactam, as well as to cefoxitin, cefotetan, and carbapenems (imipenem, faropenem, ertapenem, and meropenem). Cefoxitin MICs range from 4-64 µg/ml but generally lie within the range of 8-32 µg/ml. Thus, the *Bacteroides fragilis* group shows intermediate susceptibility to cefoxitin. It is unnecessary to test cefamycins (including cefotetan) since the response is always unpredictable except for MIC determination by the reference method.

The *Bacteroides fragilis* group is susceptible to erythromycin, clindamycin, tetracycline, tigecycline, linezolid, rifampin, chloramphenicol, 5-nitroimidazoles (metronidazole, tinidazole, ornidazole, and secnidazole), and some fluoroquinolones (gatifloxacin and moxifloxacin) (Table 4).

By the disk-diffusion technique, some *B. fragilis* strains may appear falsely susceptible to vancomycin, with MICs of 4-8 µg/ml for some "less resistant" strains which is a result of the imprecision of the diffusion method. The strain should be reported as resistant if indeed it belongs to the *Bacteroides fragilis* group.

Acquired resistance

Antimicrobial resistance rates vary in different countries and different hospitals. Clindamycin and cefotetan resistance rates have risen appreciably (3, 20). Cefotetan has lost much of its activity against species of the *fragilis* group other than *B. fragilis*. With resistance rates exceeding 30%, these two drugs can no longer be used for empirical therapy of mixed infections.

Table 2. Aid to identification of Gram-negative bacilli according to intrinsic resistance and growth in bile

Microorganism	Susceptibility or resistance to [a]:			Growth in contact with bile disk
	Vancomycin (5 µg)	Kanamycin (1 mg)	Colistin (10 µg)	
B. fragilis (group)	R[b]	R	R	+++F
Prevotella spp.	R	S	V	R
B. ureolyticus	R	S	S	R
Fusobacterium spp.	R	S	S	V
Bilophila wadsworthia	R	S	S	+++F
Selenomonas, Desulfovibrio	R	S	R	R
Porphyromonas spp.	S	R	R	R
Veillonella	R	S	S	R

[a] bioMérieux anaerodisks.

[b] F, favored; R, Resistant; S, Susceptible; V, Variable. *F. mortiferum* and *F. varium* are resistant to rifampin (15 µg disks). *Fusobacterium* grows in contact with brilliant green disks. *Fusobacterium* is nitrate reductase -. *Bilophila* and *B. ureolyticus* are nitrate reductase +.

Table 3. Comparative activity (MIC in µg/ml) of antibiotics against the main *Bacteroides fragilis* group species

Antibiotic	Data from the literature									Personal data			
	B. fragilis		*B. thetaiotaomicron*		*B. distasonis*		*B. fragilis* group		*B. fragilis*		*B. fragilis* group	
	MIC$_{50}$	MIC$_{90}$	MIC$_{50}$	MIC$_{90}$	MIC$_{50}$	MIC$_{90}$	MIC$_{50}$	MIC$_{90}$	MIC$_{50}$	MIC$_{90}$	MIC$_{50}$	MIC$_{90}$
β-lactams												
Amoxicillin	16-32	>32	64	>64	16-32	>32	8->128	64->128	16-32	64-128		
Amoxicillin + clavulanic acid	0.5-1	1-4[a]	1	1[a]	0.5-1	1[a]	0.5-2	1-8[a]	0.25	1-2		
Ampicillin	32	>64	32	>64	32	>64	32-128	>128	32	128		
Ampicillin + sulbactam (2:1)	0.25-2	4-8[a]	1-2	8[a]	4-8	16-32[a]	1-2	4-16[a]	0.25-0.5	2-4		
Ticarcillin	32-64	>128	32-64	>128	16-32	>128	32-128	>128	16-32	256		
Ticarcillin + clavulanic acid (2)	0.5-4	1-8[a]	2-4	4-16[a]	4-8	32-128[a]	1-2	4-16[a]	0.25-1	2		
Piperacillin	4-16	64-128	32-64	32->128	8-32	128->128	8-64	>128	8-16	64-128		
Piperacillin + tazobactam (8:1)	4	16[a]	8	16[a]	8	16[a]	2-8	8-32[a]	1-2	8-16		
Cefoxitin	8	16-64	32	64	16-32	64	8-16	32-64	4-16	16-64		
Cefotetan	8	32-128	128	>128	64-128	128->128	8-32	64->128	4-8	64-128		
Cefoperazone	64	>128	64-128	>128	32	>128	64	>64	32-64	>128		
Cefotaxime	4-64	>64	16	64	32	64-128	8-32	64->128	8-32	64-256		
Cefotaxime + sulbactam (8)	0.1	0.5[a]	0.25	2[a]	0.12	0.5[a]	0.5	1[a]	0.25	1		
Ceftizoxime	8-64	64-128	64	128	1-4	32-256	4-32	64->128	4-32	64-128		
Ceftazidime	16->128	>128	64	>128	128	>128	64	>128	64	1 024		
Imipenem	0.06-0.25	0.25-1[a]	0.25	0.5-2[a]	0.25-1	1-4[a]	0.125-0.25	0.5[a]	0.125-0.25	1		
Ertapenem	0.25	1	1	1	1	2	0.25-0.5	1-2	0.5	4		
Meropenem	0.125	0.25-1[a]	0.25	0.5-1[a]	0.25	0.25-0.5	0.12-0.25	0.2-0.5[a]	0.12-0.25	1		
Doripenem	0.25	0.5-1	0.25	0.5	0.5	1	0.25-0.5	1-2	0.5	2		
Other antibiotics												
Clindamycin	0.25-0.5	1-128	0.5-4	2-128	0.5-4	1-8[a]	0.5	4->128	0.25-0.5	8->128		
Metronidazole	0.5-1	1-2[a]	0.5-1	2-4	0.5-1	1-4	0.5-1	0.5-2[a]	0.5	2		
Linezolid							4	4	4	4		
Moxifloxacin	0.25-0.5	2-4	1	4	0.25-1	4	0.5	2-4	0.5	2		
Tigecycline	1-2	4-8	1-2	8	2	8	1-2	8	0.5	2		

[a] A few resistant strains have been described.

Table 4. Antibiotic activity against the *Bacteroides fragilis* group

Antibiotic	MIC₅₀	MIC₉₀	Antibiotic	MIC₅₀	MIC₉₀
β-lactamins					
Azlocillin	8	> 128	Aztreonam	> 128	> 128
Carbenicillin	32 - 64	64 - > 128	Penicillin G	16-32	64 - > 128
Mezlocillin	8 - 32	64 - 128	Cefaclor	> 64	> 64
Cefdinir	8	> 128	Cefalotin	64	> 128
Cefpirome	32	> 128	Cefadroxil	64	> 64
Cefteram	64	> 64	Cefetamet	> 128	> 128
Cefuroxime	32 - 128	> 128	Cefepime	64	> 64
Cefixime	32	> 128	Cefonicid	128	256
Cefpodoxime	128	> 128	Cefotiam	256	> 256
Latamoxef	4 - 8	32 - 128	Flomoxef	0.5 - 4	1 - 16
Clavulanic acid	32	64	Tazobactam	8 - 16	32-64
Sulbactam	16	64			
Macrolides and derivatives					
Azithromycin	2 - 32	> 64	Clarithromycin	1 - 2	< 64
Erythromycin	1 - 16	> 64	Roxithromycin	2 - 16	> 64
Spiramycin	8 - 16	16 - 128	Josamycin	0.5 - 2	> 64
Telithromycin	4	> 64	Pristinamycin	1	4
Clindamycin	0.5	> 128	Quinupristin-dalfopristin	2	2
Quinolones					
Ciprofloxacin	4 - 16	8 - 64	Nalidixic acid	128	> 128
Enoxacin	32	64	Norfloxacin	32 - 64	128
Lomefloxacin	16	32	Pefloxacin	8	32
Ofloxacin	1 - 4	4 - 16	Levofloxacin	2	8
Fleroxacin	32	32	Sparfloxacin	1 - 2	2 - 4
Moxifloxacin	0,5	2	Garenoxacin	0.25	1
Other antibiotics					
Chloramphenicol	4	8	Rifampin	1	1
Ornidazole	0.5	1	Tinidazole	0,5	1
Tetracycline	4 - 16	16 - 32	Secnidazole	1	4
Minocycline	1	4 - 32	Doxycycline	0.5 - 2	4[a]
Linezolid	4	4	Trimethoprim	16	64
Spectinomycin	160	> 160	Trospectomycin	4	16
Gentamicin	> 32		Amikacin	> 16	

β-lactams (table 5)

Intermediate-level β-lactamase hyperproduction

Strains are resistant to ticarcillin, piperacillin and cefotetan.

In most cases these strains are β-lactamase hyperproducers (36) or have decreased permeability (23). The presence of the IS*1124* insertion sequence upstream of the *cepA* gene (36) induces overproduction of the chromosomal β-lactamase, resulting in an amoxicillin MIC > 128 µg/ml and cross-resistance to ticarcillin and piperacillin. Higher inhibitor concentrations are needed to restore amoxicillin activity, e.g., 2-4 µg/ml clavulanic acid (concentrations attainable at therapeutic doses). As sulbactam is a weaker inhibitor, rare strains susceptible to amoxicillin + clavulanic acid but resistant to ampicillin + sulbactam (MIC > 16/8 µg/ml) have been described.

Cefotaxime + sulbactam is active against the majority of strains although resistant strains have been reported. In clinical practice, then, β-lactamase inhibitors should preferably be combined with a penicillin. These strains are cefotetan-resistant, cefoxitin-intermediate or resistant, but susceptible to carbapenems. Cefamycin resistance is not always the result of enzyme production and may instead be due to decreased permeability and/or lower affinity for penicillin G binding proteins. Within the *fragilis* group, *B. thetaiotaomicron* and *B. distasonis* appear less susceptible to cefotetan and cefoxitin. *B. distasonis* is less susceptible than other species to the action of β-lactamase inhibitors (Table 3). Some strains belonging to the *Bacteroides fragilis* group secrete an enzyme which inactivates cefoxitin (*cfxA* gene) but spares imipenem (25), resulting in high-level resistance to ampicillin (MIC > 256 µg/ml) and cefoxitin.

High-level β-lactamase hyperproduction

These strains are imipenem-susceptible but resistant to β-lactam + β-lactamase inhibitor combinations.

In some cases this type of resistance is due to i) alteration of outer membrane proteins which prevent penetration of the inhibitor; ii) hyperproduction of a chromosomal enzyme.

Usually, transcriptional activation of the *cepA* gene by the upstream IS*1124* insertion sequence leads to high-level β-lactam resistance and variable levels of resistance to penicillin + β-lactamase inhibitor combinations. A porin deficiency [particularly the loss of the 45 kDa porin in *B. fragilis* (23) or the 70 kDa porin in *B. thetaiotaomicron* (5)] further increases the MICs of β-lactamase inhibitor combinations. The effect is most pronounced with amoxicillin + clavulanic acid, followed by ticarcillin + clavulanic acid and piperacillin + tazobactam. In a series of *B. fragilis* strains isolated in 2008, 11% were resistant to amoxicillin + clavulanic acid but susceptible to piperacillin + tazobactam (personal data).

There have been very rare reports of β-lactamases with practically no affinity for clavulanic acid, sulbactam or tazobactam (Ki > 850 μM). Strains producing such enzymes are refractory to the combined action of β-lactams and β-lactamase inhibitors.

Imipenem resistance

This is due to the production of an Ambler class B zinc metallo-carbapenemase (30) encoded by the *cfiA* gene (or *ccrA* for cefoxitin-carbapenem resistance). Carbapenem resistance has only been described in France in the species *B. fragilis* and in Korea and Japan in *B. thetaiotaomicron*. This β-lactamase is stable to clavulanic acid, tazobactam and sulbactam. EDTA inhibition of the enzyme can be reversed by the addition of divalent cations (Ca^{2+}, Mg^{2+}, Co^{2+}, etc.). This β-lactamase has high affinity for imipenem. It hydrolyzes all the penicillins and cephalosporins including cefamycins. The *cfiA* gene is silent (26) except in the presence of upstream insertion sequences IS*1186*, IS*1187*, IS*1188*, IS*942*, and IS*612* to IS*615* which generate a strong promoter (27), in which case the level of transcription correlates with the level of resistance (29). Imipenem MICs for *cfiA*+ strains range from 1-256 μg/ml.

It is highly likely that *B. fragilis cfiA*+ strains represent a different species since DNA-DNA hybridization experiments showed only low hybridization with *cfiA*- strains (28); moreover, the chromosomal cephalosporinase *cepA* or enterofragilysin (*bft*) genes were not detected in *cfiA*+ strains (28).

Thus it is important to detect all *B. fragilis* isolates that harbor the *cfiA* gene in order to avoid inappropriate carbapenem usage which may result in the selection and emergence of high-level resistance in these strains. In addition to molecular biological data, a reduction of the carbapenem MIC by ≥ 3 dilutions in the presence of EDTA (MIC ratio ± EDTA of ≥ 8) could be interpreted as positive for metallo-β-lactamase production. This can be determined by E-test® with imipenem ± EDTA strips. Bogaerts *et al.* (7) recommend detection by E-test® with meropenem + EDTA because the antibiotic concentrations scale (0.25-16 μg/ml) is better suited to detection of low-level carbapenemase expression. In cases of off-scale results caused by high level resistance, these authors recommend imipenem + EDTA strips as a second step. In case of imipenem resistance, the following interpretive criterion should be used: cross-resistance to all β-lactams alone or combined with β-lactamase inhibitors. Concomitant resistance to macrolides and clindamycin (MLS_B resistance) and to tetracyclines is very often observed.

In *B. distasonis*, imipenem resistance is not due to a carbapenemase but rather to hyperproduction of a chromosomal cephalosporinase which is much less sensitive to the action of inhibitors; decreased permeability resulting from porin deficiency also plays a role in resistance (43). An imipenem-resistant strain is also resistant to meropenem, ertapenem, faropenem and doripenem but the opposite is not true. This is because EUCAST breakpoints for ertapenem, and imipenem are different, so a strain may test as ertapenem-resistant but imipenem-susceptible. Furthermore, Wexler *et al.* (44) noted that strains of *B. fragilis* group species required ≥ 8 μg/ml of doripenem for inhibition and suggested that overexpression of efflux pumps might contribute to the development of resistance. In this case, imipenem remains active.

Macrolides and tetracyclines

Over half of *Bacteroides* strains are resistant to macrolides (decreased permeability or target modification) and to tetracyclines (Table 4). High-level clindamycin resistance (MIC > 128 μg/ml) is observed in 30-40% of strains. In cases of inducible resistance, the strain may appear susceptible at 24 h and resistant at 48 h of incubation. It is recommended to wait 48 h before analyzing the results in case of susceptibility. Most tetracycline-resistant strains are susceptible to tigecycline.

In MLS_B resistance, cross-resistance is observed with macrolides and clindamycin. Due to the very high resistance rates currently observed for clindamycin, this drug is no longer considered active against *B. fragilis*. Several genetic determinants (*ermF, ermG,* and *ermS*) code for a methylase which displays homology to the methylases encoded by the *erm* genes of staphylococci. Transfer of these genes is frequently associated with transfer of *tet*(Q) tetracycline resistance.

Pristinamycin and telithromycin show highly variable activity and do not present any therapeutic interest.

Metronidazole

When metronidazole resistance is observed, it is necessary to check the purity of the strain and especially the anaerobiosis of the atmosphere, since metronidazole is only active in anaerobic conditions.

In Mediterranean countries and particularly in France, strains with transferable reduced imidazole cross-susceptibility have been described in the *Bacteroides fragilis* group (10). In these strains the MICs were 4-16 µg/ml whereas normally they range from 0.25-2 µg/ml. This resistance is encoded by the *nimA* to *nimE* genes located on the chromosome (*nimB*) or on plasmids (other *nim* genes) (31, 32). These genes code for a nitroreductase that reduces the NO_2 group of metronidazole to an NH_2 group, thereby preventing the formation of toxic DNA-damaging residues. *nim* genes are usually driven by a weak promoter resulting in reduced susceptibility to nitro-imidazoles (metronidazole MIC 4-16 µg/ml); their expression is increased by a strong promoter (insertion sequence IS*1168* for *nimA* and *nimB*, IS*1169* for *nimD,* and IS*1170* for *nimC*). Rare strains may be resistant to both carbapenems and metronidazole since the insertion sequence IS*1186* provides a strong promoter for both the carbapenemase *cfiA* genes (27) and the *nimA* and *nimB* genes (40). The same is true for IS*942* with respect to the *ccrA* gene. The *nim* genes can be detected by PCR with the aid of NIM-3 and NIM-5 primers (41). The effects on tinidazole and ornidazole are more pronounced than on metronidazole.

When resistance is carried on a plasmid, there are 10-20 gene copies per cell versus a maximum of two copies when resistance is chromosome-mediated (41). In a recent study (15), 24% of 206 *B. fragilis* isolates were found to harbor a *nim* gene; only 16% of these isolates were resistant to metronidazole (MIC > 16 µg/ml), with MICs ranging from 1.5-6 µg/ml in the other strains.

The following *nim* genes were detected: *nimA* (21 strains), *nimB* (7), *nimC* (6), *nimD* (3), *nimE* (7), *nimG* (1); no *nim* genes were detected in seven strains. The predominance of *nimA* has been confirmed in another study (6). On fastidious anaerobic agar (FAA) with a 5 µg metronidazole disk, the strains considered susceptible had an inhibition zone diameter of 28-30 mm, identical to that of the susceptible reference strain. For the four intermediate strains (MIC 6 µg/ml), the inhibition zone diameter was 3 mm smaller, while resistant strains (MIC 6-256 µg/ml) grew in contact with the disk. When the metronidazole MIC was between 1.5 and 6 µg/ml, inhibition zone diameters ranged from 14-30 mm. However, if incubation was prolonged to 48 and 72 h, the inhibition diameters of *nim*+ strains decreased and small colonies appeared in the inhibition zone after 5-7 days of culture. Colonies were observed in the inhibition ellipse of the E-test® strip only in *nim*+ strains (Fig. 1).

In Great Britain, resistance rates (MIC > 16 µg/ml) were 1.5% in 1995, 3.8% in 1997, and 7.5% in 1998 (8). Clinical failures have been correlated with MIC values ≥ 32 µg/ml (9, 37).

A patient with a pelvic collection remained pyrexial despite treatment with cefuroxime, gentamicin, and metronidazole 1.5 g/day; several blood cultures yielded a *B. fragilis* strain for which the MIC of metronidazole determined by E-test® was 6 µg/ml (14). This case illustrates the need to detect these reduced susceptibility strains.

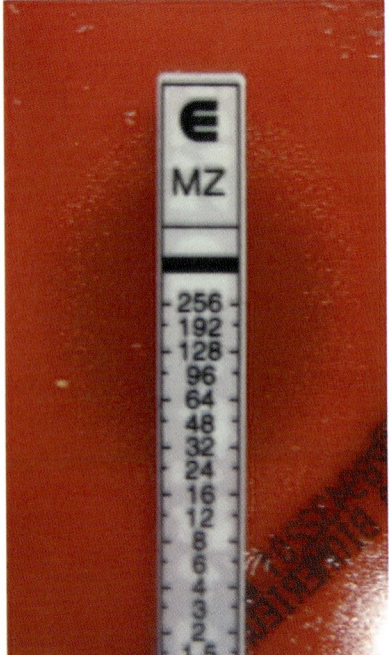

Fig. 1. Metronidazole-resistant strain: presence of colonies in E-test® ellipse after 48 h of incubation.

In France, a single metronidazole-resistant isolate (MIC 64 µg/ml) has been described (22) and shown to possess two chromosomal copies of the *nimA* gene (19). Routine detection of *nim* genes does not appear contributory since there are some resistant strains which do not possess an *nim* gene (*nim*⁻ strains) and conversely, there are *nim*⁺ strains with low MICs which remain accessible to metronidazole treatment. Based on our experience, a breakpoint of 4 µg/ml separates susceptible from resistant strains.

Fluoroquinolones

Among the fluoroquinolones, only moxifloxacin (2), gatifloxacin (13) and garenoxacin (16) are active in at least 90% of strains (Table 4). Resistance of clinical isolates, particularly to trovafloxacin, is due mainly to mutations in subunit A of DNA gyrase (1). Efflux pumps have been implicated in fluoroquinolone resistance (33); in *B. fragilis* these pumps belong to the MF, RND and MATE families and their substrates differ (24). An analysis of 12 laboratory mutants and 32 clinical isolates of *B. fragilis* detected the following resistance mechanisms: five had mutations in the QRDR of DNA gyrase subunit A, three had mutations in subunit B, and 13 strains were restored to susceptibility by CCCP (34).

Other antibiotics

Chloramphenicol resistance due to acetylation and rifampin resistance due to mutation are very rare. Linezolid is also active (4). These antimicrobials are of particular interest in light of their diffusion into brain and bone tissue. Together with moxifloxacin, they can be used against multiresistant strains expressing a carbapenemase, MLS_B resistance, and reduced metronidazole susceptibility.

Prevotella

Prevotella species are resistant to aztreonam, aminoglycosides, trimethoprim, sulfonamides, quinolones, fosfomycin, fusidic acid, and glycopeptides. Wild-type strains of *Prevotella* spp. are highly susceptible to penicillin. When a β-lactamase is detected by a nitrocefin test, penicillin G MICs determined by E-test® are higher (≥ 0.25 µg/ml) than those of non-producing strains (≤ 0.125 µg/ml). For low-level β-lactamase producers (MIC 0.5-2 µg/ml), detection tests are difficult to interpret, in contrast to E-test®. The nitrocefin test only gives a rapid positive result if the level of β-lactamase production is high (MIC > 8 µg/ml).

Two-thirds of *Prevotella* strains are β-lactamase producers; in 75% of cases the amoxicillin MIC lies between 2 and 16 µg/ml. Amoxicillin MICs are ≥ 0.5 µg/ml (≥ 0.38 µg/ml by E-test®) for β-lactamase-producing strains versus < 0.25 µg/ml for non-producing strains. Determination of the amoxicillin MIC is undoubtedly the best criterion to establish the strain's susceptibility to aminopenicillins.

Prevotella produces a cephalosporinase (18, 42) which inactivates cephalothin, cefuroxime

Table 5. β-lactam resistance phenotypes in the *B. fragilis* group (personal data)

β-lactam	Wild-type strain chromosomal β-lactamase	β-lactamase hyperproduction ± porin deficiency or silent carbapenemase gene				Carbapenemase
	78 %[a]	9 %	5 %	3 %	3 %	2 %
Amoxicillin	I/R	R	R	R	R	R
Amoxicillin + clavulanic acid	S	S	S/I	I/R	R	R
Ticarcillin	S	R	R	R	R	R
Ticarcillin + clavulanic acid	S	S	S	S	I	R
Piperacillin	S	I/R	R	R	R	R
Piperacillin + tazobactam	S	S	S	S	I	R
Cefalotin	R	R	R	R	R	R
Cefuroxime	R	R	R	R	R	R
Cefotaxime	I/R	R	R	R	R	R
Cefoxitin	I	I	I/R	R	R	R
Cefotetan	I	I/R	R	R	R	R
Imipenem	S	S	S	S	S	R

[a] Frequency (%) of resistance phenotype.

and, to a lesser extent, the aminopenicillins (like *Proteus penneri* and *Proteus vulgaris*). The enzyme is sensitive to inhibition by clavulanic acid and tazobactam. Ticarcillin is unaffected and cefamycins as well as carbapenems remain very active (Table 6).

In a study of 100 *Prevotella* isolates (12), 58% were β-lactamase producers. Ticarcillin and cefotaxime resistance rates were 8 and 12%, respectively. Non-β-lactamase-producing strains were susceptible to all β-lactams with the exception of very rare strains resistant to cefuroxime and cefixime through an unknown mechanism. β-lactamase production in *Prevotella* confers resistance to aminopenicillins, first generation cephalosporins, cefuroxime, and oral third generation cephalosporins. The activity of these drugs is restored by combination with a β-lactamase inhibitor.

The new fluoroquinolones, tigecycline, and linezolid (Tables 7 and 8) are active against *Prevotella* (4, 12).

Resistance to macrolides, clindamycin, streptogramins, ketolides, and metronidazole is very rare (11). Metronidazole resistance has been described in a few species including *P. bivia* and probably *P. melaninogenica* and *P. loeschii* (38) and the *nimA* gene has been identified in a *P. bivia* isolate (17). Clinical failure was reported in a patient with subdural empyema caused by *P. loeschii* for which the MIC of metronidazole was 12 µg/ml (38). MICs are higher for *P. bivia* than for other *Prevotella* species.

Porphyromonas

Porphyromonas species are resistant to aztreonam, aminoglycosides, trimethoprim, sulfonamides, quinolones, fosfomycin, and colistin. Rare strains of *P. asaccharolytica* produce a β-lactamase conferring amoxicillin resistance. There is no known resistance to the following antibiotics: chloramphenicol, metronidazole, penicillins + β-lactamase inhibitor combinations (Table 9). Resistance to macrolides and clindamycin is extremely rare. Fluoroquinolones, tigecycline and linezolid are active.

Fusobacterium

Fusobacterium species are resistant to aminoglycosides, trimethoprim, sulfonamides, quinolones, and macrolides (low-level for the majority of species, high-level for *F. mortiferum* and *F. varium*). *Fusobacterium* (except *F. varium*) are susceptible to fosfomycin. *F. varium* and *F. mortiferum* are resistant to rifampin. *F. varium* is also resistant to ofloxacin, ciprofloxacin, sparfloxacin, grepafloxacin, and trovafloxacin.

These species are susceptible to many antibiotics including imipenem, cefoxitin, clindamycin, streptogramins, chloramphenicol and metronidazole (Table 10).

Production of an acquired penicillinase (< 5% of strains) confers cross-resistance to penicillin G, aminopenicillins, ticarcillin and piperacillin. Sulbactam, unlike clavulanic acid and tazobactam, is a poor inhibitor of these penicillinases. Susceptibility to the new fluoroquinolones, tigecycline, and linezolid is good (Tables 7 and 8).

Bilophila wadsworthia (Table 9)

Bilophila is resistant to aztreonam, aminoglycosides, trimethoprim, sulfonamides, macrolides (low-level), quinolones, fosfomycin, and glycopeptides. Most strains are resistant to amoxicillin and piperacillin due to β-lactamase production. There are no reports of resistance to ticarcillin, ticarcillin + clavulanic acid, piperacillin + tazobactam, cefoxitin, cefotetan, imipenem, metronidazole, minocycline, sparfloxacin, trovafloxacin, or gatifloxacin. Resistance to amoxicillin + clavulanic acid, clindamycin, or ciprofloxacin has been described in some strains. MICs of penicillin and ampicillin are ≤ 0.5 µg/ml in non-β-lactamase-producing strains as compared to 1-32 µg/ml (modal MIC 2 µg/ml) for penicillin G and 2 - >64 µg/ml (modal MIC 4 µg/ml) for amoxicillin in strains that produce a β-lactamase. β-lactamase positivity can be detected by diffusion using a disk containing 2 I.U. penicillin G when the diameter is < 20 mm. β-lactamase production must be confirmed by a Cefinase® test, using *Brucella* agar supplemented with pyruvate and not taurine. The reaction is easier to read in anaerobiosis but may also be read after a 30 min incubation in aerobic conditions (39).

OTHER GRAM-NEGATIVE BACILLI

B. ureolyticus is susceptible to aztreonam, gentamicin, amikacin, amoxicillin, ticarcillin, piperacillin, third generation cephalosporins, macrolides, clindamycin, and fluoroquinolones; metronidazole susceptibility is variable.

Suterella wadsworthensis is frequently resistant to metronidazole and piperacillin + tazobactam. Clindamycin susceptibility is variable, while strains are susceptible to amoxicillin or ticarcillin

Table 6. Antibiotic activity against the main *Prevotella* species

Antibiotic	*P. melaninogenica*		Black-pigmented *Prevotella*		*P. bivia*		*P. disiens*		*P. oralis*	
	MIC$_{50}$	MIC$_{90}$	MIC$_{50}$	MIC$_{90}$	MIC$_{50}$	MIC$_{90}$	MIC$_{50}$	MIC$_{90}$	MIC$_{50}$	MIC$_{90}$
β-lactams										
Penicillin G	0.125	8[a]	0.25	4-8[a]	16	64	2	8	0.5	64
Amoxicillin	8-32	16-128	0.1-0.25	4-16[a]	8	16-128	8	16	32	256
Amoxicillin + clavulanic acid	0.06-0.5	0.5-1	0.125	1	<0.1-0.25	1-8	<0.1-0.5	0.5-1	0.25	1-8
Ampicillin	1-32	8->16	1-2	4-128	0.5-1	4	4	16		
Ampicillin + sulbactam (2:1)	2	4	0.25	4[a]	2-16	32-128	4	16	16	128
Ticarcillin	16-32	64	<0.125	0.5	2-16	32-128[a]	4	16	16	128
Ticarcillin + clavulanic acid (2)	0.25-0.5	2	<0.25	<0.25	<0.5	1-2	<0.5	1	<0.5	2
Piperacillin	1	8[a]	1	8	8	128[a]	8	32	2	8
Piperacillin + tazobactam (8:1)	0.25	0.5	0.25	0.25	0.25-1	4-8	0.12	0.25	0.25	0.5
Cefaclor	16	64	0.5-4	16-128	8	32	4	>32	0.5	
Cefoxitin	1-8	4-16	0.25-1	2-8	<0.5-4	4-8	<0.5-1	2-8	8	16
Cefotetan	4	16	0.5-1	4[a]	4	16-32	4	32	4	16
Cefoperazone	4-32	8-64			2-16	4-128	8	64		
Cefotaxime	0.25-1	4-8[a]	0.06-0.2	2-4	0.25-0.5	4-16[a]	0.5	16	0.25	4[a]
Ceftizoxime	0.25	16[a]	0.25	1	0.5	64[a]				
Cefuroxime	0.25-4	8-32[a]	0.25	16	1-4	8-32	2	8	0.25	32
Imipenem	0.06	0.06	0.03	0.03	0.06	0.12	0.5	2	0.03	0.125
Ertapenem	0.125	0.25	0.06	0.125	0.25	0.5	-	-	0.06	0.25
Doripenem	0.03	0.12	0.03	0.06	0.06	0.12	0.06	0.12	0.06	0.12
Meropenem	0.06	0.06	0.03	0.03	0.06	0.12	0.25	0.5	0.03	0
Clavulanic acid	16	32			8	32	8	8	16	32
Other antibiotics										
Doxycycline	0.25	4[a]	0.25	64	0.125	16	0.25	16	0.5	32
Metronidazole	0.5-8	4->64	0.25-0.5	0.5-1	1-2	2-8	0.5-4	2-8	0.25-2	1-4
Chloramphenicol	1-2	2-4	2	4-8	4	4	1	2	1	4
Clindamycin	<0.06	0.12-2	0.03-0.06	0.06-0.12	0.01	0.03	0.03	0.125	0.06	0.125

[a] A few resistant strains have been described.

Table 7. Activity of quinolones against Gram-negative anaerobes (excluding Bacteroides fragilis group)

Antibiotic	Prevotella spp.		Porphyromonas spp.		Fusobacterium spp.		B. ureolyticus		Veillonella spp.	
	MIC_{50}	MIC_{90}	MIC_{50}	MIC_{90}	MIC_{50}	MIC_{90}	MIC_{50}	MIC_{90}	MIC_{50}	MIC_{90}
Nalidixic acid	128	>128			128	256			128	128
Ciprofloxacin	1-2	16-32	0.5	1-2	1-8	2-32	0.03	0.06	0.25	0.5
Enoxacin	4	32			16	>32	0.25	0.25		
Garenoxacin	0.125	1	<0.06	<0.06	0.12	0.25			0.06	0.125
Levofloxacin	1	8	0.5-1	1-2	1	1	0.125	>8	0.25	0.5
Moxifloxacin	0.25	2-4	0.12	0.25	0.06	0.5	0.125	>8	0.25	0.5
Ofloxacin	2	16	1	2-4	2	4-16	0.12	0.5	0.25	0.5
Pefloxacin	8	32			8	32			1	2
Sparfloxacin	4	8-16	0.5	1-4	2	4-8	0.03	0.25	0.125	4

+ clavulanic acid combinations and to cefoxitin and imipenem.

Desulfomonas strains are resistant to amoxicillin, piperacillin, piperacillin + tazobactam and susceptible to amoxicillin + clavulanic acid, imipenem, ciprofloxacin, and metronidazole; susceptibility to ticarcillin, cefoxitin and cefotetan is variable.

Desulfovibrio strains are resistant to amoxicillin, piperacillin, piperacillin + tazobactam, cefoxitin, cefotetan, and cefotaxime, and susceptible to imipenem, clindamycin and metronidazole; susceptibility to ticarcillin, ticarcillin + clavulanic acid, amoxicillin + clavulanic acid, and ciprofloxacin is variable (21).

B. tectum is susceptible to amoxicillin + clavulanic acid, cefotaxime, erythromycin, clindamycin, doxycycline, linezolid, and metronidazole.

Tanerella forsythia (formerly *Bacteroides forsythus*) is highly susceptible to antibiotics, particularly β-lactams, macrolides, clindamycin, ketolides, tetracyclines, and metronidazole as well as levofloxacin.

Selenomonas is highly susceptible to penicillins, tetracyclines, nitro-imidazoles, and ciprofloxacin.

Anaerospirillum is susceptible to penicillin G and cefotaxime; metronidazole MICs range from 2-8 µg/ml. This genus is resistant to clindamycin.

STRICT ANAEROBIC GRAM-NEGATIVE COCCI

Most clinical isolates of strict anaerobic Gram-negative cocci belong to the genus *Veillonella*. *Veillonella* is resistant to aztreonam, aminoglycosides, trimethoprim, sulfonamides, macrolides (low-level), quinolones, and glycopeptides. These organisms exhibit low-level resistance to all the macrolides (MIC > 2 µg/ml), and to streptogramins and ketolides (telithromycin and ABT 773); clindamycin usually remains very active. Low-level resistance to ticarcillin and piperacillin has been reported and some strains are resistant to one or both of these agents (including when combined with a β-lactamase inhibitor), and to clindamycin. The *nimE* gene has been detected in a *Veillonella* isolate in France (MIC 8 µg/ml) (19).

Most strains are susceptible to all β-lactams, fluoroquinolones (including ciprofloxacin and ofloxacin), linezolid and metronidazole.

Table 8. Activity of some antibiotics against Gram-negative anaerobes (excluding *Bacteroides fragilis* group)

Antibiotic	*Prevotella* spp.		*Porphyromonas* spp.		*Fusobacterium* spp.		*B. ureolyticus*		*Veillonella* spp.	
	MIC$_{50}$	MIC$_{90}$	MIC$_{50}$	MIC$_{90}$	MIC$_{50}$	MIC$_{90}$	MIC$_{50}$	MIC$_{90}$	MIC$_{50}$	MIC$_{90}$
Macrolides and streptogramins										
Azithromycin	0.25-1	1-8	0.25	0.5*	1	2	0.25	0.5	8	16
Erythromycin	0.25-2	2-8	0.125	0.25*	1-4	8->64	0.25-0.5	0.5-1	16	32-64
Josamycin	0.25	2			0.25-32	16->64			2	8
Roxithromycin	0.5	0.5-32	0.125	0.125	2-8	16->64	0.5	2	16	32
Clarithromycin	0.25	1-2	0.06	0.125	0.12	2-128		2	32	64
Spiramycin	0.5	4-8	0.125	0.125	2-8	32	0.5	2	16	>32
Quinupristin-dalfopristin	0.12-0.5	2-4	1	4*	0.03	0.12-1		64	32	32
Virginiamycin	0.25	2	0.125	1	0.06	0.5			2	8
Telithromycin	0.125	1	0.12	0.25	1-64	16->64	1	2		
Tetracyclines										
Tetracycline	0.5-64	16-128	0.25	0.5*	0.25	0.5-16	0.06	4-8	2	32
Doxycycline	0.25-0.5	4-64	0.125	0.25	0.03	0.125	0.25	2	0.12	4
Tigecycline	0.25	0.5	0.06	0.06	0.06	0.06			0.25	1
Oxazolidinone										
Linezolid	2	2	1	2	0.5	1			0.06	0.5

Table 9. Antibiotic activity against *Bilophila* and non-*fragilis* Bacteroides

Antibiotic	*Porphyromonas spp.* MIC$_{50}$	*Porphyromonas spp.* MIC$_{90}$	*Bilophila spp.* MIC$_{50}$	*Bilophila spp.* MIC$_{90}$	*B. ureolyticus* MIC$_{50}$	*B. ureolyticus* MIC$_{90}$	*Other Bacteroides* MIC$_{50}$	*Other Bacteroides* MIC$_{90}$
β-lactam								
Amoxicillin	0.06	2	8 - 32	16 - 64	0.03	0.06	0.5	4 [a]
Amoxicillin + clavulanic acid	0.06	2	0.5	1	<0.03	<0.03	0.25	2
Penicillin G	0.06	0.25	2	4 [a]	0.03	0.03	8	16 [a]
Ampicillin	0.06	0.5	4	32	2	2 - 16	0.25	4 [a]
Ampicillin + sulbactam (2:1)	0.06	0.5	2	4	0.125	2 - 32	0.12	2 - 4
Ticarcillin	0.125	16	2 - 4	8	0.25	2	1	32
Ticarcillin + clavulanic acid (2)	0.125	16	0.06 - 0.2	0.25	0.25	2	0.125	4
Piperacillin	0.03	0.06	32	64 [a]	0.06	4	2 - 8	8 - >128
Piperacillin + tazobactam (8:1)	0.03	0.125	1 - 4	8	0.06	2	2	4
Cefoxitin	0.06 - 0.25	1 - 4	4	16	0.5	0.5	2 - 16	16 - 64
Cefotetan	0.125 - 0.25	0.5 - 8	0.5	1	1 - 4	4 - >32	4 - 8	8 - 64
Cefoperazone	0.125	8			4 - 8	16 - 128		
Cefotaxime	0.125	1	0.01	0.01	4 - 16	8 - 64		
Ceftizoxime	1	1	16	32 [a]			2	16 - 64
Imipenem	0.03	0.125	0.125	0.125	0.06	0.06 - 0.12	0.06 - 0.2	0.5
Ertapenem			0.015	0.03			0.125	0.25
Meropenem	0.03	0.06	0.008	0.008	0.016	0.06 - 0.2	0.25 - 0.5	
Aztreonam			32	128	0.5	0.5		
Other antibiotics								
Metronidazole	0.03	0.25 - 4	0.03	0.12	1 - 4	2 - 8 [a]	0.5	1 - 2 [a]
Chloramphenicol	1	2 - 4	4	4	1	2	2 - 4	4 - 8
Clindamycin	0.03	0.25 [a]	0.25	0.5 [a]	0.12	0.5 [a]	0.06 - 0.2	0.06 - 4 [a]
Gentamicin	>16	>16			2	8	0.58	>16
Amikacin					8	32	>16	
Levofloxacin	0.5	0.5	0.5	0.5	0.125	0.125 - >8	2	8
Moxifloxacin	0.5	0.5	0.5	1	0.125	0.03 - >8	1	4
Lenizolid	1	2					2	2
Vancomycin	4	8	>256	>256			>8	>8

[a] A few resistant strains have been described.

Table 10. Antibiotic activity against *Fusobacterium* and *Veillonella*

Antibiotic	*F. nucleatum* MIC$_{50}$	*F. nucleatum* MIC$_{90}$	*F. mortiferum* MIC$_{50}$	*F. mortiferum* MIC$_{90}$	*F. varium* MIC$_{50}$	*F. varium* MIC$_{90}$	*Fusobacterium* spp. MIC$_{50}$	*Fusobacterium* spp. MIC$_{90}$	*Veillonella* spp. MIC$_{50}$	*Veillonella* spp. MIC$_{90}$
β-lactams										
Amoxicillin	0.06	1	8	32	1	32	0.03-1	0.25-32	0.25	0.5
Amoxicillin + clavulanic acid	0.06	0.5	0.5-4	8	0.25	2	0.03-0.2	0.25-2^a	0.06	0.25
Penicillin G	0.125	>16	0.25-0.5	0.5-1	0.25	0.5-64	0.03-2	0.03-32	<0.25	1-4
Ampicillin	0.125-8	32	8	32	2	4	0.25-4	4-32	0.5	2
Ampicillin + sulbactam (2:1)	0.125	1	0.06-0.1	2	2	4	0.06-1	0.5-4^a	0.25-4	2-8
Ticarcillin	0.06	0.25	8	16	2	8	2	16-256	2-8	32-128
Ticarcillin + clavulanic acid	0.06	0.25	0.06-1	0.25-8	0.25	2	0.12-0.5	2-4	8	16
Piperacillin	0.06-0.2	0.12-8	0.5	8	4	32	0.06-2	1-64^a	8	16
Piperacillin + tazobactam (8:1)	0.125	1	0.125	1	4	32	0.5-2	8-16	4	8
Cefoxitin	0.06-2	2	2-4	8-16	2-4	8-16	0.5-4	0.5-64	0.5-4	4-16
Cefotetan	0.12-2	2	4	8	2	4	4	4-32^a	1-2	2-8
Cefoperazone	0.25	2	4	8	8	16	0.25-8	2-64^a	8	32
Ceftazidime	8	32	128	>256	8	256	1-32	8-64	2	4
Cefotaxime	0.06	2	16	>256	1	32	0.5	0.5->256	0.125-1	2-16
Ceftizoxime	0.25	4	16	>256	1	32	0.06-0.2	4->256	0.25-8	16-32
Imipenem	0.01-0.03	1	0.5	1	1	4	0.03-0.5	0.06-4^a	0.06-0.12	0.5-1
Ertapenem	0.03	0.25	0.125	0.25	0.125	1	0.03	0.25	0.125	1
Doripenem	0.01	0.03	0.25	1	0.125	0.25	0.01	0.25-1	1	2
Meopenem	0.01-0.03	0.1-0.5	0.25	0.5-8	0.125	0.5	0.008-0.2	0.125-8	0.03	0.06
Clavulanic acid			32	64	16	64	8-16	16->32		
Aztreonam	0.5	2	2	4			0.5	2-4		
Other antibiotics										
Metronidazole	0.12-0.2	1	0.25-1	0.5-4	0.5-1	1-4	0.03-4	0.25-8^a	<0.25	1-2
Chloramphenicol	1	4	1	4	2	4	2-4	4	0.25	1
Clindamycin	0.06-0.12	1	0.06-0.2	1-8^a	2-8	32-64	0.03-0.12	0.12->128	0.03	0.06
Moxifloxacin	0.12	1	0.25	0.5	4	8	0.12	1-8	0.25	0.5

^{a} A few resistant strains have been described.

CONCLUSION

Monitoring of antimicrobial resistance patterns is essential, including for anaerobic bacteria. It is in the *Bacteroides fragilis* group that the incidence of antimicrobial resistance is highest. Some multi-resistant strains have already proved difficult to treat, requiring recourse to drugs such as moxifloxacin, linezolid, tigecycline and even chloramphenicol.

REFERENCES

(1) **Bachoual, R., L. Dubreuil, C.J. Soussy, and J. Tankovic**. 2000. Roles of *gyrA* mutations in resistance of clinical isolates and in vitro mutants of *Bacteroides fragilis* to the new fluoroquinolone trovafloxacin. Antimicrob. Agents Chemother. **44**:1842-1845.

(2) **Behra-Miellet, J., L. Dubreuil, and E. Jumas-Bilak**. 2002. Antianaerobic activity of moxifloxacin compared with that of ofloxacin, ciprofloxacin, clindamycin, metronidazole and beta-lactams Int. J. Antimicrob. Agents **20**:366-374.

(3) **Behra-Miellet, J., L. Calvet, F. Mory, C. Muller, M. Chomarat, M.C. Bézian, S. Bland, M.E. Juvenin, T. Fosse, F. Goldstein, B. Jaulhac, and L. Dubreuil**. 2003. Antibiotic resistance among anaerobic Gram-negative bacilli: Lessons from a French multicentric survey. Anaerobe **9**:105-111.

(4) **Behra, J., L. Calvet, and L. Dubreuil**. 2003. Activity of linezolid against anaerobic bacteria. Int. J. Antimicrob. Agents **22**:28-34.

(5) **Behra-Miellet, J., L. Calvet, and L. Dubreuil**. 2004. A *Bacteroides thetaiotamicron* porin that could take part in resistance to beta-lactams. Int. J. Antimicrob. Agents **24**:135-143.

(6) **Behrendtz, S., H. Fang, M. Heldberg, and C. Hedlund**. 2003. Metronidazole resistance and *nim* genes in clinical *Bacteroides fragilis* group isolates. Anaerobe **9**:247.

(7) **Bogaerts, P., A. Engelhardt, C. Berhin, L. Bbylund, P. Ho, A. Yusof, and Y. Glupczinski**. 2008. Evaluation of a new meropenem-EDTA double–ended E-test strip for the detection of the CfiA metallo-ß lactamase in clinical isolates of *Bateroides fragilis*. Clin. Microbiol. Infect. **14**:970-981.

(8) **Brazier, J.S., S.L. Stubbs, and B.I. Duerden**. 1999. Metronidazole resistance among clinical isolates belonging to the *Bacteroides fragilis* group: time to be concerned ? J. Antimicrob. Chemother. **44**:580-581.

(9) **Chauldhry, R., P. Mathur, B. Dhawan, and L. Kumar**. 2001. Emergence of metronidazole-resistant *Bacteroides fragilis*, India. Emerging Infect. Dis. **7**:485-486.

(10) **Dublanchet, A., J. Caillon, J.P. Edmond, H. Chardon, and H.B. Drugeon**. 1986. Isolation of *Bacteroides* strains with reduced sensitivity to 5-nitroimidazoles. Eur. J. Clin. Microbiol. **5**:346-347.

(11) **Dubreuil, L., I. Houcke, and E. Singer**. 1998. Activité *in vitro* de 10 antibiotiques dont la pristinamycine et ses deux composants (RP 12536 et RP 27404) vis-à-vis des anaérobies stricts. Path. Biol. **46**:147-152.

(12) **Dubreuil, L, J. Behra-Miellet, C. Vouillot, S. Bland, A. Sedallian, and F. Mory** . 2003. β-lactamase production in *Prevotella* and in vitro susceptibilities to selected beta-lactam antibiotics. Int. J. Antimicrob. Agents **21**:267-273.

(13) **Dubreuil, L, J. Behra-Miellet, and L. Calvet**. 2003. *In vitro* evaluation of a new fluoroquinolone, gatifloxacin, against clinical anaerobic bacteria. Clin. Microbiol. Infect. **9**:1133-1138.

(14) **Elsaghier, A.A., J.S. Brazier, and E.A. James**. 2003. Bacteraemia due to *Bacteroides fragilis* with reduced susceptibility to metronidazole. J. Antimicrob. Chemother. **51**:1436-1437.

(15) **Gal, M. and J.S. Brazier**. 2004. Metronidazole resistance in *Bacteroides spp.* carrying *nim* genes and the selection of slow-growing metronidazole-resistant mutants. J. Antimicrob. Chemother. **54**:109-116.

(16) **Liebetrau, A, A.C. Rodloff, J. Behra-Miellet, and L. Dubreuil**. 2003. *In vitro* evaluation of a new desfluoro(6) quinolone, garenoxacin, against clinical anaerobic bacteria. Antimicrob. Agents Chemother. **47**:3667-3671.

(17) **Lubbe, M.M., K. Stanley, and L.J. Chakley**. 1999. Prevalence of *nim* genes in anaerobic/facultative anaerobic bacteria isolated in South Africa. FEMS Microbiol. Lett. **172**:79-83.

(18) **Madinier, I., T. Fosse, J. Giudicelli, and R. Labia**. 2001. Cloning and biochemical characterization of a class A β-lactamase from *Prevotella intermedia*. Antimicrob. Agents Chemother. **45**:2386-2389.

(19) **Marchandin, H., E. Jumas-Bilak, C. Teyssier, H. Jean-Pierre, F. Mory, M. Siméon de Buochberg, C. Carriere, and L. Dubreuil**. 2002. Detection of *nim* genes in clinical isolates of *Veillonella* and *Bacteroides fragilis* in France. Anaerobe **8**:137.

(20) **Mory, F., A. Loczniewski, S. Bland, A. Sedallian, G. Grollier, F. Girard-Pipau, M.F. Paris, and L. Dubreuil**. 1998. Survey of anaerobic susceptibility patterns: a French multicentric study. Int. J. Antimicrob. Agents **10**:229-236.

(21) **Mory, F., M. Weber, and A. Lozniewski**. 2000. In vitro activity of β-lactam antibiotics against clinical isolates of *Desulfovibrio spp*. Réunion Interdisciplinaire de Chimiothérapie Anti-Infectieuse (RICAI), Paris. Abstract 262/P2.

(22) **Mory F., J.P. Carlier, M. Thouvenin, H. Schuhmacher, and A. Losniewski**. 2004. Bacteremia caused by *Prevotella spp.* with reduced susceptibility to metronidazole. Abstract 429/81P. Int. J. Antimicrob. Agents 24 :Suppl 2:S152.

(23) **Odou, M.F., E. Singer, M.B. Romond, and L. Dubreuil**. 1998. Isolation and characterization of a porin-like protein of 45 kilodaltons from *Bacteroides fragilis*. FEMS Microbiol. Lett. **166**:347-354.

(24) **Oh, H., and C. Hedlund**. 2003. Mechanism of quinolone resistance in anaerobic bacteria. Clin. Microbiol. Infect. **9**:512-517.

(25) **Parker, A.C., and C.J. Smith**. 1993. Genetic and biochemical analysis of a novel class A β-lactamase responsible for cefoxitin resistance. Antimicrob. Agents Chemother. **37**:1028-1036.

(26) **Podglajen, I., J. Breuil, F. Bordon, L. Gutmann, and E. Collatz**. 1992. A silent carbapenemase gene in

strains of *Bacteroides fragilis* can be expressed after a one-step mutation. FEMS Microbiol. Lett. **91**:21-30.

(27) **Podglajen, I., J. Breuil, and E. Collatz**. 1994. Insertion of a novel DNA sequence, IS*1186*, upstream of the silent carbapenemase gene *cfiA*, promotes expression of carbapenem resistance in clinical isolates of *Bacteroides fragilis*. Mol. Microbiol. **12**:105-114.

(28) **Podglajen, I., J. Breuil, I. Casin, and E. Collatz**. 1995. Genotypic identification of two groups within the species *Bacteroides fragilis* by ribotyping and by analysis of PCR-generated fragment patterns and insertion sequence content. J. Bacteriol. **177**:5270-5275.

(29) **Podglajen, I., J. Breuil, A. Rohaut, C. Monsempes, and E. Collatz**. 2001. Multiple mobile promotor regions for the rare carbapenem resistance gene of *Bacteroides fragilis*. J. Bacteriol. **183**:3531-3535.

(30) **Rasmussen, B.A., Y. Gluzman, and F.P. Tally**. 1990. Cloning and sequencing the class B β-lactamase gene (*ccrA*) from *Bacteroides fragilis* TAL 3636. Antimicrob. Agents Chemother. **34**:1590-1592.

(31) **Reysset, G., A. Haggoud, W.J. Su, and M. Sebald**. 1992. Genetic and molecular analysis of pIP417 and pIP419 *Bacteroides* plasmids encoding 5 nitroimidazole resistance. Plasmid **27**:191-196.

(32) **Reysset, G., A. Haggoud, and M. Sebald**. 1993. Genetics of resistance of *Bacteroides* species to 5-nitroimidazole. Clin. Infect. Dis. **16:suppl 4**, S401-403.

(33) **Ricci, V., and L. Piddock**. 2003. Accumulation of garenoxacin by *Bacteroides fragilis* compared with that of five fluoroquinolones. J. Antimicrob. Chemother. **52**:605-609.

(34) **Ricci, V., M.L. Peterson, J.C. Rotschafer, H. Xexler, and L.J. Piddock**. 2004. Role of topoisomerase mutations and efflux in fluoroquinolone resistance of *Bacteroides fragilis* clinical isolates and laboratory mutants. Antimicrob. Agents Chemother. **48**:1344-1346.

(35) **Rogers, M.B., A.C. Parker, and C.J. Smith**. 1993. Cloning and characterization of the endogenous cephalosporinase gene, *cepA*, from *Bacteroides fragilis* reveals a new subgroup of Ambler class A β-lactamases. Antimicrob. Agents Chemother. **37**:2391-2400.

(36) **Rogers, M.C., T.K. Benett, and C.M. Payne**. 1994. Insertional activation of *cepA* leads to high level ß lactamase expression in *Bacteroides fragilis* clinical isolates. J. Bacteriol. **176**:4376-4384.

(37) **Rotimi, V.O., M. Khoursheed, J.S. Brazier, W.Y. Jamal, and F.B. Khodakhast**. 1999. *Bacteroides species* highly resistant to metronidazole: an emerging clinical problem. Clin. Microbiol. Infect. **5**:166-169.

(38) **Sandoe, J.A.T., J.K. Struthers, and J.S. Brazier**. 2001. Subdural empyema caused by *Prevotella loescheii* with reduced susceptibilty to metronidazole. J. Antimicrob. Chemother. **47**:366-367.

(39) **Summanen, P.H.** 2000. Comparison of effects of medium composition and atmospheric conditions on detection of *Bilophila wadsworthia* β-lactamase by cefinase and cefinase plus methods. J. Clin. Microbiol. **38**:733-736.

(40) **Trinh, S., A. Haggoud, G. Reysset, and M. Sebald**. 1995. Plasmids pIP419 and pIP421 from *Bacteroides*: 5-nitroimidazole resistance genes and their upstream insertion sequence elements. Microbiology **141**:927-935.

(41) **Trinh, S., and G. Reysset**. 1996. Detection by PCR of the *nim* genes encoding 5-nitroimidazole resistance in *Bacteroides* spp. J. Clin. Microbiol. **34**:2078-2084.

(42) **Valle, G., L.M. Quiros, M.T. Andres, and J.F. Fierro**. 1998. A β-lactamase belonging to group 2e from oral clinical isolates of *Prevotella intermedia*. FEMS Microbiol. Lett. **158**:191-194.

(43) **Wexler, H.M., C. Getty, and G. Fisher**. 1992. Isolation and characterisation of a major outer membrane protein from *Bacteroides distasonis*. J. Med. Microbiol. **37**:165-175.

(44) **Wexler H.M., A.E. Engel, D. Glass, and C. Li**. 2005. In vitro activities of doripenem and comparator against 364 anaerobic isolates. Antimicrob. Agents Chemother. **49**:4413-4417.

Chapter 49. MYCOBACTERIA

CNR Mycobacteries et resistance des mycobacteries aux antituberculeux

INTRODUCTION

History of antituberculous treatment

The history of antituberculous chemotherapy began in 1944 with the discovery of streptomycin (SM) (7, Table 1). The efficacy of this antibiotic in humans was demonstrated in 1948 when the first therapeutic trial was published. A first obstacle to antituberculous treatment was already identified in this publication, namely treatment failure by selection of resistant mutants under treatment.

In 1950, the combination of para-amino-salicylic acid (PAS) to SM is shown to allow recovery from tuberculosis by preventing the selection of SM-resistant mutants. In 1952, the addition of isoniazid (INH) to SM and PAS efficiently blocks the selection of resistant mutants and, provided that treatment is continued for 24 months, can lead to cure rates of 90 to 95%. In the sixties, PAS was replaced by ethambutol (EMB), which made it possible to reduce the duration of treatment (INH + SM + EMB) to 18 months. The length of treatment was mainly associated with the presence, within lesions, of a population of bacilli with slower metabolism, against which the antituberculous treatments available at that time had little effect. These populations were responsible for relapses with susceptible bacilli, a second obstacle to treatment. Towards the end of the 60's, the discovery of rifampin (RMP), with good activity against this population of bacilli with slower metabolism (often called "dormant" or "persistent"), significantly increased the efficacy of treatment and shortened its duration from 18 to 9 months (INH+RMP+EMB).

The latest advance is the addition of pyrazinamide (PZA) in the eighties. This antibiotic made it possible to shorten the treatment from 9 to 6 months thanks to its activity on slow-growing bacilli.

The standard treatment for tuberculosis, which has been recommended by WHO for more than twenty years, is based on the quadruple combination of INH+RMP+PZA+EMB for 2 months followed by the double combination of INH+RMP for the next 4 months. This treatment leads to a cure in more than 95% of tuberculosis cases with susceptible bacilli.

Active antibiotics

Tubercle bacilli (mainly *Mycobacterium tuberculosis*, *Mycobacterium bovis* and *Mycobacterium africanum*, but also other species isolated less frequently such as *M. caprae*, *M. canetti*, etc.) are naturally resistant to antibiotics active against bacterial species belonging to other genera, except for aminoglycosides, rifamycins, and fluoroquinolones. However, they are naturally susceptible to some antibiotics specifically active against tubercle bacilli. These are INH, PZA, EMB, ethionamide, and PAS. Within the *M. tuberculosis* complex, *M. bovis* is an exception, being naturally resistant to PZA.

The activity of these antibiotics is variable: some are bactericidal and others are bacteriostatic (Table 2). In the course of the tuberculosis disease,

Table 1. History of antituberculous treatment (adapted after M. Iseman)

Date	Antituberculous drug	Duration of treatment (months)
1944	Streptomycin (SM) and para-amino-salicylic acid (PAS)	
1948	Results from the 1st therapeutic trial of SM	
1950	Randomized trial of SM versus PAS versus SM + PAS	24
1952	Triple association SM + PAS + isoniazid (INH)	18
1960s	Ethambutol (EMB) replaces PAS	
1970s	Rifampin (RMP) is added to SM + EMB + INH	9
1980s	Pyrazinamide added to INH + RMP during the first 2 months	6

the bacilli's environment modulates the specific activity of each antibiotic. Only three antibiotics are bactericidal in the acid environment within macrophages and lesions undergoing caseation; the most active of these is PZA, followed by RMP and INH. In poorly oxygenated, neutral pH caseous foci, where persistent, slow-growing bacilli are found, only RMP is active. In cavitations where bacilli are actively multiplying, SM is most active, followed by INH and RMP.

The most active, easiest to administer, and best tolerated antibiotics are prescribed in first intention for standard treatment (first-line treatment) of new tuberculosis cases: these are INH and RMP (known as major antituberculous drugs), PZA and EMB. All other antibiotics, including fluoroquinolones, some of which have good bactericidal activity, are considered second-line antituberculous drugs and are only prescribed in case of resistance or major intolerance to first-line antituberculous agents.

New active molecules are under investigation, in particular a diarylquinoline drug, R207910 or TMC207 (2), two imidazoles (PA-824 and OPC-67683) and two oxazolidinones (linezolid and PNU-100480).

Mechanisms of resistance

Thanks to molecular biology techniques, much information has been gathered in the past few years on the mechanism of acquired resistance to antibiotics in mycobacteria (19). All mechanisms known to date are linked to chromosomal mutations. These mutations are localized either in the structural genes for the antibiotic target, leading to a reduction in affinity of the target for the antibiotic (RMP, fluoroquinolones, aminoglycosides, EMB), or in genes encoding activating enzymes which transform inactive antibiotic to an active metabolite (INH, PZA, ethionamide).

Isoniazid

Isoniazid (INH) is a nicotinic acid hydrazide. It is only active against mycobacteria, and almost exclusively against mycobacteria from the *tuberculosis* complex. It inhibits the synthesis of mycolic acids, major components of the cell wall of mycobacteria, and triggers the formation of free radicals, toxic for the bacterial cell.

As soon as INH started to be used, an association between resistance and loss of catalase activity was observed in resistant strains. In 1992, the *kat*G gene, encoding a catalase-peroxidase, was shown to be essential for the activation of INH in the bacterium. Conformational changes in this enzyme resulting from *kat*G mutations prevent the conversion of INH to its active form. Mutations in *kat*G are seen in 60 to 70% of INH-resistant strains and usually lead to a high level of resistance (MIC $\geq$ 1 µg/ml) with no cross-resistance to ethion-

Table 2. Activity of antituberculous antibiotics

Antibiotic	MIC[a] (µg/ml)	Route[b]	Posology (mg/kg/jour)	Serum levels (µg/ml) 3rd h	6th h	Activity
Isoniazid	0.05	orale[c]	4-5	1-2,5	0.2-1	Bactericidal
Rifampin	0.20	orale[c]	10	10	5	Bactericidal
Ethambutol	1	orale[c]	20	2.5	2	Bacteriostatic
Pyrazinamide	5 (à pH 5.5)	orale	25	40-50	40-50	Bactericidal (at acid pH)
Streptomycin	0.5	IM	15	30	10	Bactericidal
Kanamycin	0.5	IM	15	30	10	Bactericidal
Capreomycin	1	IM	15	30	-	Bactericidal
Thioamides	0.5	orale	10-20	2.5	3.5	Bactericidal
Levofloxacin	0.25	orale[c]	15	6	-	Bactericidal
Moxifloxacin	0.12	orale[c]	7	3	-	Bactericidal
Cycloserine	10	orale	10-20	40	40	Bacteriostatic
PAS	0.1	orale[c]	150-200	20-60	0.5	Bacteriostatic
Thiacetazone	0.5	orale	2-3	0.9-2.4	3	Bacteriostatic

[a] MIC: mean minimal inhibitory concentration measured in liquid medium for wild-type *M. tuberculosis* strains.
[b] Usual route of administration.
[c] Possible administration by injection.

amide. The most frequently observed mutation occurs in codon 315.

The *inhA* gene codes for a NADH-dependent enoyl-ACP reductase, an enzyme involved in long-chain fatty acid synthesis (Fas-II system). Mutations in this gene and/or its promoter were observed in 10 to 30% of INH-resistant strains, mostly in position -15 of the promoter. INH resistance through mutation in the *inhA* gene or its promoter leads to a low level of resistance (MIC > 0.2 but < 1 µg/ml) with cross-resistance to ethionamide, which shares structural similarities with INH.

Mutations in other genes (*ahpC-oxyR, kasA, mabA, furA, ndh*) were observed in INH-resistant strains, but their role in resistance remains to be demonstrated.

Rifampin

Rifampin (RMP) and the other rifamycins (rifabutin, rifapentine) block transcription initiation by binding to the ß subunit of RNA polymerase. Acquired resistance to RMP, with cross-resistance to rifabutin and rifapentine, is related to mutations in the *rpoB* gene encoding the ß subunit of RNA polymerase within a domain encompassing codons 507 to 533 (*E. coli* numbering). Most often, these are point mutations with a nucleotide change within a codon (Table 3). The most frequent of these are serine 531 mutations, observed in about half the RMP-resistant *M. tuberculosis* strains (most commonly $Ser_{531}Leu$), and histidine 526 mutations, observed in a third of the RMP-resistant strains (most commonly $His_{526}Asp$ or $His_{526}Tyr$). These mutations are associated with a high resistance level (MIC > 64 µg/ml). Other mutations are much less common (codons 511, 513, 516, 521 and 533) and may be associated with weaker resistance levels.

A critical feature of RMP-resistant strains, as opposed to INH, is that mutations in the *rpoB* gene are seen in virtually all of these strains. Thus, analysis of these mutations became the first molecular technique for rapid detection of resistance.

Pyrazinamide

Pyrazinamide (PZA), like INH, is a synthetic derivative of nicotinamide. It is very active against *M. tuberculosis* and *M. africanum*; however, *M. bovis* is naturally resistant to PZA. PZA activity requires an acid pH (optimum pH: 5.6) and an enzyme with amidase activity, the pyrazinamidase/nicotinamidase, encoded by the *pncA* gene, which metabolizes PZA to an active compound, pyrazinoic acid. The target of pyrazinoic acid remains unknown.

As early as the 1970's, an association between acquired PZA resistance and lack of pyrazinamidase activity was observed, suggesting that alterations in the pyrazinamidase gene(s) might be implicated in this resistance. In recent years, it was reported that over 80% of PZA-resistant strains contained mutations in *pncA*. These mutations are very diverse, including mostly substitutions but also deletions and insertions, and are distributed along the entire gene. The relationship between mutations and resistance has not been established for all of the described mutations.

Ethambutol

Ethambutol (EMB) is an antibiotic specifically active against mycobacteria through inhibition of mycolic acid synthesis. The target of EMB is arabinosyltransferase, an enzyme involved in linkage of arabinogalactan (one of the basic elements in the mycobacterium cell wall).

In over half of the cases, acquired resistance to EMB in *M. tuberculosis* is associated with mutations in the *embB* gene encoding arabinosyltransferase. The majority of mutations involve methionine 306 (change to isoleucine, leucine, or valine). Amino acid changes are also observed in codons 330, 406, and 630. These

Table 3. Mutations in the 507-533 region of the *rpoB* gene for the ß subunit of RNA polymerase[a]

Mutation	Leu 511	Gln 513	Asp 516	Ser 521	His 526	Ser 531	Leu 533
	Pro	Leu	Tyr	Leu	Tyr	Leu	Pro
		Pro	Val		Asp	Trp	
					Arg		
					Leu		
% mutations in RifR strains[b]			10		35	45	

[a] *Escherichia coli* numbering
[b] RifR, resistance to rifampin.

substitutions are generally associated with a high level of resistance (MIC of approximately 16 µg/ml). Other mutations, located in sequences which regulate the expression of arabinosyltransferases and lead to their overexpression, are found in strains with low-level resistance (MIC < 8 µg/ml).

Fluoroquinolones

Fluoroquinolones (FQ) inhibit type II topoisomerases which mediate DNA topology. M. tuberculosis is distinguished by its single topoisomerase, DNA gyrase, composed of two subunits, GyrA and GyrB.

Acquired resistance to FQ is, in the vast majority of cases (90%), due to a modification in DNA gyrase caused by a mutation in the *gyrA* gene. These mutations are analogous to those described in E. coli and mainly target positions 83 and 87 (E. coli numbering), defining a domain known as Quinolone Resistance Determining Region (QRDR). Mutations in position 87 (Asp) are more common (>70% of cases) and more diverse (AspGly or His or Asn or Tyr or Ala) than those in codon 83 (AlaVal). Other mutations, less frequent, can be encountered in other positions. Mutations in the *gyrB* gene (position 464) are much less common.

Aminoglycosides and related antibiotics

In mycobacteria, acquired resistance to aminoglycosides, which act at the level of protein synthesis, is most often related to target modifications. These modifications occur either in ribosomal proteins or in ribosomal RNA.

Streptomycin

Streptomycin (SM) resistance is most often (55% of cases) related to mutations in the *rpsL* gene encoding ribosomal protein S12 ($Lys_{43}Arg$ and $Lys_{88}Glu$) conferring a high-level resistance (MIC > 1000 µg/ml). Less frequently (15% of cases), it is associated with mutations in the *rrs* gene encoding 16S rRNA in loops 530 and 915. Recently, mutations in the *gidB* gene, encoding a 16S rRNA-specific methyltransferase, were shown to confer low-level resistance (16). In approximately 30% of SM-resistant strains, most of which have low-level resistance (MIC between 4 and 1000 µg/ml), the mechanism of resistance is unknown. There is no cross-resistance to kanamycin and amikacin.

Kanamycin and amikacin

Strains that are resistant to kanamycin (K) are usually cross-resistant to amikacin (AMK). Resistance to both aminoglycosides is almost always observed in multiresistant strains, and in particular resistant to streptomycin, because the former are only used after failure of the first-line treatment.

Resistance is thought to be most often linked to a mutation in the *rrs* gene, usually $A_{1401}G$ or $G_{1484}T$, which would confer high-level resistance to both aminoglycosides (MIC > 64 µg/ml) as well as resistance to capreomycin (CAP), a macrocyclic peptide related to aminoglycosides (13). Some strains resistant to K but sensitive to AMK have been described. These strains may or may not be resistant to CAP, and their *rrs* gene may or may not be mutated ($C_{517}T$ or $C_{1402}T$).

Capreomycin

Besides the mechanisms described above, resistance to CAP might also be associated to a mutation in the *tlyA* gene, encoding an rRNA methyltransferase.

Studies focusing on mutations involved in K, AMK, and CAP resistance are still too few to evaluate the relative rank of each mechanism.

Ethionamide and thiacetazone

Ethionamide (ETH) is a structural analog of INH and, likewise, acts at the level of mycolic acid synthesis. Partial cross-resistance between INH and ETH has been known for a long time (see above) and mutations in the *inhA* gene or its promoter are clearly associated with double resistance to both molecules. ETH is also structurally close to another antituberculous drug, thiacetazone, which has been used extensively, and cross-resistance between these two molecules is frequent. ETH, like INH, is a prodrug. Its activator is the EthA protein, a monooxygenase under the control of the EthR regulatory protein. The active molecule acts on the ETH target, which is also a target of INH, and is encoded by the *inhA* gene. Mutations in the *ethA* and/or its regulator *ethR* were described in some ETH-resistant strains. These mutations are scattered in the gene, with no preferential localization. Almost half are associated with mutations in the *inhA* gene or its promoter. Mutations in *ethA* have also been described in thiacetazone-resistant strains. Mutations in the *mshA* gene, encoding the first enzyme in mycothiol biosynthesis (a thiol important in the maintenance of the intracellular environment), may constitute another mechanism of ETH resistance which would not lead to INH resistance (21).

Molecular studies on ETH resistance are only beginning; therefore it is not yet possible to evaluate the frequency of the various mutations and their combinations among ETH- and INH-resistant strains. Moreover, 90% of the ethionamide-resistant strains are also resistant to INH due to mutation in the *katG* gene. This complicates any interpretation and might explain the double resistance to ETH and to INH (at high concentrations) that is often seen in multiresistant strains.

Para-amino-salicylic acid (PAS) and cycloserine

The modes of action of PAS and cycloserine in *M. tuberculosis* are poorly known, and the resistance mechanisms have not yet been identified.

PAS is thought to act on folate synthesis. Mutations in the *thyA* gene encoding thymidylate synthase, an enzyme which regulates folate levels in the cell, were described in PAS-resistant strains. They appear to be responsible for less than 40% of the resistant strains.

Cycloserine seems to act on two enzymes involved in peptidoglycan synthesis, D-alanine racemase (Alr) and D-alanine:D-alanine ligase (Ddl). Mutations in the corresponding *alr* and *ddl* genes might be implicated in resistance.

Selection of resistant mutants

In the early days of streptomycin use (1944), it became apparent that selection of resistant mutants during treatment of pulmonary tuberculosis was a major cause of failure, which could only be avoided by combining several active antibiotics. This is the principle of polychemotherapy, which became the rule for treating tuberculosis and other mycobacterial infections. Selection of resistant mutants occurred again and again during the first utilizations of each antituberculous drug in monotherapy: isoniazid, rifampin, ofloxacin. Acquired resistance to antibiotics in tuberculosis bacilli is always linked to mutations in chromosomal genes and is not transferable. No resistance plasmids or transposons have been described in *M. tuberculosis*.

In a wild-type population of *M. tuberculosis*, there is spontaneous occurrence of a few mutant bacilli which are resistant to each antituberculous drug. The proportion of resistant mutants within strains that are considered "normal" or "wild type" ranges from $1/10^5$ for isoniazid to $1/10^7$ for rifampin and ofloxacin (Table 4). This means that, before treatment, in the midst of a tuberculous cavity containing 10^8 bacilli, there are at least 1000 isoniazid-resistant bacilli and 10 rifampin-resistant bacilli. Since each mutation arises independently, the proportion of double mutants equals the product of the proportions for each mutant separately. Thus, the probability for a bacillus to be doubly resistant to isoniazid and rifampin, $1/10^5 \times 1/10^7 = 1/10^{12}$, makes this event nearly impossible. This is the reason why combining both antibiotics pre-

Table 4. Proportion method: maximal proportion of antibiotic-resistant mutants for wild-type strains of *M. tuberculosis* and critical proportions.

Antibiotic	Concentration (µg/ml) L. Jensen medium	Maximal proportion of resistant mutants	Critical proportion (%)
Isoniazid	0.2	10^{-5}	1
Rifampin	40	10^{-7}	1
Ethambutol	2	10^{-6}	1
Pyrazinamide	200	-	10
Streptomycin	4	10^{-6}	1
Kanamycin	20	10^{-6}	10
Capreomycin	20	-	10
Thioamides	20	10^{-3}	10
Ofloxacin[a]	2	10^{-7}	1
Cycloserine	30	10^{-2}	10
PAS	0.5	10^{-5}	1

[a] Result valid for other fluoroquinolones (levofloxacin, moxifloxacin).

vents the selection of mutants resistant to each. In the forms of tuberculosis that are poor in bacilli (tuberculous meningitis, primary infection), the probability that resistant mutants are present is much lower and the risk of treatment failure due to selection is minimal. In strains that are resistant to several antituberculous drugs, each resistance is acquired independently; resistance is most often acquired successively, following the antibiotics used for treatment.

Determination of susceptibility to antituberculous drugs

Objectives

Determination of susceptibility to antituberculous drugs has two objectives: individual and collective.

The first objective, individual, is to determine for each case (especially in cases of relapse and treatment failure) if the strain is susceptible to first-line antituberculous drugs. Nowadays, migratory fluxes from countries with high rates of resistance justify to perform an antibiogram for each case of tuberculosis, even for new cases in industrialized countries.

The second objective, collective, is to monitor resistance in tuberculosis bacilli at the national level. Monitoring resistance in patients without prior treatment (known as primary resistance) is essential, since the results inform on the choice of drug combinations which constitute the standard recommended treatment for all new cases of tuberculosis. Monitoring resistance in patients presenting with relapse or treatment failure (known as secondary or acquired resistance) is important, since it can be used to gauge the quality of care for tuberculosis patients.

Antibiotics to be studied

For a first attack of tuberculosis, susceptibility to antibiotics which constitute the standard first-line treatment (isoniazid, rifampin, ethambutol) is determined. Susceptibility to pyrazinamide, fourth antibiotic in the standard treatment, is not evaluated initially because the tests are very difficult to perform and can lead to interpretation errors (false resistance).

For relapses, especially in patients who have undergone several relapses and are at risk for multidrug resistance, it is also necessary to evaluate susceptibility to second-line antituberculous drugs (24), in particular to fluoroquinolones, aminoglycosides and related drugs, but also to thioamides, PAS, cycloserine, and possibly new antibiotics (linezolid). It is then critical to send the strain to a specialized laboratory with the required experience to prepare media which are not commercially available and perform result interpretation, which is often difficult.

Methods

The most widely used methods for susceptibility assays are phenotypic (antibiogram). The reference method is the proportion method on solid medium. Methods of absolute concentration (determination of the minimum inhibitory concentration which inhibit its growth) and resistance ratio (calculation of the ratio of the MIC of the tested strain to the MIC of a typically susceptible reference strain) are only used in some countries (UK, Russia and others).

For faster results, the proportion method was adapted to liquid media. Other phenotypic methods, simpler to implement and less costly, have been developed for the same goal.

In certain cases, genotypic methods are used. These methods are becoming more common in mycobacteriology laboratories.

Proportion method on solid media

Principle

The proportion method was developed in the late 50's to investigate susceptibility to isoniazid, streptomycin, PAS, kanamycin, and ethionamide (5). This method is based on the systematic bacteriological and clinical confrontation of hundreds of observations concerning treatment, failures, and new cases. Its aim is to identify bacillus strains which have become completely resistant and those which are obviously no longer "wild type" without being completely resistant. To this end, the proportion of resistant mutants within the strain is measured as accurately as possible and compared to a so-called "critical" proportion, marking a threshold above which the process of mutant selection is considered activated and indicating an increased risk for treatment failure. The strain is deemed resistant if the proportion of resistant colonies is equal to or greater than the critical population.

This critical proportion, which takes into account variations in wild-type strains and inherent to the technique, has been set much higher than the average frequency of resistant mutants in wild-type strains (50 to 2000 x as high). For ease of use, the critical population was set to a simple number: 1% for antibiotics with rapid mutant selection, and 10% for other antibiotics (Table 4).

Antibiotics are incorporated in the culture medium at a given "critical" concentration. Critical concentrations were selected to be low enough for the detection of low-level resistant strains but high enough to escape variations in susceptibility of susceptible strains and variations linked to the technique. Critical concentrations are consistent with resistance levels for strains found in patients undergoing treatment failure. They vary depending on the solid medium used (Löwenstein-Jensen medium or Middlebrook agar). When Löwenstein-Jensen medium is used, the antibiotic is added before coagulation. Partial destruction of some antibiotics at the coagulation temperature (85°F) must be taken into account. The concentrations that are said to be critical are those obtained before coagulation. Their choice is difficult, and some modifications have recently been implemented (24) (Table 4). For thermolabile antibiotics, critical concentrations are much higher than final concentrations after coagulation. Thus, for rifampin this concentration is 40 μg/ml before coagulation and 2 μg/ml after coagulation.

When performed rigorously, this method gives good results, which are reliable and reproducible. For this, three conditions must imperatively be met. The first is to use a viable and homogeneous suspension of bacilli in order to inoculate the same number in tubes with and without antibiotics, therefore allowing the determination of the proportion of resistant bacilli within the population. A homogeneous suspension is not easy to achieve due to the strong propensity of tubercle bacilli to form aggregates in culture. The second condition is to seed several different inocula, so that a satisfactory inoculum is obtained in the end, considering the intra- and inter-strain variations in viability (the inoculum should be dense enough to be able to assert that a strain is susceptible, but not too dense to be able to assert that a strain is resistant). Experience showed that, to obtain such an inoculum with all strains, three dilutions need to be seeded (with the exception of a few highly dysgonic strains: *M. africanum* or *M. bovis* strains, or multidrug-resistant *M. tuberculosis* strains). Finally, the third condition is to avoid the "reseeding" phenomenon, which leads to an overestimate of the number of colonies. To this end, it is important to allow the seeded suspensions to evaporate completely.

Implementation

The implementation of this method on Löwenstein-Jensen medium is described in detail in a seminal article from Canetti *et al.* (5). The commercial availability of kits (Bio-Rad, Becton Dickinson, Trek Diagnostics…) to test susceptibility to antibiotics used in the standard treatment facilitates the assay. Briefly, the greatest possible numbers of colonies (mature colonies but not older than 6 - 8 weeks) of the culture under study (preferably a primary culture) are sampled and placed in a sterile flask containing about thirty 5-mm glass beads. The flask is shaken for 30 s (dry) to obtain a homogeneous suspension, then 5 ml of distilled water are added and the flask is shaken again. The bacillus suspension is then transferred to a test tube and its opacity is adjusted with distilled water to that of a standard bacillus suspension with a titer of 1 mg/ml bacilli (equivalent to Mac Farland 3). Serial 10-fold dilutions are prepared from the pure suspension down to 10^{-5} mg/ml.

In order to provide enumerable colonies after culture (fewer than 100) both on positive control tubes and tubes with antibiotics for determining the proportion of resistant colonies, each of the 10^{-1}, 10^{-3} and 10^{-5} mg/ml dilutions is inoculated on two Löwenstein-Jensen tubes without antibiotics and one tube with antibiotics, using 0.2 ml/tube. After inoculation, the tubes are placed in an oven (with the cap slightly loosened), tilted so that the liquid covers the whole surface of the medium without reaching the cap to maximize evaporation. Tubes are retrieved and closed when all the liquid has evaporated.

Reading is performed on the 28th then on the 42nd day of incubation. Colonies in control tubes and in tubes with antibiotic are carefully enumerated (including the smallest ones). The proportion of resistant mutants is calculated by dividing the number of colonies in the tubes with antibiotic by the average number of colonies in the control tubes (Fig. 1 and 2). The strain is said to be susceptible if the proportion of resistant mutants is lower than the critical proportion, and resistant if it is equal to

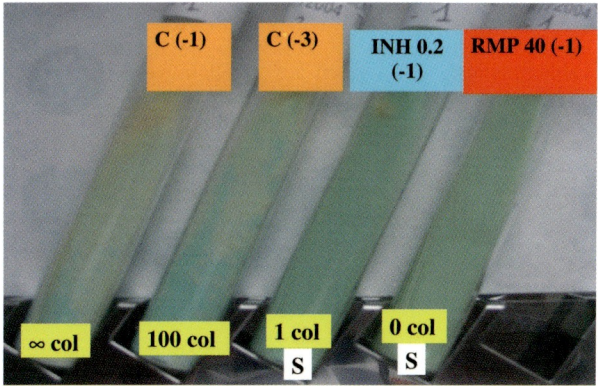

Fig. 1. Antibiogram by the proportion method. *M. tuberculosis* strain susceptible to isoniazid and rifampin. C, controls; t-1 and –3, dilutions.

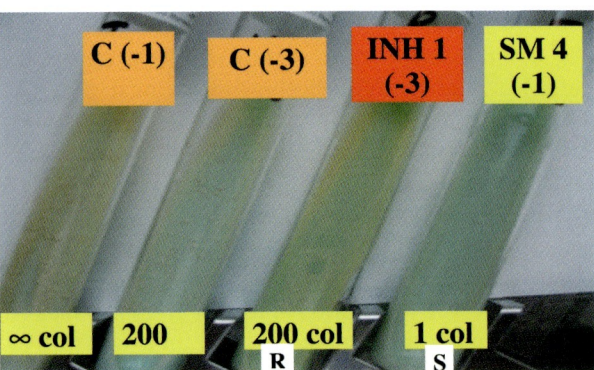

Fig. 2. Antibiogram by the proportion method. *M. tuberculosis* strain resistant to isoniazid and susceptible to streptomycin. C, controls; -1 and –3, dilutions.

or greater than the critical proportion.

Reading of results

When colonies are well-developed in control tubes and are sufficiently numerous (at least 10 in control tubes at the 10^{-5} mg/ml dilution), which is usually the case, the results can be given as early as on the 28th day of incubation. In other cases, when the strain is dysgonic or the number of colonies in control tubes is still too low, the results cannot be read until the 42nd day. The method was optimized for a definitive classification of susceptible and resistant strains after 42 days of incubation. Therefore, the results obtained at day 42 of incubation supersede those obtained at day 28.

When agar medium is used, the reading must be done after 28 days of incubation at the latest (22).

"Direct" antibiogram

Results can be obtained at the same time as the culture if the antibiogram is made from the specimen (this is known as a "direct" antibiogram). To make it likely for the direct antibiogram results to be interpretable, the specimen must be rich enough in bacilli so that a sufficient number of colonies is obtained. The specimen amount must also be large enough to inoculate all the tubes for the chosen battery of tests (see above). In actual practice, there must be more than one acid-alcohol-fast bacillus per microscope field (25 x objective) using a fluorescence microscope. The specimen is prepared as for a culture (decontamination and neutralization). Dilutions to be prepared for inoculation (and thus the specimen volume needed) depend on the bacillus density in the sample (Table 5). Tube preparation, inoculation, and reading methods are identical to the indirect test.

Special case of Pyrazinamide

Pyrazinamide is only active in acid medium, therefore the susceptibility test must be performed at acid pH (pH 5.5). At this pH, strains develop 10 to 100-fold less efficiently than at neutral pH and the results are often difficult to interpret (22). Some strains develop so poorly as to make the test invalid. Conversely, development at acid pH is sometimes identical to, or even greater than at neutral pH. In this case, it can be suspected that the pH might not be acidic enough and that, in the case of an apparent resistance, the test may be invalid.

Performance

This method gives excellent results for isoniazid and rifampin susceptibility tests, with almost 100% efficiency and reproducibility. Results are slightly less favorable with ethambutol and in particular with streptomycin (92% efficacy and 95 reproducibility). Studies led by the WHO and the International Union Against Tuberculosis (IUAT) indicated that regular implementation of external quality controls markedly improved results (11).

It is difficult to appraise the performance for second-line antituberculous drugs, because these tests are imperfectly standardized (24) and no external quality controls are used. For thermolabile

Table 5. Dilutions to perform for inoculation of a direct antibiogram for *M. tuberculosis*

No. visible AFB by microscopic examination [a]		Dilution to inoculate		Volume of sample needed[b]
Ziehl-Neelsen objective x 100	Fluorescence objective x 25	Control tubes	Tubes with antibiotic	
Less than 1 in 10 fields	< 1 per field	Do not proceed	Do not proceed	-
1 to 10 in 10 fields	1 to 9 per field	Pure and 10^{-2}	Pure and 10^{-2}	4 ml
1 to 10 per field	10 to 99 per field	Pure 10^{-2}, and 10^{-3}	Pure and 10^{-2}	4 ml
> 10 per field	> 100 per field	10^{-1} and 10^{-3}	10^{-1} and 10^{-3}	1.5 ml

[a] AFB, acid-alcohol resistant bacilli.

[b] After fluidification/decontamination to perform a standard first-line antibiogram.

antibiotics (cycloserine and thioamides), there is an important risk of false resistants.

Results of the susceptibility test for pyrazinamide are not satisfactory (see above). However, since pyrazinamide-monoresistant strains are extremely rare, this test is not essential in case of susceptibility to the other first line antituberculous drugs.

Antibiogram in liquid medium

Like the proportion method, the antibiogram in liquid medium is designed to estimate the proportion of resistant mutants within a strain of tubercle bacilli.

The media used, derived from Middlebrook medium, are commercially available as tubes (Mycobacterial Growth Indicator Tube or MGIT, Becton-Dickinson) or bottles (Bactec 460, Becton Dickinson; Versa TREK System, TREK Diagnostic System). MGIT tubes are processed manually or adapted to the automated Bactec 960 system. Versa TREK Myco bottles are used with an automated system. Bactec 460 bottles, containing radioactive carbon, are nowadays rarely used.

Necessary reagents are commercially available as kits containing isoniazid, rifampin, and ethambutol, with (BBL MGIT AST SIRE, Becton-Dickinson) or without (Versa TREK Myco Susceptibility Kit) streptomycin. The BacT/Alert SIRE Kit (bioMérieux) is no longer commercially available. Bactec MGIT 960 PZA and Versa TREK Myco PZA kits are dedicated to pyrazinamide susceptibility tests. The antibiogram in liquid media is currently being adapted for measuring susceptibility to 2nd-line antituberculous drugs (12).

Growth detection is based on various physico-chemical principles. In MGIT tubes, oxygen consumption leads to the appearance of fluorescence from a compound immobilized in silicone at the bottom of the tube (Fig. 3). In the Versa Trek System, bacterial metabolism results in a change of pressure within the bottle. In the Bactec 460 system, growth detection relies on the measurement of C^{14} released in the bottle's atmosphere.

Growth detection occurs more rapidly in liquid media than in solid media. The results of antibiograms in liquid media can be obtained in 8 to 10 days.

Principle

This method is based on determining the growth delay in liquid medium containing antibiotics compared to control media without antibiotics. With MGIT tubes, the control medium (without antibiotic) is inoculated with 100 times fewer bacilli than in media with antibiotics. If growth is detected in the antibiotic-containing tube as early as in the control tube, that means there were at least as many bacilli able to multiply (i.e., resistant to the antibiotic) as in the control tube. This corresponds to (at least) the 1% critical proportion discussed above. Antibiotic concentrations have been adapted to liquid medium. In general, they are lower than those for solid medium (Table 6).

Implementation

Procedures are carried out following the manufacturer's instructions. Briefly, an antibiogram is performed from a culture in liquid medium (kept in the incubator for a minimum of 24 h and a maximum of 5 days after the positive growth signal) or from colonies developed in solid medium (with or without prior inoculation in liquid medium). The strain is resuspended, calibrated, and inoculated in a volume of 0.5 ml in tubes containing antibiotics and in the control tube.

The antibiotics provided in the kits are reconstituted and added in volumes of 0.1 or 0.5 ml per tube, depending on the system. Media are placed in the corresponding incubator.

Reading and interpretation of results

With the Bactec 460 (semi-automated) system, the growth index is measured daily in the control bottles and in antibiotic-containing bottles. With "manual" MGIT tubes, a UV lamp is used to search for fluorescence, indicating O_2 consumption, daily starting on the 3rd day after inoculation. The strain is considered resistant to an antibiotic if

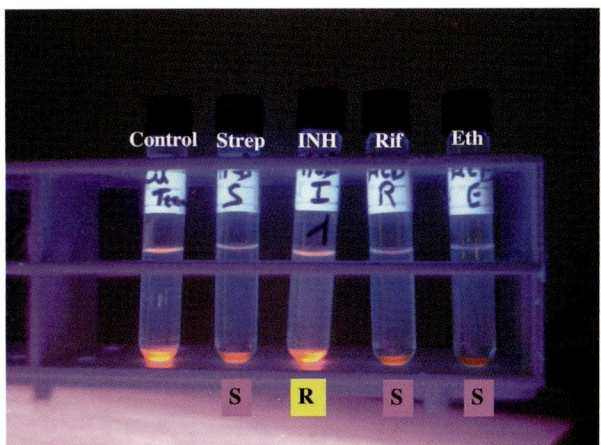

Fig. 3. Antibiogram in MGIT liquid medium. *M. tuberculosis* strain resistant to isoniazid and susceptible to rifampin, ethambutol, and streptomycin. R, resistant, fluorescent pellet; S, susceptible.

Table 6. Antibiotic concentrations (µg/ml) used for antibiogram in liquid medium

Antibiotic	MGIT AST SIRE (manual)	BACTEC MGIT 960 SIRE[a]	Versa TREK
Isoniazid	0.1	0.1	0.1
Rifampin	1	1	1
Ethambutol	3.5	5	5
Streptomycin	0.8	1	1
Pyrazinamide	100	100	ND[b]

[a] In case of resistance, confirm with a second test with higher antibiotic concentrations: isoniazid, 0.4 µg/ml; ethambutol, 7.5 µg/ml (Bactec 960) or 8 µg/ml (Versa Trek); streptomycin, 4 µg/ml.
[b] ND, not determined.

the antibiotic-containing tube is positive at the same time as the control tube or within two days following positivity in the control tube. The strain is considered susceptible if the antibiotic-containing tube remains negative or if it becomes positive over 48 h after the control tube.

With the Bactec 960 and Versa Trek systems, readings are taken almost continually by the automated detection system. The Bactec 960 system, which includes an Antibiotic Susceptibility Testing (AST) module, provides an interpretation of the results. With the Versa Trek system, the strain is considered susceptible if the antibiotic-containing bottle remains negative or becomes positive more than 72 h after the control bottles. The strain is said to be resistant if the antibiotic-containing bottle is positive at the same time as the control tube or within the next 72 h.

If controls are not positive by 15 days following the inoculation, the test is invalid; on the other hand, if one of the tubes or vials is positive within two days, a contamination must be suspected.

Performance

The antibiogram in liquid medium can be used to measure sensitivity to first-line antibiotics. Kits for second-line antibiotics are under development.

The obvious advantage of the antibiogram in liquid medium over the proportion method on solid medium is the time to response: results are obtained in 8 to 10 days instead of 28 to 42 days, making it attractive. The antibiogram in liquid medium is easier to implement than the proportion method, since it only requires the preparation of two separate inocula of the strain instead of three, and the inoculation of six tubes or bottles instead of eighteen.

Evaluation of the results obtained with the antibiogram in liquid medium (18) demonstrated a good concordance (over 97%) with those of the reference method (Table 7). Concordance is higher for manual MGIT and Bactec 960 than for Versa TREK system, with which numerous false-resistant results are seen with isoniazid. Concordance is excellent for rifampin (99.9%) which, conversely, presents very few false-resistant results. One must note that, for all four antibiotics, false-susceptible results are seen which are responsible for so-called "major" errors (1.5 to 2.5% for isoniazid and rifampin, 5 to 8% for streptomycin and ethambutol).

The Bactec 460 system has been widely used for a long time to determine susceptibility to first-line antituberculous drugs and provided very reliable results. However, due to the requirements for manipulating carbon-14, it is being supplanted by non-radioactive systems.

Due to the high risk of contamination inherent to liquid medium and the presence of antibiotic in media which may interfere with antituberculous activity, manufacturers do not recommend performing direct antibiograms in liquid media.

Other phenotypic methods

Several phenotypic methods, which are rapid, simpler to implement and much less costly than the antibiogram in liquid media, have been developed (6, 17) but are not widely used. The detection of growth is based on the utilization of a colored marker (for oxidoreduction, such as Alamar Blue, or for nitrate reduction) or on phage replication in viable cells. The FASTPlaque-Response kit (Biotec, Ipswich, UK), using phage replication, is commercially available for susceptibility testing to rifampin. Results are obtained quickly but there may be numerous false-resistant results.

Genotypic methods

Using phenotypic methods, in spite of the development of liquid media, results are obtained at best within two to four weeks after sampling,

Table 7. Sensitivity and specificity of antituberculous drug resistance detection by antibiogram in liquid medium (from published literature)

Antibiogram	Sensitivity[a]				Specificity[a]				Total concordances (%)
	INH[b] (0.1)[c]	RMP (1)	SM (1**)	EMB (5)	INH (0.1)	RMP (1)	SM (1[d])	EMB (5[d])	
MGIT manual [e]	108/111 (97.3%)	73/77 (94.8%)	68/72 (94.4%)	40/43 (93%)	196/196 (100%)	231/231 (100%)	157/167 (94%)	190/196 (96.9%)	1063/1093 (97.2%)
Bactec 960 [f]	109/109 (100%)	77/78 (98.7%)	74/78 (94.9%)	64/70 (91.4%)	203/212 (95.7%)	563/564 (99.8%)	332/343 (96.8%)	564/573 (98.3%)	1986/2027 (97.9%)
Versa TREK [f]	146/148 (98.6%)	47/47 (100%)	ND [g]		217/261 (83.3%)	362/362 (100%)	ND		772/818 (94.4%)
Total	363/368 (98.6%)	197/202 (97.5%)	142/150 (94.7%)	104/113 (92%)	616/669 (92.1%)	1156/1157 (99.9%)	489/510 (95.9%)	760/769 (98.8%)	3821/3928 (97.3%)

[a] For detection of resistance, sensitivity = resistant strain when the result is "resistant"; specificity = sensitive strain when the result is "resistant".
[b] EMB, ethambutol; INH, isoniazid; RMP, rifampin; SM, streptomycin.
[c] ( ), Final antibiotic concentration in µg/ml
[d] SM: 0.8 µg/ml and EMB: 3.5 µg/ml in manual MGIT
[e] Walters et al. (1996), Bergmann et al. (1997), Palomino et al. (1999), Palaci et al. (1996), Cambau et al. (2000).
[f] Piersimoni et al. (2006).
[g] ND, not determined.

due to the time necessary to grow bacilli in primary culture then in subculture. Molecular biology techniques offering the possibility of much faster results are thus actively considered.

Applicable antibiotics

The interest in molecular detection of resistance varies from one antituberculous drug to another, due to several factors. The essential factor is the state of current knowledge on resistance genes as well as the percentage of resistant strains where causal mutations have been identified. For a given antibiotic, this percentage will condition, for the most part, the sensitivity of the molecular detection of resistance. The number of genes involved in resistance and their size must also be taken into account for detection to be technically feasible. Finally, the therapeutic impact of resistance and difficulties encountered with the phenotypic test must be considered.

An evaluation of these various factors led to the development, in a first phase, of a molecular detection method for rifampin resistance (Table 8). This antibiotic is the best marker of multidrug resistance, and more than 95% of resistant strains present a mutation within a single gene, *rpoB*, more specifically in a small portion of this gene (Table 3). Molecular detection of isoniazid resistance, more difficult due to the large number of implicated genes, is more recent. Its implementation was markedly simplified and its performance improved with the commercial availability of the Genotype MTBDR*plus* kit, which detects nearly 90% of the causal mutations. Molecular research concerning fluoroquinolone resistance is promising, because these antibiotics are essential in case of multidrug resistance; additionally, more than 95% of resistant strains carry a mutation in a small fragment of two genes, *gyrA* and *gyrB*. Finally, sequencing the *pncA* gene for the detection of pyrazinamide resistance is attractive, because this antibiotic is essential in case of multidrug resistance, and the interpretation of the phenotypic antibiogram presents major challenges. However, exploiting the *pncA* gene sequence is difficult since there is a very large diversity in the itemized mutations and the phenotypic consequences of the mutations is not always clear.

Methods

Mutations can be identified by determining the nucleotide sequence of the amplified gene fragment or by hybridization with specific oligonucleotide probes using test strips. DNA sequencing,

Table 8. Genotypic detection of resistance in *M. tuberculosis*.

Antibiotic	% R strains with a known mutation	Number of known genes involved	Therapeutic impact	Difficulty in phenotypic methods	Priority
Isoniazid	75 à 95[a]	2	++	0	2
Rifampin	> 95	1	++++[b]	0	1
Pyrazinamide	ND[c]	1	++	++++	3
Ethambutol	50	1	+/-	+/-	
Streptomycin	70	2	+	0	
Kanamycin/Amikacin	ND	1	+	+/-	
Fluoroquinolones	> 95	2	++	+	4
Thioamides	75	2	++	+++	

[a] Depending on the study.
[b] Multidrug resistance marker.
[c] ND, cannot be determined in the current state of knowledge.

widely used in molecular biology, is now accessible to bacteriology laboratories familiar with molecular biology techniques, thanks to the advent of robots (automated sequencer) and sequence analysis software (Sescape). The hybridization technique consists in amplifying, labeling, and hybridizing a gene fragment to probes immobilized on a strip (Fig. 4). Hybrids are revealed by the development of a color. Some of the probes are specific for the wild-type allele sequence (without mutation) and the others are specific for resistant allele sequences (comprising the most frequently described mutations in resistant strains). With biochips, the amplified DNA can be hybridized to several tens of thousands of oligonucleotides grafted on a very small surface, which makes it possible to search for a great number of mutations simultaneously. This attractive method (20) will not be described, because it is not yet used in laboratories, even specialized, due to the lack of commercial materials and reagents.

Strip hybridization

The assay is performed according to the manufacturer's recommendations. Briefly, it involves the following steps: the strain to be studied is suspended in sterile water, then heat-inactivated (20 min at 95°C). The target gene fragments are ampli-

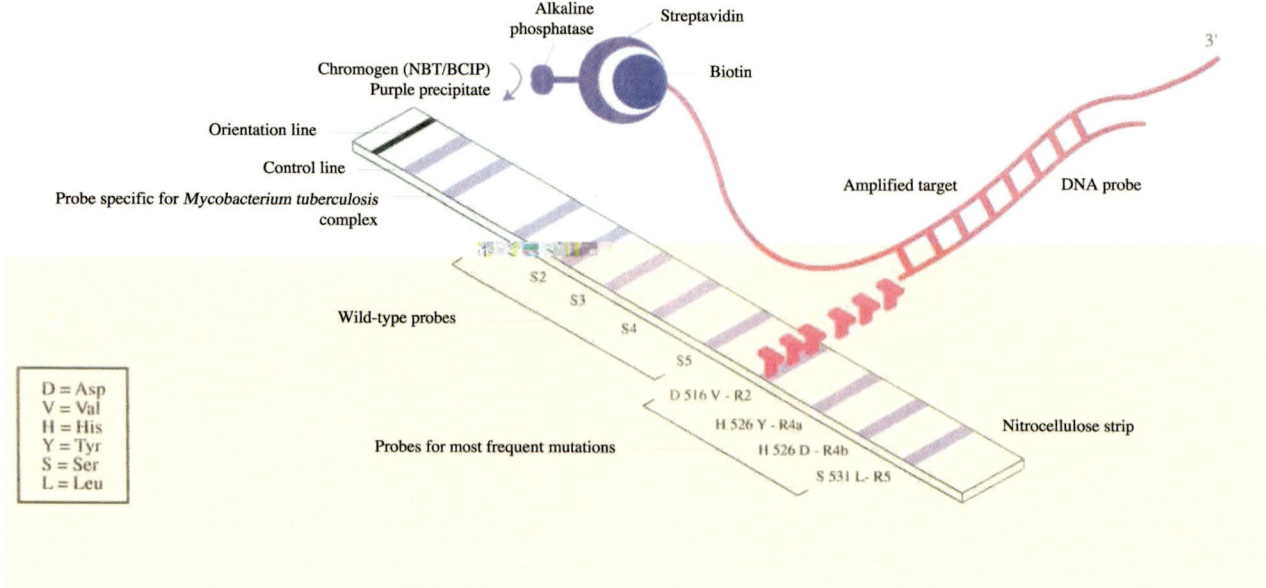

Fig. 4. Principle of the search for mutations in the *rpoB* gene by strip hybridization (example: the INNO-LiPA Rif.TB® strip).

fied with biotinylated primers, and the amplification products are denatured then hybridized to probes immobilized on the strip. Unbound fragments are removed by successive washes, and hybrids immobilized on the strip are then developed by a color reaction (brown-purple).

Reading of the results consists in detecting the color bands on the strip (Fig. 5). Two strips are commercially available: INNO-LiPA Rif.TB® (Innogenetics) and GenoType® MTBDR*plus* (Hain Science). They allow detection of mutations leading to rifampin resistance. The GenoType® MTBDR*plus* also detects isoniazid resistance.

The GenoType® MTBDR*plus* strip is designed to detect mutations in codons 506 to 533 of the *rpoB* gene, in codon 315 of the *katG* gene, as well as at positions -8, -15 and -16 of the regulator of the *inhA* gene. It contains a) probes specific for wild-type alleles of the *rpoB* gene, for position 315 of the *katG* gene and positions -8, -15 and -16 of the regulator of the *inhA* gene and b) probes specific for the most common causal mutations in rifampin resistance ($S_{531}L$, $H_{526}Y$, $H_{526}D$, and $D_{516}V$ in *rpoB*) and isoniazid resistance (two triplets leading to $S_{315}T$ mutation in *katG* and -15 CT, -16 AG, -8 TC, -8 TA in *inhA*). With this probe set, it is possible to determine if alleles are wild-type (sequence in susceptible strains) or if they are mutated. If the mutation is among the most frequent ones, it is identified by the strip. If it is not among them, its presence is indicated on the strip by the absence of hybridization with the corresponding wild-type probe, but its precise identification can only be obtained through sequencing of the corresponding gene.

A new strip, GenoType® MTBDRsl, was launched in 2009 for detecting fluoroquinolone, amikacin/capreomycin, and ethambutol resistance. It contains a) specific probes for wild-type alleles in codons 90, 91, and 94 of the *gyrA* gene (positions 83, 84, and 87 using *E. coli* numbering), of codons 1401, 1402, and 1484 of the *rrs* gene and codon 306 of the *embB* gene and b) probes specific for the most common causal mutations in fluoroquinolone, amikacin/capreomycin, and ethambutol resistance.

Performance

The strip hybridization technique is easy to implement with equipment that is now available in

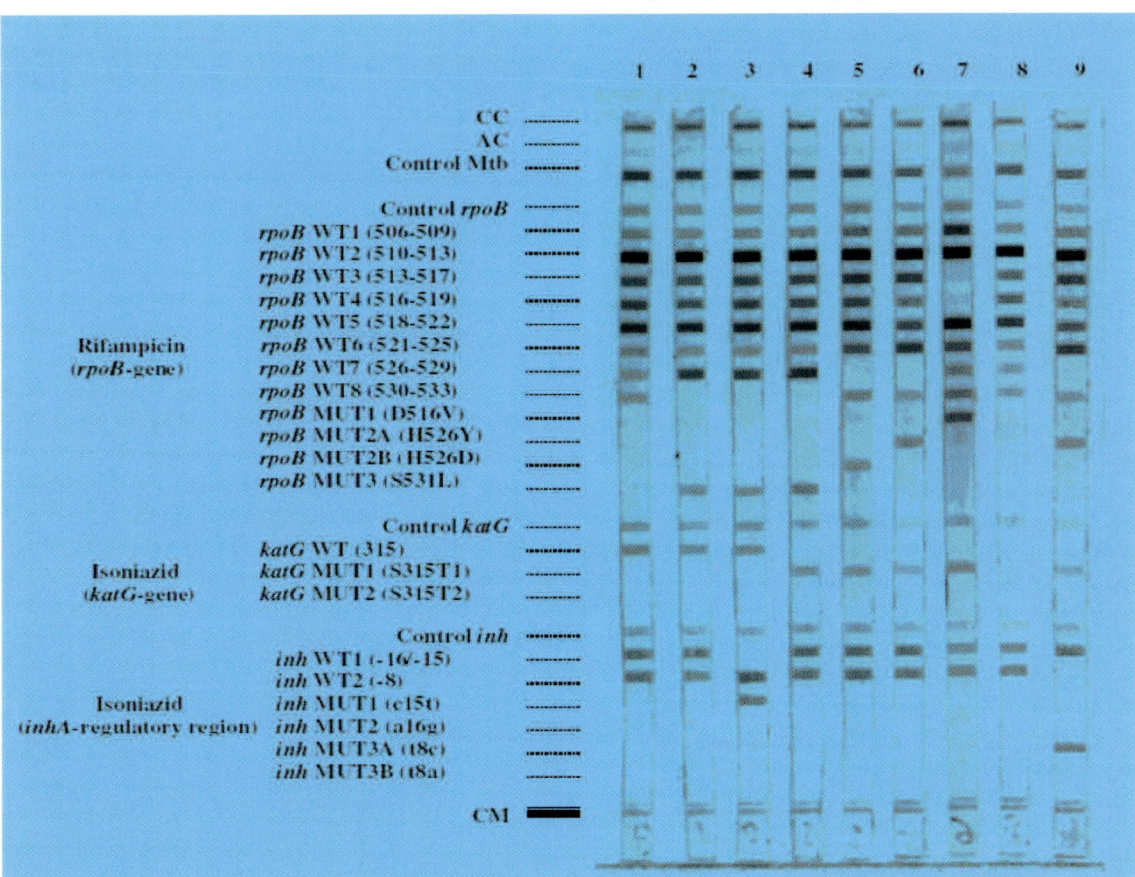

Fig. 5. Search for mutations in the *rpoB* and *katG* genes and in the *inh*A promoter by Genotype® MTBDR*plus* strip hybridization.

many bacteriology laboratories (thermocycler and shaking waterbath). In specialized laboratories, this technique can be partially automated (Hain GT-48 system). This method only takes a few hours (2 h for amplification and approximately 2 h for hybridization and detection). It can be directly applied to samples if they are rich in acid-alcohol-fast bacilli (positive microscope test). Bacilli observed under the microscope can thus be identified as belonging to the *M. tuberculosis* complex and the presence of mutations conferring rifampin resistance (and isoniazid resistance for Genotype MTBDR*plus*) within 48 to 72 h following the sampling, which is critical for the management of patients and their close contacts.

The INNO-LiPA Rif.TB®strip, which shows excellent performance but only detects rifampin resistance, was thus supplanted by Genotype® MTBDR*plus* which also detects isoniazid resistance.

The performance of the Genotype® MTBDR*plus* strip is very good, whether the technique is applied to cultures or directly to samples rich in bacilli (with positive microscopic examination) (Table 9). Sensitivity is very high (over 90%) for detecting rifampin resistance and high-level isoniazid resistance (3, 4, 8, 10, 14, 15). It is not as good for detecting low-level resistance to isoniazid, which impacts the overall sensitivity for detecting resistance to this antibiotic (from 73 to 97% depending on the study and the strain under consideration). When this technique is used for samples poor in bacilli (with negative microscopic examination) performance is much weaker.

A single evaluation of the GenoType® MTBDRsl strip has been published (9). The results are, as could be expected, good for fluoroquinolones (nearly 90% sensitivity) but much lower for amikacin (sensitivity: 75%) and insufficient for ethambutol (sensitivity: less than 40%).

Molecular detection of pyrazinamide resistance relies on sequencing the *pncA* gene. The evaluation of its performance is limited by difficulties in the phenotypic test. However, the absence of mutations seems to be correlated with pyrazinamide susceptibility.

Method selection

The method of choice to determine susceptibility depends on the case at hand.

Antibiogram

For a new case of tuberculosis in a patient coming from a region with low prevalence of primary resistance, the antibiogram in liquid medium is well suited, since the results are obtained rapidly (in 8 to 10 days) and the predictive value of susceptibility is good, or very good for the two major antibiotics (isoniazid and rifampin). Indeed, when primary resistance rates are lower than 1% for rifampin and ethambutol and around 5% for isoniazid, the negative predictive value (PV), *i.e.*, predictive of susceptibility when the method gives a "susceptible" result, is greater than 95% with manual MGIT and 98% with automated systems. The positive PV, (*i.e.*, predictive of resistance when the method gives a "resistant" result) is much weaker, in the order of 80, 50 and 30% in Bactec 960, for rifampin, isoniazid and ethambutol, respectively. For this reason, the manufacturer suggests to confirm "resistant" results with a test performed with higher antibiotic concentrations (Table 6) and the official guidelines suggest to proceed to a control using the reference method (6, 22).

For a case of tuberculosis relapse (elevated risk of secondary or acquired resistance) or a new case of tuberculosis in a patient coming from a region with high prevalence of primary resistance, the antibiogram in liquid medium presents an important risk of false susceptibility to isoniazid and rifampin, which may put the patient in jeopardy. In this case, the reference method should be preferred.

For all microscope-positive cases, the direct antibiogram on solid medium is the method of choice if the required conditions are met (see above).

Molecular biology

Molecular biology methods, attractive due to their rapidity, complement classical methods in the diagnostic workup of tuberculosis (Fig. 6), but their role must be carefully discussed. A search for mutations implicated in rifampin resistance could be useful if performed directly on respiratory secretion samples in the case of a positive microscopic examination (presence of acid-alcohol-resistant bacilli) when there is a high resistance risk, *i.e.* if the patient has already been treated for tuberculosis (particularly with multiple antecedents and poor patient compliance), is immunosuppressed, or comes from a region with high prevalence of multidrug resistance. The search for mutations can be performed during the culture step if it could not be carried out directly on the specimen.

The negative predictive value (predictive of a "no mutation" result) of molecular tests is very

Table 9. Performance of Genotype® MTBDRplus compared to phenotypic antibiogram

RIFAMPIN

	Authors	No. tested	No. valid tests [a]	No. with bacilli S	No. with bacilli R	Concordance (%)	Sensitivity (%)	Specificity (%)
Strains	Brossier et al. (France)	113	113	37	76	100	100	100
	Hillemann et al. (Germany)	125	125	50	75	99.2	98.7	100
	Lacoma et al. (Spain)	62	62	50	12	98.3	91.7	100
	Miotto et al. (Italy)	173	173	NR[e]	NR	NR	NR	NR
M + samples	Hillemann et al. (Germany)	72	71	40	31	98.6	96.8	100
	Lacoma et al. (Spain)	39	39	13	26	100	100	100
	Miotto et al. (Italy)	47	47	NR	NR	NR	NR	NR
	Barnard et al. (South Africa)	460	450	355	95	99.3	98.9	99.4

ISONIAZID

	Authors	No. tested	No. valid tests [a]	No. with bacilli S	No. with bacilli R(high level)	Concordance (%)	Sensitivity (%)	Specificity (%)
Strains	Brossier et al. (France)	113	113	18	95 (66)	88.5	86 [c]	100
	Hillemann et al. (Germany)	125	125	50	75 (71)	95.2	92	100
	Lacoma et al. (Spain)	62	62	14	48 (21)	79	73 [d]	100
	Miotto et al. (Italy)	173	173	0	173 (117)	79.2	79.2	NR
M + samples	Hillemann et al. (Germany)	72	71	30	41	94.4	90.2	100
	Lacoma et al. (Spain)	39	39	12	27	94.8	92.6 [f]	100
	Miotto et al. (Italy)	47	47	41	6	91.5	NR	NR
	Barnard et al. (South Africa)	460	450	330	120	98.2	94.2	99.7

[a] with amplification of the genes of interest.
[b] Concordance, results in agreement with antibiogram; Sensitivity and Specificity, sensitivity and specificity for detection of resistance.
[c] and [d]: 94% and 85.7% among highly resistant strains (MIC > 1 μg/ml).
[e] NR, not reported.
[f] Two false negatives from the same patient.

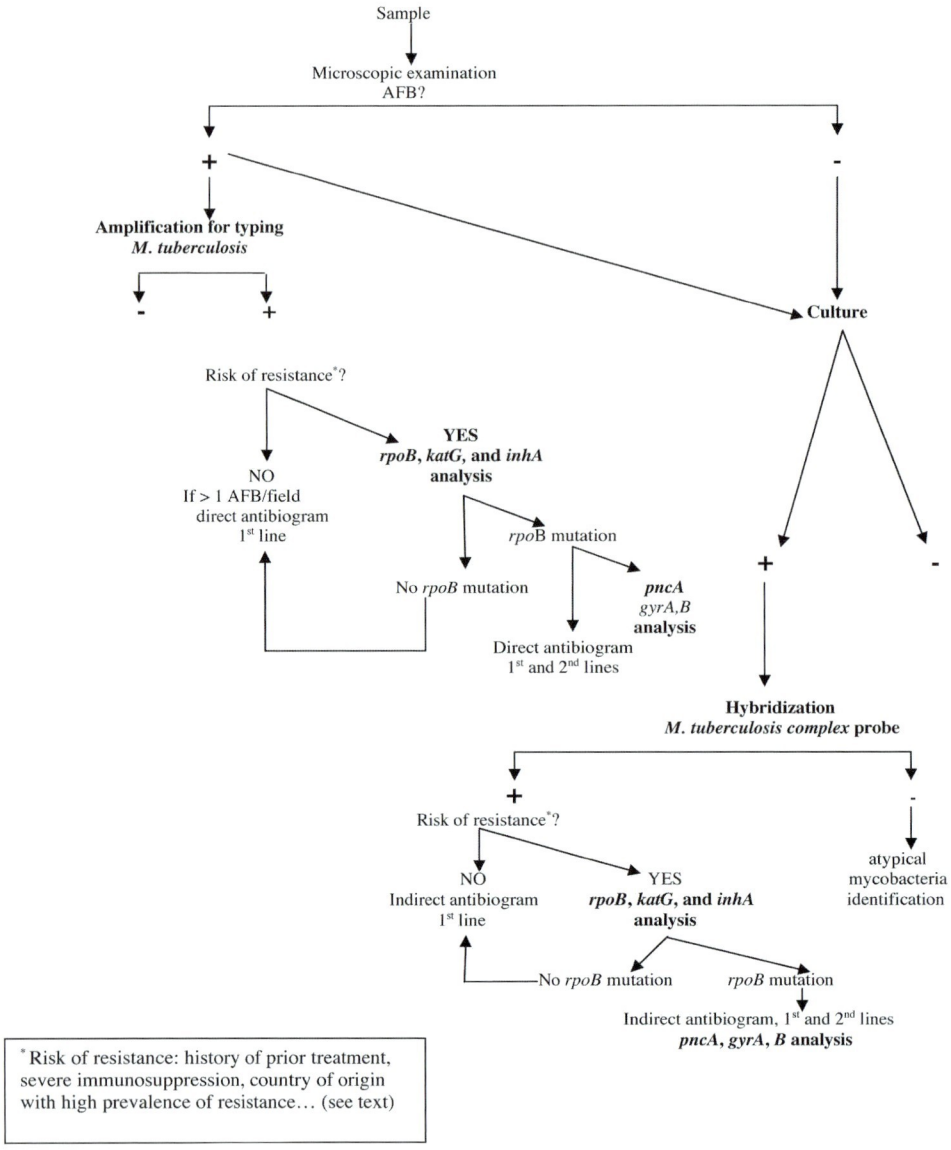

Fig. 6. Contribution of molecular biology to the bacteriological diagnostic of tuberculosis.

good for rifampin (≥ 95%). It is not as good for isoniazid (75 to 90%, depending on whether the test is performed on a patient from a region with high or low prevalence of resistance, respectively). The positive predictive value is very good for isoniazid and rifampin.

At the antibiogram step, molecular methods can be used to confirm rifampin resistance when it is not clearly expressed.

Detecting mutations in the *rpoB* gene makes it possible to quickly take appropriate steps for the patient and his close contacts (specific treatment for the patient, stricter isolation, monitoring of contacts) and to start the second-line antibiogram without delay. Of note, regardless of the step at which molecular methods are used to detect *rpoB* mutations, be it by sequencing or hybridization, the strain is simultaneously identified as belonging to the *M. tuberculosis* complex, which provides rapid confirmation of tuberculosis. This can be very important in certain situations, particularly in immunosuppressed patients which are susceptible to infections with atypical mycobacteria. This is due to the fact that the *rpoB* gene sequence is typical of the *M. tuberculosis* complex.

Detecting mutations in other genes involved in resistance (*pncA* for pyrazinamide, *gyrA* and perhaps *gyrB* for fluoroquinolones) is useful for confirmed multidrug resistance cases.

M. tuberculosis resistance in the world

Recent data on *M. tuberculosis* resistance in the world are provided by the World Health Organization and the International Union Against Tuberculosis and Lung Disease (23). These data are useful to appraise the risk of resistance to antibiotics in case of treatment failure (secondary resistance) and for new cases of tuberculosis (primary resistance) (Table 10).

The risk of resistance is much higher when the patient has received prior treatment with antituberculous drugs, stressing the importance of knowing the patient's history.

Acquired resistance

When treatment for tuberculosis is ill-conceived (*e.g.*, does not include several active antibiotics) or is not followed up regularly, it can result in the selection of resistant mutants. This is known as secondary resistance, or resistance that was "acquired" under treatment, and constitutes a hallmark of treatment failure.

Since the 1970s and the generalization of isoniazid (INH) and rifampin (RMP) use in treatment regimens for tuberculosis, therapeutic failure is less frequent and in most cases, when it occurs, bacilli remain susceptible to antibiotics. However, when resistance does occur, it frequently involves INH (nearly 30% of all cases worldwide, over 50% in Eastern Europe and up to 80% in Uzbekistan) and often INH together with the other major antituberculous drug, RMP (15% of all cases worldwide, over 30% in Eastern Europe). These cases of double resistance to INH and RMP, which are termed multidrug resistance cases, are reported in 45 countries (Table 11). Isolated resistance to RMP, without resistance to INH, is the exception (2% of cases worldwide).

Secondary resistance to streptomycin (SM) is high (20% of treatment failure cases worldwide). Resistance to ethambutol (EMB) is less frequent

Table 10. Average worldwide frequency (variance) of resistance to first-line antituberculous drugs in new cases of tuberculosis and cases with prior treatment (WHO estimates)

Resistance to	New cases (%)		Previously treated cases (%)		All cases (%)	
At least one antibiotic	17.0	(7.9[a] to 35.8[b])	35.0	(17.8[a] to 62.8[b])	20.0	(8.9[a] to 48.8[b])
Isoniazid	10.3	(5.2[a] to 25.6[b])	27.7	(13.9[a] to 52.2[b])	13.3	(6.2[a] to 38.3[b])
Rifampin	3.7	(1.1[a] to 11.4[b])	17.5	(6.7[c] to 40.9[b])	6.3	(1.9[a] to 24.7[b])
Streptomycin	10.9	(4.0[a] to 28.8[b])	20.1	(9.7[a] to 52.6[b])	12.6	(4.4[a] to 40.7[b])
Ethambutol	2.5	(0.7[a] to 10.4[b])	10.3	(3.5[c] to 31.2[b])	3.9	(1.0[a] to 19.7[b])
INH and RMP	2.9	(0.9[a] to 10.0[b])	15.3	(5.8[c] to 37.7[b])	5.3	(1.5[a] to 22.2[b])

[a] Western Europe.
[b] Eastern Europe.
[c] Africa.

Table 11. Estimated number and % of cases with multidrug resistant (MDR) tuberculosis among all cases, by WHO region (WHO report, 2008)

WHO region	Total No. cases	No. MDR cases	% MDR cases
Industrialized countries[a]	105,795	1,317	1.2
Central Europe	50,502	1,201	2.4
Eastern Europe	416,316	80,057	19.2
Latin America	349,278	12,070	3.5
Eastern Mediterranean	601,225	25,475	4.2
Africa (low HIV incidence)	375,801	8,415	2.2
Africa (high HIV incidence)	2,656,422	58,296	2.2
South East Asia	3,464,313	149,615	4.3
Western Pacific	2,173,333	152,694	7.0
All countries (N=185)	10,192,986	489,139	4.8

[a] Western Europe, USA, Canada, Japan.

(10% of cases worldwide) and almost always associated with resistance to other antibiotics, most often double resistance to INH and RMP.

Primary resistance

Patients with lung tuberculosis excreting resistant bacilli can contaminate persons they are in contact with. If they become sick, the newly infected individuals develop tuberculosis with bacilli that are resistant from the start (primary resistance) to the same antibiotics as the bacilli in the infectious carrier. Due to the generalization of standardized polychemotherapy and the relatively rare nature of treatment failure, primary resistance of tubercle bacilli to antibiotics is always weaker than secondary resistance. Because of the important reservoir of SM-resistant strains which developed in the 40's and 50's when SM was the only available antituberculous drug, the frequency of primary resistance to SM (10%) remains as high as for INH (10%). The frequency of primary resistance to RMP, multidrug resistance, and EMB resistance is lower (approximately 4, 3, and 2.5% of cases worldwide, respectively).

There are vast disparities in the frequency of primary and secondary resistance in the world. The frequency of primary resistance is very high in Eastern Europe (10% multidrug resistance and over 40% INH resistance in Baku, Azerbaijan and Tashkent, Uzbekistan) and in certain Asian countries (13% INH resistance in the Western Pacific area). At the other end of the scale, the frequency of resistance is low in Western Europe (0.9% primary multidrug resistance). These observations underline the importance of knowing the country of origin of the patients for interpreting the results of resistance monitoring, as recommended by the WHO.

Data on tuberculosis cases in HIV-positive patients are scarce but seem to support a higher risk of resistance, particularly for single resistance to RMP and multidrug resistance.

Resistance to second-line antituberculous drugs

Measuring susceptibility to second-line antituberculous drugs is a difficult exercise mastered by few laboratories only (see above). For this reason, the importance of resistance to these antibiotics is difficult to evaluate. Multidrug resistant strains, which are also resistant to fluoroquinolones and at least one second-line antituberculous drug administered by injection (kanamycin, amikacin or capreomycin), were reported in the past few years. They are called extensively drug resistant strains or XDR. Their frequency among MDR strains is variable. It is estimated at 10% worldwide, on average. It might be greater than 20% in Estonia and Japan (Table 12).

OTHER MYCOBACTERIA (ATYPICAL AND *M. LEPRAE*)

Atypical mycobacteria, found in the environment, are most often isolated as contaminants in cultures while searching for *M. tuberculosis*. Under certain circumstances, some of them can be

Table 12. Countries reporting extensively drug resistant strains (XDR) (WHO data [a])

WHO region	No. participating	No. with ≥ 1 XDR	% XDR among MDR [b]
Western Europe	19	15	0 – 8 [c]
Eastern Europe	8	8	4 – 24 [d]
America	8	8	3 [e] - 5.6
Africa	7	3	5.7 [f]
Western Pacific	8	5	1.8 – 30 [g]
South East Asia	6	5	/
Eastern Mediterranean	2	2	4.5 [h]

[a] Representative or non-representative samples.
[b] Calculated for countries reporting more than 20 multidrug resistant (MDR) strains and measuring susceptibility to 2nd-line antibiotics for more than 20% of these strains.
[c] Spain (2002-2005: 37 MDR tested).
[d] Estonia (2003-2006: 245 MDR tested).
[e] USA (200-2006: 601 MDR tested).
[f] South Africa (2004-2007: 17615 MDR tested).
[g] Japan (2002: 55 MDR tested).
[h] Israel (2003-2006: 44 MDR tested).

responsible for infections. Infections with atypical mycobacteria are mainly disseminated infections by *Mycobacterium avium* complex in severely immunosuppressed patients, pulmonary infections by *M. xenopi*, *M. kansasii*, or *M. avium* complex, cutaneous infections with fast-growing mycobacteria (*M. chelonae*...) or *M. marinum*, often following accidental inoculation. Imported cases of Buruli ulcer (*Mycobacterium ulcerans*) are among emerging pathologies in tropical countries. Infections caused by other atypical mycobacteria are even less common. Atypical mycobacterial infections are not contagious, which means there is no transmission among humans.

Some 250,000 cases of leprosy have been detected in the world in the past few years, with 70% of them in Asia. The necessary infrastructure to perform susceptibility tests *in vivo* in mice and the required delay to obtain results (10 to 12 months) have restricted their implementation to a few laboratories in the world. Kits for the molecular detection of resistance are under development (search for mutations in the *rpoB* gene for rifampin resistance, in the *folP* gene for dapsone resistance, and in the *gyrA* gene for fluoroquinolone resistance).

Resistance in atypical mycobacteria

Atypical mycobacteria are naturally highly resistant to many antibiotics, including antituberculous drugs. All of them are resistant to PAS and pyrazinamide, and almost all of them to isoniazid. *M. kansasii* is susceptible to rifampin and ethambutol and moderately susceptible to isoniazid (0.2 μg/ml < MIC < 1 μg/ml). *M. avium* complex and other slow-growing species (*M. xenopi*) are susceptible to new macrolides (clarithromycin, etc.). Fast-growing mycobacteria are susceptible to some antibiotics commonly used to treat infectious diseases: β-lactams, aminoglycosides, tetracyclines, sulfonamides, macrolides, and fluoroquinolones. *M. leprae* is susceptible to rifampin, dapsone, clofazimine, and fluoroquinolones and to a lesser extent to clarithromycin and minocycline.

In atypical mycobacteria, acquired resistance is the result of selection of resistant mutants in treated patients (secondary resistance). Since atypical mycobacterial infections are not contagious, there is no primary resistance in untreated patients. Acquired resistance to macrolides, frequent in *M. avium* complex, can develop after a few months of clarithromycin treatment. It is linked to mutations in the 23S rRNA gene. Acquired resistance to clarithromycin was also described in fast-growing mycobacteria. It is associated with the same mechanism (*M. chelonae* and *M. abscessus*) or with activation of the *erm* genes (*M. fortuitum*). Acquired resistance to fluoroquinolones is relevant to the rare fast-growing species naturally sensitive to these antibiotics (*M. fortuitum*). Acquired resistance to rifampin can be a cause of treatment failure in *M. kansasii* infections.

The susceptibility profile of strains isolated in untreated patients is homogeneous within each slow-growing species. In fast-growing mycobacteria, some strains can have a susceptibility profile different from that of the remaining of the species. These differences could be linked to the existence of sub-species which remain to be distinguished or to treatments administered to the patient for an infection other than that due to mycobacteria.

Determination of susceptibility of atypical mycobacteria

Indications

Within the scope of individual patient care, measuring the susceptibility to antibiotics of an atypical mycobacterial strain is only relevant if it is known to cause a pathology in the patient based on clinical, radiological, and bacteriological criteria (1). There is no need to perform an antibiogram for most new infection cases. However, susceptibility testing is appropriate in case of treatment failure which may be linked to the selection of a resistant mutant in the course of a first treatment. A correlation between test results and clinical response has been demonstrated for a few species and antibiotics: *M. avium* complex and clarithromycin, *M. kansasii* and rifampin, *M. chelonae* and clarithromycin, *M. fortuitum* and fluoroquinolones. Since these antibiotic susceptibility tests are not standardized, they are only carried out in a few proficient laboratories which select the antibiotics to be studied, select on the appropriate methods, and perform the test with the highest scientific rigor (22).

Selection of antibiotics and methods

The selection of antibiotics to investigate and of the test methods to use depends on the mycobacterial species. In general, as there are few active antibiotics (Table 13) there are few antibiotics to evaluate.

Slow-growing mycobacteria

For *M. avium* complex, it is recommended to evaluate clarithromycin susceptibility by determining the minimal inhibitory concentration (MIC), preferably in liquid medium (7H9 or MH supplemented with OADC, 7H12). Using microdilution plates (Sensititre® Trek Diagnostic Systems), with alleviates the need to prepare various antibiotic concentrations, and an appropriate reader (Sensititre® Vizion ™ system) facilitates considerably the implementation of this determination and of its reading.

Results depend on the pH of the medium: at pH 7.2-7.3, the MIC_{90} for this species is 4 µg/ml (variance: 0.5 to 8 µg/ml) while at pH 6.8, it is 16 µg/ml (4 to 32 g/L). The MIC for resistant strains is greater than 16 µg/ml at pH 6.8 and 8 µg/ml at pH 7.2, most often around 128 µg/ml. Results obtained for clarithromycin are also valid for azithromycin.

For *M. kansasii*, it is recommended to evaluate susceptibility to rifampin and, in case of resistance, to ethambutol and isoniazid (at concentrations of 1 and 10 µg/ml) as well as to fluoroquinolones, clarithromycin, and amikacin. Since wild-type *M. kansasii* strains are susceptible to 2 µg/ml of ethambutol and to 1 µg/ml of isoniazid, the proportion method can be used as optimized for *M. tuberculosis*. It is not advisable to use commercial kits for the antibiogram of *M. tuberculosis* in which rifampin, for stability reasons, is replaced by rifamycin SV, because *M. kansasii*, although susceptible to rifampin (MIC = 0.5 µg/ml), is naturally resistant to rifamycin SV. Strains which are susceptible to rifampin also are susceptible to rifabutin.

M. xenopi presents a very dysgonic growth; therefore, susceptibility tests are particularly difficult to implement and are rarely carried out for this species. When indicated, the MIC of clarithromycin, moxifloxacin, rifamycins, and ethambutol is determined.

For *M. haemophilum*, *M. genavense* and *M. ulcerans*, which are very difficult to grow, there are no recommendations about susceptibility tests.

For *M. marinum*, antibiotic susceptibility tests are restricted to cases of failure following several months of treatment. Rifampin, ethambutol, clarithromycin, cyclines, amikacin, and sulfonamides are investigated by MIC determination.

Fast-growing mycobacteria

Susceptibility of fast-growing atypical mycobacteria varies by species. *M. chelonae* strains are usually highly susceptible to clarithromycin and resistant to fluoroquinolones.

Table 13. Antibiotics usually active against the main atypical mycobacterial species responsible for infections

Species	Antibiotiques[a]
M. avium complex	CLA, AMK, EMB[b], RIF[b]
M. kansasii	RMP, INH[b], EMB, CLA, FQ[c]
M. xenopi	CLA, FQ[c], EMB[b], RBT
M. marinum	DOX, CLA, RMP
M. fortuitum	FQ[c], AMK, CFX, IMP, SULF, LNZ (DOX, CLA[b])
M. chelonae	CLA, AMK[b], TOB, LNZ[b] (IMP, DOX)
M. abscessus	CLA[d], AMK, CFX (IMP, LNZ[b])
M. ulcerans	RMP, AMK, SM

[a] AMK, amikacin ; CFX, cefoxitin ; CLA, clarithromycin ; DOX, doxycycline ; EMB, ethambutol ; FQ, fluoroquinolones ; IMP, imipenem ; INH, isoniazid ; LNZ, linezolid ; RIF : rifamycin (rifabutin, rifampin) ; SM, streptomycin ; SULF, sulfonamide ; TOB, tobramycin. In parentheses: antibiotics with inconstant activity.
[b] Antibiotics with poor activity.
[c] Fluoroquinolones: moxifloxacin or levofloxacin, except for *M. fortuitum*, rather ciprofloxacin.
[d] Impact of the presence of an intrinsic resistance gene is under investigation.

Table 14. Critical concentrations (µg/ml) for determination of susceptibility to antibiotics for fast-growing mycobacteria, after NCCLS (Woods 2003)

Antibiotic	MIC (µg/ml) by category		
	Susceptible	Intermediate	Resistant
Amikacin	≤ 16	32	≥ 64
Cefoxitin	≤ 16	32-64	≥ 128
Ciprofloxacin	≤ 1	2	≥ 4
Clarithromycin	≤ 2	4	≥ 8
Doxycycline	≤ 1	2-8	≥ 16
Imipenem	≤ 4	8	≥ 16
Sulfamethoxazole	≤ 32	-	≥ 64
Tobramycin	≤ 4	8	≥ 16
Linezolid	≤ 8	16	≥ 32

Conversely, *M. fortuitum* strains and related species (*M. peregrinum*, etc.) are highly susceptible to fluoroquinolones and poorly susceptible or even resistant to clarithromycin. Within a single species, there may be differences in susceptibility from one strain to another, even for strains isolated from patients who were never treated for infection by that particular mycobacterium. Thus, it is appropriate to determine the antibiotic susceptibility of all strains of fast-growing atypical mycobacteria considered to be responsible for an infection, especially when the species identity is uncertain.

Antibiotics to be included are: cefoxitin, imipenem, amikacin, tobramycin, ciprofloxacin, doxycycline, clarithromycin and sulfamethoxazole-trimethoprim. To these, moxifloxacin and linezolid can be added. Susceptibility is evaluated by determination of MIC in liquid medium in microplates (Sensititre® Trek Diagnostic Systems) using NCCLS criteria (Table 14). For all antibiotics, except for sulfonamides, MIC is defined as the concentration which inhibits all growth. For the latter, MIC is the concentration which inhibits 80% of growth. The use of E-test® strips can lead to categorisation errors (false resistance) and is not recommended.

ACKNOWLEDGMENTS

This chapter was written by Nicolas Veziris[1], Alexandra Aubry[1], Wladimir Sougakoff[1], Jérome Robert[1], Florence Brossier[1], Sylvaine Bastian[1], Emmanuelle Cambau[2], Vincent Jarlier[1] and Chantal Truffot-Pernot[1]

[1]Centre National de Référence des Mycobactéries et de la Résistance des Mycobactéries aux Antituberculeux.

[2]Laboratoire de Bactériologie-Virologie-Hygiène, Hôpital Saint-Louis, Paris.

REFERENCES

(1) **American Thoracic Society and Infectious Diseases Society of America**. 2007. Diagnosis, treatment and prevention of nontuberculous mycobacterial diseases. Am. J. Respir. Crit. Care Med. **175**:367-416.

(2) **Andries, K., P. Verhassel, J. Guillemont, H.W.H. Göhlmann, J. M. Neefs, H. Winckler, J. V. Gestel, P. Timmerman, M. Zhu, E. Lee, P. Williams, D. de Chaffoy, E. Huitric, S. Hoffner, E. Cambau, C. Truffot-Pernot, N. Lounis, and V. Jarlier**. 2005. A diarylquinoline drug active on the ATP synthase of *Mycobacterium tuberculosis*. Science **307**:223-227.

(3) **Barnard, M., H. Albert, G. Coetzee, R. O'Brien, and M. E. Bosman**. 2008. Rapid molecular screening for multidrug-resistant tuberculosis in a high-volume public health laboratory in South Africa. Am. J. Respir. Crit. Care Med. **177**:787-792.

(4) **Brossier F., N. Veziris, V. Jarlier, and W. Sougakoff**. 2009. Performance of MTBDR *plus* for detecting high/low levels of *Mycobacterium tuberculosis* resistance to isoniazid. Int. J. Tuberc. Lung Dis. **13**:260-265.

(5) **Canetti, G., N. Rist, and J. Grosset**. 1963. Mesure de la sensibilité du bacille tuberculeux aux drogues antibacillaires par la méthode des proportions. Rev. Tuberc. Pneumol. **27**:291-298.

(6) **Drobniewski, F., S. Rusch-Gerdes, and S. Hoffner**. 2007. Antimicrobial susceptibility testing of *Mycobacterium tuberculosis* (EUCAST document E. DEF 8.1)- Report on the Subcommittee on Antimicrobial Susceptibility Testing of *Mycobacterium tuberculosis* of the European Committee for Antimicrobial Susceptibility Testing(EUCAST) of the European Society of Clinical Microbiology and Infectious Diseases (ESCMID). Clin. Microbiol. Infect. **13**: 1144-1156.

(7) **Fox, W., G. A. Ellard, and D. A. Mitchison**. 1999. Studies on the treatment of tuberculosis undertaken by the British Medical Research Council tuberculosis units, 1946-1986, with relevant subsequent publications. Int. J. Tuberc. Lung Dis. **3**:S231-279.

(8) **Hillemann, D., S. Rusch-Gerdes, and E. Richter**. 2007. Evaluation of the Genotype MTBDRplus Assay for rifampin and isoniazid susceptibility testing of *Mycobacterium tuberculosis* strains and clinical specimens. J. Clin. Microbiol. **45**:2635-2640.

(9) **Hillemann D, S. Rusch-Gerdes, and E. Richter**. 2009. Feasibility of the GenoType® MTBDR*sl* Assay for fluoroquinolone, amikacin/capreomycin, and ethambutol resistance testing of *Mycobacterium tuberculosis* strains and clinical specimens. J. Clin. Microbiol. **47**:1767-1772.

(10) **Lacoma, A., N. Garcia-Sierra, C. Prat, J. Ruiz-Manzano, L. Haba, S. Roses, J. Maldonado, and J. Dominguez** 2008. GenoType MTBDR *plus* Assay for molecular detection of rifampin and isoniazid resistance in *Mycobacterium tuberculosis* strains and clinical samples. J. Clin. Microbiol. **46**:3660-3667.

(11) **Laszlo, A., M. Rahman, M. Espinal, M. Raviglione, and the WHO/IUATLD Supranational Reference Laboratory Network**. 2002. Five rounds of proficiency testing, 1994-1998. Int. J. Tuberc. Lung Dis. **6**:748-756.

(12) **Martin, A., A. Von Groll, K. Fissette, J. C. Palomino, F. Varaine, and F. Portaels**. 2008. Rapid detection of *Mycobacterium tuberculosis* resistance to second-line drugs by use of the manual Mycobacterium Growth Indicator Tube System. J. Clin. Microbiol. **46**:3952-3956.

(13) **Maus, C. E., B. B. Plikaytis, and T. Shinnick**. 2005. Molecular analysis of cross resistance to capreomycin, kanamycin, amikacin, and viomycin in *Mycobacterium tuberculosis*. Antimicrob. Agents Chemother. **49**:571-577.

(14) **Miotto, P., F. Piana, D. M. Cirillo, and G. B. Migliori**. 2007. Genotype MTBDR *plus* : a further step toward rapid identification of drug resistant

Mycobacterium tuberculosis. J. Clin. Microbiol. **46**:393-394.

(15) **Nikolayevskyy, V., Y. Balabanova, T. Simak, N. Malomanova, I. Fedorin, and F. Drobniewski.** 2009. Performance of the Genotype® MTBDR Plus Assay in the diagnosis of tuberculosis and drug resistance in Samara, Russian Federation. BMC Clinical Pathology. **9**:1-9.

(16) **Okamoto, S., S. Tamaru, C. Nakajima, K. Nishimura, Y. Tanaka, S. Tokuyama, V. Suzuki, and K. Ochi.** 2007. Loss of a conserved 7-methyl-guanosine modification in 16S rRNA confers low-level streptomycin resistance in bacteria. Mol. Microbiol. **63**:1096-1106.

(17) **Palomino, J. C., A. Martin, A. Von Groll, and F. Portaels**. 2008. Rapid culture-based methods for drug-resistance detection in *Mycobacterium tuberculosis*. J. Microbiol. Methods **75**:161-166.

(18) **Piersimoni, C., A. Olivieri, L. Benacchio, and C. Scarparo.** 2006. Current perspectives on drug susceptibility testing of *Mycobacterium tuberculosis* complex: the automated non radiometric systems. J. Clin. Microbiol. **44**:20-28.

(19) **Ramaswany, S., and J. M. Musser**. 1998. Molecular genetic basis of antimicrobial agent resistance in *Mycobacterium tuberculosis*: 1998 update. Tuber. Lung Dis. **79**:3-29.

(20) **Sougakoff, W., M. Rodrigue, C. Truffot-Pernot, M. Renard, N. Durin, M. Szpytma, R. Vachon, A. Troesch, and V. Jarlier.** 2004. Use of a high density DNA probe array for detecting mutations involved in rifampin resistance in *Mycobacterium tuberculosis*. Clin. Microbiol. Infect. **10**:289-294.

(21) **Vilcheze, C., Y. Av-Gay, R. Attarian, Z. Liu, M. H. Hazbon, R. Colangeli, B. Chen, W. Liu, D. Alland, J. C. Sacchettini, and Wr. Jacobs Jr**. 2008. Mycothiol biosynthesis is essential for ethionamide susceptibility in *Mycobacterium tuberculosis*. Mol. Microbiol. **69**:1316-1329.

(22) **Woods, G. L. , B. A. Brown-Elliott, E. P. Desmond, G. S. Hall, L. Heifets, G. E. Pfyffer, J. C. Ridderhof, R. J. Wallace Jr, N. C. Warren, and F. G. Witebsky**. Susceptibility testing of mycobacteria, nocardiae, and other aerobic actinomycetes; Approved Standard. NCCLS document M24-A (ISBN 1- 56238-500-3),Wayne, PA, USA, 2003.

(23) **World Health Organization**. Antituberculous drug resistance in the world. WHO document (WHO/HTM/TB 2008-394), Geneva 2008.

(24) **World Health Organization**. Policy guidance on drug-susceptibility testing (DST) of second line antituberculous drugs. WHO document (WHO/HTM/TB/2008.392), Geneva, 2008.

Chapter 50. *BARTONELLA, BORRELIA, BRUCELLA, FRANCISELLA, EHRLICHIA, RICKETTSIA, COXIELLA AND TREPONEMA*

Max MAURIN

The bacteria belonging to these different groups all share the ability to evade humoral immunity, either by obligate or facultative intracellular multiplication, or by antigen masking which prevents recognition by antibodies (*Borrelia, Treponema*). Specific cell-mediated immunity is the main mechanism of defense against these pathogens, as witnessed by the severe and chronic nature of these infections in patients with cellular immune deficiency. Bacteria from the genera *Rickettsia* and *Coxiella*, formerly united under the term "rickettsia" are obligate intracellular pathogens that respectively infect endothelial cells and monocytes/macrophages. *Ehrlichia* are obligate intracellular bacteria that infect granulocytes (granulocytic anaplasmosis) or monocytes/macrophages (monocytic ehrlichiosis). Species belonging to the genera *Brucella* and *Francisella* are facultative intracellular parasites of monocytes/macrophages. Lastly, bacteria from the genus *Bartonella* are facultative intracellular pathogens that infect endothelial cells and erythrocytes.

All these pathogens also share the common feature of being difficult or impossible to culture in conventional media, which precludes the use of reference methods for antimicrobial susceptibility testing. Special axenic culture media or eukaryotic cell cultures support the growth of these microorganisms and must be used if one wishes to evaluate antibiotic susceptibilities. These methods are difficult to standardize and there is little harmonization between the different laboratories which carry out such tests. This lack of standardized susceptibility testing methods has made it difficult for organizations such as EUCAST (European Committee on Antimicrobial Testing) and CLSI (Clinical and Laboratory Standards Institute) to establish technical guidance and interpretive criteria. This chapter describes the culture techniques useful for defining *in vitro* antibiotic susceptibility patterns of these microorganisms.

BARTONELLA SPP.

Bartonella spp are Gram-negative bacilli. These facultative intracellular organisms infect endothelial cells and erythrocytes. To date, the genus comprises 35 species. Humans are the only known reservoir for two of these species: *B. bacilliformis*, a species with a limited geographical distribution (Peru, Ecuador, Bolivia), is the agent of Carrion's disease, and *B. quintana*, distributed worldwide and transmitted via the body louse, causes trench fever. The other species have an animal reservoir and some are human zoonotic pathogens. *B. henselae*, a ubiquitous species whose reservoir is the domestic cat, is usually transmitted to humans by cat scratches or bites and is the causal agent of cat scratch disease. *B. quintana* and *B. henselae* can also cause septicemia, endocarditis as well as bacillary angiomatosis in immunocompromised (AIDS) patients.

Methods

Bartonella are facultative intracellular bacteria which can grow in axenic medium supplemented with hemin or blood, or else in eukaryotic cell cultures. Minimal inhibitory concentrations (MIC) have been determined in axenic medium by the dilution method in 5% horse or sheep blood agar. Plates are inoculated with 10^4-10^6 CFU/spot and read after five days of incubation in a 5% CO_2 atmosphere (4, 7, 8). *B. bacilliformis*, a slower growing species, requires six days of incubation in medium containing 10% horse blood (12). E-test® yields MICs similar to those obtained by the above methods (4, 10, 13). Bacteriostatic activity of antibiotics has also been evaluated in intracellular media, either in cell lines [human endothelial cells (9), P388D1 murine macrophages, Vero cells (5, 6)] or, more recently, in human erythrocytes (11). In these models, the cells are incubated *in vitro* in the presence of *Bartonella* for 1 hour to allow intracellular penetration of the bacteria. Intracellular growth curves are measured in the presence of different antibiotics and compared to an antibiotic-free control.

Bactericidal activity against *Bartonella* has been evaluated in axenic and cellular medium in culture conditions similar to those described above. Minimal bactericidal concentrations (MBC) are defined as the

Table 1. MICs (μg/ml) of antibiotics for *Bartonella* spp. (number of strains tested) determined by the dilution method in Columbia agar with 5-10% horse or sheep blood (4, 7, 8, 12)

Antibiotic	*B. bacilliformis* (4)	*B. quintana* (9)	*B. henselae* (3)	*Bartonella* sp. (25-31)[b]
β-lactams				
Penicillin G	0.015 - 0.03	0.03 - 0.06	0.03 - 0.06	ND[a]
Amoxicillin	0.03 - 0.06	0.03 - 0.06	0.6 - 0.12	ND
Cephalothin	4 - 8	8 - 16	8 - 16	ND
Cefotaxime	0.03 - 0.12	0.12 - 0.25	0.12 - 0.25	ND
Ceftriaxone	0.003 - 0.006	0.06 - 0.25	0.12 - 0.25	ND
Imipenem	0.5 - 1	0.12 - 1	0.5	ND
Aminoglycosides				
Streptomycin	4	ND	ND	0.12 - 8 (8)
Gentamicin	1 - 2	0.12 - 2	0.12 - 0.25	0.25 - 8 (4)
Netilmicin	ND	ND	ND	0.25 - 4 (1)
Amikacin	2 - 8	2 - 8	2 - 4	2 - 16 (8)
Tobramycin	2 - 4	0.5 - 4	0.5 - 1	0.25 - 8 (4)
Macrolide group				
Erythromycin	0.06	0.06 - 0.12	0.06 - 0.25	0.004 - 0.12 (0.12)
Roxithromycin	ND	ND	ND	0.004 - 0.12 (0.12)
Azithromycin	0.015	0.006 - 0.03	0.006 - 0.015	0.008 - 0.06 (0.03)
Clarithromycin	0.015 - 0.03	0.003 - 0.03	0.006 - 0.03	<0.002 - 0.015 (0.015)
Telithromycin	0.015	0.006	0.003	< 0.002
Fluoroquinolones				
Pefloxacin	1 - 2	2 - 8	4 - 8	ND
Levofloxacin	ND	ND	ND	0.25 - 2 (1)
Ciprofloxacin	0.25 - 0.5	0.5 - 2	0.25 - 1	0.25 - 2 (1)
Sparfloxacin	0.25	0.06 - 0.12	0.06	ND
Moxifloxacin	ND	ND	ND	0.12 - 1 (1)
Gemifloxacin	ND	ND	ND	0.06 - 0.5 (0.5)
Doxycycline	0.03 - 0.06	0.06 - 0.25	0.12	0.004 - 0.12 (0.12)
Thiamphénicol	0.25	ND	ND	ND
Rifampin	0.003	0.06 - 0.25	0.03 - 0.06	0.008 - 0.06 (0.03)
Trimethoprim/sulfamethoxazole	0.4/2 - 0.8/4	0.25/1.25 - 1/5	1/5	ND
Vancomycin	4 - 8	8 - 16	2 - 8	ND

[a] ND, not determined.
[b] Min/max MICs and (MIC90) of 25-31 isolates of *Bartonella* sp., including 21 *B. henselae* strains, 2 *B. quintana* strains, and 1 strain of each of the following species: *B. elizabethae*, *B. tribocorum*, *B. alsatica*, *B. vinsonii* subsp. *vinsonii*, *B. vinsonii* subsp. *arupensis*, *B. schoenbuchii*, *B. doshiae* and *B. grahamii*.

lowest antibiotic concentration producing a 3 Log reduction in the starting inoculum. Bacterial counts are determined by measuring colony forming units (CFU). In the cell models, bacteria are counted after lysis of the cells by heat shock.

Susceptible phenotype

In axenic medium, *Bartonella* species are susceptible to penicillin G, aminopenicillins and derivatives, third generation cephalosporins, imipenem, aminoglycosides, macrolides, phenicols, tetracyclines, co-trimoxazole, rifampin, and fluoroquinolones (Table 1). Fluoroquinolone susceptibility varies according to the molecule, with MICs ranging from 0.06-2 µg/ml for ciprofloxacin, 0.5-4 µg/ml for ofloxacin (1), 0.25-2 µg/ml for levofloxacin (4) and 1-8 µg/ml for pefloxacin (1, 4, 7, 8, 12). The modest activity of fluoroquinolones against *Bartonella* is probably related to their low affinity for DNA gyrase subunit A due to the presence of an alanine residue at position 83 instead of the usual serine present in susceptible species (1). MICs of cephalothin are higher. In contrast, glycopeptide MICs are fairly low for these Gram-negative species. The *in vitro* susceptibility of *Bartonella* to many antimicrobials is in fact a poor predictor of clinical efficacy. For example, cat scratch disease caused by *B. henselae* is characterized by chronic lymphadenopathy which may be complicated by abscess formation despite appropriate antimicrobial therapy. On the other hand, bacillary angiomatosis and/or septicemia caused by this same species respond rapidly to antimicrobial therapy, especially with a macrolide. This paradox may be related to a methodology that underestimates antimicrobial resistance in these bacteria. Clinical resistance may also be a consequence of their intracellular multiplication. Intracellular activity has been demonstrated for aminoglycosides (particularly gentamicin), macrolides and fluoroquinolones in cell models using Vero cells, endothelial cells or human erythrocytes (5, 6, 9, 11). Only the aminoglycosides, gentamicin in particular, had bactericidal activity against intracellular *Bartonella*. However, as gentamicin did not reach bactericidal concentrations inside erythrocytes, the observed bactericidal effect may occur extracellularly, preventing the spread of infection to healthy cells (11).

Phenotypes and mechanisms of resistance

Laboratory mutants resistant to macrolides have been obtained in the species *B. henselae* in the presence of erythromycin (2). Five had mutations in domain V of the 23S rRNA gene: $A_{2058}G$ (two mutants), $A_{2058}C$ and $A_{2059}G$ (two mutants). One mutant harbored two mutations - $G_{71}R$ and $H_{75}Y$ - in ribosomal protein L4 associated with 23S rRNA. Another mutant had both a $C_{2611}T$ mutation in the 23S rRNA gene and a $G_{71}R$ mutation in the L4 gene. The $A_{2059}G$ mutation was also detected by PCR amplification directly on a lymph node excised from a patient with cat scratch disease (2). This finding suggests the possibility that *B. henselae* may acquire macrolide resistance *in vivo*, in patients infected by this species and receiving therapy with a macrolide.

Mutants with high-level resistance (MIC > 32 µg/ml) to erythromycin, ciprofloxacin and rifampin have also been obtained *in vitro* in *B. bacilliformis* (3). The selected mutants harbored a mutation in the target gene of each of these antibiotics. Erythromycin resistance was due to a $A_{2058}G$ mutation in 23S rRNA; ciprofloxacin resistance was conferred by a CT transition at position 549 (*E. coli* numbering) of DNA gyrase subunit A resulting in an aspartic acid$_{87}$asparagine substitution in the GyrA protein. Rifampin resistance was related to a $G_{2868}A$ transition (*E. coli* numbering) in the RNA polymerase β subunit resulting in substitution of phenylalanine for serine at position 531. Interestingly, no gentamicin or doxycycline resistant mutants could be selected in this study. To date, no *B. bacilliformis* clinical isolates with an acquired resistance phenotype have been reported.

REFERENCES

(1) **Angelakis, E., S. Biswas, C. Taylor, D. Raoult, and J. M. Rolain.** 2008. Heterogeneity of susceptibility to fluoroquinolones in *Bartonella* isolates from Australia reveals a natural mutation in *gyrA*. J. Antimicrob. Chemother. **61**:1252-1255.

(2) **Biswas, S., D. Raoult, and J.M. Rolain.** 2006. Molecular characterization of resistance to macrolides in *Bartonella henselae*. Antimicrob. Agents Chemother. **50**:3192-3193.

(3) **Biswas, S., D. Raoult, and J.M. Rolain.** 2007. Molecular mechanisms of resistance to antibiotics in *Bartonella bacilliformis*. J. Antimicrob. Chemother. **59**:1065-1070.

(4) **Dörbecker, C., A. Sander, K. Oberle, and T. Schülin-Casonato.** 2006. *In vitro* susceptibility of *Bartonella* species to 17 antimicrobial compounds: comparison of E-test and agar dilution. J. Antimicrob. Chemother. **58**:784-788.

(5) **Ives, T.J., P. Manzewitsch, R.L. Regnery, J.D. Butts, and M. Kebede.** 1997. *In vitro* susceptibilities of *Bartonella henselae, B. quintana, B. elizabethae, Rickettsia rickettsii, R. conorii, R. akari,* and *R.*

prowazekii to macrolide antibiotics as determined by immunofluorescence-antibody analysis of infected Vero cell monolayers. Antimicrob. Agents Chemother. **41**:578-582.

(6) **Ives, T.J., E.L. Marston, R.L. Regnery, and J.D. Butts**. 2001. *In vitro* susceptibilities of *Bartonella* and *Rickettsia* spp. to fluoroquinolone antibiotics as determined by immunofluorescence-antibody analysis of infected Vero cell monolayers. Int. J. Antimicrob. Agents. **18**:217-222.

(7) **Maurin, M., and D. Raoult**. 1993. Antimicrobial susceptibility of *Rochalimaea quintana*, *Rochalimaea vinsonii*, and the newly recognized *Rochalimaea henselae*. J Antimicrob. Chemother. **32**: 587-594.

(8) **Maurin, M., S. Gasquet, C. Ducco, and D. Raoult**. 1995. MICs of 28 antibiotic compounds for 14 *Bartonella* (formerly *Rochalimaea*) isolates. Antimicrob. Agents Chemother. **39**:2387-2391.

(9) **Musso, D., M. Drancourt, and D. Raoult**. 1995. Lack of bactericidal effect of antibiotics except aminoglycosides on *Bartonella* (*Rochalimaea*) *henselae*. J. Antimicrob. Chemother. **36**:101-108.

(10) **Pendle, S., A. Ginn, and J. Iredell**. 2006. Antimicrobial susceptibility of *Bartonella henselae* using E-test methodology. J. Antimicrob. Chemother. **57**:761-763.

(11) **Rolain, J.M., M. Maurin, M.N. Mallet, D. Parzy, and D. Raoult**. 2003. Culture and antibiotic susceptibility of *Bartonella quintana* in human erythrocytes. Antimicrob. Agents Chemother. **47**:614-619.

(12) **Sobraques, M., M. Maurin, R. Birtles, and D. Raoult**. 1999. *In vitro* susceptibilities of four *Bartonella bacilliformis* strains to 30 antibiotic compounds. Antimicrob. Agents Chemother. **43**:2090-2092.

(13) **Wolfson, C., J. Branley, and T. Gottlieb**. 1996. The E-test for antimicrobial susceptibility testing of *Bartonella henselae*. J. Antimicrob. Chemother. **38**:963-968.

BORRELIA

Borrelia are helical bacilli from the family *Spirochaetaceae*. These microaerophilic, motile organisms can be visualized by dark field microscopy. Animals are the reservoir for most tick-borne borrelioses (apart from *B. duttonii*) which are transmitted to humans through the bite of *Ixodes* ticks. Their geographical distribution mirrors that of the vector. Humans are the only reservoir of *B. recurrentis*, the agent of borreliosis transmitted by the body louse and predominant in developing countries. *B. burgdorferi* sensu stricto, *B. garinii*, and *B. afzelii* are the three main agents of Lyme disease. They belong to the group *Borrelia burgdorferi* sensu lato, which currently comprises twelve species. *B. burgdorferi* sensu stricto is the only human Lyme related species in the United States; it is transmitted by *Ixodes scapularis* in the east and midwest and by *Ixodes pacificus* in the western United States. *B. burgdorferi* sensu stricto is also found in Europe where it is transmitted by the tick *I. ricinus*. *B. garinii,* and *B. afzelii* are present in Europe and Asia where the vectors are *I. ricinus* and *I. persulcatus*.

Methods

Most studies of antimicrobial susceptibility have been carried out in the *Borrelia* species responsible for Lyme disease. Susceptibility tests of *B. burgdorferi* are carried out in Barbour-Stoenner-Kelly (BSK) medium by a macro- or micro-method (13, 15). A suspension of 10^5-10^6 spirochetes per ml of BSK medium is incubated at 34°C for 3-8 days in the presence or absence of antibiotic. Growth is measured by counting spirochetes in a Petroff-Hausser counting chamber examined by dark field microscopy. The MIC is defined as the lowest antibiotic concentration at which no *Borrelia* growth is observed in comparison to an antibiotic-free control. Hunfeld *et al.* (7, 11) have developed a colorimetric method in which phenol red is added to BSK medium; during growth of *Borrelia* the medium becomes more acidic, which is manifested by a color change. An absence of acidification in the presence of different antibiotic concentrations defines the activity of the agent.

Two methods can be used to determine the MBC (8, 13, 15). In the first method, the MIC is first determined and then a sample of bacterial suspension containing an antibiotic concentration ≥ MIC is inoculated into antibiotic-free BSK medium. These subcultures are incubated for three weeks. The MBC is defined as the lowest antibiotic concentration at which no growth is observed. It should be noted that longer incubation times may result in a slight increase in MBC values (18). In the second method, 72-hour time-kill studies are carried out in BSK medium in the presence of antibiotic concentrations 2-4 times above the MIC.

Table 2. MIC and MBC of antibiotics for *B. burgdorferi sensu stricto* (4, 5, 7, 9-11, 14, 16, 19, 22) or *sensu lato* (8, 15, 17, 20)

Antibiotic	Number of isolates	MIC (µg/ml) Min/Max	MBC (µg/ml) Min/Max	Reference
β-lactams				
Penicillin G	30	0.5 - 2	1 - 4	17
	3	0.125 – 0.25	ND[a]	7
Amoxicillin	8	≤ 0.03 – 0.06	≤ 0.03 – 2	15
	8	0.015 – 0.25	0.125 – 0.5	20
Mezlocillin	3	≤ 0.06	ND	8
	11	≤ 0.06	0.125 - 2	8
Azlocillin	3	≤ 0.125 – 0.125	ND	7
Aztreonam	3	10.6 - 32	ND	8
	11	2 - > 64	16 - >64	8
Cefuroxime-axetil	5	0.03 – 0.25	4 - 32	10
Cefdinir	5	0.5 - 1	16 - 32	10
Cefixime	5	0.25 - 1	16	10
Cefotaxime	8	≤ 0.03	ND	15
Ceftriaxone	30	0.1 – 0.25	0.2 – 0.5	17
	8	0.015 – 0.06	0.06 – 0.25	20
	3	0.015 – 0.03	ND	14
	5	≤ 0.0156 – 0.0625	0.5 - 2	11
Ceftizoxime	8	0.06 – 0.5	0.25 - 1	15
Cefodizime	2	0.06	0.12	16
Cefepime	1	1	ND	5
Imipenem	3	0.125 – 0.5	32 - 64	19
Ertapenem	3	0.062	2 - 4	19
Meropenem	1	0.125	ND	5
	3	0.11 – 0.33	ND	8
	3	0.125 – 0.25	4 - 16	19
	11	0.012 – 0.5	0.5 - 32	8
Aminoglycosides				
Tobramycin	3	16 - 64	ND	7
Tetracyclines – glycylcycline				
Doxycycline	8	0.125 – 0.5	0.25 - 4	15
	8	0.25 - 4	4 - > 16	20
Minocycline	2	0.03 – 0.25	0.25 - 4	16
Tigecycline	3	0.006 – 0.012	0.095 – 0.195	22
Macrolides – azalides – ketolides				
Erythromycin	19	0.007 – 0.06	ND	4
	5	0.0039 – 0.0312	> 0.5	11
	8	≤ 0.03 – 0.06	0.06 – 0.5	15
	5	0.0075 – 0.062	ND	2
Dirithromycin	8	≤ 0.03 – 0.06	0.06 – 0.125	15
Rokitamycin	5	0.0048 – 0.115	ND	2
Azithromycin	19	0.003 – 0.03	ND	4
	8	0.008 – 0.03	0.015 – 0.06	20
	5	≤ 0.0002 - 0.0019	0.12 – 0.5	11
	2	≤ 0.003	≤ 0.003 – 0.007	16
Clarithromycin	19	0.003 – 0.03	ND	4
	5	0.0019 – 0.0156	0.25 - > 0.5	11
	8	≤ 0.03 – 0.06	0.06 – 0.25	15
14-OH clarithromycin	19	0.007 – 0.03	ND	4
	8	≤ 0.03 – 0.06	0.06 – 0.5	15
Roxithromycin	2	≤ 0.003 - 0.015	0.015 – 0.12	16
	5	0.0019 – 0.0156	0.25 - > 0.5	11
Telithromycin	5	≤ 0.0002	0.06 – 0.12	11
Cethromycin	5	≤ 0.0002	0.03 – 0.12	11
ABT-773	5	≤ 0.002	0.19 – 0.75	9
Quinupristin-dalfopristin	1	1	ND	5
Oxazilidinone				
Linezolid	1	>2	ND	5

Table 2. MIC and MBC of different antibiotics for B. burgdorferi sensu stricto (4, 5, 7, 9-11, 14, 16, 19, 22) or sensu lato (8, 15, 17, 20) (continued)

Antibiotic	Number of isolates	MIC (µg/ml) Min/Max	MBC (µg/ml) Min/Max	Reference
Quinolones				
Nalidixic acid	3	256	ND	14
Norfloxacin	3	8	ND	14
Pefloxacin	3	16	ND	14
Ofloxacin	3	4 - 8	ND	14
	8	0.5 - 2	1 - 8	15
Levofloxacin	3	2 - 4	ND	14
Ciprofloxacin	3	1 - 2	ND	14
	8	0.25 - 2	0.5 - 16	15
	2	0.03 – 0.5	0.06 - 4	16
Moxifloxacin	3	1 - 2	ND	14

[a] ND, not determined.
B. burgdorferi sensu stricto reference strains tested: B31 (5); B31, myo1 (16); B31, B31-p5, Bo12 (22); B31, LW2, PKa-I (7, 8, 14, 19); B31, LW2, PKa-I, Z25, 297 (9, 10, 11); B31, HB6, Alcaide, Myo1, Emilia (2).

Spirochetes are counted in a Petroff-Hausser counting chamber and bactericidal activity is defined as a 3 Log reduction in the starting inoculum after 72 h of incubation.

Antibiotic susceptibility of B. burgdorferi has also been studied in cell cultures, particularly in fibroblast cells including human fibroblasts, mouse keratinocytes, and cell lines (HEP-2, Vero, Caco-2 cells) (6).

The Borrelia species that cause relapsing fever are fastidious organisms and susceptibility testing has been performed by techniques similar to those used for B. burgdorferi, notably for B. hermsii, B. turicatae, B. anserina, B. bissettii and B. valaisiana (1, 7, 13).

B. recurrentis, a species long thought to be uncultivable, was isolated from an Ethiopian patient in BSK medium (3), thus allowing the antimicrobial susceptibility of the strain to be evaluated.

Susceptible phenotype

B. burgdorferi is susceptible to penicillin G (16, 17) although MICs range from 0.003 to 3 µg/ml (Table 2). The higher MICs might be the result of a methodological artefact arising from the instability of penicillin G during the long incubation times. With respect to other β-lactams, B. burgdorferi is highly susceptible to amoxicillin, third generation cephalosporins (cefotaxime, ceftriaxone), and carbapenems (imipenem, meropenem). Oral cephalosporins are less active than ceftriaxone in vitro (10). Only the most active drugs (cefuroxime-axetil, cefdinir, cefixime) are shown in Tables 2 to 5. Aminoglycosides are inactive or else have very high MICs (7, 18, 19). Tetracyclines, glycylcyclines (tigecycline) and the macrolide group (including azalides, ketolides) are also very active in vitro (2, 4, 22). Ketolides have the lowest MICs. Nalidixic acid is ineffective against B. burgdorferi (11). Fluoroquinolones show variable activity according to the strain, with MICs ranging from 0.008-64 µg/ml (14). Gemifloxacin, sitafloxacin, clinafloxacin, trovafloxacin, gatifloxacin, grepafloxacin, and sparfloxacin have the highest activity in vitro with $MIC_{90} \leq 1$ µg/ml (14).

Among the β-lactams, MBCs are similar to MICs for amoxicillin and third generation cephalosporins but markedly higher for carbapenems with respect to B. burgdorferi, B. garinii and B. afzelii (20). Macrolides are bactericidal in vitro although MBCs are much higher than MICs. Tetracyclines and fluoroquinolones are only bacteriostatic at the peak serum levels achieved in humans (14, 20).

Georgilis et al. (6) showed that ceftriaxone is inactive against B. burgdorferi cultured in the presence of fibroblast cells.

The in vitro susceptibility of B. garinii and B. afzelii is similar to that of B. burgdorferi sensu stricto (Tables 3 and 4). One major difference concerns penicillin G: the MIC for B. afzelii is ten times higher than that for B. burgdorferi and 100 times higher than that for B. garinii (7).

The Borrelia species responsible for relapsing fever all show similar susceptibility patterns, regardless of the species. B. hermsii, B. turicatae, B. anserina, B. bissettii and B. valaisiana are sus-

Table 3. MIC (μg/ml) and MBC (μg/ml) of antibiotics for *B. garinii*

Antibiotic	Number of isolates	MIC Min/Max	MBC Min/Max	Reference
β-lactams				
Penicillin G	3	0.015 – 0.03	ND[a]	7
Amoxicillin	8	0.03 – 0.25	0.5	20
Mezlocillin	3	≤ 0.006	ND	8
Aztreonam	3	2.6 – 9.3	ND	8
Cefuroxime-axetil	5	0.06 – 0.25	2 – 32	10
Cefdinir	5	0.5 – 1	16 – 32	10
Cefixime	5	0.25 – 1	16 – 32	10
Ceftriaxone	2	0.03 – 0.06	0.06 – 0.12	16
	8	0.015 – 0.03	0.06	20
	5	≤ 0.0156 – 0.062	0.5 – 2	11
	3	<0.015 – 0.03	ND	14
	8	0.015 – 0.03	ND	20
Cefodizime	2	0.06	0.12	16
Imipenem	3	0.062 – 0.125	32	19
Ertapenem	3	0.031 – 0.062	32	19
Meropenem	3	0.02 – 0.12	ND	8
	3	0.015 – 0.125	2 – 16	19
Aminoglycosides				
Tobramycin	3	16 – 32	ND	7
Tetracyclines – glycylcycline				
Minocycline	2	0.03 – 0.06	1 – 2	16
Doxycycline	8	0.25 – 1	4 – 16	20
Tigecycline	2	0.012 – 0.048	0.195	22
Macrolides – azalides – ketolides				
Erythromycin	3	0.015 – 0.03	ND	2
	5	0.0078 – 0.0625	> 0.5	11
Roxithromycin	2	0.015 – 0.03	0.03 – 0.5	16
	5	0.0039 – 0.0625	> 0.5	11
Rokitamycin	2	0.0072 – 0.056	ND	2
Clarithromycin	5	0.0019 – 0.0312	ND	11
Azithromycin	2	≤ 0.003 -0.007	≤ 0.003 – 0.015	16
	5	0.0004 – 0.0156	0.12 – >0.5	11
	8	0.008 – 0.03	0.015 – 0.03	20
Telithromycin	5	≤ 0.0002 – 0.0078	0.06 – 0.25	11
Cethromycin	5	≤ 0.0002 – 0.0019	0.03 – 0.12	11
ABT-773		≤ 0.002	0.09 – 0.25	9
Fluoroquinolones				
Nalidixic acid	3	256	ND	14
Norfloxacin	3	2 – 4	ND	14
Pefloxacin	3	8 – 32	ND	14
Ofloxacin	3	2 – 8	ND	14
Levofloxacin	3	1 – 4	ND	14
Ciprofloxacin	3	0.5 – 1	ND	14
	2	0.06 – 2	4 – 16	16
Moxifloxacin	3	0.5 – 1	ND	14
Glycopeptides				
Vancomycin	3	0.33 – 0.83	ND	8
Teicoplanin	3	4 – 6.6	ND	8
Fusidic acid	3	> 4	ND	8

[a] ND, not determined.
  B. garinii reference strains tested: PBi, VSDA (22); BITS, BL21 (16); BITS, N34, B45 (2); PTrob, G1, PSth (7, 8, 14, 19); PTrob, ZQ1, PSth, JP2, A87SB (9-11).

Table 4. MIC and MCB of antibiotics for *B. afzelii*

Antibiotic	Number of isolates	MIC (µg/ml) Min/Max	MBC (µg/ml) Min/Max	Reference
β-lactams				
Penicillin G	3	0.5 - 1	ND[a]	7
Amoxicillin	8	0.03 - 0.25	0.5 - > 0.5	20
	10	1 - 4	2 - > 4	18
Mezlocillin	3	≤ 0.06	ND	8
Aztreonam	3	17.3 - > 32	ND	8
Cefuroxime-axetil	5	0.125 - 0.5	2 - 32	10
Cefdinir	5	0.5 - 1	16 - 32	10
Cefixime	5	0.5 - 1	32	10
Ceftriaxone	2	0.03 - 0.06	0.06 - 0.12	16
	5	≤ 0.0156 - 0.0625	0.5 - 2	11
	8	0.03	0.03 - 0.06	20
	10	0.063 - 4	0.25 - 4	18
Cefodizime	2	0.06 - 0.12	0.12 - 0.25	16
Imipenem	3	0.125 - 0.25	16 - 32	19
Ertapenem	3	0.015 - 0.125	0.5 - 4	19
Meropenem	3	0.02 - 0.33	ND	8
Aminoglycosides				
Tobramycin	3	16 - 32	ND	7
Tetracyclines – glycylcycline				
Minocycline	2	0.03 - 0.12	ND	16
Doxycycline	8	0.25 - 2	4 - 16	20
	10	1 - 4	2 - 8	18
Tigecycline	2	0.012 - 0.024	0.095 - 0.195	22
Macrolides – azalides – ketolides				
Erythromycin	2	0.031 - 0.062	ND	2
	5	0.0078 - 0.0625	> 0.5	11
Rokitamycin	2	0.0097 - 0.047	ND	2
Roxithromycin	2	0.015	0.03 - 0.06	16
	5	0.0039 - 0.0625	0.12 - > 0.5	11
Clarithromycin	5	0.0039 - 0.0312	0.12 - > 0.5	11
Azithromycin	2	≤ 0.003	≤ 0.003	16
	5	0.0004 - 0.0156	0.06 - 0.5	11
	8	0.008 - 0.03	0.03 - 0.125	20
	10	0.0138 - 0.0275	0.055 - 0.22	18
Telithromycin	5	≤ 0.0002 - 0.0078	0.03 - 0.25	11
Cethromycin	5	≤ 0.0002 - 0.0078	0.03 - 0.25	11
ABT-773		< 0.002	0.002 - 0.58	9
Fluoroquinolones				
Nalidixic acid	3	128 - 256	ND	14
Norfloxacin	3	2 - 4	ND	14
Pefloxacin	3	4 - 16	ND	14
Ofloxacin	3	2 - 4	ND	14
Levofloxacin	3	1 - 2	ND	14
Ciprofloxacin	3	0.5 - 1	ND	14
	2	2 - 4	4 - 8	16
Moxifloxacin	3	0.5 - 1	ND	14
Glycopeptides				
Vancomycin	3	0.25 - 0.5	ND	8
Teicoplanin	3	3.3 - 6.6	ND	8
Fusidic acid	3	> 4	ND	8

[a] ND, not determined.
B. afzelii reference strains tested: ACA1, Pgau (22); BL3, BL31 (16); BL3, Nancy (2); EB1, EB2, Pko, FEM1 (19); EB1, FEM1, PKo (7, 8, 14); EB1, EB2, FEM1, VS461, FAC3 (9); EB1, EB2, FEM1, VS461, FAC1 (10, 11).

Table 5. MIC (µg/ml) and MBC (µg/ml) of antibiotics for B. valaisiana VS116 and B. bissettii 25015

Antibiotic	B. valaisiana		B. bissettii		Reference
	MIC	MBC	MIC	MBC	
β-lactams					
Penicillin G	0.25	ND[a]	0.125	ND	7
Mezlocillin	≤ 0.06	ND	≤ 0.06	ND	8
Aztreonam	> 32	ND	> 32	ND	8
Cefuroxime-axetil	0.125	16	0.25	8	10
Cefdinir	1	32	2	32	10
Cefixime	1	32	1	32	10
Ceftriaxone	0.0312	2	0.0312	2	11
	0.03	ND	0.03	ND	14
Imipenem	0.5	32	ND	ND	19
Ertapenem	0.031	2	ND	ND	19
Meropenem	0.20	ND	0.08	ND	8
Aminoglycosides					
Tobramycin	64	ND	32	ND	7
Tetracyclines					
Doxycycline	0.125	ND	0.25	ND	7
Macrolides – azalides – ketolides					
Erythromycin	0.0156	> 0.5	0.0312	> 0.5	11
Roxithromycin	0.0078	0.5	0.0312	0.5	11
Clarithromycin	0.0039	> 0.5	0.0078	0.5	11
Azithromycin	0.0009	0.06	0.0039	0.03	11
Telithromycin	0.0004	0.12	0.0009	0.5	11
Cethromycin	≤ 0.0002	0.006	≤ 0.0002	0.006	11
ABT-773	≤ 0.002	0.75	≤ 0.002	0.19	9
Fluoroquinolones					
Nalidixic acid	512	ND	256	ND	14
Norfloxacin	8	ND	8	ND	14
Pefloxacin	32	ND	32	ND	14
Ofloxacin	8	ND	8	ND	14
Levofloxacin	4	ND	2	ND	14
Ciprofloxacin	2	ND	1	ND	14
Moxifloxacin	2	ND	1	ND	14
Glycopeptides					
Vancomycin	0.5	ND	0.83	ND	8
Teicoplanin	> 8	ND	> 8	ND	8
Fusidic acid	> 4	ND	> 4	ND	8

[a] ND, not determined.

ceptible to penicillin G, amoxicillin, cefotaxime and ceftriaxone, doxycycline, macrolides (erythromycin, roxithromycin, clarithromycin, and azithromycin) and telithromycin (1, 7, 11, 13) (Table 5).

The B. recurrentis isolate was susceptible to tetracycline (MIC and MBC = 0.006 µg/ml), penicillin G (MIC = 0.2 µg/ml, MBC = 0.75 µg/ml), and erythromycin (MIC = 0.04 µg/ml, MBC < 0.02 µg/ml).

Phenotypes and mechanisms of resistance

Terekhova et al. (21) selected erythromycin resistance in vitro in B. burgdorferi with raised MICs (10 µg/ml) and MBCs (> 500 µg/ml). They also detected different levels of erythromycin susceptibility in 15 clinical isolates of this species. These strains were tolerant to the bactericidal effect of erythromycin with MBCs > 500 µg/ml. The mechanism of this resistance has not been elucidated. In particular, no resistance gene and no mutations in the 23S rRNA gene, known to confer macrolide resistance, have been detected.

β-lactams and tetracyclines achieve clinical cure in over 90% of acute forms of Lyme disease, particularly in patients with erythrema migrans. However, the rare clinical failures despite appropriate antimicrobial therapy suggest the possibility of *in vivo* acquired resistance in the different species of the *B. burgdorferi* complex. So far, no acquired resistance has been demonstrated in strains isolated from patients who failed treatment. Through the use of genotyping studies on *B. garinii* or *B. afzelii* strains isolated from four patients with erythema migrans who failed treatment, Hunfeld *et al.* (12) showed that each case was indeed a relapse and not a re-infection with a different strain. For each patient, the strains isolated before and after antimicrobial therapy displayed exactly the same resistance phenotype. Ruzic-Sabljic *et al.* (18) reported similar findings in three patients with recurrent erythema migrans infected with *B. afzelii*.

REFERENCES

(1) **Baradaran-Dilmaghani, R., and G. Stanek**. 1996. *In vitro* susceptibility of thirty *Borrelia* strains from various sources against eight antimicrobial chemotherapeutics. Infection **24**:60-63.

(2) **Cinco M, D. Padovan, G. Stinco, and G. Trevisan**. 1995. *In vitro* activity of rokitamycin, a new macrolide, against *Borrelia burgdorferi*. Antimicrob. Agents Chemother. **39**:1185-6.

(3) **Cutler, S.J., D. Fekade, K. Hussein, K. Knox, A. Melka, K. Cann, A.R. Emilanus, D. A. Warrell, and D.J.M. Wright**. 1994. Successful *in vitro* cultivation of *Borrelia recurrentis*. Lancet **343**:242.

(4) **Dever, L.L., J.H. Jorgensen, and A.G. Barbour**. 1993. Comparative *in vitro* activities of clarithromycin, azithromycin, and erythromycin against *Borrelia burgdorferi* Antimicrob. Agents Chemother. **37**:1704-1706.

(5) **Dever L.L, C.V. Torigian, and A.G. Barbour**. 1999. *In vitro* activities of the everninomicin SCH 27899 and other newer antimicrobial agents against *Borrelia burgdorferi*. Antimicrob. Agents Chemother. **43**:1773-5.

(6) **Georgilis, K., M. Peacocke, and M.S. Klempner**. 1992. Fibroblasts protect the Lyme disease spirochete, *Borrelia burgdorferi*, from ceftriaxone *in vitro*. J. Infect. Dis. **166**:440-444.

(7) **Hunfeld, K.P., P. Kraiczy, T.A. Wichelhaus, V. Schafer, and V. Brade**. 2000. New colorimetric microdilution method for *in vitro* susceptibility testing of *Borrelia burgdorferi* against antimicrobial substances. Eur. J. Clin. Microbiol. Infect. Dis. **19**:27-32.

(8) **Hunfeld, K.P., J. Weigand, T.A. Wichelhaus, E. Kekoukh, P. Kraiczy, and V. Brade**. 2001. In vitro activity of mezlocillin, meropenem, aztreonam, vancomycin, teicoplanin, ribostamycin and fusidic acid against *Borrelia burgdorferi*. Int. J. Antimicrob. Agents. **17**:203-208.

(9) **Hunfeld, K.P., T.A. Wichelhaus, E. Kekoukh, M. Molitor, P. Kraiczy, and V. Brade**. 2001. In vitro susceptibility of the *Borrelia burgdorferi* sensu lato complex to ABT-773, a novel ketolide. J. Antimicrob. Chemother.**48**:447-449.

(10) **Hunfeld, K.P., R. Rödel, and T.A. Wichelhaus**. 2003. In vitro activity of eight oral cephalosporins against *Borrelia burgdorferi*. 2003. Int. J. Antimicrob. Agents. **21**:313-318.

(11) **Hunfeld, K.P., T.A. Wichelhaus, R. Rodel, G. Acker, V. Brade, and P. Kraiczy**. 2004. Comparison of *in vitro* activities of ketolides, macrolides, and azalides against the spirochete *Borrelia burgdorferi*. Antimicrob. Agents Chemother. **48**:344-347.

(12) **Hunfeld, K.P., E. Ruzic-Sabljic, D.E. Norris, P. Kraiczy, and F. Strle**. 2005. In vitro susceptibility testing of *Borrelia burgdorferi* sensu lato isolates cultured from patients with erythema migrans before and after antimicrobial chemotherapy. Antimicrob. Agents Chemother. **49**:1294-1301.

(13) **Johnson, R.C., C.B. Kodner, P.J. Jurkovich, and J.J. Collins**. 1990. Comparative *in vitro* and in vivo susceptibilities of the Lyme disease spirochete *Borrelia burgdorferi* to cefuroxime and other antimicrobial agents. Antimicrob. Agents Chemother. **34**:2133-2136.

(14) **Kraiczy, P., J. Weigand, T.A. Wichelhaus, P. Heisig, H. Backes, V. Schafer, G. Acker, V. Brade, and K.P. Hunfeld**. 2001. *In vitro* activities of fluoroquinolones against the spirochete *Borrelia burgdorferi*. Antimicrob. Agents Chemother. **45**:2486-2494.

(15) **Levin, J.M., J.A. Nelson, J. Segreti, B. Harrison, C.A. Benson, and F. Strle**. 1993. In vitro susceptibility of *Borrelia burgdorferi* to 11 antimicrobial agents. Antimicrob. Agents Chemother. **37**:1444-1446.

(16) **Murgia R, F. Marchetti, and M. Cinco**. 1999. Comparative bacteriostatic and bactericidal activities of cefodizime against *Borrelia burgdorferi* sensu lato. Antimicrob. Agents Chemother. **43**:3030-3032.

(17) **Pavia C.S., G.P. Wormser, J. Nowakowski, and A. Cacciapuoti**. 2001. Efficacy of an evernimicin (SCH27899) *in vitro* and in an animal model of Lyme disease. Antimicrob. Agents Chemother. **45**:936-937.

(18) **Ruzic-Sabljic, E., T. Podreka, V. Maraspin, and F. Strle**. 2005. Susceptibility of *Borrelia afzelii* strains to antimicrobial agents. Int. J. Antimicrob. Agents. **25**:474-478.

(19) **Rödel, R., A. Freyer, T. Bittner, V. Schäfer, and K.P. Hunfeld**. 2007. In vitro activities of faropenem, ertapenem, imipenem and meropenem against *Borrelia burgdorferi* s.l. Int. J. Antimicrob. Agents. **30**:83-86.

(20) **Sicklinger, M., R. Wienecke, and U. Neubert**. 2003. *In vitro* susceptibility testing of four antibiotics against *Borrelia burgdorferi*: a comparison of results for the three genospecies *Borrelia afzelii*, *Borrelia garinii*, and *Borrelia burgdorferi* sensu stricto. J. Clin. Microbiol. **41**:1791-1793.

(21) **Terekhova, D., M.L. Sartakova, G.P. Wormser, I. Schwartz, and F.C. Cabello**. 2002. Erythromycin resistance in *Borrelia burgdorferi*. Antimicrob. Agents Chemother. **46**:3637-3640.

(22) **Yang, X., A. Nguyen, D. Qiu, and B.J. Luft**. 2009. In vitro activity of tigecycline against multiple strains of *Borrelia burgdorferi*. J. Antimicrob. Chemother. **63**:709-712.

BRUCELLA

Brucella is a genus of small, Gram-negative coccobacilli. These facultative intracellular pathogens infect monocytes/macrophages and are the causal agents of brucellosis (17). Seven species have been found in land mammals (*B. abortus*, *B. melitensis*, *B. suis*, *B. ovis*, *B. canis*, *B. neotomae* and *B. muris*) and two in marine mammals (*B. pinnipedii* and *B. ceti*). *B. abortus* and *B. melitensis* are the principal human pathogens. Transmission to humans occurs through direct contact with an infected animal (through skin, eyes or by inhalation) or indirectly by consumption of unpasteurized milk or contaminated dairy products. Brucellosis is an endemic disease in certain countries of the Mediterranean Basin, as well as in the Middle East, West Asia, Africa and Latin America. Clinically the disease progresses in three stages: an acute septicemic stage, a subacute stage with possible secondary focalizations, and a chronic stage (> 1 year).

Methods

Due to the high risk of aerosolization, laboratories working with *Brucella* should do so in a level three biosafety facility. An antibiogram can only be performed in the case where a strain can be isolated, usually from a blood culture taken during the acute stage of the disease. Antimicrobial susceptibility testing of *Brucella* requires the use of techniques suited to the slow growth of these organisms. The CLSI recommends Brucella medium pH 7.1 with a 0.5 McFarland inoculum and aerobic incubation at 35 ± 2°C for 48 h (3). Some strains may require a 5% CO_2-enriched atmosphere. CLSI has set the following susceptibility breakpoints for *Brucella*: ≤ 4 µg/ml for gentamicin, ≤ 8 µg/ml for streptomycin, ≤ 1 µg/ml for tetracycline or doxycycline, ≤ 38/2 for co-trimoxazole. E-test® (13, 21, 25) has also been used to assess the susceptibility of *Brucella* to aminoglycosides (streptomycin and gentamicin), tetracyclines (particularly doxycycline), rifampin, co-trimoxazole, fluoroquinolones (ofloxacin and ciprofloxacin), and, to a lesser extent, macrolides (particularly erythromycin).

Bactericidal activity of antibiotics against *Brucella* has been evaluated by time-kill studies in liquid medium using an inoculum of 10^5 CFU/ml. After a 48 h incubation cells are counted by the CFU method in tubes containing an antibiotic concentration above the MIC. A bactericidal effect is defined as a reduction in the inoculum of at least 3-4 Log after 48 h of incubation.

A number of cell models have been developed to study the activity of antibiotics against intracellular *Brucella*. These include mouse peritoneal macrophages, bovine uterine or testicular cells, or, most often, murine monocyte lines (J774). The human macrophage cell line Mono Mac 6 has also been used recently (28); these cells express the phenotypic and functional characteristics of mature human macrophages.

Susceptible phenotype

Brucella species show *in vitro* susceptibility to some β-lactams such as penicillins A, third generation cephalosporins (cefotaxime and ceftriaxone) and imipenem (Table 6), but these drugs are not clinically active. Macrolides have moderate activity, azithromycin being the most active *in vitro* (MIC_{90} = 0.5-2 µg/ml) (6, 8). Chloramphenicol has little activity (15) and co-trimoxazole has variable activity depending on the strain (2, 7, 13, 15, 27). The most active agents include the aminoglycosides (particularly streptomycin and gentamicin), tetracyclines, rifampin and fluoroquinolones (Table 6). Fluoroquinolones have variable and fairly modest activity, probably due to decreased affinity for DNA gyrase subunit A arising from the substitution of an alanine at position 83 in place of the serine present in susceptible species (19).

Only the aminoglycosides, tetracyclines and rifampin exhibit bactericidal activity *in vitro* (20, 22). Fluoroquinolones are not bactericidal (24).

Studies of the antimicrobial susceptibility of intracellular *Brucella* are scarce and the data are old. Streptomycin has low intracellular activity in comparison to its extracellular activity whereas rifampin retains an intracellular bactericidal effect (5). A more recent study evaluated antibiotic activity against *B. abortus* (strain 2308) in two monocyte cell lines: human Mono Mac 6 cells and J774 murine macrophages (28). After incubation of *B. abortus* cultures for 24 h in the presence of antibiotic, a bacteriostatic effect was respectively observed at 1xMIC in Mono Mac 6 cells and 4xMIC in J774 cells for tetracycline and doxycycline, at 0.25xMIC and 1xMIC for rifampin, and at 1xMIC and 4xMIC for ciprofloxacin. Gentamicin and streptomycin were not bacteriostatic in these cell systems. These antibiotics are more active when encapsulated in microspheres due to better intracellular penetration (11, 18). A modest intracellular bactericidal effect (≤ 1 Log reduction in viable cell count in the presence of antibiotic) was

Table 6. *In vitro* antibiotic susceptibility of *Brucella* spp.

Antibiotic	Number of isolates	MIC$_{90}$ (μg/ml)	MIC range (μg/ml)	Reference
β-lactams				
Penicillin G	15	4	0.25 - 8	15
Ampicillin	15	4	0.25 - 8	15
	74	2	0.09 - 3	25
Cephalothin	15	32	1 - 64	15
Cefotaxime	83	2	≤ 0.5 - 2	16
Ceftriaxone	83	1	≤ 0.25 -1	16
	24		0.06 - 0.38	13
Aminoglycosides				
Streptomycin	95	0.5	0.12 - 1	2
	86	3.1	ND[a]	20
	74	2	0.125 - 4	25
Gentamicin	15	1	0.25 - 2	15
	74	2	0.03 – 1.5	25
Tetracyclines				
Tetracycline	98	0.39	0.1 - 0.5	7
	95	0.25	0.6 - 0.25	2
	358	0.25	0.06 - 0.5	8
	74	0.5	0.03 - 1.5	25
Doxycycline	95	0.12	0.6 - 0.25	2
	24	ND	0.06 - 0.125	13
Minocycline	86	0.4	ND	20
Trimethoprim / sulfamethoxazole	98	6.4/32	1.6/8 - 25.6/128	7
	15	1/19	≤ 0.25/4.5 - 1/19	15
	24	ND	0.012/0.064	13
	74	0.75/14.2	0.03/0.6 - 1.5/28.5	25
Rifampin	98	0.5	0.06 - 1	7
	95	2	0.12 - 4	2
	24	ND	0.75 - 2	13
	74	1	0.09 - 1.5	25
Chloramphenicol	15	2	0.25 - 4	15
Macrolides azalide				
Erythromycin	62	16	0.2 - 16	6
	74	4	0.5 - 8	25
Roxithromycin	60	16	0.1 - 32	6
Clarithromycin	62	8	0.06 - 8	6
Azithromycin	59	2	0.1 - 4	6
	358		0.5 - 1	8
Fluoroquinolones				
Norfloxacin	74	3	0.125 - 4	25
Ofloxacin	86	2.5	ND	20
	160	2	1 - 2	24
Levofloxacin	160	0.5	0.5	24
	74	0.5	0.06 - 0.75	25
Ciprofloxacin	95	0.5	0.12 - 0.5	2
	160	1	0.25 - 1	24
	24	ND	0.094 - 0.5	13
Moxifloxacin	160	1	1	24

[a] ND, not determined.

observed for rifampin and ciprofloxacin (at 4x and 8xMIC) which was more pronounced in Mono Mac 6 cells than in J774 cells. Akova et al. (1) showed that in acidic culture medium (pH ~5), only doxycycline and rifampin conserved bacteriostatic activity against *Brucella* whereas streptomycin, macrolides and fluoroquinolones were inactivated. As *Brucella* multiplies within the acidic intracellular medium of phagosomes, the authors speculated that certain antibiotics were inactivated by these acidic conditions.

Phenotypes and mechanisms of resistance

Clinical experience has shown that antimicrobial therapy with a single antibiotic and/or of short duration is correlated with a high rate of treatment failure or post-treatment relapse (9, 10, 14, 22). Nonetheless, acquired antibiotic resistance among human or animal *Brucella* species currently appears to be extremely rare or nonexistent (4, 21-23).

On the other hand, it is easy to select for laboratory mutants of *B. melitensis* or *B. abortus* that are resistant to rifampin (12) or fluoroquinolones (19, 27). Rifampin resistance is conferred by mutations in the gene encoding the β subunit of RNA polymerase (12). Several different amino acid substitutions (alone or combined) in the RpoB protein confer resistance to rifampin: $Asp_{526}Tyr$ in *B. abortus*; $Val_{154}Phe$, $Asp_{526}Tyr$, $Asp_{526}Asn$, $Asp_{526}Gly$, $His_{536}Leu$, $His_{536}Tyr$, $Arg_{539}Ser$, $Ser_{541}Leu$ and $Pro_{574}Leu$ in *B. melitensis* (12). Fluoroquinolone resistance arises from the selection of mutations in the topoisomerase genes that are the targets of these antibiotics (19, 27). $Asp_{91}Tyr$ and $Ala_{87}Val$ substitutions in subunit A of DNA gyrase have been described (19, 27). Efflux pump overexpression also appears to play a role in fluoroquinolone resistance, possibly in association with the above mutations (19, 26).

REFERENCES

(1) **Akova, M., D. Gür, D.M. Livermore, T. Kocagoz, and H.E. Akalin**. 1999. *In vitro* activities of antibiotics alone and in combination against *Brucella melitensis* at neutral and acidic pHs. Antimicrob. Agents Chemother. **43**:1298-1300.

(2) **Bosch, J., J. Linares, M.J. Lopez de Goicoechea, J. Ariza, M.C. Cisnal, and R. Martin**. 1986. *In vitro* activity of ciprofloxacin, ceftriaxone, and five other antimicrobial agents against 95 strains of *Brucella melitensis*. J. Antimicrob. Chemother. **17**:459-461.

(3) **Clinical and Laboratory Standard Institute**. 2009. Performance Standards for Antimicrobial Susceptibility Testing. Nineteenth Informational Supplement. M100-S19. Vol. 29 No.3.

(4) **De Rautlin de la Roy, Y.M., B. Grignon, G. Grollier, M.F. Coindreau, and B. Becq-Giraudon**. 1986. Rifampicin resistance in a strain of *Brucella melitensis* after treatment with doxycycline and rifampicin. J. Antimicrob. Chemother. **18**:648-649.

(5) **Filice, G., G. Carnevale, P. Lanzarini, F. Castelli, G. Gorini, R. Benzi-Cipelli, and E. Concia**. 1986. Intracellular killing of *Brucella melitensis* within mouse peritoneal macrophages: influence of treatment with rifampicin. An ultrastructural study. Microbiologica **9**:189-198.

(6) **Garcia-Rodriguez, J.A., J.L. Munoz Bellido, M.J. Fresnadillo, and I. Trujillano**. 1993. *In vitro* activities of new macrolides and rifapentine against *Brucella* spp. Antimicrob. Agents Chemother. **37**:911-913.

(7) **Gutierrez Altes, A., M. Diez Enciso, P. Pena Gracia, and A. Campos Bueno**. 1982. *In vitro* activity of N-formimidoyl thienamycin against 98 clinical isolates of *Brucella melitensis* compared with those of cefoxitine, rifampin, tetracycline, and co-trimoxazole. Antimicrob. Agents Chemother. **21**:501-503.

(8) **Landinez, R., J. Linarez, E. Loza, J. Martinez-Beltran, R. Martin, and F. Baquero**. 1992. *In vitro* activity of azithromycin and tetracycline against 358 clinical isolates of *Brucella melitensis*. Eur. J. Clin. Microbiol. Infect. Dis. **11**:265-267.

(9) **Lang, R., R. Dagan, I. Potasman, M. Einhorn, and R. Raz**. 1992. Failure of ceftriaxone in the treatment of acute brucellosis. Clin. Infect. Dis. **14**:506-509.

(10) **Lang, R., and E. Rubinstein**. 1992. Quinolones for the treatment of brucellosis. J. Antimicrob. Chemother. **29**:357-363.

(11) **Lecároz, C., M.J. Blanco-Prieto, M.A. Burrell, and C. Gamazo**. 2006. Intracellular killing of *Brucella melitensis* in human macrophages with microsphere-encapsulated gentamicin. J. Antimicrob. Chemother. **58**:549-556.

(12) **Marianelli, C., F. Ciuchini, M. Tarantino, P. Pasquali, and R. Adone**. 2004. Genetic bases of the rifampin resistance phenotype in *Brucella* spp. J. Clin. Microbiol. **42**:5439-5443.

(13) **Marianelli, C., C. Graziani, C. Santangelo, M.T. Xibilia, A. Imbriani, R. Amato, D. Neri, M. Cuccia, S. Rinnone, V. Di Marco, and F. Ciuchini**. 2007. Molecular epidemiological and antibiotic susceptibility characterization of *Brucella* isolates from humans in Sicily, Italy. J. Clin. Microbiol. **45**:2923-2928.

(14) **Montejo, J.M., I. Alberola, P. Glez-Zarate, A. Alvarez, J. Alonso, A. Casanovas A., and C. Aguirre**. 1993. Open, randomized therapeutic trial of six antimicrobial regimens in the treatment of human brucellosis. Clin. Infect. Dis. **16**:671-676.

(15) **Mortensen, J.E., D.G. Moore, J.E. Clarridge, and E.J. Young**. 1986. Antimicrobial susceptibility of clinical isolates of *Brucella*. Diagn. Microbiol. Infect. Dis. **5**:163-169.

(16) **Palenque, E., J.R. Otero, and A.R. Noriega**. 1986. *In vitro* susceptibility of *Brucella melitensis* to new cephalosporins crossing the blood brain barrier. Antimicrob. Agents Chemother. **29**:182-183.

(17) **Pappas, G., N. Akritidis, M. Bosilkovski, and E. Tsianos**. 2005. Brucellosis. N. Engl. J. Med. **352**:2325-2336.

(18) **Prior, S., B. Gander, C. Lecároz, J.M. Irache, and C. Gamazo**. 2004. Gentamicin-loaded microspheres for reducing the intracellular *Brucella abortus* load in infected monocytes. J. Antimicrob. Chemother. **53**:981-988.

(19) **Ravanel, N., B. Gestin, and M. Maurin**. 2009. In vitro selection of fluoroquinolone resistance in *Brucella melitensis*. Int. J. Antimicrob. Agents **34**:76-81.

(20) **Rubinstein, E., R. Lang, B. Shasha, B. Hagar, L. Diamanstein, G. Joseph, M. Anderson, and K. Harrison**. 1991. *In vitro* susceptibility of *Brucella melitensis* to antibiotics. Antimicrob. Agents Chemother. **35**:1925-1927.

(21) **Sayan, M., Z. Yumuk, D. Dündar, O. Bilenoglu, S. Erdenlig, E. Yaşar, and A. Willke**. 2008. Rifampicin resistance phenotyping of *Brucella melitensis* by *rpoB* gene analysis in clinical isolates. J. Chemother. **20**:431-435.

(22) **Solera, J., E. Martinez-Alfaro, and A. Espinosa**. 1997. Recognition and optimum treatment of brucellosis. Drugs **53**:245-256.

(23) **Tanyel, E., A.Y. Coban, S.T. Koruk, H. Simsek, S. Hepsert, O.S. Cirit, and N. Tulek**. 2007. Actual antibiotic resistance pattern of *Brucella melitensis* in central Anatolia. An update from an endemic region. Saudi Med. J. **28**:1239-1242.

(24) **Trujillano-Martin, I., E. Garcia-Sanchez, I.M. Martinez, M.J. Fresnadillo, J.E. Garcia-Sanchez, and J.A. Garcia-Rodriguez**. 1999. *In vitro* activities of six new fluoroquinolones against *Brucella melitensis*. Antimicob. Agents Chemother. **43**:194-195.

(25) **Turkmani, A., A. Ioannidis, A. Christidou, A. Psaroulaki, F. Loukaides, and Y. Tselentis**. 2006. In vitro susceptibilities of *Brucella melitensis* isolates to eleven antibiotics. Ann. Clin. Microbiol. Antimicrob. **5**:24-27.

(26) **Turkmani, A., A. Psaroulaki, A. Christidou, G. Samoilis, T.A. Mourad, D. Tabaa, and Y. Tselentis**. 2007. Uptake of ciprofloxacin and ofloxacin by 2 *Brucella* strains and their fluoroquinolone-resistant variants under different conditions. An in vitro study. Diagn. Microbiol. Infect. Dis. **59**:447-451.

(27) **Turkmani, A., A. Psaroulaki, A. Christidou, D. Chochlakis, D. Tabaa, and Y. Tselentis**. 2008. In vitro-selected resistance to fluoroquinolones in two *Brucella* strains associated with mutational changes in *gyrA*. Int. J. Antimicrob. Agents. **32**:227-232.

(28) **Valderas, M.W., and W.W. Barrow**. 2008. Establishment of a method for evaluating intracellular antibiotic efficacy in *Brucella abortus*-infected Mono Mac 6 monocytes. J. Antimicrob. Chemother. **61**:128-134.

FRANCISELLA

Francisella are Gram-negative bacilli which are facultative intracellular parasites of monocytes/macrophages (8, 16). The genus comprises the species *F. tularensis*, *F. philomiragia,* and *F. piscicida*. *F. tularensis* comprises two subspecies which cause the disease known as tularemia: *F. tularensis subsp. tularensis* found predominantly in North America, *F. tularensis subsp. holarctica* present throughout the northern hemisphere. *F. tularensis subsp. mediasiatica* has been occasionally described in animals in central Asia. Water is the reservoir for *F. tularensis subsp. novicida* (formerly *F. novicida*) and the species *F. philomiragia* and *F. piscicida*, which have low virulence in humans. The species which cause tularemia have an animal reservoir. Human contamination occurs either through direct contact with an infected animal via bites, skin contact or consumption of contaminated food, from arthropod bite (especially tick bite), or indirectly via a contaminated environment. *Francisella* is capable of surviving for weeks or months in a wet environment, probably due in part to symbiosis with free amoebae (1).

Methods

Due to the high risk of inhalation of aerosols, laboratories working with *Francisella* should do so in a level three biosafety facility. Antimicrobial susceptibility testing of *Francisella* requires the use of techniques suited to the slow growth of these fastidious organisms, particularly the presence of L-cysteine in the culture medium. A method described in 1985 by Baker (2) uses Mueller-Hinton medium supplemented with calcium, magnesium, glucose, vitamins, L-cysteine and iron pyrophosphate. MICs are read after a 24 h aerobic incubation. More recently, the CLSI has recommended cation-adjusted Mueller-Hinton broth (CAMHB) supplemented with 2% polyvitamins (e.g. IsovitaleX®, Becton Dickinson) with incubation at $35 \pm 2°C$ for 48 h in an aerobic atmosphere (7). The CLSI has set the following susceptibility breakpoints for *Francisella*: ≤ 4 µg/ml for gentamicin, ≤ 8 µg/ml for streptomycin, ≤ 4 µg/ml for tetracycline or doxycycline, ≤ 0.5 for ciprofloxacin or levofloxacin. The CLSI method was recently used to study antibiotic susceptibility in 169 *F. tularensis* strains (including 92 subsp.

tularensis and 77 subsp. *holarctica*) isolated in the United States (19) and 71 strains of *F. tularensis* subsp. *holarctica* isolated in France (20). Brown *et al.* (6) defined MIC control limits for nine antibiotics on reference strains belonging to the species *Staphylococcus aureus*, *Escherichia coli* and *Pseudomonas aeruginosa* so as to better standardize this method. Nonetheless it remains difficult to evaluate the clinical relevance of the proposed breakpoints, especially since the incidence of tularemia is so low. E-test® has also been used for antibiotic susceptibility testing of *Francisella* spp., using either Mueller-Hinton II agar or chocolate agar supplemented with 2% IsoVitaleX™ (11, 18, 20). MIC values obtained by E-test® were similar to those obtained by the CLSI method for streptomycin, doxycycline and ciprofloxacin. The MICs of gentamicin, rifampin and chloramphenicol showed less concordance, although this did not modify the clinical categorization (susceptible, intermediate, resistant) (20). β-lactam MICs determined by E-test® were considerably higher than those obtained in liquid medium (11).

The activity of antibiotics against intracellular *Francisella* has been studied in the P388D1 murine macrophage-like cell line (14). These cells are contacted *in vitro* with a known *Francisella* inoculum for 1 h. Non-phagocytosed bacteria are eliminated by addition of an aminoglycoside to the culture supernatant for 4 h. After eliminating the aminoglycoside, the residual intracellular inoculum is counted by the CFU method after lysing the eukaryotic cells. The infected cell cultures are then incubated with fresh medium containing the antibiotic to be tested. Antibiotic activity is evaluated by counting viable intracellular bacteria after different incubation times. A bacteriostatic effect is defined as an inhibition of growth in comparison to an antibiotic-free control. A bactericidal effect corresponds to a reduction of the starting inoculum over time.

Susceptible phenotype

Bacteria belonging to the species *F. tularensis* display similar susceptibility to antibiotics with the exception of macrolides (Table 7). They are intrinsically resistant to penicillins because they harbor chromosomal Ambler class A penicillinases (4). Susceptibility to third generation cephalosporins varies in different studies and depends on the method used for MIC determination (2, 9, 15). Aminoglycosides (particularly streptomycin and gentamicin) (2, 15, 19, 20), fluoroquinolones (12, 14, 15, 17), tetracyclines (15, 19, 20), and rifampin (2, 20) have the highest activity *in vitro*. Fluoroquinolones have bactericidal activity *in vitro* (14, 17) with an MBC of 0.13 to 0.25 for ciprofloxacin. Macrolide activity varies according to the molecule. Telithromycin, a ketolide, is more active than the true macrolides. *F. tularensis* subsp. *holarctica* isolates from Eastern Europe (biovar 2) classically show intrinsic resistance while isolates from Western Europe (biovar 1) and the United States are more susceptible (18, 19). For instance, the LVS vaccine strain derived from a Russian strain of *F. tularensis* subsp. *holarctica* biovar 2 is highly resistant to erythromycin (MIC > 256 µg/ml), probably due to an $A_{2059}C$ transition in the 23S rRNA gene which is the target of these antibiotics. Interestingly, strains isolated in Spain during epidemics occurring between 1997 and 2007 appear to be particularly resistant to antibiotics, especially macrolides, although the long incubation times used in these tests (3 days) might partly explain these differences (9). Phenicols and co-trimoxazole are moderately active. *F. tularensis* has also been found to possess efflux pumps for certain antibiotics, including the AcrAB system belonging to the RND (resistance-nodulation-division) family (5) and the TolC-FtlC system (10).

Third generation cephalosporins like ceftriaxone, as well as the true macrolides, co-trimoxazole and phenocols are inactive in cell models (14), which might explain their lack of clinical efficacy. On the other hand, aminoglycosides, fluoroquinolones, tetracyclines, rifampicin and telithromycin display intracellular bactericidal activity (14). The first three classes have been successfully used in patients with tularemia. Rifampin is not used as monotherapy in humans due to the hypothetical risk of selecting resistant mutants, and the clinical interest of telithromycin has not been established.

Phenotypes and mechanisms of resistance

Acquired resistance has not been described in any human or animal strain of *F. tularensis*. Rifampin and fluoroquinolone resistance can be selected *in vitro* via mutations in DNA gyrase subunit A (3, 13).

REFERENCES

(1) **Abd, H., T. Johansson, I. Golovliov, G. Sandstrom, and M. Forsman**. 2003. Survival and growth of *Francisella tularensis* in *Acanthamoeba castellanii*. Appl. Environ. Microbiol. **69**:600-606.

Table 7. In vitro antibiotic susceptibility of *Francisella tularensis*

Antibiotic	Number of isolates	MIC$_{90}$ (µg/ml)	MIC range (µg/ml)	Reference
β-lactams				
Penicillin G	15	> 8	4 - > 8	2
	1	ND[a]	256	14
	46[b]	> 64	> 64	9
Ampicillin	15	> 8	> 8	2
	1	ND	256	14
	46[b]	> 16	> 16	9
Amoxicillin	46[b]	> 32	> 32	9
Ticarcillin	15	> 64	> 64	2
	46[b]	> 64	> 64	9
Piperacillin	15	64	≤ 0.5 - > 64	2
	46[b]	> 64	> 64	9
Cephalothin	15	> 8	≤ 0.25 - > 8	2
	46[b]	> 32	> 32	9
Cefotaxime	15	4	≤ 0.12 - 4	2
	46[b]	> 32	32 - > 32	9
Ceftriaxone	15	8	0.5 - 16	2
Ceftazidime	15	≤ 0.5	≤ 0.5 - 1	2
	46[b]	>16	4 - > 16	9
Imipenem	46[b]	> 8	> 8	9
Meropenem	46[b]	> 8	> 8	9
Aminoglycosides				
Streptomycin	15	4	≤ 0.5 - 4	2
	169	2	0.25 - 4	19
	71	ND	< 0.5 - 1	20
	46[b]	32	4 - 32	9
	38[b]	4	0.25 - 4	11
Gentamicin	15	2	0.25 - 2	2
	169	0.25	0.03 - 0.5	19
	71	ND	0.03 - 0.5	20
	46[b]	8	1 - 8	9
	38[b]	1	0.38 - 1.5	11
Tobramycin	15	2	≤ 0.12 - 4	2
	46[b]	4	2 - 8	9
Netilmicin	15	2	0.25 - 2	2
Amikacin	15	2	≤ 0.25 - 2	2
	46[b]	8	4 - 8	9
Tetracycline – glycylcycline				
Tetracycline	15	2	≤ 0.25 - 2	2
	169	1	0.25 - 2	19
	46[b]	64	4 - 64	9
	38[b]	0.38	0.094 - 0.5	11
Doxycycline	1	ND	8	14
	169	2	0.25 - 4	19
	71	ND	0.125 - 1	20
	46[b]	> 32	2 - > 32	9
Trimethoprim / sulfamethoxazole	1	ND	16/80	14
Rifampin	15	1	≤ 0.03 - 1	2
	71	ND	0.015 - 0.5	20
Chloramphenicol	15	1	≤ 0.25 - 4	2
	169	2	0.5 - 4	19
	71	ND	0.25 - 2	20
	46[b]	≤ 8	≤ 8	9
	38[b]	0.38	0.125 - 0.5	11
Thiamphenicol	1	ND	8	14
Macrolides – ketolide				
Erythromycin	15	2	0.5 - 2	2
	92[c]	0.5	0.5 - 2	19
	77[b]	2	0.5 - 4	19
	46[b]	> 4	2 - > 4	9
Clarithromycin	1	ND	8	14
Telithromycin	1	ND	0.5	14
	71	ND	0.125 - 0.25	20

Table 7. *In vitro* antibiotic susceptibility of *Francisella tularensis* (continued)

Antibiotic	Number of isolates	MIC$_{90}$ (μg/ml)	MIC range (μg/ml)	Reference
Fluoroquinolones				
Nalidixic acid	71	ND	0.06 - 2	8
Ofloxacin	1	ND	0.25	3
Levofloxacin	169	0.06	0.015 - 0.12	7
	46[b]	≤ 0.25	≤ 0.25	9
Ciprofloxacin	1	ND	0.25	3
	169	0.06	0.004 - 0.06	7
	71	ND	0.015 - 0.03	8
	46[b]	0.25	0.06 - 0.25	9
	38[b]	0.016	0.008 - 0.023	11

[a] ND, not determined.
[b] *F. tularensis* subsp. *holarctica*.
[c] *F. tularensis* subsp. *tularensis*.

(2) **Baker, C.N., D.G. Hollis, and C. Thornsberry**. 1985. Antimicrobial susceptibility testing of *Francisella tularensis* with a modified Mueller-Hinton broth. J. Clin. Microbiol. **22**:212-215.

(3) **Bhatnagar, N., E. Getachew, S. Straley, J. Williams, M. Meltzer, and A. Fortier**. 1994. Reduced virulence of rifampicin-resistant mutants of *Francisella tularensis*. J. Infect. Dis. **170**:841-847.

(4) **Bina, X.R., C. Wang, M.A. Miller, and J.E. Bina**. 2006. The Bla2 beta-lactamase from the live-vaccine strain of *Francisella tularensis* encodes a functional protein that is only active against penicillin-class beta-lactam antibiotics. Arch. Microbiol. **186**:219-228.

(5) **Bina, X.R., C.L. Lavine, M.A. Miller, and J.E. Bina**. 2008. The AcrAB RND efflux system from the live vaccine strain of *Francisella tularensis* is a multiple drug efflux system that is required for virulence in mice. FEMS Microbiol. Lett. **279**:226-233.

(6) **Brown, S.D., K. Krisher, and M.M. Traczewski**. 2004. Broth microdilution susceptibility testing of *Francisella tularensis*: quality control limits for nine antimicrobial agents and three standard quality control strains. J. Clin. Microbiol. **42**:5877-5880.

(7) **Clinical and Laboratory Standard Institute**. 2009. Performance Standards for Antimicrobial Susceptibility Testing. Nineteenth Informational Supplement. M100-S19. Vol. 29 No.3.

(8) **Ellis, J., P.C. Oyston, M. Green, and R.W. Titball**. 2002. Tularemia. Clin. Microbiol. Rev. **15**:631-646.

(9) **García del Blanco, N., C.B. Gutiérrez Martín, V.A. de la Puente Redondo, and E.F. Rodríguez Ferri**. 2004. In vitro susceptibility of field isolates of *Francisella tularensis* subsp. *holarctica* recovered in Spain to several antimicrobial agents. Res. Vet. Sci. **76**:195-198.

(10) **Gil, H., G.J. Platz, C.A. Forestal, M. Monfett, C.S. Bakshi, T.J. Sellati, M.B. Furie, J.L. Benach, and D.G. Thanassi**. 2006. Deletion of TolC orthologs in *Francisella tularensis* identifies roles in multidrug resistance and virulence. Proc. Natl. Acad. Sci. USA. **103**:12897-12902.

(11) **Ikäheimo, I., H. Syrjälä, J. Karhukorpi, R. Schildt, and M. Koskela**. 2000. In vitro antibiotic susceptibility of *Francisella tularensis* isolated from humans and animals. J. Antimicrob. Chemother. **46**:287-290.

(12) **Johansson, A., S.K. Urich, M.C. Chu, A. Sjöstedt, and A. Tärnvik**. 2002. In vitro susceptibility to quinolones of *Francisella tularensis* subspecies *tularensis*. Scand. J. Infect. Dis. **34**:327-330.

(13) **La Scola, B., K. Elkarkouri, W. Li, T. Wahab, G. Fournous, J.M. Rolain, S. Biswas, M. Drancourt, C. Robert, S. Audic, S. Löfdahl, and D. Raoult**. 2008. Rapid comparative genomic analysis for clinical microbiology: the *Francisella tularensis* paradigm. Genome Res. **18**:742-50.

(14) **Maurin, M., N.F. Mersali, and D. Raoult**. 2000. Bactericidal activities of antibiotics against intracellular *Francisella tularensis*. Antimicrob. Agents Chemother. **44**:3428-3431

(15) **Scheel, O., T. Hoel, T. Sandvik, and B.P. Berdal**. 1993. Susceptibility pattern of Scandinavian *Francisella tularensis* isolates with regard to oral and parenteral antimicrobial agents. APMIS. **101**:33-36.

(16) **Sjöstedt, A**. 2007. Tularemia: history, epidemiology, pathogen physiology, and clinical manifestations. Ann. N. Y. Acad. Sci. **1105**:1-29.

(17) **Syrjälä, H., R. Schildt, and S. Räisäinen**. 1991. In vitro susceptibility of *Francisella tularensis* to fluoroquinolones and treatment of tularemia with norfloxacin and ciprofloxacin. Eur. J. Clin. Microbiol. Infect. Dis. **10**:68-70.

(18) **Tomaso, H., S. Al Dahouk, E. Hofer, W.D. Splettstoesser, T.M. Treu, M.P. Dierich, and H. Neubauer**. 2005. Antimicrobial susceptibilities of Austrian *Francisella tularensis holarctica* biovar II strains. Int. J. Antimicrob. Agents. **26**:279-284.

(19) **Urich, S.K., and J.M. Petersen**. 2008. In vitro susceptibility of isolates of *Francisella tularensis* types A and B from North America. Antimicrob. Agents Chemother. **52**:2276-2278.

(20) **Valade, E., J. Vaissaire, A. Mérens, E. Hernandez, C. Gros, C. Le Doujet, J.C. Paucod, F.M. Thibault, B. Durand, M. Lapalus, I. Dupuis, A. Caclard, D.R. Vidal, and J.D. Cavallo**. 2008. Susceptibility of 71 French isolates of *Francisella tularensis* subsp. *holarctica* to eight antibiotics and accuracy of the E-test method. J. Antimicrob. Chemother. **62**:208-210.

EHRLICHIA

Human ehrlichioses are caused by Gram-negative, obligate intracellular bacteria of the genera *Ehrlichia*, *Anaplasma*, and *Neorickettsia*; these bacteria infect leukocytes (5, 6). *Neorickettsia sennetsu* was identified in 1953 as a causal agent of ehrlichiosis in Japan but seems to have disappeared after a few years. *E. chaffeensis* is the agent of human monocytic ehrlichiosis. *E. canis* and *E. ewingii*, which cause ehrlichiosis in dogs, rarely cause human disease. *Anaplasma phagocytophilum* causes human granulocytic anaplasmosis. *E. chaffeensis* and *A. phagocytophilum* have an animal reservoir and are transmitted to humans by the bite of the Ixodes tick (6). These ehrlichioses have been described in both the United States and Europe (1) and clinically they present as flu-like symptoms which are generally self-limiting (1, 6). Severe or even fatal disease occurs in about 3% of patients with monocytic ehrlichiosis but less than 1% of cases of granulocytic anaplasmosis (6).

Methods

Susceptibility testing of *Ehrlichia* requires the use of cell cultures. Different cell lines are used including murine macrophage-like cells (P388D1) for *N. sennetsu* (3) or *N. risticii* (11), canine monocytes (DH82) for *E. chaffeensis* (4, 12) and human granulocytes (HL60) for *A. phagocytophilum* (7, 8, 10). *Ehrlichia* have a complex life cycle that occurs in several intracellular forms which differ in their infectivity. For this reason, there is no easy method by which to titrate a suspension of these organisms. Models for studying antimicrobial susceptibility are based on the change in the percentage of infected cells over time in the presence versus absence of antibiotic. Pre-infected cell cultures are diluted with healthy cells in order to reduce the percentage of infected cells to less than 5%. After 3-5 days of incubation, this percentage approaches 100%. An antibiotic is considered bacteriostatic if the percentage of infected cells remains < 5% after this incubation period. More recently, a real-time PCR method was developed to evaluate *in vitro* susceptibilities of *Ehrlichia* (2).

Susceptible phenotype

Ehrlichia are intrinsically resistant to several classes of antibiotics (2-4, 7, 8, 10-12) (Table 8). β-lactams, aminoglycosides, macrolides and chloramphenicol are inactive. Co-trimoxazole is inactive and, as in the case of rickettsia, induces *in vitro* cell lysis by *Ehrlichia*. Fluoroquinolone activity differs according to species; *E. chaffeensis* is more resistant than *A. phagocytophila* or *N. sennetsu*. Tetracyclines and rifampin are the only agents active *in vitro* against all *Ehrlichia*, but only the tetracyclines have a recognized clinical efficacy (1, 6).

Phenotypes and mechanisms of resistance

Tetracyclines are the mainstay of treatment of ehrlichioses and no resistance to this class of antibiotic has been reported to date. *E. canis* and *E. chaffeenis* are intrinsically resistant to fluoroquinolones due to a serine$_{83}$alanine substitution (*E. coli* numbering) in subunit A of DNA gyrase (9).

REFERENCES

(1) **Blanco, J.R., and J.A. Oteo**. 2002. Human granulocytic ehrlichiosis in Europe. Clin. Microbiol. Infect. **8**:763-772.

(2) **Branger, S., J.M. Rolain, and D. Raoult**. 2004. Evaluation of antibiotic susceptibilities of *Ehrlichia canis*, *Ehrlichia chaffeensis*, and *Anaplasma phagocytophilum* by real-time PCR. Antimicrob. Agents Chemother. **48**:4822-4828.

(3) **Brouqui, P., and D. Raoult**. 1990. *In vitro* susceptibility of *Ehrlichia sennetsu* to antibiotics. Antimicrob. Agents Chemother. **34**:1593-1596.

(4) **Brouqui, P., and D. Raoult**. 1992. *In vitro* antibiotic susceptibility of the newly recognized agent of ehrlichiosis in humans, *Ehrlichia chaffeensis*. Antimicrob. Agents Chemother. **36**:2799-2803.

(5) **Dumler, J.S., A.F. Barbet, C.P. Bekker, G.A. Dasch, G.H. Palmer, S.C. Ray, Y. Rikihisa, and F.R. Rurangirwa**. 2001. Reorganization of genera in the families *Rickettsiaceae* and *Anaplasmataceae* in the order Rickettsiales: unification of some species of *Ehrlichia* with *Anaplasma*, *Cowdria* with *Ehrlichia* and *Ehrlichia* with *Neorickettsia*, descriptions of six new species combinations and designation of *Ehrlichia equi* and 'HGE agent' as subjective synonyms of *Ehrlichia phagocytophila*. Int. J. Syst. Evol. Microbiol. **51**:2145-2165.

(6) **Dumler, J.S., J.E. Madigan, N. Pusterla, and J.S. Bakken**. 2007. Ehrlichioses in humans: epidemiology, clinical presentation, diagnosis, and treatment. Clin. Infect. Dis. **15** (Suppl. 1):45-51.

(7) **Horowitz, H.W., T.C. Hsieh, M.E. Aguero-Rosenfeld, F. Kalantarpour, I. Chowdhury, G.P. Wormser, and J.M. Wu**. 2001. Antimicrobial susceptibility of *Ehrlichia phagocytophila*. Antimicrob. Agents Chemother. **45**:786-788.

(8) **Klein, M.B., C.M. Nelson, and J.L. Goodman**. 1997. Antibiotic susceptibility of the newly cultivated agent of human granulocytic ehrlichiosis: promising activity of quinolones and rifamycins. Antimicrob. Agents Chemother. **41**:76-79.

Table 8. MICs (µg/ml) of antibiotics against species of Ehrlichia, Anaplasma and Neorickettsia

Antibiotic	N. risticii	N. senettsu	E. canis	E. chaffeensis		A. phagocytophilum	
Reference	(11)	(3)	(2)	(4)	(7)	(8)	(10)
No. of isolates	1	1	1	1	6	3	8
β-lactams							
Penicillin G	ND[a]	≥ 2	ND	≥ 40	ND	ND	ND
Ampicillin	ND	ND	ND	ND	ND	ND	≥ 128
Amoxicillin	ND	ND	> 100	ND	≥ 32	≥ 32	ND
Ceftriaxone	ND	ND	ND	ND	≥ 64	≥ 64	≥ 128
Imipenem	ND	ND	ND	ND	ND	≥ 32	ND
Aminoglycosides							
Gentamicin	ND	≥ 2	≥ 100	≥ 32		≥ 50	ND
Amikacin	ND	ND	ND	ND	≥ 16	ND	≥ 64
Tetracyclines							
Tetracycline	≤ 0.01	ND	ND	ND	ND	ND	ND
Doxycycline	≤ 0.01	ND	ND	≤ 0.5	≤ 0.125	0.25	≤ 0.03
Rifampin	< 0.01	0.5	0.03	≤ 0.125	≤ 0.125	0.5	≤ 0.03
Trimethoprim/sulfamethoxazole	ND	0.8/≥ 4	0.8/≥ 4	0.8/≥ 4	ND	ND	5/≥ 25
Chloramphenicol	ND	≥ 4	≥ 4	≥ 16	≥ 16	≥ 32	2-8
Macrolides							
Erythromycin	≥ 1	≥ 4	≥ 4	≥ 8	≥ 8	≥ 8	≥ 16
Azithromycin	ND	ND	ND	ND	≥ 8	≥ 8	≥ 16
Clarithromycin	ND	ND	ND	ND	≥ 8	ND	ND
Fluoroquinolones							
Ofloxacin	ND	ND	ND	ND	≤ 2	2	ND
Levofloxacin	ND	ND	ND	ND	≤ 1		0.06 – 0.5
Ciprofloxacin	ND	ND	ND	≥ 4	ND	2	ND

[a] ND, not determined.

(9) **Maurin, M., C. Abergel, and D. Raoult.** 2001. DNA gyrase-mediated natural resistance to fluoroquinolones in Ehrlichia spp. Antimicrob. Agents Chemother. **45**:2098-2105.

(10) **Maurin, M., J.S. Bakken, and J.S. Dumler.** 2003. Antibiotic susceptibilities of Anaplasma (Ehrlichia) phagocytophilum strains from various geographic areas in the United States. Antimicrob. Agents Chemother. **47**:413-415.

(11) **Rikihisa, Y., and B.M. Jiang.** 1988. In vitro susceptibilities of Ehrlichia risticii to eight antibiotics. Antimicrob. Agents Chemother. **32**:986-991

(12) **Rolain, J.M., M. Maurin, A. Bryskier, and D. Raoult.** 2000. In vitro activities of telithromycin (HMR 3647) against Rickettsia rickettsii, Rickettsia conorii, Rickettsia africae, Rickettsia typhi, Rickettsia prowazekii, Coxiella burnetii, Bartonella henselae, Bartonella quintana, Bartonella bacilliformis, and Ehrlichia chaffeensis. Antimicrob Agents Chemother. **44**:1391-1393.

RICKETTSIA

Bacteria from the genus *Rickettsia* are Gram-negative, obligate intracellular bacilli that infect endothelial cells (10, 11). Traditionally the genus has been classified into three groups. The typhus group includes *R. prowazekii*, the agent of exanthematic or epidemic typhus for which humans are the main reservoir with human-to-human transmission via the body louse, and *R. typhi*, the agent of murine typhus which has an animal reservoir and is transmitted to humans via rat fleas. The scrub typhus group comprises only one species, *Orientia tsutsugamushi*, found throughout Asia and transmitted to humans by the bite of trombiculid larvae. The spotted fever group has many animal reservoirs and Ixodes ticks are the usual vectors of human transmission. *R. rickettsii*, which causes Rocky Mountain Spotted Fever, and *R. conorii*, which causes Mediterranean spotted fever, are the prototype bacteria of the spotted fever group. Over the past three decades this group has grown considerably with the characterization of new species and the demonstration of a pathogenic role in humans of species initially isolated in ticks. This includes the following species in particular: *R. japonica* in Japan and Korea; *R. africae* in sub-Sahara Africa and the Antilles; *R. honei* in Australia and Southeast Asia; *R. slovaca* in Europe; "*R. sibirica* subsp. *Mongolotimonae*" in China, Europe and Africa; "*R. heilongjiangensis*" in China and eastern Russia; *R. aeschlimannii* in Africa and Europe; "*R. marmionii*" in Australia; and *R. parkeri* on the American continent. The species *R. felis*, an emergent pathogen distributed worldwide, is the agent of flea-borne spotted fever.

Methods

As *Rickettsia* are obligate intracellular bacteria, antimicrobial susceptibility testing requires the use of cell models. Cell lines such as Vero cells are infected *in vitro*. The plaque assay technique is the reference method (4, 14). Intracellular multiplication of rickettsiae leads to lysis of the infected host cells and formation by cell-to-cell spread of lysis plaques which become visible to the naked eye after 7-10 days of incubation. The bacteriostatic effect of antibiotics, i.e., MICs, against rickettsiae is measured in terms of their ability to inhibit plaque formation. A simplified colorimetric method, also based on cell lysis due to rickettsial multiplication, has been developed (5). In this method, Vero cells are cultivated in microtiter plates and infected with a rickettsial inoculum so as to obtain complete lysis of the cell monolayer after 6 days of incubation. At this stage, the cell layer is incubated in the presence of a dye (neutral red), then washed. An absence of cell staining indicates cell lysis, and therefore rickettsial multiplication, in comparison with uninfected control cells. MEICs can also be determined by this method. An alternative method is based on fluorescence microscopic detection of intracellular rickettsiae in the presence of different antibiotic concentrations as compared to an antibiotic-free control (3). More recently, real-time PCR has been used to evaluate antimicrobial susceptibility of rickettsiae (8). The method measures DNA replication as a marker of intracellular growth of rickettsiae, in the presence versus absence of antibiotic. These different methods yield similar results.

Susceptible phenotype

Overall, the antibiotic susceptibilities of the different *Rickettsia* species are very similar (6) (Table 9). These microorganisms are intrinsically resistant to β-lactams and aminoglycosides, in large part because these drugs penetrate poorly into the cellular cytoplasm where rickettsial multiplication takes place. Tetracyclines, rifampin and fluoroquinolones have the highest activity *in vitro*, while phenicols are less active. Macrolide activity depends on the molecule; josamycin and telithromycin have the highest activity (5, 7). Macrolide resistance rates are higher among rickettsiae in the spotted fever group than in the typhus group. Similarly, within the spotted fever group, the species *R. massiliae*, *R. montana*, *R. rhipicephali*, *R. aeschlimannii* and the strain Bar 29 display higher intrinsic resistance to rifampin (6). Failure of rifampin therapy has been reported in Spain (1) and may be related to the existence of these more highly resistant strains (6). Co-trimoxazole is not active against rickettsiae and it amplifies *in vitro* the cell lysis effect resulting from rickettsial multiplication.

Phenotypes and mechanisms of resistance

The molecular mechanism conferring the intrinsic macrolide resistance observed in some *Rickettsia* species has yet to be elucidated (6). Weiss *et al.* (13) were able to select an erythromycin-resistant strain of *R. prowazekii in vitro* but did not identify the underlying mechanism. More recently, Rolain *et al.* (9) detected a triple amino acid difference in the conserved region of the ribosomal protein L22 which might explain the differ-

Table 9. MICs (μg/ml) of antibiotics for *Rickettsia*

Antibiotic	R. akari	R. prowazekii	R. typhi	SFGR[a]
No. of isolates	1	1	1	24
References	(3, 4, 6)	(6, 7, 13)	(6)	(6)
β-lactams				
Penicillin G	128	128	ND[b]	ND
Amoxicillin	ND	128	128	128 - 256
Aminoglycosides				
Gentamicin	8	16	16	4 - 16
Tetracyclines				
Tetracycline	ND	0.01 - 0.1	0.1	ND
Doxycycline	0.06	0.1	0.06 - 0.125	0.06 - 0.25
Rifampin	0.25 - 0.5	0.008	0.06 - 0.25	0.03 – 1c
Chloramphenicol	1	ND	1	ND
Thiamphenicol	ND	1	1 - 2	0.5 - 4
Trimethoprim / sulfamethoxazole	4/> 8	1/> 4	2/> 8	2/> 8
Macrolides – azalides – ketolides				
Erythromycin	8 - 16	0.06 - 2	0.125 - 1	1 - 8
Josamycin	1	1	0.5 - 1	0.5 - 2
Azithromycin	0.25	0.25	ND	ND
Clarithromycin	2	0.125 - 1	0.5 - 1	0.5 - 4
Telithromycin	ND	0.5	0.5	ND
Fluoroquinolones				
Ofloxacin	0.5	1	1	1
Ciprofloxacin	0.5	0.5	0.5 - 1	0.25 - 1

[a] SFGR, spotted fever group rickettsiae (including in particular *R. rickettsii* and *R. conorii*)
[b] ND, not determined.
[c] Rifampin MIC = 2-4 μg/ml for *Rickettsia* sp. strain Bar 29, *R. massiliae*, *R. aeschlimanii*, *R. Montana*, and *R. rhipicephali*.

ent macrolide susceptibilities of the typhus group as compared to the spotted fever group. Rifampin resistance in some *Rickettsia* species is conferred by mutations in the gene encoding the RNA polymerase β subunit (2). With respect to scrub typhus, clinical resistance to tetracyclines has been reported in southeast Asia (12) but no acquired resistance mechanisms have been characterized to date.

REFERENCES

(1) **Bella, F., E. Espejo, S. Uriz, J.A. Serrano, M.D. Alegre, and J. Tort**. 1991. Randomized trial of five-day rifampin versus one-day doxycycline therapy for Mediterranean spotted fever. J. Infect. Dis. **164**:433.

(2) **Drancourt, M., and D. Raoult**. 1999. Characterization of mutations in the *rpo*B gene in naturally rifampin-resistant *Rickettsia* species. Antimicrob. Agents Chemother. **43**:2400-2403.

(3) **Ives, T.J., P. Manzewitsch, R.L. Regnery, J.D. Butts, and M. Kebede**. 1997. *In vitro* susceptibilities of *Bartonella henselae*, *B. quintana*, *B. elizabethae*, *Rickettsia rickettsii*, *R. conorii*, *R. akari*, and *R. prowazekii* to macrolide antibiotics as determined by immunofluorescence-antibody analysis of infected Vero cell monolayers. Antimicrob. Agents Chemother. **41**:578-582.

(4) **McDade, J.E**. 1969. Determination of antibiotic susceptibility of *Rickettsia* by the plaque assay technique. Appl. Microbiol. **18**:133.

(5) **Raoult, D., P. Roussellier, G. Vestris, and J. Tamalet**. 1987. *In vitro* antibiotic susceptibility of *Rickettsia rickettsii* and *Rickettsia conorii*: plaque assay and microplaque colorimetric assay. J. Infect. Dis. **155**:1059-1062.

(6) **Rolain, J.M., M. Maurin, G. Vestris, and D. Raoult**. 1998. *In vitro* susceptibilities of 27 rickettsiae to 13 antimicrobials. Antimicrob. Agents Chemother. **42**:1537-1541.

(7) **Rolain, J.M., M. Maurin, A. Bryskier, and D. Raoult**. 2000. *In vitro* activities of telithromycin (HMR3647) against *Rickettsia rickettsii*, *Rickettsia conorii*, *Rickettsia africae*, *Rickettsia typhi*, *Rickettsia prowazekii*, *Coxiella burnetii*, *Bartonella henselae*, *Bartonella quintana*, *Bartonella bacilliformis*, and *Ehrlichia chaffeensis*. Antimicrob. Agents Chemother. **44**:1391-1393.

(8) **Rolain, J.M., L. Stuhl, M. Maurin, and D. Raoult**. 2002. Evaluation of antibiotic susceptibilities of three rickettsial species including *Rickettsia felis* by a quantitative PCR DNA assay. Antimicrob. Agents Chemother. **46**:2747-2751.

(9) **Rolain, J.M., and D. Raoult**. 2005. Prediction of resistance to erythromycin in the genus *Rickettsia* by

mutations in L22 ribosomal protein. J. Antimicrob. Chemother. **56**:396-398.
(10) **Parola, P., C.D. Paddock, and D. Raoult**. 2005. Tick-borne rickettsioses around the world: emerging diseases challenging old concepts. Clin. Microbiol. Rev. **18**:719-756.
(11) **Walker, D.H**. 2007. Rickettsiae and rickettsial infections: the current state of knowledge. Clin. Infect. Dis. **45** Suppl. 1:39-44.
(12) **Watt, G., C. Chouriyagune, R. Ruangweerayud, P. Watcharapichat, D. Phulsuksombati, K. Jongsakul, P. Teja-Isavadharm, D. Bhodhidatta, K.D. Corcoran, G.A. Dasch, and D. Strickman**. 1996. Scrub typhus infections poorly responsive to antibiotics in northern Thailand. Lancet **348**:86-89.
(13) **Weiss, E., and H.R. Dressler**. 1960. Selection of an erythromycin-resistant strain of *Rickettsia prowazekii*. Am. J. Hyg. **71**:292-298.
(14) **Wisseman, C.L., A.D. Waddell, and W.T. Walsh**. 1974. *In vitro* studies of the action of antibiotics on *Rickettsia prowazekii* by two basic methods of cell culture. J. Infect. Dis. **130**:564-574.

COXIELLA BURNETII

Coxiella burnetii is a Gram-negative spore-forming bacilli. This obligate intracellular pathogen infects monocytes and macrophages and is the causal agent of Q fever (8, 15), a zoonosis found worldwide. Humans are usually infected through contact with herd animals such as cattle, sheep and goats, or with domestic pets (cats in particular). Infection usually occurs by inhalation. Q fever causes an acute form of infection whose clinical manifestations are isolated flu-like symptoms, atypical pneumonia and abnormal liver tests, and a chronic form whose main complication is endocarditis. *C. burnetii* was recently shown to cause serious obstetrical complications, posing the problem of antibiotic therapy in pregnant women infected with this bacterium.

Methods

Antibiotic activity against *C. burnetii* is evaluated in cell models but only few strains have been studied. Different cell types are used including L929 mouse fibroblasts and P388D1 or J774 mouse macrophages. Two types of models are used to study the bacteriostatic or bactericidal activity of antibiotics.

In the bacteriostatic model (13), HEL fibroblasts cultured in shell vials are infected with a *C. burnetii* inoculum and incubated at 37°C for six days. Bacterial multiplication results in the formation of intracellular vacuoles which can be visualized by indirect immunofluorescence after labeling the bacteria with a fluorescein-conjugated anti-*C. burnetii* antibody. Antibiotic activity is determined by the ability to inhibit vacuole formation in comparison with an antibiotic-free control. MIC_s can thus be determined.

Yeaman *et al.* (21) were the first to describe a model for studying bactericidal activity in *C. burnetii*. L929 cells chronically infected with *C. burnetii* are exposed to different antibiotic concentrations. The percentage of infected cells, initially close to 100%, decreases if the antibiotic is active. Fluoroquinolones and rifampin were found to have a bactericidal effect in this model. The model was improved by adding cycloheximide to the incubation medium, which blocks cell division (12). This made it possible to show that the previously reported cell killing actually corresponded to a bacteriostatic effect, whereby infected cells were diluted by healthy cells that continued to multiply. More recently, a third bactericidal model was developed (6) in which P388D1 monocytes are chronically infected with *C. burnetii*, then harvested and distributed equally into culture bottles, each containing a given antibiotic concentration. The bottles are incubated at 37°C for 24 h and the bacterial inoculum before and after incubation is determined. This is done by collecting the cell monolayer, lysing the cells by heat shock, and diluting ten-fold the bacterial suspension collected. These dilutions are inoculated in healthy cultures which are incubated at 37°C for six days until intracellular vacuoles appear. The vacuoles are visualized by indirect immunofluorescence and counted by microscopy, each vacuole corresponding to one inoculated bacterium. In this manner a bacteria count can be calculated in terms of vacuole-forming infectious units. A bactericidal effect is defined as a significant reduction of the bacterial count in the presence of antibiotic relative to the starting inoculum.

More recently, real-time PCR has been used to evaluate *in vitro* susceptibilities of *C. burnetii*. The technique measures DNA replication as a marker of intracellular growth of *C. burnetii*, in the presence versus absence of antibiotic (2, 3, 17). The results are similar to those obtained with the previous methods.

Susceptible phenotype

C. burnetii is intrinsically resistant to β-lactams and aminoglycosides due its intracellular location in an acidic phagolysosomal vacuole (6). Tetracyclines, fluoroquinolones, and rifampin have the highest activity *in vitro* (1-4, 6, 7, 13, 21) (Table 10). Only tetracyclines (doxycycline in particular) and fluoroquinolones are recommended as first-line therapy in acute forms of Q fever (9, 10). Rifampin is not used as monotherapy due to the potential to select resistant mutants. Tigecycline, a glycylcycline antibiotic, is slightly more active than doxycycline (20). Susceptibility to macrolides and particularly to erythromycin varies according to the strain (13). Erythromycin and clarithromycin have little activity against *C. burnetii* and azithromycin is inactive (4, 5, 7). Telithromycin has activity similar to that of erythromycin (16, 17). Co-trimoxazole and phenocils are weakly active *in vitro*.

None of these agents is bactericidal *in vitro* against *C. burnetii* (6). Bactericidal activity has been demonstrated for the combination of doxycycline and hydroxychloroquine since the latter compound causes alkalinization of the vacuole, the site of intracellular multiplication of *C. burnetii*. This drug combination is currently recommended for Q fever endocarditis (14).

Phenotypes and mechanisms of resistance

Acquired resistance has not been described in human or animal strains of *C. burnetti*. However, Rolain *et al.* (17) recently reported large differences in the doxycycline MIC (1 to 8 µg/ml) in both human and animal isolates, and when susceptibility was evaluated after just a few subcultures. The molecular mechanism of this resistance has not been elucidated. The authors speculate that tetracycline resistance has been selected in animal strains due to the widespread use of these agents in veterinary practice.

Fluoroquinolone resistance can be selected *in vitro* and is the result of $Glu_{87}Gly$ or $Glu_{87}Lys$ substitutions in the *gyr*A gene encoding DNA gyrase subunit A (11, 18, 19). Efflux pumps have also been postulated as a mechanism of resistance although there is no formal evidence for this (19).

REFERENCES

(1) **Andoh, M., T. Naganawa, T. Yamaguchi, H. Fukushi, and K. Hirai**. 2004. *In vitro* susceptibility to tetracycline and fluoroquinolones of Japanese isolates of *Coxiella burnetii*. Microbiol. Immunol. **48**:661-664.

(2) **Brennan, R.E., and J.E. Samuel**. 2003. Evaluation of *Coxiella burnetii* antibiotic susceptibilities by real-time PCR assay. J. Clin. Microbiol. **41**:1869-1874.

(3) **Boulos, A., J.M. Rolain, M. Maurin, and D. Raoult**. 2004. Measurement of the antibiotic susceptibility of *Coxiella burnetii* using real time PCR. Int. J. Antimicrob. Agents. **23**:169-174.

(4) **Gikas, A., I. Spyridaki, A. Psaroulaki, D. Kofterithis, and Y. Tselentis**. 1998. *In vitro* susceptibility of *Coxiella burnetii* to trovafloxacin in comparison with susceptibilities to pefloxacin, ciprofloxacin, ofloxacin, doxycycline, and clarithromycin. Antimicrob. Agents Chemother. **42**:2747-2748.

(5) **Lever, M.S., K.R. Bewley, B. Dowsett, and G. Lloyd**. 2004. *In vitro* susceptibility of *Coxiella burnetii* to azithromycin, doxycycline, ciprofloxacin and a range of newer fluoroquinolones. Int. J. Antimicrob. Agents. **24**:194-196.

(6) **Maurin, M., A.M. Benoliel, P. Bongrand, and D. Raoult**. 1992. Phagolysosomal alkalinization and the bactericidal effect of antibiotics: the *Coxiella burnetii* paradigm. J. Infect. Dis. **166**:1097-1102.

(7) **Maurin, M., and D. Raoult**. 1993. *In vitro* susceptibilities of spotted fever group rickettsiae and *Coxiella burnetii* to clarithromycin. Antimicrob. Agents Chemother. **37**:2633-2637.

(8) **Maurin, M., and D. Raoult**. 1999. Q fever. Clin. Microbiol. Rev. **12**:518-553

(9) **Marrie, T.J., and D. Raoult**. 2002. Update on Q fever, including Q fever endocarditis. Curr. Clin. Top. Infect. Dis. **22**:97-124.

(10) **Marrie, T. J**. 2004. Q fever pneumonia. Curr. Opin. Infect. Dis. **17**:137-142.

(11) **Musso, D., M. Drancourt, S. Osscini, and D. Raoult**. 1996. Sequence of quinolone resistance-determining region of gyrA gene for clinical isolates and for an *in vitro*-selected quinolone resistant strain of *Coxiella burnetii*. Antimicrob. Agents Chemother. **40**:870-873.

(12) **Raoult, D., M. Drancourt, and G. Vestris**. 1990. Bactericidal effect of doxycycline associated with lysosomotropic agents on *Coxiella burnetii* in P388D1 cells. Antimicrob. Agents Chemother. **34**:1512-1514.

(13) **Raoult, D., H. Torres, and M. Drancourt**. 1991. Shell-vial assay: evaluation of a new technique for determining antibiotic susceptibility, tested in 13 isolates of *Coxiella burnetii*. Antimicrob. Agents Chemother. **35**:2070-2077.

(14) **Raoult, D., P. Houpikian, H. Tissot Dupont, J.M. Riss, J. Drditi-Djiane, and P. Brouqui**. 1999. Treatment of Q fever endocarditis. Comparison of 2 regimens containing doxycycline and ofloxacin or hydroxy-chloroquine. Arch. Intern. Med. **159**:167-173

(15) **Raoult D, T. Marrie, and J. Mege**.2005. Natural history and pathophysiology of Q fever. Lancet Infect Dis. **5**:219-226.

(16) **Rolain, J.M., M. Maurin, A. Bryskier, and D. Raoult**. 2000. *In vitro* activities of telithromycin (HMR 3647) against *Rickettsia rickettsii, Rickettsia conorii, Rickettsia africae, Rickettsia typhi, Rickettsia prowazekii, Coxiella burnetii, Bartonella henselae, Bartonella quintana, Bartonella bacilliformis*, and *Ehrlichia chaffeensis*. Antimicrob. Agents Chemother. **44**:1391-1393.

Table 10. MICs (μg/ml) of antibiotics for *Coxiella burnetii*

Antibiotic	Number of isolates	MIC range	Reference
β-lactams			
Ampicillin	1	> 4	2
Amoxicillin	13	> 4	13
Aminoglycosides			
Gentamicin	2	> 10	3
Amikacin	13	> 4	13
Tetracyclines – glycylcycline			
Tetracycline	1	≤ 4	2
	13	≤ 4	13
Doxycycline	6	0.25 - 1	1
	2	2 - 4	3
	10	1 - 2	4
	13	1 - 8	17
Minocycline	13	≤ 4	13
Tigecycline	8	0.25 - 0.5	20
Rifampin	2	4	3
	13	≤ 4	13
Trimethoprim / sulfamethoxazole	2	1.6/8 - 3.2/16	3
Chloramphenicol	1	> 8	2
	13	≥ 8	13
Thiamphenicol	2	32	3
Macrolides – azalides – ketolide			
Erythromycin	2	2-4	3
	4	> 4	7
	13	> 1	13
	13	> 8	17
Azithromycin	1	≥ 8	5
Clarithromycin	10	2 - 4	4
	4	1 - 4	7
Telithromycin	2	2	3
	13	0.5 - 2	20
Fluoroquinolones			
Ofloxacin	2	2	3
	10	1 - 2	4
	13	≤ 1	13
Levofloxacin	6	0.5 - 1	1
	2	2	3
Ciprofloxacin	6	2 - 8	1
	2	2 - 4	3
	10	4 - 8	4
Moxifloxacin	6	0.5 - 2	1
Oxazolidinone			
Linezolid	8	2 - 4	20

(17) **Rolain, J.M., F. Lambert, and D. Raoult**. 2005. Activity of telithromycin against thirteen new isolates of *C. burnetii* including three resistant to doxycycline. Ann. N.Y. Acad. Sci. **1063**:252-256.

(18) **Spyridaki, I., A. Psaroulaki, A. Aransay, E. Scoulica, and Y. Tselentis**. 2000. Diagnosis of quinolone-resistant *Coxiella burnetii* strains by PCR-RFLP. J. Clin. Lab. Anal. **14**:59-63.

(19) **Spyridaki, I., A. Psaroulaki, E. Kokkinakis, A. Gikas, and Y. Tselentis**. 2002. Mechanisms of resistance to fluoroquinolones in *Coxiella burnetii*. J. Antimicrob. Chemother. **49**:379-382.

(20) **Spyridaki, I., A. Psaroulaki, I. Vranakis, Y. Tselentis, and A. Gikas**. 2009. Bacteriostatic and bactericidal activities of tigecycline against *Coxiella burnetii* and its comparison with those of six other antibiotics. Antimicrob. Agents Chemother. **53**:2690-2692.

(21) **Yeaman, M.R., L.A. Mitscher, and O.G. Baca**. 1987. *In vitro* susceptibility of *Coxiella burnetii* to antibiotics, including several quinolones. Antimicrob. Agents Chemother. **31**:1079-1084.

TREPONEMES

Treponema are motile, helically coiled bacteria from the family *Spirochetaceae*. These obligate or preferential anaerobes can be visualized by dark field microscopy. This chapter will only address the pathogenic treponemes with a human reservoir, which cannot be cultured in axenic medium. *T. pallidum* subsp. *pallidum* causes syphilis (3), a venereal disease found worldwide. Non-venereal treponematoses are caused by *T. pallidum* subsp. *endemicum* (which causes bejel), *T. pallidum* subsp. *pertenue* (which causes yaws) and *T. carateum* (which causes pinta) (1). Bejel is rife in sub-Saharan areas of North Africa and in the Middle East (western Saudi Arabia), yaws is found in Central and West Africa, Southeast Asia and some Pacific islands, while pinta is endemic in tropical regions of Central and South America.

T. pallidum subsp. *pallidum*

Methods

Three *in vitro* models have been developed to study antimicrobial susceptibility of *T. pallidum* subsp. *pallidum*. The oldest model evaluates the ability of an antibiotic to inhibit *in vitro* motility of treponemes (4); the antibiotic concentration producing a 50% loss of motility is determined. The second model is based on radiolabeled methionine incorporation into *T. pallidum* proteins in the presence or absence of antibiotic (13). Antibiotic activity is measured as the ability to inhibit ^{35}S-methionine incorporation *in vitro* in neosynthesized *T. pallidum* proteins. Results are reported as the percent inhibition of protein synthesis in the presence of antibiotic as compared to antibiotic-free controls. The third model is based on inhibition of *T. pallidum* multiplication in cellular medium (9). *T. pallidum* multiplication can be obtained *in vitro* in SflEp cottontail rabbit epithelial cell cultures incubated at 33-34°C in the presence of 3-5% oxygen, in MEM medium supplemented with amino acids, glucose, and 20% fetal calf serum. *T. pallidum* multiplied 10-fold when incubated for 7 days and 100-fold after 12-14 days, but viability could not be maintained beyond this time in this model. Antibiotic activity is evaluated on treponemal motility and by dark field microscopic examination in a Helber bacteria-counting chamber. Using this model, Norris and Edmondson (9) determined the MICs of different antibiotics, defined as the lowest concentration which prevented multiplication of *T. pallidum* and/or inhibited treponemal motility. In a second step, samples from each cell culture were injected intradermally into healthy rabbits to determine residual virulence. This procedure determines the MBC, i.e., the lowest antibiotic concentration at which no skin lesions are seen following intradermal inoculation.

Susceptible phenotype

In vitro, *T. pallidum* Nichols strain is susceptible to penicillin G, ceftriaxone, tetracycline, chloramphenicol and macrolides (erythromycin and azithromycin) (4, 5, 10, 12, 13) (Table 11). This strain is intrinsically resistant to streptomycin, rifampin and fluoroquinolones. In the cell model, Norris *et al.* (9) reported MICs (µg/ml) for the Nichols strain of 0.0005 for penicillin G, 0.2 for tetracycline, 0.005 for erythromycin, and 0.5 for spectinomycin. MBCs for these same antibiotics were 0.0025, 0.5, 0.005, and 0.5 µg/ml, respectively. Penicillin G therefore appears to have the highest activity. However, the *in vitro* susceptibility data for spectinomycin and erythromycin contradicts experimental and clinical findings indicating that these drugs are ineffective at treating syphilis.

Table 11. *In vitro* antibiotic susceptibility of *T. pallidum* subsp. *pallidum* Nichols strain

Antibiotique	MIC ou IC_{50}[a] (µg/ml)	Reference
β-lactams		
Penicillin G	0.0005	9
	IC_{50} = 0.002	4
	IC_{50} = 0.03	12
Ceftriaxone	IC_{50} = 0.01	4
Aminoglycosides		
Spectinomycin	0.5	9
Streptomycin	IC_{50} > 50	12
Tetracyclines		
Tetracycline	0.2	9
	IC_{50} < 4	12
Rifampin	IC_{50} > 100	12
Chloramphenicol	IC_{50} < 20	12
Macrolide		
Erythromycin	0.005	9
	IC_{50} < 10	12

[a] IC_{50}: antibiotic concentration producing 50% inhibition of motility (9) or protein synthesis (12) of *T. pallidum*.

Phenotypes and mechanisms of resistance

There have been several reports of clinical resistance to penicillin G in syphilis patients (2). Furthermore, the discovery of plasmid DNA in *T. pallidum* suggests a potential for acquired β-lactam resistance in this species (8), although to date there have been no reports of *in vitro* penicillin G resistance of *T. pallidum*. An erythromycin-resistant human isolate was characterized *in vitro* (street strain 14) (12); resistance appears to be due to an adenine$_{2058}$guanine substitution (*E. coli* numbering) in both 23S rRNA genes in the resistant street strain 14 as compared to the susceptible Nichols strain (14). This same mutation was more recently detected by amplification and sequencing of 23S DNA from clinical specimens obtained from patients with azithromycin-resistant primary syphilis (6). The prevalence of this resistance has been steadily increasing among patients with sexually transmitted diseases (6, 7). Intrinsic rifampin resistance in *T. pallidum* subsp. *pallidum* has been correlated with the presence of an asparagine at position 531 (*E. coli* numbering) of the β subunit of RNA polymerase (15).

Non-venereal endemic treponematoses

Methods

The most common method of *in vitro* susceptibility testing in these organisms is the determination of ^{35}S-methionine incorporation in the presence and absence of antibiotic (11). This method has been used mainly with *T. pallidum* subsp. *pertenue*. *In vitro* susceptibility of *T. pallidum* subsp. *endemicum* has never been evaluated. Furthermore, as no *T. carateum* isolates have yet been obtained, the antibiotic susceptibility of this species is unknown.

Susceptible phenotype

In the ^{35}S-methionine incorporation model, penicillin G, tetracycline, chloramphenicol and various macrolides (erythromycin and roxithromycin, clarithromycin in particular) are bacteriostatic against the subspecies *T. pallidum* subsp. *pertenue* (Gauthier strain) (11). Streptomycin is only active at very high concentrations (500 µg/ml) and rifampin is inactive.

Phenotypes and mechanisms of resistance

Among the treponemes responsible for non-venereal endemic treponematoses, no clinical isolates resistant to penicillin G or other antibiotics have been reported to date. However, failure of penicillin G treatment in yaws has been reported in Papouasia-New Guinea and in Ecuador (1). These failures occurred in regions where disease control by massive penicillin G administration in the vulnerable populations had been attempted several times, particularly during the WHO yaws eradication campaigns between 1952 and 1964. These cases of clinical resistance may in fact be related to re-infection.

REFERENCES

(1) **Antal, G.M., S.A. Lukehart, and A.Z. Meheus.** 2002. The endemic treponematoses. Microbes Infect. **4**:83-94.

(2) **Giles, A.J.H., and A.G. Lawrence.** 1979. Treatment failure with penicillin and early syphilis. Br. J. Vener. Dis. **55**:62-64.

(3) **Golden, M.R., C.M. Marra, and K.K. Holmes.** 2003. Update on syphilis: resurgence of an old problem. JAMA. **290**:1510-1514.

(4) **Korting, H.C., D. Walther, U. Riethmuller, and M. Meurer.** 1986. Comparative *in vitro* susceptibility of *Treponema pallidum* to ceftizoxime, ceftriaxone and penicillin G. Chemotherapy **32**:352-355.

(5) **Lukehart, S.A., M.J. Fohn, and S.A. Baker-Zander.** 1990. Efficacy of azithromycin for therapy of active syphilis in the rabbit model. J. Antimicrob. Chemother. **25** (suppl A):91-99.

(6) **Lukehart, S.A., C. Godornes, B.J. Molini, P. Sonnett, S. Hopkins, F. Mulcahy, J. Engelman, S.J. Mitchell, A.M. Rompalo, C.M. Marra, and J.D. Klausner.** 2004. Macrolide resistance in *Treponema pallidum* in the United States and Ireland. N. Engl. J. Med. **351**:154-158.

(7) **Martin, I.E., R.S. Tsang, K. Sutherland, P. Tilley, R. Read, B. Anderson, C. Roy, and A.E. Singh.** 2009. Molecular characterization of syphilis infection in Canada: Azithromycin resistance and detection of *Treponema pallidum* DNA in whole blood versus ulcers. J. Clin. Microbiol. **47**:1668-1663.

(8) **Norgard, M.V., and J.N. Miller.** 1981. Plasmid DNA in *Treponema pallidum* (Nichols) : potential for antibiotic resistance by syphilis bacteria. Science **213**:553-555.

(9) **Norris, S.J., and D.G. Edmondson.** 1988. *In vitro* culture system to determine MICs and MBCs of antimicrobial agents against *Treponema pallidum* subsp. pallidum (Nichols strain). Antimicrob. Agents Chemother. **32**:68-74.

(10) **Poitevin M., M. Ly, M. Daubras, and F. Ichou.** 1988. In vivo study of the sensitivity of *Treponema pallidum* to ofloxacin. Pathol. Biol. **36**:482-7.

(11) **Stamm, L.V., and P. L. Bassford.** 1985. Cellular and extracellular protein antigens of *Treponema pallidum* synthesized during *in vitro* incubation of freshly extracted organisms. Infect. Immunol. **47**:799-807.

(12) **Stamm, L.V., J.T. Stapleton, and P.J. Bassford.** 1988. *In vitro* assay to demonstrate high-level erythromycin resistance of a clinical isolate of *Treponema pallidum*. Antimicrob. Agents Chemother. **32**:164-169.

(13) **Stamm, L.V., and E.A. Parrish**. 1990. In-vitro activity of azithromycin and CP-63,956 against *Treponema pallidum*. J. Antimicrob. Chemother. **25** (suppl. A):11-14.

(14) **Stamm, L.V., and H.L. Bergen**. 2000. A point mutation associated with bacterial macrolide resistance is present in both 23S rRNA genes of an erythromycin-resistant *Treponema pallidum* clinical isolate. Antimicrob. Agents Chemother. **44**:806-807.

(15) **Stamm, L.V., H.L. Bergen, and K.A. Shangraw**. 2001. Natural rifampin resistance in *Treponema* spp. correlates with presence of N531 in *rpo*B Rif cluster I. Antimicrob. Agents Chemother. **45**:2973-2974.

Chapter 51. *NOCARDIA*

Patrick BOIRON

The genus *Nocardia* includes strict aerobic, Gram-positive, filamentous, branching bacteria belonging to the order *Actinomycetales* and phylogenetically related to other "nocardioform" bacteria, particularly from the genera *Corynebacterium*, *Rhodococcus*, *Mycobacterium*, *Gordonia*, *Skermania*, *Tsukamurella Dietzia* and *Williamsia*. Bacteria from the genus *Nocardia* are ubiquitous. Widespread in the environment, they are found in soil, plants and compost (14).

Nocardia infections are usually acquired by inhalation and, more rarely, by direct inoculation through an open wound. Proliferation of the bacteria within the body causes a granulomatous, suppurative infection which may be localized or disseminated, known as nocardiosis (4, 21). Nocardiosis has been reported all around the world. Most cases occur in immunocompromised patients although infection in the absence of any predisposing factors is not unusual. In 80-90% of cases the etiological agent is *Nocardia asteroides*, *Nocardia farcinica* or *Nocardia nova* (these three species are still often undifferentiated and classified under the term *N. asteroides* complex); *Nocardia brasiliensis* and *Nocardia otitidiscaviarum* are a less common cause. In tropical and hot temperate regions, these bacteria can cause fistulated subcutaneous abscesses known as mycetomas. The main etiological agent is *N. brasiliensis*, while *N. asteroides* and *N. otitidiscaviarum* are less frequently incriminated.

It has now become clear that this taxonomic classification needs to be revised. Indeed, the taxonomy of the genus *Nocardia* has undergone a profound revolution over the last ten years. While only ten or so species were described between 1888 and 1996, the International Committee on Systematics of Prokaryotes now recognizes more than 50 species in the genus *Nocardia*. The identification of new species requires a periodic reassessment of the available biological data, especially in terms of their antibiotic susceptibility. Yet for a considerable number of new species there are no data available on antibiotic susceptibility. We have therefore chosen to review the "classical" species, keeping in mind that several "new" species are derived from the newly defined *N. asteroides* (*Nocardia abcessus*, *Nocardia cyriacigeorgica*, etc.) or belong to the same phylogenetic cluster as *N. nova* (*Nocardia veterana*, *Nocardia africana*, etc.) (20) and that, overall, their susceptibility profile may be similar to that of the species from which they were distinguished. Nonetheless, as more and more isolates of these species are obtained, it is important to determine the susceptibility pattern of each so as to discern any unique features.

Before the sulfonamides ushered in the antimicrobial era in 1944, *Nocardia* infections were almost always fatal. The sulfa drugs subsequently became the reference therapy for *Nocardia* infections, sometimes in association with surgical drainage of the abscess. Even today, trimethoprim-sulfamethoxazole is often used as a first-line treatment of nocardiosis since this drug combination diffuses well into lung, brain, skin, corneal tissue, etc. (9). Retrospective studies of the efficacy of trimethoprim-sulfamethoxazole illustrate the widespread success of this treatment (3).

Nevertheless, there are several reasons why it is also important to test other antibiotics both *in vitro*, in animal models and in the clinic, particularly for the species *N. asteroides*. First, different *Nocardia* species have different antibiotic susceptibilities. Moreover, there have been reports of treatment failures with sulfonamides, highlighting the need to find alternative treatments (11). In addition, it is not uncommon for sulfonamides or trimethoprim-sulfamethoxazole to cause side effects such as allergic reactions, especially during immunosuppressive therapy or in AIDS patients (15, 18), as well as hematologic toxicity, necessitating a switch to another antibiotic, the choice of which should be guided by *in vitro* susceptibility testing.

METHODS

Standardization of antibiotic susceptibility testing in *Nocardia* is problematic due to the variable growth rates of the different strains and the difficulty of obtaining a homogeneous suspension allowing standardization of the inoculum.

Cellular aggregation is the major obstacle when conducting susceptibility tests. The most efficient way to obtain a standardized, homogeneous inoculum (10^7-10^8 CFU/ml, turbidity equivalent to a 0.5 McFarland standard) is to culture the bacteria on a rotary shaker (150 rpm) in broth medium supplemented with 1/10th the volume in sterile glass beads (5 mm diameter) (8). Some authors prefer a 24 hour shaker culture in Mueller-Hinton or brain-heart broth containing one drop of Tween 80 to obtain a homogeneous inoculum. The broth is adjusted to the turbidity of a 0.5 McFarland standard and then diluted 1:100.

Under these conditions, over 90% of strains show sufficient growth within 24-48 hours on Mueller-Hinton medium at 32-37°C to be able to evaluate their susceptibility. Supplementation with 5% sheep blood, or the use of Mueller-Hinton medium containing hemolysed blood, or else culture in a 5-10% CO_2 atmosphere, enables sufficient growth of most other strains.

There is no unanimously approved method of antibiotic susceptibility testing in *Nocardia*. Dilution in cation-supplemented Muller-Hinton broth has been proposed by the Clinical and Laboratory Standards Institute (CLSI) (28), but several other methods are also possible.

Serial agar dilution with a multiple inoculator can be used for many studies but this method is fastidious in a routine testing laboratory.

The broth dilution method which, like agar dilution, allows determination of minimal inhibitory concentrations (MICs), is simple and requires only a small inoculum and few reagents when carried out in 96-well microtiter plates.

Agar diffusion methods (disk diffusion or E-test®) are the most widely used although the BACTEC method has been shown to be most reliable (2, 10). Despite the relatively slow growth of *Nocardia*, results can be read after 24-48 hours at 37°C if a small, homogeneous inoculum is used. However, the antibiogram cannot be interpreted in the same manner as for organisms with rapid growth rates: in the case of *Nocardia*, a result indicating resistance is unambiguous, but a result indicating susceptibility must be confirmed by a dilution method.

Determining the breakpoints for *Nocardia* is difficult (22).

USUAL SUSCEPTIBILITY

There is a good intra- and inter-laboratory correlation between the results obtained with different susceptibility testing methods; reproducibility is > 90% (6).

Data from the literature indicate that the antibiotic susceptibilities of *Nocardia* vary widely according to species. Nevertheless, the following general points have emerged for the most common species.

β-lactams

The majority of *Nocardia* strains have intermediate or high-level resistance to most β-lactam antibiotics (Table 1). Resistance is due in part to the presence in the large majority of species of β-lactamases, thus almost always conferring resistance to penicillin G, ampicillin and amoxicillin. One exception is *N. nova* where only half of the strains are β-lactamase producers, making this species susceptible in particular to amoxicillin (29). Clavulanic acid considerably enhances amoxicillin susceptibility in *N. farcinica* and, to a lesser extent, in *N. asteroides* and *N. brasiliensis*, but has almost no effect in *N. otitidiscaviarum*. A paradoxical effect is observed in *N. nova* where the combination of clavulanic acid and amoxicillin reduces susceptibility to amoxicillin alone (probably due to β-lactamase induction by clavulanic acid).

The majority of cephalosporins are stable with respect to the β-lactamases of this bacterial genus, but their activity is highly variable. Cefuroxime, cefotaxime and ceftriaxone are most effective against *N. asteroides* and have little activity against *N. farcinica*. It should be added that not all third generation cephalosporins can be considered equivalent. For example, ceftriaxone is active less often than cefotaxime, while ceftazidime and aztreonam are inactive.

Imipenem is the most effective β-lactam against *N. asteroides* (apart from cefmetazole), *N. farcinica* and *N. nova* (though 10-20% of strains are resistant) but is inactive against *N. brasiliensis* and *N. otitidiscaviarum* (29).

Aminoglycosides

Aminoglycoside activity differs in different *Nocardia* pathogens (Table 2) (1). Streptomycin and spectinomycin are generally inactive in all species. Kanamycin is inactive against *N. asteroides*, *N. farcinica* and *N. brasiliensis* but is effective against *N. otitidiscaviarum*. These species show intermediate to high susceptibility to gentamicin, except for *N. farcinica* which is completely resistant. Tobramycin has good activity against *N. brasiliensis* and to a lesser extent, *N. asteroides* but

Table 1. Susceptibility of *Nocardia* to β-lactams

Antibiotic	MIC$_{50}$ (µg/ml)[a]			
	N. asteroides	*N. farcinica*	*N. brasiliensis*	*N. otitidiscaviarum*
Penicillin G	6.25 - 64	> 100	8 -> 100	> 100
Ampicillin	1.56 - 64	≥ 64	≥ 64	> 100
Amoxicillin	6.25 - 64	> 100	16 - > 100	> 100
Carbenicillin	32 - > 100	> 100	64 - > 100	> 100
Ticarcillin	50 - > 100	> 100	32 - > 100	> 100
Mezlocillin	3.12 - > 100	> 100	32 - > 100	> 100
Azlocillin	3.12 - > 50	> 100	> 100	> 100
Piperacillin	50 - > 100	> 100	32 - > 100	> 100
Mecillinam	> 100	ND [b]	ND	ND
Amoxicillin + clavulanic acid	6.25 - 16	12.5	2 - 12.5	> 100
Ticarcillin + clavulanic acid	> 100	ND	ND	ND
Imipenem	0.5 - 3.12	3.12 - 4	8 - > 100	> 100
Cephalotine	62 - > 100	50 - > 100	> 64	> 100
Cefotiam	6.25 - 50	25 - > 100	> 64	> 100
Cefuroxime	4 - 50	25 - > 100	8	> 100
Cefamandole	0.78 - 50	25 - > 100	> 64	> 100
Cefoxitin	3.12 - 64	25 - > 100	> 64	> 100
Cefotaxime	0.4 - 50	25 - > 100	4	> 100
Cefmenoxime	2 - > 64	25 - > 100	> 64	> 100
Ceftizoxime	6.25 - 64	25 - > 100	2	> 100
Ceftriaxone	0.4 - 8	> 64	4	> 100
Cefoperazone	1.56 - > 100	> 64	> 64	> 100
Ceftazidime	25 - > 100	50 - > 100	> 64	> 100
Cefsulodin	6.25 - 64	25 - > 100	> 64	> 100
Latamoxef	50 - >100	50 - > 100	> 64	> 100
Aztreonam	>100	ND	ND	ND

[a] The MIC$_{50}$ value varies depending on the study.
[b] ND, not determined.

is inactive against *N. farcinica* and *N. otitidiscaviarum*. The only aminoglycosides active against all species are amikacin (12), which is the aminoglycoside to be used when bitherapy is planned, and netilmicin.

Tetracyclines, chloramphenicol, macrolides, ketolides, and lincosamides

Data on the susceptibility of *Nocardia* to these different antibiotics are conflicting (Table 3). According to our data, only minocycline and doxycycline are active in particular against *N. brasiliensis* and *N. otitidiscaviarum*.

Sulfonamides

The sulfonamides have weak *in vitro* activity which differs according to strain (Table 4). Only sulfamethoxazole has low activity against some strains of *N. asteroides*, and is more active against *N. brasiliensis*. The activity of trimethoprim-sulfamethoxazole can undoubtedly be attributed to the sulfonamide component alone, since trimethoprim alone is inactive against *Nocardia* at the recommended dosages. However, the degree of synergy *in vitro* depends on the strain, incubation time and trimethoprim/sulfamethoxazole ratio. The 1:5 ratio in the marketed drug combination is much less active than combinations containing a higher trimethoprim dose (1:1 or even 10:1 ratio), but such doses are potentially toxic *in vivo*. Susceptibility to trimethoprim-sulfamethoxazole, which is one of the classical reference treatments for nocardiosis, appears on the whole to be moderate. The correlation between the *in vitro* and *in vivo* activity of this drug combination is low, since clinical success has been achieved in patients harboring *Nocardia* isolates which tested resistant *in vitro*.

Table 2. Susceptibility of *Nocardia* to aminoglycosides

Antibiotic	MIC$_{50}$ (µg/ml)[a]			
	N. asteroides	*N. farcinica*	*N. brasiliensis*	*N. otitidiscaviarum*
Streptomycin	≥ 16	100	50	100
Spectinomycin	≥ 16	> 100	> 100	50
Kanamycin	8 - 64	≥ 64	> 100	2
Neomycin	2	ND[b]	ND	ND
Tobramycin	0.2 - 8	> 16	0.05	25
Dibekacin	0.1 - 8	> 16	0.05	0.1
Amikacin	≤ 0.25 - 1	1	0.78	1.56
Gentamicin	0.78 - 8	16 -> 100	0.2	0.2
Sisomicin	0.2 - 4	25	0.2	0.2
Netilmicin	0.1 - 16	0.4	0.05	0.1

[a] The MIC$_{50}$ value varies depending on the study.
[b] ND, not determined.

Table 3. Susceptibility of *Nocardia* to tetracyclines, phenicols, macrolides, ketolides, and lincosamides

Antibiotic	MIC$_{50}$ (µg/ml)[a]			
	N. asteroides	*N. farcinica*	*N. brasiliensis*	*N. otitidiscaviarum*
Tetracycline	≥ 25	50	25	25
Chlortetracycline	50	> 100	25	50
Oxytetracycline	50	100	50	> 100
Demethylchlortetracycline	25	100	12.5	12.5
Doxycycline	2 - 6.25	25	6.25	1.56
Minocycline	1 - 6.25	4 - 6.25	6.25	3.12
Chloramphenicol	16 - 50	25	100	50
Thiamphenicol	> 100	> 100	> 100	> 100
Erythromycin	16 -> 100	32 -> 100	50	> 100
Oleandomycin	16 - > 100	32 - > 100	> 100	> 100
Clarithromycin	0.25 - > 128	> 128	ND[b]	> 128
Spiramycin	0.25 - > 128	> 128	ND	> 128
Lincomycin	0.25 - > 128	> 128	ND	> 128
Clindamycin	8 - > 100	> 128	ND	6.25
Pristinamycin	50	100	50	100
Cethromycin	0.25 - > 128	128	ND	64 - > 128

[a] The MIC$_{50}$ value varies depending on the study.
[b] ND, not determined.

Quinolones

The quinolones have little activity against *N. asteroides*, with the exception of ciprofloxacin which has an MIC similar to the serum levels obtained *in vivo* (Table 5). Garenoxacin [desfluoro(6)quinolone] is active against 90% of *N. asteroides* isolates at a concentration of 8 µg/ml and 50% of *N. asteroides* and *N. brasiliensis* isolates at concentrations of 0.13 and 1 µg/ml, respectively (24). Sparfloxacin is more active than ciprofloxacin against *N. asteroides* (12).

Oxazolidinone

Linezolid is the first antibiotic active against all the medically relevant species of *Nocardia* (5, 9), particularly *N. brasiliensis*, a common cause of actinomycetoma (25). It has proved to be particularly effective, alone or in combination therapy, in

Table 4. Susceptibility of *Nocardia* to sulfonamides, fosfomycin, and vancomycin

Antibiotic	MIC$_{50}$ (µg/ml)[a]			
	N. asteroides	N. farcinica	N. brasiliensis	N. otitidiscaviarum
Sulfonamides (except sulfamethoxazole)	> 100	> 100	3.12 -> 100	> 100
Sulfamethoxazole	≤ 1 - 16	4	1.56	> 100
Trimethoprim	> 100	> 100	> 100	> 100
Sulfamethoxazole + trimethoprim	1 - 20	ND[b]	ND	ND
Fosfomycin	> 100	> 100	> 100	> 100
Vancomycin	32 -> 100	> 100	> 100	> 100

[a] The MIC$_{50}$ value varies depending on the study.
[b] ND, not determined.

Table 5. Susceptibility of *N. asteroides* and *N. farcinica* to quinolones

Antibiotic	MIC$_{50}$ (µg/ml)[a]	
	N. asteroides	N. farcinica
Nalidixic acid	> 100	ND[b]
Pipemidic acid	≥ 100	> 100
Norfloxacin	4 - 32	ND
Pefloxacin	4 - 32	ND
Ofloxacin	≥ 4	ND
Ciprofloxacin	4	1
Cinoxacin	> 64 a	ND
Enoxacin	32	ND
Amifloxacin	≥ 64	ND
WIN 35439	16	ND

[a] The MIC$_{50}$ value varies depending on the study.
[b] ND, not determined.

the treatment of central nervous system infection and disseminated disease (17), although it can cause side effects necessitating the discontinuation of treatment (16).

RESISTANCE PHENOTYPES AND AID AS FOR IDENTIFICATION

Antibiotic susceptibility testing has a twofold interest. Obviously, it can be used to evaluate the activities of antibiotics with a potential therapeutic effect (13, 18, 23), but it also aids in the identification of species having a specific resistance profile.

Generally, the resistance phenotype of *N. asteroides*, *N. brasiliensis* and *N. otitidiscaviarum* strains allows rapid identification to the species level. Susceptibility tests also enable presumptive speciation of the newly classified *N. asteroides*, as well as *N. farcinica* and *N. nova*. Wallace et al. (26, 27) report that *N. farcinica* isolates are resistant to cefamandole, cefotaxime and tobramycin. *N. nova* isolates are susceptible to ampicillin and erythromycin and resistant to carbenicillin and tobramycin. Only *N. asteroides* isolates display a heterogeneous resistance phenotype which results from either interspecies variability or a taxonomic classification that is not sufficiently precise. The combination of amoxicillin susceptibility and clavulanic acid resistance points to the species *N. nova*.

IN VITRO SUSCEPTIBILITY AND CHOICE OF TREATMENT

Despite their controversial *in vitro* efficacy, the sulfonamides (with or without trimethoprim) are still widely considered to be the treatment of choice for nocardiosis. Although the trimethoprim-sulfamethoxazole ratio on the market is not ideal, its observed clinical efficacy can be explained by the fact that trimethoprim levels reached in tissues are higher than those of sulfamethoxazole, whose tissue concentrations remain lower than in serum, thus reestablishing *de facto* an optimum ratio.

Nonetheless, the indications of this treatment are limited because it is poorly tolerated and only minimally active against *N. brasiliensis* and certain *N. asteroides* isolates (15). As far as other species are concerned, several recent reports propose alternative treatments that are almost always based on a multidrug combination. Besides the classic amoxicillin-clavulanic acid + amikacine combination, imipenem + amikacin is increasingly used to treat infections caused by sulfonamide-resistant *N. asteroides* and *N. farcinica*. Other β-lactams: cefuroxime, cefotaxime and ceftriaxone have also been used in combination with amikacin. *N. otitidiscaviarum* infections should be treated with a combination of an aminoglycoside (kanamycin, gentamicin, etc. with the exception of tobramycin) and doxycycline or minocycline. Other combinations, including sulfonamide + aminoglycoside or sulfonamide + β-lactam have also been used. In spite of variable *in vitro* activity against *Nocardia*, some authors report the successful use of monotherapy with amikacin, minocycline, erythromycin, second generation quinolones or chloramphenicol.

In conclusion, the treatment of nocardiosis remains problematic. In the absence of controlled clinical trials, empirical guidelines must be relied upon. Depending on the site of infection and the patient, surgery completed by appropriate antibiotics can contribute to a favorable outcome.

While clinical improvement is usually observed after about ten days of treatment, there is a general consensus about the need for a prolonged course of antibiotics, although the optimum treatment duration has yet to be clearly established. Indeed, the treatment duration depends on several factors: severity of infection, immune status of the patient, virulence of the bacterium and risk of relapse. No prospective studies have specifically examined these albeit crucial factors in the treatment of nocardiosis. Primary cutaneous forms require at least three months of antibiotics; pulmonary infection is classically treated for six months, while disseminated disease or immunocompromised patients require at least twelve months of therapy which may need to be continued indefinitely. Inadequate treatment durations incur the risk of relapse which, in some published series, has been observed in 10-30% of patients (7).

REFERENCES

(1) **Alvirez-Freites, E., A.E. Yeo, M.S. DeStefano, and M.H. Cynamon.** 2004. In vitro susceptibility of nocardia species to cethromycin, clarithromycin and amikacin. Eur. J. Clin. Microbiol. Infect. Dis. **23**:69-70.

(2) **Ambaye, A., P.C. Kohner, P.C. Wollan, K.L. Roberts, G.D. Roberts, and F.R. Cockerrill, III.** 1997. Comparison of agar dilution, broth microdilution, disk diffusion, E-test, and BACTEC radiometric methods for antimicrobial susceptibility testing of clinical isolates of the *Nocardia asteroides* complex. J. Clin. Microbiol. **35**:847-852.

(3) **Beaman, B.L., and L. Beaman.** 1994. *Nocardia* species: host-parasite relationships. Clin. Microbiol. Rev. **7**:213-264

(4) **Boiron, P.** 2000. Nocardiose. pp. 54-56. *In* A. Eyquem, J. Alouf, and L. Montagnier (ed), Traité de microbiologie clinique. Piccin Nuova Libraria, Padova, Italia.

(5) **Brown-Elliott, B.A., S.C. Ward, C.J. Crist, L.B. Mann, R.W. Wilson, and R.J. Wallace, Jr.** 2001. In vitro activities of linezolid against multiple *Nocardia* species. Antimicrob. Agents Chemother. **45**:1295-1297.

(6) **Brown, J.M., and M.M. McNeil.** 2003. *Nocardia, Rhodococcus, Gordonia, Actinomadura, Streptomyces*, and other aerobic actinomycetes, p. 502-531. *In* P.R. Murray, E.J. Baron, M.A. Pfaller, F.C. Tenover, and R.H. Yolken (ed.), Manual of Clinical Microbiology, 8th ed. American Society for Microbiology, Washington, D.C.

(7) **Burgert, S.J.** 1999. Nocardiosis: a clinical review. Infect. Dis. Clin. Pract. **8**:27-32.

(8) **Carroll, G.F., J.M. Brown, and L.D. Haley.** 1977. A method for determining in-vitro drug susceptibility of some *Nocardia* and *Actinomadurae*. Results with 17 antimicrobial agents. Amer. J. Clin. Path. **68**:279-283.

(9) **Cockerill, F.R., and R.S. Edson.** 1991. Trimethoprim-sulfamethoxazole. Mayo. Clin. Proc. **66**:1260-1269.

(10) **Glupczynski Y., C. Berhin, M. Janssens, and G. Wauters.** 2006. Determination of antimicrobial susceptibility patterns of *Nocardia* spp. from clinical specimens by E-test. Clin. Microbiol. Infect. **12**:905-912.

(11) **Hitti, W., and M. Wolff.** 2005. Two cases of multidrug-resistant *Nocardia farcinica* infection in immunosuppressed patients and implications for empiric therapy. Eur. J. Clin. Microbiol. Infect. Dis. **24**:1442-1444.

(12) **Kanemitsu, K., H. Kunishima, T. Saga, H. Harigae, S. Ishikawa, H. Takemura, and M. Kaku.** 2003. Efficacy of amikacin combinations for nocardioses. Tohoku J. Exp. Med. **201**:157-163.

(13) **Laurent, F., E. Casoli, A. Couble, and P. Boiron.** 2001. Sensibilité aux antibiotiques des bactéries appartenant au genre *Nocardia* et traitement des nocardioses. Antibiotiques **3**:104-110.

(14) **Laurent, F., J. Freney, and P. Boiron.** 2003. *Nocardia* et actinomycètes aérobies apparentés. pp. 1-21. *In* J. Freney, F. Renaud, W. Hansen, and C. Bollet (ed.), Actualités en bactériologie clinique théorique et pratique. ESKA, Paris.

(15) **Lederman, E.R., and N.F. Crum.** 2004. A case series and focused review of nocardiosis: clinical and microbiologic aspects. Medicine (Baltimore) **83**:300-313.

(16) **Lewis, K.E., P. Ebden, S.L. Wooster, J. Rees, and G.A.J. Harrison.** 2003. Multi-system infection with *Nocardia farcinica*. Therapy with linezolid and minocycline. J. Infect. **46**:199-202.

(17) **Moylett, E.H., S.E. Pacheco, B.A. Brown-Elliott, T.R. Perry, E.S. Buescher, M.C. Birmingham, J.J. Schentag, J.F. Gimbel, A. Apodaca, M.A. Schwartz, R.M. Rakita, and R.J. Wallace, Jr.** 2003. Clinical experience with linezolid for the treatment of *Nocardia* infection. Clin. Infect. Dis. **36**:313-318.

(18) **Peraira, J.R., J. Segovia, R. Fuentes, J. Jimenez-Mazuecos, R. Arroyo, B. Fuertes, P. Mendaza, and L.A. Pulpon.** 2003. Pulmonary nocardiosis in heart transplant recipients: treatment and outcome. Transplant Proc. **35**:2006-2008.

(19) **Rivero, A., M. García-Lázaro, I. Pérez-Camacho, C. Natera, M. Del Carman Almodovar, A. Camacho, J. Torre-Cisneros.** 2008. Successful long-term treatment with linezolid for disseminated infection with multiresistant *Nocardia farcinica*. Infection **36**:389-391.

(20) **Roth, A., S. Andrees, R.M. Kroppenstedt, D. Harmsen, and H. Mauch.** 2003. Phylogeny of the genus *Nocardia* based on reassessed 16S rRNA gene sequences reveals underspeciation and division of strains classified as *Nocardia asteroides* into three established species and two unnamed taxons J. Clin. Microbiol. **41**:851-856.

(21) **Saubolle, M.A., and D. Sussland.** 2003. Nocardiosis: review of clinical and laboratory experience. J. Clin. Microbiol. **41**:4497-4501.

(22) **Tomlin, P., C. Sand, and R.P. Rennie.** 2001. Evaluation of E-test, disk diffusion and broth microdilution to establish tentative quality control limits and review susceptibility breakpoints for two aerobic actinomycetes. Diagn. Microbiol. Infect. Dis. **40**:179-186.

(23) **Tripodi, M.F., L.E. Adinolfi, A. Andreana, G. Sarnataro, E. Durante Mangoni, M. Gambardella, R. Casillo, C. Farina, and R. Utili.** 2001. Treatment of pulmonary nocardiosis in heart-transplant patients: importance of susceptibility studies. Clin. Transplant. **15**:415-420.

(24) **Valera L., E. Gradelski, E. Huczko, T. Washo, H. Yigit, and J. Fung-Tomc.** 2002. *In vitro* activity of a novel des-fluoro(6) quinolone, garenoxacin (BMS-284756), against rapidly growing mycobacteria and *Nocardia* isolates. J. Antimicrob. Chemother. **50**:137-148.

(25) **Vera-Cabrera L., A. Gomez-Flores, W.G. Escalante-Fuentes, and O. Welsh.** 2001. In vitro activity of PNU-100766 (linezolid), a new oxazolidinone antimicrobial, against *Nocardia brasiliensis*. Antimicrob. Agents Chemother. **45**:3629-3630.

(26) **Wallace, R.J., Jr, M. Tsukamura, B.A. Brown, V.A. Steingrube, Y.S. Zhang, and D.R. Nash.** 1990. Cefotaxime-resistant *Nocardia asteroides* strains are isolates of the controversial species *Nocardia farcinica*. J. Clin. Microbiol. **28**:2726-2732.

(27) **Wallace, R.J., Jr, B.A. Brown, M. Tsukamura, J.M. Brown, and G.O. Onyi.** 1991. Clinical and laboratory features of *Nocardia nova*. J. Clin. Microbiol. **29**:2407-2411.

(28) **Woods, G.L., B.A. Brown-Elliott, E.P. Desmond, G.S. Hall, L. Heifets, G.E. Pfyffer, M.R. Plaunt, J.C. Ridderhof, R.J. Wallace, Jr., N.G. Warren, and G.F. Witebsky.** 2003. Susceptibility testing of *Mycobacteria*, *Nocardiae*, and other aerobic actinomycetes; approved standard M24-A, vol. 23, no. 18. NCCLS, Wayne, PA, USA.

(29) **Yazawa, K., Y. Mikami, K. Otozai, J. Uno, and T. Arai.** 1989. In vitro susceptibility of pathogenic *Nocardia* to beta-lactam antibiotics, especially imipenem, a carbapenem antibiotic. J. Antibiotics **42**:2354-2362.

Chapter 52. ANTIBIOGRAM IN VETERINARY PRACTICE

Frank M. AARESTRUP

The introduction of antimicrobial agents in human medicine and animal husbandry was one of the most significant achievements of the 20th century. Antimicrobial agents have literally changed our way of living. Already in the beginning of the "antibiotic era" antimicrobial agents gained widespread use in food animal production for treatment of infectious diseases, in eradication programmes, and for non-therapeutic usage for prevention of diseases and as a growth promoter (1). Today antimicrobial agents have become an integrated part of modern food animal production and even though there is only limited data on antimicrobial consumption for animals, the available data suggest that more antimicrobial agents are used for food animals than for humans (10). Sale of antimicrobials for use in swine production are reported to be worth an estimated 1.7 billion dollars, equal to 34% of the global animal health antimicrobial market followed by poultry (33%) and cattle (26%) (17).

The largest usage of antimicrobial agents is non-therapeutic for prevention and growth promotion and thus, entirely based on empiric experiences and no guidance from susceptibility testing. In contrast to human medicine where the individual person has a value, infections control and antimicrobial therapy is in most cases targeting larger groups or even entire herds or farms. Thus, laboratory diagnostic is mainly used for monitoring and thereby guidance of empiric treatment rather than for guidance of treatment of the individual animal (one exception might be bovine mastitis in cattle). Thus, a much more limited number of samples are handled in food animal medicine compared to human medicine, but much more data are desired from those samples. Consequently, the few isolates obtained are often tested towards a larger panel of antimicrobial agents and MIC determinations have relatively more widespread use in veterinary medicine.

The use of antimicrobial susceptibility testing in veterinary medicine has closely paralleled that of human medicine. The pathogens causing infections in animals and human are often the same and the test methods developed for human medicine provide equivalent results for isolates from animals. However, the use of these methods have caused problems for some animal specific pathogens as have the use of human interpretative criteria for some disease conditions in animals. Furthermore, a number of antimicrobial agents are only used in veterinary medicine. Thus, some attempts to develop animal specific guidelines and interpretative criteria have been done especially by the Clinical and Laboratory Standards Institute (CLSI) through the forming of a veterinary sub-committee and publications of veterinary specific standards (4). Most focus has, however, been on newly developed antimicrobial agents, whereas the older compounds have not gained the same attention. Thus, much still needs to be done before a global standard has been developed.

This chapter provides some examples of animal specific bacteria, antimicrobial agents, and disease conditions and the importance in relation to susceptibility testing and interpretative reading.

MODE OF ACTION OF ANTIBIOTICS

Most antimicrobial agents approved for treatment of infections in animals are the same substances as those approved for treatment of infections in humans. However, a number of drugs have been developed exclusively for animal use but all belong to classes also approved for human usage. An overview is given in Table 1.

It is not the same antimicrobial agents which are approved for use in animals in all countries globally. Thus, the antimicrobial agents used and tested differ therefore considerable between countries. However, some common antimicrobial agents are used and can therefore be recommended for testing in all countries.

In veterinary medicine it has, in many laboratories, become tradition to test for susceptibility towards the specific compound used for therapy. With an increasing number of compounds belonging to the same classes this has become increasingly difficult. Thus, in many laboratories class representatives are now used; *e.g.* ciprofloxacin to represent all fluoroquinolones. In the recommendations below I have chosen to follow this in the suggested compounds to be tested.

Table 1. Susceptibility of various bacterial species towards antimicrobial agents almost exclusively used for treatment of infections in animals

Class	Antimicrobial agent	Site of action	Examples of target pathogen and MICs (µg/ml)					Reference
			E. coli	S. aureus	A. pleuropneumoniae	S. suis	B. hyodysenteriae	P. multocida	
Aminoglycosides	Apramycin	30S ribosomal subunit	1 – 8	-	-	-	-	-	www.danmap.org
	Neomycin		1 – 8	-	-	-	-	-	
Cephalosporins	Ceftiofur	Transpeptidase	0.125 – 1	0.125 – 1	≤0.015 – 0.03	0.03 - 0.125	-	≤0.015	www.eucast.org
	Cefquinome		-	-	-	0.03 – 0.125	-	-	(3)
Macrolides	Tilmicosin	50S ribosomal subunit	-	-	2 - 16	-	-	0.5 – 16	www.eucast.org
	Tylosin		-	-	-	0.25 - 4	≤2 - 16	-	(5, 6, 16)
	Tulathromycin		-	-	8 - 32	-	-	0.25 - 2	
Amphenicols	Florfenicol	Peptidyl transferase	2 - 16	2 - 8	0.125 - 2	0.5 - 4	-	0.25 - 1	www.eucast.org
Pleuromutilin	Tiamulin	Peptidyl transferase	-	0.25 - 2	-	-	≤0.015 - 2	-	www.eucast.org
	Valnemulin		-	-	-	-	≤0.015 - 2	-	(5)

ANIMAL SPECIFIC BACTERIAL SPECIES AND DISEASE CONDITIONS

The bacterial species causing infections in animals are to a large extent the same or belongs to the same groups as those infecting humans. Thus, in many cases the methods for susceptibility testing and interpretative criteria have traditionally been the same. However, a few diseases differ as outlined below and specific recommendations for those are available (Table 2).

Gastro-intestinal infections

Lawsonia intracellularis

Lawsonia intracellularis is an important cause of intestinal infections in pigs. However, the bacteria can only be grown in cell cultures and no routine procedure for susceptibility testing has been developed. Currently, pleuromutelins, tetracycline, macrolides seems to be efficient in controlling the disease. The effect and potential development of resistance have to be observed though clinical experience and potential treatment failure.

Brachyspira spp.

Brachyspira hyodysenteriae and *Brachyspira pilosicoli* are important causes of diarrhoea in pigs and seemingly the only clinically efficient drugs against infections with these bacteria are the pleuromutilins, macrolides, and lincosamides (5). There are currently no approved standards for antimicrobial susceptibility testing of these fastidious spirochetes. Different methods including disk diffusion, agar MIC determination and broth dilution have been used. However, the method with greatest reproducibility seems to be micro-broth dilution which also has been evaluated in an interlaboratory study where MIC quality control ranges for six antimicrobial agents for the type strain of *B. hyodysenteriae* were established (12). Because of the difficulties in growing these bacteria and the need for strict anaerobic growth conditions, susceptibility testing is normally performed on a few selected samples in a reference laboratory. The antimicrobial agents to be tested should be tiamulin, valnemulin, tylosin, and lincomycin (Table 2).

The resistance mechanisms observed in *Brachyspira* spp. have so far mainly been due to mutations. Resistance to macrolides and lincosamides is due to mutations in adenine 2058 of the 23S rDNA gene (*E. coli* numbering). This gives rise to a change in MIC of tylosin from a susceptible range from 2 to 16 µg/ml to a resistant population with MICs above 64 µg/ml. Resistance to pleuromutelins develop in a stepwise manner. The susceptible strains seem to have MICs of tiamulin below 2 µg/ml, whereas non-susceptible isolates have MICs ranging from 4 and above. There are some indications that these MICs might already be a shift towards higher MIC values (12, 13).

Gram-negative species

Escherichia coli in particular, but also other *Enterobacteriaceae* are very frequent causes of diarrhoea in swine, cattle, and poultry. The method for susceptibility testing is as for humans using Mueller-Hinton II, but the agents tested might differ because of the animal specific drugs that are approved (Table 2). The aminoglycosides apramycin and neomycin are not used in human medicine. The susceptible isolates have MICs ranging from 1 to 8 µg/ml of both antimicrobials, whereas isolates with acquired resistance have MICs 32 µg/ml and above.

Clostridium

Clostridium perfringens is an important cause of intestinal infections in swine and poultry. In swine, infections are mainly controlled by vaccination, but treatment might be required. So far *C. perfringens* has been universally susceptible to the penicillins and, thus, no routine susceptibility testing is required. *Clostridium difficile* has recently emerged as a pathogen in swine. Most likely, as in humans, antimicrobial associated due to the routine use of antimicrobials. Limited information on the susceptibility of this pathogen from infections in animals is available, but susceptibility testing towards macrolides, tetracycline and the penicillins seems appropriate.

Respiratory and generalised infections in swine, ruminants, and poultry

Some bacterial species belonging to the *Pasteurellaceae* grow poorly in the most commonly used growth media for susceptibility testing of human pathogens. Thus, for broth micro-dilution veterinary fastidious medium and for disk diffusion chocolate Mueller-Hinton agar is recommended (4). These media work well for *Actinobacillus pleuropneumoniae*, *Haemophilus parasuis*, *Mannheimia haemolytica*, and *Histophilus somni* (2, 9). *Pasteurella multocida* might give a number of different infections in swine, cattle, and poultry, but can be tested using Mueller-Hinton II agar or broth. Penicillin G or ampicillin will, in most cases, be effective against these organisms, even though resistance due to β-lactamase activity has emerged in some countries. Only one of these two drugs needs to be tested. Other effective drugs include florfenicol, tulathromycin, tilmicosin, tetracycline, co-trimoxazole, ceftiofur, and the fluoroquinolones. Even though tulathromycin and tilmicosin belong to the macrolides, there is still insufficient knowledge regarding potential mechanisms of resistance. It is, thus, advisable to test both. A suggested standard panel for testing is ampicillin, ceftiofur, ciprofloxacin, co-trimoxazole, florfenicol, tetracycline, tilmicosin, and tulathromycin. It should be noted that due to human health concerns the use of ceftiofur and fluoroquinolones is not recommended. The resistance mechanism found in *Pasteurellaceae* are to a wide extent the same as those observed in other Gram-negative species (7).

Staphylococci and streptococci are also common causes of generalized infections in animals. Streptococci are generally susceptible to the penicillins. However, reduced susceptibility seems to emerge in *Streptococcus suis*, even though the mechanism and clinical importance has not been elucidated. Thus, for this species routine susceptibility testing towards penicillin G might be advisable. *Staphylococcus aureus* is a common cause of multiple different infections in all animal species and *Staphylococcus hyicus* of skin infections in pigs. The procedure for susceptibility testing is as for all other staphylococci and the recommended drugs to test are listed in Table 2.

Clostridium septicum and *Clostridium sordelli* give serious infections in cattle and sheep. However, as for *C. perfringens* they appear susceptible to the penicillins. *E. coli* can also be a cause of generalized infections, especially in poultry. The procedure for susceptibility testing is as for intestinal infections, but the antimicrobial agents to be tested differ.

Bovine, porcine, and ovine mastitis

Mastitis is one of the most common and economically important infections in dairy cattle and also important in lactating sheep and goats. The infections can be clinical or sub-clinical and, even though a large number of bacterial species can be implicated in the disease, most cases are caused by a limited number of bacteria. In most countries clinical bovine mastitis is mainly caused by *E. coli* followed by *S. aureus* and streptococci. In countries/regions where *Streptococcus agalactiae* is

Table 2. Suggested antimicrobial agents to test for different animal and bacterial species and disease conditions

Disease complex and animal species	Bacterial group	Method	Routine antimicrobial agents to test	Comment
Gastro-intestinal infections				
Swine	*Lawsonia intracellularis*	None developed		Treatment has to be based on clinical experience
Swine	*Brachyspira* spp.	Microbroth with brain-heart infusion	Lincomycin Tiamulin Tylosin Valnemulin Penicillin G	
Swine, poultry	*Clostridium perfringens*			Universally susceptible to penicillins
Swine, ruminants, poultry	Gram-negatives	Mueller-Hinton II	Ampicillin Apramycin Ciprofloxacin Colistin Co-trimoxazole Gentamicin Neomycin Tetracycline	
Respiratory and generalized infections				
Swine	Streptococci	Mueller-Hinton II supplemented with blood	Cefoxitin Erythromycin Oxacillin Penicillin G Tetracycline	Streptococci almost always susceptible to penicillins. Cefoxitin represents cephalosporins. Erythromycin represents macrolides.
All animal species	Staphylococci	Mueller-Hinton II	Cefoxitin Co-trimoxazole Erythromycin Penicillin G Tetracycline	Cefoxitin represents cephalosporins cephalosporins and antistaphylococcal penicillins. Erythromycin represents macrolides.
All animal species	Gram-negatives	Mueller-Hinton II	Ampicillin Apramycin Ceftriaxone or cefuroxime Ciprofloxacin Colistin Co-trimoxazole Florfenicol Gentamicin Neomycin Tetracycline	
Swine and cattle	*Actinobacillus pleuropneumoniae* *Haemophilus parasuis* *Histophilus somni*	Veterinary fastidious medium or chocolate agar	Ampicillin Ceftriaxone or cefuroxime Ciprofloxacin Co-trimoxazole Florfenicol Gentamicin Tetracycline Tilmicosin Tulathromycin	Ceftriaxone or cefuroxime represent cephalosporins. Ciprofloxacin represents fluoroquinolones.

Table 2. Suggested antimicrobial agents to test for different animal and bacterial species and disease conditions (continued)

Disease complex and animal species	Bacterial group	Method	Routine antimicrobial agents to test	Comment
Mastitis				
Cattle, swine, sheep	Staphylococci	Mueller-Hinton II	Cefoxitin Co-trimoxazole Erythromycin Penicillin G Tetracycline	Cefoxitin represents cephalosporins and antistaphylococcal penicillins. Erythromycin represents macrolides. Penicillin G is always efficient
Cattle, swine, sheep	Streptococci	Mueller-Hinton II with blood	Not necessary	
Cattle, swine, sheep	Gram-negatives	Mueller-Hinton II	Ampicillin Ceftriaxone or cefuroxime Co-trimoxazole Streptomycin Tetracycline	Ceftriaxone or cefuroxime represent cephalosporins.

controlled the most common cause of sub-clinical mastitis is *S. aureus*, followed by coagulase negative staphylococci and streptococci (*Streptococcus dysgalactiae* and *Streptococcus uberis*). A similar bacterial patterns seems to be the case with sheep and goats.

Penicillin G is highly effective against streptococci and since penicillin-resistant isolates have never been confirmed, no susceptibility testing is required. Penicillin G is also highly efficient against β-lactamase negative staphylococci. However, the prevalence of penicillin resistance varies greatly between countries and other antimicrobials can be necessary. Cloxacillin is widely used in many countries for treatment of dairy cattle during the dry period. Methicillin-resistant staphylococci have become more common in recent years and it seems indicated to routinely examine for the presence of such isolates. Several studies have shown that cefoxitin is superior to other cephalosporins as well as oxacillin and cloxacillin in detecting such isolates. The suggested panel to test is listed in Table 2.

It should be noted that in real life the choice of treatment depends mainly on economy and not concern of the individual animals. Thus, since the 3rd generation cephalosporin ceftiofur has no withdrawel time and the loss due to discard of milk production is very limited this drug has become the drug of choice in many countries.

Mastitis in sows is often part of a disease complex normally referred to as mastitis-metritis-agalactiae (MMA). This disease is more generalized in nature and often with multiple bacterial species involved. Thus, treatment has to be mainly based on empiric experience.

CONCLUSIONS

Compared to human medicine much less is known about the clinical efficacy of antimicrobial agents in veterinary medicine. Furthermore, for many compounds the interpretative criteria are based on those developed in human medicine. In 1993 the CLSI formed a subcommittee on Veterinary Antimicrobial Susceptibility Testing (V-AST) with the task of developing veterinary specific antimicrobial susceptibility testing standards (4). This committee has, since then, in particluar for novel compounds, developed animal specific interpretative criteria. Much work is, however, still lacking for older generic compounds and data on clinical efficacy are to a large extent missing.

Table 3. Examples of most common mechanisms of resistance towards antimicrobial agents almost exclusively used for treatment of infections in animals

Antimicrobial agent	Resistance gene, mechanism, and bacterial species	Examples of bacterial species	Reference
Apramycin	*aac(3)-IVa*	Gram-negative	15
Ceftiofur, cefquinome	β-lactamases with extended spectrum (CTX, TEM, SHV, CMY)	Gram-negative	14
	pbp2	*Staphylococcus*	
Tilmicosin, tylosin, tulathromycin	*erm*	Gram-positive	14
	Mutations in 23S rDNA	*Brachyspira, Campylobacter*	
Oxolinic acid, flumequine, danofloxacin, enrofloxacin, ibafloxacin, marbofloxacin, orbifloxacin, sarafloxacin	Point mutations and transferable quinolone mechanisms similar to those in humans pathogens	Gram-negative Gram-positive	14
Florfenicol	*floR*	Gram-negative	14
	fexA	*Staphylococcus*	
	cfr	*Staphylococcus*	
Tiamulin, valnemulin	Mutations in L3 and 23S rDNA	*Brachyspira*	5, 8
	cfr	*Staphylococcus*	

REFERENCES

(1) **Aarestrup, F. M.** 2005. Veterinary drug usage and antimicrobial resistance in bacteria of animal origin. Basic Clin. Pharmacol. Toxicol. **96**:271-281.

(2) **Aarestrup, F. M., A. M. Seyfarth, and Ø. Angen.** 2004. Antimicrobial susceptibility of *Haemophilus parasuis* and *Histophilus somni* from pigs and cattle in Denmark. Vet. Microbiol. **101**:143-146.

(3) **Burton, P. J., C. Thornsberry, Y. Cheung Yee, J. L. Watts, and R. J. Yancey Jr.** 1996. Interpretive criteria for antimicrobial susceptibility testing of ceftiofur against bacteria associated with swine respiratory disease. J. Vet. Diagn. Invest. **8**:464-468.

(4) **Clinical and Laboratory Standards Institute.** 2008. Performance standards for antimicrobial disk and dilution susceptibility tests for bacteria isolated from animals, approved standard – Third edition. CLSI document M31-A3. Wayne, PA: Clinical and Laboratory Standards Institute.

(5) **Franklin, A., M. Pringle, and D. J. Hampson.** 2006. Antimicrobial resistance In *Clostridium* and *Brachyspira* and other anaerobes. pp 127-144. In F.M. Aarestrup (ed.), Antimicrobial resistance in bacteria of animal origin. American Society for Microbiology Press, Washington DC.

(6) **Godinho, K. S.** 2008. Susceptibility testing of tulathromycin: interpretative breakpoints and susceptibility of field isolates. Vet. Microbiol. **129**:426-432.

(7) **Kehrenberg, C., R. D. Walker, C. C. Wu, and S. Schwarz.** 2006. Antimicrobial resistance in members of the family *Pasteurellaceae*. pp 167-186. In F.M. Aarestrup (ed.), Antimicrobial resistance in bacteria of animal origin. American Society for Microbiology Press, Washington DC.

(8) **Long, K. S., J. Poehlsgaard, C. Kehrenberg, S. Schwarz, and B. Vester.** 2006. The Cfr rRNA methyltransferase confers resistance to phenicols, lincosamides, oxazolidinones, pleuromutilins, and streptogramin A antibiotics. Antimicrob. Agents Chemother. **50**:2500-2505.

(9) **McDermott, P. F., A. L. Barry, R. N. Jones, G. E. Stein, C. Thornsberry, C. C. Wu, and R. D. Walker.** 2001. Standardization of broth microdilution and disk diffusion susceptibility tests for *Actinobacillus pleuropneumoniae* and *Haemophilus somnus*: quality control standards for ceftiofur, enrofloxacin, florfenicol, gentamicin, penicillin, tetracycline, tilmicosin, and trimethoprim-sulfamethoxazole. J. Clin. Microbiol. **39**:4283-4287.

(10) **Moulin, G., P. Cavalié, I. Pellanne, A. Chevance, A. Laval, Y. Millemann, P. Colin, C. Chauvin.** 2008. A comparison of antimicrobial usage in human and veterinary medicine in France form 1999 to 2005. J Antimicrob Chemother. Sep;62(3):617-25.

(11) **Priebe, S., and S. Schwarz.** 2003. *In vitro* activities of florfenicol against bovine and porcine respiratory tract pathogens. Antimicrob Agents Chemother. **47**:2703-2705.

(12) **Pringle, M., F. M. Aarestrup, B. Bergsjø, M. Fossi, E. Jouy, A. Landén, D. Mevius, K. Perry, C. Teale, J. Thomson, T. Skrzypczak, K. Veldman, and A. Franklin.** 2006. Quality-control ranges for antimicrobial susceptibility testing by broth dilution of the *Brachyspira hyodysenteriae* type strain (ATCC 27164T). Microb. Drug Resist. **12**:219-221.

(13) **Rohde, J., M. Kessler, C. G. Baums, and G. Amtsberg.** 2004. Comparison of methods for antimicrobial susceptibility testing and MIC values for pleuromutilin drugs for *Brachyspira hyodysenteriae* isolated in Germany. Vet. Microbiol. **102**:25-32.

(14) **Schwarz, S., A. Cloeckaert, and M. C. Roberts.** 2006. Mechanisms and spread of bacterial resistance

to antimicrobial agents. pp 73-98. *In* F.M. Aarestrup (ed.), Antimicrobial resistance in bacteria of animal origin. American Society for Microbiology Press, Washington DC.

(15) **Shaw, K. J., P. N. Rather, R. S. Hare, and G. H. Miller.** 1993. Molecular genetics of aminoglycoside resistance genes and familial relationships of the aminoglycoside-modifying enzymes. Microbiol. Rev. **57**:138-163.

(16) **Shryock, T. R., J. M. Staples, and D. C. DeRosa.** 2002. Minimum inhibitory concentration breakpoints and disk diffusion inhibitory zone interpretive criteria for tilmicosin susceptibility testing against *Pasteurella multocida* and *Actinobacillus pleuropneumoniae* associated with porcine respiratory disease. J. Vet. Diagn. Invest. **14**:389-395.

(17) **Vivash-Jones, B.** 2000. COMISA report. The year in review. COMISA, Brussels, Belgium.

Third Part:

PROTOCOLS FOR STUDY OF ANTIBIOTICS
(P. COURVALIN, R. LECLERCQ and L. DUBREUIL)

Procedure 1. ANTIBIOTICS BY CLASSES AND GROUPS

INHIBITORS OF PEPTIDOGLYCAN SYNTHESIS

β-lactams – I. Penams, carbapenems, and oxapenams (or clavams)

Penams

Group penicillin G
- Penicillin G (benzylpenicillin)
- Long acting penicillins
- Procaïne-penicillin
- Benethamine-penicillin
- Clemizole-penicillin
- Benzathine-penicillin
- Oral penicillins
- Penicillin V (phenoxymethylpenicillin)
- Clometocillin

Penicillins antistaphylococci
- Methicillin
- Oxacillin
- Cloxacillin
- Dicloxacillin
- Nafcillin

Penicillins with a broad spectrum
- Ampicillin
- Pro-ampicillins
- Bacampicillin
- Pivampicillin
- Metampicillin
- Hetacillin
- Equivalent
- Amoxicillin
- Carboxypenicillins
- Carbenicillin
- Ticarcillin
- Ureido-penicillins
- Azlocillin
- Mezlocillin
- Piperacillin

Amidino-penicillins
- Mecillinam
- Pivmecillinam (pro-mecillinam)

Penicillins-sulfones
- Sulbactam ⎱ β-lactamase inhibitors
- Tazobactam ⎰
- Ampicillin + Sulbactam
- Piperacillin + Tazobactam

Carbapenems
- Imipenem (N formimidoyl thienamycine)
- Meropenem
- Ertapenem
- Faropenem

Oxapenams or Clavams
- Clavulanic acid (β-lactamase inhibitor)

Used in combination with amoxicillin or ticarcillin

β-lactams – II. Cephems and oxacephems

1st generation injectable cephalosporins
- Cephalothin
- Cefaloridin
- Cefacetril
- Cefazolin
- Cefapirin

2nd generation injectable cephalosporins
- Cefamandol
- Cefuroxim
- Cefoxitin (cephamycin)

3rd generation injectable cephalosporins
- Cefotaxime
- Cefmenoxime
- Ceftizoxime
- Ceftriaxone
- Latamoxef (oxacephem)
- Ceftazidime
- Cefpirome
- Cefepime

Other injectable cephalosporins
- Cefoperazone
- Cefotiam
- Cefotetan (cephamycin)

Procedure 1. ANTIBIOTICS BY CLASSES AND GROUPS

- Cefsulodine *(exclusively against P. aeruginosa)*

Oral cephalosporins

- Cefadroxil
- Cephalexine
- Cefradine
- Cefaclor
- Cefatrizine
- Loracarbef
- Cefotiam-hexetil
- Cefuroxime-axetil
- Cefixime
- Cefpodoxime-proxetil

β-lactams – III. Monobactams

- Aztreonam

Fosfomycin

- Fosfomycin
- Fosfomycin-trometamol

Glycopeptides

- Vancomycin
- Teicoplanin
- Telavancin
- Oritavancin
- Dalbavancin

Bacitracin

ANTIBIOTICS ACTIVE AGAINST MEMBRANES

Polymyxins

- Polymyxin B
- Polymyxin E or Colistin

Gramicidins and tyrocidine

Lipopeptides

- Daptomycin

Depsipeptides

- Fusafungin

PROTEIN SYNTHESIS INHIBITORS

Aminoglycosides (aminocyclitols)

- Streptomycin and Dihydrostreptomycin
- Deoxystreptamines

4-5 disubstituted

- Neomycin
- Framycetin
- Paromomycin

4-6 disubstituted

- Kanamycin
- Tobramycin
- Dibekacin
- Amikacin
- Isepamicin
- Gentamicin
- Sisomicin
- Netilmicin
- Micronomicin
- Ribostamycin
- Spectinomycin

Macrolides – Ketolides – Lincosamides – Streptogramins (MLS)

Macrolides (atoms)

- Erythromycin (14)
- Roxithromycin (14)
- Oleandomycin (14)
- Dirithromycin (14)
- Clarithromycin (14)
- Azithromycin (15)
- Spiramycin (16)
- Midecamycin (16)
- Josamycin (16)
- Rokitamycin (16)

Ketolide

- Telithromycin

Lincosamides

- Lincomycin
- Clindamycin

Streptogramins

- Pristinamycin
- Virginiamycin
- Quinupristin-Dalfopristin

Tetracyclines

- Tetracycline
- Lymecycline
- Oxytetracycline
- Chlortetracycline
- Demethyl-Chlortetracycline
- Rolitetracycline
- Methylenecycline
- Doxycycline
- Tigecycline
- Aminomethylcycline

Chloramphenicol group

- Chloramphenicol

Procedure 1. ANTIBIOTICS BY CLASSES AND GROUPS

- Thiamphenicol

Fusidic acid

Oxazolidinone

- Linezolid

INHIBITORS OF NUCLEIC ACIDS

Rifamycins

- Rifamycin SV
- Rifamycin
- Rifaximin

Quinolones

- Nalidixic acid
- Pipemidic acid
- Oxolinic acid
- Piromidic acid
- Cinoxacin
- Flumequin
- 6-fluoroquinolones
- Pefloxacin

- Ofloxacin ⎫
- Levofloxacin ⎬ systemic
- Ciprofloxacin ⎭

- Norfloxacin ⎫
- Enoxacin ⎬ urinary
- Lomefloxacin ⎭

- Sparfloxacin ⎫
- Moxifloxacin ⎪
- Gatifloxacin ⎬ respiratory
- Gemifloxacin ⎪
- Trovafloxacin ⎭

- Garenoxacin
- Rosoxacin (gonorrheae)

Novobiocin

5-nitroimidazoles

- Metronidazole
- Ornidazole
- Secnidazole
- Tinidazole

Nitrofurans

For urinary tract infections

- Nitrofurantoïn
- Hydroxymethylnitrofurantoïn

For intestinal infections

- Furazolidone
- Nifuroxazide

INHIBITORS OF FOLATE SYNTHESIS

Sulfonamides

- Sulfacetamine
- Sulfadiazine
- Sulfafurazole
- Sulfamoxole
- Sulfamethoxazole
- Sulfamethizol
- Sulfaguanidine
- Succinylsulfathiazol
- Sulfadoxine
- Sulfanilamide

2-4-diaminopyrimidines

- Trimethoprim

Combinations sulfonamides-diaminopyrimidines

- Sulfamethoxazole-trimethoprim (co-trimoxazole)
- Sulfamoxole-trimethoprim
- Sulfametrole-trimethoprim

" ANTISEPTICS " URINARY AND INTESTINAL

8-hydroxyquinolines

- Nitroxoline
- Tilbroquinol
- Broxyquinoline

ANTITUBERCULOSIS AGENTS

- Ethambutol
- Ethionamide
- Isoniazid
- Pyrazinamide
- Rifabutin
- Rifampin
- Streptomycin

ANTILEPROSY AGENTS

- Clofazimine
- Dapsone

663

Procedure 2. ANTIBIOTICS BY INTERNATIONAL COMMON DENOMINATION

International Common Denomination (ICD)	Class or Group
Fusidic acid	Steroid
Nalidixic acid	Quinolones
Pipemidic acid	Quinolones
Piromidic acid	Quinolones
Amikacin	Aminoglycosides
Amoxicilline	Aminopenicillins
Amoxicillin + clavulanic acid	β-lactams
Ampicillin	Aminopenicillins
Ampicillin + sulbactam	β-lactams
Apalcillin	Acylpenicillins
Arbekacin	Aminoglycosides
Azithromycin	Macrolides
Azlocillin	Ureidopenicillins
Aztreonam	Monobactams
Bacampicillin	Aminopenicillins
Bacitracin	Polypeptides
Benzathine-benzylpenicillin	Penicillin G
Carbenicillin	Carboxypenicillins
Cefacetrile	Cephalosporins 1 oral
Cefaclor	Cephalosporins 1 oral
Cefadroxil	Cephalosporins 1 oral
Cefalexin	Cephalosporins 1 oral
Cefaloridine	Cephalosporins 1
Cefalothin	Cephalosporins 1
Cefamandole	Cephalosporins 2
Cefapirine	Cephalosporins 1
Cefatrizine	Cephalosporins 1
Cefazolin	Cephalosporins 1
Cefepime	Cephalosporins 3
Cefixime	Cephalosporins 3 oral
Cefmenoxime	Cephalosporins 3
Cefoperazone	Cephalosporins 3
Cefotaxime	Cephalosporins 3
Cefotetan	Cephalosporins 2
Cefotiam	Cephalosporins 3 oral
Cefoxitin	Cephalosporins 2
Cefpirome	Cephalosporins 3
Cefpodoxime	Cephalosporins 3 oral
Cephalexin	Cephalosporins 1
Cephalothin	Cephalosporins 1
Cephradine	Cephalosporins 1 oral
Cefoxitin	Cephalosporins 2
Cefsulodin	Cephalosporins
Ceftazidime	Cephalosporins 3
Ceftizoxime	Cephalosporins 3
Ceftriaxone	Cephalosporins 3
Cefuroxime	Cephalosporins 2
Chloramphenicol	Phenicols
Cinoxacin	Quinolones
Ciprofloxacin	Quinolones
Clarithromycin	Macrolides
Clindamycin	Lincosamides
Clofazimine	Antileprosy
Clometocilline	Phenoxypenicillins
Cloxacillin	Isoxazolylpenicillins
Colistin	Polymyxins
Cotrimoxazole	Sulfonamides and diaminopyrimidine
Dalbavancin	Lipoglycopeptides
Dapsone	Antileprosy
Daptomycin	Lipopeptides
Dibekacin	Aminoglycosides
Dicloxacillin	Isoxazolylpenicillins
Dihydrostreptomycin	Aminoglycosides
Difloxacin	Quinolones
Dirithromycin	Macrolides
Doripenem	Carbapenems
Doxycycline	Tetracyclines
Enoxacin	Fluoroquinolones
Ertapenem	Carbapenems
Erythromycin	Macrolides
Ethambutol	Antituberculosis
Ethionamide	Antituberculosis
Faropenem	Carbapenems

Procedure 2. ANTIBIOTICS BY INTERNATIONAL COMMON DENOMINATION

International Common Denomination (ICD)	Class or Group
Fleroxacin	Quinolones
Flumequine	Quinolones
Fosfomycin	Phosphonic antibiotic
Fosfomycin-trometamol	Phosphonic antibiotic
Framycetin	Aminoglycosides
Furazolidone	Nitrofurans
Fusafungin	Polypeptides
Garenoxacin	Fluoroquinolones
Gatifloxacin	Fluoroquinolones
Gemofloxacin	Fluoroquinolones
Gentamicin	Aminoglycosides
Gramicidin	Polypeptides
Hetacillin	Aminopenicillins
Imipenem + cilastatin	Carbapenems
Isepamicin	Aminoglycosides
Isoniazid	Antituberculosis
Josamycin	Macrolides
Kanamycin	Aminoglycosides
Latamoxef	Cephalosporins 3
Levofloxacin	Fluoroquinolones
Lincomycin	Lincosamides
Linezolid	Oxazolidinones
Lomefloxacin	Fluoroquinolones
Lymecycline	Tetracyclines
Meropenem	Carbapenems
Metampicillin	Aminopenicillins
Methylenecycline	Tetracyclines
Methicillin	Dimethyloxybenzyl-penicillins
Metronidazole	Imidazoles
Mezlocillin	Ureidopenicillins
Midecamycin	Macrolides
Micronomicin	Aminoglycosides
Miloxacin	Quinolones
Minocycline	Tetracyclines
Moxifloxacin	Fluoroquinolones
Mupirocin	Pseudomonic acid
Nafcillin	Naphtamidopenicillins
Neomycin	Aminoglycosides
Netilmicin	Aminoglycosides
Nifuratel	Nitrofuranes
Nifurtoïnol	Nitrofuranes
Nifuroxazide	Nitrofuranes
Nitrofurantoïn	Nitrofuranes

International Common Denomination (ICD)	Class or Group
Nitroxoline	Oxyquinolines
Norfloxacin	Quinolones
Ofloxacin	Quinolones
Oleandomycin	Macrolides
Oritavancin	Lipoglycopeptides
Ornidazole	Imidazoles
Oxacillin	Isoxazolylpenicillins
Oxytetracycline	Tetracyclines
Paromomycin	Aminoglycosides
Pefloxacin	Quinolones
Penicillin G	Penicillins
Phenoxymethylpenicillin	Phenoxypenicillins
Phtalylsulfathiazole	Sulfonamides
Piperacillin	Ureidopenicillins
Piperacillin + tazobactam	Ureidopenicillins
Pivampicillin	Aminopenicillins
Pivmecillinam	Amidinopenicillins
Polymyxin B	Polymyxins
Pristinamycin	Streptogramins
Pyrazinamide	Antituberculosis
Quinupristin-Dalfoprisitne	Streptogramins
Ramoplanin	Lipoglycodepsipeptides
Rifabutin	Antituberculosis
Ribostamycin	Aminoglycosides
Rifampin	Rifamycins, Antituberculosis
Rifamycin	Rifamycins
Rifaximin	Macrolides
Rokitamyxin	Macrolides
Rolitetracycline	Tetracyclines
Rosoxacine	Quinolones
Roxithromycin	Macrolides
Salazosulfapyridine	Sulfonamides
Sisomicin	Aminoglycosides
Sparfloxacin	Fluoroquinolones
Spectinomycin	Aminocyclitol
Spiramycin	Macrolides
Streptomycin	Aminoglycosides, Antituberculosis
Succinylsulfathiazol	Sulfonamides
Sulfacetamide	Sulfonamides
Sulfadiazine	Sulfonamides
Sulfadoxine	Sulfonamides
Sulfafurazole	Sulfonamides
Sulfaguanidine	Sulfonamides
Sulfamethizole	Sulfonamides
Sulfamethoxazole	Sulfonamides

Procedure 2. ANTIBIOTICS BY INTERNATIONAL COMMON DENOMINATION

International Common Denomination (ICD)	Class or Group
Sulfamoxole	Sulfonamides
Sulfanilamide	Sulfonamides
Teicoplanin	Glycopeptides
Telavancin	Lipoglycopeptides
Telithromycin	Ketolides
Temafloxacin	Quinolones
Tetracycline	Tetracyclines
Thiamphenicol	Phenicols
Ticarcillin	Carboxypenicillins
Ticarcillin + clavulanic acid	Carboxypenicillins
Tinidazole	Imidazoles
Tobramycin	Aminoglycosides
Tosufloxacin	Quinolones
Trimethoprim	Diaminopyrimidine
Trimethoprim + sulfamethoxazole	Diaminopyrimidine + sulfonamides
Trimethoprim + sulfametrole	Diaminopyrimidine + sulfonamides
Trimethoprim + sulfamoxole	Diaminopyrimidine + sulfonamides
Troleandomycin	Macrolides
Tygecycline	Tetracyclines
Vancomycin	Glycopeptides
Virginiamycin	Streptogramins

Procedure 3. PREPARATION OF SERIAL DILUTIONS OF ANTIBIOTICS

Example: Prepare a 2560 µg/ml stock solution

$$\frac{v \times 2560}{1\,000} = \text{mg of powder} \times \text{titer}$$

v = ml H2O or solvent to be added to prepare a 2560 µg/ml solution. This volume must be at least 5 ml.

Stock solution (µg/ml)	Stock solution (ml)		Water (ml)	Concentration obtained (µg/ml)	Final concentration in culture medium[a] (µg/ml)
2 560	2	+	2	1 280	128
	1	+	3	640	64
	0.5	+	3.5	320	32
	0.5	+	7.5	160	16
160[b]	2	+	2	80	8
	1	+	3	40	4
	0.5	+	3.5	20	2
	0.5	+	7.5	10	1
10[b]	2	+	2	5	0.5
	1	+	3	2.5	0.25
	0.5	+	3.5	1.25	0.125
	0.5	+	7.5	0.625	0.0625
0,625[b]	2	+	2	0.312	0.0312
	1	+	3	0.156	0.0156
	0.5	+	3.5	0.08	0.008

[a] Add 2 ml of the range to 18 ml of Mueller-Hinton agar.

[b] These solutions are the last of the previous serial dilutions.

Procedure 4. KINETICS OF BACTERICIDAL ACTION

PRINCIPLE

The kinetics of the bactericidal activity of antibiotics is determined by enumerating the surviving bacteria cultured in the presence of the antibiotic at defined time intervals. At least four bacterial counts must be performed during the first 6 to 8 hours to study the early phase of bactericidal activity. One or two samples taken at the 24th or 48th hour are used to characterize the late phase.

PREPARATION OF ANTIBIOTIC SOLUTIONS

Concentration ranges must be tenfold higher than the desired final ranges.

METHOD

1st day

- Prepare an exponential phase of culture of the bacterial strain to be studied : subculture 0.1 ml (Gram-negative bacillus), 0.3 ml (*Enterococcus*, *Staphylococcus*, *P. aeruginosa*) or 0.6 ml (*Streptococcus*) of an 18-hour culture in 10 ml of Mueller—Hinton (M-H) medium.
- Place in a shaking water-bath at 37°C for 3 to 5 h until slight opalescence (5 to 10^7 bacteria/ml).
- If the tube used has an outer diameter of 17 mm and a flat bottom, verify the bacterial density with an API ATB 1550® nephelometer.
- Dilute the inoculum to 1/10 in M-H medium previously heated to 37°C.
- Verify the purity of the inoculum by isolation on a plate of M-H medium at the end of manipulation.
- Distribute 9 ml of bacterial suspension in a number of tubes equal to the number of concentrations of antibiotics studied plus one control tube.
- Add 1 ml of each antibiotic dilution and 1 ml of sterile distilled water to the control tube.
- Enumerate the inoculum in the control tube by performing 1/10 serial dilutions (from 10^{-1} to 10^{-5}). Inoculate 0.1 ml of these dilutions by smearing them with an inoculation loop or glass spheres on M-H agar.
- Incubate the tubes at 37°C (with stirring if possible).
- Depending on the periodicity selected, perform subsequent counts in an identical way to the initial count.
- Incubate the plates for 18 h at 37°C.

Note

The importance of the "carry over" effect (transfer of antibiotic onto the subculture medium, which inhibits growth of the survivors) can be assessed by performing the same test with the same inoculum and the same antibiotic concentrations, but by immediately counting the bacteria by the same method. If this carry over effect is excessive, it prevents counting of the surviving bacteria. The carry over effect can be minimized by counting bacteria at higher dilutions, by introducing substances that inhibit the activity of antibiotics into the agar (for example *Bacillus cereus* penicillinase 0.3 BU/plate for penicillins, 1% SPS + 0.01 M cysteine for aminoglycosides) or by using a spiral inoculator (Spiral system®).

2nd day

- Count the colonies. The bacterial concentration per milliliter is obtained by multiplying the result by 10 and by the dilution factor used. Only plates with a colony count between 30 and 300 are taken into account.

REFERENCE

(1) **Carlier, C., and P. Courvalin**. 1990. Emergence of 4′,4″-aminoglycoside nucleotidyltransferase in enterococci. Antimicrob. Agents Chemother. **34** : 1565-1569.

Procedure 5. ANTIBIOTIC COMBINATIONS

PRINCIPLE

Indications

Four essential circumstances can motivate the use of antibiotic combinations.
- Emergency treatment of a serious undiagnosed infection: the combination of two antibiotics with a complementary activity spectrum should be initiated after having taken the samples necessary for diagnosis and should be modified, if necessary, as a function of the bacteriology results.
- Infections due to multiple bacteria, in which a single antibiotic cannot be active on the entire bacterial population.
- The risk of selection of resistant mutants: the treatment of tuberculosis constitutes a typical example; but other clinical circumstances also illustrate this situation, whenever there is a dense bacterial population and when certain molecules with an increased risk (rifamycins, novobiocin, fusidic acid) are used.
- The main reason for using a combination of antibiotics is to obtain a synergistic effect and a rapid bactericidal action. This increased therapeutic efficacy has been demonstrated experimentally and/or confirmed by clinical experience in the treatment of serious infections such as septicemia, endocarditis, osteomyelitis, septic arthritis, infections in immunodepressed subjects, etc.
- The research of a synergistic combination, apart from established treatment regimens, often requires in each case, specific studies that the microbiologist should be able to decide in collaboration with clinicians.

Definition of interactions

Antibacterial effects of antibiotic combinations are generally defined by the four following interaction possibilities:
- **Indifference**: the activity of one of the antibiotics of the combination is not affected by the presence of the other.
- **Addition**: the activity of a combination of antibiotics is equal to the sum of the effects of each antibiotic studied separately at the same concentration as in the combination.
- **Synergy**: the effect is significantly greater than the sum of the effects of each antibiotic alone at the same concentration.
- **Antagonism**: the combination decreases the activity of one of the antibiotics. Its activity is less than the sum of the effects of each antibiotic studied separately.

In vitro characterization of these interactions depends on the precision of the method used, which is why indifferent and additive effects, reflecting a low interaction, are not always distinguished.

Synergistic combinations

Various mechanisms can explain the synergistic interactions of antibiotics, for example:
- synergy of combinations of β-lactams and aminoglycosides, glycopeptides and aminoglycosides, related to increased permeability of the bacterial wall to aminoglycosides.
- synergy of β-lactams possessing various PBP (penicillin-binding protein) binding sites: pivmecillinam and amoxicillin.
- synergy by competitive affinity for a β-lactamase: penicillin or amoxicillin and cloxacillin, amoxicillin and clavulanic acid.
- synergy by sequential inhibition of the same metabolic pathway: sulphamethoxazole and trimethoprim.

Antagonistic combinations

Antagonistic effects can result from the following interactions:
- the combination of bacteriostatic antibiotics, such as tetracyclines or chloramphenicol, with a β-lactam antibiotic decreases the bactericidal activity of the β-lactam.
- the combination of chloramphenicol and a macrolide, which induces competition of these molecules for the same binding site on the 50S subunit of the ribosome.

- the combination of an aminoglycoside, a tetracycline or chloramphenicol, in which antagonism would be related to inhibition of active transport of the aminoglycoside in the bacterium.
- certain combinations of β-lactams are antagonistic when one of the β-lactams is an inducer of the production of a β-lactamase.

ANTIBIOTIC COMBINATIONS TO BE STUDIED

The choice of antibiotics depends on:
- the bacterium and its resistance phenotype;
- the capacity of antibiotics to diffuse into the site of infection;
- the desired route of administration;
- toxic risks;
- possible adverse effects;

CHECKERBOARD TECHNIQUE

Principle

This technique allows quantification of the interaction of two antibiotics A and B by realizing the combination of a range of concentrations of A and B according to Table 1. These concentrations must include the effective humoral concentrations established for each antibiotic.

The concentrations prepared usually represent a 1:2 serial dilution, but a 1:1.5 serial dilution may be necessary for more precise quantification of interactions.

Methodology

According to the example shown in Table 1.

1. Prepare 10 rows of 10 sterile hemolysis tubes on a square rack.
2. Prepare each concentration of antibiotic A and antibiotic B in 10 ml of Mueller-Hinton (M-H) broth by preparing a range with a fourfold higher concentration than the desired final concentration: 256 to 1 µg/ml for antibiotics A and B (Table 1).
3. Dispense 0.5 ml of sterile M-H broth to each tube of the first column and each tube of the last row. These tubes will only receive antibiotics A and B, respectively.
4. Horizontally dispense 0.5 ml of each concentration of A in the corresponding rows I to IX. The Xth row is used for antibiotic B only. The same pipette can be used to dispense the checkerboard from top to bottom, i.e. from the lowest to the highest concentration.
5. Vertically dispense 0.5 ml of each concentration of antibiotic B in the corresponding columns 2 to 10 (the first column contains antibiotic A only). As in step 4, the same pipette can be used to dispense from right to left (from the 10th to the 2nd column).
6. Preparation and counting of the inoculum: dilute, in 100 to 150 ml of M-H broth, an exponential phase culture of the bacterial strain to be examined to obtain a suspension of about 2×10^6 bacteria/ml. Enumerate the inoculum by dilution and inoculate as in the previous technique. Incubate for 18 h at 37°C and store this control plate.
7. Dispense 1 ml of inoculum into each tube. Final concentrations of each antibiotic (64 to 0.25 mg/l) are fourfold lower than the initial concentrations.
8. Shake well and incubate at 37°C.
9. After 18 h, read the bacteriostatic results obtained. An example is given in Table 2.

Table 1. Antibiotic dispensing chart (final concentrations)

ANTIBIOTIC A (µg/ml)		1	2	3	4	5	6	7	8	9	10
	I	0.25	0.25/64	0.25/32	0.25/16	0.25/8	0.25/4	0.25/2	0.25/1	0.25/0.5	0.25/0.25
	II	0.5	0.5/64	0.5/32	0.5/16	0.5/8	0.5/4	0.5/2	0.5/1	0.5/0.5	0.5/0.25
	III	1	1/64	1/32	1/16	1/8	1/4	1/2	1/1	1/0.5	1/0.25
	IV	2	2/64	2/32	2/16	2/8	2/4	2/2	2/1	2/0.5	2/0.25
	V	4	4/64	4/32	4/16	4/8	4/4	4/2	4/1	4/0.5	4/0.25
	VI	8	8/64	8/32	8/16	8/8	8/4	8/2	8/1	8/0.5	8/0.25
	VII	16	16/64	16/32	16/16	16/8	16/4	16/2	16/1	16/0.5	16/0.25
	VIII	32	32/64	32/32	32/16	32/8	32/4	32/2	32/1	32/0.5	32/0.25
	IX	64	64/64	64/32	64/16	64/8	64/4	64/2	64/1	64/0.5	64/0.25
	X	0	64	32	16	8	4	2	1	0.5	0.25

ANTIBIOTIC B (µg/ml)

10. Count the survivors in tubes not presenting any visible growth, by streaking onto agar medium with a calibrated platinum loop (5-cm long streak, up to 10 streaks on a plate). Incubate for 18 h at 37°C.
11. After this period of time, determine the percentage of survivors in each tube compared to the control plate prepared in 6 (Fig. 1).

Interpretation of the results

Bacteriostatic activity

The results shown in Table 2 (A + B combination) can be plotted on arithmetic or logarithmic coordinates in the form of isobolograms (Fig. 1)

- Note the first tube containing A + B in each row with no visible growth: II-4, III-6, IV-7, V-7 of Table 1.
- Determine, in each of these tubes, the Fractional Inhibitory Concentration (FIC) of A and B, i.e. FIC_A and FIC_B, which represent the coordinates of each tube.
- Plot the curve representing the effect of the combination, by indicating these coordinates (logarithmic or arithmetic) on the respective axes (Fig. 2).
- The value of the combination is quantified by the FIC index:

$$FIC = FIC_A + FIC_B = \frac{\text{MIC of A with B}}{\text{MIC of A alone}} + \frac{\text{MIC of B with A}}{\text{MIC of B alone}}$$

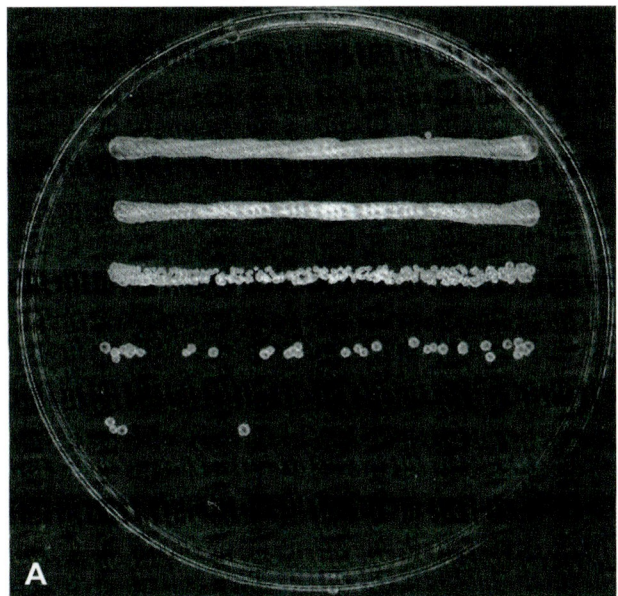

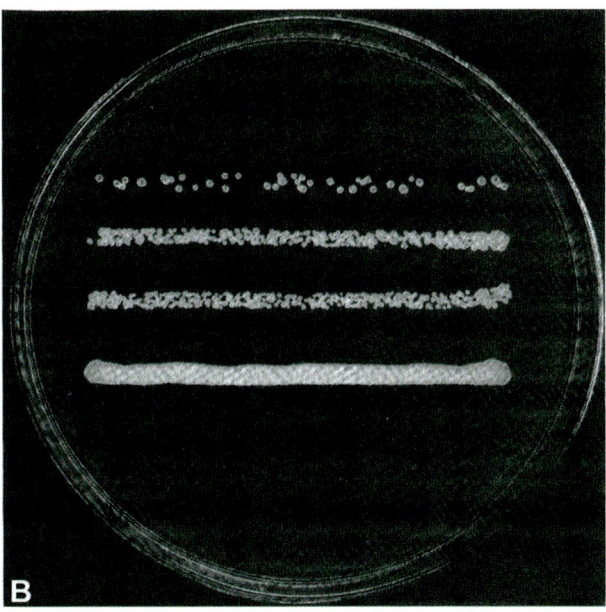

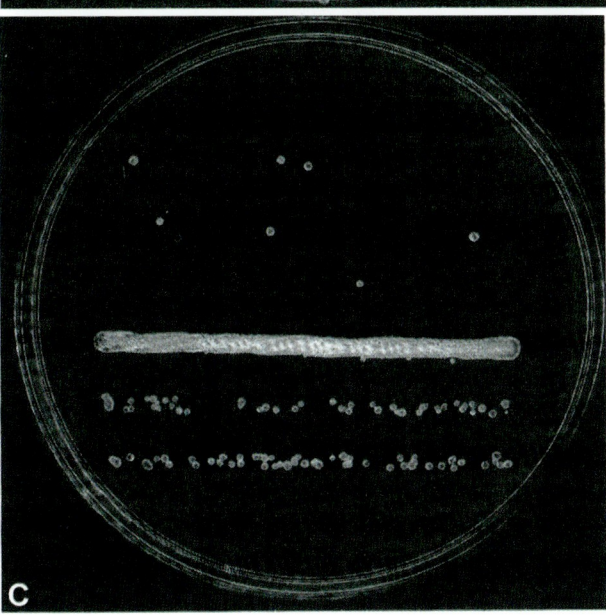

Fig. 1. Example of enumeration of survivors

A. Control inoculum (from top to bottom). Pure inoculum, 100% of survivors; 10-1 dilution, 10% of survivors; 10-2 dilution, 1% of survivors; 10-3 dilution, 0.1% of survivors; 10-4 dilution, 0.01% of survivors.

B. Isolated antibiotics (from top to bottom). Antibiotic A, 0.1% of survivors; antibiotic B, 1% of survivors; antibiotic C, 1% of survivors; antibiotic D, 10% of survivors.

C. Antibiotic combinations (from top to bottom). A + B, 0.01% synergy; A + C, 0.01%, synergy; A + D, 0.01%, synergy; B + C, 100%, antagonism; B + D, 0.1%, synergy; C + D, 0.1%, synergy; B + C is antagonist and non-bactericidal; B + D and C + D, although synergistic, are insufficiently bactericidal.

Procedure 5. ANTIBIOTIC COMBINATIONS

Table 2. Bacteriostatic and bactericidal results of the A and B antibiotic combination expressed as a percentage of survivors. + bacterial growth

FIC_A	Antibiotic A µg/ml						MIC B							
	0.25	+		+	+	+	+	+	+	+	+			
0.06	0.5	+		+	1	+	+	+	+	+	+			
0.125	1	+		+	0.01	0.1	1	+	+	+	+			
0.25	2	+		+	0.01	0.01	0.01	0.1	+	+	+			
0.5	4	+		+	0.01	0.01	0.01	0.01	+	+	+			
1	8	—	—	—	—	—	—	—	—	—	—	—	—	MIC A
	16	0.01												
	32	0.01												
	64	0.01												
	0	+	0.01	0.01	+	+	+	+	+	+	+			
		0	64	32	16	8	4	2	1	0.5	0.25	µg/ml		
				1	0.5	0.25	0.125	0.06				FIC_B		

Antibiotic B

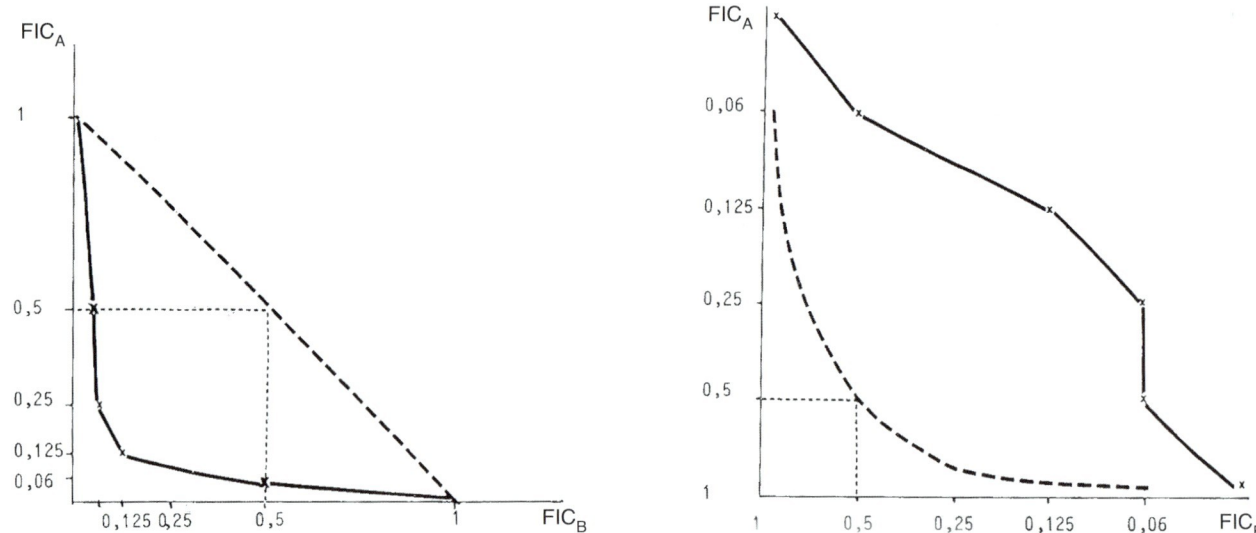

Fig. 2. Left, isobologram in arithmetic coordinates; right, isobologram in logarithmic coordinates

Addition

Addition is represented in Fig. 2 by the curve joining all points for which the FIC index $FIC = FIC_A + FIC_B = 1$. Example: 0.25 + 0.75; 0.5 + 0.5; 0.75 + 0.25, etc.

Synergy

It is usually defined by a FIC index ≤ 0.75. The most favorable point of the curve gives the value of the FIC index of the combination. In this example, the A + B combination is synergistic with FIC = 0.25 (tube III-6: $FIC_A + FIC_B = 0.125 + 0.125$).

Antagonism

It corresponds to a FIC index > 2.

Indifference

It comprises all values of FIC between $1 < FIC < 2$.

Bactericidal activity

In contrast with the bacteriostatic activity, the bactericidal activity is generally not proportional to the antibiotic concentration and the number of survivors can remain stable over a large concentration range. It is therefore usually impossible to define the interaction of two antibiotics as fractions of active concentration or calculate an "index" as in the previous case. These interactions can nevertheless be interpreted in the following way:

Indifference

The number of survivors is equal to that obtained with the more active antibiotic.

Addition or synergy

The number of survivors is less than that obtained with the more active antibiotic.

Antagonism

The number of survivors is equal to or greater than that obtained with the less active antibiotic.

Comments

This technique is considerably facilitated by the use of 8 x 12 microtiter plates in which dispensing and dilution of solutions can be automated using a multipoint inoculator.

In practice, this technique can also be simplified by limiting the study to two or three concentrations of each antibiotic.

KINETICS OF BACTERICIDAL ACTIVITY OF ANTIBIOTICS AND ANTIBIOTIC COMBINATIONS (TIME-KILLING CURVE)

Principle

The antibacterial activity of isolated antibiotics and antibiotic combinations is determined by enumerating the surviving bacteria at defined time intervals. The growth curves obtained can be used to assess the kinetics of the observed effects. A technical modality of assessment of the bactericidal and bacteriostatic activity of two antibiotics alone or in combination allows kinetic analysis of the various types of interactions. This technique overcomes some of the defects described for the previous protocol. For two antibiotics or combinations with a similar bactericidal effect (0.01% survivors after 18 h of contact), a major difference may be identified concerning the kinetics of the bactericidal effect and the presence of synergy between the two antibiotics. Observation of the bactericidal effect during the first hours of culture avoids phenomena related to bacterial regrowth or degradation of antibiotics in the culture medium.

Technique

1. *Preparation of antibiotic solutions*
   The concentration of antibiotic solutions must be tenfold higher than the desired final concentration.
2. *Preparation of the inoculum*
   Dilute, in M-H broth, an exponential phase culture of the bacterial strain to be examined to obtain a suspension of about 10^6 bacteria per ml.
3. Dispense 8 ml of this suspension into 4 tubes numbered from 1 to 4:
   - Add 1 ml of the solution of antibiotic A to tubes 1 and 3.
   - Add 1 ml of the solution of antibiotic B to tubes 2 and 3.
   - Add 2 ml of distilled water to tube 4 and 1 ml to tubes 1 and 2.
4. *Bacterial count*
   - At time 0, take 0.5 ml from tube 4 and perform 1/10 dilutions (0.5 ml in 4.5 ml of distilled water from 10^5 to 10^6. Inoculate by streaking 0.1 ml onto agar medium in Petri dishes. Incubate these Petri dishes for 18 h at 37°C.
   - Incubate tubes at 37°C, preferably after shaking, and proceed in a similar way for subsequent counts performed after 2, 4, 6 and 18 h of incubation.
5. Plot curves representing the number of viable bacteria (expressed in Log) as a function of contact time (h) with each antibiotic and their combination.

Interpretation of the results (Fig. 3)

Synergy

The effect of the combination is greater than that of the more effective antibiotic.

Indifference or addition

The effect of the combination is comparable to that of the more effective antibiotic.

Antagonism

The combination is less active than the more effective antibiotic.

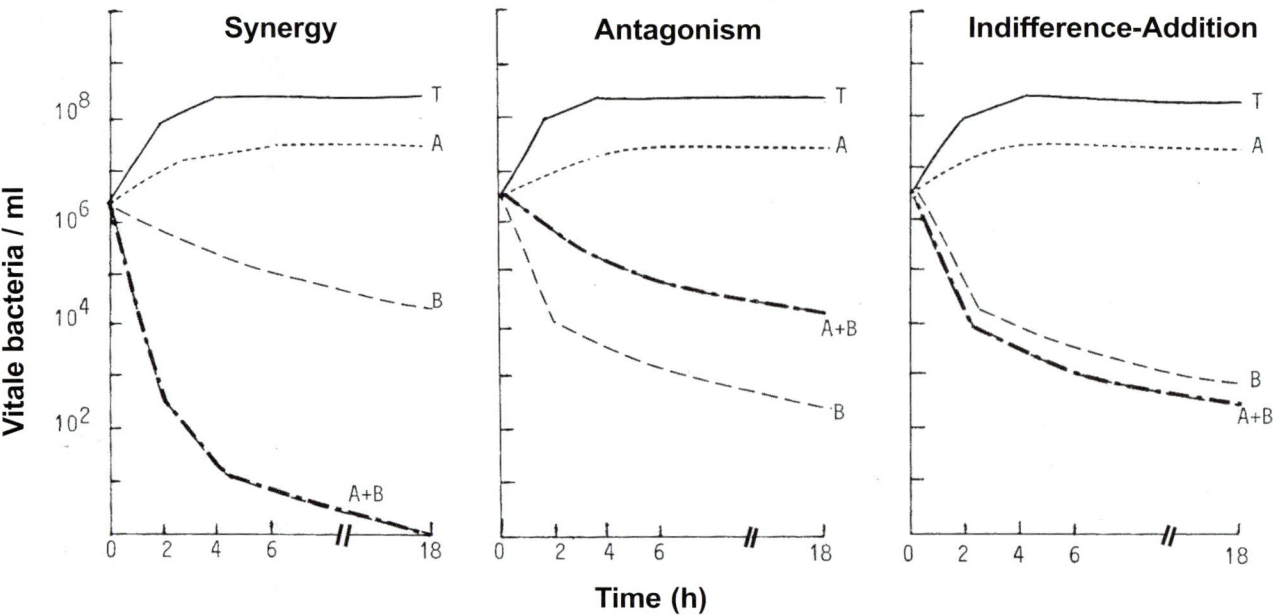

Fig. 3. Kinetics of the activity of antibiotic combinations. A, B and A + B, growth curves in the presence of antibiotic A, antibiotic B, and the A + B combination; C, control without antibiotic.

CONCLUSIONS

The advantages and limitations of the various techniques described determine the choice of technique, which essentially depends on:
- the practicability of the technique,
- the objective of the test, which can be:
  - selection of a bactericidal combination,
  - characterization of a synergistic effect,
  - to obtain an early bactericidal effect.

The checkerboard method allows precise determination of the synergistic effects observed for a large range of concentrations of the antibiotic combination.

However, simultaneous study of several combinations, each requiring a separate examination, represents a considerable workload, usually reserved for the choice of treatment for serious infection (septicemia, endocarditis, meningitis, osteomyelitis) due to multiresistant bacteria. The use of microtechniques constitutes a major progress for routine clinical practice.

Synergy techniques can also be performed by using E-test® strips.

The kinetic study of the bactericidal activity of an antibiotic combination (time-killing curve) requires a large number of manipulations over a considerable period of time. In practice, its use is limited when several types of combinations are studied simultaneously. Interpretation of the observed interactions may vary as a function of the concentrations of the two antibiotics studied in combination.

REFERENCES

(1) **Courvalin, P., F. Golstein, A. Philippon, and J. Sirot**. 1985. Fiches techniques d'étude pratique des antibiotiques, pp. 165-250. In Courvalin, P., F. Golstein, A. Philippon, and J. Sirot (ed.), L'Antibiogramme. MPC-Videom, Paris, Bruxelles.
(2) **Pillai, S.K., R.C. Moellering Jr., and G.M. Eliopoulos**. 2005. Antimicrobial combinations, pp. 365-440. In V. Lorian (ed.), Antibiotics in Laboratory Medicine. Lippincott Williams & Wilkins, Philadelphia.

Procedure 6. SUSCEPTIBILITY TESTING OF ANAEROBES

AGAR DILUTION AND DIFFUSION

Inoculum

Prepare the inoculum by suspending overnight colonies grown on Columbia agar + 5% blood, or Brucella agar + vitamin K1 (1 μg/ml) + 5% blood (or else a Brucella or Schaedler broth culture), in Brucella or Schaedler broth to a turbidity matching a McFarland 0.5 standard for the dilution method (1.5 x 10^8 CFU/ml) or a McFarland 1 standard (3 x 10^8 CFU/ml) for the diffusion method. All broth media should be prereduced before use.

For some slow-growing species (> 72 h), prepare a suspension in Brucella or Schaedler broth to a turbidity equivalent to a McFarland 1 standard for the dilution method and a McFarland 2 standard for the diffusion method.

Medium

Wilkins Chalgren agar with 5% blood, or Brucella agar with vitamin K1 (1 μg/ml) + 5% blood. For some species, other supplements are used (sodium bicarbonate 1 μg/ml, hemin 5 μg/ml).

Brucella medium for anaerobes supports the growth of a larger number of species and is recommended by many international authorities.

Difco dehydrated powder for Brucella medium (broth or agar)

Pancreatic digest of casein	10 g
Peptic digest of animal tissue	10 g
Glucose	1 g
Yeast extract	2 g
Sodium chloride	5 g
Sodium bisulfite	0.1 g

Add 15 g of agar to the 28 g of dehydrated powder.

Brucella broth (anaerobic)

Powder for Brucella broth	28 g
Hemin solution (5 mg/ml)	1 ml
Vitamin K1 solution (1 mg/ml)	1 ml
Bicarbonate solution (20 mg/ml)	5 ml
Water	900 ml

Boil to completely dissolve. Sterilize at 121°C for 15 min.

Cool to ≤ 48-50°C and add 100 ml lysed horse blood (a V/V mixture of defibrinated horse blood and distilled water).

Store at 4-8°C.

Prepare the hemin solution by dissolving 0.1 g hemin in 2 ml of 1N sodium hydroxide (40 g sodium hydroxide in 1 liter distilled water). Dilute to 20 ml with distilled water and autoclave at 121°C for 15 min. The solution may be stored at 4-8°C protected from light for a maximum of 1 month.

Prepare the vitamin K1 stock solution by dissolving 0.2 ml vitamin K1 (3-phytylmenadione) in 20 ml of 95% ethanol. The solution may be stored in a refrigerator for up to 1 year. Add 1 ml stock solution to 9 ml distilled water to obtain a 1 mg/ml solution which is added to the dehydrated media as indicated above. This solution may be stored in a refrigerator for 1 month.

Brucella agar (anaerobic)

Powder for Brucella agar	43 g
Hemin solution (5 mg/ml)	1 ml
Vitamin K1 solution (1 mg/ml)	1 ml
Distilled water	1000 ml

Boil to completely dissolve. Autoclave at 121°C for 15 min.

Cool to ≤ 48-50°C and add 50 ml lysed sheep blood.

Store at 4-8°C.

If blood is not added the media may be stored in tubes or bottles. Melt the agar at 48-50°C before use. Add 5 ml sheep blood per 100 ml bottle or 1 ml per 20 ml tube.

Lysed blood is obtained by freezing at –20°C followed by slow overnight thawing at 2-8°C or rapid thawing in a water bath at 35-37°C. Adjust the temperature of the blood to 48-50°C before adding it to the Brucella medium.

Inoculation

Dilution method: apply 2-3 μl of the inoculum suspension (McFarland 0.5) equivalent to approximately 10^5 CFU per spot.

Diffusion method: inoculate by swabbing the inoculum suspension (McFarland 1).

E-test® inoculum: proceed as directed for the agar diffusion method.

Dry the plates for several minutes, then invert and incubate under conditions of anaerobiosis.

Reading

Read after 48 h of incubation at 35-37°C in an anaerobic atmosphere (chamber or jar) if growth is adequate. For clindamycin, it is essential that results be read after 48 h of incubation.

With the diffusion method, metronidazole plates should be read a second time after 4-5 days of anaerobic incubation in order to detect reduced susceptibility strains growing in the inhibition zone.

ANTIBIOTICS TO BE TESTED

Table 1. Antibiotics to be tested against anaerobes

Standard list	Additional list
Amoxicillin	Ticarcillin (H) or piperacillin (H)
Amoxicillin + clavulanic acid	Ticarcillin / clavulanic acid (H)
Imipenem	or piperacillin / tazobactam
Clindamycin	Cefoxitin[b]
Metronidazole	
Vancomycin 30 µg	Pristinamycin[c]
Chloramphenicol	Spiramycin[d]
Colistin 10µg[a]	Levofloxacin[e]
Kanamycin 1000 µg[a]	Moxifloxacin[f]
Vancomycin 5 µg[a]	Linezolid[f]
	Rifampin

Disk concentrations are indicated when special concentrations are used.

(H), dispensed in hospitals.

[a] Aid to identification of Gram-negative bacilli. *Bacteroides fragilis* group strains are resistant to kanamycin, colistin and vancomycin; *Prevotella* is resistant to kanamycin and vancomycin, colistin susceptibility varies according to species; *Porphyromonas* is susceptible to vancomycin and resistant to kanamycin and colistin; *Fusobacterium* is susceptible to kanamycin and colistin, resistant to vancomycin.

[b] Do not use the diffusion method to test cefoxitin or cefotetan against the *Bacteroides fragilis* group (moderately susceptible species, antibiotic used as prophylaxis in abdominal surgery)

[c] In case of dental or skin infection with the exception of *Bacteroides fragilis*

[d] In case of dental infection.

[e] For *Propionibacterium* spp. and some strains of *Peptostreptococcus* spp. isolated in severe infections (bone or brain).

[f] In case of multiresistance or insufficient antibiotic concentrations at infection site.

bioMérieux ATB ANA® system

In the API 20A medium tube, prepare a suspension having a turbidity equivalent to a McFarland 3 standard. Transfer 200 µl to ATB S medium. Inoculate 135 µl per well. Incubate under conditions of anaerobiosis for 24-48 h at 36°C 2°C.

Table 2. Concentrations (µg/ml) present in the wells of the ATB ANA® device

Amoxicillin (Gram-negative)	0.5	1
Amoxicillin (Gram-positive)	4	16
Amoxicillin + clavulanic acid	4/2	16/2
Ticarcillin	16	64
Ticarcillin + clavulanic acid	16/2	64/2
Piperacillin	16	64
Piperacillin + tazobactam	16/2	64/2
Cefoxitin		32
Cefotetan		32
Imipenem	4	8
Chloramphenicol	8	16
Levofloxacin	2	4
Moxifloxacin	1	2
Clindamycin	2	
Vancomycin	4	
Rifampin	4	16
Metronidazole	4	16

INTRINSIC RESISTANCE

Before any interpretation of the antibiogram, it is necessary to control the intrinsic resistances of the anaerobes. If the findings are discordant, identification is necessary. If the identification is correct, interpret as follows:

Table 3. Intrinsic resistance in anaerobes

Anaerobes: Aminoglycosides (except *Bacteroides ureolyticus* and gentamicin, aztreonam (except *Fusobacterium*), trimethoprim, quinolones, fosfomycin (except *Fusobacterium*).

Bacteroides fragilis group: aminopenicillins, 1st generation cephalosporins, cefamandole, cefuroxime, colistin, polymyxin B, glycopeptides, fosfomycin.
Prevotella: glycopeptides, fosfomycin.
Porphyromonas: fosfomycin, colistin, polymyxin B.
Fusobacterium: macrolides (low-level).
Fusobacterium varium - Fusobacterium mortiferum: rifampin.

Clostridium – Eubacterium – Peptostreptococcus: colistin, polymyxin B, fosfomycin.
Clostridium difficile: cephalosporins.
Clostridium clostridioforme: teicoplanin, daptomycin, ramoplanin.
Clostridium innocuum: cefoxitin, cefotetan (low-level vancomycin), daptomycin.
Clostridium ramosum: vancomycin, linezolid, daptomycin.

Actinomyces – Propionibacterium: 1st generation cephalosporins, nitroimidazoles.
Mobiluncus: nitroimidazoles.
Veillonella: macrolides (low-level), glycopeptides.

INTERPRETIVE READING

Table 4. Rules for interpretive reading of the results of antibiogram of anaerobes

1. In *Fusobacterium*, β-lactamase production detected by a chromogenic test done at isolation confers resistance to penicillin G, amino-, carboxy- and ureido-penicillins. Activity is restored by addition of a β-lactamase inhibitor.
2. In *Prevotella*, β-lactamase production confers resistance to penicillin G, amino-penicillins, 1st generation cephalosporins, cefuroxime and oral 3rd generation cephalosporins. Activity is restored by addition of a β-lactamase inhibitor. Any strain for which the MIC of amoxicillin is > 0.5 µg/ml (0.38 µg/ml by E-test®) is considered a β-lactamase producer.
3. In *Clostridium butyricum*, *C. clostridioforme* and *C. ramosum*, β-lactamase production is detected by a chromogenic test at isolation. Only the *C. butyricum* β-lactamase is inhibited, at therapeutic concentrations, by β-lactamase inhibitors.
4. Imipenem resistance has been described in Europe in *Bacteroides fragilis* (carbapenemase) and *B. distasonis*. Cross-resistance is seen for all β-lactams even when combined with β-lactamase inhibitors.
5. For some *Clostridium*, dissociated resistance between the different glycopeptides may be observed (see Intrinsic resistance).

Table 5. Acceptable ranges of MICs (µg/ml) for quality control anaerobic strains (agar dilution method)[a]

Antibiotic	Bacteroides fragilis ATCC 25285	Bacteroides thetaiotaomicron ATCC 29741	Clostridium perfringens ATCC 13124	Eggerthella lenta ATCC 43055
Amoxicillin + clavulanic acid (2:1)	0.25/0.125-1/0.5	0.5/0.25-2/1	0.25/0.125-1/0.5	NR[b]
Ampicillin	16-64	16-64	1-4	-
Ampicillin + sulbactam (2:1)	0.5/0.25-2/1	0.5/0.25-2/1	0.25/0.125-4/2	0.25/0.125-2/1
Cefotaxime	8-32	16-64	-	64-256
Cefotetan	4-16	32-128	-	32-128
Cefoxitin	4-16	8-32	-	4-16
Ceftriaxone	32-128	64-256	-	NR
Chloramphenicol	2-8	4-16	-	-
Clindamycin	0.5-2	2-8	2-8	0.06-0.25
Doripenem	-	-	0.5-4	-
Ertapenem	0.06-0.25	0.25-1	-	0.5-2
Faropenem	0.03-0.25	0.125-0.5	-	1-4
Garenoxacin	0.06-0.5	0.25-1	0.5-2	1-4
Imipenem	0.03-0.125	0.125-0.5	-	0.125-0.5
Linezolid	2-8	2-8	1-4	0.5-2
Meropenem	0.03-0.25	0.125-0.5	0.5-4	0.125-1
Metronidazole	0.25-1	0.5-2	0.125-0.5	-
Moxifloxacin	0.125-0.5	1-4	1-4	0.125-0.5
Penicillin G	8-32 or (16-64 U.I./ml)	8-32 or (16-64 U.I./ml)	1-4	-
Piperacillin	2-8	8-32	4-16	8-32
Piperacillin + tazobactam	0.125/4-0.5/4	4/4-16/4	4/4-16/4	4/4-16/4
Tetracycline	0.125-0.5	8-32	-	-
Ticarcillin	16-64	16-64	16-64	16-64
Ticarcillin + clavulanic acid (2 µg/ml)	-	0.5/2-2/2	16/2-64/2	16/2-64/2
Tigecycline	0.12-1	0.5-2	0.125-1	0.06-0.5
Vancomycin	-	-	0.5-4	-
Personal data:				
Amoxicillin	16-32	32-64	-	0.25-1
Amoxicillin + (2 µg/ml) clavulanic acid	0.06-0.5	0.25-1	-	0.5-1
Secnidazole	0.25-1	0.25-1	-	0.125-0.5

[a] Adapted from CLSI document M11A7 (Methods for Antimicrobial Susceptibility Testing of Anaerobic Bacteria; Approved Standard—Seventh Edition, Clinical and Laboratory Standards Institute, 940 West Valley Road, Suite 1400, Wayne, Pennsylvania 19087-1898 USA, 2007 and personal data when not provided by CLSI)

[b] NR, no recommendation.

Fourth Part:

APPENDICIES

DEFINITIONS

Addition: the activity of a combination of antibiotics is equal to the sum of the effects of each antibiotic studied separately at the same concentration as in the combination.

Antagonism: the activity of a combination of antibiotics is less than the sum of the effects of each antibiotic studied separately at the same concentration as in the combination. The combination decreases the activity of one of the antibiotics.

Bactericidal activity: activity of an antibiotic which induces death of the bacteria (3 or 4 Log reduction). It depends on the antibiotic concentration and its duration of action.

Bacteriostatic activity: reduction of bacterial growth without cell death. At maximum bacteriostatic activity, the bacterial count remains equal to that of the inoculum.

Co-resistance: combination of various resistance mechanisms in the same bacterial strain.

Concentration-dependent: the bactericidal activity of an antibiotic, determined during the early phase, is a function of the concentration. The duration of action has a limited impact at high concentrations. Concentration-dependent bactericidal activity is usually rapid (example: aminoglycosides).

Minimum Bactericidal Concentration (MBC): lowest antibiotic concentration at which there are only 0.1 or 0.01% of surviving bacteria.

Minimum Inhibitory Concentration (MIC): lowest antibiotic concentration at which there is no visible growth.

Indifference: the activity of one of the antibiotics of a combination is not affected by the presence of the other.

Cross-resistance: a resistance mechanism which confers resistance to several antibiotics of the same class or, in the case of efflux or ribosomal methylation, to antibiotics of various classes.

Synergy: bacteriostatic or bactericidal effect of a combination of antibiotics is greater than simple addition of the effects of each antibiotic alone.

Time-dependent: the bactericidal activity of an antibiotic, determined during the early phase, is influenced by the duration of action. It increases only slightly or not at all with the antibiotic concentration (beyond a cut-off of 4 times the MIC) when the antibiotic is bactericidal. Time-dependent bactericidal activity is usually slow (example: β-lactams).

STRAIN STORAGE

Various techniques have been developed for the storage of strains. We recommend the following methods.

SHORT-TERM STORAGE

Most bacteria can be stored for 1 to 2 weeks on the surface of an agar medium. Petri dishes must be stored at 4°C, upside down and hermetically sealed with Parafilm®.

Mutations usually represent errors during replication and plasmids and transposons are not perfectly stable. Therefore, in order to minimize inevitable genetic drift, it is advised, whenever possible, to use the storage tube. A practical solution for frequently used *E. coli* strains is storage in $MgSO_4$ at 4°C. An overnight culture is centrifuged (3,500 rpm for 10 min.) and the pellet is resuspended in half the volume of 0.001 M $MgSO_4$. Strains stored under these conditions can be kept for up to one month.

LONG-TERM STORAGE

Two main techniques are available and should be used simultaneously.

Stab in deep agar

Most bacteria can be stored for one to several years in this way. Incubation of the storage tube is not recommended. Immediately after inoculation, the tube must be closed and sealed with Parafilm®. Tubes must be stored at room temperature and protected from light. This technique is not recommended for strains harboring plasmids, especially in multiple copies, and transposons.

Freezing at -80°C

This is the most reliable method for long-term storage of bacteria. Strains are stored in screw-cap tubes in a medium containing 15% glycerol.
1) Inoculate and incubate an agar slope or Petri dish at 37°C for 16 to 18 h.
2) Flood the surface of the agar slope with 4 to 5 ml of brain-heart broth containing 15% glycerol and mix (Vortex®) or prepare a dense suspension from the surface of the Petri dish.
3) Dispense about 1 ml into each of two labelled screw-cap tubes. A variant consists of tubes containing spheres, which allows the spheres to be used individually to harvest frozen bacteria.
4) Immerse in a mixture of dry ice and ethanol for 5 min.
5) Store in the freezer at -80°C.

Storage in two freezers is recommended. One tube constitutes the working stock and the other constitutes the permanent stock. Tubes can be melted and frozen many times with no marked loss of viability. However, when harvesting bacteria, it is recommended to scrape the surface of the frozen tube using a sterile platinum loop rather than allowing the whole tube to melt.

ABBREVIATIONS AND ACRONYMS

AAC	aminoglycoside *N*-acetyltranferase
DNA	deoxyribonucleic acid
ANT	aminoglycoside *N*-nucleotidyltransferase
APH	aminoglycoside *O*-phosphotransferase
ATCC	American Type Culture Collection
AUC	area under the curve
AUIC	area under inhibitory curve $\frac{AUC}{MIC}$
BHI	brain heart infusion
Bla	beta-lactamase
BLNAR	β-lactamase negative, ampicillin resistant
BORSA	*S. aureus* with diminished susceptibility to methicillin by hyperproduction of beta-lactamase (Bordeline *S. aureus*)
bp	base pair
BSAC	British Society for Antimicrobial Chemotherapy
C	High critical concentration
c	Low critical concentration
CA.MRSA	community acquired MRSA
CAT	chloramphenicol acetyltransferase
CDC	Centers for Disease Control and Prevention
CFU	colony forming unit
CIP	Collection de l'Institut Pasteur
CLSI	Clinical and Laboratory Standards Institute (formerly NCCLS)
C_{max}	serum maximal concentration
CoA	coenzyme A
ECQ	external quality control
DHFR	dihydrofolate reductase
DHPLC	Denaturing high performance liquid chromatography
DHPS	dihydropteroate synthetase
DIN	Deutsches Institut für Normung
DTNB	5,5'-Dithiobis-2-nitrobenzoïque
EARSS	European Antimicrobial Resistance Surveillance System
ECCLS	European Committee for Clinical Laboratory Standards
EDTA	ethylene diaminetetraacetate
EMEA	European Medicines Agency
Em_c	erythromycin constitutive resistance
Em_i	erythromycin inducible resistance
Ere	erythromycin resistance esterase
erm	erythromycin resistance methylase
ESBL	extended-spectrum β-lactamase

EUCAST	European Committee on Antimicrobial Susceptibility Testing
FDA	Food and Drug Administration
GISA	glycopeptide intermediate *Staphylococcus aureus*
GRE	glycopeptide resistant *Enterococcus*
HPLC	high performance liquid chromatography
H.MRSA	hospital MRSA
HTM	*Haemophilus* Test Medium
I	intermediate resistance to antibiotics
ICD	international common designation
ICQ	internal quality control
ICS	international collaborative study
IFU	inclusion forming unit
Ip	isoelectric point
IQ	inhibitory quotient $\frac{C_{max}}{MIC}$
IRT	inhibitor resistant TEM
IS	insertion sequence
ISO	International Organization for Standardization
kb	kilo base pairs
kDa	kilodalton
KPC	*Klebsiella pneumoniae* carbapenemase
Lin	lincosamide inactivation nucleotidylation
log	logarithm 2 basis
Log	natural logarithm 10 basis
LPS	lipopolysaccharide
lsa	lincosamides and streptogramins A resistance
MDR	multidrug resistant
MH	Mueller-Hinton medium
MBC	minimal bactericidal concentration
MIC	minimal inhibitory concentration
MIC_{50}	minimal concentration inhibiting 50 % of the strains
MIC_{90}	minimal concentration inhibiting 90 % of the strains
MLS	Macrolides-Lincosamides-Streptogramins
MRSA	methicillin resistant *Staphylococcus aureus* (by production of PBP2')
MSSA	methicillin susceptible *Staphylococcus aureus*
MW	molecular weight
NAD	nicotinamide adenine dinucleotide
NCCLS	National Committee for Clinical Laboratory Standards (now CLSI)
NCTC	National Collection of Type Cultures
OD	optical density
PAB	para aminoenzoïque acid
PCR	polymerase chain reaction
PD	pharmacodynamic
PK	pharmacokinetic
PBP	penicillin binding protein
PNSP	*Streptococcus pneumoniae* with diminished susceptibility to penicillin G
QA	quality assurance
QC	quality control
QRDR	quinolone resistance-determining region

®	registered
R	antibiotic resistance
RCP	summary of product characteristics (SmPc)
RF	running front
RFLP	restriction fragment length polymorphism
RNA	ribonucleic acid
rpm	revolution per minute
S	antibiotic susceptibility
S100	supernatant of a 100.000 x g ultracentrifugation of a bacterial lysate
SDS	sodium dodecyl-sulfate
SFM	Société Française de Microbiologie
Sg	streptogramin resistance
SSCP	single strand conformation polymorphism
T_{max}	time necessary to obtain C_{max}
Tn	transposon
Tris	tris (hydroxymethyl) aminomethane
TSB	trypticase soy broth
UV	ultra violet
VISA	vancomycin intermediate *Staphylococcus aureus*
VRE	vancomycin resistant *Enterococcus*
VRSA	vancomycin resistant *Staphylococcus aureus*
WT	wild type
WHO	World Health Organization
xg	multiple of terrestrial gravity
XGC	X generation cephalosporin

LITERATURE

- **Bryskier, A.**. 2005. Antimicrobial Agents. American Society for Microbiology, Washington D.C. 1426 p.
- **Gillespie, S.H.** 2001. Antibiotic Resistance. Methods and Protocols. Humana Press, Totowa, New Jersey. 287 p.
- **Lorian, V.** 2005. Antibiotics in Laboratory Medicine. 5th edition. Lippincott Williams & Wilkins, Baltimore, Maryland. 889 p.
- **Murray, P.R.** 1999. Manual of Clinical Microbiology. 7th edition. American Society for Microbiology, Washington D.C. 1773 p.
- **Courvalin, P., H. Drugeon, J.P. Flandrois et F. Goldstein** (ed.). 1990. Bactéricidie. Maloine, Paris.

WEB SITES

APUA (Alliance for the Prudent Use of Antibiotics)
http://www.tufts.edu/med/apua/

ATCC-LGC Promochem (ATCC collection)
http://www.lgcpromochem.com/atcc

BSAC (British Society for Antimicrobial Chemotherapy)
http://www.bsac.org.uk

CASFM (Comité de l'Antibiogramme de la Société Française de Microbiologie)
http://www.sfm.asso.fr/

CDC (Center for Diseases Control)
http://www.cdc.org

CIP (Collection de l'Institut Pasteur)
http://www.crbip.pasteur.fr

CLSI (The Clinical and Laboratory Standards Institute)
http://www.clsi.org/

EARSS (Eupean Antimicrobial Resistance Surveillance System)
http://www.earss.rivm.nl

EUCAST (European Committee on Antimicrobial Susceptibility Testing)
http://www.eucast.org

EUROSURVEILLANCE (Peer-reviewed European information on communicable disease surveillance and control)
http://www.eurosurveillance.org

FDA (Food and Drug Administration)
http://www.fda.gov

NARSA (Network on Antimicrobial Resistance in *Staphylococcus aureus*)
http://www.narsa.net

ROAR (Reservoirs of Antibiotic Resistance Network)
http://www.tufts.edu/med/apua
puis cliquer sur l'onglet « ROAR »

SRGA (The Swedish Reference Group of Antibiotics)
http://www.srga.org

USDA FSIS (United States Department of Agriculture, Food Safety and Inspection Service)
http://www.fsis.usda.gov

WHO (World Health Organization)
http://www. who.int

INDEX

A

A site, 21, 225-226, 357, 365
A. actinomycetemcomitans, 541-542, 544, 546-547, 549
A. baumannii, 27, 181, 193, 206, 231, 233-234, 237, 239, 334, 336, 368, 371, 407-419, 421-424
A. denitrificans, 175, 192-193, 196
A. faecalis, 175, 179, 192, 195
A. xylosoxydans, 175, 179, 181, 191, 193, 196
AAC, 17-18, 30, 32-33, 48-49, 67, 69, 71-73, 152, 184, 186, 209, 213, 215-217, 219-224, 227-232, 234-242, 267-267, 274, 417, 421-422, 425, 435, 482-483, 518, 656, 687
ABC transporter, 309, 314, 384, 387, 526
Abiotrophia defectiva, 110
acetylase, 309, 316
Achromobacter, 175, 191-196, 207-208, 210, 370
Acinetobacter, 15, 27, 34-35, 49, 53-54, 56, 58, 73, 91, 93, 138, 154, 173, 194-195, 200, 225, 229-232, 236-237, 241, 264, 271-272, 328, 331-333, 335, 337, 348, 350, 353-354, 358, 360-363, 369, 370-371, 407-409, 411, 416-417, 419-426
acquired resistance, 27, 50, 67, 99-100, 104, 127-128, 135-136, 141, 158, 163-164, 176, 184, 187, 190-191, 193-195, 199-200, 213, 232, 263, 288, 307, 330, 335, 349, 351-352, 363, 369, 374, 376-377, 381, 393, 402-403, 430-431, 434, 436, 441, 443, 446, 451-453, 456-457, 480, 488, 492, 497-498, 501, 510, 514-515, 519, 522-523, 527, 529, 536-537, 547-548, 578, 594-598, 606, 609, 611, 617, 624, 629, 635, 637, 653
ACT, 148, 435
Actinobacillus, 59, 332, 431, 541, 550-551, 653-654, 656-657
Actinomyces, 333, 341, 348, 365, 567, 570-573, 576, 681
Actinoplanus, 303
AdeABC, 231, 233-234, 237, 241, 334, 336-337, 360, 411, 415, 421-423, 425
Aeromonas, 56, 59, 332, 368, 509-518
Aeromonas salmonicida, 517-518
Alcaligenes, 175-176, 191-192, 195-196, 207-210, 332, 370
amidase, 26, 35, 159, 595

amikacin, 48-50, 54, 69, 73, 80-81, 85-86, 88, 91, 152, 180, 182, 185, 188, 193, 196-197, 200-202, 204-205, 213-225, 227-233, 235, 237-241, 375, 381, 399, 401, 407, 409-410, 416-417, 419, 421-423, 425, 436, 493, 501, 506, 577, 580, 584, 588, 596, 604-606, 610, 612-613, 616, 630, 633, 638, 645-648, 662, 665
aminocyclitol, 213, 224-225, 241, 666
aminoglycoside, 17-19, 22-23, 30, 33, 48, 50, 54, 64, 69-70, 72-73, 80, 85, 87-88, 92, 132-133, 184, 187, 210, 213, 215-218, 220-225, 227-233, 237-242, 268, 274, 285, 290, 294, 337, 376, 381, 385, 387, 401, 403, 407, 413, 415, 417, 419-422, 425-426, 436, 455, 483, 487, 489, 493, 500, 544, 629, 644-645, 648, 657, 671, 674, 687
amoxicillin, 27, 52, 72, 86, 100-101, 104-105, 110, 112-113, 115-117, 120, 122-123, 128-133, 135-136, 142-146, 148, 150, 176-177, 179-183, 185, 187-204, 206, 222, 373-375, 377, 380, 384-386, 391-393, 399, 402-404, 409-410, 412-414, 427-428, 430-433, 437-438, 443-445, 447, 451, 453-454, 459-463, 465, 467-469, 471-473, 477, 484-485, 491-492, 494-498, 502, 505-506, 511-515, 535, 544-549, 555-556, 559, 561-565, 567-568, 578-581, 583-586, 588-589, 616, 619-620-623, 630, 63, 635, 638, 644-645, 647, 661, 665, 673, 680-682
amoxicillin-clavulanate, 100, 110, 155, 122-123, 427-428, 430-433, 437
ampC, 21, 26-27, 35, 64, 138-140, 146-150, 153-154, 158-159, 198-199, 208, 274, 409, 411-413, 416-419, 516, 518
ampD, 26-27, 35, 159, 171
ampG, 26
ampR, 26-27, 158, 186, 198
ampicillin, 30-31, 39, 52, 63, 76, 91, 93, 99-102, 104-105, 109-100, 115-117, 121-123, 125, 127-133, 135-136, 150, 180-182, 185-186, 188, 193, 196-197, 200, 206, 294, 344, 361, 373-376, 380, 384, 386, 391-392, 398-399, 401, 403-404, 408-409, 419, 428, 430-433, 436-439, 443-445, 447, 451, 453, 463, 482, 484, 491-496, 498, 502, 506, 510, 516-517, 544-546, 548-549, 556, 568-569, 572, 579-580, 588-589, 626, 630, 633, 638, 644-645, 647, 653-655, 661, 665, 682, 687

anaerobic, 584-585
Anaerococcus, 341, 567
ANT, 17-18, 48-49, 69, 103, 215-224, 227-228, 232, 234-238, 240, 242, 417, 421, 483, 687
Antimicrobial Susceptibility Testing, 37-38, 42, 44-45, 55, 58-59, 61-62, 65-66, 89-90, 94, 124, 136, 153-154, 158, 172, 176-177, 179, 187, 195, 205-206, 208-209, 223, 272-273, 276, 283, 293-294, 303-304, 325, 330, 372, 389, 396, 400, 405, 408, 424, 427, 437, 439, 442, 447-448, 456-458, 476-477, 480, 486, 488, 490, 499, 501, 508, 510, 520, 538-539, 541, 550, 553-555, 557, 559, 561, 563, 565, 567, 574, 576, 613, 615, 618, 627-628, 631, 634, 648, 651-652, 655-656, 682, 688
APH, 17-18, 48-49, 69, 184, 213, 215-223, 227-230, 232-233, 235-237, 417, 421, 436, 483, 489, 493, 687
apramycin, 54, 227, 230-232, 237, 239, 421, 653
Arcanobacterium haemolyticum, 381, 385-386
*arm*A, 20, 226, 236, 240-241, 417, 419
Arthrobacter, 379-383, 386
AST, 61, 89-94, 601-602, 655
attC, 76, 303
AUC, 41-43, 87, 281, 687
AUIC, 687
automated, 49, 51, 55, 59-61, 64, 67-68, 72-73, 81, 90-91, 94, 136, 152-153, 278 279, 283, 288, 292-293, 297, 312, 325, 340, 396, 408, 429, 460, 510, 601-602, 604, 606, 614, 677
azithromycin, 42, 76, 195, 305, 307, 310, 313, 317, 321, 323, 324, 375, 381, 427-428, 436, 439, 442, 446, 452-453, 456, 458, 467, 479, 482, 497, 504-508, 521-522, 524-529, 532-538, 544-545, 549-550, 555, 565, 612, 623-656, 627, 637, 639-641
aztreonam, 49, 135, 137-139, 143, 147, 149-150, 152, 158-165, 168, 170, 176-177, 179, 182, 184, 187, 191, 193, 196, 198, 200, 204-205, 373-374, 380, 409-410, 412-415, 428, 545-548, 577-578, 583-584, 586, 624, 644, 681

B

B. cepacia, 53, 58, 175, 179-181, 184-185, 187, 190, 206, 239, 360, 368
β-lactams, 27, 91, 99-102, 104-106, 109-112, 114-116, 120, 122-123, 157-168, 174-175, 177, 181-182, 185-187, 189-196, 198-210, 361, 367, 378, 407, 409, 411, 415, 419, 427-428, 430-432, 454, 457, 461, 465, 483-484, 504-505, 611, 665, 673-674, 681
B. pseudomallei, 58, 175, 179-180, 186-188, 190-191, 368
Bacillus, 36, 53, 56, 59-60, 76-77, 157, 187, 196, 215, 217, 223-224, 229, 243-244, 246, 248, 255, 258-259, 296, 306, 308, 329-330, 333, 342, 348-349, 354, 360, 367, 369, 389-397, 493, 597-600, 671
Bacillus clausii, 223, 306, 308
Bacillus subtilis, 36, 77, 224, 246, 296, 360
bacterial population, 48, 143, 532, 536, 673
bacteriophage, 28, 35
Bacteroides, 18, 19, 27, 35, 54, 59, 210, 223, 264, 308, 332, 334-335, 340-341, 348, 350, 358-359, 361-362, 366, 369, 371, 528, 547, 551, 553-555, 557, 559, 562-565, 576-582, 586-588, 590-591, 680-682
Bartonella, 56, 330, 348, 350, 615-619, 621, 623, 625, 627, 629, 631, 633, 635, 637, 639, 641
BCYE, 272, 503
BES, 146
beta hemolytic streptococci, 340
beta-lactamase inhibitor, 185, 408, 502, 681
Bifidobacterium, 333, 567, 572
Bilophila wadsworthia, 371, 553-554, 562-564, 577-578, 584, 591
blaR1, 31, 101, 103
blaZ, 103, 128
BLNAR, 428-433, 436, 438, 687
borderline, 102, 104, 149, 343
Borrelia, 15, 329-330, 348, 366, 615, 617-621, 623-625, 627, 629, 631, 633, 635, 637, 639, 641
BPS, 176, 190, 208
Brachyspira, 652, 654, 656
Branhamella, 232, 242, 350, 491-493, 495, 497, 499-500
Brevibacterium, 379-384
BRO, 492-493, 498-500
Brucella, 53, 57-60, 67, 198, 303, 329, 330, 348, 350, 368, 371, 460, 542-543, 554-555, 557-559, 561, 584, 615, 617, 619, 621, 623, 625-629, 631, 633, 635, 637, 639, 641, 679
BSYE, 503
Burkholderia, 15, 53, 56, 60, 175-176, 179-180, 184-191, 207-211, 231-232, 240-241, 330, 348, 352, 355, 357, 360-362, 370

C

C. acidovorans, 175-176, 179, 200-202, 209-211, 370
C. amalonaticus, 139
C. butyricum, 554, 562, 568, 575, 681
C. clostridioforme, 341, 553-554, 562, 568-569, 574, 681
C. coli, 479, 481, 483-486, 488
C. difficile, 300-301, 303, 568-573, 576
C. freundii, 53, 140-141, 147-149, 152, 236
C. hominis, 542, 544, 547
C. indologenes, 175, 203, 205
C. innocuum, 553, 562, 568-569, 572
C. jeikeium, 365, 379-385

C. jejuni, 59, 264, 479, 481-485, 487
C. koseri, 139, 150, 369
C. meningosepticum, 179, 181, 203
C. perfringens, 301, 555, 558, 561, 564, 568-570, 573, 653
C. pneumoniae, 531-537
C. ramosum, 553, 562, 568, 681
C. sedlakii, 145
C. tertium, 568
C. trachomatis, 335, 531-537
Campylobacter, 53, 56, 71, 74, 229-230, 232, 241, 264, 271-272, 306, 332, 335, 348, 350, 353, 360, 368, 372, 479-490, 577, 656
Capnocytophaga, 332, 541, 543, 545-551
CARB, 69, 138, 143, 159-160, 164-165, 174, 193-194, 411, 510, 512, 516-518
carbapenemase, 35, 60, 64, 91-93, 139, 145, 149, 152-154, 159, 162, 166, 173, 190, 205, 210, 371, 411, 413-414, 510, 513-514, 517-518, 581-583, 590-591, 681, 688
carbapenems, 18, 20-23, 35, 47-49, 53, 90-91, 100, 106-107, 110, 112, 115, 119, 129, 135, 138-139, 141-143, 145, 147, 149-150, 152-153, 157-161, 163, 170, 173-174, 187, 191, 194-195, 198, 200, 202, 204, 336, 393, 398, 407, 411, 413, 415, 420, 423, 430, 452, 549, 564, 567-568, 572-573, 578, 580, 582, 584, 620, 661, 665-666
carbenicillin, 157-158, 174, 392, 484, 510-511, 517, 580, 645, 647, 661, 665
carboxypenicillins, 140-143, 147, 149, 158, 195-196, 391, 501, 661, 665, 667
Cardiobacterium hominis, 541, 550-551
cassette, 20, 68, 102-103, 107, 172-173, 186, 196, 210, 224, 309, 254, 387, 483, 486, 510, 514, 518, 526
ccr, 103, 107
CdiA, 139
cefaclor, 116-117, 123, 399, 428, 431, 491, 493, 495, 497, 580, 585, 662, 665
cefadroxil, 110, 580, 662, 665
cefamandole, 53, 99-102, 140, 150, 182, 193, 195, 199, 201, 204, 206, 399, 410, 412-414, 484, 546, 578, 645, 647, 665, 681
cefazolin, 86, 91, 110, 123, 181, 197, 199, 399, 484, 661, 665
cefdinir, 110, 115-117, 120, 123, 580, 619-623
cefepime, 78, 83, 86, 91, 100, 110, 116-117, 121-123, 126, 135, 137-138, 142, 144-146, 148-150, 152, 155, 157-168, 170-172, 177, 182, 184-185, 192-194, 196-199, 201, 204-206, 209, 375, 398, 408-414, 416-419, 422-423, 428, 576, 578, 580, 619, 661, 665
cefixime, 117, 142, 144-146, 148, 150, 188-189, 199, 399, 428, 431, 433, 437, 451, 453-458, 491, 497, 499, 502, 543-544, 548, 563, 578, 580, 584, 619-623, 662, 665
cefotaxime, 45, 48-49, 53-54, 78, 83, 86, 99-102, 110, 113-114, 116-117, 120-123, 126, 130-133, 135, 137, 142, 144-148, 150, 152, 158, 160, 162-165, 168, 177, 179-182, 185-189, 192-197, 199, 201-202, 204-206, 362, 364, 373, 375, 380, 385-386, 398-399, 401-402, 404, 409-410, 412-414, 419, 423, 427-428, 431-433, 437, 443-445, 447-448, 452, 454, 456-457, 482, 484, 491, 496-497, 499, 502, 511-514, 544-549, 556, 569, 571-572, 575, 578-580, 583-586, 588-589, 616, 619-620, 623, 625-626, 630, 644-645, 647, 649, 661, 665, 682
cefoxitin, 27, 49, 53, 92, 102, 104-107, 135, 139-150, 158, 161, 177, 179-180, 182, 185, 188, 191-201, 203-204, 206, 392, 399, 410, 412-414, 484, 496-497, 506, 511-513, 544-548, 553, 555-556, 561, 564-565, 568-569, 571-572, 578-581, 583-586, 588-590, 612-613, 645, 654-655, 661, 665, 680-682
cefpirome, 87, 100, 126, 135, 138, 142, 144-146, 148, 150, 152, 154-155, 158-165, 168, 185, 201, 205, 209, 399, 413, 484, 580, 661, 665
cefpodoxime, 110, 116-117, 123, 150, 152, 197, 427-428, 431-432, 453, 502, 563, 578, 580, 662, 665
cefoperazone, 157-158, 160, 162-163, 165, 168, 182, 184-185, 188, 193-194, 197, 202, 483-484, 512, 579, 585, 588-589, 645, 661, 665
cefquinome, 652, 656
ceftiofur, 197, 274, 652-653, 655-656
ceftriaxone, 54, 76-77, 86, 90-91, 100, 110, 113-114, 116-117, 120-123, 125-127, 150, 180-181, 188-189, 191, 193, 195, 197, 205, 211, 364, 373, 380, 392, 398-399, 402, 409, 427-428, 431, 433, 443-444, 446-448, 451-458, 491, 496, 502, 516, 548-549, 563, 572, 616, 619-627, 629-630, 633, 639-640, 644-645, 647, 654-655, 661, 665, 682
cefuroximase, 140, 189
Cellulomonas, 379
cephamycins, 48-49, 135, 137-138, 140, 143, 145, 147, 149-150, 196, 204
cephalexin, 110, 463, 665
cephalosporinase, 21, 34, 51, 78, 139-140, 147-149, 152, 158-159, 163-164, 166, 168, 186, 190, 194, 198-199, 391, 409, 412-413, 418-420, 510, 512-514, 516, 518, 581, 583, 591
cephalosporins, 17, 21, 26-27, 47, 50-51, 53, 69, 76, 78, 91-92, 100, 103, 106-107, 110, 112, 115, 118-119, 125, 127, 130, 135-139, 143, 147, 150, 152, 154, 157-161, 164, 168, 177, 181-182, 184-187, 189-191, 193-196, 198-200, 202-204, 210-211, 225, 285, 374, 377, 384, 391-393, 398, 401-402, 407-409, 411, 413, 415, 417-418, 427,

430, 432-433, 436, 439, 443-445, 452-455, 457-458, 479, 483, 491, 495, 497-499, 501-502, 505-506, 510, 512, 515, 518, 543-548, 550, 565, 568, 571, 576, 578, 581, 584, 617, 620, 624-625, 627, 629, 644, 652, 654-655, 661-662, 665-666, 681

cephalothin, 91, 123, 135, 142, 144-146, 148, 192, 199, 201, 411, 484, 510-516, 544-548, 563, 583, 616-617, 626, 630, 661, 665

cfiA, 559, 581-582, 590-591

cfr, 19, 23, 343-344, 359-360, 656

CfxA, 547, 580

CGB, 176, 205-207

Chlamydia, 67, 306, 327, 335, 348, 350, 357, 362-363, 372, 528, 531-533, 535, 537-539

chloramphenicol, 17, 19, 23, 51, 78, 109, 124, 137, 150, 164, 180-182, 184-188, 190-191, 193, 197, 201, 204-205, 246, 264, 267, 269-270, 331, 339, 343-345, 352, 357-361, 363, 365, 367, 369, 371-377, 383-384, 388, 392, 394, 400-404, 410, 415-416, 422, 428, 430-431, 435-436, 441, 443-445, 447-449, 451-453, 456, 461, 465, 482, 485, 490-492, 497-498, 501, 511, 513, 515, 517, 521-522, 527, 543-549, 556, 561, 563-564, 569-570, 574-545, 578, 580, 583-585, 588-590, 625-626, 629, 630, 632-633, 635, 638-640, 645-646, 648, 662, 665, 673-674, 680, 682, 687

Chryseobacterium, 161, 175-177, 200, 202-205, 207-211, 340, 370

Citrobacter amalonaticus, 139

Citrobacter freundii, 53, 140, 150, 240, 242, 263, 364, 369

Citrobacter koseri, 139

Citrobacter sedlakii, 140

CjBla2, 484

CKO, 139

clarithromycin, 305-307, 310, 313, 317, 321, 323-324, 344, 375, 381, 392, 400, 427-428, 436, 459-461, 463-464, 467-477, 491, 493, 497, 504-508, 522, 534-535, 537-538, 549, 580, 587, 611-613, 616, 619, 621-624, 626, 630, 633, 635, 637-638, 640, 646, 648, 662, 665

clavulanate, 99-100, 110, 115-117, 120, 122-123, 125, 137-150, 152, 155, 184, 408-409, 417, 419, 427-428, 430-433, 437-438, 484-485, 491, 565, 568

clavulanic acid, 27, 48, 52-53, 76-77, 86, 101-102, 105, 110, 113, 123, 128-132, 137, 157-163, 165, 167-168, 170, 173, 176-177, 179-206, 211, 391, 408-414, 416-418, 443, 454, 491, 493, 495-499, 501-502, 505-506, 508, 511-514, 545-549, 555-557, 559, 561, 563, 568, 578-581, 583-586, 588-589, 644-645, 647, 661, 665, 667, 673, 680, 682

clinafloxacin, 182, 205, 244, 374-375, 506, 620

clindamycin, 33-34, 42, 48, 50, 60, 64, 83, 86, 89, 91-92, 127, 188, 203, 205, 305-306, 310-325, 344, 373-375, 377, 381, 383, 386, 392-394, 398-400, 402-404, 479, 482, 522, 524, 527, 544-548, 555-556, 558-559, 561-562, 567-569, 571-574, 578-582, 584-586, 588-590, 646, 662, 665, 680, 682

clinical categorization, 37, 39, 41, 43-45, 48, 201, 275-276, 278-280, 292, 385, 447, 457, 629

Clostridium, 53, 89, 95, 213, 223, 298, 308, 330, 333, 335, 340-341, 343, 345, 350, 359, 362, 365-366, 553-555, 557, 559, 562-564, 567-568, 570, 572-576, 653-654, 656, 681-682

CME, 204, 206-207, 210, 482-483

CmeB, 482-483, 489

cmeABC, 360, 482-488, 490

CMT, 143, 146

CMY, 148, 656

co-trimoxazole, 179-180, 182, 184-185, 188, 193, 195, 199, 201, 205, 208, 347-348, 350, 353-354, 375, 392, 419, 435, 495, 498, 501, 548, 617, 625, 627, 629, 632, 634, 637, 653-655, 663

colistin, 20, 53, 61, 76, 78, 93, 179, 181-182, 184-185, 193, 199-201, 204, 269-270, 358, 361, 367-372, 407-408, 410, 41-420, 423-425, 493-494, 506, 511, 513-516, 535, 544, 578, 584, 654, 662, 665, 680-681

Com, 81, 691

Comamonas, 200, 202, 209-210, 370

composite, 30-33, 35, 226, 241, 317-319

composite transposon, 30-31, 226, 241

concentration dependent, 41, 77, 85, 225, 244, 300, 394, 685

conjugation, 29, 31, 196, 321, 493, 500, 575

conjugative, 30-31, 34-35, 143, 145, 148, 159, 196, 274, 277, 287, 331, 334, 337, 377, 434, 449, 452, 456, 485, 488, 515-516, 518, 523, 546, 570-571

conservative, 29-30, 42

co-resistance, 47-48, 52, 493, 685

Corynebacterium, 59, 224, 300, 308, 325, 333, 342, 345, 362, 365-366, 378-383, 386-388, 404, 575, 643

Coxiella, 329, 342, 344, 348, 350, 358, 532, 615, 617, 619, 621, 623, 625, 627, 629, 631, 633, 635-639, 641

cross-resistance, 19, 47, 49-52, 129, 137, 185, 190, 231, 237, 247, 265, 277, 295, 305, 307-308, 319-320, 339-340, 354, 360, 363, 366, 369, 371-372, 384-385, 393, 403, 443, 454-455, 464, 467, 470, 482, 523-524, 526, 569, 574, 580-582, 584, 594-596, 685

cryptic, 230, 233, 241, 334, 535

CTX-M, 137, 144, 146, 149, 153-154, 161-162, 171-173, 184, 209-210, 411, 413, 419, 512, 514, 518

D

D-Ala-D-Ala, 110-112, 135, 285, 288, 300

D-Ala-D-Lac, 286-287, 290
D-Ala-D-Ser, 112, 287-288
dalbavancin, 295, 298, 300-304, 344, 384, 575, 662, 665
dalfopristin, 42, 93, 205, 305-307, 310, 312, 315-317, 321, 323-326, 343-344, 375, 382, 386, 400-404, 504-505, 507-508, 522, 524-526, 575, 580, 587, 619, 662
danofloxacin, 656
daptomycin, 17, 39, 42, 54, 57-60, 91, 93, 95, 291, 295-298, 300, 303-304, 344-345, 384, 392-393, 395, 399, 401-402, 404, 575, 662, 665, 681
Dermabacter, 342, 379-383
2-deoxystreptamine, 213, 225
dfrD, 376
DHA, 148
DHfR, 18, 21, 348, 351-353, 435, 687
DHPS, 18, 348, 351-352, 435, 687
difloxacin, 665
dihydrofolate reductase, 18, 21, 348, 354-355, 376, 393, 435, 484, 687
dirithromycin, 305, 310, 344, 508, 619, 662, 665
DNA gyrase, 21, 23, 33, 49, 71, 184, 190, 258-259, 262, 265-266, 268, 273-274, 422, 434, 455, 457, 466, 526, 528, 537, 570, 583, 596, 617, 625, 627, 629, 632-633, 637
DNA topoisomerase IV, 262, 266
donor, 28-30, 80, 465-466
doxycycline, 88, 180-182, 185, 187-188, 190, 195, 197, 205, 327-329, 331, 344, 357, 374-375, 382, 386, 392-395, 400, 409, 419, 423, 425, 455, 465, 479-480, 484, 488, 491, 502, 506, 521-524, 527, 534-537, 574, 580, 585-587, 612-613, 616-617, 619, 621-623, 625-630, 633, 635, 637-638, 645-646, 648, 662, 665
Dysgonomonas, 541, 543, 546-548, 550

E

E. aerogenes, 140, 147-150, 369, 514
E. avium, 128, 285, 287, 306
E. breve, 175, 205
E. casseliflavus, 52, 128, 222, 285-289, 306
E. cloacae, 26, 140, 147, 149, 237, 268-269, 271, 336
E. corrodens, 542, 545, 547
E. durans, 128-129, 285, 287, 297, 306
E. faecalis, 28-31, 127-132, 213, 217, 222, 245-246, 248, 253, 279, 287, 289, 296-300, 302, 306, 324, 340-343, 353, 403
E. faecium, 20, 31, 35, 127-132, 217, 222, 246, 287, 289-290, 292, 296-300, 302, 306-307, 324, 341, 343
E. gallinarum, 128-129, 222, 285-290, 306
E. hirae, 128, 306
E. persicina, 145

Eagle, 129
EDTA, 75, 137, 138, 149, 152-153, 163, 168, 170, 182, 194, 204-205, 370, 391-392, 417-418, 581, 590, 687
efflux, 17-18, 21-23, 27, 33, 48, 50, 51, 64, 70-71, 136-137, 154, 158, 163-166, 168, 172-174, 176, 181-184, 186, 190-191, 198, 207-211, 224, 231-234, 236-242, 244, 246-255, 258-259, 263, 265, 267-268, 274, 306, 309-310, 312, 314, 316, 321-322, 325-326, 330-337, 339, 348, 351-352, 354-355, 359-360, 367, 369, 374, 376, 377, 384-387, 393, 407, 411, 415-416, 420-425, 433-437, 446, 454-456, 458, 463, 465-466, 481-490, 501, 506, 515, 517, 522-523, 526, 529, 546, 570, 581, 583, 591, 627, 629, 631, 637, 685
Ehrlichia, 348, 615, 632-633, 635, 637
Eikenella corrodens, 53, 59, 541, 549, 550-551
Empedobacter, 175, 200, 207, 370
enrofloxacin, 268, 482, 656
Enterobacter aerogenes, 136, 140, 155, 517
Enterobacter cloacae, 34, 78, 140, 155, 240, 263, 273-274, 364, 369
Enterococcus, 20, 28, 34-36, 50-53, 56, 58, 64, 70, 72, 93, 132-133, 224, 238, 241, 244, 258-259, 283, 285, 291, 293-294, 297, 301, 304, 306, 308, 325, 329, 331, 333-334, 339-341, 344-345, 348, 354, 359-364, 366, 372, 377, 403, 404, 483, 546, 571, 575, 671, 688, 689
ere, 19, 309
erm(A), 34, 308-310, 319-322,
erm(B), 308-310, 319-322, 324-325, 570
erm(C), 34, 308-310, 312, 319, 376-377, 403
erm, 19, 33-34, 64, 70, 72, 92, 306-310, 312, 316-317, 319-322, 324-325, 333, 340, 376-377, 384, 386, 393, 403, 446, 456, 481, 546, 570, 582, 611, 656, 687
ertapenem, 115, 117, 123, 125-126, 152-153, 158, 177, 484, 572, 574, 576, 578, 581, 624
Erwinia persicina, 140
Erysipelothrix rhusiopathiae, 362, 397-398, 402-403, 405,
erythromycin, 19, 30-31, 33, 34, 40, 48-49, 64, 70, 72-73, 89, 92, 101, 103, 124, 164, 184, 188, 203, 205, 305-326, 367, 373-379, 381, 383-387, 392, 398-400, 404-405, 415-416, 428, 431, 436, 451, 453-454, 456, 460, 463-464, 467, 469, 473, 479-482, 485, 487-491, 493-495, 497-499, 502-508, 521-522, 524-525, 527-529, 534-537, 544-548, 550-551, 555, 568, 571-572, 574, 578, 580, 586-587, 616-617, 619, 621-626, 629-630, 633-640, 646-648, 654- 655, 662, 665, 687
ESBL, 17, 32, 64, 139, 144-147, 149-150, 152, 155, 160-161, 165, 166, 176, 182, 184, 187, 189-190, 194-195, 204, 412-413, 417-419, 427, 432, 438, 687

Escherichia hermanni, 139
ESCMID, 44-45, 104, 129, 157-158, 172, 442, 613,
esterase, 367, 687
ethambutol, 593, 598, 600-603, 605-606, 609, 611-613
Eubacterium, 332-333, 341, 362, 567, 571-573, 681
excision, 31, 34, 102, 575
extended spectrum β-lactamase, 160-161, 168, 171-172, 174, 176, 194-195, 205, 207, 209-210, 362, 413, 427, 438
external quality control, 687

F

F. johnsoniae, 175, 205
fexA, 359, 656
Finegoldia, 341, 567
fitness, 363, 366
Flavobacterium, 175, 200, 205, 207-211, 340, 370
floR, 359, 656
florfenicol, 19, 23, 31, 197, 344, 357-360, 372, 515, 652, 653, 654, 656,
fluoroquinolone, 23, 33, 35-36, 48, 72, 83, 94, 206, 211, 225, 230, 244, 247-248, 250, 258-259, 261, 265, 268-271, 273-274, 362, 374, 377, 381, 385-386, 395, 422, 430, 434, 438-439, 446, 448, 452-453, 455, 457-459, 465, 468-469, 472, 475, 477, 479, 481-490, 493, 498-499, 501, 506-507, 515, 517, 519, 526-528, 537-538, 548, 550, 574, 576, 583, 590-591, 603, 605, 611, 613, 617, 618, 627-629, 632, 637,
fortimicin, 23, 232, 237-239, 421
fosfomycin 17, 19, 22, 76-77, 86, 193, 196, 199, 204, 269-270, 340, 358, 361-365, 367, 372,374, 377, 380, 394, 401-402, 409-410, 436, 438, 461, 521, 546, 583-584, 647, 662, 681
FOX, 142, 144-146, 148, 177, 179, 204, 410, 412-414, 511, 513, 516
fusidic acid, 21, 76, 83, 136, 203, 340, 344, 358-359, 365-367, 372, 385-386, 395, 401-402, 415, 430, 577, 583, 624, 663, 673
Fusobacterium, 332, 335, 340-341, 363, 366, 371, 553-554, 557-559, 562-563, 565, 577-578, 584, 586-587, 589, 680-681

G

gatifloxacin, 182, 184, 188, 205, 243-246, 248, 261-264, 344, 374-375, 395, 472, 507, 522, 526-527, 535, 570, 574, 578, 583-584, 590, 620, 663, 666
GCN5 acetyltransferase, 230
Gemella, 74, 109-110, 333
generalized, 28, 49, 653-655
genomic islands, 536, 538
gentamicin, 30-31, 34-35, 48-49, 53-54, 64, 69, 80-81, 85-86, 88, 91, 101, 110, 129, 180, 182, 185, 188, 190, 193, 195-198, 200-202, 204-205, 213, 215-225, 227-233, 235, 237-241, 248, 289-290, 293, 325, 340, 344, 373-377, 381-382, 385-386, 392-394, 397-399, 401-404, 407, 409-410, 417, 419, 421-423, 436, 479, 483, 485, 487-488, 495, 498, 501, 506, 517, 522, 535, 544-545, 577, 580, 582, 584, 588, 616-617, 625-630, 633, 635, 638, 644, 646, 648, 654, 656, 662, 666, 681
GES, 73, 145-146, 149, 155, 161, 166, 170-171, 173-174, 411, 413, 415, 419-420
GISA, 21, 44, 67, 83-84, 277-279, 281, 283-284, 295, 297-302, 688
glycolipodepsipeptide, 303
glycopeptide, 21-22, 32, 34, 44, 51, 64, 67, 70, 72, 84, 129, 132, 222, 275-296, 298-300, 302-303, 362, 376, 401, 403-404, 617, 688
GOB, 176, 205-206
Granulicatella, 57-58, 110
GRE, 295, 299-300, 302-303, 688
group A streptococci, 39, 123, 351
gyrA, 21, 49, 71, 73, 74, 248, 255, 258-259, 262, 265-266, 269-270, 272, 381, 385, 387, 393, 422, 425-426, 434-435, 438, 446, 455, 463, 466, 477, 482-483, 485, 487-488, 490, 501-502, 506, 517, 526, 528, 537, 539, 569, 574, 590, 596, 603, 605, 608, 611, 617, 628, 637
GyrA, 21, 243-244, 246-248, 250-251-255, 259, 262, 266, 422, 434-435, 458, 515, 569, 596, 617
gyrB, 21, 71, 73, 262, 266, 393, 434-435, 466, 477, 506, 510, 518, 526, 569, 574, 596, 603, 608
GyrB, 21, 243, 262, 266, 435, 482, 570, 596

H

H. alvei, 140, 147
H. aphrophilus, 59, 541-544, 546-547, 549-551
H. influenzae, 18, 20, 40, 58, 60-61, 125, 232, 264, 266, 271-273, 331, 335, 340, 342, 350, 352, 357-359, 361, 368, 427-439, 441, 499-501, 541-543, 546, 549
H. pylori, 18-20, 58, 67, 70, 309, 329-330, 368, 372, 459-477, 488
HACEK, 59, 541, 543, 545, 547-551
Haemophilus, 20, 40, 51, 53, 56-57, 60-62, 64, 87, 125, 232, 264, 332, 335, 340, 342, 353, 357, 359-361, 363, 427, 431-433, 436-439, 441, 499-501, 541-542, 549-551, 653-654, 656, 688
Haemophilus aphrophilus, 541, 549-551
Hafnia alvei, 140, 158, 369
Helicobacter, 19, 56, 62, 67, 70, 306, 309, 329-330, 348, 350, 368, 459, 476-477, 483, 488
HER-1, 139
heterogeneous, 69, 80, 105-106, 138, 176, 200, 202, 238, 282-284, 437, 446, 536, 541, 569, 571, 575, 647
high-level cephalosporinase, 147-148
Histophilus, 653-654, 656
homogeneous, 39, 82, 364, 599, 611, 643-644

homologous recombination, 29
horizontal transfer, 50, 258, 366, 441, 485, 509, 514
hyperOXY, 147

I

IBC, 146, 161
ICE, 686
IMI, 149, 415
imipenem, 22, 27, 34, 40-41, 75-76, 78, 83, 86, 91, 99-101, 115-117, 120-123, 126-129, 131, 133, 135, 137-140, 142, 144-146, 148-150, 152-155, 157-160, 162-168, 170, 174, 177, 179-183, 185, 187-194, 196-199, 201-206, 340, 344, 362, 364, 374, 375, 391-393, 398-399, 401-404, 407-410, 412-419, 421, 428-429, 433, 437, 439, 484, 496, 505-506, 510-516, 544-549, 553-559, 561-565, 567-569, 571-573, 578-581, 583-586, 588-589, 612-613, 616-617, 619-625, 630, 633, 644-645, 647, 649, 661, 666, 680-682
IMP, 138, 149, 159, 161, 166, 170, 172-173, 176, 179, 194, 209, 410-419, 515, 517, 612
impossible phenotypes, 52
incompatibility, 226
incompatibility group, 226
IND, 176, 205-206
inducible resistance, 27, 33, 51, 64, 285, 308, 319-320, 333, 368, 581, 687
INH, 19, 21, 26, 593, 597, 603, 609-610, 612
inhibitory quotient, 84-85, 269, 688
inhibitor-resistant TEM, 138
initiation complex, 26, 339
inoculum effect, 84, 157, 275, 278, 307, 321, 367, 390, 503, 512, 557, 536
insertion sequence, 29, 31, 35-36, 68, 171, 224, 387, 421, 466, 567, 580-582, 591, 688
integrase, 30, 32, 210
integration, 31-32, 102
integron, 19, 23, 30, 171-173, 184, 196, 210, 224, 232, 241, 353, 359, 361, 384, 420, 422, 424-425, 483, 486-487, 510, 512, 514-515, 517-518
internal quality control, 437, 688
interpretative reading, 54, 176, 230, 232, 240, 451, 651
intrinsic activity, 17, 49, 238, 261, 263, 358, 417, 430-431, 527
IRKO, 143
IS, 27, 29-30, 32, 35, 553, 688

J-K

josamycin, 305, 307, 310, 318, 323-324, 386, 430, 469, 505, 521, 524-525, 527, 534, 536, 634
K. ascorbata, 145-146, 369
K. cryocrescens, 145-146
K. oxytoca, 139, 143, 147-148, 150, 369

K. pneumoniae, 53, 76-77, 93, 139, 145, 148-150, 152-153, 264, 266-268, 270, 335-336, 352, 368, 371
kanamycin, 30-31, 35, 48-49, 53, 103, 182, 185, 188, 195, 204, 213-219, 221-223, 225, 227-229, 231-233, 237, 367, 371-372, 375, 381, 385, 392, 399, 401, 410, 419, 421-423, 436, 483, 486, 488-490, 493, 577-578, 594, 596-598, 604, 610, 613, 644, 646, 648, 662, 666, 680
ketolide, 73, 305, 325, 378, 395, 405, 524, 527, 538, 624, 629-630, 638, 662
Kingella kingae, 541, 549-551
Klebsiella oxytoca, 139, 155, 263
Klebsiella pneumoniae, 21, 32, 35, 90, 95, 136, 139, 145, 149, 154-155, 161, 173, 227, 263, 274, 337, 364, 369, 425, 688
Kluyvera ascorbata, 140
Kluyvera cryocrescens, 140, 369
Kluyvera georgiana, 140
KPC, 32, 64, 149, 153-155, 162, 171, 415, 688

L

L. monocytogenes, 223, 363, 373-378
L3, 656
L4, 20, 70, 306, 309, 316, 323, 326, 343, 345, 436, 482, 485, 524-525, 617
L22, 20, 70, 306, 309, 316-317, 323, 326, 436, 482, 485, 524-525, 536, 634, 636
Lactobacillus, 53, 56, 59, 308, 325, 333, 342, 397-400, 402-405
Lawsonia intracellularis, 652, 654
LEN-1, 139
Leuconostoc, 53, 59, 342, 397-405
linA, 313
lincomycin, 48-49, 64, 70, 306, 310-321, 323-325, 339, 381, 384, 386-387, 521-522, 544-545, 652
lincosamides, 19, 23, 30, 33, 47, 49, 64-65, 70, 72, 109, 127, 305-307, 310, 312-313, 317, 319, 321, 324-325, 343, 360, 375, 381, 384, 386, 401, 403, 415, 430, 443, 453, 456, 461, 501, 506, 521-522, 524-525, 645-646, 652, 656, 662, 688
linezolid, 19, 26, 35, 42, 76, 91, 339, 342-345, 367, 374, 383, 386, 394, 401, 404, 430, 521, 564, 573-575, 578, 584, 586, 590, 594, 598, 612-613, 648-649, 681
lipid I, 303
lipid II, 303
lipodepsipeptide, 295
lipopeptide, 295, 297, 299, 393, 662, 665
Listeria, 20, 53, 56, 224, 298, 333, 342, 350, 362, 373-375, 377-379
lnu(A), 310, 312-313, 321
lnu(B), 321, 324
lnu(C), 321, 325
lnu, 70, 309

LSA, 306, 321, 688
lyases, 70, 309, 316

M

M. avium, 611-612
M. catarrhalis, 59, 264, 273, 368, 491-498
M. hominis, 335, 519-529
M. leprae, 366, 610-611
M. morganii, 140-141, 151, 335-336, 364-365, 368
M. odoratimimus, 175, 205
M. odoratus, 175, 203
M. pneumoniae, 335, 344, 463, 519-527
M. tuberculosis, 72, 363, 463, 466, 593-597, 599-601, 604, 606, 608-610, 612
macrolides, 17-20, 23, 30, 33, 42, 47-49, 64, 70, 72, 74-76, 81, 84, 109, 136, 190-191, 305-315, 317-321, 323-326, 333, 339, 343-345, 352, 357, 360, 374-377, 381-382, 384-386, 393-395, 398, 401-403, 405, 427, 430, 436, 444, 446, 453-454, 456, 460-461, 463-464, 467, 469, 481-483, 488, 491-494, 499, 501-502, 504-508, 519, 521-522, 524, 527, 529, 534, 537-538, 543-545, 549, 554-555, 567, 570-571, 581-582, 584, 586-587, 611, 617, 619, 623-627, 629-630, 632-633, 635, 637-640, 645-646, 652-655, 662, 665-667, 681, 688
Major Facilitator Superfamily, 137, 186, 268, 309, 360, 374, 377
Mannheimia, 332
marbofloxacin, 656
MBC, 57, 129, 157, 220-221, 277, 314, 362, 365, 381, 463, 465, 505, 520, 531, 615, 618-623, 629, 639, 685, 688
MDR, 109, 184, 331, 359-360, 407-408, 413, 415-416, 482, 609-610, 688
mdrL, 374
mecillinam, 137, 150, 177, 196, 204, 374, 409, 419, 430, 645, 661, 666, 673
mef(A), 64, 70, 309, 321-325, 334
meropenem, 100, 110, 114-117, 120-123, 125-126, 135, 153, 155, 157-160, 162-168, 180-182, 184-185, 187-188, 190-191, 193, 197-198, 200-202, 205-206, 375, 395, 407-410, 412-416, 419, 427-428, 430-431, 443-444, 447, 479, 483-485, 488, 549, 556, 563, 578-579, 581, 585, 588, 590, 619-624, 630, 661, 666, 682
metalloenzyme, 69, 137-138, 209, 363, 392-393
methicillin, 20, 22, 45, 47-48, 51, 53, 57-58, 66-69, 73, 89, 95, 99-100, 102-103, 105, 107, 248, 277, 280, 282-283, 295, 298-302, 304, 310, 325, 334, 341, 343-344, 349, 351, 353-354, 359, 362, 364-366, 493, 655, 661, 666, 687-688
methylation, 19, 23, 70, 226-227, 238, 241, 274, 307-308, 310, 312, 319, 322, 325, 343-344, 417, 420-421, 463, 685

metronidazole, 18-19, 23, 53, 83, 400, 402, 459-463, 465-477, 535, 541, 544-546, 555-556, 558-565, 567-569, 571-572, 575, 578-579, 582-586, 588-591, 663, 666, 680, 682
MexXY-OprM, 164-166, 168, 172, 231, 233, 241, 335
MFS, 137, 186, 268, 309, 321, 352, 360, 377
Microbacterium, 379-384, 386
Micrococcus, 53, 77, 308, 342
Micromonas, 341, 567
microscan, 60-61, 155, 281, 292, 298, 408, 558
midecamycin, 305, 494, 521-522, 662, 666
minimal bactericidal concentration, 463, 615, 688
minocycline, 30, 53, 180, 182, 184, 187-188, 205, 327-331, 334-335, 374, 376-377, 393, 400-401, 409, 422-423, 435, 438, 442-444, 447, 455, 465, 491, 493, 504, 506, 522-524, 527, 534, 535, 580, 584, 611, 619, 621-622, 626, 638, 645-646, 648, 666
mobile element, 19, 28, 31, 35, 128, 424
mobilizable, 28, 159, 517, 570
Mobiluncus, 572, 576, 681
MODSA, 103
molecular, 11-12, 17, 22-23, 34-35, 47, 51, 69, 72-74, 89, 99-101, 105, 107, 111, 135-140, 150, 153-155, 171-175, 207-211, 224, 242, 246, 259, 262-263, 274, 278, 303, 325, 336, 362, 367, 369-370, 372, 376, 379, 384, 391-392, 395, 404-405, 416-417, 420, 425-426, 437-439, 445, 448, 457, 464, 467, 474-477, 485-486, 488-489, 499-500, 502, 516-517, 519-521, 525-526, 528, 531-532, 536-537, 559, 574-575, 581, 591, 594-595, 597, 603-604, 606, 608, 611, 613-614, 617, 627, 634, 637, 640, 657, 688
Moraxella, 56, 64, 264, 306, 332, 335, 340, 342, 359, 366, 439, 491-493, 495, 497, 499-500
Moraxella catarrhalis, 64, 264, 306, 335, 340, 342, 359, 366, 439, 491, 499-500
Morganella morganii, 140, 263, 335, 337, 362-363, 369
mosaic, 28, 36, 68-69, 111-112, 248, 443, 445, 455, 458, 465
MOX, 148, 158, 160, 162-163, 165, 177, 179, 204, 264, 272, 410, 412-414
moxalactam, 48-49, 107, 158, 160, 162-163, 165, 168, 198, 410, 412-414, 484, 497
moxifloxacin, 184, 243-244, 247-254, 258-259, 262-264, 272, 343-344, 374-375, 377, 381, 385, 387, 401, 423, 428, 438, 473, 497, 505-508, 526-528, 535, 537, 561, 569-570, 573-575, 578, 583, 590, 597, 612-613
mph, 19, 70, 309, 317
MRSA, 66, 68, 89, 92, 93, 95, 99, 100, 102-103, 107, 277, 295, 298, 300-302, 361, 364, 367, 687-688

msr(A), 309-310, 312, 317
MSSA, 100, 277, 361, 364, 367, 688
mtr, 454, 458, 560
MtrCDE, 454-456
MUS, 162, 176, 205, 209
mutant, 33, 68, 76, 83-84, 103, 129, 138, 143-144, 147-148, 154, 164, 168, 172, 181-182, 184, 191, 200, 202, 213, 222, 229-231, 233, 239, 241, 244, 246-247, 249-250, 258-259, 265-269, 278, 289-290, 294, 296-297, 299-300, 302, 309-318, 321-323, 336, 339, 342-343, 352, 355, 363-364, 366-367, 369, 384-385, 393, 395-396, 422-423, 436, 453, 463-464, 466-467, 475, 482, 506, 514, 517, 519, 524-526, 528-529, 533, 536-539, 569, 583, 590-591, 593, 597-599, 601, 609-611, 617, 627, 629, 631, 637, 673
mutation, 11, 17-22, 25-27, 32-35, 39, 48-49, 51, 68-74, 102-103, 106, 111-112, 124, 128, 133, 135, 138, 143, 145, 147, 148, 154-155, 158-159, 181, 184, 190-191, 211, 213, 217, 222-223, 225-227, 229-232, 237-238, 240-241, 244, 246-248, 251-253, 258-259, 262, 265-274, 278, 289, 296, 299, 307, 309, 312, 316-318, 321, 323-326, 331, 333-335, 339, 342-345, 351-352, 354-355, 359-360, 363-364, 366-367, 369, 376, 381, 384-385, 387, 391, 393, 395, 407, 422, 425-426, 432-436, 438-439, 441, 446, 448, 453-458, 463-466, 469-470, 474-477, 481-490, 492, 501, 506, 508, 512, 515, 517-521, 523-529, 536-538, 569-571, 574, 583, 590-591, 594-597, 603-606, 608, 611, 614, 617, 623, 627-629, 635-636, 641, 652, 656, 686
Mycobacterium, 18, 20, 23, 26, 67, 70, 72-73, 89, 95, 226, 306, 309, 330, 333, 335, 340, 342, 358, 344, 350, 362, 366, 463, 593, 595, 611, 613-614, 643
Mycoplasma, 18, 20, 55, 71, 327, 329, 330, 333, 335, 340, 342, 344, 358, 362, 507, 519-529
Myroides, 175, 200, 203, 209, 370

N

N. gonorrhoeae, 58, 264, 266, 271-273, 331, 336, 451-457
N. meningitidis, 58, 360-362, 366, 441-448
N-acetyltransferase, 50, 54, 72, 184, 213, 227, 230-232, 240-242, 274, 425
Neisseria, 6, 9, 20, 28, 51, 53, 54, 56, 64, 71, 93, 226, 232, 241, 264, 332, 345, 340, 348, 350, 351, 358, 359, 361, 366, 368, 371, 372, 434, 441, 443, 445, 447-449, 451, 453, 455, 457, 458, 491, 492, 528, 547, 551
neomycin, 197, 213-220, 225, 227-229, 231-233, 237, 381, 421, 483, 493, 646 652-654, 662, 666
netilmicin, 48, 50, 69, 80, 81, 85, 152, 182, 188, 193, 195, 199-201, 204, 205, 213, 215-223, 225, 227-233, 237-240, 375, 381, 399, 401, 409, 410, 417, 419, 421-423, 616, 630, 645, 646, 662, 666
nimB, 567, 576, 582
NMC, 148, 149, 415
NMC-A, 148, 149
Nocardia, 6, 53, 325, 333, 340, 342, 344, 348, 350, 358, 366, 614, 643-649
non-conjugative, 143, 159, 570, 571
nucleotidyltransferase, 17, 18, 48, 52, 59, 70, 215-217, 223, 227, 228, 309, 313, 321, 417, 483, 671, 687

O

O. anthropi, 175, 179, 181, 196-199
OCH, 176, 198, 199
Ochrobactrum, 176, 196, 198, 208, 210, 211, 370
Oerskovia, 209, 384, 385, 387
oleandomycin, 305, 646, 662, 666, 667
Omp, 411
OmpD2, 27
O-nucleotidyltransferase, 52, 227, 313
O-phosphotransferase, 184, 187, 213, 227, 231, 687
OprD2, 163-165
oral streptococci, 245-248, 252, 323
oritavancin, 295, 298-303, 662, 666
outer membrane porin, 135, 415
OXA, 17, 32, 69, 138, 139, 143, 149, 158-166, 170-176, 190-194, 200, 201, 208-210, 411-420, 484, 485, 487, 512, 516
oxacillin, 21, 49, 58, 72, 76, 83, 86, 92, 99-106, 114, 116, 122, 123, 127, 138, 158, 168, 174, 367, 380, 384, 387, 399, 403, 417, 430, 445, 502, 512, 544, 545, 654, 655, 661, 666
oxacillinase, 138, 139, 143, 158-168, 171, 172, 186, 190-194, 200, 210, 411, 413, 415, 416, 418-420, 512, 513
oxazolidinone, 5, 17, 18-23, 35, 73, 339, 341, 343-345, 360, 375, 377, 567, 573, 587, 594, 638, 646, 649, 656, 663, 666
OXY, 139, 147

P

P. acnes, 571, 573
P. aeruginosa, 18, 20, 22, 27, 33, 49, 50, 53, 56, 77, 85, 87, 91, 138, 157, 158-171, 181, 185, 193-196, 206, 226, 227, 231, 233-239, 263, 264, 266, 267, 271, 272, 328, 335, 336, 350, 352, 353, 359-364, 368, 369, 371, 413, 415, 514, 662, 671
P. agglomerans, 140
P. mirabilis, 41, 139, 141, 143, 145, 148, 150, 152, 264, 266, 270, 335, 336, 350, 364, 369, 413
P. penneri, 140, 141, 143, 145, 369
P. rettgeri, 140, 369
P. stuartii, 140, 235, 268
P. vulgaris, 53, 140, 141, 143, 145, 369
PAB, 688

Pantoea agglomerans, 140, 369
parC, 21, 71, 243-255, 258, 259, 262, 266, 267, 269, 270, 272, 393, 422, 425, 426, 434, 435, 438, 455, 457, 458, 482, 501, 502, 506, 515, 517, 526, 528
parE, 21, 71, 243-248, 251-253, 258, 259, 262, 266, 267, 434, 435, 482, 526, 528
Pasteurella, 6, 53, 56, 59, 77, 329, 330, 332, 335, 340, 350, 362, 368, 431, 434, 501, 502, 653, 656, 657
Pasteurellaceae, 431, 434, 653, 656
PBP, 17, 18, 20, 21, 28, 35, 68, 69, 99, 102, 103, 107, 110-114, 123, 124, 127-139, 163, 278, 374, 411, 427, 431-433, 437, 438, 443, 445, 454, 455, 465, 492, 535, 567, 568, 656, 673, 688
PBP2a, 20, 99, 107, 111
Pediococcus, 53, 59, 325, 397-405
penA, 176, 186, 190, 191, 208, 211, 443-445, 448, 454, 455, 458, 487, 627
PENA, 186, 190, 191
penB, 454, 457
penicillin G, 17, 39, 40, 49, 51, 99-105, 109-123, 127-132, 135, 199, 222, 349, 351, 359, 369, 373-375, 380, 381, 384, 390-394, 397-404, 409, 430, 432, 441, 443,-456, 463, 493-497, 535, 544-549, 556, 563, 564, 568, 580, 583-589, 616-623, 626, 630, 633, 635, 639, 640, 644, 645, 653-655, 661, 665, 666, 681, 682, 688
penicillin V, 116, 117, 121, 661
penicillinase, 11, 17, 40, 49-52, 54, 69, 78, 100-107, 128, 133, 137-145, 159, 168, 186, 187, 190-196, 199, 211, 385, 393, 395, 411-413, 443, 448, 452-454, 457, 492, 496, 510-514, 517, 547, 559, 584, 629, 671
penicillins, 28, 47, 49, 51, 57, 78, 83, 100-110, 112, 118, 122, 123, 127-129, 135-138, 140-143, 147, 149, 157, 158, 181, 182, 186-198, 200, 204, 222, 373, 374, 376, 385, 391, 398, 407, 408, 411, 413, 429, 443, 453, 483, 492, 493, 501, 506, 510, 535, 547, 567, 568, 571, 572, 574, 578, 581, 584, 586, 625, 629, 653-655, 661, 666, 671, 681
penicillin-binding protein, 17, 107, 125, 132, 133, 154, 172, 378, 407, 415, 427, 431, 437, 439, 448, 458, 483, 535, 546, 673
peptidoglycan, 18, 20, 21, 32, 34, 99, 100, 110, 111, 127, 132, 133, 135, 136, 213, 278, 285-290, 298, 300-303, 361, 362, 372, 374, 403, 404, 432, 443, 448, 465, 535, 538, 568, 597, 661
Peptococcus, 365, 366, 567
Peptoniphilus, 341, 567
Peptostreptococcus, 333, 335, 340, 341, 362, 366, 558, 559, 561, 563, 567, 572, 573, 575, 576, 680, 681
PER, 146, 159, 160, 165, 166, 170-173, 195, 209, 210, 240, 411, 413, 419, 512, 514, 517, 518

permease, 26
pharmacodynamic, 368
pharmacokinetic, 26, 38, 40-45, 50, 55, 75, 82, 83, 87, 88, 90, 112, 115, 124, 125, 261, 295, 302, 304, 305, 329, 347, 349, 350, 368, 372, 394, 407, 427, 443, 447, 453, 457, 480, 536, 688
pheromone, 28
phoenix, 60, 61, 155, 279, 281, 283, 292, 293, 298, 310, 325, 326, 408
phosphotransferase, 17, 18, 19, 48, 50, 69, 70, 184, 187, 210, 213, 216, 217, 223, 224, 227-231, 241, 309, 317, 360, 385, 417, 425, 483, 487, 489, 490, 687
pilus, 28
piperacillin, 39, 40, 45, 86, 91, 100, 101, 105, 115, 125, 128-131, 135, 141-146, 148, 150, 157-168, 177, 179-189, 191-202, 204-206, 364, 391, 392, 399, 401, 408-410, 412-414, 419, 428, 432, 484, 511-514, 545, 546, 548, 555, 556, 561, 578-589, 630, 645, 661, 666, 680, 682
piperacillin-tazobactam, 86, 100, 125, 130, 408, 409, 428
PK/PD, 40-45, 394, 427, 428, 436, 447, 457, 502, 556
plasmid, 11, 19, 20-23, 28-30, 32, 35, 36, 64, 67, 73, 101, 102, 104, 138, 148, 149, 154, 155, 159, 161, 173, 174, 182, 192, 196, 199-201, 207, 210, 222-227, 229, 239-242, 265, 267, 268, 269, 272-274, 287, 293, 317, 325, 326, 337, 343, 350-354, 359, 363, 366, 376-378, 384, 385, 387, 388, 396, 403-405, 415, 422, 425, 435, 436, 439, 443, 447, 449, 451-456, 481-486, 489, 490, 493, 494, 510, 512, 514-518, 547, 551, 570, 582, 590, 640
Plesiomonas, 6, 59, 509-518
pneumococcus, 352, 4275, 109, 243, 309, 319, 320, 323, 343, 345, 352, 427
polymyxins, 5, 17, 18, 20, 21, 176, 184, 185, 187, 190, 191, 202, 207, 357, 359, 361, 363, 365, 367-372, 407, 409, 424, 425, 443, 453, 461, 515, 521, 662, 665, 666
ponA, 127, 454, 455, 458
population analysis, 278, 280, 281, 284
porA, 386, 441, 482, 489
porin, 18, 22, 27, 51, 135-137, 150, 163-166, 172, 241, 263, 267, 333, 370, 384, 415, 434, 441, 454, 456, 457, 489, 581, 583, 590,
Porphyromonas, 332, 335, 341, 362, 366, 369, 371, 554, 557, 558, 562, 577, 578, 584, 586-588, 680, 681
post antibiotic effect, 41, 42, 85, 87, 505,
PPNG, 453, 454
Prevotella, 332, 335, 341, 362, 366, 371, 547, 554, 557, 558, 562-565, 577, 578, 583-587, 590, 591, 680, 681

pristinamycin, 2, 78, 305, 306, 310-325, 344, 382, 385, 400, 401, 404, 493, 498, 499, 522, 527, 536, 580, 582, 590, 646, 662, 666, 680
promoter, 27, 30, 68, 141, 147, 148, 230, 246, 288, 327, 333, 335, 421, 435, 493, 498, 559, 567, 581, 582, 595, 596, 605, 651
Propionibacterium, 20, 53, 335, 341, 365, 567, 570-576, 680, 681
Proteus penneri, 140, 584
Proteus vulgaris, 53, 140, 186, 584
Providencia rettgeri, 140
Providencia stuartii, 140, 274, 358, 369
pyrazinamid, 18, 19, 23, 71, 593-598, 600-604, 606, 608, 611, 663, 666
PSE, 159, 165, 171, 172, 193, 194, 361, 510, 517
Pseudomonas, 5, 15, 19, 23, 35, 36, 50, 53, 54, 56, 73, 76, 83, 85, 87, 91, 93, 107, 154, 155, 157, 159-163, 165, 167, 169, 171-174, 177, 181, 184, 186, 207-211, 225, 229, 230, 232, 241, 242, 244, 261, 263, 272, 331-333, 340, 348, 352, 358, 360, 361, 363-366, 370, 372, 407, 424, 493, 629

Q

Qnr, 18, 21, 23, 33 34, 71-73, 268, 269, 271, 273, 274, 422, 482, 515, 516, 518
QRDR, 21, 244, 247, 265, 422, 434, 466, 501, 526, 537, 583, 596, 688
quality assurance, 283, 688
quality control, 38, 44, 50, 52, 56, 60, 62, 65, 114, 279, 283, 312, 353, 372, 390, 398, 429, 430, 437, 452, 460, 480, 488, 555, 557, 563, 600, 631, 649, 652, 656, 682, 687, 688
quinupristin, 42, 93, 205, 305-307, 310, 312, 315-317, 321, 323-326, 343, 344, 375, 382, 386, 400-404, 499, 504, 505, 507, 508, 522, 524-526, 575, 580, 587, 619, 662, 666

R

R. aquatilis, 145
R. pickettii, 175, 190-191
rahnella, 140, 369
Ralstonia, 175, 191-192, 208, 210-211, 370
ramoplanin, 291, 295, 303-304, 574, 666, 681
recipient, 28-30, 199, 201, 206, 271, 484, 648
recombinase, 102
recombination, 18, 26, 29, 34, 35, 69, 111, 343-344, 441, 443-444, 448
reference strain, 76, 353, 390, 430, 442, 451-452, 504, 521, 526, 532-533, 536, 582, 598, 620-622, 629
regulation, 27, 31-35, 102-103, 158-159, 164, 182, 185, 207-208, 232, 296, 331, 333-334, 336, 355, 512
regulator, 23, 45, 211, 230-231, 259, 335, 422, 517, 596, 605
repeat sequence, 486

replication origin, 404
replicative transposition, 30
replicative, 29-30, 531
resistance frequency, 466
Resistance Nodulation Division, 163, 184, 208, 360, 367, 415, 422, 629
resolvase, 29-30
ribosomal mutation, 72, 217, 312, 316, 318, 321, 323-326, 342, 359, 376, 384, 456, 482
ribosomal subunit, 225, 339, 357, 455
Rickettsia, 55, 67, 306, 327, 329, 348, 350, 358, 615, 617, 619, 621, 623, 625, 627, 629, 631-637, 639, 641
rifampin, 17-19, 21, 23, 25-26, 34, 71-73, 76, 86, 95, 136, 184, 191, 198, 205, 264, 269-270, 344, 364, 367, 371, 373-375, 377, 381-382, 385-386, 392-394, 400-402, 404, 408-410, 415-416, 419, 422, 425, 436, 441, 443-444, 446-448, 470, 491, 493, 503-508, 521, 534-539, 543-549, 561, 578, 580, 583-584, 593-595, 597-609, 611-614, 616-617, 625-627, 629-630, 632-641, 663, 666, 680-681
rmtA, 20, 226
rmtB, 20, 226, 268
RNA 16S, 328, 331
RNA polymerase, 18, 21, 25, 72, 296, 393, 422, 436, 466, 521, 539, 595, 617, 627, 635, 640
RND, 33, 137, 163, 184, 186, 190, 231, 241, 333, 335-337, 360, 415, 422, 424-425, 583, 629, 631
ROB, 431-432, 435, 437-439, 501-502
Rothia, 379-380, 382-383, 386
roxithromycin, 305, 307, 310, 428, 500, 505, 508, 522, 534-535, 555, 623, 640
rplD, 70, 312, 316, 343
rpoB, 25, 35, 71-72, 296-297, 393, 436, 446, 463, 466, 476, 506, 508, 521, 536, 538, 595, 603-605, 608, 611, 628, 635, 641

S

S. agalactiae, 109-110, 121-123, 217, 245, 300, 321, 341
S. anginosus, 109-110, 121, 341
S. aureus, 18-21, 26, 28-30, 33, 42, 44, 51-53, 68-70, 76, 83-84, 87, 89-90, 92-93, 95, 99-106, 128, 215, 217-220, 244-246, 248-250, 275-282, 295-302, 306, 309-319, 334, 336, 339, 341-343, 349, 353, 359-361, 364-367, 369, 390, 442, 504, 652-653, 655, 687
S. cohnii, 53, 306
S. maltophilia, 58, 175, 179, 181, 184, 206, 232-233, 239, 264, 267, 328, 350, 368, 371
S. marcescens, 140, 147-149, 229-231, 234, 237, 364, 368
S. milleri, 109, 121
S. mutans, 109, 341

S. oneidensis, 175, 200-201
S. oralis, 109, 252, 323, 341
S. pneumoniae, 18, 20, 28, 30, 49, 58, 70, 84, 90, 92, 109-116, 118-120, 122-123, 213, 222, 243-248, 250-251, 253-254, 297-299, 301-302, 319-324, 331, 341, 343, 359, 361, 364
S. putrefaciens, 175, 199, 201
S. pyogenes, 89, 109-110, 121-122, 245, 298-301, 308, 319-323
S. salivarius, 109, 341
S. sanguis, 109, 252, 341
S. sciuri, 306, 314
S. xylosus, 53, 306
Salmonella enterica, 72, 94, 230, 240, 369, 372, 515, 517
Salmonella, 20, 27, 72, 92, 94, 136, 139, 146, 148, 154, 230, 240-241, 265-266, 273, 332, 351-352, 354, 359-361, 363, 369, 372, 377, 407, 479, 482-483, 515, 517
serratia fonticola, 140
S. fonticola, 139-140, 145, 149
serratia marcescens, 73, 85, 91, 140, 150, 154, 158, 223, 229-230, 241-242, 263, 363
SFC, 149
SfC-1, 149
SfO-1, 140
Shewanella, 21, 175, 199-201, 208-210, 370
Shigella, 136, 139, 146, 332, 351-352, 359, 363, 369, 479
SHV, 17, 69, 73, 137-139, 141, 143, 145, 149, 154, 161, 166, 170, 173, 411, 413, 419, 656
SHV-1, 137, 139, 141, 143, 145
SME, 91, 149, 415
SOS, 509, 516
specialized, 466, 507, 531, 598, 604, 606
spiramycin, 305, 310-320, 322-324, 400, 430 493-494, 504-505, 507, 521-522, 534, 564, 580, 587, 646, 662, 666
Staphylococcus, 17, 22-23, 26, 34-36, 39-40, 45, 48-54, 56, 58, 64-67, 69-70, 72-73, 76-77, 87-89, 92-95, 99, 103, 105, 107, 224, 243, 258-259, 263, 275, 277, 279, 282-284, 291, 293, 303-304, 306, 308, 313, 325-326, 329, 331, 333-334, 337, 339-340, 343-345, 347, 351, 354, 359-366, 369, 372, 376, 442, 483, 493, 502, 504, 629, 653, 656, 671, 688-689, 691
Staphylococus hyicus, 337, 653
Stenotrophomonas, 56, 78, 93, 161, 171, 175, 181-183, 207-211, 232, 241, 264, 332, 335, 348, 354, 361-362, 370
streptidine, 213, 225
streptomycin, 18, 20, 31, 48-49, 64, 73, 129, 196-197, 213, 215-218, 220-223, 226, 228, 231-232, 236, 238, 241, 289-290, 353, 357, 361, 375-377, 381, 385, 399, 401, 403, 417, 452, 483, 511, 513, 515, 518, 547, 593-594, 596-598, 600-604, 609, 612, 614, 616, 625-630, 639-640, 644, 646, 655, 662-663, 666
streptothricin, 483, 487
Streptococcus, 20, 23, 28, 35-36, 40, 45, 48, 53-54, 56, 58, 61-62, 64, 70, 72, 74, 87-90, 92-93, 95, 107, 109, 116, 123-126, 133, 217, 222-224, 243, 258-259, 298, 308, 319, 323, 325-326, 329, 333-334, 336-337, 340-341, 343, 345, 351, 355, 358-359, 361, 363, 366, 377, 398, 403, 433, 439, 441-442, 499-500, 502, 547, 567, 575, 653, 655, 671, 688
Streptococcus suis, 653
sub-inhibitory concentration, 506
sulfonamides, 17-18, 71, 78, 109, 184, 186, 193, 197, 200, 204, 269-270, 347-353, 355, 361, 391, 400-402, 424, 429, 435, 437, 441-444, 446-447, 484, 492-494, 501, 506, 511, 513, 515, 521, 536, 547, 583-584, 586, 611-613, 643, 645, 647, 663, 665-667
synergy, 48, 64, 129, 131, 139-140, 144-150, 152, 154, 168, 170, 177, 179, 181-182, 184, 186-187, 191, 193, 195-196, 200, 202-204, 221-222, 229, 285, 289, 310-311, 313, 316-317, 340, 348-351, 353, 364, 367, 371, 373, 376, 397, 401-402, 416-419, 425, 472, 485, 502, 514, 548, 571, 645, 673, 675-678, 685

T

telithromycin, 87, 305, 307, 309-311, 313-325, 344, 374-375, 381-382, 386, 392-393, 400-402, 404, 428, 430-431, 436-437, 479, 493, 497-498, 521-522, 524-525, 527, 534-535, 538, 580, 582, 586-587, 616, 619, 621-623, 629-630, 633-635, 637-638, 662, 667
TEM, 17, 30, 69, 72-73, 137-138, 141, 143, 145, 152, 159, 161, 165-166, 170, 172, 184, 195, 207-208, 411-413, 419, 431-432, 435, 437, 439, 443, 452-453, 465, 501-502, 510, 514, 516-517, 547, 551, 656, 688
telavancin, 295, 298, 300-304, 404, 662, 667
tet(A), 384, 422, 425
tet(B), 331-332, 422, 434-435, 493, 546
tet(K), 103, 332-334, 546
tet(M), 18, 21, 332-335, 376-377, 393, 403, 422, 425, 435, 447, 456-457, 519, 523-525, 528, 547, 571, 576
tetracycline, 19-22, 30-31, 39, 53, 71-72, 83, 103, 109, 164, 180, 182, 185, 188-189, 197, 199, 201, 224, 328-331, 333-337, 354, 361, 367, 373-378, 382-387, 394, 396, 399-400, 403-405, 409-410, 415-416, 423-424, 428, 430-431, 434, 437, 444, 447, 449, 451-461, 463, 465, 467-468, 472-473, 479-480, 482, 484-491, 495, 497-500 502, 506, 511, 513, 515, 517, 519-520, 522-524, 527-528,

536, 538, 546-549, 558, 569-572, 578, 580-582, 587, 623, 625-628, 630, 633, 635, 637-640, 646, 652-656, 662, 667, 674, 682
therapeutic efficiency, 107
tiamulin, 652-654, 656
ticarcillin, 101, 105, 115, 125, 129, 135, 138, 141-142, 144-145, 146, 148, 150, 157-160, 162-168, 170, 172, 176-177, 179-185, 187-202, 204-206, 399, 401, 407-410, 412-414, 416, 419, 423, 484, 498, 511-515, 548, 556, 559, 561, 563, 565, 578-581, 583-586, 588-589, 630, 645, 661, 667, 680, 682
tilmicosin, 652-654, 656-657
time-dependent, 41, 84-85, 277, 340, 685
tobramycin, 48, 54, 69, 80-81, 85, 91, 103, 152, 180, 182, 185, 187-188, 190, 193, 196-202, 204-205, 213-223, 225, 227-233, 236-241, 372, 376, 381, 399, 401, 409-410, 417, 419, 421, 423, 436, 438, 483, 487, 511, 513, 612-613, 616, 619, 621-623, 630, 644, 646-648, 662, 667
topoisomerase, 21, 28, 33, 71, 243-244, 250, 258-259, 262, 265-267, 274, 395, 422, 425, 434, 455, 457, 466, 482, 486, 506, 517, 526, 528, 538, 591, 596, 627
transduction, 28
transformation, 28, 243, 343, 351, 441, 453, 463, 465-466, 481, 487
transpeptidase, 99, 111, 127, 129, 132-133, 135, 374, 432, 652
transposase, 29-30
transposition, 29-30, 148, 334, 388, 425, 518
transposon, 19, 29-31, 34-35, 67, 171, 207, 223, 226, 241, 277, 287, 321, 334, 353, 359, 376, 384-385, 388, 413, 415, 425, 434, 456, 502, 512, 514-515, 518, 523, 528, 570-571, 575, 689
trapping, 227, 231, 237
Treponema, 15, 332, 348, 615, 617, 619, 621, 623, 625, 627, 629, 631, 633, 635, 637, 639-641
TRI, 26, 288-289
trimethoprim, 17-18, 21, 31, 51-53, 71, 76, 78, 93, 109, 150, 164, 181-182, 184-187, 190-191, 193, 195-201, 204, 206, 211, 269-270, 347-355, 373-374, 376-377, 390-391, 393, 395, 400-402, 409, 415, 423-424, 428-431, 435, 437, 442-444, 447, 453, 461, 484, 486, 491-492, 494, 501-502, 511, 513, 515-518, 521, 536, 539, 545-546, 549, 577, 580, 583-584, 586, 613, 616, 626, 630, 633, 635, 638, 643, 645, 647-648, 656, 663, 667, 673, 681

trimethoprim-sulfamethoxazole, 93, 109, 184, 187, 190-191, 193, 195, 198-199, 206, 354-355, 377, 390, 401, 423, 428, 430, 444, 447, 491, 501-502, 516, 549, 643, 645, 648, 656
tulathromycin, 652-654, 656
Turicella, 379-383
Tween, 379, 644
tigecycline, 43, 60, 65, 126, 181-182, 184-185, 205, 327-331, 335-337, 344, 374-375, 382-383, 386, 407-410, 419-420, 423-425, 435, 522, 556, 573-575, 578-579, 581, 584, 587, 590, 619-622, 624, 637-638, 662, 682
tylosin, 305, 309, 482, 652, 654, 656

U-V

ubiquitous, 107, 181, 231, 482, 509, 615, 643
Ureaplasma, 71, 330, 333, 335, 340, 342, 344, 519-529
ureidopenicillins, 101, 127, 130, 135, 138-143, 147, 149, 158, 183, 187, 196, 498, 501, 665-666

V

valnemulin, 652, 654, 656
vanA operon, 30, 70, 277-278, 285, 288, 385
vanB operon, 33
vanC operon, 289
vat(A), 316
VEB, 146, 159, 161-162, 166, 170, 172, 174, 176, 194, 210, 411, 413, 416, 418-420
vga(A), 310, 314, 316
vga(B), 316
Vibrio, 31, 34, 53, 56, 58, 332, 334, 354, 359, 361-362, 509-518
VIM, 138, 149, 154, 159, 161, 163, 166, 170-174, 176, 194, 210, 242, 411, 415, 417, 419, 515, 517
virginiamycin, 305-306, 587, 662, 667
viridans group streptococci, 74, 109-110, 112, 120-125, 258, 301, 345
virulent, 197
VISA, 21, 44, 277-282, 689
VITEK 2, 60, 107, 154, 292-294, 326, 408
VRSA, 276-278, 281-282, 295, 298, 301-302, 689

W-X-Y-Z

Y. enterocolitica, 140
Yersinia enterocolitica, 140, 186, 369
Zinc, 137-138, 163, 181, 392, 514, 581